Amphetamine Use Disorders
Amphetamine Dependence
Amphetamine Abuse

Amphetamine-Induced Disorders
Amphetamine Intoxication
Amphetamine Withdrawal
Amphetamine Intoxication Delirium
Amphetamine-Induced Psychotic Disorder
Amphetamine-Induced Mood Disorder
Amphetamine-Induced Anxiety Disorder
Amphetamine-Induced Sexual Dysfunction
Amphetamine-Induced Sleep Disorder
Amphetamine-Related Disorder Not Otherwise Specified

Caffeine-Induced Disorders
Caffeine Intoxication
Caffeine-Induced Anxiety
Caffeine-Induced Sleep Disorder
Caffeine-Related Disorder Not Otherwise Specified

Cannabis Use Disorders
Cannabis Dependence
Cannabis Abuse

Cannabis-Induced Disorders
Cannabis Intoxication
Cannabis Intoxication Delirium
Cannabis-Induced Psychotic Disorder
Cannabis-Induced Anxiety Disorder
Cannabis-Related Disorder Not Otherwise Specified

Cocaine Use Disorders
Cocaine Dependence
Cocaine Abuse

Cocaine-Induced Disorders
Cocaine Intoxication
Cocaine Withdrawal
Cocaine Intoxication Delirium
Cocaine-Induced Psychotic Disorder
Cocaine-Induced Mood Disorder
Cocaine-Induced Anxiety Disorder
Cocaine-Induced Sexual Dysfunction
Cocaine-Induced Sleep Disorder
Cocaine-Related Disorder Not Otherwise Specified

Hallucinogen Use Disorders
Hallucinogen Dependence
Hallucinogen Abuse

Hallucinogen-Induced Disorders
Hallucinogen Intoxication
Hallucinogen Persisting Perception Disorder
Hallucinogen Intoxication Delirium
Hallucinogen-Induced Psychotic Disorder
Hallucinogen-Induced Mood Disorder
Hallucinogen-Induced Anxiety Disorder
Hallucinogen-Related Disorder Not Otherwise Specified

Inhalant Use Disorders
Inhalant Dependence
Inhalant Abuse

Inhalant-Induced Disorders
Inhalant Intoxication
Inhalant Intoxication Delirium
Inhalant-Induced Persisting Dementia
Inhalant-Induced Psychotic Disorder

Inhalant-Induced
Inhalant-Induced
Inhalant-Related

Nicotine Use Dis
Nicotine Depende

Nicotine-Induced Disorder
Nicotine Withdrawal
Nicotine-Related Disorder Not Otherwise Specified

Opioid Use Disorders
Opioid Dependence
Opioid Abuse

Opioid-Induced Disorders
Opioid Intoxication
Opioid Withdrawal
Opioid Intoxication Delirium
Opioid-Induced Psychotic Disorder
Opioid-Induced Mood Disorder
Opioid-Induced Sexual Dysfunction
Opioid-Induced Sleep Disorder
Opioid-Related Disorder Not Otherwise Specified

Phencyclidine Use Disorders
Phencyclidine Dependence
Phencyclidine Abuse

Phencyclidine-Induced Disorders
Phencyclidine Intoxication
Phencyclidine Intoxication Delirium
Phencyclidine-Induced Psychotic Disorder
Phencyclidine-Induced Mood Disorder
Phencyclidine-Induced Anxiety Disorder
Phencyclidine-Related Disorder Not Otherwise Specified

Sedative, Hypnotic, or Anxiolytic Use Disorders
Sedative, Hypnotic, or Anxiolytic Dependence
Sedative, Hypnotic, or Anxiolytic Abuse

Sedative-, Hypnotic-, or Anxiolytic-Induced Disorders
Sedative, Hypnotic, or Anxiolytic Intoxication
Sedative, Hypnotic, or Anxiolytic Withdrawal
Sedative, Hypnotic, or Anxiolytic Intoxication Delirium
Sedative, Hypnotic, or Anxiolytic Withdrawal Delirium
Sedative-, Hypnotic-, or Anxiolytic-Induced Persisting Dementia
Sedative-, Hypnotic-, or Anxiolytic-Induced Persisting Amnestic Disorder
Sedative-, Hypnotic-, or Anxiolytic-Induced Psychotic Disorder
Sedative-, Hypnotic-, or Anxiolytic-Induced Mood Disorder
Sedative-, Hypnotic-, or Anxiolytic-Induced Anxiety Disorder
Sedative-, Hypnotic-, or Anxiolytic-Induced Sexual Dysfunction
Sedative-, Hypnotic-, or Anxiolytic-Induced Sleep Disorder
Sedative-, Hypnotic-, or Anxiolytic-Related Disorder Not Otherwise Specified

Polysubstance-Related Disorder
Polysubstance Dependence

Abnormal Psychology

INTEGRATING PERSPECTIVES

G. Terence Wilson
Rutgers University

Peter E. Nathan
The University of Iowa

K. Daniel O'Leary
State University of New York at Stony Brook

Lee Anna Clark
The University of Iowa

ALLYN AN BACON
Boston • London • Toronto • Sydney • Tokyo • Singapore

Vice-President, Publisher: Susan Badger
Associate Publisher: Mylan Jaixen
Editorial Assistant: Susan Hutchinson
Executive Marketing Manager: Joyce Nilsen
Developmental Editors: Mark Palmer, Carolyn Smith
Editorial-Production Administrator: Annette Joseph
Editorial-Production Service: Susan Freese, Communicáto
Text Designer and Page Layout: Karen Mason
Photo Researcher: Laurie Frankenthaler
Composition and Prepress Buyer: Linda Cox
Manufacturing Buyer: Megan Cochran
Cover Administrator: Linda Knowles
Cover Designer: Studio Nine

A previous edition was published as *Abnormal Psychology,* by G. Terence Wilson, K. Daniel O'Leary, and Peter Nathan, copyright 1992.

Library of Congress Cataloging-in-Publication Data

Abnormal psychology : integrating perspectives / G. Terence Wison . . .
  [et al.].
    p.   cm.
   Includes bibliographical references and indexes.
   ISBN 0-205-17578-3
   1. Psychology, Pathological.   I. Wilson, G. Terence.
RC454.W543   1995
616.89—dc20
                                         95-40374
                                           CIP

Printed in the United States of America
10 9 8 7 6 5 4 3 2 1   00 99 98 97 96 9!

PHOTO CREDITS

Chapter-Opening Art

Art courtesy of Very Special Arts Gallery: Chapter 1, p. xii, *Home Free,* © JAH. Oil on canvas, 24" x 30", 1989; Chapter 3, p. 68, *Step 12,* © Jan Gerus. Acrylic on canvas, 16" x 31", 1984; Chapter 19, p. 600, *Friends,* © Jane Gerus. Arylic on canvas, 22" x 28", 1986; Chapter 21, p. 646, *The Arrival,* © Jane Gerus. Acrylic c canvas, 5' x 7', 1989.

Art courtesy of HAI, photographed by Donna McAdam: Chapter 2, p. 26, *Checkerboard* by George Knerr. Watercolor and pencil on paper, 11-/8" x 15"; Chapter 4, p. 102, *Four Faces* by Donna Caesar. Watercolor and pencil on pape 11" x 15"; Chapter 5, p. 132, *Woman with Big Hair* by Irene Phillips. Ink and ball point pe on paper, 9-7/8" x 12-7/8"; Chapter 6, p. 166, *Four Women* by Jennie Maruki. Acrylic o paper, 14-7/8" x 22"; Chapter 7, p. 190, *Happy Heart Day* by Mercedes Jamison. Watcolor and marker on paper,

Credits continue on page 775, which constitutes a continuation o e copyright page.

Brief Contents

Contents

PART ONE INTRODUCTION

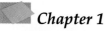
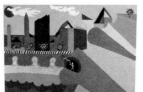
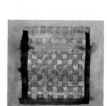

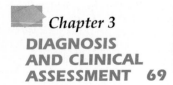
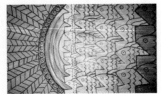

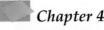
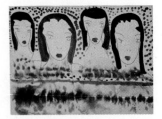

*P*ART *T*WO　*P*SYCHOLOGICAL *D*ISORDERS

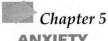
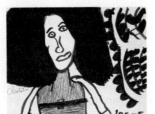

Chapter 6
SOMATOFORM AND DISSOCIATIVE DISORDERS 167

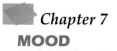

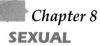

Chapter 7
MOOD DISORDERS 191

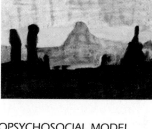

Chapter 8
SEXUAL DISORDERS 235

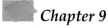

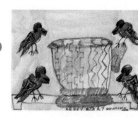

Chapter 9
SUBSTANCE-RELATED DISORDERS 271

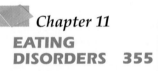

Chapter 10
PSYCHOLOGICAL FACTORS AFFECTING HEALTH   321

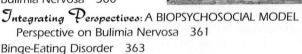

Chapter 11
EATING DISORDERS   355

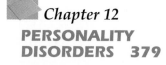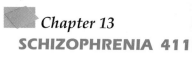
 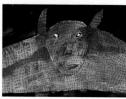
PART THREE   DEVELOPMENTAL AND LIFE SPAN DISORDERS

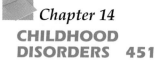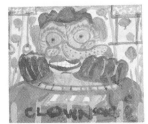

x   Contents

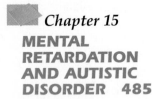

Chapter 15
MENTAL RETARDATION AND AUTISTIC DISORDER   485

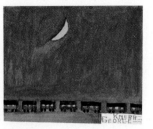

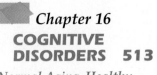

Chapter 16
COGNITIVE DISORDERS   513

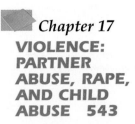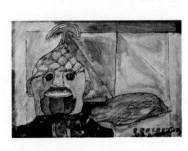

Chapter 17
VIOLENCE: PARTNER ABUSE, RAPE, AND CHILD ABUSE   543

PART FOUR   TREATMENT

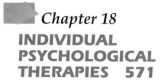
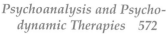

Chapter 18
INDIVIDUAL PSYCHOLOGICAL THERAPIES   571

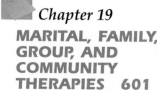
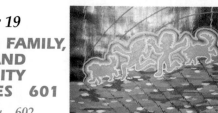
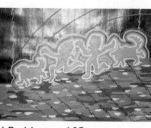

Chapter 19
MARITAL, FAMILY, GROUP, AND COMMUNITY THERAPIES   601

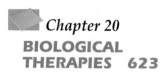
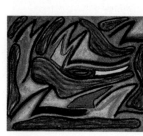

Chapter 20
BIOLOGICAL THERAPIES   623

*P*ART *F*IVE   *L*EGAL AND *E*THICAL *I*SSUES

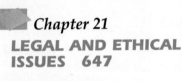

Chapter 21
LEGAL AND ETHICAL ISSUES   647

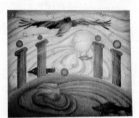

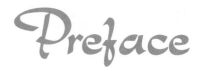

The study of abnormal psychology has changed significantly. In the past, investigators typically concentrated on single theoretical perspectives. They adopted a behavioral, psychodynamic, or humanistic model and approached all clinical disorders from this single perspective. Genetic and biological factors were frequently de-emphasized or totally ignored by many psychologists. And all too often, social and cultural influences were neglected by other scientists, who focused on the role of genetics and a fundamentally biological approach.

Advances in research over the last two decades have made this "one-track" thinking obsolete. It's now clear that the study of clinical disorders necessarily involves an understanding of the full range of biological, psychological, and socio-cultural factors. This approach—commonly called the *biopsychosocial perspective*—is a central feature of this book.

OUR INTERACTIVE APPROACH

Throughout this text, we emphasize the interactive influence of biological, psychological, and social factors in the development, course, and modification of abnormal behavior. Some interactions among these factors may surprise you and even stimulate you to think about abnormal psychology in new ways.

Consider, for example, the role of social support in reducing stress and maintaining good health. The quantity of social support a person enjoys is a function of the social environment. But did you know that *how* a person perceives the quality of that social support is strongly influenced by genetic factors? This intriguing finding suggests that the positive effect of social support on health is a product not only of environmental events but also of genetic factors that influence what environments people select and how they interpret them.

Similarly, in discussing posttraumatic stress disorder (PTSD), we consider how a psychosocial event—a traumatic experience—can cause biological changes in brain chemistry that, in turn, make the person more vulnerable to psychological stressors. Here is a case of biology being altered by behavior. In the past, we thought only in linear terms—of biological abnormalities causing behavioral problems. Now, we are more aware of the complex interactions among different influences on abnormal functioning.

Given this new insight, it's time to stop debating whether a particular disorder is a product of genetic *or* environmental determinants. Both sets of factors contribute to the development of the clinical disorders described in this text. Genetic predispositions have been firmly established for many clinical disorders. But the very evidence that documents the importance of genes also emphasizes the critical importance of nongenetic factors. Most studies have shown that genetic factors account for less than 50 percent of the variance in any behavioral trait or clinical disorder. These findings highlight the importance of nongenetic factors, particularly environmental forces, in determining abnormal behavior.

ORGANIZING THE CONTENT

We have divided this book into five parts. Part I, Chapters 1 through 4, lays the foundation for our study of psychopathology. In these chapters, we look at different perspectives on abnormal behavior, models of conceptualizing behavior, diagnosis and assessment, and research methods.

In Parts II and III, Chapters 5 through 17, we examine the major disorders. For each, we carefully analyze its causes, nature, diagnosis, and implications for treatment. Of special interest, we have included two chapters on topics currently of great interest. The first, **eating disorders,** is of particular relevance and interest to young women in college. This topic also provides an informative example of how sociocultural forces can help cause a major clinical disorder (see Chapter 11). The second hot topic we look at is **violence.** We devote a whole chapter to violence because we believe it's useful to provide an organized and concentrated analysis of the violent phenomena that clinicians are often called on to address, including child abuse, spouse abuse, and rape (see Chapter 17). For these and the other topics covered, our goal is to provide the most up-to-date and accurate information. You'll find throughout this book a high frequency of work published in the 1990s. Moreover, we provide critical analyses of the latest research findings.

Part IV, Chapters 18 through 20, concentrates on treatment, considering individual therapies; marital, family, and social therapies; and biological therapies. Although aspects of treatment are also addressed in other chapters, greater detail is provided in this part of the book.

Lastly, Part V of the book contains Chapter 21 on legal and ethical issues relevant to abnormal behavior.

Integrating Multicultural and Gender Influences

Our goal as authors has been to present the most up-to-date view of the field. We recognize that scientific advances are taking place in a multicultural world. The racial/ethnic composition of the United States is changing; one-quarter of the population is now defined as belonging to an ethnic minority (U.S. Bureau of the Census, 1990). Predictions are that this proportion will increase as the demographics of the country continue to change.

The growing cultural diversity of the United States has important implications for the study of abnormal psychology. Accordingly, we address the relevance of multicultural issues in all chapters. We have included a similar focus on the role of gender in clinical disorders, in view of its profound impact on several important kinds of psychopathologies.

Integrating Therapy

Our own clinical work with individuals, couples, and families has given us an extensive body of knowledge about the possibilities and limitations of therapy. We have therefore carefully integrated methods of treatment with the discussion of the nature and causes of each disorder. By doing so, we create a more cohesive view of the disorder. And because there is a great deal of additional information available about the various therapies, we have provided three integrative chapters on biological, psychological, and social treatments (Chapters 18 through 20).

Special Features

A number of special features make this book more interesting and, at the same time, easier to use than many texts:

Cases   Each chapter opens with a case study featuring an actual person. For the most part, these cases are drawn from our own clinical experience. At various points in the chapter text, we extend the opening case by including additional clinical material relevant to the topic at hand. We identify that additional case material with a thin, blue, vertical line in the margin. Strategically weaving this case study through the chapter not only helps illustrate the material but also provides greater continuity and structure.

To portray further the human side of psychopathology, additional cases on other individuals are embedded in the chapters. We think this "minicase" material as well as the opening cases will do much to enhance your understanding of the causes, diagnoses, and treatments of the various disorders.

High-Interest Boxes   As we reviewed the material for each chapter, we found many really interesting topics that we wanted to include and certain themes or patterns emerged. For example, we pointed out earlier that we integrated relevant material on multicultural aspects of psychopathology in the chapter narratives. Yet we found ourselves wanting to direct the spotlight on particularly interesting aspects of the issue. To achieve this goal, we created high-interest boxes entitled Thinking about Multicultural Issues. These boxes appear in chapters in which the content calls for additional elaboration.

We faced the same challenge with research issues, gender issues, social issues, and controversial issues. Accordingly, throughout this book, you will find "thinking about" boxes addressing these issues. As with the multicultural boxes, we let the chapter content determine which types of feature boxes were appropriate. Not all chapters include all types of boxes.

DSM-IV Tables   One of the major challenges in studying abnormal psychology is judging whether behavior is normal or abnormal, healthy or pathological. Currently, mental health professionals use the fourth edition of the *Diagnostic and Statistical Manual of Mental Disorders (DSM-IV)*, published in 1994 by the American Psychiatric Association, as a guide in diagnosing what is abnormal. To help convey the role of the *DSM-IV* in defining the major disorders, we integrate into our discussions *DSM-IV* tables, listing the diagnostic criteria.

Critical Thinking   Another prime goal of this book is to engage readers in thinking more reflectively about the subject matter and its implications. In an effort to help guide that thinking, we have developed an elaborate critical thinking feature, consisting of several elements. First, at the end of each major section in each chapter, you will see a short boxed section called Focus on Critical Thinking. It contains one or more questions designed to help you recall information, synthesize new material with your existing knowledge, and stimulate you to make informed judgments about the scientific nature of the data. Second, at the end of each high-interest box, we include a question or two designed to encourage you to think about the issue. Then, at the end of each chapter, we have created a Critical Thinking Exercise. Each exercise uses a minicase plus questions to help you draw conclusions about the implications of what you have read in the chapter.

Biopsychosocial Application   Earlier in this preface, we explained why we adopted the biopsychosocial approach in this book. You will notice in all chapters that we show the striking connections among the biological, psychological, and sociocultural factors as we try to understand the causes, diagnoses, and treatments of clinical disorders. To enhance that message, we have created a full-page visualization of our integrative approach in each of the chapters in Parts II and III, called Integrating Perspectives: A Biopsychosocial Model. This pedagogical feature focuses on a specific disorder; lists the key biological, psychological, and social factors; and ends with a brief minicase and analysis. By presenting all this information in this consistent format, we hope to help you envision the convergence of the three perspectives.

Written Style   In reading this book, you may note that the written style is more informal than is typical of most texts. Our aim was to make the discussion lively and engaging, conveying our enthusiasm for this fascinating subject. You may also note that when single individuals are discussed in general terms, the use of pronouns alternates between *he* and *she*. We have used this style to avoid sexist language; it does not mean that certain comments apply only to males or females.

Finally, in writing and editing this book, we have striven to avoid stigmatizing people with disorders. Thus, we have eliminated the use of negative labels and emphasized that these are, above all, *people*. For instance, in most cases, we discuss *people with schizophrenia*, rather than *schizophrenics*. We encourage you to follow this style in your own writing. Consider that the very words you choose to express yourself convey your attitudes and values, not just your knowledge.

Supplements

An extensive array of supplements for instructors and students accompany this book:

Instructor's Resource Manual   This resource consists of detailed lecture outlines, teaching suggestions, additional materials for lectures and class handouts, sources for elaborative information, and transparency masters. This valuable instructional aid was assembled by Maureen Sullivan and Frank Collins of Oklahoma State University.

Transparencies   Over 100 transparencies have been made from the text and other sources. These acetates will be useful to instructors as they introduce and reinforce key principles of abnormal psychology and as they examine the results of research.

Test Item File   This file contains over 2,000 multiple-choice test questions, designed to test factual recall as well as higher-order learning. The test item file is available both as hard copy and as software for PC and Macintosh computers. The computerized testing versions allow users to select or edit existing items, insert additional questions, and choose from a range of printing and scrambling options. The test item file was also created by Maureen Sullivan and Frank Collins.

A call-in and FAX testing service is also available. If an instructor calls in a request, the testing center will send a finished, ready-to-duplicate test within 48 hours or FAX a test for rush service.

Student Study Guide   Maureen Sullivan and Frank Collins have also prepared a valuable learning supplement. Consisting of chapter objectives, reviews, outlines, and practice tests, this learning aid will help students master the content. Also included are additional critical thinking exercises and other applications.

Case Book   Additional case material is available in *Case Studies in Abnormal Behavior*, third edition (1996), by Robert Meyer and Yvonne Hardaway Osborne.

Two to four cases are provided for each category in the *DSM-IV*. This rich collection ranges from classic cases to those involving people currently in the news.

Washington Post Reader   This collection of recent articles from *The Washington Post* was assembled by Martin Heesacker, University of Florida, and The Washington Post Writers Group. This book complements the mission of the textbook by featuring contemporary developments in the field and by exemplifying the dynamic nature of scientific discovery and the advance of knowledge.

CNN Video   This video runs 60 minutes in length. Linked to important topics in the text, these film clips are great for launching lectures, sparking classroom discussion, and encouraging critical thinking. A CNN Video User's Guide integrates the video segments with the text.

Allyn and Bacon Video Library   This library offers an impressive selection of videos from such sources as *Films for the Humanities* and *Annenberg/CPB* for qualified adopters of this text.

America Online (AOL)   For instructors who adopt this text, AOL membership will be waived for the first 2 months. Thus, instructors can use this introductory membership to access a wide range of interactive services, online readings, and educational information, providing a fast and easy gateway to the Internet. Additionally, instructors will have access to Simon & Schuster's College Online, a service with material of specific interest to psychology students, researchers, and faculty.

Just-In-Time (JIT) Custom Publishing   This exciting custom publishing program gives instructors the option of building textbooks or supplements to fit their specific instructional needs. Instructors may select materials from the JIT database or from their own materials.

$\mathcal{A}$CKNOWLEDGMENTS

Creating a book of this magnitude involves a number of people, whose contributions come at different times. We wish to acknowledge those individuals and express our appreciation for their efforts.

First, we want to convey our sincere thanks to the reviewers who read chapters of this book during the writing phase.

Kelly D. Brownell
Yale University

David Cohen
University of Texas at Austin

W. Edward Craighead
University of Colorado at Boulder

Linda W. Craighead
University of Colorado at Boulder

Joan F. DiGiovanni
Western New England College

Donald D. Evans
Drake University

Don C. Fowles
The University of Iowa

James H. Geer
Louisiana State University

Dashiel J. Geyen
University of Houston–Downtown

Daniel Houlihan
Mankato State University

Karen H. C. Huang
Stanford University

William G. Iacono
University of Minnesota

Rolf G. Jacob
University of Pittsburgh Medical Center

Steven R. Kubacki
University of Wyoming

Jennifer Langhinrichsen-Rohling
University of Nebraska–Lincoln

Robert J. McCaffrey
State University of New York, Albany

Linda Musun-Miller
University of Arkansas at Little Rock

Ron Prinz
University of South Carolina

Paul G. Retzlaff
University of Northern Colorado

R. Kevin Rowell
The University of Central Arkansas

Kathleen Sheridan
University of Missouri, Columbia

Norris D. Vestre
Arizona State University

We were fortunate to have Maureen Sullivan and Frank Collins, of Oklahoma State University, write the instructor's manual, student study guide, and test item file for our book. Their creativity and many hours of work have resulted in fine instructional tools. Also, we want to acknowledge Shirley Glynn, West Los Angeles Veterans Medical Center, and Don Fowles, The University of Iowa, for their assistance in developing the chapter on schizophrenia.

We wish to thank our colleagues and staff at our respective universities. A special thank-you is in order for Barbara Honig, Terry Wilson's secretary. We owe our gratitude to Jeffrey Vittengl, of The University of Iowa, for methodically checking the entire set of page proofs for this book. Likewise, we thank Pam Brown, of SUNY at Stony Book, for her help in finalizing galleys and pages.

Several key people behind the scenes had an impact on the book. We thank Mark Palmer for his early work as a developmental editor and Carolyn Smith for her later work on the manuscript. And we thank Sue Freese, our copyeditor, for her diligent and attentive work. At Allyn and Bacon, our thanks go to: Annette Joseph, who guided the manuscript through the book production process; Susan McIntyre, for her insightful work on the biopsychosocial applications; Susan Duane and Laurie Frankenthaler, for their work on the photo program; and Megan Cochran, who found shortcuts at the printing and binding stage. We acknowledge Joyce Nilsen for her fine work in coordinating the marketing campaign on behalf of this book.

We are also greatly appreciative of Susan Badger, Vice-President and Publisher at Allyn and Bacon, for her unfailing support, which was instrumental in bringing this project to fruition. We especially want to thank our editor, Mylan Jaixen, for his guidance, good humor, wisdom, and support. His patience and perseverance, often under the most difficult circumstances, went beyond the call of duty.

Finally, special acknowledgment and appreciation go to our families for bearing with us and for providing support through the arduous task of writing a major text. It is to them that we dedicate this book.

T. W.
P. N.
D. O.
L. A. C.

About the Authors

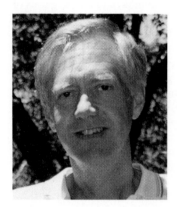

TERRY WILSON, after receiving his Ph.D. at the State University of New York at Stony Brook in 1971, moved to Rutgers University in New Jersey, where, in 1985, he was appointed Oscar K. Buros Professor of Psychology. In addition to teaching undergraduate and graduate students, he is a practicing clinical psychologist. Terry Wilson has co-authored or co-edited a number of books, including *Behavior Therapy: Application and Outcome* (with K. D. O'Leary), *The Effects of Psychological Therapy* (with S. Rachman), *Annual Review of Behavior Therapy: Theory and Practice* (with C. M. Franks), and *Binge Eating: Nature, Assessment and Treatment* (with C. G. Fairburn). A past president of the Association for Advancement of Behavior Therapy, his academic honors include fellowships at the Center for Advanced Study in the Behavioral Sciences at Stanford (1976–77 and 1990–91); the Distinguished Scientific Contributions to Clinical Psychology award from Division 12 of the American Psychological Association (1994); and the Distinguished Contributions to Applied Scientific Psychology award from the American Association of Applied and Preventive Psychology (1995).

PETER E. NATHAN received his A.B. in Social Relations with Honors from Harvard College in 1957 and a Ph.D. in Clinical Psychology from Washington University in 1962; after that, he joined the faculty of Harvard Medical School (1962–69) and the staff of Boston City Hospital and began his research into the causes of alcoholism. At Rutgers University (1969–90), he established the Alcohol Behavior Research Laboratory and chaired the Graduate Department of Clinical Psychology. In 1983, he was appointed director of Rutgers' Center of Alcohol Studies and Henry and Anna Starr Professor of Psychology. From 1987 to 1990, he was on partial leave from Rutgers to serve as senior health program officer for the MacArthur Foundation in Chicago. In January 1990, Dr. Nathan was appointed Vice President for Academic Affairs, Dean of the Faculties, and University of Iowa Foundation Distinguished Professor of Psychology at The University of Iowa. In July 1993, his title was changed to Provost. Dr. Nathan served as a member of the *DSM-IV* Work Group considering new diagnostic criteria for the substance use disorders as well

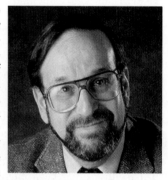

as a member of the Task Force on *DSM-IV*, which oversaw the whole *DSM-IV* process. He served eight years as Associate Editor of *American Psychologist*, seven years as Executive Editor of *Journal of Studies on Alcohol*, and four years as Associate Editor of *Contemporary Psychology*. He is a past president of the Division of Clinical Psychology of the American Psychological Association.

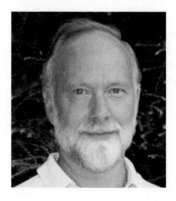

DANIEL O'LEARY is Distinguished Professor of Psychology and past chairman of the Psychology Department at the University at Stony Brook, New York. He received his Ph.D. from the University of Illinois at Urbana in 1967 and has been at Stony Brook throughout his career. He received the Distinguished Scientist Award from the Clinical Division of the American Psychological Association and is a member of the National Academies of Practice. Dr. O'Leary has written seven books, including *Behavior Therapy: Application and Outcome* (with Wilson), *Mommy I Can't Sit Still: Coping with the Aggressive and Hyperactive Child*, *Assessment of Marital Discord*, and *Marital Therapy: Treatment for Depression* (with Beach and Sandeen). He has published numerous articles on the relationship between marital problems and childhood psychopathology, the treatment of aggressive and hyperactive children, and the assessment and treatment of partner (wife) abuse.

LEE ANNA CLARK is a Professor of Psychology at The University of Iowa. After receiving her Ph.D. in Clinical Psychology from the University of Minnesota in 1982, she completed a two-year Postdoctoral Fellowship at Washington University in St. Louis. From 1984–1993, Dr. Clark was on the faculty of Southern Methodist University in Dallas, serving for five years as Director of Clinical Training. Dr. Clark's research interests in personality and psychopathology led her to develop the Schedule for Nonadaptive and Adaptive Personality, a unique self-report instrument for assessing traits relevant to personality disorder. She is also co-translator of the Japanese version of the MMPI-2 and maintains an interest in cross-cultural psychology. Dr. Clark served on a *DSM-IV* Anxiety Work Group subcommittee and as an advisor to the *DSM-IV* Work Group on Personality Disorders; she was selected as a panel participant for the first American Psychological Association video-teleconference, Highlights of the *DSM-IV*. Dr. Clark is currently an Associate Editor of the *Journal of Abnormal Psychology* and has served on the editorial boards of *Psychological Assessment* and the *Journal of Personality Disorders*.

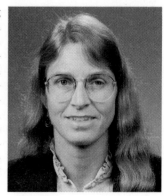

About the Artists

The art featured on our chapter-opener pages has been kindly provided by HAI (Hospital Audiences, Inc.) and Very Special Arts. We extend our thanks to these organizations and to the artists, adults with mental disabilities, for sharing their works. Each piece has been carefully selected to provide a thought-provoking illustration of the chapter's theme.

HAI (Hospital Audiences, Inc.), a nonprofit arts organization dedicated to providing cultural access to the disabled and disadvantaged, was founded by Executive Director Michael Jon Spencer in 1969. The HAI participatory Arts Workshop Program brings professional artists to work with mentally disabled adults in community based programs throughout New York City. Through the Arts Workshop Program, HAI discovered talented artists who live with major mental illness. HAI assists these mentally ill artists in bringing their work to the public through exhibition and sale.

Since its inception, eight million have attended HAI's broad range of events. HAI events take individuals to live, professional musical and theatrical performances and sporting events; professional performances are also presented on site at institutions and facilities. Other HAI programs include the Omni*Bus which transports people in beds to cultural events in the community; Describe! which provides audio description of live theatrical events to visually impaired people. The Prevention/Education Program utilizes the theatrical improvisation technique to bring HIV prevention issues to young people.

The work of Dona Ann McAdams, photographer of these HAI paintings, has been internationally recognized. She has taught Photography Workshop for HAI since 1982. She has been the archive photographer at Performance Space 122 in New York City since 1983. She has exhibited at The Museum of Modern Art, New York City; The Museum of Contemporary Art, Los Angeles; and La Primavera Fotographica, Barcelona. She is represented by Galeria H2O, Barcelona. A monograph documenting 15 years of her performance photography will be published with the Aperture Foundation in 1996. Her most recent portfolio, The Garden of Eden, documents her work with the mentally ill and homeless in Coney Island, Brooklyn, New York.

The Very Special Arts Gallery in Washington, D.C. represents emerging and professional artists with disabilities from around the country. Through informative and engaging exhibitions, the not-for-profit Very Special Arts Gallery creates opportunities for the public to enjoy and purchase artwork of the highest quality, including limited edition prints, original paintings, and sculpture. Exhibitions present a wide variety of genres, ranging from abstraction to realism to American folk art.

In support of its mission, the Very Special Arts Gallery also maintains an extensive artists registry of images and information on over 700 artists with disabilities. The gallery helps to connect these artists with art patrons, collectors and exhibition opportunities across the country. Proceeds from art sales benefit the artists and programs of Very Special Arts.

The Very Special Arts Gallery is also an educational resource. Each year, visitors learn about the wealth of talent that exists amongst a growing pool of artists with disabilities. Educational displays help explain both the important role of the arts in the lives of individuals with disabilities, and the programs of Very Special Arts.

Very Special Arts is an international non-profit organization that offers learning opportunities through the arts for people with disabilities, especially children and youth. Founded in 1974 by Jean Kennedy Smith as an affiliate of The John F. Kennedy Center for the Performing Arts, the organization offers educational programs in dance, drama, music, creative writing, and the visual arts. The Very Special Arts Gallery represents an important extension of the organization's mission to promote worldwide awareness of the importance of arts-based education for children, youth, and adults with disabilities.

Donna Caesar, Chapters 4 and 16 (b. 1927, Bronx, New York)

Caesar's early works were usually a single female, elongated face, styled in the look of the 1920s or 1930s. Simple, idiosyncratic touches of color—such as purple hair and matching purple lipstick—embellished the drawings. Written comments in Spanish, Patois, or English completed the drawings. More recently, Caesar has been working in acrylic paint and her style has become bolder and reflective of Caribbean influences.

Jane Gerus, Chapters 3, 19, and 21 (St. Paul, Minnesota)

Originally from Cleveland, Ohio, Jane Gerus moved to Minnesota fifteen years ago for drug addiction treatment. She became sober, but then had to be hospitalized for schizophrenia and asthma. During her long stay, Jane produced her first pictures. She needed to capture her dreams and visions with bright colors, so she drew daily with magic markers on paper mats.

Jane continued to draw with markers for several years, then taught herself to paint using acrylics on posterboard. These paintings opened the door to Jane's survival with chronic illness.

William Gonzalez, Chapter 12 (b. 1927, Brooklyn, New York)

Gonzalez embellishes his finely drawn paintings with written text. His comments reflect objects and ideas which relate to his idiosyncratic thought patterns and are charged with deeply personal meanings and emotional energy. Gonzalez spent fifteen years in a state mental hospital and now lives independently in the community with the help of his devoted sister.

Carl Greenberg, Chapter 14 (b. 1917, Brooklyn, New York)

Greenberg has been a prolific painter, but now works only as his health permits. Greenberg assigns a theatrical relationship to his subjects, although the subjects themselves are not necessarily related to the theater. He includes representations of the stage, such as footlights and a proscenium. He adds rich details relating to the main subject of each work. He is pleased that his work is exhibited and that he has earned profits from sales, but he has declined to attend exhibits of his work.

Ray Hamilton, Chapters 17 and 18 (b. 1920, North Carolina)

Hamilton's early works were creations of quasi-human figures and subjects from his environment. He structured complex compositions involving multiple divisions of the page and used a delicate but vibrant palette. More recent choices of subject are animals—perhaps reflecting Hamilton's youth on a Carolina farm. Whether painted in watercolor or drawn in ball-point pen, the animals retain the delicacy of his earlier works. Hamilton, now living in a skilled healthcare facility, continues to paint following a stroke. Alert and interested, Hamilton enjoys visitors and trips to see his work exhibited.

JAH, Chapter 1 (Glen Ridge, New Jersey)

The Haas brothers often collaborate on work, yet each creates distinctly unique images in very individual styles. John, diagnosed with schizophrenia, began painting at age nineteen. He paints alongside his brother Henry, who attended art school and has been painting for more than twenty years. Henry is overcoming challenges developed from carpal tunnel syndrome. Their father and two other brothers, Michael and James, all follow the family painting tradition.

John and Henry, working under the name JAH, use painting as a means of therapy. Their bold and playful images suggest an escape from an often insensitive world.

Mercedes Jamison, Chapter 7 (b. 1933, Queens, New York)

Jamison has a lengthy history of mental illness. She now lives in a group residence. She paints erratically, needing assistance in focusing her attention. She is currently in an active phase, drawing regularly and completing most works. Her works—landscapes, animals, or faces—are composed of many fragmented elements and usually include a wildly smiling sun. She will use any medium that is available to her, but she is currently working effectively in acrylic and favoring the color yellow.

George Knerr, Chapters 2 and 15

Knerr constructs highly ordered figurative and abstract works. Shapes combine to create geometrically formed animals, flowers, or landscapes. Abstract works appear sophisticated and distinctive; his sense of design and color is distinctive. Knerr now resides in a skilled healthcare facility and continues to paint regularly.

Helen Kossoff, Chapters 10 and 13 (1922–1994, Bronx, New York)

Kossoff found her subject matter—animals and people—in photographs from newspapers and magazines. After Kossoff transformed the subjects to her own vision, the images bore minimal resemblance to their source. All her subjects seem to have happy personalities. Kossoff filled her paintings with vibrant traditional as well as psychedelic colors and she completed the backgrounds of her paintings with dense geometric patterns. Sometimes the pattern crossed the subject entirely. Kossoff enjoyed success with her art and took pleasure in using her profits from sales to add to her wardrobe and to go to the beauty parlor.

Kenny McKay, Chapter 9 (b. 1941, Mt. Vernon, New York)

McKay, who spent more than twenty-five years in state mental institutions, has a fine intellect and a creative sense of humor. His humor has recently been incorporated into his paintings by writing jokes, puns, and word plays on his paintings. McKay lives in a group residence in the community and takes a special interest in food. His earliest source of inspiration for painting was the coffee cup, which he painted in endless variations. He also paints a unique bird—blue and slightly demonic—regularly. McKay has taken an interest in the Renaissance and has painted related subjects. He is currently painting contemporary popular icons, such as Mickey Mouse, Bugs Bunny, and Marilyn Monroe. McKay's transparent, overlapping forms are the result of his technique of drawing fluid outlines, followed by scrubbing watercolor onto the page, thereby blurring the final images.

Jennie Maruki, Chapter 6 (b. 1917, Florin, California)

As a Japanese-American who was interred during World War II, Maruki moved from California to New York after the war. After being hospitalized for mental illness for many years, Maruki now lives in a group residence in the community. She is a cheerful, hard working woman, who contributes her efforts to group projects and activities regularly. When Maruki broke her right (dominant) arm, she continued to paint by using her left hand. Her work retained its distinctive style, but became considerably emboldened. Now again painting with her right hand, the same boldness sometimes surfaces, distinct from her usual delicate paintings of female figures. Maruki shows a fondness for blue colors.

Wally C. Nicholson, Chapters 11 and 20 (b. 1939, Jamaica, West Indies)

Nicholson's religious beliefs preclude painting the human figure. Nicholson's abstract designs and recognizable landscapes reflect his preference for decorative patterns. Nicholson's early works, sensual, densely colored forms, were exclusively in oil crayon. Recently, Nicholson has begun working in acrylic paint. Nicholson is quite isolated and goes through prolonged periods when he does not paint.

Irene Phillips, Chapter 5 (b. 1925, Virginia)

A prolific painter, Phillips' subjects frequently come from her imagination. She also paints animals, and people she knows. She has recently taken an interest in painting Native Americans in her bold, spontaneous, free-flowing style. Phillips was in a state mental institution for twenty-three years. She now lives in a group residence and regularly visits her sister's nearby home. Phillips is active and energetic and enjoys diverse artistic activities. She is an excellent singer. She has been pleased by the recent success of her art work, including its regular exhibition and sale.

James Prendergast, Chapter 8

Prendergast's diverse subjects included the predatory birds that he loved, erotic animals and landscapes. Watercolor was freely applied over line drawings, resulting in imagery often floating through a fluid environment. His paintings frequently used black; his choice of yellow and orange skies may be reflective of his interest in Van Gogh. Prendergast died in 1989.

Chapter 1
PERSPECTIVES ON ABNORMAL BEHAVIOR

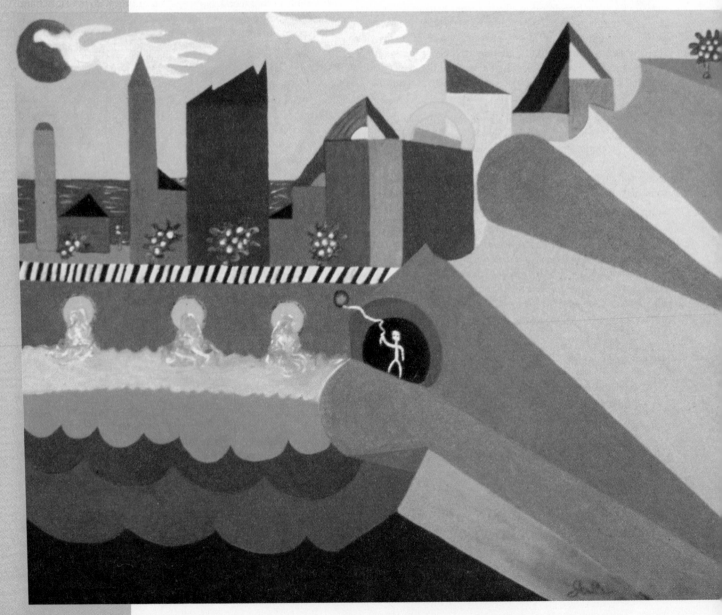

JAH, **Home Free,** 1989, Very Special Arts Gallery

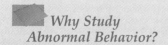
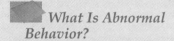
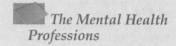
The young woman called at dinnertime. After giving her name, she said she was calling people in Saint Louis and asking them to participate in a national survey on mental health and mental illness, sponsored by the National Institute of Mental Health (NIMH), an agency of the federal government. Elizabeth H. had been randomly selected to participate in a face-to-face interview. The young woman went on to explain that the federal government wanted to get a clear picture of the mental health needs of healthy, functioning people in order to decide whether the nation's mental health dollars were being spent as efficiently as possible.

Although she was a little apprehensive about talking about such personal things with a stranger, Elizabeth decided it was in the country's best interest to know more about mental health and mental illness. And besides, her family would clearly come across as being normal. As far as she knew, no one in the family had ever gone to a psychiatrist or to a mental hospital.

Sure, over the years, her husband had been drinking heavily, and he'd occasionally been abusive to her and the children. And Elizabeth still had her "spells" every once in a while, when she couldn't get out of bed and didn't have the energy to go to work or care for her children as well as she usually did. All these problems seemed to be getting better, though. So Elizabeth told the young woman she'd see her, and they set up an appointment for the following Friday, after work.

Throughout history, we've been fascinated by the abnormal behavior of others and preoccupied with signs of abnormality in ourselves. So it's not surprising that today, many of us are interested in studying the subject, as undergraduate students of abnormal behavior or as graduate or professional students of clinical psychology, psychiatry, psychiatric nursing, or social work. Our fascination with this subject also plays a role in the design of surveys like the NIMH study in which Elizabeth H. was asked to participate. (We'll review some of the NIMH findings and Elizabeth's role in the study later in the chapter.)

This chapter puts the subject *abnormal behavior* into proper perspective. We'll look at the many ways in which abnormality has been defined and review findings from recent epidemiologic surveys, including the NIMH study that Elizabeth participated in. You may be surprised to find that mental health problems are even more prevalent and impactful than you had imagined. The next section is an overview of the history of efforts to understand, describe, and treat mental disorders. We'll conclude the chapter with an overview of the mental health professions, since many of you may be interested in becoming mental health professionals.

WHY STUDY ABNORMAL BEHAVIOR?

Human beings have always noticed abnormality and wanted to understand it better. The ancient Greeks developed elaborate scientific theories to explain abnormality, and the ancient Romans and Chinese tried to treat it. During the Inquisition, people who were insane were tortured and scorned because they presumably conversed with the devil. Shakespeare wrote plays in the seventeenth century in which characters exhibit mental disorders recognizable to us today. In the nineteenth century, composers of operas wrote scenes in which their heroines were insane—screaming and sobbing hysterically—which allowed these performers to show off their voices. And in this century, television programs and movies regularly portray such disorders as multiple personality, paranoia, autism, schizophrenia, and depression. Abnormal behavior is so commonly discussed now that the technical language of psychology has become pervasive in everyday speech. We might say, "He's a sadist" or "She's neurotic," knowingly using terms such as *narcissistic, paranoid, compulsive,* and *phobic.*

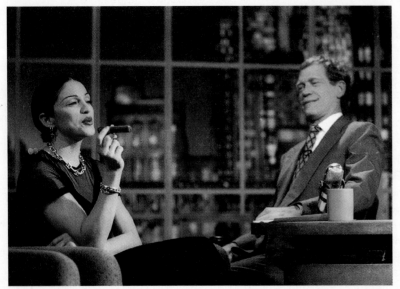

Both Madonna and David Letterman seem to take great delight in their eccentricities. But are they abnormal?

We've all asked ourselves, usually during periods of stress, whether we're going to "lose it" or "go off the deep end." And who hasn't wondered whether an aunt, a cousin, or even a rock star is abnormal, eccentric, or just plain weird? The normal strains of life inevitably create situations that cause us pain and anxiety. Despite the turmoil we may be in, though, our bouts with depression, anxiety, and fear usually play out and then disappear, without leaving significant effects or meriting formal diagnoses. Even when we decide to seek help during particularly troublesome periods—for instance, when we end important relationships, have difficulties with our parents or friends, or make tough vocational choices—we're often surprised later to realize that living through the distress was a necessary step toward greater self-understanding and maturity.

Perhaps you've witnessed firsthand the impact of mental disorder on a close friend or relative. Alcoholism and drug abuse, depression and anxiety, and even the serious mental disorder we call **psychosis** (which is synonymous with **insanity**) are sufficiently common that most of us know someone who suffers from one or another of them. Psychosis involves an actual break with reality; it's typically accompanied by **delusions** (i.e., false beliefs) and **hallucinations** (i.e., false perceptions).

Learning about these conditions will give you some understanding of how they originate, are diagnosed, and can be treated. You'll also develop a better sense of whether the circumstances of your life, as well as your family's history of medical or psychiatric disorders, increase or decrease your chances of developing a mental disorder. By learning about these conditions, you'll likely come to appreciate that definitions of abnormality can vary with time and culture.

psychosis Serious form of mental disorder, involving an actual break with reality.

insanity Synonym for psychosis.

delusions Common symptom of psychosis that involves false or unusual beliefs; common delusions include persecution, romance, grandeur, and control.

hallucinations Abnormal auditory, gustatory, kinesthetic, olfactory, or visual perceptions that are common symptoms of psychosis; most common are those in which voices are heard or objects are seen that don't exist.

We also hope that by studying this material you'll come to appreciate—perhaps for the first time—the vital interplay of biology, psychology, and the environment in determining behavior. We stress repeatedly throughout this book that all behavior—normal and abnormal—is affected by many influences. We think it's important to share with you this **biopsychosocial perspective.** This term is used throughout to highlight the simultaneous impact on behavior of:

- *biological factors*—normal biology and disease processes as well as genetic influences
- *psychological factors*—our thoughts, feelings, and perceptions
- *social and environmental factors*—features of the social environments we live in

To understand psychopathology, we believe you must understand the biopsychosocial perspective.

Focus on Critical Thinking

1. Think of a few behaviors that you consider normal but that your grandparents or their grandparents would have considered abnormal. What are possible reasons for these differences between generations?

WHAT IS ABNORMAL BEHAVIOR?

How do we decide whether our own behavior or that of others is normal or abnormal? In some cases, the symptoms are so dramatic or unusual that there's little doubt that a person is no longer behaving normally. For instance, a young man who believes that his thoughts are being broadcast by the local radio station or that a fraternity brother plans to wire his car with explosives is clearly no longer thinking normally. Similarly, a young woman who regularly converses aloud with deceased members of her family as she sits in class has, to some degree, lost touch with reality.

But other cases are more subtle. What about the individual who becomes so upset over a supervisor's criticism that she quits her job, causing her and her family great financial hardship? What about someone who's firmly convinced that a fortune-teller can predict the future? What about the man who occasionally enjoys dressing up in women's clothing, although he's happily married and seems, in all other respects, an average, well-adjusted person? For that matter, what about people who continue to smoke cigarettes or athletes who continue to take steroids, even though they know the substantial health risks they're running? As these examples suggest, it's not always easy to decide when behavior is abnormal.

The case material that follows makes the same point. In reading about Billy Ainsworth, you'll find yourself asking whether he suffered from mental illness at all or just had a few rough months. Was his behavior abnormal or just troubled for a brief period?

Billy Ainsworth was a 21-year-old senior at a university in the southwestern United States when he came to the university's counseling center following the end of a relationship three months earlier with a young woman, Jill, with whom he had had a lengthy relationship. Even though, in his words, they had shared a real love relationship, they had ultimately decided to date other people. After doing so for a time, Jill had found someone else she preferred to Billy.

After their breakup, life at the university changed dramatically for Billy. His interest in his schoolwork, previously very high, diminished substantially, in part because he began finding it harder and harder to concentrate properly, both during class and when he wanted to study. Billy also found it more and more difficult to get to sleep; and even when he was able to do so, he would often awaken early in the morning, unable to fall back to sleep. His waking thoughts centered on his role in the loss of his relationship with Jill. Interestingly, though he felt sad when he thought about what they had had together, there were times when he could enjoy himself with friends and get involved again in politics and sports, his special interests.

biopsychosocial perspective *View stressing the vital interplay of biology, psychology, and the social environment in determining normal and abnormal behavior.*

Compounding his turmoil and adding to his reasons for coming to the counseling center were Billy's problems making choices among his career options. Although he was within a few months of graduating from the university, he had still not decided what he wanted to do after graduation. Should he find a job and begin a business career or, instead, remain a student for a few additional years? And, if he chose the graduate school route, should it be law school or business school?

This was the agenda Billy brought to his first appointment with a counselor at the university counseling center. (adapted from Spitzer, Skodol, Gibbon, & Williams, 1983, p. 195)

Billy's problems interfered enough with living a normal life that he sought professional help to deal with them. One of the most common reasons people seek help for psychological problems is that their problems have begun to interfere with their school, job, or family life. (As a general rule, if and when you come to believe you need help with emotional problems, you probably do!)

Billy Ainsworth's behavior raises a number of questions: Is it abnormal to be so sad following the loss of a valued relationship that it interferes with regular functioning? When do sadness and the experience of loss become depression? When should someone who's depressed seek help, and who should he turn to? Since we all experience periods of depression (most of them, fortunately, of brief duration), it's clear that only some depressive experiences merit professional attention. Finally, when should someone seek professional help for other emotional or psychological problems, either for himself or for a friend or loved one? Answers to these questions will be offered throughout the rest of this chapter and book.

How Should We Judge Behavior?

We use a variety of standards to judge whether behavior—our own and that of others—is normal or abnormal, healthy or pathological. These judgments are important to us. During times of stress, grief, or illness, for example, we may worry that our behavior has become so disturbed or unusual that taking care of ourselves, receiving solace from friends, or just letting time pass may not be enough. Professional consultation may be required. Billy Ainsworth came to this conclusion, but only after several months of suffering.

Judgments of behavior (including our own) are difficult to make because the standards we use to determine adequacy or appropriateness vary a lot from person to person and group to group within our multifaceted society. These standards vary even more between societies, cultures, and nations that are separated by time, climate, and distance. Consider how much things have changed in the United States over the past few generations. For example, today, we consider the harsh physical punishments once routinely imposed on children to be child abuse. And although divorce is common today, only a couple of generations ago, it was considered shockingly deviant. Similarly, in the 1940s and 1950s, the idea of a coed dormitory would have been considered scandalous. In light of these changes in what's considered *normal*, no wonder it's so difficult to label someone's actions *abnormal*.

The fourth edition of the ***Diagnostic and Statistical Manual of Mental Disorders (DSM-IV)*** (American Psychiatric Association, 1994)—the current, authoritative listing of mental disorders used by U.S. mental health professionals—solves the problem of judging what's abnormal by adopting a very broad definition. The *DSM-IV* conceptualizes *mental disorder* as "a clinically significant behavioral or psychological syndrome or pattern . . . associated with either a painful symptom or impairment in one or more important areas of functioning."

Billy Ainsworth's condition meets this definition. However, as our detailed discussion of the *DSM-IV* in Chapter 3 will show, the individuals who drafted this instrument and its immediate predecessors were criticized for adopting an overinclusive definition of mental disorder, which means that the *DSM* includes some

Diagnostic and Statistical Manual of Mental Disorders (DSM-IV) Current authoritative listing of mental disorders in use in the United States.

behaviors that not everyone agrees should be considered mental disorders. For example, these critics would claim that Billy Ainsworth's reaction to the loss of his relationship with Jill doesn't warrant inclusion because its impact on his life was likely to be brief and of little long-term consequence.

Seven Views of Abnormal Behavior

Wakefield (1992) describes seven different views of abnormal behavior. Even though each is thought provoking, none completely defines the concept *abnormal behavior*. Collectively, however, these definitions nicely establish the limits of the concept.

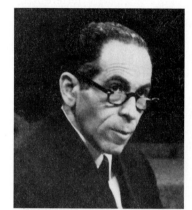

THOMAS SZASZ *proposed the revolutionary notion more than 35 years ago that mental illness is a myth. What was Szasz trying to convey in taking this position?*

Mental Disorder as Myth   More than thirty years ago, psychiatrist Thomas Szasz (1960) expressed the idea that schizophrenia is not a disease. (His views are discussed more fully in Chapter 13.) Even today, Szasz is considered psychiatry's best-known critic for his belief that mental disorders don't exist and that the concept *mental disorder* was invented by psychiatrists to justify their exercise of power and social control over others. Critiquing this view that mental disorders are myths, Wakefield cites a wide range of data that demonstrate the real, undoubted existence of mental conditions that harm individuals and interfere with their ability to function in society. Wakefield and most other authorities, including the authors of this text, now accept the very substantial empirical evidence that mental disorders do exist.

Mental Disorder as Violation of Social Norms   Can mental disorders be the product of social norms? Can those behaviors a group considers unacceptable be labeled abnormal? In fact, some of the behaviors a group chooses to condemn might be defined as mental disorders, even though groups with different norms might not define them this way. As an example, some groups in U.S. society still consider homosexuality a form of mental disorder, even though most behavioral and biological scientists have rejected this view (as explained in Chapter 8).

In suggesting this view of mental disorder, Wakefield acknowledges that social norms do play an important role in defining certain behaviors as normal or abnormal. Previous generations would certainly have found a great deal in contemporary society to take issue with. Nonetheless, as Wakefield also notes, many of the most serious mental disorders have been considered problems by people of every society, regardless of when they lived or what values they had, which suggests that social values must yield to objective reality in these instances.

mental disorder as myth Mental disorders don't exist; the concept of mental disorder was invented by psychiatrists to justify their exercise of power.

mental disorder as violation of social norms Mental disorder is largely a product of social norms that determine the behaviors a group finds acceptable and unacceptable.

mental disorder as whatever professionals treat Mental disorder is best defined as whatever professionals decide to treat.

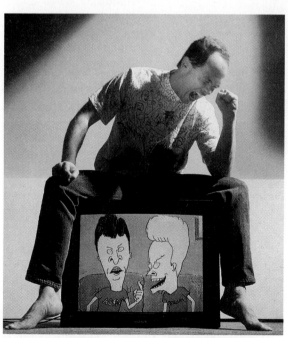

How could someone as normal as Mike Judge think up characters as bizarre as Beavis and Butt-Head?

Mental Disorder as Whatever Professionals Treat Perhaps mental disorder should be defined as whatever professionals decide to treat

Thinking about CONTROVERSIAL ISSUES   Creativity and Madness

It's common knowledge that creativity and mental disorder go together. But do they?

This belief is not a new one. Aristotle, in the fourth century B.C., asked, "Why is it that all men who are outstanding in philosophy, poetry or the arts are melancholic?" Three hundred years ago, poet John Dryden rhymed, "Great wits are sure to madness near allied / And thin partitions do their bounds divide." How valid are these beliefs?

If several prominent authorities, writing recently on the subject, are to be believed, the ties linking creative genius and madness are extremely strong. In a recent review of two books exploring this link, Angier (1993) concludes that these volumes' authors have assembled exceptionally convincing cases. Jamison's *Touched with Fire: Manic Depressive Illness and the Artistic Temperament* (1993) examines the lives of a long list of distinguished authors who suffered from manic depressive disorder

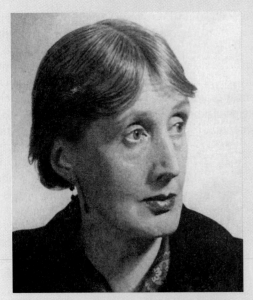

Although Virginia Woolf experienced serious mental illness throughout her life, she wrote some of the twentieth century's most distinguished fiction. How might creativity and madness be linked?

(which is a serious psychosis), including Lord Byron, Herman Melville, Virginia Woolf, and Robert Lowell. Jamison claims the rate of manic depression and major depression among distinguished artists such as these is 10 to 30 times the rate in the population at large. Ludwig's *The Price of Greatness* (1994) explores psychiatric disorders in 1,004 eminent women and men, finding that these disorders are much more common among artists than other prominent people. For example, 60 percent of actors and 41 percent of novelists suffered from alcoholism, as compared to only 3 percent of physical scientists and 10 percent of military officers.

Schildkraut, Hirshfeld, and Murphy (1994) report that the relationship between creativity and mental disorder is as valid for contemporary creative geniuses as for artists and writers of the past. Fifteen mid-twentieth-century abstract expressionist artists of the New York School were studied, including such famous individuals as Franz Kline, Willem de Kooning, Jackson Pollock, and Mark Rothko. More than half were found to have "some form of psychopathology, predominantly mood disorders, and preoccupation with death, compounded by alcohol abuse" (p. 482).

Angier offers this explanation for the link between mood disorders and creativity: "Because manic-depressive patients are ever riding the biochemical express between emotional extremes, their brains end up more complexly wired and remain more persistently plastic than do the brains of less mercurial sorts" (1993, p. B6).

Regardless of why it happens, lifelong emotional turmoil may be the price paid by some creative geniuses to have their gifts.

Think about the following questions:

1. Why might mood disorders be linked more closely to artistic creativity than to scientific creativity?
2. Is it possible that the link between creativity and madness is valid only for exceptional creativity and severe madness? How would you test this hypothesis?
3. Think about your most creative high school or college friends. Have any experienced emotional turmoil? If so, did it help or harm their creativity? How so?

(assuming, of course, that professionals know best what mental disorder is and how it should be treated). This suggestion has an obvious flaw, however, since mental health professionals are often called on to treat troubling behavior that clearly does not represent mental disorder. Difficulties with marriage, childrearing, and finding meaning in life are all troubling issues, but they aren't mental disorders.

Mental Disorder as Statistical Deviance   Defining mental disorder as statistical deviance would have us consider only behaviors that are statistically deviant (that is, unusual and rare). However, many conditions that are generally agreed to be mental disorders aren't unusual. Suicide is all too common—in fact, it's the third-leading cause of death among young people—but it's not normal. Moreover, as Wakefield points out, exceptional levels of intelligence, energy, and talent are rare, but no one thinks they're signs of mental disorder.

Mental Disorder as Biological Disadvantage   It's also tempting to define mental disorder in terms of its impact on reproduction, given the great personal importance reproduction has to us, as well as its significance to our species from an evolutionary perspective. Defining mental disorder as biological disadvantage labels as mental disorders those behaviors that interfere seriously with an individual's reproductive capacities. A number of serious mental disorders affect their victims' reproductive capacity adversely (including schizophrenia, some mood disorders, and developmental disabilities), even though many others do not. Homosexuality also affects reproduction, even though few psychologists or psychiatrists today consider it a mental disorder.

Mental Disorder as Unexpectable Distress or Disability   Defining mental disorder as unexpectable distress or disability is attractive because doing so comes reasonably close to the *DSM-IV* definition. According to this view, if your behavior causes you distress or disability that you don't expect, it meets the definition of mental disorder. However, as Wakefield observes, many conditions that simply can't be anticipated also cause distress or disability but are clearly not disorders (for example, extreme ignorance and plain misfortune, as well as poverty and discrimination).

Mental Disorder as Harmful Dysfunction   The view of mental disorder as harmful dysfunction is Wakefield's choice as the most accurate and helpful definition. It also happens to come closer than any of the other six to the definition of mental disorder in the *DSM-IV*.

There are two crucial elements in this definition. The first is that the concept *harmful* is a value term based on social norms. That is, what's considered harmful behavior varies from society to society. Some societies consider behaviors such as premarital sex, drug use, and certain antisocial actions to be harmful, whereas other societies consider them harmless. The second crucial element in this definition is *dysfunction*, which Wakefield considers to be a scientific term that refers to the failure of our "mental mechanism" (responsible for our emotional and cognitive selves) to perform the function it was designed for.

In sum, Wakefield values this definition of mental disorder above the others because it requires both scientific validation and consideration of social values.

mental disorder as statistical deviance Behaviors that are statistically deviant, rare, and unusual should be considered mental disorders.

mental disorder as biological disadvantage Behaviors that interfere with reproduction and evolution should be considered mental disorders.

mental disorder as unexpectable distress or disability Mental disorder is best defined as unexpectable distress or disability.

mental disorder as harmful dysfunction Mental disorder is best defined as harmful dysfunction.

Focus on Critical Thinking

1. Based on what you've read and discussed in class thus far, which view or definition of mental disorder do you most agree with? Why?

2. What separates weird or eccentric behavior from abnormal behavior? What consistent rules could you use to separate one from the other? Or is doing so possible? Have you known eccentric people? Did you judge them to be abnormal? Why?

Because of the complexity of judging behavior, most modern societies depend on mental health professionals to differentiate psychopathology from eccentricity, cultural deviance, or lifestyle variations. On their clinical judgments rest such vital decisions as whether someone ought to receive psychological or psychiatric treatment, where it should occur, and what it should consist of. Near the end of this chapter, we'll consider who these professionals are, how they're trained, and what each field contributes to understanding and treating people with mental disorders.

ABNORMAL BEHAVIOR IN THE CONTEMPORARY UNITED STATES

How many people in the United States suffer from mental disorders? What are the most common forms of mental illness? Is psychopathology increasing or decreasing in U.S. society? Do age, gender, race, income, lifestyle, or living conditions influence abnormal behavior? What about creativity or artistic temperament? How is abnormal behavior affected by natural catastrophes, such as floods and hurricanes, or environmental disasters, like the *Exxon Valdez* oil spill?

In March 1989, the supertanker *Exxon Valdez* spilled 11 million gallons of crude oil into the waters of Prince William Sound in Alaska, killing millions of sea birds, mammals, and fish; despoiling one of the nation's most pristine natural settings; and disrupting the economy of a large region of southern Alaska. A year later, an epidemiologic survey investigated the social and psychological consequences the event and its cleanup had on 599 residents of 13 communities in the region surrounding Prince William Sound (Palinkas, Petterson, Russell, & Downs, 1993).

Although significantly higher rates of both physical and psychiatric disorders have been reported following other disasters, the *Exxon Valdez* calamity was different in that its victims were never in physical danger or felt physically threatened. Nonetheless, the psychiatric consequences caused by this event and its cleanup were formidable. Of the residents who participated in the study, 30 percent met the diagnostic criteria for anxiety disorder, including posttraumatic stress, and 15 percent met the criteria for depressive disorder. These rates were between two and three times higher than those for Alaskans who had not been exposed to the oil spill and its consequences.

Women in the sample reported higher rates of depression and anxiety than men, whereas Inuits (Native Alaskans) reported higher rates of depression than non-Inuits. Previous research has reported women to be more vulnerable than men to the psychological consequences of disasters (Breslau, Davis, Andreski, & Peterson, 1991), but the reasons for this difference aren't obvious. Palinkas et al. (1993) speculate that the increased psychological vulnerability of Native Alaskans to the oil spill may reflect high rates of alcohol abuse before the spill as well as the traumatic effects of seeing these special lands spoiled. As the authors point out, "When the *Exxon Valdez* ran aground in Prince William Sound, it spilled oil into a social as well as a natural environment" (p. 1522).

Determining what impacts environmental events have on behavior is one of the primary tasks of mental health professionals. Much of the training of clinical psychologists, psychiatrists, psychiatric social workers, and psychiatric nurses is devoted to learning how to evaluate and diagnose (as shown in our overview of professional education, later in this chapter). Yet only in the last two decades have standardized diagnostic interviews enabled clinicians to achieve diagnostic agreement. These new, more reliable diagnostic tools have made it possible to reach greater consensus on the **incidence** and **prevalence** of psychopathology in the United States. The prevalence of a disorder is the total number of people within a given population who suffer from it, and the incidence is the number of people within a given population who have acquired the disorder within a specific time period (usually, a year).

It's surprising that agreement on the extent of psychopathology in the United States has only been reached so recently, given that five landmark **epidemiological surveys** of psychiatric disorder have been conducted since World War II, along with many smaller-scale epidemiologic investigations, such as the *Exxon Valdez* study. An epidemiological survey examines a carefully defined group of people to answer questions relating to the incidence, prevalence, and causation of disorder. The landmark surveys of psychiatric epidemiology include the Stirling County

incidence Number of people within a given population who have acquired a disorder or condition within a specific time period, usually a year.

prevalence Total number of people within a given population who suffer from a disorder or condition.

epidemiological surveys Studies of the incidence, prevalence, and often causation of specific disorders in particular groups or populations.

Study (Hughes, Tremblay, Rapaport, & Leighton, 1960), the Baltimore Morbidity Survey (Pasamanick, Toberts, Lemkau, & Krueger, 1962), the Midtown Manhattan Study (Srole, Langner, Michael, Opler, & Rennie, 1962), the New Haven Study (Weissman, Myers, & Harding, 1978), and the NIMH Epidemiologic Catchment Area (ECA) Study (Eaton, Anthony, Tepper, & Dryman, 1992; Regier et al., 1984). Each is considered a landmark study because its authors drew on the best survey methodology of their day to design a study that would yield data that could be generalized to populations across the United States.

The comparison that follows of data from the two most recent large-scale epidemiologic surveys of mental health and mental disorder in the United States (the Midtown and ECA surveys), as well as data from a more restricted survey of depression (Blazer, Kessler, McGonagle, & Swartz, 1994), shows the overall scope of the problem of mental disorder in this country.

Abnormal Behavior in Midtown Manhattan: 1952–1960

The **Midtown Manhattan Study** surveyed the mental health problems and resources in New York City between 1952 and 1960 (Srole et al., 1962). At the time, it was the most ambitious survey ever undertaken of mental health and mental illness in the United States. Interviews, based on a 200-item questionnaire, were given to 1,660 residents of mid-Manhattan who were selected to represent the 750,000 residents of the area as closely as possible in age, sex, race, ethnicity, and socioeconomic status.

The mental health of Midtown residents was categorized on a 6-point scale. Figure 1.1 shows the percentages of Midtown residents who fell into each category. These judgments were made by two psychiatrists after reading the completed interviews.

Only 18.5 percent of the persons surveyed were considered "well," or free from psychopathology. By contrast, more than 23 percent fell into one of the three severity categories: "marked," "severe," and "incapacitated." An individual given one

Midtown Manhattan Study Investigation of mental health problems and resources in New York City between 1952 and 1960; revealed substantially more psychiatric impairment in residents than anyone expected.

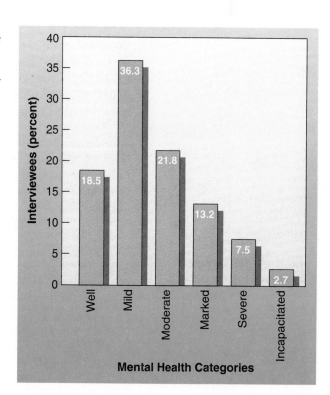

FIGURE 1.1 Prevalence of psychopathology in Midtown Manhattan

To almost everyone's surprise, only 18.5 percent of the people interviewed in the Midtown survey were considered to be free from psychopathology (those in the "well" category). More than 23 percent (those in the "marked," "severe," and "incapacitated" categories) were considered to have significant impairment.

SOURCE: From *Mental Health in the Metropolis: The Midtown Manhattan Study* by L. Srole et al., 1962. New York: McGraw-Hill. Reprinted by permission of the author.

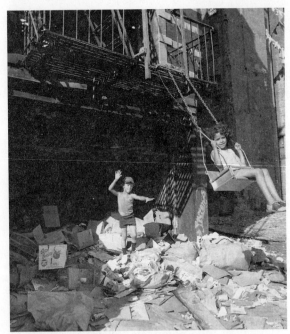

The Midtown study's most controversial finding—that the poor are most likely to be considered impaired psychologically—has since been repeatedly replicated, most recently by the ECA study. What are some of the factors that cause poverty and psychopathology to be associated with one another?

of these ratings had at least some difficulty working, going to school, meeting ordinary family obligations, and the like. Since these interviewees were representative of the entire New York metropolitan area, the study's unexpected major finding was that almost one-quarter of the several million people living and working there were emotionally impaired.

The Midtown study generated additional controversy when subsequent analysis of its findings showed that lower-class, or poor, Midtown residents were much more likely to be judged impaired than middle- or upper-middle-class residents. Since a principal aim of the study was to examine the effects of urban stress on psychopathology, the obvious conclusion from these findings was that urban stress disproportionately burdens people who are poor. Publication of these findings brought charges ranging from racism on the part of the interviewers, because the poor in Midtown were mainly African American and Hispanic, to insensitivity on the part of the politicians, who were accused of systematically ignoring the plight of these people.

Similar findings have emerged from subsequent epidemiological studies, leading to the conclusion that racism and discrimination against people who are poor appear to have a disproportionate impact on psychopathology in American society. The *social consequence model of psychopathology*, which is informed by findings like these, is considered in detail in Chapter 2.

Abnormal Behavior in Five U.S. Cities: 1981–1983

The **NIMH Epidemiologic Catchment Area (ECA) Study** surveyed the psychiatric status of more than 20,000 persons residing in five U.S. cities and towns in the early 1980s (Eaton et al., 1992; Regier et al., 1984). The ECA study assessed rates of specific mental disorders, rather than the more general rates of impairment the Midtown study reported (Regier & Burke, 1987). The development of a standardized interview schedule, the Diagnostic Interview Schedule (DIS) (Robins, Helzer, Croughan, & Ratcliff, 1981) (described in Chapter 3), enabled interviewers to make diagnostic judgments this specific. The DIS could also be administered by trained nonprofessionals, making a large-scale diagnostic study economically feasible.

The size, diversity, and representativeness of the ECA sample population was an additional strength. Drawn from five sites (Baltimore, Maryland; Durham, North Carolina; Los Angeles, California; New Haven, Connecticut; and Saint Louis, Missouri), survey subjects were almost as diverse geographically, economically, socioculturally, and ethnically as the United States as a whole.

Major findings from the ECA survey included the following:

- Significantly more major depressive episodes and drug abuse/dependence were found among residents of the city of Durham, North Carolina, than those living in rural areas outside Durham. However, alcohol abuse/dependence was a greater problem for inhabitants of the rural areas (Blazer et al., 1985). These findings reinforce the idea, first suggested by the Midtown survey, that the social environment people live in affects both the rates of psychopathology and the forms it takes.
- Hispanics, most of them Mexican Americans, displayed significantly higher rates of brain damage than non-Hispanic whites in the Los Angeles sample. By contrast, non-Hispanic whites had higher rates of drug abuse/dependence than either Mexican Americans in Los Angeles or interviewees at

NIMH Epidemiologic Catchment Area (ECA) Study Surveyed the psychiatric status of more than 20,000 persons residing in five U.S. cities and towns in the early 1980s; reported even higher rates of psychiatric disorder than the Midtown Manhattan Study.

TABLE 1.1 Lifetime Prevalence Rates of DIS/DSM-III Disorders (in percent)			
Disorders	**New Haven**	**Baltimore**	**Saint Louis**
Any disorder	28.8	38.0	31.0
■ Substance use disorders	15.0	17.0	18.1
■ Schizophrenic/schizophreniform	2.0	1.9	1.1
■ Affective disorders	9.5	6.1	8.0
■ Anxiety/somatoform disorder	10.4	25.1	11.1
■ Eating disorder	0.0	0.1	0.1
■ Antisocial personality	2.1	2.6	3.3
■ Cognitive impairment—severe	1.3	1.3	1.0

Source: From Robins et al. (1984), "Lifetime Prevalence Rates of DIS/DSM-III Disorders," *Archives of General Psychiatry, 41,* p. 952. Copyright 1984 American Medical Association.

other ECA sites (Burnam et al., 1987). These findings reinforce the growing conviction that race and ethnicity play an important role in the development of psychopathology, a finding that data from the Midtown study implied but couldn't confirm.

■ As Table 1.1 indicates, about one-third of the persons studied in the three ECA communities of New Haven, Baltimore, and Saint Louis met interview criteria for one or more of nine common diagnoses at some time during their lives—from a low of 28.8 percent in New Haven to a high of 38.0 percent in Baltimore (Robins et al., 1984). These figures are even higher than the impairment figures reported by the Midtown study.

Overall, the ECA study confirms that many Americans suffer significant impairment from stress, distress, and emotionally related problems. Men and women demonstrate comparable prevalence rates, which vary with age, socio-economic status, race, ethnicity, and environment. Relatively few individuals, however, seek treatment for their disorders, and of those who do, even fewer go to adequately trained mental health professionals.

Remember Elizabeth H. from the scenario at the beginning of the chapter? She'd been asked to participate in an ECA study conducted by NIMH. Let's take a look at Elizabeth H.'s interview.

Elizabeth's interview didn't begin exactly as she thought it would. Because she arrived back home late from work, the young woman who was to interview her was waiting by her door when she got off the elevator. So Elizabeth had no time to get her children settled or to change into more comfortable clothes before sitting down in the living room for the interview.

Most of the questions were what Elizabeth expected (it helped that she'd been a psychology major in college!), but there were more of them and they covered a broader range of thoughts, feelings, and behaviors than she'd anticipated. They also got pretty personal at times, such as when she was asked about her sexual preferences and drug and alcohol use. The only times Elizabeth actually got flustered, though, were when she was asked about her husband's drinking (along with the anger that sometimes accompanied it) and her "spells" of lethargy and sadness.

Although she may have been especially sensitive to these questions, Elizabeth thought the interviewer pushed a bit more about these subjects, asking a few more probing questions than she had to. But later that evening and then several more times during the days that followed, when Elizabeth reflected on the interview, she began to feel differently. Maybe those issues were ones she hadn't ever been able to view objectively. Maybe she'd been fooling herself a bit. The interviewer, with her objectivity and established interview style, was only doing what she was supposed to be doing.

Elizabeth concluded that the experience had been interesting, worthwhile, a bit daunting, but ultimately valuable. She thought some more about her "spells" and her husband's drinking and decided that she should come to better terms with them. She wondered whether she ought to ask a friend at work for the name of a counselor she could talk to about them.

Depression in a National Sample: 1990–1992

Depression is a very common, sometimes disabling psychiatric condition. Based on results of a recent survey, involving a national sample of 8,098 persons, 15 to 54 years of age, from the 48 mainland U.S. states, Blazer and his colleagues report a current rate of major depression of about 5 percent (Blazer et al., 1994). Women, young adults, and individuals with less than a college education showed the highest rates. Lifetime prevalence for major depression was about 17 percent, with the same groups (women, young adults, and individuals with less than a college education) demonstrating the highest lifetime prevalences.

When called on to explain these rates, which are substantially higher than estimates from the ECA and Midtown studies (which were themselves surprisingly high), Blazer and his co-workers point to a more sensitive diagnostic questionnaire and a younger sample, from which higher rates of major depression could be expected. As the product of a methodologically sound, large-scale epidemiologic study, these findings confirm that depression, in its several forms, has become one of the major mental health problems in the United States, especially among women.

Speculating on reasons for women's heightened vulnerability to depression, Strickland (1992) concludes that because both biological and psychosocial factors are involved, a biopsychosocial perspective on the problem makes the most sense. She cites three factors relevant to the biological side of the equation: (1) gender differences in neurophysiological functioning, (2) the premenstrual mood changes some women experience, and (3) the use of oral contraceptives by some women. Psychosocial factors include gender-role socialization patterns, the economic realities that face most single mothers, and the high levels of sexual and physical violence against women in this country. The heightened risk of depression for women is a highly important clinical and methodological issue and will be discussed in greater detail in Chapter 7.

> ### Focus on Critical Thinking
>
> 1. Consider the similarities and differences between your home community and the communities studied in the epidemiologic surveys discussed in this section. Using the numbers reported in those studies as a basis, estimate the incidence and prevalence of mental disorder in your community.

natural forces As causes of mental disorder, include genetic factors, disease processes, and environmental and psychological factors.

supernatural forces Long thought responsible for mental disorder; demonic possession was an especially common explanation for psychosis.

ABNORMAL BEHAVIOR THROUGH HISTORY

Our earliest ideas about abnormal behavior have been lost in prehistory. We have no way of knowing whether our distant ancestors attributed strange behavior to **natural forces,** such as sickness or a blow to the head, or to **supernatural forces,** like demonic possession or punishment from the gods. Perhaps they accepted both kinds of explanation, as some people still do today.

Throughout recorded history, natural and supernatural explanations for abnormal behavior have competed for acceptance. Only during the last century have most people come to recognize that mental disorders are caused by natural forces, rather than supernatural ones. Today, we know these natural forces include biological, psychological, and social factors. But even in the relatively recent and enlightened past, people believed that the gods caused every event beyond human understanding or control, including natural events (such as earthquakes, hurricanes, pestilence, famine, eclipses, and seasons) as well as personal disorders (such as psychosis, mental retardation, and epilepsy).

Many of the disorders that ancient and medieval peoples attributed to supernatural forces were psychotic disorders, or psychoses. We can easily understand why ancient peoples were frightened by such behavior, which they couldn't understand. Since they lacked the knowledge provided by modern science, they created mythic explanations to account for abnormal behavior and employed harsh measures to treat it. In like manner, the behavioral abnormalities associated with **mental retardation** and **epilepsy** caused people with these conditions to be socially isolated and even persecuted.

The Ancient World

Not all ancient societies accepted the prevailing supernatural explanations for psychiatric and behavioral disorders. During the seventh century B.C., for example, Chinese physicians concluded that an imbalance in the essential natural forces they called *yin* and *yang* shared responsibility for physical and mental illness.

The ancient Greeks held a similarly naturalistic view of the causes of disease. Hippocrates (460–377 B.C.), the father of medicine, suggested that disease (mainly brain disease) was responsible for mental disorders. He believed that most common mental disorders were due to an imbalance in the four essential fluids, or *humors,* circulating through the body: blood, phlegm, yellow bile, and black bile. For example, too much black bile caused depression, and too much yellow bile caused anxiety and irritability. Hippocrates prescribed natural treatments for these conditions, including rest, solitude, good food and drink, and abstinence from sexual activity.

Hippocrates' theory of imbalance in the body's chemistry foreshadowed the discovery of biological components of mental disorders made centuries later by modern science. Hippocrates also recognized other natural causes of abnormality—including stress, diet, heredity, head injury, and family problems—and contributed to the diagnoses of medical and psychiatric disorders. Although the most rudimentary diagnostic instruments had not yet been invented and knowledge of human anatomy was extremely primitive, Hippocrates described a number of mental disorders that are familiar to us today, including mania, melancholia (depression), and paranoia. His careful observation of patients, which was by itself innovative, permitted him to describe these conditions with great accuracy.

Although Plato (429–347 B.C.) and Aristotle (384–322 B.C.) were philosophers, not physicians, they were influential in promoting a naturalistic approach to treating mental disorders. They also believed that people with mental disturbances were ill; accordingly, they were to be treated humanely and not to be held accountable for their actions. In addition, the ancient Greeks recognized the behavioral effects of pathological aging, describing the symptoms of what we now call Alzheimer's disease as well as the psychological and behavioral effects of alcohol abuse.

The Middle Ages

Greek views of mental disorder persisted into Roman times, but after the fall of the Roman empire in the fifth century, efforts such as those by Hippocrates and Galen

mental retardation Condition of subaverage general intellectual functioning which originates in the developmental period and is associated with impairments in adaptive behavior.

epilepsy Chronic brain disorder manifested by recurrent seizures.

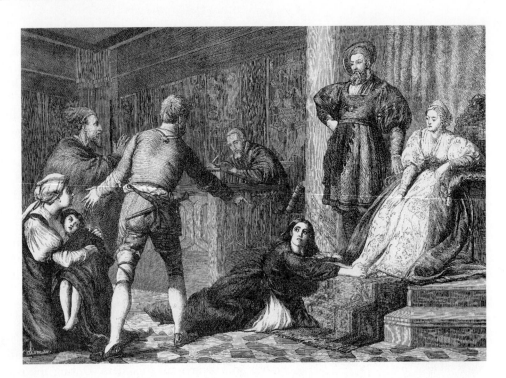

This contemporary woodcut shows the inquisition of an unfortunate young woman accused of witchcraft during the Middle Ages.

(c. A.D. 130–200) to discover natural causes for abnormal behavior virtually stopped. During the Middle Ages, religion dominated all aspects of European life, and people explained episodes of mental disorder in supernatural terms. Persons who were troubled were supposedly being punished for their sins or possessed by demons. Although some of these individuals were considered to be sick and were humanely cared for at home, others were horribly persecuted. Exorcisms were performed on some disturbed individuals, in an attempt to drive out the devils possessing them, and others were shouted at, deprived of food, flogged, or tortured.

During the late years of the Middle Ages, the stable medieval world began to change. Wars, peasant revolts, and finally the Black Death convinced people of the idea that powerful evil forces existed. One result of this thinking was the phenomenon known as the *witch craze.*

The Renaissance

During the Renaissance (1400s–1600s), people who were insane, poor, and epileptic were treated more humanely. Swiss physician and philosopher Paracelsus (1493–1541) criticized the notion that demons possess people. He proposed instead that the stars and planets affect the actions of the brain—specifically, that the phases of the moon play an important role in the development of abnormal behavior. This idea is preserved today in the word *lunatic,* which refers to an insane person. (*Luna* is the Latin word for *moon.*)

After personally witnessing the torture and death of several supposed witches, German physician Johann Weyer (1515–1588) wrote a treatise published in 1563, in which he argued that many of the people put to death were mentally unbalanced and thus couldn't be held responsible for their actions. Although the Catholic Church banned his work, a few academics and intellectuals shared Weyer's skepticism. One such individual was Englishman Reginald Scot (1538–1595), who published *Discovery of Witchcraft* in 1584, arguing that mental disorders were caused by illness, rather than demons and devils.

Asylums and Reforms

The earliest institutional care for people who were mentally disturbed was provided by religious orders, who sometimes sheltered them in monasteries. Hospitals occasionally accepted mental patients, too. By the mid–sixteenth century, institutions

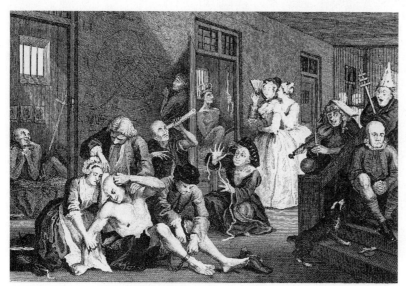

This famous engraving by William Hogarth (1697–1764) captures seventeenth-century England's attitude toward the human misery of the inmates of London's Bethlehem Hospital. How are contemporary attitudes toward mental patients different from those of seventeenth-century England? How are they similar?

known as *asylums,* or madhouses, were established specifically to house the mentally ill. Perhaps the best known was London's Bethlehem Hospital, whose name was commonly contracted to *Bedlam,* a term that has come to mean chaos and confusion. Residents were chained to walls and otherwise subjected to a variety of mistreatments; the public purchased tickets to see them, as if they were animals in a zoo. "Bedlam" and other contemporary asylums were more like prisons than hospitals. In the United States, the first asylums were established in the mid-1700s. Conditions in these institutions weren't much better than those in Europe.

Reform in the care of mental patients followed the American (1776) and French (1789) Revolutions, which both spread ideas about individual rights and human dignity. The first notable reform occurred at La Bicêtre, a large asylum in Paris. Conditions improved through the efforts of Philippe Pinel (1745–1826), physician-in-chief at La Bicêtre, and his staff. Pinel unchained patients, allowed them outdoor exercise, ordered their cells cleaned, and prohibited attendants from beating them.

While Pinel was instituting his reforms, Englishman William Tuke (1732–1822) set up York Retreat, an asylum in a country house in northern England. A Quaker, Tuke believed that a haven of rural quiet and considerate treatment would benefit mental patients. At York Retreat, patients prayed and worked together, took walks, and rested. Many apparently recovered and went home.

In America, the most prominent mental health reformer was Benjamin Rush (1745–1813), who's known as "the father of American psychiatry." While associated with the Pennsylvania Hospital in Philadelphia, Rush wrote the first American treatise on psychiatry and established the first medical course in psychiatry. His medical theories were primitive; for instance, he believed that the positions of the stars influenced the brain and regularly employed bloodletting, believing that too much blood in the brain caused disturbed behavior. But Rush's interest in the scientific study of his patients and his insistence on humane treatment were positive influences on the field.

Another American reformer, Dorothea Dix (1802–1887), was a Massachusetts schoolteacher. Her work teaching women inmates in prison made her aware of the conditions in the asylums of her day. Hoping to improve conditions inside mental institutions and to raise money to build new ones, Dix began to travel around her state and then across the country. Through her efforts, more than 30 mental hospitals were built.

The Rise of the Scientific Model

The founding of insane asylums toward the end of the eighteenth century meant that, for the first time, sizable groups of mental patients were brought together. In

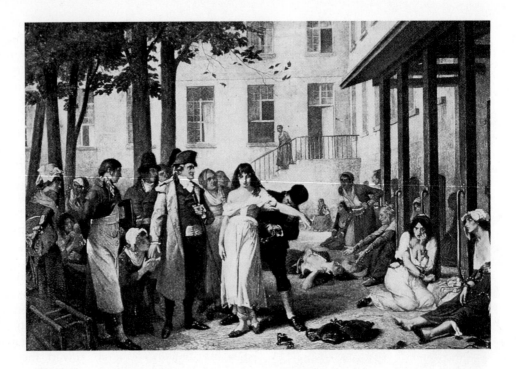

This contemporary painting shows Philippe Pinel freeing La Bicêtre's patients from their chains, thereby ushering in a more enlightened era for hospitalized mental patients throughout Europe and America.

addition to providing humane conditions for patients, asylums also gave physicians their first opportunity to observe, contrast, and study the behavior of large groups of individuals with serious disorders. These studies laid the groundwork for the scientific model of mental disorder, which was soon to follow.

melancholia Term used by Pinel to refer to severe depression; rarely employed today to describe that condition.

mania Part of Pinel's classification system; today refers to periods of marked agitation, elation, and grandiose thinking.

delirium Part of Pinel's classification system; used today to describe an acute brain disorder chiefly characterized by profound disorientation.

dementia Part of Pinel's classification system; used today to refer to chronic cognitive disorder affecting memory, personality, and judgment.

idiotism Component of Pinel's classification system; no longer used to refer to mental retardation.

schizophrenia Most common psychosis; characterized by hallucinations, delusions, profound problems in thinking, and bizarre behavior.

Pinel's Classification System   Philippe Pinel was one of the first to take advantage of this new opportunity for research. After making detailed observations of patients, he divided their disorders into the following categories:

■ **melancholia** (severe depression)
■ **mania** (marked agitation, grandiose thinking, and elation) without **delirium** (lost awareness of the environment, time, and self)
■ mania with delirium
■ **dementia** (a chronic disabling disorder marked by memory loss, personality change, and deterioration in judgment and personal habits)
■ **idiotism** (mental retardation)

This classification system, based on Pinel's careful clinical observations, was one of the first modern psychiatric nomenclatures.

Kraepelin and the German Classifiers   German physicians working in the latter half of the nineteenth century, about 60 years after Pinel's reforms, led a growing effort to develop more systematic methods for classifying and categorizing mental disorders. The availability of large groups of patients in mental hospitals made the effort possible.

The most influential of these workers was Emil Kraepelin (1856–1926). He combined previously separate diagnostic conditions into a single diagnostic category, which he called *dementia praecox* (literally, "premature dementia"). Kraepelin used this term to describe the decline in cognitive functioning he saw in adolescents suffering from the disorder, which resembled the decline found in some elderly people. Kraepelin described this common disorder in detail and carefully described its subtypes. Swiss psychiatrist Eugen Bleuler (1857–1939) subsequently renamed the condition **schizophrenia,** which it's known as today.

The emergence of dementia praecox, or schizophrenia, as a single, recognized disorder constituted a great advance. It marked the first time that a clinician taking a scientific approach had investigated in detail a common and serious psychiatric disorder. In his *Psychiatry: A Textbook* (1913), Kraepelin argued persuasively that many of the most common mental disorders are disorders of the brain—for instance, dementia praecox, manic-depressive psychosis (now called *bipolar affective disorder*), and disorders of the central nervous system. Kraepelin's views on the causes of mental disorders were revolutionary. In fact, his views and practices continue to influence mental health professionals today, including his detailed medical and psychiatric histories of patients, his development of the mental status examination (to assess more completely the patient's mental state), his emphasis on thorough behavioral observation of patients' symptoms to establish diagnoses, and his consideration of the psychoses as, first and foremost, diseases of the brain.

Also during the mid-nineteenth century, French physician Louis Pasteur (1822–1895) postulated the germ theory of disease. He was the first to prove that tiny organisms and viruses infect the body, ultimately producing physical symptoms. Ultimately, bacterial diseases with behavioral consequences received scientific attention; syphilis, a sexually transmitted disease with many serious consequences, was among the first to be studied. The causal agents of these diseases were identified and effective antibacterial treatments were found for some of them, with discoveries continuing well into the present century. Acceptance of the idea that bodily diseases had identifiable, biological causes supported the notion that mental problems might also prove to be diseases, with known causes and effective treatments.

Freud's Psychoanalytic Revolution

Another influential view on mental illness emerged at the end of the nineteenth century and, like that of Emil Kraepelin, still affects us today. Psychoanalytic theory was developed by Viennese physician Sigmund Freud (1856–1939). As a young man, Freud studied in Paris with the famous neurologist Jean-Martin Charcot (1825–1893), who was interested in the role of emotional factors in neurological disorders. Charcot and his associates found that patients lost their neurological symptoms when they were hypnotized. Freud concluded that patients lost their symptoms during hypnosis because psychological factors, not bodily disease, had caused them.

Returning to Vienna, Freud began working with neuropsychiatrist Josef Breuer (1842–1925), who had begun to treat psychiatric patients with hypnosis. Breuer revealed to Freud that even very disturbed patients recovered when they talked about their problems under hypnosis. He called this approach the *cathartic method,* or "talking cure," since hysterical patients seemed to undergo an emotional catharsis, or cleansing, while talking about their problems under hypnosis (Jones, 1953). After trying Breuer's method for a time, Freud abandoned hypnosis and began to simply encourage his patients to talk freely in his presence. He believed that the emotional conflicts behind patients' problems would eventually reveal themselves during verbal free association, when patients were asked to talk about whatever came to mind.

Together, Breuer and Freud wrote *Studies in Hysteria,* published in 1895, and launched the psychoanalytic revolution. Their book put forth several revolutionary ideas:

- Psychological factors affect behavior in powerful ways.
- "Talking treatments" could be more effective for treating disordered behavior than the harsh physical and moral treatments then in use.
- Behavior is influenced by thought patterns, impulses, and wishes that individuals are largely unaware of.

■ Nonpsychotic behavioral disorders, such as anxiety and phobic behavior, are worthy of attention and treatment by psychiatrists.

These tenets of psychoanalytic theory (considered in greater detail in Chapter 2) dominated the treatment of mental disorders in the early and mid–twentieth century. That's no longer the case, largely because a variety of other views of psychopathology have been developed since that time. Nonetheless, psychoanalytic theory continues to influence the views of mental health professionals regarding some conditions.

Adolf Meyer's Psychobiology

During the 1920s and 1930s, clinicians jarred by the horrors of World War I and its psychiatric casualties began to play a significant role in the development of psychiatry. One such figure was Adolf Meyer (1866–1950), a German psychiatrist who had emigrated to the United States. His conviction that organic, psychological, and environmental factors all contribute to psychopathology greatly influenced the clinical methods and procedures of his era. Meyer succinctly summarized his primary thesis as follows: "All life is a reaction, either to stimuli of the outside world or of the various parts of the organism. We recognize death by the absolute absence of these reactions" (Meyer, 1994, p. 44).

At the time, Meyer's *psychobiology* influenced generations of psychiatrists in training and countered the emphasis that psychoanalytic theory placed on the primacy of unconscious factors in determining behavior. Today, the influence of psychobiology (called the *biopsychosocial perspective* in this book) can be seen in a number of developments: in the nearly universal practice of clinicians, who take detailed personal, social, psychiatric, and family histories of all patients; in the multiaxial, biopsychosocial approach of the *DSM-IV* to diagnosis; and in the increasingly prevalent idea that one-dimensional perspectives on etiology (for instance, entirely biological or entirely psychological) are less productive than biopsychosocial views.

Contemporary Developments

Research on Etiology　Kraepelin, Freud, and Meyer all proposed theories of **etiology,** or explanations of the causes, of psychiatric disorders. These theories still influence many mental health workers.

The advances made in recent decades in understanding the etiology of mental disorder have outpaced those of any other time. Making these advances required the development of new investigative techniques and procedures, such as neuroimaging, genetics, molecular biology, and longitudinal research. Consequently, the etiologies of such common, profoundly disabling disorders as schizophrenia, bipolar affective disorder, alcoholism, and some cognitive disorders are now much better understood. Etiologic understanding, in turn, will almost certainly lead at some point to more effective prevention and treatment.

Advances in Treatment　Psychiatric patients have been offered treatment, rather than punishment, only since the late 1700s, when Pinel brought reform to psychiatric institutions. During most of the 1800s, however, until Freud's time, treatment consisted mainly of ineffective physical measures, such as special diets, baths, and bloodletting, even in mental hospitals that prided themselves on their humane care of patients. Dr. Samuel Woodward described one such treatment for mania in 1850:

As a means of exciting nausea, in violent cases of mania, the circular swing was recommended by the highest medical authority. Dr. Darwin speaks well of it and Dr. Cox relies upon it almost exclusively to remove maniacal excitement. It is a very

etiology Cause or causes of disorders and diseases, including mental disorders.

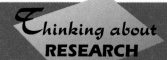

Thinking about RESEARCH   **Effects of the Gulf War on Israeli Civilians**

What are the short- and long-term consequences of profound stress on human beings? This remains an enduring, unanswered research question, in part because of the difficulty of setting up a study that would provide useful data. Ethical standards prohibit behavioral researchers from subjecting humans to intense stress for experimental purposes. As a result, some stress researchers have subjected animals to stress, which presents its own ethical problems as well as those involved in generalizing behavioral findings from animals to humans. Other researchers have prepared research teams to take advantage of naturally occurring environmental stressors, when and where they occur.

A team of psychiatrists and psychologists from Israel and the United States (Weizman et al., 1994) chose the latter research strategy to study the effects of the stress on civilians before, during, and after the Gulf War missile bombardment of Tel Aviv. (The Gulf War started with Iraq's invasion of Kuwait in January 1992. Iraq later retaliated against Israel for U.S. involvement.) In Study 1, levels of subjective anxiety and plasma cortisol and growth hormone (both of which reflect the effects of stress on the body) were assessed in 15 men and 11 women between the ages of 28 and 59 years before, during, and after the war. All these individuals were medical personnel from a mental health center in Tel Aviv. Study 2 involved 13 healthy residents of Tel Aviv (6 women and 7 men) between 25 and 59 years old. Their anxiety levels and levels of cortisol and growth hormone were assessed three times a day (morning, noon, and night) at two points, during and after the war.

In both studies, the subjective anxiety levels of the Israeli citizens were found to be significantly higher

before and during the war than afterward (by a factor of about 3). Anxiety levels tended to peak at night, which wasn't surprising, since most of the Iraqi missile attacks on Tel Aviv took place then. Unexpectedly, this marked increase in subjects' subjective feelings of anxiety wasn't accompanied by increases in the levels of plasma cortisol or growth hormone, which remained at constant levels before, during, and after the war. Moreover, the stress of the war didn't affect the normal daily variation of these measures. The authors of the studies concluded that these findings reflected the body's adaptation to continuous stress.

These findings are important, in part, because they contradict the assumption that subjective anxiety in response to a continuous stressor will be accompanied by similar increases in physiological measures of stress. The fact that the subjects reported marked anxiety but didn't show bodily changes in response to continuous stress documents a most important capability of the body to cope with intense, ongoing stress. And if these findings are confirmed and extended, they may prompt a change in the common view of the effects of chronic stress on the body, much of which is based on research with animals.

Think about the following questions:

1. What are some other examples of varying subjective and bodily responses to environmental stimuli?
2. Does this research convince you that some kinds of psychological research require the use of human subjects? If so, describe what kinds of research.
3. What are some of the implications these findings have for the assessment and treatment of mental disorders?

effective means of producing sickness, vertigo, and vomiting, and usually prostrates the system remarkably. It is not always a safe remedy. It is extremely unpleasant to the patient, and always regarded as a punishment, rather than a means of cure. (Woodward, 1994, p. 222)

Following Freud's development of the "talking therapies," psychological treatments were more widely used. After Freud proposed his psychoanalytic theory, a continuing stream of theorists and clinicians modified this theory and its techniques. These developments are summarized in Chapter 2, along with other psychological theories of abnormal behavior. Most notably, the behavioral model is discussed, since it has also strongly influenced contemporary psychological treatment methods.

Recent advances in pharmacotherapy (the use of drugs to treat psychopathology) have restored many persons suffering from psychoses to independent living. Newly developed drug treatments for schizophrenia, bipolar affective disorder, and major depression have permitted some patients to leave the hospital permanently after years of institutionalization. Also promising is the use of psychoactive

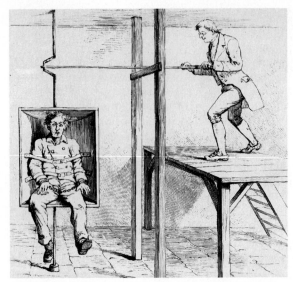

In its day, the circulating swing was considered a humane treatment for dealing with mania. How effective would this approach have been in curing the patient?

drugs to treat less severe disorders, including nonpsychotic but troubling conditions like mild and moderate depressive disorders and attention-deficit, obsessive-compulsive, and anxiety disorders. Used in combination with brief, intensive, inpatient treatment lasting two or three weeks, these new drugs help patients return far more quickly to their families and jobs than was possible before. Overall, the average length of a hospital stay for treating a mental disorder has been shortened dramatically, in part because of advances in drug therapy and in part because lengthy stays are too costly. Contemporary approaches to the physical treatment of psychiatric and behavioral disorders, which have been developed mainly during the last 30 years, are discussed in Chapter 20.

Another exciting development, even more recent than the development of effective physical treatments for psychiatric and behavioral disorders, has been the emergence of health psychology and its effort to find effective psychological treatments for physical disorders. Although still in its relative youth, the field of health psychology (discussed in the next section and Chapter 10) holds great promise for the fuller understanding and more effective treatment of some of our most burdensome physical disorders, including cancer and heart disease (Chesney, 1993).

Developments in Diagnosis and Classification   As mentioned earlier, advances in treating patients with mental disorders were made following the recognition that some of these individuals behaved differently from others in predictable ways. Based on careful observations, patients could be classified according to which symptoms they showed. With the realization that distinctive psychological disorders existed came awareness of the value of careful diagnosis. Accurate diagnosis is crucial, since, as with physical disease, proper treatment depends on correct identification and evaluation of the problem.

A psychiatric classification system designed specifically for use in the United States was first developed in the mid-1930s by an association of state hospital superintendents. Previously, almost every hospital that cared for psychiatric patients had its own diagnostic system. The lack of a standard system created enormous communication difficulties among professionals working in different hospitals. The new system predictably served the pressing needs of the large state psychiatric hospitals, which cared for most of the country's mental patients.

After the United States entered World War II in 1941, the need for a new classification system became clear, as many American soldiers developed behavioral symptoms under the profound stress of combat that couldn't be diagnosed by the existing system. A system was needed to categorize the psychiatric casualties of war, one that emphasized disorders reactive to the stress of combat rather than chronic psychosis. The U.S. War Department undertook the task.

In 1946, shortly after the end of World War II, representatives of the state hospitals, the War Department, and the Veterans Administration met to discuss creating a contemporary diagnostic system—a system that would be as useful for diagnosing people whose disorders seemed to be reactions to the stresses of modern life as it was for diagnosing long-term psychotic patients. The result was publication of the first edition of the *Diagnostic and Statistical Manual of Mental Disorders (DSM-I)* by the American Psychiatric Association in 1952. The *DSM-I* has been followed by the *DSM-II* (1968), *DSM-III* (1980), *DSM-III-R* (1987), and, most recently, *DSM-IV* (1994). Chapter 3 discusses the historical and clinical context of these instruments.

All four editions of the *DSM* show Kraepelin's influence. Each calls for the careful observation of signs and symptoms of psychiatric disorder, assumes that many of these disorders derive from central nervous system damage, and separates the major psychotic disorders into subtypes based on the same signs and symptoms Kraepelin identified. Meyer's psychobiology has also influenced the *DSM*.

By introducing a diagnostic system that enabled all mental health professionals in the United States to employ a common language, the first two editions of the *DSM* represented a great step forward. But once in use, its serious deficiencies became obvious. These slim volumes provided only a brief description of each disorder, together with one or two short paragraphs listing distinguishing signs and symptoms. This information wasn't detailed enough to enable clinicians to make reliable diagnoses. The third edition of the *DSM*, published in 1980, made marked advances in diagnoses (M. Wilson, 1993), giving clinicians and researchers a more reliable diagnostic system.

Focus on Critical Thinking

1. Why did so many ancient peoples believe abnormal behavior stemmed from the supernatural? What contemporary attitudes may remain from earlier beliefs in supernatural influences on mental illness?

2. Why did enlightened views on the treatment of mental patients likely coincide with the American and French Revolutions?

THE MENTAL HEALTH PROFESSIONS

Four distinct professions—clinical psychology, psychiatry, psychiatric social work, and psychiatric nursing—provide care for patients suffering from mental disorders. Differences in education, training, and experience ensure that each of these professions makes a unique contribution to the understanding and care of people with mental disorders.

Clinical Psychology

The first work in clinical psychology was conducted in the early 1900s by experts on the assessment of intelligence and personality. But it wasn't until the psychiatric casualties of World War II overwhelmed existing mental health resources that the field of clinical psychology began to grow in earnest. Beginning with a handful of clinical psychologists in 1945, the field had grown to more than 60,000 members by 1994.

Although men still make up the majority of clinical psychologists, increasing numbers of women have been attracted to the field during the past 20 years; in fact, more than half the graduate students in clinical psychology are now women. Historically, the clinical psychologist's major contributions to the mental health team have been skills in the assessment of intelligence, personality, and psychopathology as well as research skills. Clinical psychologists in training now receive more extensive education than other mental health professionals in psychotherapy and behavior therapy, so in many clinical settings, they have become authorities on the "talking therapies."

Because clinical psychologists have responded to the growing body of research that points to psychological and environmental factors in the etiology of a number of physical disorders, they have played an important role in establishing the new field of **health psychology** (Carmody & Matarazzo, 1991). Health psychologists assess the role of psychological factors in physical diseases and apply psychological treatments to people with those diseases. Health psychologists also carry out research on the relationship between psychological and biological factors in specific physical diseases in an effort to develop more effective psychological assessment and treatment methods.

health psychology
Developed from clinical psychology, this new field employs psychological methods to assess and treat physical diseases.

Neuropsychology is another recently developed branch of clinical psychology (Jones & Butters, 1991). Neuropsychologists study, evaluate, and diagnose patients with suspected or actual brain injury, using the neuropsychological test batteries and, increasingly, the imaging techniques detailed in Chapter 3. Neuropsychologists have also begun to develop remediation strategies to help patients with these types of injuries regain as many of their cognitive abilities as possible.

Like all health professionals, clinical psychologists have been challenged by the profound changes in health care delivery patterns currently under way in the United States, in which the goal is to provide a broader range of services at lower costs (Dial et al., 1992). For clinical psychologists, whose traditional roles are as mental health assessment and treatment specialists, this means shorter, more focused, more intensive assessment and treatment. One new role involves directly admitting psychiatric patients to hospitals and assuming primary responsibility for them while they're in the hospital (Dorken, 1993). Another role change calls for the clinical psychologist to develop a close working relationship with the family physician; in this role, the psychologist becomes the primary resource to diagnose, evaluate, and treat the psychological problems that influence patients' decisions to consult their family doctors (Schmittling, 1993; Wiggins, 1994).

On graduating from a four-year college, usually with a major in psychology or another social or natural science, the clinical psychologist-to-be enters a Ph.D. (doctorate in philosophy) or Psy.D. (doctorate in psychology) program in clinical psychology. Both require four or five years of academic work, plus a minimum one-year clinical internship. Programs awarding the Ph.D. provide more extensive training in research, while those awarding the Psy.D. offer more comprehensive training in practice.

Psychiatry

The special contributions psychiatrists make to the mental health team stem from their education and training as physicians, which gives them special skills in recognizing the impact of physical health and disease on both normal behavior and psychopathology. Since physical disorders masquerade as behavioral or psychiatric conditions and behavioral and psychiatric disorders share symptoms with some physical illnesses, these diagnostic skills are essential. Moreover, psychiatrists study **psychopharmacology** (the use of drugs to treat psychopathology) as part of their training as physicians and with special emphasis during their psychiatric residencies. During the past 30 years, effective drug treatments for several serious psychiatric disorders have been developed. The ability to prescribe the right drug for a certain condition, as well as knowing when a drug is not the treatment of choice, is an invaluable part of the psychiatrist's role and an essential element in the contemporary treatment of psychiatric patients.

A recent survey of the professional practice patterns of psychiatrists (Olfson, Pincus, & Dial, 1994) revealed that psychiatry, unlike the other three mental health professions, remains predominantly a private, rather than public, practice profession. More than 75 percent of psychiatrists now work primarily in private hospitals, clinics, and offices. In comparison, a substantially larger percentage of clinical psychologists work primarily in public service settings, and relatively few psychiatric social workers and psychiatric nurses work independently in private settings.

Psychiatry is a branch of medicine. As a result, the person intent on becoming a psychiatrist must first complete four years of college, followed by four years of medical school, a year of internship in a medical setting, and then three or more years in a psychiatric residency. During their residencies, psychiatrists-in-training assume increasing responsibility for the care of both inpatients, most of them seri-

neuropsychology Branch of clinical psychology devoted to the evaluation and diagnosis of brain injury.

psychopharmacology Use of drugs to treat psychopathology.

ously disturbed, and outpatients. As part of their residencies, psychiatrists learn how to diagnose psychiatric disorders, differentiate them from physical disorders they may share symptoms with, and treat them both psychotherapeutically and somatically (by physical means, including drugs). Psychiatric residents are also trained extensively in consultation skills, because consultation has become an increasingly important part of the role of the psychiatrist. Consultation involves conferring with other physicians and health professionals on the diagnosis and treatment of patients with physical disorders influenced by psychological factors.

Psychiatric Social Work

Psychiatric social workers bring strengths in group work to the mental health team—specifically, in assessing and treating the problems experienced by families, married couples, and groups in the urban United States. Psychiatric social workers trained in group psychotherapy devote much of their workday to providing psychotherapeutic services to couples, families, and groups. Not surprisingly, psychiatric social workers in poor, inner-city neighborhoods frequently suffer from burnout from having to care for too many patients with few individual resources.

Social workers also use their detailed knowledge of resources available in the community to help bring people badly in need of those resources to the mental health team. This knowledge enables psychiatric social workers to make sure that their patients receive the financial and social support from community programs that they may qualify for. Given their involvement in the community, it's not surprising that psychiatric social workers are often experts on the impact of environmental factors (such as substance abuse, poverty, crime, and homelessness) on patients' abilities to benefit from treatment.

Psychiatric social workers must complete four years of college and then two additional years at a university-based school of social work, from which they receive the master of social work (M.S.W.) degree. During their two years of graduate training, social work students learn about group and social processes and development, public policy and social organization, research methods, and the various kinds of programs federal, state, and local governments develop to help persons who can't help themselves. While in training, social workers may also study psychology, sociology, and other social science disciplines.

Psychiatric Nursing

Nurses trained in university settings generally receive a B.S. (bachelor of science) degree and a diploma in nursing upon graduation from the four-year nursing curriculum. After passing the required examination, graduates of these programs are then licensed as registered nurses. Psychiatric nursing students spend an additional two years in college pursuing a master's degree in psychiatric nursing, during which time they study psychopathology, diagnosis, and treatment. Special emphasis is given to psychopharmacology; nurses are usually responsible for ensuring that the powerful medications given to psychiatric inpatients are both effective and as free from side-effects as possible.

Extensive practicum training during the master's program, frequently with patients in inpatient settings, ensures that psychiatric nursing students acquire therapeutic skills. Psychiatric nurses have contributed to family therapy substantially. Another contribution has been to the *therapeutic milieu*, also termed the *therapeutic community*. Helped and supported by the nursing staff, psychiatric patients in a therapeutic community establish and enforce the rules governing their unit and regulating their interactions with each other. Many professionals believe

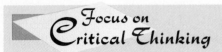

1. Weigh your own skills and interests objectively to determine which, if any, of the four mental health professions best suits you. Explain your answer.

that this approach helps even seriously disturbed patients to start reassuming responsibility for their own behavior and reestablishing social relations. Psychiatric nurses frequently have the task of ensuring the smooth functioning of the inpatient unit; for this reason, more and more psychiatric nurses are obtaining the management skills necessary for their roles as unit administrators.

SUMMARY

Why Study Abnormal Behavior?

■ One reason for studying abnormal behavior is that we all have frequent contacts with family, friends, and others whose behavior is abnormal.

■ Another reason for studying abnormal behavior is the perspective it gives us on the vital interplay among biology, psychology, and the environment as they affect normal and abnormal behavior.

What Is Abnormal Behavior?

■ The symptoms of abnormal behavior are sometimes obvious, sometimes obscure. Reflecting this fact, a variety of definitions of mental disorder have been adopted. The authoritative American listing of mental disorders, the *DSM-IV*, intentionally chose a very broad definition of mental illness, whereas some of the definitions suggested in a recent article by Wakefield (1992) are much more narrow.

Abnormal Behavior in the Contemporary United States

■ Epidemiological studies provide data on the incidence and prevalence of mental disorder for use in planning prevention and treatment. The three large-scale studies reviewed in this chapter all found much higher rates of impairment and disorder than expected. Urban, poor people and members of racial and ethnic minority groups demonstrated the highest rates of mental disorder; women were especially prone to depression.

Abnormal Behavior through History

■ Only during the last century have people become convinced that mental disorders are caused by natural, rather than supernatural, forces.

■ Reforms in the care of mental patients following the French and American Revolutions were led by Pinel, Tuke, and Dix.

■ Toward the end of the nineteenth century, Kraepelin developed systematic methods for categorizing mental disorder that continue to influence diagnostic practice today.

■ A decade later, Freud launched the psychoanalytic revolution.

■ Marked advances in research on etiology, in treatment, and in diagnosis and classification have been made in the last 20 years.

The Mental Health Professions

■ Four distinct professions—clinical psychology, psychiatry, psychiatric social work, and psychiatric nursing—provide care for patients suffering from mental disorders. Differences in education, training, and experience ensure that each profession makes unique contributions to the understanding and care of people with mental disorders.

KEY TERMS

biopsychosocial
perspective, **p. 3**
delirium, **p. 16**
delusions, **p. 2**
dementia, **p. 16**
*Diagnostic and Statistical
Manual of Mental
Disorders (DSM-IV),*
p. 4
epidemiological surveys,
p. 8
epilepsy, **p. 13**
etiology, **p. 18**
hallucinations, **p. 2**
health psychology, **p. 21**
idiotism, **p. 16**
incidence, **p. 8**

insanity, **p. 2**
mania, **p. 16**
melancholia, **p. 16**
mental disorder as biological disadvantage, **p. 7**
mental disorder as harmful
dysfunction, **p. 7**
mental disorder as myth,
p. 5
mental disorder as statistical deviance, **p. 7**
mental disorder as
unexpectable distress or
disability, **p. 7**
mental disorder as
violation of social
norms, **p. 5**

mental disorder as what-
ever professionals treat,
p. 5
mental retardation, **p. 13**
Midtown Manhattan Study,
p. 9
natural forces, **p. 12**
neuropsychology, **p. 22**
NIMH Epidemiologic
Catchment Area (ECA)
Study, **p. 10**
prevalence, **p. 8**
psychopharmacology, **p. 22**
psychosis, **p. 2**
schizophrenia, **p. 16**
supernatural forces, **p. 12**

$\mathcal{C}$RITICAL THINKING EXERCISE

As you've probably guessed, there were details of both her own behavior and her husband's that Elizabeth H. didn't really want to reveal to the ECA interviewer— or to herself. However, the diagnostic instrument the interviewer used was sensitive enough to register both diagnoses.

The ECA instrument diagnosed Elizabeth's husband's drinking problem as alcohol abuse. Over the course of an average month, he put away more than a case of beer. Even though 24 bottles of beer isn't excessive when consumed over 30 days, Elizabeth's husband tended to concentrate his drinking, so that when he drank, he drank enough to become very intoxicated. And when he did, he sometimes became abusive verbally and even physically to his wife and children. He had also been arrested twice for drunken driving and once for picking a fight in a bar.

Elizabeth H.'s "spells" were diagnosed by the ECA instrument as recurrent brief depressive disorder. Every three or four weeks, Elizabeth experienced a couple of days or more of low energy, insomnia, problems with concentration, and subjective feelings of sadness and lowered self-esteem. These "blue" periods sometimes interfered with her relationships at work and home.

1. Why did Elizabeth find it so difficult to admit that these two conditions existed and affected her and her family?

2. Why didn't Elizabeth seek help for herself or her husband for one or both of these conditions? She never failed to seek medical advice when she, her husband, or one of her children became physically sick.

*C*hapter 2
MODELS OF
ABNORMAL BEHAVIOR

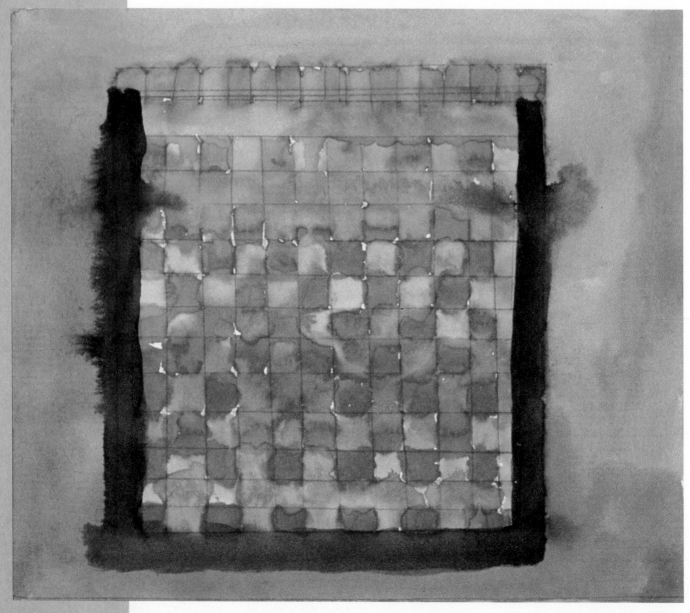

George Knerr, **Checkerboard,** HAI

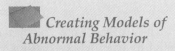
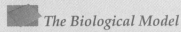
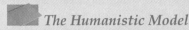
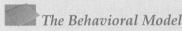
Malcolm Little was born in 1925 in Omaha, Nebraska, the son of the Reverend and Mrs. Earl Little. Reverend Little was a traveling Baptist minister and volunteer organizer for Marcus Garvey's Universal Negro Improvement Association; he was a passionate apostle for black justice, a cause that had few followers 70 years ago. Malcolm's mother, Louise, was born in the British West Indies to a black mother and white father; she was a gentle soul whose emotional instability affected Malcolm throughout his life. It was from his mother that Malcolm inherited the light skin and reddish hair that he ultimately grew to detest. Malcolm had seven siblings: two older brothers, an older sister and a younger sister, and two half brothers and a half sister from his father's previous marriage.

Malcolm's earliest memories were of fierce arguments between his father and mother. They often started when his mother began to criticize his father's emotional insensitivity and lack of ambition, and they frequently ended in violence. Malcolm remembered his father being gruff and impatient with his brothers and sisters and that he beat the older ones "almost savagely if they broke any of his rules." But his father never beat Malcolm. As an adult, Malcolm explained it this way:

> Nearly all my whippings came from my mother. I've thought a lot about why. I actually believe that as anti-white as my father was, he was subconsciously so afflicted with the white man's brainwashing of Negroes that he inclined to favor the light ones, and I was his lightest child. Most Negro parents in those days would almost instinctively treat any lighter children better than they did the darker ones. (Malcolm X, 1964, p. 4)

His father's sudden, violent death—which occurred when Malcolm was 6—became his most enduring early memory. The Reverend's body was discovered late one evening, lying across streetcar tracks in downtown Lansing, Michigan, where the family was then living. It was cut almost in half, and the skull was crushed in. Although no one knew for sure, most people were convinced that the Reverend had been killed by white vigilantes because of his civil rights "agitation."

The study of abnormal behavior gives insight to a broad range of human experience. Some abnormal behaviors deviate so slightly from what's considered normal that only a skilled diagnostician can identify them; others are so grossly abnormal that a child can recognize them as such. But the study of abnormal behavior, like the contents of this textbook, doesn't focus solely on the behavior of people with mental disorders. It also examines the complex causes of mental disorders as well as efforts to prevent and treat them.

CREATING MODELS OF ABNORMAL BEHAVIOR

We attempt to make sense of the puzzle of psychopathology by creating **models** that help us understand how abnormal behavior develops and how it might be treated or prevented. The first two models of mental disorder were developed long ago. One stressed the role of supernatural influences in the development of abnormal behavior, and another attributed these abnormalities to natural influences. Today, we term the latter the *biological model*. Models developed more recently emphasize the impact of social factors and psychological factors on psychopathology.

Models of abnormal behavior have changed greatly through the centuries, as we have acquired more factual information and relied less on speculation and superstition. In fact, during the past half century, we have learned more about abnormal behavior than in all the earlier centuries combined. Yet even today, new models are proposed because they are still useful.

This chapter considers in detail six contemporary models of psychopathology. Despite how much we have learned about mental disorder, these models focus on the same three broad factors: the biological, the social, and the psychological. Even scientists and philosophers exploring models of abnormal behavior centuries ago would have recognized these factors.

Each of the six models of abnormal behavior reviewed in this chapter has strong support among contemporary scientists and clinicians, and each has contributed to our current understanding of psychopathology. The *biological* model emphasizes the role of disordered brain metabolism in determining the causes of and influencing the treatments for psychopathology. The *psychodynamic* and *humanistic* models stress the impact of disturbed psychological processes on maladaptive thinking, feeling, remembering, and acting. The *social consequence* model and the *behavioral* model focus on the reciprocal interaction of social and psychological factors to understand etiology (causation) and treatment. Finally, the *biopsychosocial* model emphasizes the interaction of all three factors—social, psychological, and biological—to explain abnormal behavior. In this text, we endorse the biopsychosocial model, which we believe explains abnormal behavior most fully.

Focus on Critical Thinking

1. Think of someone you know who either suffers from a mental disorder or behaves abnormally at times. Does thinking about this person's behavior in terms of one of the models of abnormal behavior help you better understand it? Explain your answer.

models Approximations of real-world phenomena designed to help clarify and explain them.

biological model Assumes the principal causes of and most effective treatments for abnormal behavior are biological.

THE BIOLOGICAL MODEL

The **biological model** of mental disorder assumes that the principal causes of and most effective treatments for abnormal behavior are biological. Specifically, the model suggests that one or more neurobiological dysfunctions of the brain are responsible for mental disorders and that correcting these dysfunctions with drugs will treat these conditions.

Because this model likens abnormal behavior to the symptoms of physical disease, it has been called the **disease model.** We prefer the term *biological model,* however, because the analogy to disease is not always appropriate. For example, genetic factors such as extreme shyness and aggression have been shown to cause several kinds of psychopathology, yet they don't influence behavior solely by producing disease. Likewise, abnormal behavior may be caused by an injury to the brain, which isn't the result of disease.

As we learned in Chapter 1, the history of the biological model of abnormal behavior is an ancient one. This model was strongly supported by the ancient Romans and Greeks, even though their understanding of the biological causes of psychopathology turned out to be largely incorrect. The biological model was sustained by Chinese and Arab physicians during the Middle Ages. But in the Western world, people believed in the supernatural model, assuming that demons and devils, rather than biological dysfunction, caused mental disorder.

The biological model regained influence in the West in the seventeenth and eighteenth centuries, which marked the beginning of modern science. Support for this model reached a peak with the work of Emil Kraepelin (1856–1926) and his coworkers in the latter part of the nineteenth century. Their focus on the role of the diseased brain in mental disorder coincided with critical discoveries in the studies of bacteria and infectious disease. These discoveries further supported the view that diseases of the brain cause serious disorders, such as dementia praecox and the **manic-depressive disorders** (which are now termed the **bipolar disorders**).

Current Understanding of Brain Disorders

When we look at the underlying assumptions of the biological model of mental disorder, we find striking similarities between those first stated by the ancient Greeks almost 2,500 years ago and those held by modern neurobiologists today. Those assumptions are as follows:

1. Impairment or dysfunction of the brain is responsible for mental disorder.
2. Accurate diagnosis of mental disorder requires identifying the impairment in brain function causing the abnormality.
3. Proper treatment involves efforts to modify or eliminate the brain dysfunction (today, generally with drugs).

The cognitive disorders are a distinct group of serious mental disorders characterized by provable disturbance in brain function. They are grouped in the *Diagnostic and Statistical Manual of Mental Disorders (DSM-IV)* and collectively termed **delirium, dementia, and amnestic and other cognitive disorders** (American Psychiatric Association, 1994). Some of these conditions are marked by progressive deficits in memory and planning, reasoning, and problem-solving skills, which makes it impossible for people with cognitive disorders to live independently. These serious brain disorders are associated with pathological aging, the abuse of drugs and alcohol, and injury, infection, and diseases that directly affect brain function. Twenty years ago, cognitive disorders could only be confirmed by postmortem (after-death) examination of the brain, but today, they can almost always be diagnosed in the living brain using new technological procedures.

In our own times, especially over the past 30 years, there has been an explosive increase in our understanding of the brain mechanisms responsible for a wide range of mental disorders. Previously, some of these disorders were thought to be of psychological or environmental origins. Exploration of biological origins has been furthered by dramatic advances in investigative techniques, especially neuroimaging (Damasio & Frank, 1992; Resnick, 1992) and behavioral and molecular genetics (Coryell & Zimmerman, 1988; Plomin & McClearn, 1993). As a result, the biological model has become an extremely influential perspective on mental disorder.

disease model Suggests that metabolic brain dysfunction is the likely cause of several common mental disorders; synonymous with the biological model.

manic-depressive disorder Serious psychiatric disorder that (like schizophrenia) involves psychotic behavior; now called bipolar disorder.

bipolar disorders Psychoses characterized generally by recurrent mood extremes, ranging from mania to severe depression; formerly called manic-depressive disorders.

delirium, dementia, and amnestic and other cognitive disorders Conditions involving deterioration in cognitive abilities such as memory, reasoning, and planning; sometimes short lived, sometimes long lasting and progressive.

One of the most characteristic symptoms of people with schizophrenia is hearing voices inside their heads. Those voices may forcefully remind schizophrenics of their inadequacies, tell them to do things they wouldn't otherwise consider, or convince them that friends or family are plotting to harm or kill them. It turns out that the voices heard by people with schizophrenia come from the same location in the brain we all depend on when we speak or think in words.

An innovative use of a neuroimaging procedure called *positron emission tomography (PET)* permits us to see brain activity in the living brain. (PET is described in Chapter 3, along with the other neuroimaging procedures.) P. K. McGuire and his colleagues, of King's College Hospitals in London, studied cerebral bloodflow, a sensitive measure of brain activity. Their subjects were schizophrenic men. Bloodflow was measured both when the subjects were and were not having auditory hallucinations (that is, hearing voices) (Goleman, 1993b). During periods of hallucinatory activity, the greatest brain activity was in *Broca's area,* which is the brain's speech center and the region most heavily involved when we speak or think in words. Looking at this finding, one prominent neuroscientist observed, "Broca's area is a surprise, since that's

where you make sounds, not where you hear them. . . . This finding suggests that, in terms of unusual brain activity, auditory hallucinations have more to do with the generation of words in the brain than listening to them" (Goleman, 1993b, p. B9).

Many of the studies we've reviewed in this book have reported similar findings, localizing the brain abnormalities responsible for some of the most important mental disorders. This latest finding about Broca's area indicates that some abnormalities are generated in the very areas of the brain where normal functions reside. This remarkable discovery was only recently made possible by neuroimaging, which permits scientists to study the living brain. Studies like this have obvious significance for the development of more effective approaches to treating and preventing these disorders as well as to better understanding their etiology.

Think about the following questions:

1. What significance does this finding have for the treatment and prevention of schizophrenia?
2. How do these findings help us better understand the cause or causes of schizophrenia?

These studies of brain dysfunction have revolutionized our understanding of etiology. It now seems certain that such major disorders as schizophrenia (Buchsbaum, 1990), several of the mood disorders (Baxter, 1991), and alcohol and drug abuse/dependence (Cadoret, O'Gorman, Troughton, & Heywood, 1985) are linked to disturbances in brain function, to some degree. Even obsessive-compulsive behavior and the anxiety disorders may be caused, at least in part, by disturbed brain functioning (Baxter, Schwartz, Guze, Bergman, & Szuba, 1990; Nordahl et al., 1990). This would be a remarkable finding, since as recently as 20 years ago, nearly all researchers believed that these disorders were psychological responses to difficult or otherwise stressful environments.

Biological Bases of Normal and Abnormal Behavior

To appreciate the advances in recent biological research on psychopathology that are highlighted throughout the text, you need to know something about the structure and function of the nervous system.

The Nervous System The nervous system controls our every thought and movement. When functioning properly, the nervous system allows us to perceive the environment, integrate our perceptions with memories of prior experiences, and then make appropriate and timely responses to what we have seen and heard.

neurons *Nerve cells; the brain is composed of billions of these cells.*

Neurons and Neurotransmitters Our nervous system contains many billions of nerve cells, or **neurons.** These specialized cells serve two crucial functions:

FIGURE 2.1   A nerve cell, or neuron

Nerve impulses are transmitted across the synapse between the axon terminal of one neuron and the dendrite tip of the next neuron by a chemical neurotransmitter. The nerve impulse then travels through the cell body of the next neuron to its axon terminal, where neurotransmission occurs across the next synaptic gap.

SOURCE: From Neil R. Carlson, *Psychology: The Science of Behavior,* 4th edition. Copyright © 1993 by Allyn and Bacon. Reprinted by permission.

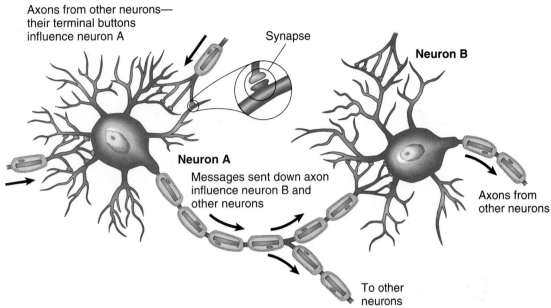

Axons from other neurons— their terminal buttons influence neuron A

Synapse

Neuron B

Neuron A
Messages sent down axon influence neuron B and other neurons

Axons from other neurons

To other neurons

sensory receptors Receive information from the environment for transmission to the central nervous system; for instance, the eyes, ears, and skin.

dendrites Extensions of neurons that receive nerve impulses from the axons of other neurons.

axons Extensions of the neuron that transmit nerve impulses to the dendrites of other neurons.

synapse Minute space between one neuron and another across which nerve impulses are sent.

neurotransmitter Chemical substance in the brain responsible for communication of nerve impulses among brain cells; excesses and deficits are responsible for a number of serious mental disorders.

central nervous system (CNS) The brain and spinal cord; all sensory nerve impulses are transmitted to the CNS, and all motor impulses are sent from the CNS.

1. They receive information from **sensory receptors** (which include the eyes, ears, and skin) as well as from specialized receptors that obtain information on the states of internal organs.
2. They transmit messages to other neurons or to muscles and glands by means of central nervous system interconnections. (The central nervous system is discussed later in this section.)

Figure 2.1 shows typical neurons, which consist of a cell body, branched extensions called **dendrites** (which receive nerve impulses from other neurons), and other extensions called **axons** (which transmit nerve impulses to other neurons). The minute space between the axon of one neuron and the dendrite of another is called the **synapse.** A nerve impulse is conveyed across the synapse when a chemical called a **neurotransmitter** is released from the axon tip and travels across the synapse to the dendrite tip. On making contact, the neurotransmitter excites the dendrite, thereby sending the nerve impulse along the new neuron.

In measuring these transmissions, neuroscientists today use instruments and procedures that are much more sensitive than those used as recently as a decade ago. Research has confirmed the central importance of neurotransmitters to the coordinated functioning of the nervous system. It now seems clear that different regions of the brain control different bodily functions and contain concentrations of different neurotransmitters. For example, researchers are reasonably certain that regions of the brain regulating the autonomic nervous system (discussed later), which is responsible for the expression of emotion, are high in concentrations of at least two neurotransmitters, acetylcholine and norepinephrine.

Neuroscientists have also found that excesses or deficits of the neurotransmitters norepinephrine, serotonin, and dopamine are responsible, in large part, for the symptoms of schizophrenia and the mood disorders. And to everyone's surprise, two common gases—carbon monoxide and nitric oxide—have also been found to function as neurotransmitters. This finding has been one of the most exciting in neuroscience in recent years, opening up a whole new area of research.

The Central and Peripheral Nervous Systems   As Figure 2.2 indicates, the nervous system is divided into the **central nervous system (CNS)** and the

---

FIGURE 2.2   Components of the nervous system

The brain and the spinal cord comprise the central nervous system (CNS). The peripheral nervous system includes the somatic nervous system (which serves the skeletal muscles) and the autonomic nervous system. The autonomic nervous system (ANS) includes sympathetic and parasympathetic divisions; both control the activities of the heart, glands, blood vessels, and other internal organs.

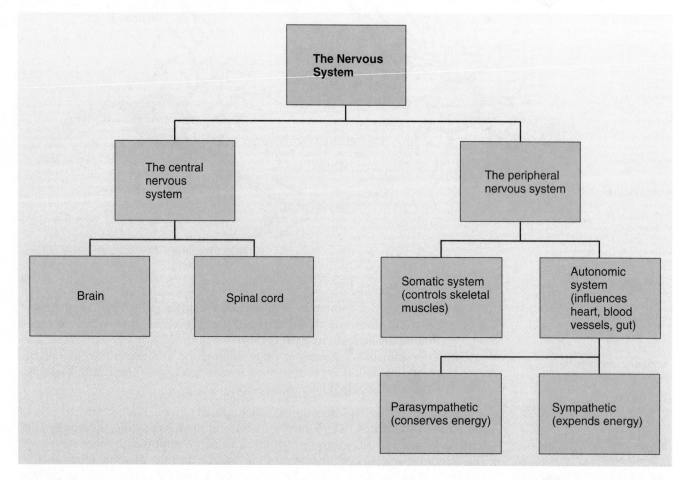

peripheral nervous system. The brain and the spinal cord make up the central nervous system. They receive and process information on the internal and external environment received from sensory receptors and, when necessary, transmit instructions for response.

The peripheral nervous system is also divided into two parts. The **somatic nervous system** serves the skeletal muscles, which control voluntary movements such as walking and talking. The **autonomic nervous system (ANS)** regulates the glands, heart muscle, blood vessels, and other internal organs.

The autonomic nervous system is divided into **sympathetic** and **parasympathetic divisions,** which link the brain and spinal cord to many of the same organs of the body. These two divisions act cooperatively most of the time, but on occasion, they act in opposition by means of different nerve pathways, especially during times of stress (see Figure 2.3). During those times, the sympathetic nervous system energizes or activates the organs to enable the body to respond to emergency situations. Consider your body's physical and emotional reactions to a near-miss auto accident. Your sympathetic nervous system responds as it would to any potential threat to the body: Your heart beats faster, you breathe more quickly, you begin to perspire, and you feel shaky, lightheaded, and anxious. These are all sympathetic nervous system responses to the threat posed to you by having a close call.

FIGURE 2.3 The sympathetic and parasympathetic divisions of the autonomic nervous system

The sympathetic division prepares internal organs to respond to stress. After the stress ends, the parasympathetic division resumes its control of the normal functioning of the organs.

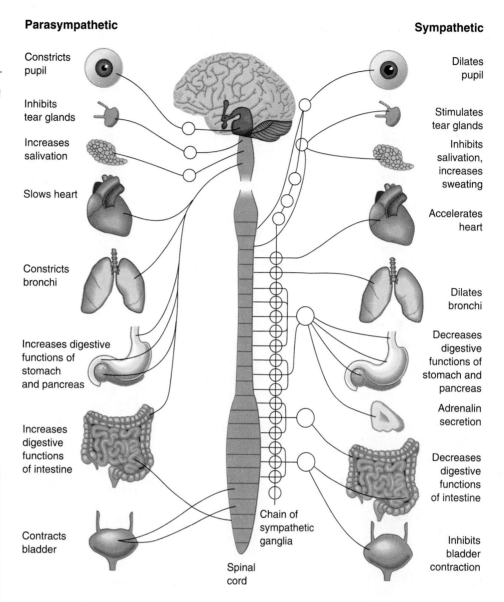

Constricts pupil

Inhibits tear glands

Increases salivation

Slows heart

Constricts bronchi

Increases digestive functions of stomach and pancreas

Increases digestive functions of intestine

Contracts bladder

Dilates pupil

Stimulates tear glands

Inhibits salivation, increases sweating

Accelerates heart

Dilates bronchi

Decreases digestive functions of stomach and pancreas

Adrenalin secretion

Decreases digestive functions of intestine

Inhibits bladder contraction

Chain of sympathetic ganglia

Spinal cord

sympathetic division
Division of the ANS that energizes or activates organs to enable the body to respond in times of stress.

parasympathetic division
Division of the ANS that regulates normal bodily functions, such as digestion and heartbeat; the "housekeeping" functions.

hindbrain Part of the brain that controls autonomic nervous system functions.

midbrain Part of the brain that contains most of the reticular activating system (RAS); the sleep-wake center; also mediates attentional processes.

forebrain Part of the brain that controls our abilities to speak, think, plan, and remember.

reticular activating system (RAS) Brain's "sleep-wake" center; also mediates attentional processes.

By contrast, the parasympathetic division regulates normal bodily functions, such as digestion and heartbeat. During an emergency, the activity levels of these "housekeeping" functions *decrease,* corresponding to the *increase* in activity of the sympathetic division. So in stressful situations, when your heart races and your body perspires (sympathetic activities), you may also feel a knot in your stomach, due to reduced digestive functioning (a parasympathetic activity).

The Brain   Composed of billions and billions of densely packed neurons, the brain is the most complex organ in the nervous system. It's divided into three parts: the **hindbrain,** the **midbrain,** and the **forebrain.**

The hindbrain controls autonomic nervous system functions, such as heartrate and digestion. The midbrain contains the **reticular activating system (RAS),** which also extends down into the hindbrain. The RAS—the brain's "sleep-wake" center—also mediates attention processes and may play a role in such devastating psychiatric disorders as childhood autism.

The forebrain enables us to speak, think, plan, and remember. It follows, then, that nearly all mental disorders with known biological causes involve some kind of forebrain dysfunction. For instance, infants born without a forebrain, a rare condition

thalamus With the hypothalamus and parts of the cerebral cortex, this part of the forebrain controls the experiences of emotion, pain and pleasure, and aggression.

hypothalamus With the thalamus and parts of the cerebral cortex, this part of the forebrain controls the experiences of emotion, pain and pleasure, and aggression.

cerebrum Outer layer of this part of the forebrain, called the cerebral cortex, mediates our ability to think, feel, perceive, and reflect.

cerebral cortex Outer layer of the cerebrum; this part of the brain mediates such human abilities as thinking, feeling, perceiving, and reflecting.

limbic system Composed of the thalamus and hypothalamus; along with parts of the cerebral cortex, responsible for the physical expression of emotion.

sensory function Cerebral cortex function that receives information from the sense organs and processes it for later recall or immediate response.

motor function Function of the cerebral cortex that controls movements of our muscles.

associational function Function of the cerebral cortex that links its parts, facilitating the reasoning, planning, memory, creativity, and problem-solving skills that are uniquely human.

hemispheres Symmetrical halves of the cerebral cortex.

temporal lobes Part of the cerebral cortex that controls visual information processing, long-term memory, emotional experience, and sound recognition.

called *anencephaly,* "often can maintain vegetative and other basic functions. Indeed, these infants can even learn primitive conditioned responses. One anencephalic boy was able to regulate his body temperature and maintain respiration and displayed near-normal fear and startle responses" (Willerman & Cohen, 1990, p. 201). Because they do not have a forebrain, however, these infants cannot think, speak, or display any other distinctively human behaviors. Sadly, nearly all these children die before such behaviors can develop.

The forebrain consists of the **thalamus** and **hypothalamus** (together commonly termed the *diencephalon*) and the **cerebrum** (also called the *telencephalon*). The thalamus and hypothalamus, together with parts of the **cerebral cortex** (the outer layer of the cerebrum, discussed in the following paragraph), mediate the experiences of emotion, pain and pleasure, and aggression. These structures comprise the **limbic system.** The actions of this system are markedly affected by many varieties of psychopathology because the limbic system is the center of emotion and such basic drives as hunger, thirst, sex, and aggression.

The cerebrum is the largest part of the human brain. Its outer layer, the cerebral cortex, is the locus of our ability to think, feel, perceive, and reflect. Thus, the cerebral cortex is responsible for many of our most human intellectual and emotional capabilities. With the development of neuroimaging techniques, described earlier (and in detail in Chapter 3), the time may finally have come to test the assumption that the size and structure of the brain influence intelligence.

Such a test was conducted by pioneering neuroscientist Nancy Andreasen and her colleagues at the University of Iowa (Andreasen et al., 1993). They measured the volume of a number of brain structures by using magnetic resonance imaging (MRI) in 67 normal, healthy volunteer women and men; subjects were also given a standard intelligence test, the Wechsler Adult Intelligence Scale. Results indicated that the greater the size of the skull cavity, the higher the IQ. Full-scale and verbal IQs were also related positively and significantly to the size of other brain structures, especially to the volume of the grey matter of the cerebral cortex; this is where associational neurons are concentrated. Performance IQ was related to brain volume measures to a lesser extent.

Although these findings are significant, the statistical relationships shown are rather modest. So, in sum, the size of the brain can be considered only one factor in determining intelligence. Andreasen and her colleagues (1993) estimate that between 12 percent and 31 percent of the variation in human intelligence is accounted for by brain size; the volume of associational neurons is most highly related to intelligence.

The Cerebral Cortex   The human cerebral cortex controls our sensory, motor, and associational functions. Its **sensory function** is to receive information from our sense organs and direct it either to storage in memory or for immediate response. The **motor function** of the cerebral cortex is to direct the movements of our muscles. The **associational function,** however, is the most complex and uniquely human function of the cerebral cortex. In it, all the parts of the cerebral cortex are linked in a massive system of interconnections that far surpasses the complexity of the telephone system in any of the world's largest cities. Because of these interconnections, we can reason, plan, remember, create, innovate, and problem solve.

The cerebral cortex is divided into symmetrical halves called **hemispheres.** Each hemisphere contains four lobes (see Figure 2.4). The **temporal lobes** control our visual information processing, long-term memory, emotional experience, and sound recognition. The **parietal lobes** control our touch recognition, for the most part; a portion of the left parietal lobe is also involved in speech. The **occipital lobes** are primarily concerned with our visual perception. The **frontal lobes** are the locus of problem solving, a uniquely human capability that calls on high-level reasoning and remembering. The frontal lobes are also involved in *social cognition,* which is our

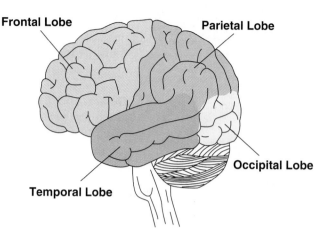

FIGURE 2.4 *The human brain (side view)*

The cerebral cortex is divided into four lobes: frontal, parietal, occipital, and temporal.

Frontal Lobe

Parietal Lobe

Occipital Lobe

Temporal Lobe

SOURCE: From Neil R. Carlson, *Physiology of Behavior,* 5th edition. Copyright © 1994 by Allyn and Bacon. Reprinted by permission.

parietal lobes *Portion of the cerebral cortex that mediates touch recognition; a portion of the left parietal lobe is also involved in speech production.*

occipital lobes *Division of the cerebral cortex that controls visual perception.*

frontal lobes *Part of the cerebral cortex that enables us to solve problems flexibly; also appears to be involved in social cognition.*

pituitary gland *Triggers the activities of many other glands by releasing hormones into the bloodstream that affect them; the "master gland."*

thyroid gland *Endocrine organ that produces hormones that affect the body's metabolism rate.*

adrenal gland *Endocrine organ that produces hormones; secretes cortisone and corticosterone, which help regulate metabolism and control inflammation; also secretes epinephrine and norepinephrine, sympathetic nervous system stimulants.*

gonadal gland *Endocrine organ that produces sex hormones responsible for the development of secondary sexual characteristics and influential in determining the pattern of sexual behavior.*

endocrine organs *Endocrine glands secrete hormones into the bloodstream, which stimulates a variety of physiological functions.*

hormones *Chemical substances secreted into the bloodstream by endocrine organs; serve as chemical messengers in much the same way that neurons convey nerve impulses.*

knowledge of the rules that govern social conduct. As you read this book, you'll learn that many of the people who display abnormal behavior have mental disorders rooted in neurotransmitter dysfunctions centered largely in the frontal lobes.

Although the two hemispheres of the brain appear to be identical, they control different cognitive functions and thus play different roles in the development of psychopathology. Both hemispheres are capable of carrying out learning, memory, and perceptual functions independently. However, the left hemisphere, which is dominant in most right-handed people, is responsible for the analytic, cognitive, and language-based processes most essential to our functioning as intelligent beings. By contrast, the right hemisphere is more involved in global perceptions and language comprehension, rather than expression. For most of us, the ability to express language resides in the left hemisphere, and imagery and spatial relations reside in the right hemisphere.

The relevance of these hemispheric differences in function to psychopathology remains uncertain. Yet recent research (Resnick, 1992) suggests that children with autism may have a severe left-hemisphere dysfunction, since so many of their significant behavioral deficits are controlled by that hemisphere. People who are schizophrenic also show behavioral deficits and excesses that point to left-hemisphere damage; these individuals also show more left- than right-hemisphere activation (Resnick, 1992).

The Endocrine System   The **pituitary, thyroid, adrenal,** and **gonadal glands** are all **endocrine organs.** Each produces substances called **hormones,** which are chemical messengers secreted by the endocrine glands directly into the bloodstream and sent throughout the body to act on other organs. Among many other functions, hormones help regulate our physiological processes and coordinate internal bodily processes with external events. They function very much like nerve impulses, except that they are transmitted through the bloodstream rather than across neurons.

Prolonged stress, including that associated with significant psychopathology, can cause temporary or permanent dysfunction in the endocrine system. When this happens, psychiatric patients experience more stress-induced physical and emotional distress. Stress can also impair the functioning of the immune system, making us more susceptible to disease. (See Chapter 10 for a thorough discussion of this complex relationship.)

Genetic Factors in Normal and Abnormal Behavior

The role of genetic dysfunction in such major disorders as schizophrenia (Gottesman, 1993), the mood disorders (McGuffin & Katz, 1993), autism (Rutter,

genes Basic chemical units of heredity; millions align along the 46 human chromosomes.

chromosomes Humans have 46 chromosomes (23 pairs), along which millions of genes are aligned.

gamete Sperm cell or ovum.

sperm cell Male gamete; when it fertilizes an ovum, develops into an embryo.

ovum Female gamete, which, when fertilized by a sperm cell, develops into an embryo.

identical twins Twins who develop from a single fertilized ovum; also called monozygotic twins.

monozygotic twins Twins who develop from a single fertilized ovum; also called identical twins.

fraternal twins Twins who develop simultaneously from two fertilized ova; also called dizygotic twins.

dizygotic twins Twins who develop simultaneously from two fertilized ova; also called fraternal twins.

dominant gene One of a pair of genes that determines a particular physical or psychological characteristic in the phenotype.

recessive gene Gene that must be paired with one identical to it to determine a trait in the phenotype.

phenotype Observable characteristics, such as hair color and height.

genotype Array of genes a person possesses, which is hereditary.

diathesis-stress theory Meehl's theory that although some people inherit or develop predispositions (diatheses) to particular disorders, they will not emerge until or unless environmental stressors convert the predispositions into actual disorders.

Bailey, Bolton, & Le Couteur, 1993), and alcoholism (McGue, 1993) has been studied intensively in recent years. In this section, we'll review the mechanisms of genetic transmission and outline recent advances in the investigative techniques used in genetics research.

Genes and Chromosomes   Everything we inherit from our parents and their parents is transmitted by many millions of genes, which are the chemical units of heredity. **Genes** are arranged in a specific order along **chromosomes,** almost like numbered beads on a string. Most of us have 46 chromosomes. All the cells in the body contain identical sets of chromosomes, except the sperm and ova, which have only half the usual number. In every other cell, the 46 chromosomes are grouped into 23 pairs, with 1 member of each pair coming from each parent.

When we reach adolescence, our testes or ovaries produce **gametes** (**sperm cells** or **ova**). Each of these reproductive cells receives only 1 member of each pair of chromosomes. So the union that occurs between an ovum and a sperm during reproduction restores the full human set of 46 chromosomes to the developing embryo.

The only time two people inherit exactly the same genetic material is when **identical twins** are created. Identical twins develop from the same fertilized ovum, or *zygote* (the union of two gametes). As a result, identical twins are also called **monozygotic twins.** They differ genetically from **fraternal,** or **dizygotic, twins,** who are conceived simultaneously but grow from separate fertilized ova. One percent of all children born are twins, and one in three sets of twins are identical. The identical genetic makeup of monozygotic twins makes them very useful to scientists investigating the effects of heredity and environment on development and psychopathology.

Phenotype and Genotype   If you inherit the gene for brown hair from one parent and the gene for blond hair from the other parent, you will have brown hair. This always happens because the gene for brown hair is **dominant** over the gene for blond hair, which is **recessive.** When you inherit a dominant gene and a recessive gene, you will end up with the feature conveyed by the dominant gene, even though your chromosomes will also contain the recessive gene. This pattern explains why brown-haired people can have blond-haired children. Regardless of their own hair color, if each parent contributes the gene for blond hair, their child will inherit two recessive genes for blond hair.

To describe the difference between actual physical appearance and heredity, we use the terms *phenotype* and *genotype*. A **phenotype** is an observable characteristic, such as hair, eye, and skin color; height and weight; as well as temperament and personality. A **genotype** relates to the array of genes a person possesses, which is hereditary. The transmission of a recessive characteristic like blond hair is unimportant in studying psychopathology; however, a number of serious mental disorders are transmitted recessively, including some of the psychoses and certain kinds of mental retardation. We must keep in mind that most traits are inherited by *multiple* gene pairs, rather than by *single* gene pairs.

Nonhereditary factors also influence phenotype. Take weight, for example. We each inherit the predisposition to be lean or heavy, but our environment—including factors such as diet, family eating patterns, and socioeconomic status—has a lot to do with whether we follow that tendency. It seems highly likely that a similar relationship between phenotype and genotype affects the expression of certain forms of psychopathology. Some persons are born with or later develop predispositions to particular kinds of psychopathology. Whether they actually develop these conditions, though, may depend a great deal on their environment and life experiences.

This assumption, termed the **diathesis-stress theory,** was first argued by Meehl (1962). He suggested that some people inherit or develop predispositions (diatheses) to disorders such as schizophrenia and substance use disorders.

However, these disorders will not emerge unless or until environmental stressors (death, divorce, serious interpersonal or vocational problems, etc.) or biological stressors (disease or injury) become intense enough to convert the genetic predispositions into actual disorders. Since Meehl first proposed the diathesis-stress theory, scientists have developed a variety of powerful research strategies to explore the all-important issue of gene-environment interaction in the etiology of mental disorder (McClearn, 1993; Plomin, 1993).

Behavioral Genetics and Gene-Environment Interactions

Four techniques for studying gene-environment interactions have been developed over the years: the family method, the pedigree method, the twin method, and the adoption method.

Family studies were the initial focus of genetic factors in mental illness. They were based on the assumption that even if a mental disorder does not obey the established laws of inheritance, it is hereditary if it occurs more often in the families of **index cases,** or **probands.** (*Index cases* and *probands* are equivalent terms for "affected patients.") The family method is useful because it establishes which disorders run in families and to what extent. But this method is inadequate as a means of separating the influences of heredity and environment. For example, emotional disorders run in families for hereditary reasons, for environmental reasons, or for both.

Pedigree studies trace the distribution of disorders among close and distant relatives of index cases. This information shows whether a certain disorder is distributed according to established laws of inheritance and, if so, whether the gene or genes responsible for the disorder are dominant, recessive, or sex linked. Pedigree studies are frequently used in conjunction with molecular genetic studies of the genes responsible for specific disorders. When a disorder such as depression, schizophrenia, or alcohol dependence is found throughout a family's ancestry, genetic "markers" that help localize the gene or genes responsible for the disorder can sometimes be found in the genetic material of affected individuals. Figure 2.5 shows a striking family pedigree that has helped researchers at the National Institutes of Mental Health explore genetic factors in several mental disorders.

Twin studies have special value for genetics researchers because the genetic makeup of the two groups of subjects can be known for certain. Identical, or monozygotic, twins share 100 percent of their genetic material (because they developed from a single fertilized ovum), and fraternal, or dizygotic, twins share only some genetic material—on average, 50 percent (because they developed from separately fertilized ova). It follows that **concordance** for genetically transmitted disorders will be significantly more among identical twins than fraternal twins. (That is, identical twins will be more likely to both have the disorder.) Because twins generally grow up in the same home, an advantage of twin studies is that the environment can be kept constant. In other words, it's unlikely that environmental influences could account for differences in twins' likelihood to develop mental disorders. Given that, researchers can focus on the varying degrees of genetic transmission of certain disorders (between the 100 percent of identical twins and the 50 percent average of fraternal twins).

Twin studies have provided convincing data on the heritability (likelihood of inheriting) of schizophrenia, depression, alcoholism, and autism (a serious developmental disorder that affects very young children). Identical twins have been found much more concordant than fraternal twins for schizophrenia (Gottesman, 1991), alcoholism (Kendler, Heath, Neale, Kessler, & Eaves, 1992; McGue, Pickens, & Svikis, 1992), depression (Tsuang & Faroane, 1990), and autism (Bailey et al., 1991; Steffenberg, 1991). (These findings are reviewed in greater detail in Chapters 7, 9, 13, and 15.)

Adoption studies, the newest method for research on genetic factors in mental disorders, have been especially useful in the study of alcoholism. Several studies

family studies Genetic studies that assume that even if a mental disorder does not obey the laws of inheritance, it is hereditary if it occurs more often in the families of index cases.

index cases Patients who suffer from the disorder being studied; synonymous with probands.

probands Patients who suffer from the disorder under study; synonymous with index cases.

pedigree studies Genetic research involving families in which substantial numbers of members are affected with the disorder under study.

twin studies Genetic studies that depend on the differences in shared genetic material between monozygotic (identical) and dizygotic (fraternal) twins.

concordance Likelihood of individuals sharing a quality or condition; twins who both have a mental disorder are concordant for that disorder.

adoption studies Genetic studies that examine relationships between the psychopathology of biological and adoptive parents and that of adopted children after they become adults.

FIGURE 2.5   Pedigree chart

Starting from the top, this hierarchy shows that a woman who had bipolar affective disorder had two normal children as well as a son who developed bipolar affective disorder and a son who developed unipolar depression. The woman's children had 16 grandchildren; 13 of them had from unipolar depression, bipolar affective disorder, alcohol and drug abuse/dependence, and other psychiatric disorders.

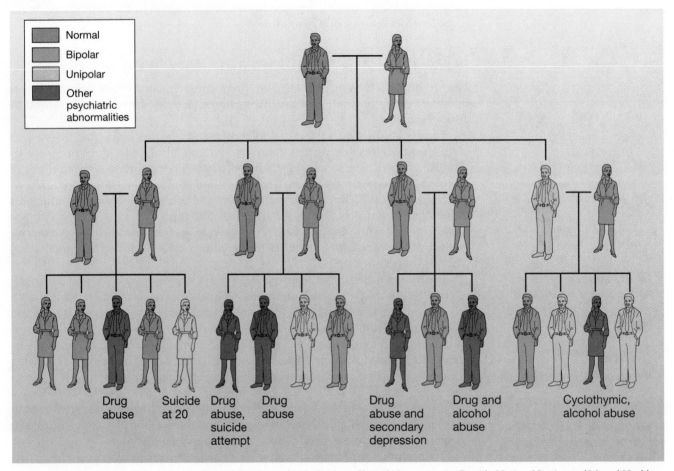

Source: Courtesy of E. S. Gershon, Clinical Neurogenetics Branch, National Institute of Mental Health.

compared Danish and Swedish adults with and without family histories of alcoholism who, as children, had been adopted away from their biological families (Cloninger, Bohman, & Sigvardsson, 1981; Goodwin, Schulsinger, Hermansen, Guze, & Winokur, 1973). Subjects who had alcoholic biological parents were significantly more likely than those without alcoholic biological parents to develop alcohol problems of their own as adults.

More recently, essentially the same findings have been reported for schizophrenia. Several studies examined Danish adoptees who had been diagnosed with schizophrenia as adults (Kendler et al., 1994; Kety et al., 1994). Researchers found that the adoptees' biological parents and other blood relatives were much more likely to have schizophrenia and related disorders than the parents and other relatives of adoptees who were not schizophrenic.

Carey and DiLalla (1994) have recently surveyed the literature on genetics and personality in relation to psychopathology. They conclude that between 30 percent and 60 percent of the responsibility for personality traits such as sociability, psychological flexibility, self-control, and self-acceptance stems from genetic, rather than environmental, factors. Linking the genetic transmission of personality traits to the development of psychopathology, these researchers argue that people with certain types of personalities tend to develop specific kinds of psychopathology. For this reason, they suggest, we need to pay more attention to the role of genetics in inheriting *personality types* because doing so will provide more information on the role of genetics in inheriting psychopathology.

Advances in Molecular Genetics

Genetics researchers have begun locating the gene or genes responsible for certain mental disorders, due to advances made in molecular genetics. Although the work has been long and hard, much progress has been made in identifying first, the location of the chromosome, and more recently, the gene for Huntington's chorea, a devastating cognitive disorder. Advances have also been made in localizing the gene or genes for Alzheimer's disease, manic-depressive illness, and schizophrenia, but completing this work will probably take years (Plomin & McClearn, 1993).

Once the gene or genes responsible for a disorder have been identified, their biochemical composition can then be studied to learn about the nature of the brain dysfunction they are responsible for. Molecular genetics research, which localizes the genes causing psychiatric disorders, working in partnership with behavioral genetics research, which initially established the heritability of these disorders, is an especially promising approach. It will speed the discovery of the causes of mental disorders as well as hasten the development of effective prevention and treatment methods.

Contributions and Shortcomings

When Kraepelin reintroduced the biological model of mental disorder a little over 100 years ago, it represented a distinct step forward. Viewing mental patients as sick, rather than immoral, eased the moral stigma that had been attached to mental disorder through the ages. The biological model represented a humane advance. The ties of the biological model to medicine, moreover, encouraged empirical inquiry, careful observation of abnormal behavior, and respect for reliable diagnosis. As a result, scientific research that tried to uncover the causes of disorders and then find treatments for them became highly valued.

Recent advances in understanding how disturbances in brain functioning are related to some psychiatric disorders have led to marked improvements in diagnosis and treatment. A prominent example is new research on neurotransmitter dysfunctions in the brain. Insights from these studies have led to improved treatments by guiding psychopharmacologists to develop drugs that have specific effects on certain neurotransmitter systems (Andreasen & Black, 1991).

These advances would represent a problem, however, if they led us to view *all* behavioral and psychiatric disorders through the lens of the disease model. The biopsychosocial perspective on mental disorder, on the other hand, encourages recognizing the diverse factors that contribute to the causes of and treatments for these conditions. Poverty and discrimination, for example, are commonly linked to drug and alcohol abuse/dependence, antisocial personality disorder, and conduct and learning problems among children. But to look at these human problems simply as *diseases* makes it too easy to conclude that societal variables don't influence their development. What's more, taking this view makes it too easy to avoid taking responsibility for change.

A strong case can be made for the influences of biological, social, and psychodynamic factors in the life of Malcolm X. Let's consider now what we know about biological factors that may have affected him.

Malcolm X's *Autobiography* paints a compelling picture of the young black man from tragic beginnings who became a historic figure in the continuing struggle of African American people for their share of the American dream. In young

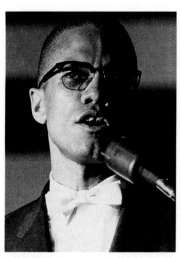

MALCOLM X

adulthood, Malcolm became an alcoholic and a drug addict, and he suffered from depression throughout his life. All these conditions involve neurobiological brain disturbance, and genetic transmission is involved in the etiology of all three, as well. What do we know of Malcolm's family history that would help us speculate on the role of biological factors in his substance abuse and depression problems?

Malcolm's mother, Louise Little, bore five children, looked after a total of eight, and managed to live with an abusive husband until he was killed. But she was nervous, prone to extreme moodiness, and given to "visions" of things to come. His mother's instability was a constant feature of Malcolm's childhood. He writes of seeing his family on the verge of disintegration, after caring for eight fatherless children had finally taken its toll on Louise's fragile temperament:

> We children watched our anchor giving way. It was something terrible that you couldn't get your hands on, yet you couldn't get away from. It was a sensing that something was going to happen. . . . Eventually my mother suffered from a complete nervous breakdown, and the court orders were finally signed. They took her to the State Mental Hospital at Kalamazoo. . . . My mother remained in the same hospital in Kalamazoo for about twenty-six years. Later, when I was still growing up in Michigan, I would go to visit her every so often. Nothing that I can imagine could have moved me as deeply as seeing her pitiful state. (Malcolm X, 1964, pp. 19, 21)

Malcolm's brutally honest writing in his *Autobiography* makes it possible for us to identify crucial biological factors in the development of his substance abuse and depression. He had a severely disturbed mother, at least later in her life, and an abusive, angry father. Both parents almost certainly passed along genes to Malcolm and his siblings that greatly predisposed them to mental disorders.

Even while focusing on the substantial family history that might account for Malcolm's psychopathology, we must also acknowledge his profound strengths—the gifts that ultimately made him the dynamic, visionary leader many people remember. We can't ignore the foundations of some of his greatest strengths while searching for factors that better explain his psychopathology.

psychodynamic model
Based on the belief that human behavior is influenced, in large part, by unconscious factors that we are largely unaware of.

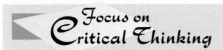

Focus on Critical Thinking

1. The stress-diathesis model links biological/genetic and environmental factors influential in the etiology of certain mental disorders. Think about the troubled behavior of a family member or friend. As best you can, explain the behavior according to the stress-diathesis model.
2. From what you have read of him so far, could the stress-diathesis model help explain Malcolm's psychopathology as a child and adolescent? Explain your answer.

THE PSYCHODYNAMIC MODEL

unconscious psychological processes Psychological conflicts, impulses, desires, and motives that influence behavior we are largely unaware of.

conscious psychological processes Thoughts, feelings, and memories we are aware of that influence our behavior.

structural theory of personality Divides the psyche into three parts: the ego, id, and superego; each is responsible for a distinct set of psychological operations.

The **psychodynamic model** is based on the belief that human behavior is strongly influenced by **unconscious psychological processes** that we are largely unaware of—in other words, internal conflicts, impulses, desires, and motives. The psychodynamic model assumes that all behavior, normal and abnormal, results from the interaction of genetic and environmental factors and that both types of factors affect behavior by influencing unconscious as well as **conscious psychological processes**. Finally, psychodynamic theorists stress the crucial importance of our earliest years, believing that childhood events have lifelong effects on our psychological states.

Freud's Psychoanalytic Theory

The Structure of Personality Sigmund Freud (1856–1939) was the first and most prominent psychodynamic theorist, and his ideas continue to influence other psychodynamic theorists. His **structural theory of personality** (1961, 1963b)

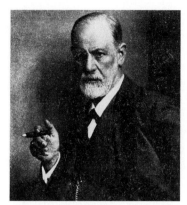

SIGMUND FREUD *(1856–1939), founder of the psychoanalytic movement*

id Reservoir of primitive drives and desires untouched and unaffected by the real world; strongly influences infant behavior.

libido Life instinct of the id; composed primarily of sexual drives and impulses.

thanatos Death instinct of the id; composed of aggressive and destructive impulses.

primary-process thinking Characterized by sexual preoccupations and fantasies, anger, jealousy, selfishness, and envy; guides the id's impulses.

pleasure principle To maximize pleasure and reduce tension without concern for morality or reality; the sole aim of the id.

ego Part of the psychic apparatus that tempers and controls the id's primitive drives and impulses so they conform more closely to the realistic demands of the environment.

reality principle To recognize society's realistic demands; guides the ego "by observing the rules."

secondary-process thinking Mode that employs reason and logic; used by the ego.

superego Earliest source of what we call conscience; our ability to distinguish right from wrong.

divides what he called the *psychic apparatus* into three parts: the id, ego, and superego. Freud believed that each entity is responsible for a distinct set of psychological operations.

The **id** is the source of inherited, primitive drives and desires that are untouched and unaffected by the real world and its so-called civilizing influence. The id is dominant during the earliest months of life, when these drives and desires strongly influence the infant's behavior. Thus, the id is the first psychic element to influence behavior. Two basic drives color id impulses. The first is the life instinct, or **libido,** composed primarily of sexual impulses and drives. The second is the death instinct, or **thanatos,** including aggressive and destructive drives. In the id, as in human behavior overall, life instincts, which are generative, oppose death instincts, which are regressive.

Psychodynamic theory suggests that the id and the infant—both unsocialized, primitive, and selfish—are jointly preoccupied with gratifying basic instincts. They are engaged in **primary-process thinking,** which is largely characterized by sexual preoccupations and fantasies, anger, jealousy, selfishness, and envy. To satisfy its desires, the id's operations are guided by the **pleasure principle,** which aims to maximize pleasure and reduce tension without concern for morality or reality. Not surprisingly, the id's impulses repeatedly conflict with society's rules and expectations.

Freud believed that the basic ingredients of the id are present in every infant—in other words, that babies and young children have strong sexual and aggressive feelings. This view involved Freud in a great deal of controversy; he outraged many of his contemporaries. But consider when Freud lived. He proposed his theory in the midst of the prim and proper Victorian era, when even adult sexual impulses were largely denied or ignored.

The second part of the psychic apparatus is the **ego,** which tempers and controls the id's primitive drives and impulses so they conform more closely to the demands of the environment. Freudian theory teaches that the ego emerges from the id after a few months of life, when the infant must begin to respond and adapt to the realities of her external environment. This is the time when the infant begins to notice that all her needs for food, comfort, and warmth are not gratified immediately, even though her unsocialized id demands immediate gratification.

The ego gradually assumes the prime responsibility for making the id's primitive impulses conform more closely to society's moral and ethical standards. As such, the ego is the principal means by which we, as human beings, meet these societal standards, while we struggle to adapt id impulses to the demands of reality.

The ego is guided by the **reality principle,** which recognizes society's realistic demands. In "observing the rules," the ego employs **secondary-process thinking**—reason and logic—rather than the primary-process thinking used by the id. Anything that impairs the reality principle, which the ego depends on (for instance, drugs or alcohol or serious emotional disturbance), lessens the ego's capacity to assess the real world accurately. When that happens, the ego is weakened and the id is strengthened.

The ego has been called the "executive" of the personality because it manages the functioning of the person just as a chief executive officer (CEO) manages the functioning of a corporation. This metaphor is especially appropriate. The ego must balance the demands of the real world with the energies of the id, just as the CEO must coordinate and channel the energies and talents of the company's employees in order for it to compete successfully.

As the child grows, the ego assumes an additional role: It must deal with the **superego,** which is the earliest source of what we call *conscience*—our ability to distinguish right from wrong. The superego emerges gradually, as the child starts to learn the rules his parents use to interpret society's expectations. Parents serve the essential function of conscience until the child evolves his own internal set of standards.

The superego also makes demands, however, which the ego must manage. For a child raised by extremely critical, punitive, and judgmental parents, these demands can be excessive. In such cases, the superego may become so restrictive that it prevents the child from enjoying the normal, innocent pleasures of childhood. When children with punitive superegos become adolescents and encounter the great increase in sexual feelings and desires that accompany puberty, they may have even greater difficulty handling the demands of the superego. Freud believed that anxiety and depression commonly accompany excessively strong superego demands.

According to the psychodynamic model, the ego, id, and superego naturally conflict because they have different goals and methods. If the id or superego becomes strong enough to overwhelm the ego, the result is internal conflict and psychological symptoms. Freudian theory teaches that if this conflict among the ego, id, and superego remains unresolved, it can lead to mental disorder.

Many of Freud's most influential writings were case histories of patients from whom he drew the clinical insights that led to the development of psychoanalytic theory. One of the most important of these was the early case of Frau Elisabeth von R. (Breuer & Freud, 1895), which illustrates a number of the concepts we have just discussed:

> Frau Elisabeth, 24 years old, was referred because of crippling pains in her leg. Freud initially hoped hypnosis would uncover her repressed memories concerning the origin and fluctuations of her symptoms, but her lack of responsivity to this procedure forced him to abandon direct hypnotic suggestion and further pursue the free association method. . . . Frau Elisabeth's leg pains, which specifically radiated to her right thigh, were traced to the exact place upon which her father's swollen leg rested every morning while she changed his bandages. In free associating, Frau Elisabeth revealed how her happy feelings of her first love (for her father) commingled with her sadness about her father's illness. . . . After further free association, Freud helped her recognize that a secondary experience leading to her painful symptoms related to the death of her nearest older sister. Frau Elisabeth had always been fond of her brother-in-law, and after her sister's death, she was greatly troubled by her wish to benefit from his new freedom by becoming his wife. Once her memories had been liberated by Freud's interpretation of her love for her brother-in-law, her symptoms were "spoken away." (Liff, 1992, p. 573)

The Stages of Psychosexual Development   Freud's **theory of psychosexual development** (1953, 1955) portrays the development of personality in distinct, successive stages, each characterized by a different means of gratifying libidinal (sexual) needs. The five stages are the oral stage, the anal stage, the phallic stage, the latency stage, and the genital stage.

The **oral stage** of psychosexual development extends from birth to about 18 months. The infant's major physical need during this period is for the food necessary to sustain rapid growth. As a consequence, the infant's mouth, lips, and tongue become sources of libido, so that eating gives great pleasure. Freud believed this would ensure that the infant would want to eat and thus be nourished.

Freud also recognized that distinctive forms of psychological and cognitive growth take place during each psychosexual stage. In the oral stage of development, for example, infants learn that they are not the center of the universe, that they will not be fed, held, or comforted whenever they wish. In short, they learn that their ability to influence the world around them (including their parents) has clear limits.

theory of psychosexual development Freud's portrayal of the development of personality in distinct, successive stages; each is characterized by a different means of gratifying libidinal (sexual) needs.

oral stage First stage of psychosexual development, extending from birth to about 18 months; the infant's mouth, lips, and tongue are invested with libido, so that eating gives great pleasure.

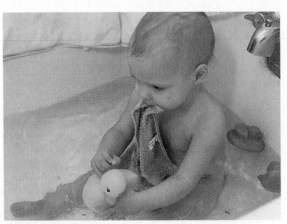

During the oral stage of psychosexual development, the mouth, lips, and tongue give great pleasure. That pleasure is often experienced when the infant eats, or sometimes it is enjoyed during a bath.

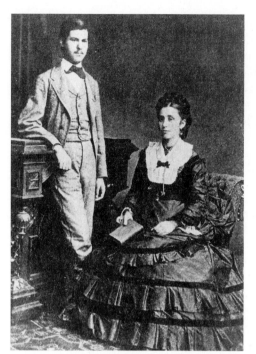

One of the roots of Freud's strong interest in the events of the Oedipal period may have been his exceptionally close relationship with his own mother, Amalia Freud, shown here with her eldest son, Sigmund.

anal stage Second psychosexual stage, during which the child derives pleasure from the anal and urinary sphincters and learns new ways to control his parents.

phallic stage Third stage of psychosexual development; libido is invested in the genitals, and the child works through her feelings about her parents.

Oedipus complex Psychosexual challenge that boys experience during the phallic period; requires the resolution of conflicting sexual and aggressive feelings about parents.

Electra complex In Freudian theory, a common feature of girls' efforts during the phallic stage to deal with conflicting sexual and aggressive feelings toward their parents.

latency stage Extended period of psychosexual calm; age 6 to about 12 years.

The second stage of psychosexual development—the **anal stage**—lasts from about 18 months to 3 years old. The focus of attention (and thus pleasure) shifts to the anal and urinary sphincter muscles, which control the elimination of urine and feces. During this stage, the child learns that it's pleasurable to withhold and expel feces and urine. Freud believed that experiencing this pleasure is nature's way of focusing the child's attention on these basic bodily skills. And while acquiring them, the child learns new ways to manipulate her parents' behavior, as she realizes her parents cannot control certain parts of her body (the bladder and bowels) and behavior (urination and defecation).

The third stage of psychosexual development is the **phallic stage,** which lasts from 3 to 6 years of age. One of Freud's most hotly debated suggestions was that during this stage, children's principal source of pleasure comes from their genitals. Freud also believed that during this period, boys face the challenge of the well-known **Oedipus complex,** which is why many clinicians refer to these years as the *Oedipal period.* Freud was impressed by how many of his patients recalled childhood memories or fantasies of incest with the opposite-sex parent, accompanied by jealous, sometimes murderous, rage at the same-sex parent. Accordingly, he named this scenario for the mythical Greek King Oedipus. As a youth, Oedipus is told he is doomed to play out a great tragedy, by killing his father and marrying his mother. Despite his best efforts to prevent the tragedy, the forecast comes true.

During the phallic period, Freud observed, the young boy becomes preoccupied with power and strength as well as the size and functioning of his penis. He wants to become stronger, bigger, and more powerful and, symbolically, to take his father's place in his mother's bed. Loving his father yet fearing his wrath, the boy must repress his longing for his mother. The crucial lesson of the phallic stage of development is learned when the boy resolves his conflicting feelings of love and anger for his father along with his feelings of dependence and desire for his mother.

Freud also speculated on a counterpart to the Oedipus complex in girls who are 3 to 6 years old. He called it the **Electra complex,** after another Greek tragedy. Recognizing that she does not have a penis, like her brother and father, a girl of this age wishes symbolically to possess her father and thereby gain a penis. She resolves this conflict when she realizes she will ultimately have a man (a mate) and a baby, which will substitute for a penis. Freud's description of the Electra complex and so-called *penis envy* has been strongly criticized in recent years by both women and men. Many feel these ideas are sexually demeaning as well as an inaccurate description of the feelings of women and girls in our time.

Between the ages of 6 and 12, children enter the **latency stage,** an extended period of psychosexual calm. During this time, children consolidate the psychological and interpersonal lessons they have learned during the preceding psychosexual stages.

The onset of puberty marks the beginning of the **genital stage,** when adolescents learn the pleasures and dangers of adult sexuality. How much of each the adolescent experiences depends on how successfully he has progressed through the earlier developmental periods. The belief that the lessons learned during the stages of psychosexual development—especially the first three—largely determine both the personality and the emotional status of the adult is central to psychoanalytic theory.

What does psychoanalytic theory—especially the theory of psychosexual development—teach us about Malcolm X?

The Oedipal period, always tumultuous, was especially so for Malcolm X. It was toward the end of this period of Malcolm's life that his father met his shocking end, presumably murdered by the Black Legion, a group of white vigilantes. The events of the day his father was killed were indelibly etched in Malcolm's memory:

> One afternoon in 1931 when Wilfred, Hilda, Philbert, and I came home, my mother and father were having one of their arguments. There had lately been a lot of tension around the house because of Black Legion threats. Anyway, my father had taken one of the rabbits which we were raising, and ordered my mother to cook it.... My mother was crying. She started to skin the rabbit, preparatory to cooking it. But my father was so angry he slammed on out of the front door and started walking up the road toward town.... It was then that my mother had this vision. She had always been a strange woman in this sense, and had always had a strong intuition of things about to happen.... She told me later, my mother did, that she had a vision of my father's end. All the rest of the afternoon, she was not herself, crying and nervous and upset.... When my father was not back home by our bedtime, my mother hugged and clutched us, and we felt strange, not knowing what to do, because she had never acted like that.... I remember waking up to the sound of my mother's screaming again. When I scrambled out, I saw the police in the living room; they were trying to calm her down. She had snatched on her clothes to go with them. And all of us children who were staring, knew without anyone having to say it that something terrible had happened to our father. (Malcolm X, 1964, pp. 9–10)

Traumatic events of this magnitude—the sudden, shocking death of a father, the emotional disintegration of a mother—have long-lasting effects on us, regardless of how old we are when they take place. But when they occur during the Oedipal period, before a young boy like Malcolm has resolved his conflicting feelings about his mother and father, they have a particularly profound impact. In particular, they affect our feelings about ourselves, especially our ability to love and be loved, to trust and be trusted.

The Ego's Mechanisms of Defense   Freud believed we experience **anxiety** when the ego comes under attack from the environment or by the id or superego. We feel **neurotic anxiety** when id impulses threaten to overwhelm the ego. Anxiety caused by guilt and shame, which are both products of a harsh and punitive superego, is called **moral anxiety**. **Objective anxiety** is the apprehension we experience when we are confronted by real danger.

In normal day-to-day functioning, the ego handles stress through reasoning and intellect according to the reality principle. The healthy ego is able to meet id demands, superego restraints, and environmental pressures without much difficulty. But when any combination of stress from these three sources increases, reasoning and intellect may not be enough to reduce tension. In such an instance, the ego will call on one or more of a variety of defense mechanisms to protect itself.

Freud described a few of these strategies of defense, but his daughter Anna developed the concept much more fully in a classic 1936 book called *The Ego and the Mechanisms of Defense*. In this book, Anna Freud stressed the importance of the ego to our psychological lives and thus the importance of protecting and nurturing it. She also examined the elaborate set of defense mechanisms the ego employs to protect its central position within the psychic apparatus.

The ego's protective tactics operate beyond our conscious control or awareness. However, we might sometimes realize when we use defense mechanisms—for instance, when we deny that a recent argument with a loved one has upset us, that we

---

genital stage Puberty marks the beginning of this psychosexual stage.

anxiety Emotion experienced when the ego is threatened by the environment or attacked by the id or superego.

neurotic anxiety Experienced when id impulses threaten to overwhelm the ego.

moral anxiety Generated by guilt and shame; product of a punitive superego.

objective anxiety Realistic apprehension we feel when confronted by real danger.

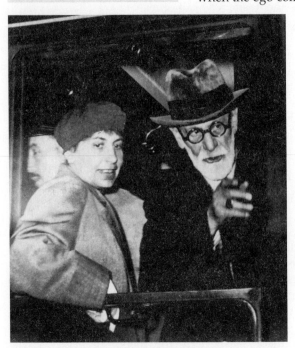

Anna Freud, with her father, Sigmund. Her book The Ego and the Mechanisms of Defense *(1936), which emphasized the role of the ego in health and illness, laid the groundwork for subsequent developments in ego psychology.*

TABLE 2.1   Some of the Ego's Defense Mechanisms

Defense Mechanism	Description	Example
Regression	Avoids the experience of painful thoughts and feelings from the past by returning psychologically to an earlier, less stressful period.	Common and harmless regressions include crying and childlike expressions of anger and resentment when frustrated or traumatized; the development of hallucinations and delusions in response to insoluble life problems reflects more dangerous regressions.
Fixation	Keeps potentially threatening thoughts and feelings that are aroused by environmental or psychological stressors from consciousness by remaining at an earlier, less threatening stage of psychological maturity.	The young man "who has never grown up" and continues to evade adult responsibility, like Peter Pan.
Repression	Prevents painful, potentially disruptive thoughts, feelings, memories, and impulses from reaching consciousness (although they may still be experienced in dreams, as slips of the tongue, or during psychoanalysis).	The young woman in psychoanalysis who suddenly recalls the guilt she felt over her sexual feelings for her father during childhood.
Identification	Defends against threatening feelings aroused by the behavior of another person by experiencing a strong sense of psychological linkage between that person and oneself.	Willy Loman, the salesman in Miller's tragic play *Death of a Salesman*, identifies with the ambitious, magnetic, and successful peers he has never been able to be like.
Projection	Denies the existence of an emotion or feeling that one fears or finds threatening in oneself by attributing it to another person.	The college student who believes that every other student is out to do better than him academically, by fair or unfair means; he is attributing motives to his classmates that he finds difficult to admit to in himself.
Reaction Formation	Avoids the turmoil aroused by conflicting feelings about someone by excluding the negative feelings about her from consciousness and focusing on the positive ones.	The young man who emphasizes his love for and pride in his father's achievements avoids having to deal with feelings of competition and rivalry with him.
Sublimation	Transforms the psychological energy associated with threatening sexual or aggressive feelings and impulses into socially acceptable pursuits, such as art, music, politics, or intellectual activities.	The local politician who devotes himself to the welfare of his constituents may be defending himself against anxiety from unconscious sexual or aggressive conflicts.
Rationalization	Avoids confronting irrational motives for behavior by invoking an "after the fact" set of rational and logical reasons for it.	Rationalization is a favorite defense of college students (and their professors); it sometimes produces heated arguments that protect participants from anxiety-arousing, competitive emotions because they focus on the intellectual and the scholarly.

have displaced anger from one person onto another, or that we have lost all memory for a particularly painful incident. Do any of the common ego defenses described in Table 2.1 sound familiar?

Using the ego's defense mechanisms to adjust to the inevitable pressures of life isn't always healthy. Relying extensively on defense mechanisms can become self-perpetuating, making it more difficult for us to deal directly and effectively with our problems, both minor and major. This is especially true with such mal-adaptive defenses as fixation and regression. Anna Freud was convinced that many of the signs and symptoms of emotional disorder (including anxiety, depression, and the behaviors indicative of psychosis) stem from undue reliance on these defensive maneuvers.

Vaillant (1977, 1992) and Vaillant, Bond, and Vaillant (1986) developed a nine-point scale designed to assess the maturity (essentially, the effectiveness) of the most common ego defenses. Descriptions of adaptive human behavior in times of crisis were converted into realistic scenarios, each illustrating one of fifteen different defenses. Each defense was then categorized by a panel of experienced psychoanalysts as "immature," "intermediate," or "mature."

Validity studies of the questionnaire revealed that the maturity of these defenses in 307 middle-aged men (Vaillant, Bond, & Vaillant, 1986) and 188 older men (Vaillant & Schnurr, 1988) correlate strongly with independently assessed measures of maturity. These results have led Vaillant (1994) to argue that a thorough knowledge of defense mechanisms is as important to understanding a psychiatric patient as an accurate diagnosis.

Other Contributors to Psychodynamic Theory

Defectors from Freud's Inner Circle   Carl Gustav Jung (1875–1961), Alfred Adler (1870–1937), and Otto Rank (1884–1939) were young psychiatrists who worked closely with Freud during the first two decades of the twentieth century, when he developed psychoanalytic theory. But none of these individuals could accept Freud's view that infants and young children have unconscious sexual feelings for their parents that lead to mental disorder when left unresolved. For that reason, each of the three developed an alternative psychodynamic theory to explain the development of psychopathology:

- Jung believed that mental disorder should be traced to problems that the patient's parents experienced when she was a child.
- Adler emphasized the negative consequences of feelings of inferiority that every child has in relation to bigger, wiser, more powerful adults.
- Rank conjectured that the emotional consequences of the trauma of birth (the infant's shock at having to give up the security of the womb for the uncertainty of the external world) were responsible for psychopathology.

All three of these influential neo-Freudian theories have founded schools of psychotherapy that have substantial numbers of followers. They all offer alternatives to Freudian psychoanalysis today.

The Impact of Culture and Society on Personality   During the early 1930s, while economic depression gripped most of the world, Europeans began to see signs of the fascism of Adolf Hitler, including the denial of rights for many Germans. With the threat of Nazism in mind, a group of European personality theorists modified psychoanalytic theory to emphasize the impact of culture and society on the development of personality and psychopathology. These theorists included Karen Horney (1885–1952), Erich Fromm (1900–1980), and Erik Erikson (1902–1994).

Karen Horney based her theory on the belief that anxiety and depression, both common signs of psychopathology, develop following one of three basic interpersonal conflicts: *moving toward people, moving against people,* and *moving away from people.* These conflicts relate to problems we all experience in loving, expressing anger, and losing loved ones. Like Jung, Adler, and Rank, Horney rejected Freud's assumptions about the pervasiveness of sexual motives in children. She desexualized the Oedipus complex by reinterpreting it as primarily a disturbed parent/child rela-

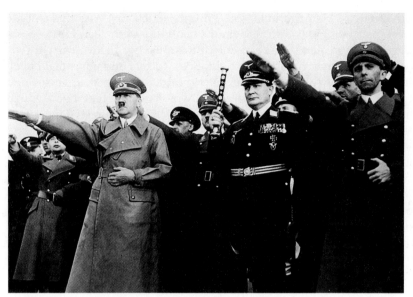

Erich Fromm's Escape from Freedom *(1941) explained the appeal of fascism to many Europeans during the 1920s and 1930s by referring to their distress at having to choose among the many new opportunities available to them during that time. Why might these new-found freedoms have been frightening to so many people?*

tionship. Specifically, she believed that a childhood characterized by parental coldness, insecurity, and feelings of isolation in an unfriendly world would lead to anxiety and depression later on. In this way, Horney linked a hostile environment with the etiology of psychopathology.

Erich Fromm's most famous book, *Escape from Freedom,* was published in 1941 at the height of the Nazi threat to the world. Puzzled by the appeal of fascism to many of his fellow Central Europeans, Fromm concluded that the problem in modern society was the boundless opportunity for choice in lifestyle and individual freedom. Based on what he observed, Fromm believed that some citizens of free countries, such as prewar Germany and Austria, were so uncomfortable with their unlimited opportunities that they chose to "escape from freedom" and embrace Hitler's totalitarian regime.

Erik Erikson also emphasized the role of social and cultural factors in personality and behavior. He suggested that personality continues to grow and change through a series of eight developmental stages, from the beginning to the end of life:

1. *infancy:* basic trust vs. mistrust
2. *early childhood:* autonomy vs. shame, doubt
3. *play age:* initiative vs. guilt
4. *latency:* industry vs. inferiority
5. *adolescence:* identity vs. role confusion
6. *young adulthood:* intimacy vs. isolation
7. *adulthood:* generativity vs. stagnation
8. *maturity:* ego integrity vs. despair

This concept is especially appealing to many people, perhaps because each stage presents a different challenge and a fresh opportunity for growth. Erikson noted that we face social and psychological conflicts in each stage of our lives, requiring that a distinct dilemma be resolved. Our success in doing so influences the development of personality and psychopathology, just as it determines our success in life.

The Ego Psychologists   A third group of neo-Freudian psychodynamic theorists—Heinz Hartmann (1894–1970), Rene Spitz (1887–1974), and Margaret Mahler (1897–1985)—are called *ego psychologists* because their theories stress the importance of the ego and its defenses to personality development and psychopathology. These theorists were strongly influenced by Anna Freud's *The Ego and the Mechanisms of Defense* (1936), mentioned earlier. They emphasize the role of the strong, mature ego in enabling adults to adapt effectively to changing external environments as well as internal challenges from the id and superego.

Margaret Mahler emphasized the importance for normal development of the separation of the child's ego from the mother's during early childhood; the child achieves this essential goal, in part, by relying on the mother's example to make sense of the world. Mahler's theory has influenced subsequent views of normal as well as pathological child development. Especially influential is her concept of *psychological birth,* which occurs later than physical birth, corresponds to the emergence of the child's individuality, and is facilitated by maternal encouragement.

Kohut's Self-Theory Heinz Kohut (1913–1981) extended psychoanalytic theory beyond the ego psychologists' emphasis on the centrality of the ego for development. In doing so, he created *self-theory*, one of the most productive current psychoanalytic views of human nature. To Kohut, both normal and abnormal development depend on how realistically the individual assesses her successes and failures in confronting life's inevitable ups and downs. Rejecting Freud's belief that psychopathology results only from intrapsychic conflict, Kohut stressed the role of *self-defects*, or developmental flaws in the individual's view of herself in relation to others. These defects play an important role in the development of anxiety, depression, and other signs and symptoms of psychopathology.

Kohut was especially concerned with what he calls the "narcissistically disturbed," including persons who have been diagnosed with narcissistic personality disorder in the *DSM-IV* (American Psychiatric Association, 1994). Kohut believed both (1) that these individuals become fixated at an early developmental stage on a parent or other love object and (2) that their greatest fear is the loss of the object. For such individuals, the psychoanalytic transference relationship (the relationship between therapist and patient) is crucial for therapeutic growth.

Contributions and Shortcomings

Freud's psychoanalytic theory represents a lasting contribution to the understanding of human behavior. His theory of psychosexual development is ingenious in the way it ties the physical and emotional tasks of childhood to the organs of the body that must carry them out. The theory also alerts clinicians to the crucial impact of childhood experiences, including childhood sexuality, on later development and psychopathology.

Freud's readiness to acknowledge the impact of the unconscious on human behavior was courageous; he was strongly criticized by contemporaries for taking this essentially unproven position. By explaining both normal and abnormal behavior as the result of unconscious interaction among the id, ego, and superego, he stressed the continuity of normality and abnormality. In doing so, Freud demystified mental illness at a time when its causes were virtually unknown. In addition, though, Freud has been heavily criticized for his exclusive emphasis on the role of unconscious processes in determining behavior and his corresponding deemphasis on biological factors in psychopathology.

Freud was a keen observer of clinical phenomena, and his insights have influenced generations of psychotherapists. Of particular influence are his insights into the interpersonal phenomena that characterize psychotherapy relationships—the thoughts and feelings patients and therapists develop for each other, termed **transference** and **countertransference.** When his detailed clinical narratives were published, they added immensely to the existing store of chronicles of psychotherapeutic studies. A number of the psychoanalytic techniques Freud developed were quickly incorporated into the existing clinical methodology and continue to be used today.

Freud developed psychoanalytic theory from his observations of his own patients. Yet these very origins have made psychoanalytic theory resistant to empirical investigation. Because Freud thought clinically, not empirically, it has proven extraordinarily difficult to translate the key elements of psychodynamic theory into operational terms and researchable topics. Researchers have been unable to agree on how to *operationalize* psychoanalytic concepts—that is, how to redefine and reconstruct them so they can be subjected to empirical examination.

Perhaps because Freud developed his theory in the consulting room, rather than the laboratory, his view emphasizes psychological abnormality, rather than health. The theory is clear in its vision of how psychopathology develops but less certain about how early life events and childrearing practices affect psychological health. As a result, psychodynamic theory has contributed little on prevention or

transference In psychoanalytic theory, the feelings a patient has for his psychotherapist; may be central to the course of therapy.

countertransference In psychoanalytic theory, the feelings a psychotherapist develops for his patients.

Focus on Critical Thinking

1. Think about your own behavior today. What specific actions or thoughts are primarily influenced by id functions? by ego functions? by superego functions? Explain your choices.

2. Which of Freud's insights into human nature are still valid today? Which are no longer valid? For instance, Freud's views on the inevitability of the Oedipus complex were based on observations of middle-class Viennese children made 100 years ago. Are these views as descriptive today of urban children, their working mothers, and the single-parent families so many of them live in? Why or why not?

early intervention methods. Psychodynamic theorists have also been faulted for their pessimism about human nature as well as their apparent unwillingness to acknowledge that people can change and grow emotionally on their own.

Freud's conviction that the interpersonal phenomena he observed were universal through time and place has also been questioned. Are the stages of psychosexual development and the Oedipus complex invariable features of children everywhere, as Freud believed? Or were they mainly the products of the time and place he lived in? Are Freud's century-old observations of the psychological lives of children and their parents as valid in the 1990s as they were in the 1890s?

THE HUMANISTIC MODEL

The **humanistic model,** developed shortly after World War II, emphasizes the uniqueness of human consciousness and the importance of understanding each person's individual perception of reality (Rice & Greenberg, 1992). The model highlights the uniqueness and worth of each person—the special qualities each of us has, regardless of our status, position, power, or influence. Another major element of the humanistic tradition is the optimistic belief that most human beings have the capacity to grow emotionally and intellectually and to realize their full potential if they work at it.

The humanistic model reacted against and thus differs sharply from the psychodynamic model. The humanistic model is optimistic and future oriented. It stresses our capacity to look after our own welfare and act in our own best interests. The humanistic model also contrasts strongly with the biological model, which insists that behavior and fate are determined at birth by a genetic inheritance we have no control over. The humanistic model affirms that we can achieve our potential by hard work, perseverance, and personal insight.

Rogers's Person-Centered Theory of Personality

The **person-centered theory of personality** of Carl Rogers (1902–1987) assumes that personality and behavior develop from our perceptions and interpretations of the world as well as from biological factors and learning (Zimring & Raskin, 1992).

humanistic model
Emphasizes the uniqueness of human consciousness and the importance of understanding each person's singular perception of reality; highlights the uniqueness and worth of each of us.

person-centered theory of personality Rogers's humanistic theory emphasizing each of our value, worth, and individuality; also stresses our potential to improve ourselves and our personal environment.

Rogers's humanistic theory emphasizes our potential to improve ourselves and our personal environment (Rogers, 1942, 1961).

Signs of Rogers's great respect for the worth, dignity, and power of the individual are evident throughout the person-centered theory. Even the name he chose for his theory reflects this conviction. It emphasizes the central importance of the *person* in understanding behavior. Rogers focuses on a few such key beliefs in his writings. The following summary of the 14 principles underlying person-centered theory (and the therapy that developed from it) also represents Rogers's philosophy of living:

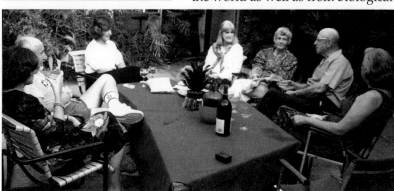

CARL ROGERS *(1902–1987), shown here conducting a group therapy session, stressed his belief in the uniquely human ability to achieve full potential by working hard and striving to develop personal insight.*

1. In my relationships with persons I have found that it does not help, in the long run, to act as though I were something that I am not.
2. I find I am more effective when I can listen acceptantly to myself, and can be myself.
3. I have found it of enormous value when I can permit myself to understand another person.
4. I have found it enriching to open channels whereby others can communicate their feelings, their private perceptual worlds, to me.
5. I have found it highly rewarding when I can accept another person.
6. The more open I am to the realities in me and in the other person, the less do I find myself wishing to rush to "fix things."
7. I can trust my experience.
8. Evaluation by others is not a guide for me. . . . Only one person can know whether what I am doing is honest, thorough, open, and sound, or false and defensive and unsound, and I am that person.
9. Experience is, for me, the highest authority. . . . It is to experience that I must return again and again, to discover a closer approximation to trust as it is in the process of becoming to me.
10. I enjoy the discovering of order in experience.
11. The facts are friendly. . . . Painful reorganizations are what is known as learning.
12. What is most personal and unique in each one of us is probably the very element which would, if it were shared or expressed, speak most deeply to others.
13. I have come to feel that the more fully the individual is understood and accepted, the more he tends to drop the false fronts with which he has been meeting life, and the more he tends to move in a direction which is forward.
14. Life, at its best, is a flowing, changing process in which nothing is fixed. (Rogers, 1961, pp. 16–27)

Maslow's Theory of Self-Actualization

Abraham Maslow (1908–1970), like Carl Rogers, was a psychologist and humanist who believed that people are basically good. As a personality theorist, Maslow prescribed the means people can use to achieve their unrealized potential, despite the frustrations and anxieties of modern life. He called this **self-actualization.**

Maslow's major theoretical contribution was his description of the **hierarchy of needs** of human beings (Maslow, 1954) (see Figure 2.6). At the base of the hierarchy are physiological needs for food, water, sex, shelter, safety, and security. These needs must be met before all others to ensure survival of the self and the species. Further up the hierarchy are social needs, such as friendship and affiliation. And at the top of the hierarchy are the most complex, difficult, and human of needs: love, self-esteem, and self-actualization. According to Maslow, the self-actualized person has successfully ascended the hierarchy of needs and satisfied her most complex, most human needs.

self-actualization Term used by Abraham Maslow to describe how human beings can achieve their unrealized potential, despite the inevitable frustrations of life.

hierarchy of needs Concept developed by Maslow describing the hierarchy of physiological, social, and complex human emotional needs people progress through to reach self-actualization.

Contributions and Shortcomings

As you may already have noticed, the optimism of Rogers's and Maslow's theories (a feature of all humanistic theories of behavior) contrasts sharply with the relative pessimism of both the biological and psychodynamic models, discussed earlier. Both of the latter models attribute most of the responsibility for our successes and failures to factors beyond our control. As a theory of personality and a basis for

FIGURE 2.6 Maslow's
hierarchy of needs

At the base of the hierarchy are our physiological needs for food, water, sex, and shelter. At midpoint are our social needs for friendship and affiliation. At the top are our most complex and human needs for love, self-esteem, and self-actualization.

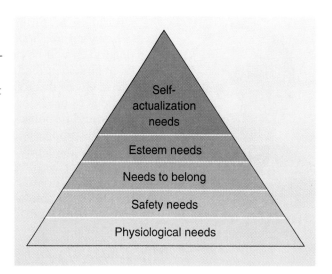

psychotherapy, however, the humanistic model encourages us to take advantage of every human capability in trying to fully realize our potential.

The humanistic model is not an elaborate or comprehensive theory of personality. For that reason, it should be viewed differently from the other models reviewed in this chapter. Perhaps the best way to view the humanistic model is as a set of uniquely personal theories of living created by humane men and women with great optimism about humans' potential to realize their full value in life. It would be a mistake to see the humanistic model as a scientifically based framework for understanding behavior, to which facts and data are added as they accumulate (as is the case with the other models covered in this chapter).

> ## Focus on Critical Thinking
>
> **1.** We stated that the biological and psychodynamic models are pessimistic, whereas the humanistic model is optimistic. Do you agree with this conclusion? If so, give examples of the pessimism of the first two models and the optimism of the third. If you don't agree, explain why.

behavioral model Assigns learning the key role in the development of behavior.

introspectionism Subjective analysis of consciousness, introduced and intensively pursued by Wilhelm Wundt.

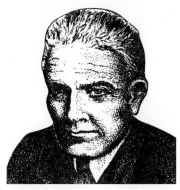

JOHN B. WATSON *(1878–1958),*
founder of behaviorism

THE BEHAVIORAL MODEL

John B. Watson (1878–1958), a founder of behaviorism, defined the **behavioral model** in 1913: "Psychology as the behaviorist views it is a purely objective experimental branch of natural science. Its theoretical goal is the prediction and control of behavior. . . . It needs introspection as little as do the sciences of chemistry and physics" (Watson, 1913, p. 158).

In this famous behavioral manifesto, Watson rejects **introspectionism,** or the subjective analysis of consciousness. This concept was introduced and intensively pursued by Wilhelm Wundt (1832–1920), who founded the first experimental psychology laboratory in Leipzig in 1879. By rejecting the most influential psychological method of his time, Watson sought to redirect the infant science of psychology away from thoughts and feelings—the objects of introspectionism—because they could not be measured with precision. Instead, Watson wanted psychologists to focus on behavior, which was observable, quantifiable, and objectifiable, just like chemical and physical phenomena.

The behavioral model of personality and psychopathology contrasts sharply with the biological and psychodynamic models, suggesting that learning plays the key role in the development of behavior. Three principal modes of learning are

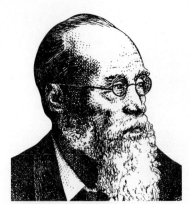

WILHELM M. WUNDT
(1832–1920), founder of the first experimental psychology laboratory

classical conditioning
Form of learning in which an unconditioned stimulus and a conditioned stimulus are repeatedly paired to produce a conditioned response.

unconditioned stimulus (UCS) In classical conditioning, a stimulus naturally capable of eliciting a UCR.

unconditioned response (UCR) In classical conditioning, the natural response elicited by a UCS.

conditioned stimulus (CS) In classical conditioning, a formerly neutral stimulus that comes to elicit the CR after repeated pairing with the UCS.

conditioned response (CR) In classical conditioning, the response elicited by the CS.

crucial to acquiring new behavior and modifying existing behavior: *classical (respondent) conditioning*, *operant (instrumental) conditioning*, and *observational learning*. (Each will be discussed in a following section.) These three learning modes were first identified in psychological laboratories by studying the behavior of animals. Given this foundation, the behavioral model relies heavily on direct observations of behavior that are obtained in studying the stimuli, reinforcing conditions, and responses that make up the learning sequence.

This emphasis on observable data in the behavioral model is quite different from the psychodynamic model's reliance on hypothetical constructs (structures that cannot be directly observed, such as the id, ego, and superego). And even though the current biological model is built on data (like the behavioral model), not too long ago, philosophers and physicians had to assume that biological factors existed because they could not be confirmed with the instruments then available.

Classical Conditioning

Ivan Pavlov (1849–1936) was a professor of physiology at the Military Medical Academy of St. Petersburg in Russia between 1895 and 1924. During the early years, Pavlov completed the research on digestive secretions and emotion for which he was awarded one of the first Nobel Prizes given in medicine and physiology in 1904. Later, as almost an afterthought to his award-winning research, Pavlov reflected on the strong influence environmental events appeared to have on gastric and salivary secretions in dogs, who started salivating (showing that they were anticipating the food) when they first heard the footsteps of and then saw the laboratory assistants who brought the meat powder they were given. This reaction occurred well before the dogs could see or smell the meat. To explore the topic, he undertook a series of experiments that ultimately established the principles of what is now called **classical conditioning,** one of the three principal ways in which humans and other animals learn.

The Classical Conditioning Process The classical conditioning process begins when an **unconditioned stimulus (UCS)** elicits an innate, unlearned behavior called an **unconditioned response (UCR)** (see Figure 2.7). In Pavlov's original experiment, the UCS was meat powder; it elicited the UCR of salivation in the dogs. When a **conditioned stimulus (CS)** that bears a significant association with the UCS is then introduced, the UCR is ultimately elicited by the CS and becomes a **conditioned response (CR)**. In Pavlov's experiment, the CS was the

Ivan Pavlov's research at the turn of the century on the conditioned reflex of dogs led to establishing the principles of classical conditioning.

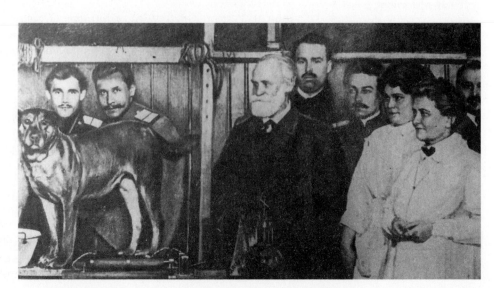

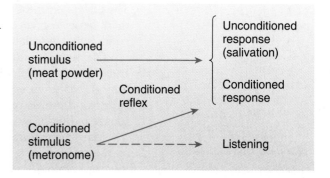

FIGURE 2.7   Classical conditioning experiment

Pavlov demonstrated the principles of classical conditioning by repeatedly pairing the sound of a metronome (the conditioned stimulus, or CS) with meat powder (the unconditioned stimulus, or UCS) to elicit salivation (before conditioning, the unconditioned response, or UCR; after conditioning, the conditioned response, or CR) from his dogs.

Source: From P. E. Nathan and S. L. Harris (1980), *Psychopathology and Society*, 2nd ed. Copyright 1980 by McGraw-Hill, Inc. Reproduced with permission of McGraw-Hill, Inc.

sound of the metronome that always occurred immediately before the meat powder was given to the dogs (the UCS). Pavlov concluded that the repeated pairing of the sound of the metronome and the appearance of meat powder ultimately caused his dogs to salivate as soon as they heard the metronome.

Generations of researchers who study learning have believed that *contiguity* (a close temporal or spatial relationship between the CS and UCS) is crucial to the classical conditioning process. Yet two recent articles by Robert Rescorla (1988, 1992), a leading researcher, report convincing evidence that these and some other long-held beliefs about how and why classical conditioning occurs are probably wrong. For example, Rescorla concludes that the simple temporal pairing of two events—for example, the sound of the metronome and the sight of meat powder in Pavlov's experiment—is not a sufficient explanation for the development of classical conditioning. Instead, Rescorla claims, classical conditioning really involves learning the relations and contingencies among events. According to Rescorla, Pavlov's dogs learned a complete sequence of events, not just the simple sequence of bell/laboratory assistant/meat powder. They also learned that three other events—the sound of a step or a bell and their experience of hunger—all had certain contingent relations to the appearance of meat powder. All three of the former events reliably predicted the latter event.

Rescorla (1988, 1992) and others are now convinced that classical conditioning is far more complex than previously believed. It is not invariably automatic and beyond awareness. Instead, it may involve a range of processes that previously were thought to be bypassed by this mode of learning. In humans, for example, cognitive processes may be involved in classical conditioning. Baker and his colleagues (1987) distinguish between *automatic* conditioning (fear conditioning in humans may be of this kind) and *controlled* conditioning (the more complex kind involving awareness and other cognitive processes).

Conditioned responses are acquired gradually. The speed with which a response is acquired and the strength of the conditioning depend on three principal factors:

1. whether the conditioning trials are massed (presented one right after another) or spaced (spaced trials usually induce a stronger relationship between stimulus and response)
2. the value of the UCS to the organism (food, water, and sex are the most effective unconditioned stimuli)
3. whether the CS is relevant to the UCS (the more relevant the CS is to the UCS, the more predictable the conditioning)

A number of real-life illustrations demonstrate how much the relevance of the CS to the UCS affects conditioning. For instance, cancer patients who experience one of the common side effects of radiation therapy—nausea and vomiting—typically begin to have those feelings when they again see the hospital where they receive radiation treatment. Seeing other hospitals sometimes brings on those feelings, too.

The relevance of the side effects of radiation treatment to cancer patients (the treatment tends to preoccupy their lives) clearly influences the development of a strong conditioned association between the hospital and the experience of nausea.

Classically conditioned behaviors are eliminated by a process called **extinction.** Pavlov's dogs gradually stopped salivating at the sound of the metronome after it was sounded repeatedly but not followed by meat powder. Stated technically, conditioned responses become extinguished when the CS and UCS are no longer paired or when the relevance of the CS to the UCS has been lost.

Many behavioral clinicians believe that anxiety and fear are acquired by classical conditioning (Lang, 1985). A number of behavioral methods for treating anxious and phobic behavior try to extinguish the association between the experience of fear and the objects in the environment responsible for it. The appearance of a stimulus or stimuli relevant to the fear-inducing stimulus (for example, a person, an animal, or a situation) can produce the thoughts and feelings associated with fear even when the original fear stimulus is not present.

Using **stimulus generalization,** some conditioned responses are linked both to the conditioned stimuli they were first associated with and to similar stimuli not originally part of the conditioning. Stimulus generalization is responsible for the development of phobic and anxious behavior (McNally, 1987). Once the cognitive, subjective, and physiological sensations of fear and anxiety become related to one or more conditioned stimuli (for example, a punitive father or a critical mother), they can generalize to all males, all females, or all people. The result is a generalized phobia that seriously interferes with normal functioning.

Higher-order conditioning, in essence, converts a CS into a UCS when a second-order conditioned association forms. Higher-order conditioning occurs when the UCS (the experience of anxiety, for instance) generalizes from the stimulus object itself (that punitive father or critical mother) to thoughts or memories of the object. For example, assume that a woman has acquired an association between the experience of fear and anxiety and the sight of her abusive ex-husband. That negative association might eventually generalize to all men who remind her of him. Through higher-order conditioning, even her ex-husband's first name or words such as *husband* or *man* might prompt the fear and anxiety previously associated only with his physical presence.

Operant Conditioning

In 1911, Ivan Pavlov was in the midst of exploring classical conditioning in dogs and John B. Watson was about to describe psychology as the science of behavior. The same year, Edward L. Thorndike (1874–1949) announced the discovery of the **law of effect,** which states that behaviors associated with satisfying consequences are strengthened by those consequences and thus more likely to be repeated, whereas those linked to unsatisfying consequences are weakened and thus less likely to be repeated. For instance, the college student who is acknowledged and praised by her professor for speaking in class will be more likely to ask questions again, and the student whose questions are ignored or minimized will be less likely to inquire next time.

Watson and Thorndike both strongly influenced Burrhus F. Skinner (1904–1990) who, in the early 1930s, established the principles of **operant conditioning** (so named because operant behavior "operates on" the environment). B. F. Skinner did more than any other psychologist to promote the behavioral revolution that occurred in psychology from the 1950s through the 1970s (Lattal, 1992).

Skinner recorded the basic principles of operant (instrumental) conditioning in his classic research monograph *The Behavior of Organisms,* published in 1938. At the beginning of the monograph, Skinner responded to the well-known statement attributed to Pavlov that animals and humans learn only by classical conditioning. Skinner observed instead that "there is a large body of behavior that does not seem to be elicited, in the sense in which a cinder in the eye elicits closure of the lid" (1938, p. 19). The "large body of behavior" Skinner referred to in his statement is operant learning.

extinction In classical conditioning, the disappearance of the CR when it is no longer paired with the UCR.

stimulus generalization In classical conditioning, when a CR is linked both to the CS with which it was first associated and to similar stimuli not originally part of the conditioning.

higher-order conditioning In classical conditioning, when a CS effectively becomes a UCS following the formation of a second-order conditioned association.

law of effect Thorndike's theory that behaviors associated with satisfying consequences are strengthened and thus more likely to be repeated whereas those linked to unsatisfying consequences are weakened and less likely to be repeated.

operant conditioning Mode of learning in which behavior is acquired, maintained, and eliminated as a function of its consequences.

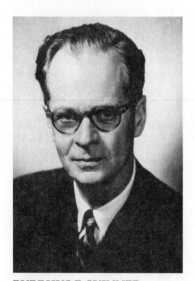

BURRHUS F. SKINNER
(1904–1990), who recorded the principles of operant conditioning in The Behavior of Organisms *(1938), was one of the world's most revered psychologists at the time of his death.*

Skinner's ultimate goal for operant conditioning was to use it in predicting and controlling behavior to make a better world. Through the work of others, that goal has been achieved, at least in part. In the 60 years since publication of *The Behavior of Organisms,* the theory of operant learning has had a profound impact on experimental and clinical psychology, psychiatry, education, social and community planning, and law enforcement and corrections. Upon his death in 1990, Skinner was one of the most revered figures in American psychology (Dinsmoor, 1992; Greenwood et al., 1992).

Another of Skinner's lasting legacies is the **single-case design,** his prime research strategy. It involved the repeated, intensive study of single animals under varying environmental conditions; this method permitted the systematic exploration of the environmental factors influencing the animal's operant behavior. Behavioral researchers studying human psychopathology use single-case designs to do essentially the same thing. For example, to study a child with an emotional disorder, researchers first modify one and then another part of the child's environment. By studying the effects that these changes have on the child's maladaptive behavior, researchers learn what controls the behavior and how it might be changed for the better.

The Operant-Conditioning Process   As Thorndike's law of effect predicts, in the operant conditioning process, reinforced behaviors tend to increase in frequency and punished or ignored behaviors tend to decrease in frequency. The initial term in Figure 2.8, **discriminative stimulus (SD),** refers to the information our environment provides us about the likelihood that our responses will be rewarded, ignored, or punished. The second term, **operant response (R),** refers to our behaviors in anticipation of these consequences. The third term, **reinforcing stimulus (SR),** refers to the consequences—the reinforcing or punishing results of our behavior.

Most of the discriminative stimuli humans must interpret are subtle and complex. A smile, a frown, a nod of the head—each lets us know the likelihood that our behavior will be rewarded by the person who provides the **social cue** (a term describing many discriminative stimuli, or SDs). To be sure, our environments have their formal SDs: red and green stoplights, course grades, and so on. But most of the information we receive from our environment consists of social cues. As a result, one of the key tasks of childhood is to learn to read and understand these cues. Perceiving social cues accurately is one of the earliest human capacities that breaks down under the strain of serious mental disorder.

Operant responses produce one of the two following consequences, or reinforcing stimuli (SRs):

1. **Reinforcement** occurs when a pattern of responses is followed by satisfying consequences; this tends to increase the likelihood that the pattern of response will be repeated. When an instructor praises a piece of written work, for instance, the student is more likely to produce writing of the same kind again. And when a child is rewarded for good behavior, he is more likely to repeat that behavior.

single-case design Intensive study of single subjects over time under systematically varied environmental conditions.

discriminative stimulus (SD) In operant conditioning, the information the environment provides about the likelihood that a response will be reinforced, ignored, or punished.

operant response (R) Voluntary response that operates on the environment and produces reinforcement or punishment.

reinforcing stimulus (SR) In operant conditioning, the positive or negative consequences of a response that determine its subsequent frequency.

social cue Human discriminative stimulus that informs us whether a particular social behavior is likely to be reinforced or punished.

reinforcement In operant conditioning, presentation of a rewarding stimulus or removal of an aversive stimulus following a response; increases the probability that a response will recur.

FIGURE 2.8   Operant conditioning experiment

In one of Skinner's early operant conditioning experiments, pigeons learned to peck repeatedly at a disk lit by a green light to obtain grain. In the example shown, the green disk served as the discriminative stimulus, signaling that the operant response (key pecks of the disk) would produce grain (the reinforcing stimulus).

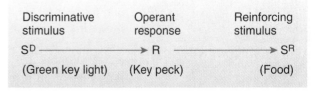

Discriminative stimulus	Operant response	Reinforcing stimulus
SD ⟶	R ⟶	SR
(Green key light)	(Key peck)	(Food)

Source: From P. E. Nathan and S. L. Harris (1980), *Psychopathology and Society,* 2nd ed. Copyright 1980 by McGraw-Hill, Inc. Reprinted with permission of McGraw-Hill, Inc.

2. Punishment takes place when a response is followed by an aversive or unwelcome behavioral consequence; this tends to decrease the likelihood of a similar pattern of responses in the future. In the dating world, it generally takes only a single "no" from a person we want to date to convince us that we should focus our attention elsewhere. A poor grade on a midterm exam can cause a radical decrease in partying behavior, if we decide we want to do better on the final.

Psychopathology and Operant Conditioning   Operant mechanisms play a role in the etiology and maintenance of a number of the disorders discussed in this book (Gewirtz & Pelaez-Nogueras, 1992). Moreover, operant conditioning has had a significant impact on the design of therapeutic programs (Schreibman, 1994; Whitman, 1994). Many of those that train parents and teachers to modify the behavior of children who are aggressive, mentally retarded, or psychotic, for example, use operant principles (Kazdin, 1994). (Some of these programs are described in Chapters 14 and 15.) By teaching when and how to reward children such as these for appropriate behavior, behavioral clinicians have helped countless parents and teachers who previously wondered if they would ever bring their children's behavior under control (Greenwood et al., 1992).

Contributions and Shortcomings

Supporters of the behavioral model put a lot of emphasis on research and empirical data, which has convinced other mental health professionals to move in the same direction. Even those with primary allegiances to other models of psychopathology have accepted the usefulness of this view.

The behavioral model emphasizes environmental and learning variables in explaining behavior, but it does not ignore biological and individual factors. Because of its greater openness to a range of explanations for behavior, the model has served as a counterforce to the predominant emphases of the biological model on biological mechanisms and the psychodynamic model on intrapsychic ones.

Critics of the behavioral model fault its stress on learning and environmental determinants of behavior, especially in view of current findings that point to the role of genetics in disorders such as alcoholism and depression, once widely thought to be environmental problems. Others criticize behavioral researchers and clinicians for deemphasizing cognitive and self-control in their efforts to demonstrate the power of the environment to affect behavior. (**Cognition** refers to the uniquely human mental processes of thinking and reasoning, perceiving and recognizing, judging and conceiving.) In response to these concerns, primarily during the 1970s and 1980s, cognitive concepts and strategies were energetically incorporated into the framework of what is now termed *social-learning theory* (Hawkins, Kashden, Hansen, & Sadd, 1992).

Social Learning Theory

Observational Learning   Until the early 1960s, most learning theorists believed that classical and operant conditioning were responsible for essentially all human and animal learning. At that time, Albert Bandura and his colleagues at Stanford University began to study what they called **observational learning,** or **modeling.** Observational learning is now recognized as a basic mode of learning, distinct from both classical and operant conditioning. Bandura's early research on observational learning demonstrated that children acquired entirely new response patterns by simply watching others engaging in various kinds of behaviors (Bandura, 1973, 1977). One of the earliest experiments on modeling reported that children who observed aggressive models were more likely themselves to act aggressively toward other children (Bandura, Ross, & Ross, 1961, 1963).

The research findings on observational learning have had many therapeutic applications. Initially, application focused on the usefulness of observational

punishment In operant conditioning, presentation of an aversive stimulus or removal of a reinforcing stimulus following a response; decreases the probability that the response will recur.

cognition Uniquely human mental processes of thinking and reasoning, perceiving and recognizing, judging and conceiving.

observational learning Mode of learning in which you watch others engaging in various kinds of behavior, without engaging in them yourself.

modeling Synonym for observational learning.

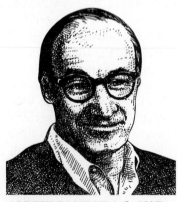

ALBERT BANDURA *(b. 1925), whose research on observational learning has strongly influenced the development of social learning theory. In what ways did data from Bandura's studies of observational learning impact the principles of social learning theory?*

learning in modifying or eliminating fearful behaviors of phobic children and adults. More recently, application has expanded to a variety of situations in which the unwanted behaviors of primates (Mineka & Cook, 1986) and children (Thase & Moss, 1976) have been modified by exposing them to models demonstrating more appropriate, adaptive behavior. For example, Mineka and her colleagues (1984) and Cook and his co-workers (1985) studied the acquisition of emotional behavior in animals. Rhesus monkeys raised in laboratories generally don't fear snakes. But after watching monkeys who were born in the wild show strong, innate reactions of fear to snakes, the domestic monkeys also become fearful.

The impact of modeling on the development of psychopathology in humans has focused on alcohol consumption. Research has shown that the intensity of alcohol consumption by a drinking companion strongly influences the intensity of one's own drinking, although neither person is apparently aware of this influence (Larimer & Marlatt, 1994).

Self-Control   The concept of **self-control,** or **self-regulation,** developed from Bandura's empirical and conceptual work (Bandura, 1977). Kanfer (1977) also made key contributions to self-control theory. The concept of self-control grew out of the recognition that behavior is not simply a function of external rewards and punishments, whether experienced directly or by watching others. We can learn to regulate our own behavior. (This is a central feature of the cognitive-behavioral approach to treatment, described later.) We can make active choices from among behavioral alternatives, choosing to pursue one and ignore the others. We self-regulate when we establish rewards and punishments that we earn, depending on our ability to meet our own performance standards.

The self-control concept derives from a three-stage model (Bandura, 1977). The first stage is *self-observation,* which is the capacity to view our own behavior as it occurs. Next is *self-evaluation,* which involves two tasks: (1) setting standards for evaluating the adequacy of our behavior and (2) monitoring our behavior continuously and consciously, according to those standards, in order to evaluate how much we do or do not meet them. The third stage, *self-reinforcement,* depends on both preceding self-control strategies; we reward or punish ourselves based on how we've judged our performance.

Reciprocal Determinism   Bandura's belief in the reciprocal interaction of behavior, cognitive factors, and environmental influences is known as **reciprocal determinism** (1977, 1989). The concept highlights his recognition that people both affect and are affected by their environment and that behavior is the result of factors that both influence and are influenced by each other. Bandura's concept of self-efficacy (1977, 1989), described in the following section, is derived from his views on reciprocal determinism.

self-control Central feature of this social learning concept is the recognition that we can learn to regulate our own behavior.

self-regulation Synonym for self-control.

reciprocal determinism Describes Bandura's belief in the reciprocal interaction of behavioral, cognitive, and environmental influences.

self-efficacy Bandura's term for beliefs about our ability to exercise control over events that affect our lives.

Self-Efficacy   Bandura defines **self-efficacy** as "people's beliefs about their capabilities to exercise control over events that affect their lives" (1989, p. 1175). Those beliefs influence motivation, including the motivation to undertake a difficult or novel task; the attitudes and expectations associated with taking on the task; and the actions necessary to complete the task. Bandura also reminds us that reciprocal determinism ensures that the outcome of the effort to complete a task—that is, the relative success or failure of the effort—influences our continuing reassessment of self-efficacy.

As some of the discussions on treatment later in this book show (see Chapters 18–20, in particular), it's important to assess self-efficacy before and during treatment for a number of conditions, including substance-related disorders, eating disorders, depression, and the sexual disorders. People entering treatment who believe they have a good chance to control or change their behavior are more likely to succeed at doing so than those who are pessimistic about their ability to change. Increasingly, clinicians want to know their patients' self-efficacy for behavioral change *before* trying to induce change (Craighead, Craighead, Kazdin, & Mahoney, 1994).

Contributions and Shortcomings

Social learning theory emphasizes the powerful role that our thoughts and feelings about ourselves play in the choices we make. For example, psychiatric patients have attitudes and expectations about how their disordered behavior developed and how likely they will be able to change it. Clinicians who do not explore these beliefs (and, if necessary, dispute them) ignore a factor that has a lot of influence on the outcome of their efforts. When the insights of social learning theory are combined with the environmental and learning factors emphasized by the behavioral model, an impressively comprehensive view of normal and abnormal behavior results.

Even so, some behavioral critics of social learning theory question its emphasis on the role of cognitive factors in behavior because those factors are not observable and cannot be easily measured. From a different perspective, supporters of the biological model, who criticize the behavioral model's neglect of the role of genetic and biological factors in psychopathology, take the same critical position toward social learning theory.

Cognitive-Behavioral Approaches to Treatment

Cognitive-behavioral treatment methods draw on insights and data from behavioral and social learning theories. Both stress precise definition and, when possible, operationalization of concepts. Likewise, both stress the importance of subjecting treatment methods to empirical study and retaining only those that can be experimentally supported.

Cognitive-behavioral treatments call on two uniquely human capacities. The first is our ability to self-regulate our own behavior. This skill is central to cognitive-behavioral treatment because many programs teach self-control strategies. As noted earlier, for example, retraining in self-evaluation and self-reinforcement is an important component of cognitive-behavioral treatment for depression in adults (Hollon & Carter, 1994).

Another important aspect of cognitive-behavioral treatment is our ability to manipulate *symbolic events* (the thoughts and feelings we attach to past, present, and future experiences). **Attributional processes,** which are significant symbolic events, are the explanations we offer ourselves of past successes and failures. Attributing a failure to events beyond our control is clearly more constructive personally than blaming it on our own shortcomings. Attributing a success to our own actions, similarly, is more positive than attributing it to circumstances we had no control over. Attributional processes influence many psychopathological conditions, including both depression and responses to stress.

attributional processes
Explanations we use to explain our successes and failures to ourselves.

The principal goal of cognitive-behavioral treatment is to help people make the changes in their behavior they want to make by teaching them more adaptive ways to relate to their social environments (Craighead et al., 1994). Learning more effective problem-solving techniques is an especially important part of cognitive-behavioral treatment. This type of treatment is time limited; its goals are mutually agreed on by patient and therapist. Unlike other therapies, during cognitive-behavioral treatment, patient and therapist collaborate to identify problems, plan treatment strategies, and evaluate outcomes.

Focus on Critical Thinking

1. The behavioral model has been criticized for neglecting the biological factors involved in psychopathology. Do you agree with this criticism? If so, how might behavioral theorists incorporate biological factors in their model? If you disagree with this criticism, why?

2. Which of the three principal modes of learning—classical conditioning, operant conditioning, or modeling—has played the most important role in our efforts to explain abnormal behavior from the behavioral perspective? Why?

Che Social Consequence Model

The social consequence model emphasizes the impact that belonging to certain groups in society has on group members. Supporters of the model believe that societal attitudes and behavior toward certain persons because of their gender, ethnicity, race, or socioeconomic status, for example, affect both their behavior and the risk they run of developing certain kinds of psychopathology.

Epidemiological Survey Data

In the Midtown Manhattan Study (also reviewed in Chapter 1), poor residents, most of whom were African American or Hispanic, were much more likely to be judged psychologically impaired by interviewers than were middle- or upper-middle-class residents (Srole, Langner, Michael, Opler, & Rennie, 1962). One interpretation of this finding is that the stress of urban poverty increases the risk of psychopathology. Another is that Midtown interviewers were more inclined to see the behavior of poor residents as being abnormal than they were that of middle-class residents. Both explanations support the view that biased attitudes toward poverty and race help define or determine psychopathology.

Data from the NIMH Epidemiologic Catchment Area (ECA) Study (Eaton et al., 1984; Regier et al., 1984) (also reviewed in Chapter 1) provide added support for the social consequence model. The survey revealed systematic differences in disorder prevalence rates between urban and rural residents as well as between Mexican American and non-Hispanic respondents. Major depression and drug abuse/dependence were diagnosed most frequently in urban residents, many of whom were poor members of minority groups. And alcohol abuse and dependence were substantial problems among people living in the country. Mexican Americans experienced high rates of cognitive disorder, and non-Hispanics living in the same area had high rates of drug abuse and dependence. Both sets of findings confirm that place of residence and ethnicity have a strong influence on psychopathology.

Gender and Psychopathology

Many studies, including some reviewed later in this text, have found comparable differences between men and women in rates of specific disorders. One of the most consistent gender-related findings is a higher rate of depression among women than men. The 1981–83 ECA study (Eaton et al., 1992) found systematic differences between men and women in rates of depression, alcohol and drug abuse/dependence, and antisocial behavior. And the 1990–92 national survey of major depression (Blazer et al., 1994) reported significantly higher rates of major depression among women than men.

Throughout this text, we look carefully at gender-linked differences in rates of psychopathology. Although we take account of gender-related biological and psychological differences that affect behavior and psychopathology, we also weigh the effects of society's different attitudes toward and treatment of men and women.

Race and Psychopathology

How can attitudes toward race affect psychiatric status? The *Autobiography* of Malcolm X (1964) offers repeated, eloquent testimony to the mechanisms linking the two. Throughout his life, Malcolm X remained convinced that welfare workers conspired to take him and his brothers and sisters away from their mother and place them in foster care, thereby destroying the family. He also remained convinced that the true reason behind this effort was that welfare workers believed the worst about his mother's ability to care for her children because she was poor and African American.

Throughout his *Autobiography*, Malcolm returns again and again to the same theme: the impact of institutional racism in the United States on his own life and the lives of his parents, siblings, friends, and fellow African Americans. It seems reasonable to assume that Malcolm was strongly affected by the pervasive prejudice against African Americans he witnessed during his youth, including the resulting limitations on educational, social, and vocational opportunities. But how did seeing and enduring discrimination affect his psychopathology? Consider the following excerpt from the earliest pages of his *Autobiography:*

> Meanwhile, the state Welfare people kept after my mother. By now she didn't make it any secret that she hated them, and didn't want them in her house. But they exerted their right to come, and I have many, many times reflected upon how, talking to us children, they began to plant the seeds of division in our minds. . . . I think they felt that getting children into foster homes was a legitimate part of their function, and the result would be less troublesome, however they went about it. . . . And when my mother fought them, they went after her—first, through me. I was the first target. I stole; that implied that I wasn't being taken care of by my mother. . . . I'm not sure just how or when the idea was first dropped by the Welfare workers that our mother was losing her mind. . . . They were as vicious as vultures. They had no feelings, understanding, compassion, or respect for my mother. They told us, "She's crazy for refusing food." Right then was when our home, our unity, began to disintegrate. (Malcolm X, 1964, pp. 17–21)

Throughout his entire, short life, Malcolm carried the weight of being the family's "bad boy." As such, he thought he had contributed to the dissolution of his family and his mother's subsequent descent into psychosis. That burden—accompanied by memories of his father's violent death and his dismay at having been unable to prevent the welfare agency from splitting up his family—clearly played a causal role in the development of his psychopathology. When Malcolm used alcohol and narcotics, he could blot out both the rage he felt for his family's persecutors and the depression and regret he felt at his inability, as a young child, to hold the family together.

Lex (1985) and others have examined elevated rates of drug abuse/dependence and antisocial behavior among minority groups. Researchers asked whether these behaviors might demonstrate ways these groups have chosen to deal with the discouraging social and psychological conditions many of them live in. Unfortunately, efforts to explain such differences as a function of race have been held back because too few studies exploring racial effects are available in the psychological literature. A recent content analysis of six leading journals in psychology revealed "a declining representation of African-American research in the journals" (Graham, 1992). Moreover, those few articles that did study African Americans tended to lack methodological rigor, so their findings are suspect.

We conclude that the available data support the view that racial identity influences risk for some kinds of psychopathology, but how this influence is exerted is unclear. Several important questions still need to be answered:

- How much do society's biased attitudes and reactions toward certain minority groups directly influence their risks for certain kinds of psychopathology?
- How much do differences in socioeconomic status between members of minority and nonminority groups impact those rates?
- What roles do biological and sociocultural differences play?

Poverty and Psychopathology

The social consequence model also asks whether a relationship exists between poverty and psychopathology. Anthropologist Oscar Lewis (1961, 1969) is closely

hy have so many Vietnam veterans become homeless? What factors are associated with their homelessness? Are African American and Hispanic veterans at special risk?

These questions have become increasingly important as the number of homeless people in our cities continues to swell. If we can understand the problem of homelessness among Vietnam veterans, perhaps we will be better able to understand it for all people living in this condition.

A recent study of 1,460 male veterans who participated in the National Vietnam Veterans Readjustment Study (Rosenheck & Fontana, 1994) provides answers to some of these questions. Unexpectedly, the strongest direct effects on homelessness arose following, rather than during, military service. These effects included the strong sense of social isolation and lack of social support many Vietnam veterans experienced on their return from combat, mental disorder undiagnosed during military service, and substance abuse, which often developed while in Vietnam. War-related experiences did not seem to play a substantial role in the later development of homelessness. However, certain childhood experiences turned out to be quite influential, including foster care placement, physical or sexual abuse, and other early traumas. (Schizophrenia, a common accompaniment of homelessness, was not assessed in this sample; as a result, the relation between psychiatric disorder and homelessness was probably underestimated.)

One of the study's most surprising findings was that childhood poverty and minority racial or ethnic status were not associated with homelessness, even though many more Vietnam veterans are members of minority groups than the proportion of minorities in the U.S. population would predict. As our review of the data in support of the social consequence model of psychopathology indicates, poverty and minority group status are strongly linked to a range of adverse health and social consequences. Yet neither predicted homelessness in this study. One explanation for this finding is that fewer minority group members may have chosen to participate in the national survey this study was part of. Another explanation is the usual socioeconomic status of individuals in the military. As the authors of the study note, "Men in the military services, while similar to other Americans in many ways, tend to come less frequently from the high and low socioeconomic extremes of society."

You've probably recognized that some of the same social factors that predict psychopathology and support the social consequence model of psychopathology also influence the development of homelessness in Vietnam-era veterans. Keep in mind, though, that the military is different enough from U.S. society as a whole that findings based on military subjects will not be exactly representative. (For example, the military enlists fewer men and women from the socioeconomic extremes of society and substantially fewer women overall.) Nonetheless, it's clear that social factors play an important role in one of society's greatest current challenges: the problem of homelessness in our cities.

Think about the following questions:

1. If you compared homeless male Vietnam veterans with other groups of homeless individuals, what social and psychological differences might you find? Explain your answer.
2. Why do you think childhood traumas (such as physical and sexual abuse and foster care placement) were associated with developing homelessness in this group of veterans?
3. Why do you think war-related experiences were *not* associated with developing homelessness in this group?

---

identified with this question. In the 1960s, he convinced many that a **culture of poverty** had arisen among poor people in U.S. society that tended to keep these people living in poverty. Lewis linked the traits of the culture of poverty to a variety of social ills and also to psychopathology and physical illness. According to Lewis, the social and psychological traits of poverty include crowded quarters, violence, little sense of history, and strong feelings of marginality, helplessness, and dependency. Other traits include resignation and fatalism, relatively high death rates, and high tolerance for psychological pathology. All these traits of poverty are clearly precursors to abnormal behavior.

Contributions and Shortcomings

The social consequence model forces us to consider the impact that our treatment of and attitudes toward women, people who are poor, and members of racial and

culture of poverty Concept that suggests that the social and psychological traits of people who are poor maintain their poverty and contribute to their high rates of psychopathology.

61

ethnic minorities have on their behavior and psychopathology. In doing so, the social consequence model counterbalances an exclusive biological or psychodynamic understanding of the development of psychopathology. The model does not rely solely on biological factors, such as neurotransmitter dysfunction, or psychodynamic factors, such as inadequate ego defenses. Instead, the social consequence model asks us, as members of the society in which we live, to accept some of the responsibility for its problems.

Even though volumes of data have been accumulated during recent decades in support of the social consequence model, how it exerts its influence has been difficult to trace. For instance, relationships between poverty and greater risks for some kinds of physical and psychological disorders have been demonstrated repeatedly, but they do not prove that poverty causes psychopathology. As noted earlier, sometimes it may be the other way around. Perhaps people afflicted with certain forms of psychopathology are less able to earn a living than those who are not. Or perhaps middle-class interviewers are simply more likely to judge the behavior of poor people as abnormal because it differs so much from their own.

Systematic, controlled research is needed to identify the means by which social factors exert their influence on psychopathology. Meanwhile, the social consequence model focuses important attention on the substantial contribution of society to psychopathology.

Focus on Critical Thinking

1. A number of studies show hard evidence of the relationship between social factors, such as gender and poverty, and greater risk for physical and psychological disorders, such as depression and drug and alcohol abuse/dependence. What could be done to reduce this relationship in U.S. society?

THE BIOPSYCHOSOCIAL MODEL

In this chapter, we have presented a lot of strong evidence in support of the role of biological factors in the causes of some of the most serious and disabling mental disorders. Data from multiple sources point to the role of biological and genetic factors in schizophrenia, the major affective disorders, and the substance use disorders, among others.

The significance of learning in the development of psychopathology has also strongly been supported by data reviewed in this chapter. The behavioral and social learning models of psychopathology give convincing empirical evidence for the belief that learning factors influence the development of some of the depressive disorders, the anxiety disorders, the stress disorders, and the substance use disorders.

Much of the epidemiological evidence presented in Chapter 1 attests to the impact of social factors on the development of some forms of psychopathology. Society's attitudes toward race, ethnicity, gender, and socioeconomic status clearly influence our chances of becoming mentally ill. By helping determine whom we work and live with, how we treat each other, how satisfied we are with ourselves, and how others feel about us, these social group memberships have powerful effects on our behavior.

The psychodynamic and humanistic models of abnormality are not as well supported empirically as the behavioral, social consequence, and biological models. Nonetheless, several generations of clinicians have concluded that psychological processes have the power to create *and* remediate disordered behavior.

Despite the compelling logic that supports each of these five models of abnormal behavior, none seems sufficient by itself to explain the development of even a single distinct disorder. Consider the following examples:

A young woman, Julia, has been the victim of a serious automobile accident. She has suffered substantial brain damage, causing severe memory loss and marked behavioral deterioration. Yet Julia is surprisingly responsive to the world around her. She is still capable of caring for family and friends, enjoys social situations and behaves appropriately in them, and readily feels and expresses emotions such as happiness and sadness. She benefits a great deal from having a supportive, understanding family. Their continued involvement in Julia's life has helped her remain productive, maintain an optimistic attitude, and work hard at rehabilitation.

Gary is a middle-aged man, a Vietnam veteran, who suffers from posttraumatic stress disorder (PTSD). This disabling condition, characterized by severe anxiety and depression, is a reaction to the profound environmental stress Gary experienced during the 13 months he spent in combat 25 years ago. Complicating his condition are a variety of physical symptoms, which is surprising, since his PTSD appears to have been caused entirely by environmental and psychological factors. Among other symptoms, Gary complains of a perpetually hyperaroused autonomic nervous system that makes him feel, he says, like "it's Vietnam inside me all over again."

How much can you say about each person? What seems to be causing Julia's behavior? What about Gary's behavior? Why does Gary suffer so much more than Julia?

The point of this contrast is to emphasize the difficulty of fully understanding the behavior of either person without focusing on the interaction among the social, psychological, and biological systems that jointly influenced his or her behavior. A single model of behavior is insufficient to permit full understanding of their conditions, unless it gives weight to all three systems.

The same can be said of efforts to understand Malcolm X. It's a gross oversimplification to say he simply inherited or acquired the depression or substance abuse that afflicted him most of his days; likewise, these are not suitable explanations for the strengths of leadership, resolve, and intelligence that he demonstrated. To produce the three-dimensional view of Malcolm X that is most revealing, we must appreciate the interaction of biological, psychological, and social factors—as woven throughout his life—that produced the man.

In the last few years, several investigators have reported empirical findings that support the biopsychosocial position. Behavioral geneticist Robert Plomin has gathered convincing data that point to the interactive role of genetic inheritance and environmental factors in determining many of the behaviors that make us uniquely human (Plomin & Neiderhiser, 1992). Social psychologist John Cacioppo has also reported data that support the interaction of brain functions and psychological and social processes. Regarding this work, he notes, "Our understanding of the function of hormones would be far more rudimentary if not for analyses of their effects on social behavior and for the effects of social behavior on hormonal changes" (Cacioppo & Berntson, 1992, p. 1020). And in the clinical arena, Andersen, Kiecolt-Glaser, and Glaser (1994), among others, have documented the substantial impact that the environment, whether stressful or unthreatening, has on cancer progression and regression. (Previously, researchers thought that cancer was influenced only by biological factors.)

Another prominent researcher, Robert Cloninger, has argued that the biopsychosocial model is the most complete explanation for alcoholism, one of the most serious social problems in the United States. Earlier in the chapter, we reviewed Cloninger's previous work on the genetic component of alcoholism (Cloninger, Bohman, & Sigvardsson, 1981). More recently, Cloninger has published several empirical reports, bringing together diverse data and proposing a biopsychosocial theory of alcoholism that he believes is also relevant to other disorders (Cloninger,

1987; Cloninger, Svrakic, & Przybeck, in press; Svrakic, Whitehead, Przybeck, & Cloninger, in press).

Cloninger has examined data that separate alcoholics into two groups, based on family history of alcoholism and signs and symptoms of the disorder. He has concluded that the two groups may also differ systematically along biological, psychological, and social dimensions. Cloninger has observed that the brain's principal neurotransmitters (dopamine, serotonin, and norepinephrine) modulate three categories of brain/behavior relationships: behavioral activation, inhibition, and maintenance. These three brain systems, in turn, respond with greater sensitivity to different social stimuli (for instance, stimuli that encourage or support novelty seeking, harm avoidance, reward dependence, and persistence) to produce different social and behavioral consequences. Cloninger believes that genetic factors determine which neurotransmitter is most influential in a particular person's life. He suggests that this interactive system may help explain other serious mental disorders as well as healthy and productive behavior.

Cloninger's biopsychosocial theory proposes that the alcohol-related problems that distinguish the two groups of alcoholics result from different patterns of interaction among biological, psychological, and social factors. Although biological factors (that is, a predominance of one neurotransmitter system over another) are extremely important, by themselves, they are not sufficient to produce different alcohol-related problems. What's more, alcoholism has distinct social and psychological consequences: fights and arrests during periods of intoxication, loss of control, and guilt and fear about alcohol dependence. These are all clearly behaviors whose presence or absence affects how other people react to alcoholics as well as how they view themselves.

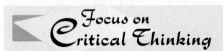

Focus on Critical Thinking

1. Think of two or three behavioral patterns that others would say are most characteristic of you. What biological, social, and psychological factors influenced the development of these behaviors? Explain your answers.

SUMMARY

Creating Models of Abnormal Behavior

■ Models help us clarify and organize our thinking about complicated phenomena. They are especially useful when our knowledge of such phenomena contains gaps.

The Biological Model

■ The biological model of mental disorder assumes that the principal causes of abnormal behavior involve neurobiological dysfunction of the central nervous system.

■ Over the past 20 years, a great deal of data has been gathered relating neurotransmitter excesses or deficits to the etiology of many mental disorders; a number of these neurotransmitter dysfunctions are transmitted genetically.

■ Marked advances in behavioral and molecular genetics have aided these investigations, as have increasingly sophisticated neuroimaging techniques.

The Psychodynamic Model

■ The psychodynamic model teaches that our behavior is strongly influenced by unconscious factors that we are largely unaware of, including internal conflicts, impulses, desires, and motives.

■ Freud's structural theory of personality divided the psychic apparatus into three parts: the id, ego, and superego.

■ According to Freud, a different region of the body gives libidinous pleasure and different kinds of cognitive and psychological growth take place during each stage of psychosexual development: oral, anal, phallic, latency, and genital.

■ The ego's mechanisms of defense, which vary in both maturity and effectiveness, defend it against the threat of attack by the id or the superego.

The Humanistic Model

■ The humanistic model emphasizes the worth of each individual and teaches that each of us has the capacity to realize our full intellectual, social, and emotional potential.

The Behavioral Model

■ The behavioral model assigns learning the key role in the development of behavior.

■ Three principal modes of learning are crucial to acquiring new behavior and modifying existing behavior: classical (respondent) conditioning, operant (instrumental) conditioning, and observational learning.

■ Social learning theory, which developed from early research on modeling, reflects the view of many behavioral scientists today that cognitive learning (including self-control) plays an important mediating role in all three principal modes of learning.

The Social Consequence Model

■ The social consequence model suggests that societal attitudes and behaviors toward groups of persons based on gender, ethnicity, race, socioeconomic status, or other distinguishing characteristics affect both individuals' behavior and the risks they run of developing particular kinds of psychopathology.

The Biopsychosocial Model

■ The biopsychosocial model teaches that the most comprehensive explanation for normal and abnormal behavior lies in understanding the interaction among the biological, psychological, and social factors that contribute to behavior.

KEY TERMS

adoption studies, **p. 37**

adrenal gland, **p. 35**

anal stage, **p. 43**

anxiety, **p. 44**

associational function, **p. 34**

attributional processes, **p. 58**

autonomic nervous system (ANS), **p. 32**

axons, **p. 31**

behavioral model, **p. 51**

biological model, **p. 28**

bipolar disorders, **p. 29**

central nervous system (CNS), **p. 31**

cerebral cortex, **p. 34**

cerebrum, **p. 34**

chromosomes, **p. 36**

classical conditioning, **p. 52**

cognition, **p. 56**

concordance, **p. 37**

conditioned response (CR), **p. 52**

conditioned stimulus (CS), **p. 52**

conscious psychological processes, **p. 40**

countertransference, **p. 48**

culture of poverty, **p. 61**

delirium, dementia, and amnestic and other cognitive disorders, **p. 29**

dendrites, **p. 31**

diathesis-stress theory, **p. 36**

discriminative stimulus (SD), **p. 55**

disease model, **p. 29**

dizygotic twins, **p. 36**

dominant gene, **p. 36**

ego, **p. 41**

Electra complex, **p. 43**

endocrine organs, **p. 35**

extinction, **p. 54**

family studies, **p. 37**

fixation, **p. 45**

forebrain, **p. 33**

fraternal twins, **p. 36**

frontal lobes, **p. 34**

gamete, **p. 36**

$\mathcal{C}$RITICAL THINKING EXERCISE

No one who knew Malcolm Little as a child or young adult would have predicted that he would become a dynamic, visionary leader. Why? Because Malcolm's life was filled with events and issues that put him at risk for a life of crime as a child, and ultimately, severe psychopathology as an adult. Think about what Malcolm experienced: extreme poverty; a loving but fragile mother who ultimately descended into chronic psychosis; an abusive father who was murdered when Malcolm was 6 years old; racial and economic oppression by the so-called system; abusive foster parents; a pattern of petty crime early in life and more serious crime later; and substance abuse beginning in early adolescence.

Is it any wonder that virtually everyone who knew Malcolm as a child or young adult expected the worst for him? Yet Malcolm X became one of the most influential U.S. leaders of the twentieth century. Admittedly controversial, out-spoken, and troubling to many, Malcolm X exerted greater influence—most of it for good—than all but a few leaders of his time.

We make much in this text of the ample data that allow us to predict the development of psychopathology from what we know about the biological, psychological, and social factors affecting a person. Most of the time, we can do so with fair precision. But in the case of Malcolm X, predictions based on the usual sources are virtually worthless. Although Malcolm didn't remember his childhood as having been so terrible, it seems that way to us when we read about it in his *Autobiography*. How did Malcolm Little become Malcolm X?

1. Reread the information on Malcolm X presented throughout this chapter. You may want to borrow or purchase *The Autobiography of Malcolm X*. (We suggest that you read its early chapters.) First, list the sources of strength and support in Malcolm's early life that could have countered the turmoil and chaos that were so prevalent. Then develop a set of hypotheses to explain Malcolm's later strengths, based on what you have concluded about his early life. Your goal is to explain the evolution of Malcolm X from Malcolm Little.

Chapter 3
DIAGNOSIS AND CLINICAL ASSESSMENT

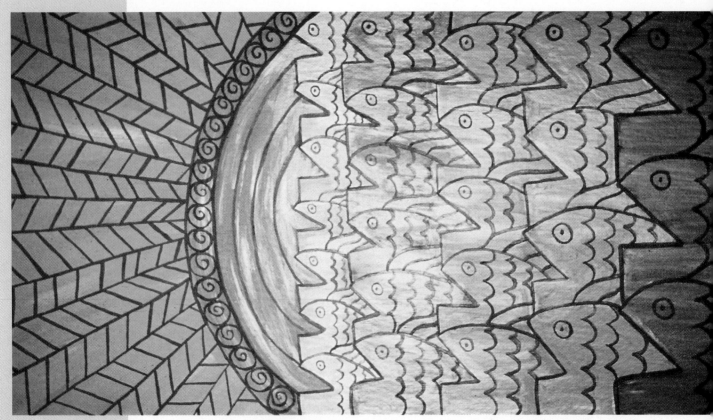

Jane Gerus, **Step 12,** 1984, Very Special Arts Gallery

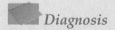
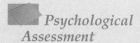
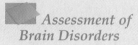
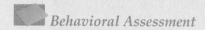
I t took Anne M. more than a year to decide she needed help.

It wasn't as though she didn't know she was in trouble. For years—since ninth grade, in fact—she'd known that she was unhappy more often and for longer times than her friends. She also knew that she sometimes had problems sleeping and even eating, on occasion, and that her self-esteem often hovered around zero. But she'd settled into a reassuring routine at home, and she had a few friends she could share her concerns with. So she did nothing about her feelings, even though they burdened her terribly all through high school.

When Anne started college, though, things became even more difficult. She went away to school, at the large state university that was a two-hour drive from her home, so she was on her own for the first time. She missed her family and close friends. Her mood problems were compounded by the other predictable stresses of college life: academics, dating, managing time and money. Anne began to worry constantly: Could she measure up to her fellow students? Could she keep up with the demanding preengineering curriculum she'd chosen? Would she make friends, maybe even find a sorority she'd fit into? Would she find a boyfriend, someone she could be close to?

Things became even more difficult for Anne the spring of her sophomore year. In the midst of breaking up with the guy she'd dated for well over a year, she learned from her mother that her parents had decided to separate. They had reached this painful decision after many years of unhappiness, mutual abuse, and alcohol and drug use. Anne wondered whether her parents' troubles were really her fault— maybe they would have been better off without having her as their daughter.

At this point, Anne knew she was in trouble. So early in April of her sophomore year, she called the university counseling center to make arrangements to see someone. The woman who answered assured Anne that she could get in to see someone right away. When she asked why Anne wanted counseling, Anne surprised herself (but not the woman at the other end of the telephone) by bursting into tears. In a torrent of words, Anne described her desperate unhappiness, her conviction that things were not going to get better fast enough, and her fear that her despair and hopelessness might cause her to hurt herself.

How do psychologists and psychiatrists make sense of such a puzzling array of feelings and behaviors as those of Anne M.? What do clinicians need to know to

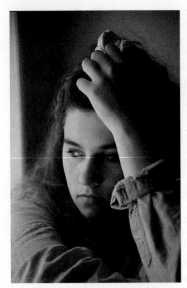

How can we make sense of Anne M.'s array of feelings and behaviors?

plan treatment for someone like Anne? How do they try to understand the causes of Anne's behavior or predict its future directions? All these issues are part of diagnosis and clinical assessment.

DIAGNOSIS

Diagnosis is the act of identifying and naming a disorder or disease by using a system of categorization that has been agreed on. **Clinical assessment** is the process clinicians use to gather the information they need to diagnose, determine causes, plan treatment, and predict the future course of a disorder. In undertaking a clinical assessment, clinicians gather detailed information on each patient's personal, medical, psychiatric, and family history. A thorough physical examination is usually included to determine if physical disease plays a role in the patient's condition; this exam might even involve exploration of the structure and function of the central nervous system.

Once they've gathered this information, researchers use *classification systems* to organize and share their knowledge. These systems allow scientists to communicate their observations without having to specify every distinguishing characteristic of every subject under study. If they didn't use classification systems, scientists would have no way of organizing and drawing conclusions from their observations. The best known classification systems were developed centuries ago to categorize animals, plants, chemical elements, and other natural phenomena. Without plant classifications, for example, plants would fall into a single, impossibly broad category: "organisms that live, grow, and die but do not move independently." Animals would fit into another essentially useless category: "organisms that live, grow, die, and move independently."

A classification system must be based on a set of *criteria*, or typical characteristics. In diagnosing a physical disease, for example, classification is based on past and present signs and symptoms. A **sign** is a characteristic feature of a disease that is observed by the clinician but probably not the patient, such as elevated temperature, increased count of white blood cells, or swollen glands. A **symptom** is a disease characteristic that the patient recognizes and perhaps complains about, such as a sore throat, a headache, or blurred vision.

In order to diagnose, clinical psychologists and psychiatrists typically perform a clinical assessment. In doing so, they look for behavioral and psychological as well as physical signs and symptoms. Collectively, this group of characteristics of disease is termed *psychopathology*. Some kinds of psychopathology, such as disorders of the brain, are characterized by changes in blood chemistry or electroencephalographic (EEG) brainwave patterns; these signs would be explored in a physical examination. However, diagnosis of behavioral disorders is more often made from present behavior, which the clinician might observe by interviewing the patient. Important aspects of past behavior might be determined by a medical history (which reviews the person's physical health history) or psychosocial history (which traces the person's family and friendship relationship patterns). An interview with a family member or friend might provide additional information about past behavior.

Gathering all this information—using a variety of sources and means—is vital to painting a complete picture of the individual's psychopathology. Think of diagnosis as a two-stage process: After gathering detailed biological, neurophysiological, and behavioral data on signs and symptoms of psychopathology, the clinician must also find some way of organizing and summarizing his observations. Just as physicians apply a set of disease labels to particular sets of physical signs and symptoms, psychiatrists and clinical psychologists use a system for classifying behavioral disturbances. That system, first developed in 1952, is called the *Diagnostic and Statistical Manual of Mental Disorders*, or *DSM*.

diagnosis Formal act of identifying and naming a disorder or disease.

clinical assessment Process clinicians use to gather the information needed to diagnose a disorder, determine its causes, plan treatments for it, and predict its future course.

sign Characteristic feature of a disorder a patient may be unaware of.

symptom Feature of a disease that a patient recognizes and may complain of.

The Diagnostic and Statistical Manual of Mental Disorders (DSM)

The fourth edition of the *Diagnostic and Statistical Manual of Mental Disorders (DSM-IV)* (American Psychiatric Association, 1994) has improved on two diagnostic features—*operational criteria* and *multiaxial diagnosis*—originally developed by its predecessors, the *DSM-III* and *DSM-III-R* (American Psychiatric Association, 1980, 1987, respectively). Other improvements include the *DSM-IV*'s increased reliance on empirical findings and greater sensitivity to cultural differences in diagnosis (Frances, Pincus, Widiger, Davis, & First, 1994).

Operational Criteria   The **operational criteria** in the *DSM-IV* outline and briefly describe the signs and symptoms considered in the diagnosis of each disorder listed. In most instances, these criteria are based on substantial empirical, scientific findings.

The case material that follows presents the *DSM-IV* operational criteria for dysthymic disorder, a depressive mood disorder that sometimes afflicts college students (American Psychiatric Association, 1994).* Consider how accurately these criteria describe the behavior of Anne M., the 20-year-old college student introduced at the beginning of this chapter.

A. Depressed mood for most of the day, more days than not, as indicated either by subjective account or observation by others, for at least 2 years.
    Anne admitted that she'd felt unhappy most of the time she'd been in college and for several years before that. When she compared her moods to those of her friends, Anne almost always concluded that her friends were happier more often than she was.

B. Presence, while depressed, of two (or more) of the following:
    (1) poor appetite or overeating
    (2) insomnia (difficulty sleeping) or hypersomnia (abnormally long sleeping)
    (3) low energy or fatigue
    (4) low self-esteem
    (5) poor concentration or difficulty making decisions
    (6) feelings of hopelessness
    Anne frequently complained of "having no pep," especially when she had to get up in the morning after a poor night's sleep. She also clearly suffered from low self-esteem. She was especially critical of her ability to do good academic work, to make and keep friends, and to measure up to her parents' expectations of her. Finally, Anne often became exasperated when she tried to do her homework; she couldn't concentrate long enough to read and understand assignments.

C. During the two-year period of the disturbance, the person has never been without the symptoms in Criteria A and B for more than 2 months at a time.
    Even though Anne hadn't kept a detailed record, over the past few years, she couldn't recall more than a day or two when she hadn't felt at least a little sad. Her therapist agreed with this observation. During the short time she had known Anne, Anne had been depressed virtually the entire time, although her depression had increased and decreased unpredictably during that time.

D. No Major Depressive Episode has been present during the first two years of the disturbance.
    Anne had never shown the symptoms of this condition, which causes marked impairment in functioning in virtually every area.

E. There has never been a Manic Episode, a Mixed Episode, or a Hypomanic Episode, and criteria have never been met for Cyclothymic Disorder.
    Anne had never shown any of the symptoms of these conditions, which involve markedly increased activity levels and pronounced feelings of euphoria and elation (see Chapter 7).

F. The disturbance does not occur exclusively during the course of a chronic Psychotic Disorder, such as Schizophrenia or Delusional Disorder.

operational criteria Signs and symptoms of each DSM-IV diagnosis are organized as a set of operational criteria, which outlines and fully describes the behaviors characteristic of the diagnosis.

*Diagnostic criteria A–H are from *DSM-IV,* 1994, p. 349

Anne had never shown any of the symptoms of **psychosis,** *such as* **hallucinations, delusions** *(false beliefs), or disordered thinking (see Chapter 13).*

G. The symptoms are not due to the direct physiological effects of a substance (e.g., a drug of abuse, a medication) or a general medical condition.

Anne has never used any substance abusively. She is in excellent physical health.

H. The symptoms cause clinically significant distress or impairment in social, occupational, or other important areas of functioning.

Anne's sadness, low self-esteem, difficulty concentrating, and problems sleeping upset her a lot. They also make it harder for her to complete coursework assignments, participate actively in class discussions, and concentrate on examination questions. She also finds it difficult to maintain friendships and other close relationships; when she's feeling depressed, it's very difficult for Anne to be attentive to and supportive of others. In other words, her symptoms impair several important areas of functioning.

Multiaxial Diagnosis   The drafters of the *DSM-IV* and its predecessors *DSM-III* and *DSM-III-R* developed **multiaxial diagnosis** to improve the usefulness of diagnosis. Using multiaxial diagnosis, the clinician evaluates each patient along five distinct behavioral dimensions, or axes. With earlier editions of the *DSM*, the clinician used only one dimension: abnormal behavior. Consequently, the clinician now has much more information about each patient to use in planning treatment.

The multiaxial diagnostic system divides abnormal behavior itself into two axes. Axis I is used to report all mental disorders except the personality disorders and mental retardation, which are reported on Axis II. This division was made because the drafters of the *DSM-III* worried that clinicians might give most of their attention to the often dramatic Axis I disorders, rather than to the less striking, long-lasting symptoms of mental retardation and especially the personality disorders.

Axis III codes medical diseases or conditions that may be relevant to understanding or treating the mental disorders reported on Axes I and II. For instance, the details of Anne M.'s multiaxial diagnosis report a relationship between her Axis I diagnosis of dysthymic disorder and the series of viral infections she suffered during early adolescence. Those infections clearly delayed Anne's transition to high school and probably played a role in her depressive symptoms.

Axis IV permits clinicians to record psychosocial and environmental problems affecting the diagnosis and treatment of the patient's Axis I and Axis II conditions. Axis IV calls attention to the important role played by environmental factors in many of the *DSM-IV* disorders. Using this dimension could help clinicians decide whether the early stages of treatment for an Axis I condition should focus on removing a specific environmental stressor. On completing Anne M.'s multiaxial diagnosis, for example, her therapist concluded that Anne needed to reduce some of the stress in her life before she would be able to deal effectively with her self-esteem problems.

Axis V, the Global Assessment of Functioning (GAF) Scale, is used to assess the patient's overall level of functioning, on a scale from 1 to 100. This dimension is especially useful to clinicians who want to measure treatment-induced behavioral changes. During treatment, as Anne's depression lifted, she and her therapist could compare her original score of 60 on the GAF (which reflected moderate behavioral impairment) to improvements made in functioning.

Anne M.'s multiaxial diagnosis provides a more complete picture of her situation than did the Axis I diagnosis of dysthymic disorder alone. This additional information gave her therapist data on Anne's pretreatment functioning, helpful initial ideas on where to focus treatment, and insight into prior and current causal factors.

Axis I—Clinical Disorders   Dysthymic disorder, early onset (before age 21 years).

■ Anne met most of the operational criteria for dysthymic disorder, listed earlier.

■ Anne did not meet the criteria for any other Axis I disorder.

Axis II—Personality Disorders and Mental Retardation   No diagnosis; obsessive-compulsive personality features.

psychosis Serious form of mental disorder, involving an actual break with reality.

hallucinations Abnormal auditory, gustatory, kinesthetic, olfactory, or visual perceptions that are common symptoms of psychosis; most common are those in which voices are heard or objects are seen that don't exist.

delusions Common symptom of psychosis that involves false or unusual beliefs; common delusions include persecution, romance, grandeur, and control.

multiaxial diagnosis Complete DSM-IV multiaxial diagnosis requires the clinician to evaluate the patient along five behavioral dimensions, or axes.

- Anne was not mentally retarded, and she did not meet the criteria for personality disorder. However, she did show some of the features of obsessive-compulsive personality disorder, although not enough to merit the diagnosis. These behaviors included the following: a self-imposed expectation of perfect performance that sometimes prevented Anne from completing a less than perfect assignment; a preoccupation with her academic responsibilities that sometimes prevented her from enjoying a social life; an unwillingness to let others do something for her unless they agreed to do it her way; and sporadic episodes of inappropriate rigidity and stubbornness.

Axis III—General Medical Conditions Potentially Relevant to Understanding the Individual's Mental Disorder   Recurrent viral infections during ninth grade.

- Recurrent viral infections forced Anne to miss almost half of ninth grade. As a result, she had a lot of difficulty keeping up with her schoolwork and making friends during that crucial schoolyear. It is significant that she dates the onset of her symptoms of depression to that year.
- Anne's recurrent illnesses may also have affected her central nervous system functioning enough to interfere with her ability to concentrate, focus on her schoolwork, and participate fully in extracurricular activities at school.

Axis IV—Psychosocial and Environmental Problems   Problems with primary support group: impending parental divorce; problems related to the social environment: stresses of college life.

- During her first two years in college, Anne experienced the intense but predictable social stresses of college life. In her case, these included ending a 15-month relationship with a boyfriend and moving from an on-campus residence hall and leaving the good friends she'd made there to live in an off-campus apartment with other friends. Anne also spent most of the first year knowing that her parents might divorce, after many years of a rocky marriage. While these stresses didn't *cause* Anne's depression (which clearly began much earlier), her therapist thought they may well have made her symptoms worse.

Axis V—Global Assessment of Functioning (GAF)   Rating of 60 on a 100-point scale. Anne is functioning reasonably well, although she continues to experience mild to moderate depressive symptoms.

- Although she continues to experience a variety of depressive symptoms, Anne still does better than average work at school, has a few good friends, provides support to her parents and siblings during difficult times for them, and manages the everyday details of her life reasonably well. At the same time, both she and her therapist are convinced that Anne would function substantially better were she not burdened by depression.

The developers of the *DSM-IV* maintained the number of diagnostic categories available to diagnosticians in the *DSM-III-R,* which put a stop to the trend of the two previous editions to greatly increase the number of categories. Table 3.1 lists the major diagnostic categories and some of the most important diagnoses included in Axes I and II of the *DSM-IV.*

Issues in Diagnosis and Classification

Diagnostic reliability, diagnostic validity, and *diagnostic bias* are extremely important issues. Every diagnostic system must confront and resolve them.

Diagnostic Reliability   A reliable diagnostic system produces diagnoses that clinicians agree on. If clinicians can't agree with each other on which signs and symptoms signal a specific disorder or on how to observe or define them, they won't be able to study the condition's causes, develop appropriate treatments for it, or predict its outcome. Thus, **diagnostic reliability** is vital in clinical diagnosis.

diagnostic reliability
Degree to which a diagnostic system fosters diagnostic agreement among clinicians.

TABLE 3.1 Major Diagnostic Categories in the DSM-IV

Disorders Usually First Diagnosed in Infancy, Childhood, or Adolescence	This broad array of disorders includes the physical, psychological, and behavioral conditions that first appear in infancy, childhood, and adolescence. Among them are mental retardation, learning and motor skills disorders, communication disorders (which include stuttering), pervasive developmental disorders (including autism), attention-deficit disorder (often affecting hyperactive children), conduct and oppositional disorders, and feeding and eating disorders. These disorders are considered in Chapters 11, 14, and 15.
Delirium, Dementia, and Amnestic and Other Cognitive Disorders	These disorders involve impaired thinking or remembering that substantially affects functioning and represents a deterioration from previous levels. Causes include physical injury or disease; a substance, which could include one or more of the drugs of abuse, a medication, or a poison; or both. *Delirium* is associated with substantial disturbance in consciousness and deterioration in thinking ability. *Dementia* involves multiple deficits in thinking, especially memory impairment. *Amnestic disorder* is characterized by impairment in memory without other deficits in thinking. These conditions are discussed in Chapter 16.
Substance-Related Disorders	These conditions all involve the use of one or more substances of abuse, of medications with side effects, or of poisons. Abused substances include alcohol, amphetamine, caffeine, cannabus, cocaine, nicotine, the opiates, and the sedatives. The substance-related disorders include substance abuse, dependence, intoxication, and withdrawal, among others; all can substantially disrupt functioning, and some can threaten life. The substance-related disorders are reviewed in Chapter 9.
Schizophrenia	Schizophrenia is a psychotic disorder. The defining features of psychosis are delusions (misrepresentations of reality) and hallucinations (false perceptions). Additional symptoms of schizophrenia include disorganized speech and profoundly disorganized or stereotyped behavior. Schizophrenia is typically a long-lasting disorder; it can have a catastrophic impact on the ability to function independently. Schizophrenia is considered in Chapter 13.
Mood Disorders	A disturbance in mood is the predominant feature of these disorders. They include a range of depressive disorders that vary in severity and involve periods of depressed mood and loss of interest or pleasure in usual activities; manic or hypomanic disorders characterized by periods of abnormally elevated or irritable mood and accompanying behavior; and disorders that include periods of depression and periods of mania or hypomania. The mood disorders are examined in Chapter 7.
Anxiety Disorders	This large group of diverse disorders share the common experience of **anxiety.** Included among these conditions are the panic disorders (during which individuals experience the sudden onset of intense feelings of apprehension, fearfulness, or terror accompanied by parallel physical sensations) and the phobic disorders (in which persons develop an unreasoning fear of situations or objects which they must then avoid). Other conditions in this diverse group of disorders are the anxiety disorders (characterized by the pervasive, sometimes disabling, physical and subjective sensations of anxiety), obsessive-compulsive disorder (in which individuals experience the insistent, unwanted influence of **obsessions, compulsions**), or both. The anxiety disorders are studied in Chapter 5.
Somatoform Disorders	These disorders share the feature of troubling physical symptoms that cannot be explained by physical disease, the effects of a substance, or another mental disorder. These symptoms sometimes appear to serve a psychological need or purpose. These conditions are discussed in Chapter 6.
Dissociative Disorders	The essential feature of this group of disorders is the disruption of the customarily organized and sequenced pattern of consciousness, memory, identity, or environmental perception. Individuals with one of these conditions may be unable to remember important events in their past that may have been associated with trauma and cannot be explained as ordinary forgetting. Individuals may suddenly travel away from home or work, be unable to remember their pasts, and assume new identities, or they may develop two or more distinct and compelling personality states. These puzzling conditions are examined in Chapter 6.

TABLE 3.1   continued

Sexual and Gender-Identity Disorders	These disorders include the sexual dysfunctions, the paraphilias, and the gender-identity disorders. The first involves a disturbance in sexual desire as well as in the pattern of psychophysiological changes that accompany the sexual response cycle; individuals may experience less sexual desire than they wish, choose to avoid sexual contact despite being troubled by having to do so, be unable to complete the sex act despite wanting to do so, or experience a consistent delay in or the absense of orgasm following a normal sexual sequence. The second group of disorders is characterized by strong sexual desires or behaviors causing significant distress that involve unusual objects, behaviors, or situations. Individuals in the third group strongly identify with the opposite sex and are unhappy with their own biological sex. These conditions are reviewed in Chapter 8.
Eating Disorders	These behaviors all entail severe disturbances in eating. Anorexia nervosa comprises an inability or unwillingness to maintain normal body weight, and bulimia nervosa involves a recurrent pattern of binge eating and self-induced vomiting, fasting, or use of laxatives to compensate for the binges. The eating disorders are detailed in Chapter 11.
Personality Disorders	These disorders represent long-lasting patterns of behavior that substantially deviate from societal expectations. They affect behavior and personality very broadly, are difficult to modify, and cause distress or impairment. Personality disorders begin in adolescence or young adulthood and are relatively unchanging. They are examined in Chapter 12.

anxiety An uncomfortable experience of worry, fear, and apprehension accompanied by various bodily sensations, including palpitations and increased arousal.

obsessions Repetitive, intrusive thoughts, images, or impulses that are distressing and unwanted.

compulsions Repetitive, stereotypical acts that the person feels compelled to carry out, despite recognizing that it's unreasonable.

diagnostic validity Ability of a diagnostic system to identify and predict disorders accurately.

concurrent validity Diagnostic system's ability to identify and categorize current disorders accurately.

predictive validity Describes a diagnostic system's capacity to predict future mental disorders.

diagnostic bias Biases or prejudices by diagnosticians that affect the reliability and validity of the diagnostic process.

In one of the first studies to report higher diagnostic reliability for the *DSM-III*, Spitzer and two colleagues (Spitzer, Forman, & Nee, 1979) conducted field trials in which 274 mental health clinicians evaluated 281 adult patients in a variety of treatment settings. These clinicians reached significantly higher levels of diagnostic agreement than had been reached in reliability studies of the *DSM-I* and *DSM-II*. This finding was one of the first of many to confirm the superior diagnostic reliability of the operational criteria introduced in the *DSM-III* (and an important feature of the *DSM-III-R* and *DSM-IV,* as well). This was achieved by establishing a common structure and an agreed upon set of signs and symptoms for each disorder (Shrout, Spitzer, & Fleiss, 1994).

Diagnostic Validity   The capacity of a diagnostic system like the *DSM* to identify and predict behavioral and psychiatric disorders accurately is known as **diagnostic validity.** A diagnostic system's ability to categorize current disorders accurately is termed **concurrent validity;** its capacity to predict future conditions is called **predictive validity.** The reliability and the validity of diagnosis are closely related: The more reliable a diagnostic system is, the more likely it will lead to valid diagnoses.

The diagnostic validity of the *DSM-III-R* has been confirmed for some forms of schizophrenia and the personality disorders (Herron, Schultz, & Welt, 1992; Widiger, 1993). Moreover, research has also demonstrated the capacity of the *DSM-III* to distinguish depressed from nondepressed individuals (Fabrega, Mezzich, Mezzich, & Coffman, 1986), hypochondriacal from nonhypochondriacal medical outpatients (Barsky, Wyshak, & Klerman, 1986), and people dependent on alcohol or drugs from those who are not (Rounsaville, Kosten, Williams, & Spitzer, 1987).

Diagnostic Bias   The *DSM-III, DSM-III-R,* and especially the *DSM-IV* were each carefully examined for **diagnostic bias** that might affect its validity (Rogler, 1994). Nonetheless, some bias remains. In trying to tie psychiatry more closely to medicine, for example, the *DSM-III* may have overemphasized the organic view of causes and a medical orientation to treatment (Schacht & Nathan, 1977) when the available data did not support such a position (Schacht, 1985). Similar concerns have been voiced about the *DSM-III-R* and *DSM-IV* (Nathan, 1994a; Wakefield, 1992). The Thinking about Social Issues box that follows raises a similar question: When is a deviant behavior a mental disorder, and when is it a reflection of "diagnostic imperialism"?

*A*n op-ed (opinion-editorial) piece appearing in the *New York Times* in May 1994, just after the *DSM-IV* was published, takes the drafters of the instrument to task for a whole list of shortcomings, saying that it "is poorly organized, has no scientific breakthroughs, makes no major changes from earlier editions, presents its material in turgid prose and costs $55."

The critics—social workers Stuart A. Kirk and Herb Kutchins—save their most scathing criticism, however, for the diagnostic imperialism they think the instrument is most guilty of. As Kirk and Kutchins put it, "Insomnia, worrying, restlessness, getting drunk, seeking approval, reacting to criticism, feeling sad, and bearing grudges are all considered possible signs of a psychiatric illness." The authors make the same point when they note that, between the 1952 and 1994 editions of the *DSM*, the number of mental disorders listed has risen from 106 to more than 300. Does this mean that U.S. society is generating that much more mental illness now than was the case 42 years ago? That's possible but unlikely.

When we read beyond the authors' excessive rhetorical latitude, we find that Kirk and Kutchins raise an important question: When is a behavior a symptom of an underlying disorder or disease, and when is it simply unpleasant and annoying but nothing more? For example, do poor use of grammar, terrible spelling, and bad handwriting characterize a mental disorder? Are children who lose their tempers, argue with adults, annoy people, and act touchy, angry, or spiteful mentally disturbed? Are cigarette smokers and coffee drinkers addicts and thus, like cocaine addicts and heroin addicts, dangerous to society? Or have the drafters of the *DSM-*

IV gone too far in labelling these behaviors, among others, mental disorders?

Kirk and Kutchins don't fault the drafters just for overexpanding the limits of mental illness. They also find fault with the drafters' trying to justify their actions in the name of science, when, in fact, they have completely confused science and social values. Kirk and Kutchins note the American Psychiatric Association's previous "battles with gay activists, who succeeded in having homosexuality dropped from the manual; demonstrations by Vietnam veterans, who had posttraumatic stress disorder included; skirmishes with feminists, who campaigned successfully to have self-defeating personality disorder deleted." According to the authors, these disputes embarrassed the association because they showed how much political pressures affects what is presented as science.

Is the *DSM-IV* a scientific document, a political statement, or a social contract? Those who helped create it stress its scientific base; those who criticize it emphasize its political and social meanings.

Think about the following questions:

1. What do you think? Do you agree that the *DSM-IV* is a political document as well as a scientific one? Why? If so, how would you suggest dealing with the problems that Kirk and Kutchins raise? Try to produce a definition of *mental disorder* that would reduce the political problems that Kirk and Kutchins complain of.

2. Do you think alcoholism is a mental disorder? What about cigarette smoking? What about coffee drinking? All three are included in the *DSM-IV*. If you think that one is a disorder and the others are not, explain why.

Another source of bias stems from the diagnosticians themselves. Apparently, diagnosticians are more likely to give certain diagnoses to patients whose sex, race, and socioeconomic status conform to their expectations about the kinds of people who have such disorders. For example, Warner (1978) asked 175 mental health professionals of both sexes to diagnose a patient from a written case history. Some subjects were told the patient was male; others were told that she was female. The sex of the patient made a substantial difference in the diagnosis given. When subjects thought the patient was female, they were more likely to diagnose hysterical personality, a so-called woman's disorder; when they thought the patient was male, the more likely diagnosis was antisocial personality, believed to be a man's condition.

Unfortunately, psychiatrists and psychologists are not free from prejudice and bias regarding qualities such as race, sex, and socioeconomic status (Pavkov, Lewis, & Lyons, 1989; Wakefield, 1992). Investigating this issue, Morey and Ochoa (1989) asked 291 psychologists and psychiatrists to diagnose a composite patient with symptoms of borderline personality disorder (so named because its symptoms place it on the borders of several psychiatric disorders). As we will discuss in Chapter 12, borderline personality disorder is one of the most commonly misdiagnosed (and most controversial) of the personality disorders. Its symptoms include unstable and intense interpersonal relationships, impulsiveness, rapid shifts in mood, inability to

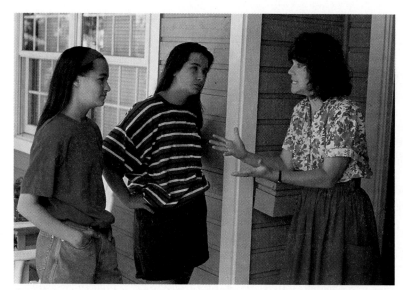

Can adolescents who lose their tempers, resist their parents, and annoy teachers and other adults be considered mentally ill? Some critics of the DSM-IV say it encourages drawing that diagnostic conclusion for a number of behaviors that are typical of the developmental period yet not actually signs of mental disorder. What do you think?

control anger, chronic feelings of emptiness and boredom, and recurrent suicidal threats, gestures, or behaviors.

Morey and Ochoa (1989) found that inexperienced, female, and psychodynamically oriented clinicians were more likely than others to overdiagnose the imaginary patient as borderline. This was particularly likely if the patient was described as poor, white, or female. Male clinicians were less likely to diagnose a patient as borderline, particularly if the patient was described as wealthy. These findings indicate that the identity of the imaginary patient—male or female, black or white, rich or poor—as well as the identity of the diagnostician—male or female, psychologist or psychiatrist, experienced or inexperienced, psychodynamic or behavioral—strongly influenced the diagnosis given. Clearly, the clinicians who were subjects in this study did not respond just to the patient's signs and symptoms in making their diagnoses. They responded to their own diagnostic biases, as well.

Diagnosis to Plan Treatment and Conduct Research

Diagnoses enable clinicians to convey a great deal of information about patients in a concise, widely accepted form. But this function of the diagnostic process is not the only reason clinicians diagnose. They also do so because a valid diagnosis leads to the most effective treatment, when research on outcomes of treatment has already established a link between a diagnosis and its treatment. Conditions that can be treated using psychoactive medication benefit from accurate and prompt diagnoses (for example, bipolar disorder, serious depression, and schizophrenia). Similarly, accurate and timely diagnoses are essential for planning effective uses of psychotherapy or behavioral therapy, which are appropriate for the anxiety disorders and some of the childhood disorders.

Valid diagnoses are also indispensable for the study of etiology (the search for the cause or causes of a disorder). Consider the design of a study for testing the theory that being unable to learn to read plays a role in childhood depression. For subjects, the clinical researcher would want to select a group of patients diagnosed with childhood depression and, for comparison purposes, another group identical to the depressed patient group except in that diagnosis. That way, if it turned out that only the children with depression had trouble learning to read, the logical explanation would be that reading problems play a causal role.

Finally, research on prevention also requires accurate diagnosis. When the diagnosis of a specific disease is confirmed in individuals who share a particular sex, age, lifestyle, or behavioral pattern, epidemiologists can focus prevention efforts on the population at greatest risk. A recent example is research leading to the identification of lifestyle patterns associated with increased risk of contracting HIV (human immunodeficiency virus), the virus that causes AIDS.

Focus on Critical Thinking

1. How are the depressive behaviors of Anne M. and Billy Ainsworth (the case in Chapter 1) similar? How are they different? Which person's depression interfered more with his or her life? Which person is more likely to experience troubled behavior in the future? Why?

2. Assume that you are a mental health professional about to diagnose a young woman, an older man, an African American individual, and a person who is homeless. What influence might each of these designations have on your diagnosis of the individual? If you were influenced in any of these ways, how valid would your diagnosis be?

$\mathcal{P}$SYCHOLOGICAL $\mathcal{A}$SSESSMENT

diagnostic interview
Designed to gather information on past and present behaviors that have specific value for diagnosis.

assessment interview
Focuses on a wide range of topics, including assessment of personality, interpersonal behavior, and family functioning.

Interview Methods

Interviews are invaluable tools for the mental health professional (Matarazzo, 1992; Wiens, 1991). A **diagnostic interview** provides information on the patient's past and present behavior—both normal and abnormal—that may not be available from another source. An **assessment interview** can be used for many purposes, including the assessment of personality, interpersonal behavior, and the functioning of family units.

An **individual therapy interview** brings together the patient and therapist in an ongoing, extended relationship. That relationship is based on the patient's willingness to recall and reevaluate past and present behaviors, feelings, and attitudes and the therapist's agreement to use what she learns to try to help the patient. Actually, individual therapy interviews are a sequence of assessment interviews, during which both patient and therapist gather more and more data on the patient's memories, thoughts, beliefs, and behaviors. One of the most important ingredients in the success of individual therapy is the rapport that develops between the patient and therapist early in the relationship. The patient must feel secure in a close and trusting relationship in order to reveal things about himself.

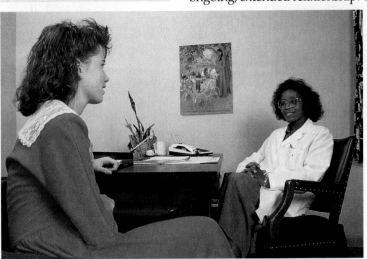

Developing a good rapport between patient and therapist is an important ingredient for successful individual therapy.

Some interviews are highly **structured;** they contain a detailed set of questions that are prepared and tested before the interview and always asked in the same order. One such interview, the Diagnostic Interview Schedule, or DIS (Robins, Helzer, Croughan, & Ratcliff, 1994), can produce the full range of the *DSM-III* Axis I and Axis II diagnoses.

The DIS poses the following initial question about panic and anxiety symptoms: "Have you ever had a spell or attack when all of a sudden you felt frightened, anxious, or very uneasy in situations when most people would not be afraid?" Interviewees who answer this question "yes" are then asked, "During this spell: Did your heart pound? Did you have tightness or pain in your chest? Did you sweat? Did you tremble or shake?" Because it always gathers diagnostic information from precisely the same questions, asked in precisely the same order, the DIS yields very reliable diagnoses (Antoni, Levine, Tischer, Green, & Millon, 1987; Robins et al., 1994). Given this consistent format, nonprofessional interviewers can be trained to administer the DIS reliably.

individual therapy interview Basic element of the therapeutic relationship; requires therapists to be good listeners and insightful and skilled commentators; requires patients to be willing to remember and reproduce past and present behaviors, feelings, and attitudes.

structured interview
Guided by a detailed set of questions prepared and tested before the interview and always presented in the same order; generally more reliable, which explains their expanding use for research purposes.

semistructured interview
Follows an outline but does not prescribe specific questions or require a particular ordering of questions.

Some interviews are **semistructured;** they follow an outline but do not prescribe specific questions or require that the questions be in a particular order. Table 3.2 outlines a typical mental status examination, which is a semistructured interview intended to establish the current status of a patient's thinking, feeling, sensing, and perceiving. The results of mental status examinations are used primarily for two purposes: to diagnose (because mental status is a key factor in diagnosing such conditions as schizophrenia and the mood and anxiety disorders) and to plan treatment (because intact mental status is necessary for "talking therapies" to work).

Let's look at the first few minutes of a semistructured diagnostic interview: Dr. S.'s initial assessment interview with Anne M. As you can see, Dr. S.'s questions and comments seem to focus on determining which of the *DSM-IV* criteria for the depressive disorders Anne meets. However, the exact forms of the questions and the order she asks them in are determined largely by Anne's responses.

TABLE 3.2	Outline for a Mental Status Examination

General Appearance and Manner
- Is the patient clean and neat?
- Does he or she show peculiarities of posture (the way the patient stands) or movement?
- How easily and appropriately does the patient interact with the inteviewer?

Speech Characteristics
- Does the patient show abnormalities of speech, such as making up words or repeating the same word or phrase over and over?

Mood
- Is the patient's mood excessively happy, sad, or somewhere in between?
- Is it appropriate to what is being discussed?

Content of Thought
- Does the patient dwell on a particular topic or topics, excluding others?
- Is the patient delusional (having false beliefs), or does he show paranoid thinking (believing someone or something wishes one harm)?

Orientation, Memory and Learning, Attention and Concentration, and Information
- Does the patient know who and where he is and what time and date it is?
- Does the patient pay attention to the interview?
- Does he have an adequate store of information on current and past events?
- Is the patient's memory intact?

Insight and Judgment
- Does the patient have insight into his behavior?
- Do his decisions reflect sound judgment?

Dr. S.: Anne, could you tell me a bit about what led you to come to the counseling center today?

Anne M.: Actually, I've been meaning to come for over a year, but I just kept putting it off, hoping things would get better. But they haven't. Actually, they've gotten worse—and I'm feeling worse. That's what finally convinced me to come in.

Dr. S.: Tell me what's been happening.

Anne M.: I guess I've been pretty depressed for several years. I'm down a lot of the time, and I don't get much pleasure even out of things I should feel good about. I'm pretty down on myself, too, even though, objectively, I'm doing OK. Lately, I've begun having trouble getting to sleep, and even when I do, I wake up in the middle of the night and can't get back to sleep.

Dr. S.: You say you've experienced these feelings for several years?

Anne M.: Yes, only lately they're getting worse. My sleep and my concentration are worse now than before, and I don't feel like spending much time with my friends. That's new. And it's harder to study now than it used to be, even though I'm still a very conscientious student.

Dr. S.: Can you trace back to when these feelings of depression started? Can you remember a time when you didn't have them?

Anne M.: Well . . . kind of. Even as a young girl, I was more serious, maybe even more pessimistic, than my friends. So maybe it's always been part of me. But when I remember really noticing it was in ninth grade.

Dr. S.: Ninth grade. That would be six years ago.

Anne M.: Yeah. I was sick a lot that year, some kind of virus that kept me out of school twice, for more than a month each time. My schoolwork suffered and my social life, too. As a result, I guess, I started feeling bad about myself, whether I'd ever have the friends and the grades my parents expected of me.

Dr. S.: It sounds like that virus really set you back at a crucial time . . .

Anne M.: I guess it did. Just when I was beginning to make some friends and feel good socially. So that's what kind of laid the groundwork, I think, for what's happened last year and now.

Psychotherapy interviews are **unstructured.** In treatment sessions, the therapist generally tries to assess the patient's current concerns and preoccupations. This is true regardless of the therapist's theoretical orientation. However, most therapists respond to their patients in a manner that is consistent with that orientation. For example, psychoanalysts are almost always less active during therapy sessions than behavior therapists (see Chapter 18). But no therapist knows for sure what issues a patient will want to discuss before a particular session or the order in which he will want to discuss them.

Personality Measures

What traits of character, skills, abilities, and competencies make one person different from another? For example, better or worse at adjusting to adversity? more or less successful in a particular job? vulnerable or resistant to mental disorder? a suitable adoptive parent or an unsuitable one?

A variety of answers have been given to these questions through the years, reflecting the diversity of views on what we mean by **personality.** Psychologists use the term to mean the basic, lasting qualities that make us who we are. This concept has fascinated psychologists since the late 1800s, the first days of the discipline, and philosophers, theologians, and others pondered the mystery of personality several thousand years before that. A form of psychological assessment was practiced in both ancient China and Greece as early as 2,000 to 2,500 years ago; it was based on individual differences in intellectual, personality, and physical traits (Matarazzo, 1992; McReynolds, 1986).

Assessing personality is useful in diagnosis and clinical assessment because our past and present behavior often predict our future behavior (Loevinger, 1993; Meehl, 1992). The personality measures reviewed in the following sections aim to capture individual character and, in doing so, understand and predict behavior over time.

The Projective Tests   The **Rorschach Inkblot Test** is the most familiar of the **projective tests,** which share one common feature: They ask respondents to impose their own structure and meaning on unstructured, ambiguous test stimuli. The theory is that in doing so, respondents reveal underlying needs and conflicts they may be unaware of.

Hermann Rorschach (1884–1922), a Swiss psychiatrist, was influenced by the description of personality types created by psychoanalytic pioneer Carl Gustav Jung (1875–1961). According to Jung (1923), **introverted** people tend to be quiet, shy, and uncomfortable in social settings, whereas **extraverted** individuals are gregarious, social, and open. In 1921, in the effort to separate his patients according to these two Jungian personality types, Rorschach developed the Rorschach Test. It was made of inkblots—some black and white, some color, but all sufficiently ambiguous that no two viewers would see precisely the same thing. Rorschach's aim was to study people's *projections* (the meanings they gave the ambiguous inkblots) to gain insight into the unconscious determinants of their behavior. Since this test had no obvious right or wrong answers, Rorschach hoped people would respond from the depths of their personalities, revealing how their behavior was influenced by introversive or extraversive personality factors.

Shortly after they began using the Rorschach instrument, clinicians began to consider certain responses as signs of specific mental disorders. Respondents who looked at the inkblots and saw people with both male and female characteristics, for example, were assumed to have homosexual tendencies. Individuals who preferred the black-and-white cards to the colored ones were considered to be depressed. Ultimately, the test began to be used mainly as a diagnostic instrument (e.g., Beck,

unstructured interview
Does not follow an outline but occurs spontaneously.

personality According to psychologists, enduring traits of character—the basic, lasting qualities that make us who we are.

Rorschach Inkblot Test
Projective measure of personality that consists of 10 cards, each showing a different inkblot design.

projective tests Measures of personality based on the assumption that individuals call on enduring traits of character to structure otherwise unstructured test stimuli.

introverted personality type Jung's personality type describing persons who tend to be quiet, shy, and uncomfortable in social situations.

extraverted personality type Jung's personality type for persons who tend to be gregarious, social, and emotionally open.

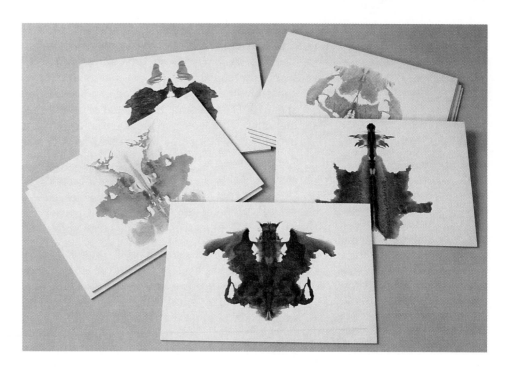

What you see in these Rorschach cards and how you see it gives psychologists trained in projective testing information on personality and psychopathology.

1938; Blatt, 1986; Piotrowski, 1937), despite considerable research evidence that it was not ideal for that purpose.

A new means of interpreting and scoring Rorschach responses, The Comprehensive System (Exner, 1993), has restored respect for empirical findings among clinicians using the Rorschach. Exner's scoring system produces greater reliability than other Rorschach scoring systems (Greiner & Nunno, 1994). Moreover, The Comprehensive System is based on large, standardized samples of respondents of diverse age, sex, diagnostic category, and personality. Thus, the validity of clinical judgments and personality assessments made from Rorschach responses scored by this system may turn out to be superior to those made from other systems.

Early findings from application of The Comprehensive System seem to accurately reflect personality changes associated with treatment (e.g., Abraham, Lepisto, Lewis, Schultz, & Finkelberg, 1994; Blatt, 1992) and diagnostic distinctions that stem from abuse during childhood (Nash, Hulsey, Sexton, Harralson, & Lambert, 1993; Zivney, Nash, & Hulsey, 1988). Moreover, studies of the Rorschach and the Minnesota Multiphasic Personality Inventory (MMPI) (Meyer, 1992, 1993) show less overlap in the aspects of personality they reflect than was previously thought to exist. As a result, some personality researchers have concluded that projective tests, like the Rorschach, and personality inventories, like the MMPI, provide information on personality that is complementary, rather than contradictory (Lovitt, 1993; Weiner, 1993). Based on that conclusion, these researchers have suggested that these types of measures be used together to provide a fuller picture of personality.

Thematic Apperception Test (TAT) Projective measure of personality consisting of 31 cards; 30 portray an ambiguous scene that often includes people, and the remaining card is blank.

The **Thematic Apperception Test (TAT)** is one of the most widely used projective tests in the world (Piotrowski & Keller, 1989; Sweeney, Clarkin, & Fitzgibbon, 1987). It was created by psychologist Henry Murray in 1938 and, like

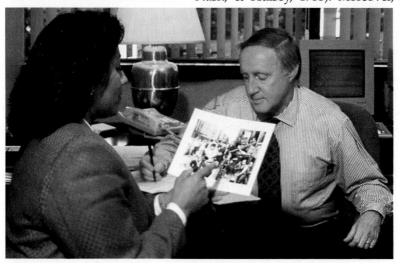

Some psychologists believe that the stories people tell about TAT pictures reveal important traits of personality that are accessible in few other ways.

the Rorschach, was designed to uncover personality traits and mental processes that may not be accessible to consciousness.

The TAT consists of 31 stimulus cards. Thirty are drawings of ambiguous scenes that mostly involve people; the remaining card is blank. Up to 20 cards are chosen with the respondent's age and sex in mind. Then they're shown to her, one at a time. The respondent is to "tell as dramatic a story as possible" about each card, including what led up to the event in the picture, what's happening now, what the people in the story are thinking and feeling, and what will happen next.

Murray (1938) made two important assumptions about TAT responses:

1. The behaviors and feelings respondents attribute to the main character in a TAT story represent their own tendencies toward such behaviors and feelings.
2. Respondents react to those aspects of the pictures that are most similar to important aspects of their own environments.

Murray proposed a scoring system to evaluate every TAT story along two dimensions: the respondent's *needs* (for food, affection, dominance, sex, and the like) and *presses* (for example, poverty, lack of emotion, discrimination because of race or sex, and so on). He maintained that presses prevent people from meeting their needs and that the TAT can reveal a respondent's key needs and presses.

Despite extensive research on the TAT, as both a diagnostic instrument (Weiner, 1983) and a measure of personality (Atkinson, 1983; McClelland, 1980), its usefulness for either purpose has been questioned (Lanyon, 1984). The most important reason for this doubt is the difficulty psychologists have had in developing a reliable system for categorizing and scoring TAT responses (Entwisle, 1972; Lundy, 1985). Recently, however, Weston (1991; Weston, Lohr, Silk, Gold, & Kerber, 1990) proposed a new method of scoring TAT responses that appears to give measures of reliability and validity at the levels of those for the MMPI.

Other projective tests include a variety of **sentence-completion tests** (e.g., Lanyon & Lanyon, 1980) that ask respondents to complete sentences beginning with such open-ended phrases as "My mother was . . ." or "The happiest time was . . ." It's assumed that in answering these loosely structured questions, respondents will guard their answers less than when asked more structured questions on the same topics.

Another type of projective test asks people to draw familiar objects or people (Gynther & Gynther, 1983; Sutker & Allain, 1988). The assumption behind **projective drawings** is that the content and form individuals give to pictures made without explicit instruction will provide uncensored information about their personality traits (Stricker & Healey, 1990). The validity of this method is unproven, at this time.

Personality Inventories Personality inventories investigate personality by asking questions about respondents' behaviors, attitudes, experiences, and beliefs. Most of these inventories have been normed and standardized. This means that before publication, they were administered to large groups of subjects, whose responses were analyzed according to age, sex, socioeconomic status, diagnosis, and the like. General patterns are observed and established as what is considered normal for members of certain groups; these patterns are called *norms*.

Standardization of personality inventories means two things:

1. The questions asked in the inventories are written directly and clearly, increasing the likelihood that they will be understood and that respondents will be able to answer them reliably and accurately.
2. It is easier to determine whether respondents' responses are valid because they can be compared to the responses of similar individuals in the standardization sample.

Personality inventories share features and assumptions about how to measure personality. In completing one of these inventories, the respondent gives direct and objective responses to questions about memories, attitudes, beliefs, and feelings

sentence-completion tests Projective devices that ask respondents to complete incomplete sentences, thereby imposing structure on unstructured test stimuli.

projective drawings Assessment technique in which respondents are asked to draw objects; based on the assumption that they reveal important traits of character by what they draw and how they draw it.

standardization Process in which the validity of an assessment device has been analyzed for age, sex, education, socioeconomic status, or other relevant variables to yield quantifiable indices of validity.

about past, present, and future behaviors. (That's why personality researchers consider these instruments *self-report measures*.) The clinician takes the individual's responses, looks for patterns among them, and compares those patterns to the norms established for the instrument. In doing so, the clinician determines how closely the individual's responses resemble those of persons of his age, sex, socioeconomic status, or diagnosis. Based on this determination, the clinician can assess the individual's personality and predict his behavior.

The most widely used self-report measure of personality and behavior is the Minnesota Multiphasic Personality Inventory, or MMPI (Hathaway & McKinley, 1943, 1951); it was revised extensively in 1989, producing the MMPI-2 (Butcher, Dahlstrom, Graham, Tellegen, & Kaemmer, 1989). Other well-known personality tests include the California Psychological Inventory (Gough, 1969), the Sixteen Personality Factor Questionnaire (Cattell & Stice, 1957), the Eysenck Personality Inventory (Eysenck & Eysenck, 1969), and the Edwards Personality Inventory (Edwards, 1967). Newer objective measures of personality include the Millon Clinical Multiaxial Inventory (MCMI and MCMI-II) (Millon, 1983, 1987) and the NEO Personality Inventory (NEO-PI) (Costa & McCrae, 1985, 1989).

The **Minnesota Multiphasic Personality Inventory (MMPI)** asks respondents to answer "true" or "false" to each item in a lengthy series of statements about themselves. The first version of the MMPI contained 566 items (Hathaway & McKinley, 1943), which were selected from an original pool of 1,000. The items were chosen because they differentiated among eight different diagnostic groups as well as a control group of nonpatients (Buchanan, 1994).

The MMPI was revised in 1989—creating the MMPI-2—for several important reasons: to modify or eliminate some questions and add others and to restandardize the resulting instrument (Butcher et al., 1989). In the 50 or so years between the original standardization of the MMPI and the standardization of the MMPI-2, responses to questions changed and developments in U.S. society made some of the original questions inappropriate. What's more, it had become clear over the years that the original normative sample was not ideal.

The MMPI-2 added new items, removed old items, and modified many of the original 566 items to create a revised test of 567 items. The standardization sample was increased to a representative nationwide group of 2,600 adults, including substantial numbers of African Americans and Hispanics.

Like the MMPI, the MMPI-2 contains 10 basic clinical scales (see Table 3.3). As the case material that follows will demonstrate, these scales correspond to some of the most important classifications of diagnostic signs and symptoms. So a respondent's pattern of scores on the clinical scales can be compared against those of like individuals in the standardization sample with one or another of the *DSM* diagnoses.

The MMPI contained three validity scales; the MMPI-2 contains those three and three more, as well. These scales reveal the respondent's attitude toward test taking—specifically, whether she read the questions carefully and answered them truthfully. Examiners rely on these scales in deciding whether the conclusions they draw are likely to be valid.

Anne M. completed the MMPI-2 as part of the diagnostic process at the counseling center. The intern in clinical psychology who administered the instrument to Anne drew the following conclusions:

- Anne took a great deal of time—more than two hours—to answer all 567 questions. The fact that she took so long and answered every question suggests that she was conscientious and careful in taking the test, thereby increasing the likelihood that her responses are valid reflections of her current experiences.
- Anne's scores on the validity scales of the MMPI-2 supported this conclusion. Specifically, they indicated that Anne had tried hard to answer questions truthfully, that she had not tried to appear more healthy psychologically than she was, and that, in fact, she may have been more willing than most respondents to reveal unpleasant or unacceptable thoughts or feelings.

Minnesota Multiphasic Personality Inventory (MMPI) *Most commonly used objective, self-report measure of personality; used to explore personality and aid in diagnosis; revised test is the MMPI-2.*

TABLE 3.3   **Eight of the Clinical Scales of the MMPI**

Eight of the MMPI's ten clinical scales and sample items from them are shown below. A plus sign after an item means that persons in the 1943 standardization sample diagnosed with the disorder associated with the clinical scale were likely to endorse the item; a minus sign means that they were unlikely to do so.

Hypochondriasis   This condition is characterized by excessive concern with bodily functions and imagined illness.

- I do not tire quickly. (–)
- The top of my head sometimes feels tender. (+)

Depression   The term *depression* is used in the conventional sense to imply strong feelings of "blueness," despondency, and worthlessness.

- I am easily awakened by noise. (+)
- Everything is turning out just as the prophets of the Bible said it would. (+)

Hysteria   The development of physical disorders such as blindness, paralysis, and vomiting as an escape from emotional problems is termed *hysteria*.

- I am not likely to speak to people until they speak to me. (+)
- I get mad easily and then get over it soon. (+)

Psychopathic Deviance   An individual who lacks "conscience," who has little regard for the feelings of others, and who gets into trouble frequently is called a psychopathic deviate.

- My family does not like the work I have chosen. (+)
- What others think of me does not bother me. (+)

Paranoia   Extreme suspiciousness to the point of imagining elaborate plots is paranoia.

- I am sure I am being talked about. (+)
- Someone has control over my mind. (+)

Psychasthenia   The term *psychasthenia* indicates strong fears and compulsions.

- I become impatient with people easily. (+)
- I wish I could be as happy as others seem to be. (+)

Schizophrenia   Bizarre thoughts and actions, out of communication with the world, characterize schizophrenia.

- I have never been in love with anyone. (+)
- I loved my mother. (–)

Hypomania   Overactivity and inability to concentrate on one thing for more than a moment are typical of hypomania.

- I don't blame people for trying to grab everything they can get in this world. (+)
- When I get bored, I like to stir up some excitement. (+)

Source: From "Self-Report Measures of Personality Traits," by J. C. Nunnally. In N. S. Endler and J. M. Hunts (Eds.), *Personality and the Behavior Disorders*, pp. 221–260. Copyright © 1984 John Wiley & Sons, Inc. Reprinted by permission of John Wiley & Sons, Inc.

- The most prominent feature of Anne's performance on the clinical scales was the marked elevation of the Depression scale. This suggests that Anne is currently experiencing a great deal of emotional pain and distress. The Psychasthenia scale, which reflects the presence of fears, worries, and anxiety as well as obsessions and compulsions, was also significantly elevated, as was the Hypochondriasis scale, which asks questions tapping concern about bodily functions, including eating and sleeping.
- Overall, Anne's MMPI-2 portrays a person suffering a good deal from depression, low self-esteem, and concerns about her ability to meet very high, self-generated standards. This pattern of responses—signaled by elevations of the Depression, Psychasthenia, and Hypochondriasis scales—is consistent with the diagnosis of mood disorder.

The broader and more representative standardization sample of the MMPI-2, along with substantial improvements in items and scoring procedures, are expected to increase both the reliability and validity of the instrument (Finn & Butcher, 1991). Findings of early research suggest that the reliability of the MMPI-2 is as high or higher than that of the MMPI (e.g., Clavelle, 1992; Edwards, Morrison, & Weissman, 1993) and that the validity of the revised instrument will also be comparable to or better than that of the original (Hargrave, Hiatt, Ogard, & Karr, 1994). The MMPI is also considered more reliable than most projective measures of personality because it asks direct, understandable questions, demanding equally direct answers (Werner & Pervin, 1986).

Nonetheless, Helmes and Reddon (1993) remain critical of the MMPI-2's capacity to aid substantially in diagnosis, in part, because it relies on self-reports of behavior, thoughts, and feelings, which respondents can modify to suit their needs. Burisch (1984) is also uncertain about the MMPI's validity and usefulness. Although it distinguishes between broad diagnostic groups, it is much less accurate in making finer diagnoses. For example, the instrument has not been able to differentiate sex offenders from other violent and nonviolent criminals (Levin & Stava, 1987), alcoholics from nonalcoholics (Nathan, 1988; Preng & Clopton, 1986), or among patients with different schizophrenia diagnoses (Young, 1972).

The **Millon Clinical Multiaxial Inventory (MCMI)** (Millon, 1983) and its revision, the MCMI-II (Millon, 1987), are objective measures of personality designed specifically for diagnostic purposes; their major focus is on diagnosing the personality disorders. Both instruments are 175-item, true-false questionnaires. In designing the MCMI and MCMI-II, researchers took special care to avoid the problems that have burdened the MMPI in clinical settings. Test items in the MCMI and MCMI-II correspond directly to the *DSM-III* diagnoses, whereas the MMPI's clinical scales relate only broadly to the diagnostic categories of the *DSM-I* (published nine years after the MMPI first appeared). The MCMI, like the MMPI, has both clinical and validity scales; unlike the MMPI, however, the MCMI has scales that parallel Axis I and Axis II diagnoses.

The MCMI and MCMI-II have been used extensively in recent years, in large part because they are sensitive to diagnostic differences among certain types of the personality disorders (Retzlaff, Ofman, Hyer, & Matheson, 1994; Widiger & Sanderson, 1987). The MCMI has been criticized, though, because it consistently underestimates the severity of depressive syndromes (Patrick, 1988) and overdiagnoses personality disorders (Piersma, 1987). Some clinicians think that the MMPI and MCMI should be used together, based on the assumptions that the MMPI is especially useful in diagnosing Axis I disorders and that the MCMI is most useful in identifying Axis II disorders (Smith, Carroll, & Fuller, 1988).

The **NEO Personality Inventory (NEO-PI)** (Costa & McCrae, 1985, 1989) is another objective measure of personality, although it differs markedly from both the MMPI and MCMI. Whereas these older measures were designed for use primarily with clinical populations and for diagnostic purposes, the NEO-PI was designed to study normal personality development (Ben-Porath & Waller, 1992). Specifically, the NEO-PI was created to study what are termed the *"big five"* personality traits: Extraversion, Agreeableness, Neuroticism, Conscientiousness, and Openness to Experience.

These traits are called the "big five" because extensive research has suggested that they explain a great deal of the variability in human behavior (Wiggins & Pincus, 1989). Although some psychologists have questioned the relevance of traits of normal behavior to psychopathology, others have applauded the effort to study both normal development and abnormal behavior with the same instrument.

The developers of the NEO-PI report that the instrument is as reliable and valid for clinical populations as it is for nonclinical samples. Early data lead them to suggest that the instrument may be useful clinically for several purposes:

1. to put patients' behavior in environmental and temporal perspective
2. to suggest a range of possible diagnoses

Millon Clinical Multiaxial Inventory (MCMI) Objective measure of personality designed specifically for diagnostic purposes; major focus is on diagnosis of personality disorders; revised test is the MCMI-II.

NEO Personality Inventory (NEO-PI) Objective measure of personality designed to study normal personality development, specifically, the "big five": Extraversion, Agreeableness, Neuroticism, Conscientiousness, and Openness to Experience.

3. to provide insights into personality that will help therapists establish empathy and rapport with patients early in therapy

4. to produce data to assist therapists in considering possible courses of therapy (Costa & McCrae, 1992a)

Although these possible uses are intriguing, much more evaluation is needed to determine the validity and reliability of the NEO-PI with both clinical and nonclinical groups.

Intelligence Measures

Intelligence plays a crucial role in how successfully we relate to our environment. The specific role of intelligence in our ability to adapt to the complexities of modern life is a key theme in the recently developed theories of intelligence that we will review in this section.

Pursuing an ongoing interest in human heredity, English biologist Sir Francis Galton (1822–1911) undertook one of the first scientific studies of intellectual ability in 1883. He attempted to compare and contrast aspects of intelligence in people who were biologically related and unrelated. Based on his findings, Galton ultimately concluded, as we do today, that intelligence runs in families.

Galton also concluded that *sensory discrimination* (the ability to perceive and respond quickly to environmental stimuli) is the most valid measure of intelligence. He studied simple reaction time, or the speed with which subjects responded to a tone or a flash of light. He also asked subjects to discriminate between tones, weights, and painful stimuli of different intensities. Galton's conviction about the significance of sensory intelligence foreshadowed today's renewed interest in physiological measures of intelligence.

At the beginning of the twentieth century, French psychologist Alfred Binet (1857–1911) developed a series of tests that continue to influence our thinking about the nature and measurement of intelligence. These tests were intended to determine which Parisian schoolchildren would benefit from a public school education and which required special schooling. Binet believed that children's intelligence grows and develops as they do: The older they are, the better their ability to reason and understand, make judgments, and come to rational decisions.

Binet evaluated intelligence by comparing children's performance on tests of judgment, comprehension, and reasoning to norms from a large, standardized sample of children. The Binet Scale produced an estimate of intelligence called the **intelligence quotient,** or **IQ.** It was calculated by dividing the child's **mental age** (which corresponded to the number of age-grouped tests and problems the child was able to pass) by his or her **chronological age** and then multiplying by 100. For example, a child with a mental age of 12 years and a chronological age of 10 years would have an IQ of 120 ($^{12}/_{10}$ × 100). Although the **Stanford-Binet Scales** have been extensively revised through the years and are now in their fourth edition (Terman & Merrill, 1960, 1973; Thorndike, Hagen, & Sattler, 1986), they are still widely used to test children's intelligence (Laurent, Swerdlik, & Ryburn, 1992).

About 40 years after Binet began his work, psychologist David Wechsler (1896–1981) devised new tests of intelligence to replace the Binet Scales (Wechsler, 1939, 1955, 1958). He did so for two reasons. First, the Binet Scales were originally developed to test the intelligence of children. Second, the single score that the Binet tests yield—the IQ—does not highlight an individual's intellectual strengths and weaknesses.

---

intelligence quotient (IQ)
Estimate of intelligence produced by dividing mental age by chronological age and multiplying by 100; first associated with the Binet Scales.

mental age Refers to the number of age-grouped tests and problems passed in the Binet Scales; mental age divided by chronological age multiplied by 100 determines IQ.

chronological age Age in years; used to determine IQ on the Binet Scales.

Stanford-Binet Scales
Series of intelligence tests for children originally developed by Alfred Binet at the beginning of the twentieth century; their form, content, and philosophy continue to influence the field of intellectual assessment.

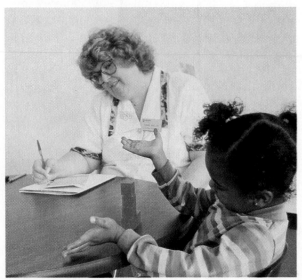

A young girl puzzles over the solution to a block design problem in the Wechsler Intelligence Scale for Children.

In 1939, Wechsler published the first of his new tests, the Wechsler Adult Intelligence Scale, or WAIS (1955). It was the first test to permit the separate examination of the diverse intellectual abilities that most experts believe constitute intelligence. It was also the first intelligence test designed specifically for adults. Average intelligence on all the Wechsler intelligence tests is 100. Scores below 70 suggest mental retardation, and those above 130 indicate exceptional intellectual performance. Fewer than 5 percent of persons tested score lower than 70 or higher than 130 on the Wechsler tests.

The latest of Wechsler's tests for adolescents and adults is the **Wechsler Adult Intelligence Scale-Revised (WAIS-R),** published in 1974. It tests eleven separate abilities: six verbal and five performance. The six verbal measures assess general information, abstract thinking, short-term memory, arithmetic ability, the capacity to recognize and act on well-learned societal rules and expectations, and vocabulary. The five performance measures test the capacities to solve puzzles, reproduce designs, and manipulate objects, symbols, and numbers (Kramer, 1990; Waller & Waldman, 1990).

As a part of the assessment process at her university's counseling center, Anne M. completed the WAIS-R. It was administered by an intern in clinical psychology at the center, who wrote an extensive report on Anne's performance. What follows is a portion of the summary of that report:

> Anne cooperated fully in the testing process, although, at times, she appeared downcast. During subtests that required concentration (such as those asking her to immediately recall numbers or words), she recognized her apparent impairment in concentration and became quite critical of her performance. At other times, Anne seemed preoccupied, almost in another world. Nonetheless, I believe that Anne tried hard to do her best during the administration of this test. Accordingly, I believe the results represent a valid measure of Anne's current intellectual functioning. As I point out below, however, I am convinced that her intellectual capacity is almost certainly higher than her current level of functioning.
>
> Anne's performance on the Vocabulary and Information subtests of the WAIS-R was in the "superior" range, suggesting that her ability to remember well-learned information and to recall the meanings of words at successively greater levels of difficulty remains intact.
>
> Anne did substantially less well on the Digit Span subtest, in which she had to remember and recall lists of numbers read to her, and on the Arithmetic subtest, in which she had to concentrate on the details of an arithmetic problem that was read to her and then work out its solution in her head. These subtests require good concentration and immediate memory to a far greater extent than either Vocabulary or Information. Anne's performance on these tests was in the "average" range.
>
> Anne's performance on the Block Design and Picture Arrangement subtests, which required her to problem solve, concentrate, and coordinate hand and eye movements, was in the "bright normal" range. This finding suggests that her performance on these subtests was also affected by her evident problems with concentrating.
>
> In summary, I estimate Anne's intelligence to fall within the "superior" range; she is clearly capable of excellent academic work in her demanding curriculum at the university. Her scores in the "superior" range on the Vocabulary and Information subtests, which are both resistant to impairment as a result of psychological difficulties, suggest that she remains capable of high-level intellectual functioning. However, her performance on several subtests sensitive to concentration, memory, and problem-solving deficits was less adequate, suggesting that her current intellectual functioning is affected by the mood disorder responsible for those deficits. The anxiety and depression accompanying such a disorder could be expected to interfere with Anne's concentration, short-term memory, and problem solving, while leaving longer-term memory, conceptual ability, and intellectual potential more or less intact.

Besides the WAIS-R, there are two other current Wechsler measures of intelligence: the **Wechsler Intelligence Scale for Children-III (WISC-III),** published in

Wechsler Adult Intelligence Scale-Revised (WAIS-R) Revision of first test to permit the separate examination of the diverse intellectual abilities that most experts believe constitute intelligence; the first intelligence test designed specifically for adults.

Wechsler Intelligence Scale for Children-III (WISC-III) Latest edition of the intelligence test designed for children between 5 and 16; based on the notion that intelligence is the sum of many separate abilities.

1991 and designed for children between 5 and 16 (Wechsler, 1991), and the **Wechsler Preschool and Primary Scale of Intelligence (WPPSI),** published in 1967 and intended for preschool children (Wechsler, 1967). Like the WAIS-R, these other measures are based on the notion that intelligence is the sum of many separate abilities—some verbal, others performance.

New Developments in the Assessment of Intelligence   Psychologist Joseph Matarazzo, a national authority on intellectual assessment, recently predicted that future efforts to assess intelligence will likely include physiological measures along with the verbal and performance measures we have traditionally depended on (Matarazzo, 1992). Matarazzo thinks that two physiological measures are excellent candidates for possible use in assessing intelligence:

- *reaction time measures,* which reflect the time it takes to see or hear a stimulus and then react to it
- *measures of evoked potential,* which track the brain's processing time from the instant a stimulus is perceived to when it completes traveling through the brain

In support of these measures, Matarazzo cites two recent demonstrations of strong, positive relationships between intelligence, as measured by standard verbal tests, and auditory-evoked potential measures (Oken, 1989; Reed & Jensen, 1991).

Performance on intelligence tests is a function of two factors. Environmental influences include the adequacy of our schooling and the intellectual stimulation available in our homes. Genetic factors include the genes governing cognitive functioning that we inherit from our parents and their parents and grandparents (Chipuer, Rovine, & Plomin, 1990; Loehlin, 1989). Most of us assume that the relative importance of genetic and environmental influences on our performance on intelligence tests remains more or less constant as we age. However, questions about that assumption have been raised by the results of a recent study (Pedersen, Plomin, Nesselrode, & McClearn, 1992), which suggests that the likelihood of inheriting general cognitive ability may increase significantly with age.

Pedersen and colleagues (1992) studied 46 pairs of identical twins who were separated at an early age and reared apart, 67 pairs of identical twins reared together, 100 pairs of fraternal twins reared apart, and 89 pairs of fraternal twins reared together. The purpose of the study was to determine the heritability of intelligence. The researchers found that the heritability in these Swedish twins, whose average age was 65, was much higher (80 percent) than estimates typically made earlier in life (about 50 percent). In other words, as we age, genetic influences on intelligence appear to increase and environmental influences appear to decrease. More research is necessary to show whether this surprising finding can be replicated (proven again experimentally) and, if it can, why these environmental effects hold true.

Two New Concepts of Intelligence   In recent years, experts have questioned widely held notions of intelligence, including those underlying the tests of Binet and Wechsler. Interestingly, these new theories go back to some of the thinking of the late 1800s that led Galton to consider sensory responses as good measures of intelligence. Psychologists Howard Gardner and Robert Sternberg have views on intelligence that owe as much to Galton as they do to Binet and Wechsler.

Gardner (1983, 1986) believes that the best way to understand intelligence is to study the spontaneous thought processes that accompany our efforts to adapt to our everyday environment. As a result, he has developed a **theory of multiple intelligences,** which emphasizes the existence of several independent intelligences. Gardner has identified seven intelligences: linguistic, logical-mathematical, musical, spatial, bodily kinesthetic, interpersonal, and intrapersonal. He believes our individual patterns in these diverse intelligences determine how successfully we interact with the world. He also thinks the best way to assess intelligence is in the real world, as we struggle to achieve our goals and make our mark. Even Gardner's def-

Wechsler Preschool and Primary Scale of Intelligence (WPPSI) Intelligence test for preschool children; based on the notion that intelligence is the sum of many separate abilities.

theory of multiple intelligences Conceives of seven independent intelligences that interact with the environment to determine success in it; proposed by Howard Gardner.

Psychologist Janet Helms has recently reviewed the scientific research on how genetic and environmental factors affect performance on intelligence tests (Helms, 1992). She acknowledges that most authorities in the field explain test performance as a function of both these factors, but she takes a very different position. She believes that neither the genetic perspective (which views the quality of performance mainly as a product of inheritance from parents and grandparents) nor the environmental perspective (which suggests that performance is shaped by intellectual resources available in the environment) explains the meaning of intelligence test scores for diverse racial and ethnic groups. Helms urges us, instead, to adopt the *culturalist perspective* in investigating influences on tests of cognitive ability.

Suppose a psychologist wants to understand the meaning of intelligence test items to an African American. In order to do so, she must appreciate the effects of both "European-centered values and beliefs," which have influenced the development of virtually all tests of cognitive ability, and "African-centered values and beliefs," which underlie the responses of many African Americans to tests of cognitive ability. These two sets of values and beliefs are often at odds with one another. As a result, test-taking behavior that is highly valued by one culture may not be valued at all by the other.

Consider the following European-centered values and beliefs and their likely impact on test taking by African Americans:

Rugged individualism: Individual achievement is most highly valued. The person[s] with the highest test scores is [are] entitled to the most privileges. . . .

Communication: White English is best. Tests are written in White English. . . .

Competition: One is either a winner or a loser. High test scores mean that a person is intelligent and meritorious; low scores mean the converse. . . .

Time: Time is a valuable commodity. The faster one obtains "right" answers, the brighter one is. . . .

Aesthetics: The best music and art come from European culture. Test content is likely to reflect European culture. (Helms, 1992, p. 1095)

Helms believes that each of these values and beliefs clashes with African-centered cultural values, making it difficult for African Americans to approach test taking in a way that will maximize test performance. In contrast to the Eurocentric emphasis on rugged individualism, for example, the African-centered value is *communalism,* or valuing your group more than the individuals in it. And contrary to the Eurocentric acceptance of time as a valued commodity, the African view is that "time is measured by socially meaningful events and customs"; so finishing a test on time is not as important as obtaining a "socially-meaningful" answer (Helms, 1992, p. 1096).

Helms's views on this matter are unlikely to replace the prevailing emphasis on the roles of genetic and environmental influences on intelligence test performance; the impact of these factors has been documented repeatedly. Publication of a recent book on the subject, *The Bell Curve* (Herrnstein & Murray, 1994) has caused a great deal of controversy, however, because in it, genetic factors are assigned a more important role in test performance than that given by many testing experts. Helms's cultural perspective makes us ask whether, in fact, a third set of influences—cultural factors—helps explain test performance.

Think about the following questions:

1. Do you think a combination of genetic and environmental factors best explains performance on IQ tests, or do you think cultural factors influence performance, as well? Regardless of your answer, give examples of the sources of influence on intelligence test performance that you are aware of.

2. Whatever your racial or ethnic identity, imagine for a moment that you are something else. (For instance, if you are African American, imagine that you are Caucasian. If you are Caucasian, imagine that you are African American.) Now imagine that you are taking an intelligence test. How might your performance on the test be affected—for better or for worse—by the Eurocentric values and beliefs listed above? Explain your answer.

inition of intelligence makes this point: "Intelligence is the capacity to solve problems or to fashion products that are valued in one or more cultural settings" (Gardner & Hatch, 1989, p. 5).

Gardner also assesses intelligence in a cultural setting, or context. Depending on the demands of the culture we live in, one or another of the separate intelligences will be most important to our success in that culture. For instance, our Western Eurocentric culture values linguistic and logical-mathematical competence; other cultures value interpersonal abilities or bodily kinesthetic ones.

Depending on which of these intelligences we have the most skills in, we will succeed or fail in our respective cultural environments. This position is also similar in important ways to Helms's culturalist position on intelligence testing (1992), discussed in the Thinking about Controversial Issues box (see page 89).

Robert Sternberg believes that intelligence determines three things: (1) where and how we choose to live, (2) how we adapt our lives to those choices, and (3) how we shape our choices to suit how we want to live (Sternberg, 1984a). His **triarchic theory of human intelligence** (Sternberg, 1984b, 1985) emphasizes the central role of intelligence in helping us adapt to the world.

The first aspect of Sternberg's triarchic theory is what he calls the *componential* aspect of intelligence. It includes the mental processes or skills emphasized by most theories of intelligence, and it determines how well we learn to do things and acquire new knowledge. The second aspect of his theory, the *experimental* aspect, helps us adjust to new intellectual demands, explore and use new concepts, and adjust quickly to new situations and challenges. Finally, the *contextual* aspect of intelligence enables us to choose environments we can succeed in, adapt to if necessary, and structure to fit our own needs. Sternberg also calls the third aspect of intelligence *tacit knowledge,* which he defines as "the practical know-how one needs for success on the job. Often it is not openly expressed or stated, and it usually is not taught directly" (Sternberg & Wagner, 1993, p. 2).

Both Gardner's and Sternberg's theories of intelligence demand that we judge the ultimate worth of our intelligence according to our success in the real world. They also require that we consider the cultural demands that the world places on our intelligences. In a society such as that of the United States, which values success and distinct cultures equally, these theories have much to offer.

Focus on Critical Thinking

1. Projective tests have been criticized for their lack of reliability and validity. How might these problems be addressed so these measures could be more widely used?

2. The MMPI-2 asks direct questions about thoughts and feelings in order to assess personality and psychopathology. Under what circumstances might you find it difficult to respond to these questions in an open and honest way?

3. Why is intelligence testing so often a component of psychological assessment? Even though we know that IQ doesn't affect the likelihood of acquiring most mental disorders, we routinely measure intelligence when we assess and diagnose mental disorders. Why?

ASSESSMENT OF BRAIN DISORDERS

Virtually every type of brain disorder affects behavior. Minor changes in brain function—such as those caused by having two or three drinks of alcohol—cause barely perceptible, short-lived changes in thinking and behavior. And major brain disturbances—strokes, tumors, and infections, for example—produce profound, permanent changes. Clinicians working with individuals who may have brain damage must be able to assess changes in the brain accurately, both to plan treatment and to try to prevent further deterioration.

Most brain disorders cannot be diagnosed in the way that most behavioral disorders are diagnosed—that is, using diagnostic interviews. The overlap in signs and symptoms between disorders affecting the brain and behavioral disorders is too great. As a result, if a brain disorder is suspected, diagnostic information must be obtained from multiple assessment sources: diagnostic and specialized interviews, neuropsychological tests, electroencephalograph (EEG), and neuroimaging techniques.

Neuropsychological Assessment

Neuropsychological assessment of disordered brain function involves evaluating memory, problem-solving, and psychomotor tasks. The individual's performance

triarchic theory of human intelligence Stresses the role of intelligence in helping us adjust to new situations and environments; proposed by Howard Sternberg.

on these tasks may reveal subtle brain damage before it begins to affect behavior. Sometimes, identifying difficulties with these tasks also helps in localizing damage to a specific region of the brain (Benton, 1994).

Several subtests of the WAIS and WAIS-R (Block Design, Digit Span, Digit Symbol) are able to determine the existence of brain damage (Reitan & Wolfson, 1992; Spreen & Strauss, 1991). When confirmation is needed of the extent of the deficit in memory, reasoning, or problem solving, specialized neuropsychological batteries are used (Jones & Butters, 1991). The two neuropsychological tests most widely used in the United States today are the Halstead-Reitan Neuropsychological Battery (Halstead, 1947; Reitan, 1959; Reitan & Davison, 1974) and the Luria-Nebraska Neuropsychological Battery (Golden, Hammeke, & Purisch, 1980).

The **Halstead-Reitan Neuropsychological Battery,** published almost 50 years ago, was developed by Ralph Reitan, a student of pioneering neuropsychologist Ward Halstead. Reitan was strongly influenced by Halstead's research in the 1920s and 1930s, which represented the first systematic study of the neuropsychological consequences of brain injuries.

Karl Lashley, who, like Halstead, was an influential leader in the new science of neuropsychology, put Halstead's groundbreaking research in perspective in 1951 with the following words:

> Dr. Halstead's work represents what is almost the first attempt to explore in a systematic way a great variety of possible defects arising from localized injury in the brain. He has been engaged for a number of years in devising tests for almost every imaginable function and trying them, as to their effectiveness in revealing defects. . . . Earlier studies depended pretty largely on chance observations of defects, without systematic investigation to determine what functions may be correlated in the defects produced by localized brain injury. (Lashley, 1951, p. 272)

Reitan used Halstead's findings—including data from a large number of auditory, visual, psychomotor, and verbal tests of brain function—to create a neuropsychological battery, which he later normed and standardized.

Despite the development of newer neuropsychological tests, the Halstead-Reitan remains the most widely used means of assessing the cognitive and behavioral consequences of brain damage (Reitan, 1994). The instrument assesses the full range of cognitive functions affected by brain damage.

The newer **Luria-Nebraska Neuropsychological Battery** is based on concepts and techniques developed by Aleksander Luria (1902–1977), a well-known Soviet neuropsychologist. It assesses cognitive functioning in 14 domains. This instrument reflects Luria's conviction that, whereas local areas of the cerebral cortex control specific skills, even the simplest human behavior calls on a variety of such skills and must accordingly be connected to several cortical centers. The neuropsychologist must therefore look across brain areas and specific skills to produce the most accurate picture of disturbances in brain structure and function.

Electroencephalography

Electroencephalography (EEG) is a technique for measuring the electrical activity of the brain. It involves placing pairs of electrodes in 16 locations on an individual's scalp; the electrodes send signals corresponding to the differences measured in voltage between the pairs to one of the EEG's recording channels.

Before the development of neuroimaging techniques, the EEG was the technique of choice for studying abnormalities in brain activity that resulted from injuries, tumors, or seizures. Neuroimaging techniques are able to create an image of brain structure, which the EEG does not provide. Nonetheless, the EEG remains the simplest, cheapest, and fastest method of evaluating seizures, drug effects, and metabolic disturbances in the brain.

The EEG of a normal, conscious, relaxed adult shows regular, oscillating waves (waves that move up and down in a regular pattern) of between 8 and 12 cycles per

Halstead-Reitan Neuropsychological Battery Most widely used measure of the cognitive and behavioral consequences of brain damage; developed more than 50 years ago.

Luria-Nebraska Neuropsychological Battery Tests cognitive functioning in 14 areas; some, such as memory and problem solving, are also tapped by the Halstead-Reitan Battery; others, such as writing, are not.

electroencephalography (EEG) Technique that measures the electrical activity of the brain; EEG waves can indicate brain injury or damage.

FIGURE 3.1 Alpha and delta waves

Alpha waves are regular and oscillating, between 8 and 12 cycles a second; they represent the EEG patterns of normal, conscious, relaxed adults. Delta waves, by contrast, are irregular and much slower, about 4 cycles a second; they often signal localized brain damage.

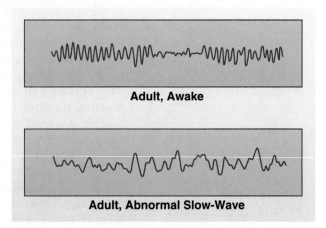

Adult, Awake

Adult, Abnormal Slow-Wave

second; they are called **alpha waves** (see Figure 3.1). Other patterns of electrical activity replace alpha waves when the person becomes excited, sleeps, suffers a brain injury or disease, or falls into a deep coma. These conditions are frequently (but not always) associated with distinct EEG patterns. For example, irregular, slow waves (less than 4 cycles per second), known as **delta waves,** are typically recorded from damaged or dying localized areas of the brain. By contrast, an epileptic seizure may be signaled by extremely rapid, irregular "spikes," which are dramatic portrayals of the disorganized activity of the brain during a seizure.

Most forms of psychopathology are not associated with specific EEG patterns, so this technology has very limited value in diagnosing mental disorders. Even known disorders of the brain do not always produce positive EEG findings, unless they are caused by or associated with localized brain damage or specific kinds of epilepsy (Rebok & Folstein, 1994). The EEG remains useful for other purposes, though, including the investigation of sleep patterns (e.g., Kupfer, Buysse, Nofzinger, & Reynolds, 1994; Regestein, 1994). The EEG is also sensitive to metabolic disturbances and to the effects of some drugs. In fact, an abnormal EEG may be the first indication that a person's increasing agitation and confusion is due to a metabolic disturbance, caused by either a drug or a toxin (Andreasen & Black, 1995).

Neuroimaging Techniques

Computerized Tomography   A dramatic advance in brain-imaging technology moved clinical radiology ahead in the early 1970s. Before that, the brain had been X-rayed using a procedure called **angiography.** It involves injecting a contrasting substance (like a dye) into the bloodstream; that substance shows up on film, outlining the blood vessels of the brain. This procedure had been used successfully to diagnose circulatory diseases in the brain. It had not been useful, however, in localizing brain lesions because the contrast in substance could not reveal differences in tissue densities.

Early in the 1970s, **computerized axial tomography (CAT)** revolutionized the clinical investigation of many brain diseases. This procedure uses sophisticated, high-speed computers—capable of solving many equations simultaneously—to look at multiple X-rays of the brain from different angles. To begin, a radioactive substance is injected into the bloodstream; as with angiography, this substance shows up on X-rays. A radiation scanner rotates 360 degrees around the body, measuring the different densities of tissue, bone, and water. Multiple views of the brain are filmed and then combined, producing a single, reconstructed image. The computer can then look at a "slice," or cross-section, of the brain. This technology is sensitive enough to show relationships among structures of the brain, such as differences in tissue densities.

alpha waves Regular, oscillating waves of 8 to 12 cycles a second; represent the EEG pattern of a normal, conscious, relaxed adult.

delta waves EEG pattern involving a slow brainwave pattern of less than 4 cycles a second; normally recorded when a person is deeply asleep; may also signal localized brain damage.

angiography Imaging procedure in which a contrasting substance injected into the bloodstream shows an outline of the blood vessels in the brain, which is visible on an X-ray; enables diagnosis of circulatory diseases affecting the brain.

computerized axial tomography (CAT) Brain-imaging technique in which multiple views of the brain are X-rayed and then combined, producing a single, reconstructed image.

One of the first achievements made through CAT technology was confirmation of a long-held suspicion about people with schizophrenia: namely, that their brains have enlarged spaces on the inner and outer surfaces. These enlargements correspond to an overall reduction or shrinkage in the volume of brain tissue. This condition—called **cortical atrophy**—may involve shrinkage in the volume of brain neurons, an actual loss of neurons, or both. Precisely what is responsible for cortical atrophy is unclear, as is how these changes in brain tissue affect behavior. But in addition to people with schizophrenia, this condition has been observed in aged persons, especially those with Alzheimer's disease (although to a lesser extent), and in some people with alcoholism, anorexia nervosa, and the mood disorders. Males appear to be more vulnerable than females to cortical atrophy.

Magnetic Resonance Imaging   One very new neuroimaging technique, available only since the early 1980s, is called **magnetic resonance imaging (MRI).** It might ultimately displace CAT as the preferred neuroimaging technology for portraying structural (anatomical) abnormalities in the brain (Andreasen & Black, 1995). MRI produces a finely detailed visual reconstruction of the brain by analyzing the nuclear magnetic movements of ordinary hydrogen nuclei in the body's water and fat.

In addition to the more detailed image it provides, MRI also has several other advantages over the earlier technologies. Unlike X-rays and CAT scans, MRI does not expose subjects to radiation, so repeated tests can be made without having to worry about overexposure. Moreover, MRI is a *noninvasive procedure,* which means that nothing is injected or otherwise put into the body; this substantially reduces the risk of side effects from the procedure.

MRI studies have provided important data on the role of brain damage in schizophrenia (Andreasen, 1989). In a landmark study at the University of Iowa, the brains of 38 patients with schizophrenia were compared to those of 49 normal control subjects (Andreasen, Hoffman, & Grove, 1985). The investigators ultimately focused their MRI imaging studies on the frontal lobe because many schizophrenic behaviors resemble those of patients with known frontal lobe damage (for instance, decreased spontaneity and fluency of speech, reduced voluntary motor behavior, and difficulties with mood and emotions, including apathy, indifference, and emotional shallowness). Comparing the sizes of the frontal lobes of the two groups, the researchers reported that the schizophrenic subjects had significantly smaller frontal lobes than did the control subjects (Andreasen et al., 1985). In recent years, MRI studies have also revealed brain abnormalities in the cerebellum in autistic children and tiny areas of tissue loss, scattered through the brain, in patients with bipolar affective disorder (Andreasen & Black, 1995).

Positron Emission Tomography   As technology has developed—from X-ray to CAT scan to MRI—it has provided successively more precise representations of brain *structure.* But one of the newest neuroimaging techniques—**positron emission tomography (PET)**—permits direct access to information on brain *function* for the first time (Fischbach, 1992). In this procedure, a chemical medium is injected into the bloodstream of the subject; that medium carries radioactive isotopes, which interact with electrons in the brain to generate gamma rays. Depending on the isotopes used, the PET technique can provide information on a range of metabolic, neurochemical, and physiological processes in the brain, making it an extremely valuable research tool.

When used in conjunction with CAT or MRI, PET helps clinicians localize structural abnormalities in specific regions of the brain and then test for possible causes of those abnormalities, such as reduced bloodflow or impaired use of oxygen. The initial application of PET has been to study how glucose is used in the brain, since this is a direct measure of brain activity. Clinical findings show abnormal metabolic patterns of glucose uptake in individuals with seizure disorders,

cortical atrophy Reduction in brain volume.

magnetic resonance imaging (MRI) Noninvasive imaging technique that produces a finely detailed visual reconstruction of the brain that looks like a three-dimensional "slice"; does so by analyzing the nuclear magnetic movements of ordinary hydrogen nuclei in the body's water and fat.

positron emission tomography (PET) Neuroimaging technique that relies on scanning receptors of gamma emissions from selected brain areas; capable of high-resolution reflection of both the structure and function of the brain.

tumors, stroke, Alzheimer's disease (see Chapter 16), schizophrenia (see Chapter 13), bipolar affective disorder, and obsessive-compulsive disorder.

In several instances, PET has provided answers to important questions that have gone unanswered for decades, even centuries. For example, researchers at Washington University in Saint Louis have localized bloodflow in different parts of the brain as a function of the specific intellectual tasks that subjects are doing: hearing words, seeing words, speaking words, and generating words (Fischbach, 1992). The same research group has also localized the brain areas associated with the range of emotions experienced in reaction to different arousing stimuli.

Focus on
Critical Thinking

1. How might neuroimaging and neuropsychological techniques be used together clinically? Select a disorder or group of disorders, and propose a diagnostic application of these techniques.

BEHAVIORAL ASSESSMENT

Behavioral assessment focuses on those specific aspects of a person's behavior that led her to seek treatment—perhaps fearful behavior, stressful or troubled interpersonal relationships, inadequate social skills, or unassertiveness. Behavioral assessment approaches do not try to assess the whole person, as do some of the psychodynamically oriented personality measures; that "big picture" would not be specific enough to help the behavior therapist plan treatment. Instead, behavioral assessment seeks detailed information on the following:

■ **target behaviors**—the disturbed or disturbing behavior or behaviors as well as the thoughts and feelings that accompany them
■ **antecedents**—the events and circumstances (including thoughts and feelings) that typically precede development of the target behaviors
■ **consequences**—the events and circumstances (including thoughts and feelings) that typically follow the target behaviors

Behavioral Interviews and Direct Observation Methods

Behavioral clinicians have developed specific assessment instruments for many conditions and disorders. They do not assume that a single battery of tests can adequately describe the behavior of every person and every condition (Bellack & Hersen, 1988; Haynes, 1991).

These beliefs about assessment mirror the assumptions psychodynamic and behavioral clinicians make about intervention. Psychodynamic clinicians stress the power that traumatic childhood events have in causing unconscious conflict, emotional distress, and even emotional disorder later on. Based on this theory, psychodynamic assessment tends to focus as much on personal history and unconscious factors as on present issues. Behavioral clinicians believe that a person's distress or disorder results from the interaction of environmental stressors, the person's learning history, and associated constitutional factors (such as energy level, intelligence, physical attractiveness, and the like). Consequently, behavioral assessment focuses very much on present issues in an effort to identify relevant antecedents and consequences of the distress or disorder.

A behavioral interview is usually the first step in this assessment process. The interviewer gathers information on the sequence of events that came before and after the person's problems developed and data on the target behaviors themselves, too. As the case material that follows suggests, Anne M.'s therapist chose to organize her behavioral assessment interview around the three elements of behavioral analysis that many behavioral clinicians have found useful: target behaviors,

target behaviors In behavioral assessment, the disturbed and disturbing behaviors themselves as well as the thoughts and feelings that accompany them.

antecedents In behavioral assessment, the events and circumstances that typically precede the target behaviors.

consequences In behavioral assessment, the events and circumstances that typically follow the target behaviors.

antecedents, and consequences. Based on the assessment of these elements, Anne's therapist also recommended a treatment plan.

Target Behaviors   When she is with her friends or parents and begins to feel anxious and depressed, Anne withdraws emotionally and, when possible, physically. When she cannot avoid being with others, she speaks much less than usual. She laughs or jokes rarely at those times. Following disturbing social encounters, Anne avoids her friends for a day or more. With her parents, Anne becomes visibly more childlike during these disturbing times, permitting her mother to do things Anne has long since done for herself.

During Anne's self-critical periods, when her self-esteem seems to be under attack, she criticizes herself severely and continuously for her imagined faults: social incompetence, unattractiveness, inability to do coursework, and failures as a friend and a daughter.

Antecedents   Anne M. possesses a full and adequate behavioral repertoire. She is interpersonally skilled, sensitive to others' feelings, appropriately assertive, conscientious, hard working, bright, and energetic. But in certain circumstances and mood states, she recedes dramatically into the background. When this occurs (which is now once or twice a week), she withdraws from friends and family; her withdrawal is typically accompanied by self-critical thoughts and feelings of depression and worthlessness.

Meeting someone new, especially a person of her own age, sometimes precipitates social withdrawal and self-deprecatory feelings. These feelings, according to Anne, depend on who the person is, how the person behaves, and who else Anne is with. When the new person appears brighter, more skilled interpersonally, more attractive, or more interesting than she is, Anne is most likely to feel inadequate and to withdraw. While Anne rarely meets people who are more competent than she is, she doesn't feel this is the case.

When Anne is with her parents for any time, she reexperiences some of the feelings of incompetence she felt as a child. Anne says that, even now, her parents tend to treat her like the sick child she was in ninth grade, not like the competent, independent adult she has become.

Anne's social withdrawal, self-critical behavior, and depressive and anxious moods began in earnest her first year of high school, when she missed a good deal of school because of recurrent viral infections. She says a doctor told her parents at the time that she may also have suffered a period of acute, reversible brain damage following these infections. This time, she feels, marked the beginning of her inability to concentrate and complete her schoolwork. Since then, in academic settings and with peers, Anne has told herself that she doesn't measure up, either intellectually or socially.

Consequences   By withdrawing from others when she is troubled, Anne avoids the possibility of ever learning how inaccurate her assessment of her intellect, social skills, interpersonal appeal, and maturity is. That is because, when she withdraws, Anne's friends respect her wish to be alone, although they sometimes ask if they can help. Anne rarely shares her negative feelings about herself with friends. When she does, they are quick to disagree with her view of herself as incompetent and unworthy.

At home, however, Anne's parents strongly reinforce her view of herself as delicate, sickly, and socially inept.

Treatment Plan   Anne's behavioral treatment should include cognitive restructuring: that is, direct and repeated feedback on the very positive impact she has on others, their clear desire to spend time with her, and the strength of her academic record. Consistent repetitions of these observations will make it more difficult for Anne to persist in denying them. Her therapist should use cognitive restructuring to help Anne change her negative self-perceptions and to bring them into better alignment with others' positive assessment of her. Behavioral family therapy sessions are also strongly recommended, in order to align Anne's parents' perceptions of her with her current skills and achievements.

Behavioral clinicians also try, whenever possible, to observe their patients' troubled behaviors directly. Techniques have been developed for observing the behaviors of a wide range of clinical populations. For instance, methods for systematically observing troubled children and their parents help identify the environmental variables that may elicit the problems, including actions of parents, siblings, and friends (Arnold, O'Leary, Wolff, & Acker, 1993; Greenbaum, Dedrick, Prange, & Friedman, 1994). Valid observational systems have also been developed to identify the behaviors of partners in troubled marriages (Bradbury & Fincham, 1993) and adolescents and adults suffering from various kinds of behavioral disorders (Clark et al., 1994; Cox, Swinson, Parker, Kuch, & Reichman, 1993) and health-related disorders (Cooper, 1994).

Self-Monitoring and Self-Report Measures

Usually, the best way to gather information about people is to ask them for it. As we discussed earlier in this chapter, interviews are a useful way to gather information. So are **self-reports,** which are essentially individuals' observations of their own behavior. For example, behavior therapists treating substance abusers asked them to keep detailed records of cigarettes smoked, drinks consumed, and drug "hits" made—when, where, and with whom—along with the feelings and thoughts that accompany their use (Foy, Cline, & Laasi, 1987; Shiffman, Kassel, Paty, Gnys, & Zettler-Segal, 1994). Behavioral clinicians investigating substance use/abuse and sexual risk asked their adolescent subjects to report how often they had unsafe sex after using drugs or drinking (Cooper, Peirce, & Huselid, 1994).

Behavior therapists treating people who were depressed asked their clients to **self-monitor** thoughts and feelings to help them become aware of the sequence of events leading to their self-defeating or self-damaging cognitions. (You may remember that Anne's therapist asked her to self-monitor her depressive thoughts.) And behavioral health psychologists used self-report techniques to investigate relationships between daily life stressors and gastrointestinal symptoms (Suls, Wan, & Blanchard, 1994) and between middle-aged women's following recommendations for regular mammograms and their believing in the value of preventive health practices (Aiken, West, Woodward, & Reno, 1994).

Behavioral clinicians have also begun to track therapeutic progress through self-report measures. Improved self-esteem was demonstrated by individuals' self-reported decreases in making negative self-statements and increases in making positive self-statements; for instance, individuals reported saying "I could never do that" less often and thinking or saying "Maybe I should at least give it a try" more often (Lewinsohn & Lee, 1981). Self-reports are also useful in identifying target problems for behavioral treatments (Nezu & Nezu, 1993), their antecedents (Haynes, Spain, & Oliveira, 1993), and the patients' perceptions of how successful treatment has been (Mash & Hunsley, 1993).

The validity of self-reports may be questionable at times. Psychologist Linda Sobell and her colleagues have examined the reliability of self-reports of drinking by alcoholics and problem drinkers (Sobell & Sobell, 1990). They conclude that if individuals sense that giving an accurate self-report might cause something bad to happen—like a forced return to treatment—their reports will probably be inaccurate. This raises an all-important question regarding persons in treatment for any of a number of disorders: Do they give their therapists accurate self-reports when they believe that doing so will disappoint the therapist or lead to other unwanted consequences (Babor, Brown, & Del Boca, 1990)?

self-reports Individual accounts of the frequency of target behaviors, along with descriptions of their antecedents and consequences.

self-monitoring Behavioral assessment method that asks people to observe and record their own behavior over time.

Assessment of Physiological Functioning

Behavioral clinicians rely on measures of bodily functioning—primarily, autonomic nervous system (ANS) activity and muscle tension—to track treatment responses, plan interventions, and sometimes actually intervene. Behavior can be expressed in three ways (Lang, 1969; Zinbarg, Barlow, Brown, & Hertz, 1992):

1. the overt behavior itself—our words and deeds
2. subjective feelings and attitudes about it—how we interpret the behavior for ourselves
3. our body's accompanying physiological responses—how the ANS and other bodily systems reflect the behavior

Since behavior is expressed in these ways, it's typically measured using them, as well. To get an accurate picture, it's important to measure all three types of responses. Sometimes, they are in agreement, showing consistency among how we act, how we feel about it, and how it affects us physically. But sometimes, our responses are not consistent. For example, we might subjectively experience a fear of heights and show phobic behavior when we're more than two floors above the ground; even so, we may not necessarily experience the physical ANS changes characteristic of stress and fearfulness.

Measures of ANS activation reflect stress levels. Heart and respiration (breathing) rates, galvanic skin response (measuring perspiration), and blood pressure are all measured to reflect stress. In one common measurement situation, the patient listens to a description (and may see a still or moving picture) of objects or situations that the therapist believes are particularly stressful to him, while the therapist takes several measures of ANS response. When confronted with fear-inducing stimuli, phobic patients may show dramatic increases in level of autonomic activity (Nay, 1986); this increase can help clinicians identify which stimuli to focus on in treatment. Another recent development is *ambulatory monitoring* of psychophysiological indicators of stress; with this type of monitoring, patients are allowed to go about their everyday lives while being studied. Given this real-world setting, ambulatory monitoring promises greater correspondence between stress and stressors (Haynes, Falkin, & Sexton-Radek, 1989).

Another valuable procedure is *electromyographic assessment*, in which the level of activation of certain voluntary muscle groups is measured. Patients suffering from chronic pain, for example, may react to the description of a particular situation by tensing those muscle groups that exacerbate their pain. Electromyographic feedback of this kind indicates which situations help maintain the chronic pain and thus enables the clinician to focus therapy more effectively (Blanchard, 1981).

Reliability and Utility

Because behavioral clinicians believe that direct observation and behavior therapy go hand in hand, they developed the methods for each simultaneously. The fact is, behavioral assessment methods were designed for planning and evaluating a treatment's success or failure.

A reliable method of behavioral observation would enable clinicians to observe the behavior of a group of disturbed children and agree on what they see. A reliable self-report of smoking behavior would accurately reflect the number of cigarettes smoked. In short, an assessment's usefulness is based on the assistance it provides clinicians in planning or evaluating treatment.

To make sure that assessment techniques would not suffer from the reliability problems found in some personality measures, behavior therapists developed measures that focus very closely on target behaviors, rather than requiring patients to interpret their own behavior, respond to ambiguous test stimuli, or give responses to open-ended questions. Consequently (and predictably), individuals being assessed tend to give the same answers to behavioral assessment instruments, despite the passage of time. Exceptions occur in these situations:

- when individuals are asked questions about behaviors targeted for therapeutic change—as we observed earlier, drug addicts don't always give accurate self-reports on drug use
- when the behavior assessed occurs across too vast a timespan—for example, asking a depressed person what his mood was like six months earlier
- when the behavior is too complex to capture in words—for instance, expecting a person to describe in complete detail a lengthy interaction with another person

Another problem relates to the measurement process itself. This is an issue for psychologists who use behavioral assessment methods as well as those who use personality assessment procedures. The direct observation of a person's problem behavior can be costly and impractical; consider what's involved in observing someone who's afraid of flying. Because of practical limitations, clinicians may have to plan assessments in situations that are *comparable* to patients' actual environments. Despite their similarities, the assessment and real-life situations may be different enough so that the resulting assessment will not be valid. For instance, an individual may seem to be appropriately assertive, based on the results of a paper-and-pencil test of assertiveness, which asks her to respond to a series of situations that call for assertiveness. But the situations included in the test may actually have little to do with those in which the person usually lacks assertiveness. If that's the case, the test results will not be valid.

The usefulness of behavioral assessment also depends on whether the clinician shows *observational bias*. Without knowing or recognizing it, we all introduce our own biases into what we hear and see, no matter how hard we try not to. Thus, assessment—filtered through the clinician's perspective—may not be completely valid.

Focus on **Critical Thinking**

1. How do behavioral assessment and personality assessment share similar goals, and how do their goals differ? How might behavioral assessment and personality assessment complement each other in the comprehensive assessment of a person?
2. What kinds of information are provided uniquely by behavioral assessment? by personality assessment? Is one approach more valuable than the other in assessing certain mental disorders? Explain your answer.

SUMMARY

Diagnosis

- Diagnosis involves identifying and naming a disorder or disease using an agreed upon system of categorization. Clinical assessment is the process of gathering diagnostic information to determine what causes a disorder, how to treat it, and what future course it might take.
- To diagnose physical diseases, physicians most often rely on physical signs and symptoms. Mental health clinicians base their diagnoses on behavioral and psychological as well as physical signs and symptoms, collectively termed *psychopathology*. The biopsychosocial model of psychopathology holds that important diagnostic and treatment decisions require thorough examination of the psychological, social, and biological factors present in all behavioral disorders.
- The *DSM-IV* (American Psychiatric Association, 1994) is the latest version of the *Diagnostic and Statistical Manual of Mental Disorders*. In comparison to previous versions, the *DSM-IV* offers improvements in two diagnostic features—operational criteria and multiaxial diagnosis—both of which enhance diagnostic reliability and diagnostic validity. The mental health professionals who

developed the *DSM-IV* were much more representative of U.S. society than their predecessors in terms of number, sex, disciplinary bases and work settings, and racial and ethnic diversity. As a result, the instrument is substantially more sensitive to individual differences affecting diagnosis; this reduces the possibility of diagnostic bias.

Psychological Assessment

■ Mental health professionals use several types of interviews: diagnostic, assessment, and therapy. Some interviews are highly structured; the Diagnostic Interview Schedule (DIS) is one such interview. Diagnostic interviews can also be semistructured. Therapy interviews are typically unstructured.

■ Psychologists use the term *personality* to mean enduring traits of character—in other words, the basic, lasting qualities that make us who we are. Based on that belief, psychologists study past and present behaviors, assuming that they often predict future behaviors.

■ Projective tests ask respondents to impose their own structure and meaning onto unstructured, ambiguous test stimuli, thereby supposedly revealing underlying personality traits. The Rorschach Inkblot Test is the most familiar of the projective tests. Although the reliability and validity of Rorschach responses have been questioned, Exner's new, empirically based system for interpreting and scoring Rorschach responses has attracted attention. The Thematic Apperception Test (TAT), another widely used projective test, appears to have similar problems of reliability and validity.

■ The Minnesota Multiphasic Personality Inventory (MMPI) is the most commonly used objective measure of personality; it recently underwent extensive revision. The new test, the MMPI-2, is a 567-item, self-report questionnaire that asks subjects to mark statements "true" or "false," as appropriate. The instrument contains 10 basic clinical scales and 6 validity scales. The MMPI-2 was standardized on a large, national sample, so its validity is stronger than that of the MMPI. Other prominent personality inventories include the Millon Clinical Multiaxial Inventory (MCMI and MCMI-II) and the NEO Personality Inventory (NEO-PI).

■ Intelligence is the best predictor of adaptation to all kinds of environments, although it isn't the only one. Central figures in the history of intelligence testing include Sir Francis Galton, who believed that sensory discrimination is the most valid measure of intelligence; Alfred Binet, who developed a series of intelligence tests that introduced the concepts of intelligence quotient (IQ), mental age, and chronological age; David Wechsler, who created the Wechsler Adult Intelligence Scale and the Wechsler Intelligence Scale for Children, both of which were designed to measure the diverse intellectual abilities most experts believe constitute intelligence; and Robert Sternberg and Howard Gardner, who have recently proposed, respectively, the triarchic theory of human intelligence and the theory of multiple intelligences.

Assessment of Brain Disorders

■ The instruments used for neuropsychological assessment of disordered brain function involve memory, problem-solving, and psychomotor tasks to reveal subtle brain damage before it begins to affect behavior. Several subtests of the WAIS-R are able to detect brain damage. However, when greater specification of a neuropsychological deficit in memory, reasoning, or problem solving is required, the Halstead-Reitan Neuropsychological Battery is generally used; it includes 10 subtests to evaluate the cognitive and behavioral functions most affected by central nervous system disease. The Luria-Nebraska Neuropsychological Battery is also used for this purpose.

■ Electroencephalography (EEG) is a means of measuring the electrical activity of the brain. The EEG of a normal, conscious, relaxed adult shows regular, oscillating waves of between 8 and 12 cycles per second, called *alpha waves*. Irregular, slow waves of less than 4 cycles per second, known as *delta waves*, are typically recorded from damaged or dying cells in the brain. An epileptic seizure may be signaled by extremely rapid, irregular EEG "spikes."

■ Marked advances have been made in recent years in procedures for examining the structure and function of the brain. The two techniques most often used today to examine brain structure are computerized axial tomography (CAT) and magnetic resonance imaging (MRI). A newer technology, positron emission tomography (PET), permits direct imaging access to information on the functioning of the brain.

Behavioral Assessment

■ Behavioral assessment focuses on the person's current environment and behavior, thoughts, feelings, and attitudes. Behavioral clinicians need to determine when and how often a disturbed or disturbing behavior occurs and the conditions that precede and follow it.

■ Behavioral clinicians typically emphasize three sources of data: target behaviors, the disturbed behaviors themselves as well as the thoughts and feelings that accompany them; antecedents, the events and circumstances that typically precede the target behaviors; and consequences, the events and circumstances that typically follow the target behaviors.

■ Behavioral clinicians have developed assessment instruments for specific conditions and disorders, since they don't believe that a single battery of tests is suitable for every condition.

■ A behavioral interview is usually the first step in behavioral assessment. Behavioral clinicians also try, whenever possible, to observe their patients' troubled behaviors directly.

■ Usually, the best way to gather information about people is to ask them for it. Clinicians rely on this premise in employing interviews and self-report measures.

■ Behavioral clinicians also rely on measures of bodily functioning—primarily autonomic nervous system activity and muscle tension—to track therapeutic success, plan interventions, and sometimes actually intervene.

KEY TERMS

alpha waves, **p. 92**
angiography, **p. 92**
antecedents, **p. 94**
anxiety, **pp. 74–75**
assessment interview, **p. 78**
chronological age, **p. 86**
clinical assessment, **p. 70**
compulsions, **pp. 74–75**
computerized axial tomography (CAT), **p. 92**
concurrent validity, **p. 75**
consequences, **p. 94**
cortical atrophy, **p. 93**
delta waves, **p. 92**
delusions, **p. 72**
diagnosis, **p. 70**
diagnostic bias, **p. 75**
diagnostic interview, **p. 78**

diagnostic reliability, **p. 73**
diagnostic validity, **p. 75**
electroencephalography (EEG), **p. 91**
extraverted personality type, **p. 80**
hallucinations, **p. 72**
Halstead-Reitan Neuropsychological Battery, **p. 91**
individual therapy interview, **p. 78**
intelligence quotient (IQ), **p. 86**
introverted personality type, **p. 80**
Luria-Nebraska Neuropsychological Battery, **p. 91**

magnetic resonance imaging (MRI), **p. 93**
mental age, **p. 86**
Millon Clinical Multiaxial Inventory (MCMI), **p. 85**
Minnesota Multiphasic Personality Inventory (MMPI), **p. 83**
multiaxial diagnosis, **p. 72**
NEO Personality Inventory (NEO-PI), **p. 85**
obsessions, **pp. 74–75**
operational criteria, **p. 71**
personality, **p. 80**
positron emission tomography (PET), **p. 93**
predictive validity, **p. 75**
projective drawings, **p. 82**

CRITICAL THINKING EXERCISE

Much of what we know of Anne M.'s psychopathology can be understood using the biopsychosocial model. Her eating and sleeping problems, for example, and perhaps her depressive feelings as well were primarily influenced by biological factors (although they were also affected by social and psychological influences). Similarly, Anne's anxiety and self-esteem difficulties were primarily psychological in nature. Her social withdrawal during periods of depression, however, was largely a response to environmental pressures, although these behaviors also clearly have other biopsychosocial determinants.

We can divide the multiple causes of Anne's condition along the same lines. The viral infection she had early in high school and the impact it may have left on her central nervous system are clearly biological factors. Social factors include the interpersonal pressures she was under during that crucial first year in high school and her parents' reaction to her illness. Among the psychological factors affecting her that year was her understandable (but complicating) emotional reaction to the infection and the effects it had at school and at home.

1. Reexamine the comprehensive psychological assessment of Anne M. in this chapter, looking specifically at its biopsychosocial findings. Which assessment instruments and techniques identified signs and symptoms primarily of biological origin? of psychological origin? of social origin?
2. Which assessment measures best reflected the interaction of these three factors in Anne's behavior?

Chapter 4
RESEARCH METHODS IN THE STUDY OF ABNORMAL BEHAVIOR

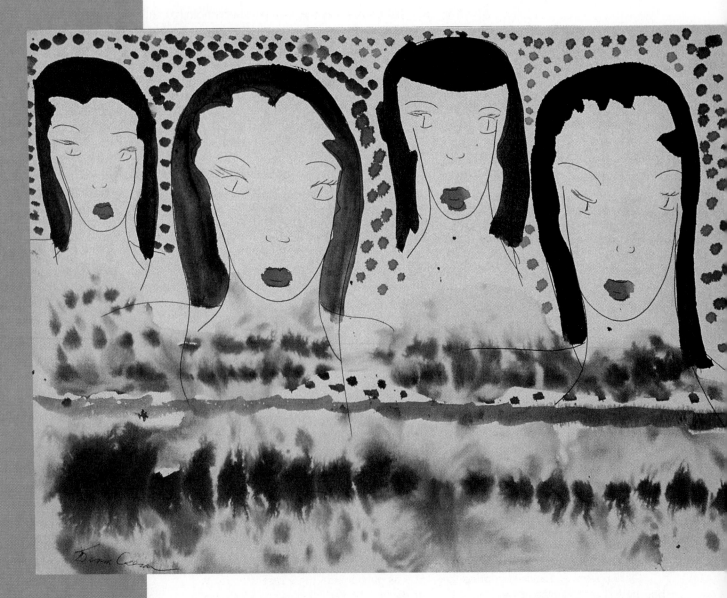

Donna Caesar, **Four Faces,** HAI

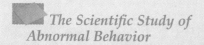
L aura sat in the waiting room, thinking about the therapy session she was going to have with Dr. Paul at the Eating Disorders Unit of the New York State Psychiatric Institute. She had come to Manhattan a year ago as a 22-year-old-college graduate, ready to pursue her goal of becoming a fashion model.

It had been a struggle. Laura was always short of money. To make ends meet, she had taken a variety of temporary jobs and shared a small apartment with an aspiring actress. The two women had little in common and went their separate ways. Laura had a boyfriend, but he insisted on dating other women and would not make an emotional commitment to her.

The stress and loneliness in Laura's life made her eating disorder worse. Actually, this had been a problem, on and off, over the last five years. She would binge eat several times a week and then try to get rid of the food by vomiting. She always felt ashamed and guilty when she did this, but she was even more scared of gaining weight and jeopardizing her modeling prospects.

Feeling trapped and increasingly hopeless, Laura finally confided in a friend at the modeling agency. The friend had seen other young models with eating disorders and knew this was a serious problem. She suggested that Laura see a therapist. Laura remembered reading about a free treatment program for eating disorders at a prominent psychiatric institute in New York City.

Laura made an appointment. During her first visit, she met with a research assistant, who had her complete several questionnaires and two lengthy interviews. The questions asked were designed to see if she met the selection criteria for the treatment program, which was being offered as part of a major research study on **bulimia nervosa,** funded by the National Institute of Mental Health.

Laura was accepted for treatment, but she wasn't sure what to expect as a research subject. Her concerns were soon put to rest. Laura liked the friendly and cheerful young research assistant who coordinated all the data collection. And she was impressed with the psychotherapist, Dr. Smith; she seemed to really care and immediately understood the problems Laura was having with eating. Laura trusted Dr. Smith and found it easy to open up and talk. The psychiatrist assigned to Laura was a young man, Dr. Paul. He had a gentle, encouraging manner and always made her feel welcome; he was attentive whenever he assessed Laura's reactions to the medication she was taking.

Only once was Laura reminded that she was participating in a research study. She had seen a therapist on a TV talk show who claimed that eating disorders result from traumatic experiences in childhood. Laura disclosed that bad things had happened to her as a child and that she was considering joining a support group for individuals with similar experiences. She mentioned this to Dr. Paul, who reminded her that one of the criteria for her being part of the study was that she not be involved in any other form of treatment. Dr. Paul encouraged her to devote all her energy to the therapy she was in now, dealing with her eating disorder. He promised to discuss any ideas Laura might have about additional treatment at the end of the 20-week program.

Laura was just about to have her twelfth session. As she waited, she thought about the progress she had made. Her eating had improved, and the pattern of binge eating and vomiting had virtually stopped. She felt less depressed and much more hopeful about the future, despite continuing problems with her boyfriend. She wondered if her improvement was due to the drug or the sessions with Dr. Paul. The truth was, she wasn't even sure that she was *on* the drug. But more and more, she suspected that she was because of general feelings of fatigue as well as dryness in her mouth. She had been informed that these were common side effects of the medication. (In fact, Laura *was* receiving the medication, not a *placebo*, or so-called sugar pill, which contains no active substance.) Whatever the case, she was glad she had been accepted for treatment. She hadn't solved all her problems, but she was on the right track.

Laura's experience is representative of subjects in clinical trials that assess the effectiveness of psychological and pharmacological (drug) treatments. In this chapter, we will discuss the details of this type of study, plus a variety of other research strategies for investigating the causes and treatments of clinical disorders.

THE SCIENTIFIC STUDY OF ABNORMAL BEHAVIOR

The scientific study of abnormal behavior tries to discover patterns and trends that can be used as the foundation for general laws that explain apparently diverse bits of behavior.

For example, you may have noticed that when your friends drink alcohol, they often behave in very different ways. Some become aggressive, even mean; others become talkative and social; and still others become amorous, maybe looking for sex. How can the same substance—alcohol—have such varying effects on us?

It makes sense if you understand the effects that alcohol has on the brain. Research has shown that when we drink alcohol, we do things we wouldn't usually do. Normally, we have *inhibitions*—behaviors that are held in check by a common brain mechanism. One of the effects of alcohol is to reduce our inhibitions and release those behaviors from control. So all these apparently unrelated effects of drinking can be explained by a single mechanism: reduced inhibitions (Gray, 1985). This gives us a general principle that links and explains otherwise unrelated instances of behavior.

Two important concepts in scientific research are reliability and validity. *Reliability* means that a psychological measure, such as a test or questionnaire, produces consistent results; its findings can be replicated, or obtained again, in further experimentation. *Validity* means that a psychological measure accurately captures what the researcher wanted to study; the test or survey measures what it was supposed to measure.

In the following sections, we will look at reliability and validity in regard to assessment, diagnosis, and research.

bulimia nervosa Eating disorder characterized by binge eating and extreme weight-control behaviors, such as self-induced vomiting; rooted in abnormal attitudes about the importance of body shape and weight.

Reliability

To meet scientific standards, a diagnosis or finding must be reliable. At a minimum, it must be consistent and replicable. **Reliability** can be established in different ways. Suppose that you want to find out whether a clinical interview is a reliable means of diagnosing depression. One strategy would be to have two different clinicians conduct interviews with the same patient and then compare notes, determining how much they agree on the diagnosis. A second strategy would be to have the same clinician interview the patient on two different occasions and then compare his observations for consistencies. Whatever approach is used, the extent to which the findings from the two interviews are consistent would provide a measure of reliability.

Before they can be accepted, research results must be repeated under carefully specified conditions—ideally, by different investigators in different research centers. To ensure reliability, researchers must describe and define the phenomena they study in precise terms that other investigators can clearly understand. For example, *anxiety* can have several different meanings, ranging from arousal of the autonomic nervous system (for instance, increased heartrate and blood pressure) to subjective self-reports of fear (such as "I feel uptight"). Using these different operational definitions of *anxiety,* we could make reliable and useful measurements: one of heartrates and the other of self-reports of fear (Rachman, 1990). But we would be assessing two separate things.

Thus, individual researchers must clearly define and describe the phenomena they study to ensure reliability. Otherwise, their findings have no legitimate basis for comparison.

Validity

Validity refers to the accuracy of a test or measure—as mentioned earlier, how well it does what it was intended to do. There are several types of validity. Let's look at some examples involving eating disorders.

Suppose we want to determine the validity of a clinical interview as a means of assessing bulimia nervosa. To be valid, the interview should discriminate patients with this eating disorder from patients with other disorders and also from normal subjects. This is called *discriminant validity.* Using a particular model, or theoretical framework, we might also want to determine how much the results of the interview overlap with the findings of other measures of behavior. For example, to be valid, the findings of the interview should correlate with those from other measures of disturbance in eating behavior and attitudes toward body weight and shape. This is known as *construct validity. Predictive validity* refers to the ability of the interview to predict the future course of the patient's disorder.

When we discuss specific research designs, later in this chapter, you will understand how validity applies to experimental designs and the accuracy and usefulness of the findings they yield.

Theory

A scientific **theory** is an explicit and formal statement of a set of propositions designed to explain a particular phenomenon. A theory must meet three criteria:

1. It should clearly explain and integrate the information currently known about the phenomenon in question.
2. It must be testable, using rigorous experiments designed to either support or refute it.
3. It should stimulate research leading to new findings.

reliability Consistency or replicability of a test, measure, or finding.

validity Degree to which a test or measure accurately captures what it was intended to.

theory Formal statement of a set of propositions designed to explain a particular phenomenon.

One practical consequence of theory is that it can guide research and help determine what will be discovered. Consider another example about eating disorders. By the mid-1980s, three facts had become clear about bulimia nervosa. First, it had come to the attention of clinicians during the 1970s. Second, the disorder occurs predominantly in women. And third, it strikes mainly in adolescence and young adulthood (Fairburn, Hay, & Welch, 1993). Why? To make sense of these different facts, behavioral and social scientists came up with a theory.

Striegel-Moore and her colleagues (Striegel-Moore, Silberstein, & Rodin, 1986) proposed that cultural norms about female beauty changed at the end of the 1960s. *Thin* became *in*. And because physical attractiveness is more important for women than men in U.S. society, women came under intense social pressure to conform to the new ideal body weight and shape. But not all women felt this pressure in the same way. Researchers theorized that adolescents and young adults would experience the greatest pressure to look like the slim, "hard body" models on magazine covers. Being popular and dating is especially important to adolescent girls, and looking attractive is a big part of achieving that goal. To make themselves look the right way, young women increasingly resorted to rigid and unhealthy dieting. And it was hypothesized that this unhealthy dieting—driven by the cultural pressure to be thin—put women at risk for bulimia nervosa.

If you review what's been said about theory thus far, you'll see that this one about bulimia nervosa meets all the criteria. First, it explains the facts known about bulimia nervosa, as described above. Second, the theory is testable. For instance, researchers could test the observation that people usually start the pattern of binge eating and purging after a period of rigid dieting. Another testable prediction is that the women who are under the most pressure for thinness—for instance, fashion models, gymnasts, and ballet dancers—have especially high rates of eating disorders. (We discuss the cases of several prominent gymnasts in Chapter 11.)

Finally, a theory should be *heuristic*, meaning that it should stimulate new ideas and innovative research. This theory about bulimia nervosa has done just that. One new study (Heffernan, in press) has examined the theory that bulimia nervosa occurs less often in lesbians than heterosexual women. This theory assumes that lesbians reject the traditional feminine role and emphasis on physical attractiveness. Hence, lesbians should be less vulnerable to these cultural pressures and less likely to diet to influence body weight and shape. The results of this study show that lesbians do reject the feminine role, in general, but not its emphasis on the importance of body weight. Lesbians are as likely to report problems with eating as heterosexual women.

A second practical use of theory is in guiding therapists in clinical practice as they try to understand their patients' problems and devise useful assessment and treatment strategies. For example, the theory about the cause and effect of bulimia nervosa led to development of the currently most effective treatment for this disorder (Fairburn & Wilson, 1993). (This treatment is described in Chapter 11.)

The Importance of Research and Research Training

Throughout this book, we give examples of how research has improved the everyday lives of people with clinical disorders. The antidepressant drug Prozac, which is

Thinness is an important feature of the ideal body among adolescent and young adult white women in U.S. culture. The body shape and weight of the models in women's magazines is part of a cultural emphasis on the perfect body shape and weight that is believed to be one of the causes of eating disorders among young women.

used to treat anxiety and mood disorders, has helped countless people live happier and more productive lives. Prozac is an example of a high-tech, "designed drug" (Kramer, 1993) that was developed according to a theoretical blueprint. Based on their knowledge about the biology of depression (see Chapter 7), researchers set out to develop a drug that would have a specific effect. They wanted to single out serotonin, one of the neurotransmitters in the brain, without altering other neurotransmitters, so that the side effects would be fewer. Their success in doing so marked a new era in the development of drugs to treat abnormal behavior (see Chapter 20).

Scientific research is also important in establishing the truth about abnormal behavior. Research has shown, again and again, that some popularly held beliefs about abnormal behavior are simply not true. In many cases, these beliefs have come from well-meaning clinicians, who jump to unfounded conclusions. As we'll describe later in this chapter, erroneous and even damaging beliefs about abnormal behavior flourish in the absence of well-validated theories and systematic feedback about their value (Dawes, 1994).

For example, until the 1960s, it was widely assumed that autism in children was largely caused by cold, inexpressive parents who did not provide their children with the affection required for normal development (see Chapter 15). Imagine the personal suffering this assumption caused families who were already devastated by having an autistic child. Sadly, this anguish was unnecessary. We know today that childhood autism is caused by biological factors, which parents have no control over.

Despite the progress that's been made, the complex nature of major clinical disorders remains something of a mystery. Given this uncertainty, we need to approach the study of abnormal behavior in an open, questioning manner. In response to any theory about the cause or cure of a disorder, we should say "Prove it." And the best way to do this is through research and research training.

Focus on Critical Thinking

Bulimia nervosa was first diagnosed in the 1970s, with the start of the social pressure on young women to be thin in order to be considered attractive and popular. The women who were adolescents at that time are now in their thirties and forties. Most have probably gone on to get married, and given divorce rates, many have probably gotten divorced or will eventually. As a result, they are or will be single again in middle age. Keeping all this in mind, critique the theory that bulimia nervosa may increase among middle-aged, divorced women. Does it meet the criteria of a scientific theory? Why or why not?

RESEARCH STRATEGIES

Controlled Experiments

Experimental methods are needed to establish that one event causes another. In an experimental study, one variable—called the **independent variable**—is manipulated, or controlled, by the researcher in order to measure the effects on another variable or variables—called **dependent variables.** An experimental effect is demonstrated when manipulating the independent variable produces reliable effects on one or more of the dependent variables.

Consider another example about the effects of anxiety. Based on uncontrolled case studies, clinicians have long hypothesized that anxiety interferes with or decreases sexual arousal (Masters & Johnson, 1970). David Barlow and his colleagues tested this hypothesis with a laboratory experiment (Barlow, Sakheim, & Beck, 1983). The subjects were three groups of normal, male college students who watched an erotic film; afterward, their sexual arousal was assessed by measuring penile erection (see Figure 4.1). The men in group 1 were told that if they did not become sexually aroused, they stood a 60 percent chance of receiving an electric

independent variable Variable manipulated by the researcher in an experiment by randomly assigning subjects to treatment conditions.

dependent variable Variable the researcher expects to be influenced by the independent variable in an experiment.

FIGURE 4.1 The effects of anxiety on sexual arousal

Sexual arousal was measured as average penile circumference change in millimeters for each 15-s epoch during each of three conditions: contingent shock threat, non-contingent shock threat, and no shock threat.

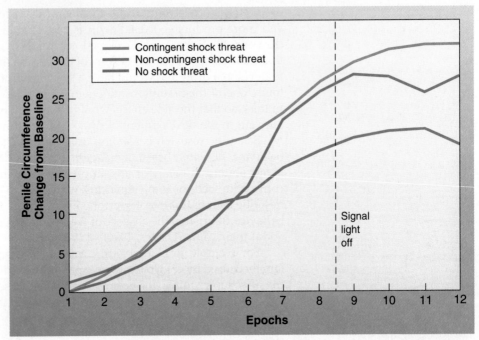

Source: From "Anxiety Increases Sexual Arousal" by D. H. Barlow, D. K. Sakheim, and J. G. Beck, *Journal of Abnormal Psychology, 92,* p. 52. Copyright © 1983 by the American Psychological Association. Reprinted by permission.

shock to the hand. The group 2 subjects were told that they might be shocked, regardless of whether they became sexually aroused. The subjects in group 3 were not exposed to the threat of shock. Contrary to the researchers' hypothesis, anxiety did not decrease sexual arousal; instead, it increased arousal (see Chapter 8).

In the Barlow experiment, anxiety was the independent variable. To manipulate this variable in the laboratory, the experimenters defined anxiety in terms of the threat of receiving an electric shock. This is an example of an **operational definition.** (No subject was ever actually shocked; it was the threat of receiving a shock that was manipulated.) Sexual arousal was the dependent variable; it was defined as a change in penile erection.

Hypotheses   Simply put, the **hypothesis** is what an experiment is designed to test. Because it leads to new experiments and observations, the hypothesis is the main intellectual instrument in research. It must be testable in order to specify conditions under which it can be disproved. We test a hypothesis by specifying an independent variable to manipulate in the experiment, as just described in the Barlow study.

Researchers generate hypotheses in different ways. Systematic observation of behavior by clinical researchers and practitioners has been a principal source of hypotheses in the study of abnormal behavior. For example, psychodynamically oriented investigators have produced a wealth of hypotheses from their clinical observations of individual patients. Other researchers derive hypotheses from reading the published literature. The creativity and critical thinking involved in generating testable hypotheses is illustrated in the Thinking about Research box.

Internal Validity   The **internal validity** of a study is the degree to which change in the dependent variable (or variables) is due to manipulation of the independent variable. Ruling out alternative explanations of the results increases the internal validity of the experiment and enables the researcher to conclude that the independent variable caused the change.

Suppose we need to test the hypothesis that a particular psychological therapy cures depression. We select a sample of individuals who are depressed and assess

operational definition
Description of a construct in objective, measurable terms.

hypothesis What an experiment is designed to test.

internal validity Degree to which change in the dependent variable is due to manipulation of the independent variable.

In 1964, as a first-year graduate student in experimental psychology at the University of Pennsylvania, Martin Seligman helped conduct a study on the transfer of learning about fear in dogs (Seligman, 1991). The first phase of the research consisted of Pavlovian conditioning; accordingly, the dogs were repeatedly exposed first to a tone and then to a brief shock. The idea was to get the dogs to associate the neutral tone with the noxious shock—to pair them—so that later, when the dogs heard the tone, they would react to it with fear—as if it were a shock.

In the second phase, the dogs were taken to a large shuttle box, divided into two compartments by a low wall. The investigators wanted to see if the dogs would react to the tones in the same way they would to the shock—that is, by jumping the wall to enter the other compartment. If the dogs would do this, it would show that emotional learning could transfer across different situations. The dogs first had to learn to jump over the barrier to escape the shock, something they typically learn easily. After that, they could be tested to see if the tones alone evoked the same reaction. The problem was that the dogs didn't even try to get away from the shocks. They just lay there, whimpering while receiving the shocks.

Seligman's insight was that the dogs had learned that they couldn't do anything to stop the shocks. During phase 1, the Pavlovian conditioning, they had felt the shocks go on and off, regardless of whether they struggled, jumped, barked, or did nothing at all. They had concluded, or *learned,* that their attempts to escape were futile. Seligman described his excitement at this realization as follows: "I was stunned by the implications. If dogs could learn something as complex as the futility of their actions, here was an analogy to human helplessness, one that could be studied in the laboratory."

Seligman and fellow graduate student Steve Maier designed an experiment to see if dogs could learn helplessness. Seligman and Maier (1967) used what is known as a *yoked-control design.* One group of dogs received escapable shocks, which they could turn off by pushing a panel with their noses. In other words, they had control over their environment. A second group of dogs was "yoked" to the first. These dogs received exactly the same shocks as those in the first group, but nothing they did had any effect on the shocks. They had no control; they were helpless. A third group of dogs received no shocks at all.

Following this experience, the dogs were placed in the shuttlebox. The crucial test was whether they would learn to escape from the shocks by easily jumping over the barrier

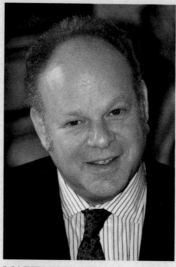

MARTIN SELIGMAN

into the other compartment. The results showed that two groups of dogs easily learned to jump over the barrier: those who had learned that they could control the shocks and those who had received no shocks. But the dogs who found that nothing they did mattered made no effort to escape. They gave up and lay down, despite being regularly shocked.

These findings about learned helplessness were so compelling that they were published in the *Journal of Experimental Psychology,* one of the most prestigious journals in experimental psychology (Seligman & Meier, 1967). The results directly contradicted the behaviorist view (which was dominant at the time) that learning occurs only when a response produces a reward or punishment. Seligman and Maier showed that the dogs had learned to expect that their actions were futile.

Seligman then went on to apply his findings to people. With his colleagues, he showed that on laboratory tasks, most people gave up when confronted with outcomes they had no control over—but not all. Roughly one-third persevered, instead of giving up. With the help of Lyn Abramson, a graduate student, and John Teasdale, a colleague from Oxford, Seligman reformulated the theory of learned helplessness (Abramson, Seligman, & Teasdale, 1978). These researchers argued that the key to learned helplessness is the way people explain to themselves the things that happen to them.

The way we explain these things to ourselves—our *explanatory style*—is based on three factors:

1. *Endurance*—Is the success or failure permanent or only temporary?
2. *Universality*—Is the success or failure general or specific?
3. *Causation*—Is the success or failure due to my actions or the result of circumstances?

In explaining personal failures and other bad experiences, people who view the causes as being temporary, specific, and outside themselves tend to be optimists. Those who view their setbacks as permanent, universal, and brought on by themselves tend to be pessimists. Not surprisingly, the first group—the optimists—are less vulnerable to depression and physical illness than the second group—the pessimists.

Think about the following question:

1. Reflect on your own reactions to life events—your failures and successes. What is your explanatory style? Are you usually an optimist or a pessimist?

the extent of their depression. This is known as *pretreatment assessment.* For the next four months, we treat the subjects using the therapy we're testing. Next, we reassess the subjects on the same measures as before; this is the *posttreatment assessment.* We find that the subjects are significantly less depressed at posttreatment than they were at pretreatment. Did the therapy cause the improvement?

Our results are consistent with the hypothesis that this particular therapy is effective in curing depression. But success could also be attributed to other factors. For example, over the four-month treatment period, the subjects may have improved by themselves. There is good evidence that **spontaneous remission** such as this happens (Rachman & Wilson, 1980). In fact, the possibility of spontaneous remission occurring during this hypothetical experiment is quite good. Depression is a cyclical disorder. Perhaps at the time of the posttreatment assessment, patients were at the point in their cycle when depression was declining.

Another possible explanation of the result of this hypothetical experiment is that repeated testing of the subjects may have had some unintended therapeutic effect. Perhaps the testing prompted patients to reflect on their problems and become more aware of the thoughts and activities that made them depressed. This valuable insight might have enabled the individuals to make some changes in their lives, thus decreasing their depression. The point is that we must consider these alternative explanations of the causes of experimental results. The results could be due to variables other than the independent variable, called **confounds,** which undermine the internal validity of the experiment.

Use of a control group rules out confounds and alternative causal explanations of the hypothesis. A **control group** is functionally the same as the experimental (treatment) group on all relevant dimensions except the one being manipulated. Refer back to the Barlow et al. (1983) experiment on anxiety and sexual arousal. In it, the control group consisted of subjects of the same age, sex, and college status as those in the two experimental groups. The only difference between the control and experimental groups was that the latter were exposed to the threat of an electric shock.

To improve on the hypothetical study of the treatment of depression, depressed patients would be assigned to an experimental or a control group on a random basis. **Random assignment** means that each subject has an equal chance of being in either the experimental or control group. When the number of subjects is sufficiently large, this method is frequently used to ensure that there are no differences between subjects in the experimental and control groups before the experimental treatment or manipulation.

During posttreatment assessment, researchers would evaluate whether individuals in the experimental (treatment) group were significantly more or less depressed than those in the control group. If the experimental group were significantly less depressed, we would have strong evidence that the therapy caused the improvement. We could eliminate the possible confounding role of spontaneous recovery or the effects of repeated testing. Also, by randomly assigning individuals to groups, we could rule out any explanation based on subjects' having different characteristics prior to treatment.

Control Groups Researchers employ different types of control conditions, depending on the independent variable being manipulated. Studies of the effects of drugs on behavior illustrate several of the issues that investigators must consider in choosing appropriate control groups.

To analyze the effects of alcohol and other drugs on behavior, studies usually compare the given drug with a placebo (or chemically inert drug, discussed earlier in this chapter). Figure 4.2 shows this comparison as group I versus group II, in which the experimenter's goal is to hold everything constant except the active chemical agent: alcohol (Marlatt & Rohsenow, 1980). The subjects in group II are led to believe that they're consuming the real thing, which allows researchers to

spontaneous remission Improvement in the patient's condition over time in the absence of formal therapy.

confounds Factors other than the independent variable that could explain changes in the dependent variable.

control group Group of subjects that is functionally the same as the experimental group on all dimensions except the one being manipulated.

random assignment Procedure for assigning subjects to treatment groups such that each subject has an equal chance of being in either the experimental or control group; improves the chances that subjects' characteristics will be equally distributed across treatment conditions in an experiment.

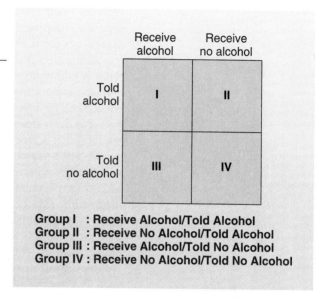

FIGURE 4.2 The effects of alcohol and expectations about those effects

Group I   : Receive Alcohol/Told Alcohol
Group II : Receive No Alcohol/Told Alcohol
Group III : Receive Alcohol/Told No Alcohol
Group IV : Receive No Alcohol/Told No Alcohol

control for the subjects' expectations and beliefs about alcohol's effects. If the results of the experiment show that group I differs from group II, this difference can be attributed to the effects of alcohol.

But what if the researcher thinks that variables such as expectations about the drug affect behavior independently or interact with the drug? To answer this question, it's necessary to test expectations. Figure 4.2 illustrates the *balanced placebo,* which allows us to evaluate the separate and interactive effects of alcohol and the subject's expectations (Marlatt & Rohsenow, 1980). Doing so requires the addition of groups III and IV to the traditional comparison between alcohol and a placebo drink. The subjects in these two groups are led to believe that they have consumed a nonalcoholic beverage, whereas those in groups I and II believe they have consumed alcohol. In this design, both the actual consumption of alcohol and beliefs about its effects are experimentally manipulated.

Use of the balanced placebo design has produced surprising and important findings (see also Chapter 9). Investigators have used this design to study the effects of alcohol on sexual arousal. Clinical and survey findings show that acts of sexual aggression are often correlated with intoxication (Wilson, 1981). To better understand this, Briddell and his colleagues (1978) conducted an experiment in which they randomly assigned male college students to the four groups of the balanced placebo design. All subjects listened to one audiotape portraying mutually enjoyable heterosexual intercourse and another portraying forcible rape. Sexual arousal was measured by degree of penile erection while subjects listened to the tapes.

The study found that changes in subjects' sexual arousal was produced by the *belief* that they had been drinking but not by actual alcohol consumption. As might be expected, subjects who believed that they were sober showed substantial arousal to the audiotape depicting mutually consensual sex and little arousal to the tape depicting forcible rape. In contrast, subjects who believed they had been drinking showed almost the same level of sexual arousal to both tapes. These disturbing findings led researchers to conclude that normal heterosexual males who believe that they've been drinking can show a pattern of sexual responsiveness that is similar to that of rapists (Briddell et al., 1978).

Although the balanced placebo design has helped encourage experimental analysis of individual expectations in alcohol research, this approach has one major limitation: It works well only when subjects are given low doses of alcohol—the equivalent of one or two drinks. At higher doses, it's very difficult to convince subjects who actually receive alcohol that they have simply been given a nonalcoholic placebo. In other words, at higher doses, it seems virtually impossible to completely separate the pharmacological effects of the alcohol from the person's knowledge that he has consumed alcohol (Sayette, Breslin, Wilson, & Rosenblum, 1994).

A common practice in conducting experimental studies of drug effects is to use what is known as a **double-blind strategy.** This involves preventing both subjects and researchers from knowing who has received the drug versus the placebo; in effect, both groups are "blind" to the manipulation. In theory, double-blind control prevents the researcher from inadvertently giving subjects clues about whether they are receiving active treatment. In practice, however, this ideal is rarely achieved.

Recent research on the use of antidepressant drugs has shown that both patients and their psychiatrists typically know whether an active drug or placebo was given. Moreover, psychiatrists can even accurately distinguish among different types of medication (Margraf et al., 1991). All drugs have side effects that affect some patients more than others. Presumably, these side effects can lead both patients and their psychiatrists to identify who is receiving the real medication. Remember that Laura, from the chapter-opening case, didn't know whether she was receiving the antidepressant drug or a placebo; she suspected the former because of side effects such as a dry mouth and general fatigue.

This failure of control poses a serious threat to the internal validity of drug studies. Specifically, the pharmacological effects of the drug being studied are confounded with subjects' expectations about their likely consequences. Using placebos that have active side effects might improve the internal validity of studies and ultimately lead to more effective treatment. However, the scientific benefits of such a strategy would have to be balanced against the risks of deliberately inducing negative physical reactions in patients receiving only placebos.

As discussed throughout this book, research on abnormal behavior often involves complex ethical issues, such as this. They have to be decided by careful judgment of the ratio of relative risk to benefit for the subject or patient. We'll return to consider ethical issues in psychological research later in this chapter.

External Validity The **external validity** of a study is the degree to which its findings can be generalized to other individuals in different settings. For example, it's unclear whether the findings from the Briddell et al. (1978) study, described earlier, and other similar laboratory experiments can be applied to behavior in the real world. Sexual arousal in a laboratory—an artificial setting—might not adequately reflect individuals' typical responses in more natural settings.

Conducting experimental research in real-life settings—sometimes referred to as **field research**—would seem to solve some of these external validity problems. Yet field research is exceedingly more complex and costly than research done in a laboratory. External validity is vital for research on the effects of treatment of abnormal behavior. The most direct way to study the effects of treatment would be to design an experiment in which experienced therapists treated actual patients under clinical conditions. This would be difficult to do, for several reasons. From a methodological point of view, experimenters find it hard to conduct highly controlled research in service-delivery settings. From a practical point of view, recruiting experienced therapists who have the time and desire to participate in such research is difficult. Finding large enough numbers of patients with common problems and other characteristics is another formidable task. Finally, from an ethical point of view, it's inappropriate to assign clients to control groups that will not receive the most effective form of treatment, particularly if their disorder is serious.

An alternative research strategy to studying the clinical situation directly is to evaluate specific treatment methods that have been applied to well-defined problems under controlled laboratory conditions. This is commonly called **analogue research.** For example, subjects who have intense anxiety (phobias) about small animals are used to study the nature of anxiety and its treatment. This approach

double-blind strategy Administration of medication in an experiment in which neither the patient nor the therapist knows whether the medication is an active drug or a pill placebo.

external validity Degree to which the findings of a particular experiment can be generalized to other subjects under other circumstances.

field research Research design in which subjects are randomly assigned to treatment conditions in natural settings.

analogue research Experimental treatment research conducted in the laboratory under highly controlled conditions with carefully selected subjects.

ntil recently, there was a clearcut pattern among researchers in selecting subjects for the study of clinical disorders. In the past, samples were primarily young, white males, and findings from these studies were generalized to the larger population. As a result, relatively little was learned about the nature and prevalence of clinical disorders among women and people from ethnic and racial groups. And perhaps worse yet, inaccurate assumptions were made in believing that these research findings could be generalized.

This lack of research and knowledge is an incredible disparity, considering that over half the U.S. population is female and another 25 percent is made up of ethnic and racial minorities (United States Bureau of the Census, 1990). Moreover, as U.S. demographics change, the proportion of minorities will likely increase rapidly. Certainly, the increasing cultural diversity of the United States has important implications for research. We cannot assume that conclusions drawn from research using samples of young, white males necessarily apply to other groups.

In fact, there is growing evidence that ethnic and racial minorities may differ in their compliance with and response to antidepressant medication (Muñoz, Hollon, McGrath, Rehm, & Vandenbos, 1994). For example, Hispanic patients may require less antidepressant med-

ication and report more side effects at lower doses than white patients (Mendoza, Smith, Poland, Lin, & Strickland, 1991).

In response to these concerns, federal guidelines now require that all proposals for research grants include truly representative samples: males and females, individuals from ethnic and racial minorities, and the young and old. The goal is to ensure that findings will benefit all people at risk for the particular disorder being studied. The guidelines do allow researchers to exclude one sex or to study only one ethnic group if a compelling rationale is given for doing so. For instance, it is acceptable to use only young, female subjects in a study of the treatment of eating disorders because these disorders are associated almost exclusively with that group; eating disorders occur only rarely in males and older women (Hsu, 1990).

Think about the following questions:

1. By requiring greater diversity among subject samples, the federal government is emphasizing the importance of what kind of validity? Explain your answer.

2. In requiring greater diversity among research subjects, is the federal government simply being politically correct, or does this initiative have genuine scientific merit? Explain your answer.

has several advantages. First, the treatment method can be standardized, and a wide range of subjective and objective measures of behavioral change can be obtained. And second, by selecting a homogeneous subject population with the same problem behavior, researchers can evaluate the particular problem the specific treatment is best suited for.

Recruiting subjects by advertising a program and contacting physicians and other appropriate treatment facilities has been a common tactic in research on treatment effectiveness. Critics charge that subjects who are recruited this way are by nature different from individuals who seek therapy on their own. However, studies have failed to show differences in treatment effects between individuals recruited for clinical research and those who initiated treatment on their own (O'Leary & Wilson, 1987).

Whether the findings of a research study can be generalized to therapeutic situations applies to all clinical research, including studies conducted with patients in actual therapeutic settings. In evaluating therapy outcome research, the critical question is: How much do the conditions of the study approximate the clinical situation? The generalizability of a study needs evaluation along several different dimensions, including the kind of problem being studied or treated, the type of subject, subject motivation for treatment, therapist characteristics and training, nature of the treatment method and how it might vary from the way it's usually administered in clinical practice, assessment of treatment effects, and so on (Kazdin & Wilson, 1978). Researchers generally assume that the more similar the study is to the clinical situation, the greater the generalizability of the results.

Quasi-Experimental Methods

By randomly assigning sufficient numbers of subjects to different groups, we ensure—at least in principle—that the experimental and control groups are alike on all relevant dimensions except the one being manipulated, or tested. In reality, however, it's often impossible to randomly assign subjects to experimental and control groups. Imagine, for example, a study of the effects that being a child of an alcoholic parent (COA) has on cognitive functioning. A child cannot randomly be made the biological offspring of an alcoholic or a nonalcoholic. Preexisting subject characteristics—specifically, being a COA—inevitably confound the experiment. A true experiment—which demands random assignment to the experimental variable—cannot, therefore, be conducted.

Quasi-experimental methods are used to study preexisting individual differences. In a quasi-experiment, membership in a class or category defines the experimental group. Typical groups in research on abnormal psychology are subjects who are COAs; subjects who share specific psychopathologies, such as schizophrenia; and subjects who have experienced common life events, such as divorce or bereavement.

The control group in a quasi-experiment is selected to match the experimental group on known personal characteristics that might confound interpretation of results, except for the independent variable. In studying the effects that being a COA has on cognitive functioning, then, a control group of non-COAs would match the experimental COA group in terms of age, sex, socioeconomic status, current drinking status, and degree of psychopathology, among other factors. The case-control design is an example of a quasi-experimental design.

Even with a carefully chosen control group, there is no guarantee that the two groups are identical, except with respect to the independent variable. Thus, even if COAs (the independent variable) score more poorly on a test of cognitive functioning (the dependent variable) than non-COAs, being a COA cannot be inferred as the cause. The experimental and control groups may have differed in terms of another, unknown confounding variable.

A good example of a quasi-experimental study is the Stanford Five-City Project (Farquhar et al., 1990) (see also Chapter 10). It was designed to reduce risk factors for heart disease in an entire community—for instance, encouraging people to stop cigarette smoking, reduce their blood pressure, and decrease their intake of dietary fat. The psychosocial intervention program (the independent variable) aimed at changing these health-related behaviors was implemented in two rural communities; three other communities served as the control groups. Before the intervention began, the five communities were carefully matched on relevant dimensions, such as frequency of cigarette smoking, blood pressure, and dietary patterns. Because subjects were not randomly assigned to the independent variable, however, we cannot rule out the possibility that the communities were different in one or more ways.

A quasi-experimental design does not allow strong inferences about causation. Confidence in the finding obtained will ultimately depend on eliminating the effects of group differences that may have correlated with the observed result. Eliminating these effects requires repeated replication of the basic finding by different research groups using different samples. If the result is replicated under these varying conditions, there is greater confidence that the result has not been confounded with some unknown, correlated variable.

Criteria for subject selection are essential in interpreting the results of any study. As discussed, if the experimental and control groups differ in any way other than the experimental manipulation, there is a confound across the two groups. But depending on the subject-selection criteria, a confound may also exist within the experimental group. For example, researchers comparing COAs with non-COAs try to select only those subjects who don't show a drinking problem. If one or more subjects did have a drinking problem, it would make it impossible for researchers to attribute any difference observed between COAs and non-COAs to the influence

quasi-experimental methods Studies in which membership in a class or category defines the experimental group; for example, a case-control design.

of having an alcoholic parent. Yet Sher (1985) has shown that by excluding COAs who are problem drinkers, researchers diminish their chances of demonstrating real differences between COAs and non-COAs. By eliminating individuals showing drinking problems as young adults, those particular high-risk subjects who were the initial focus of experimental interest may be lost.

Correlational Designs

Correlational designs assess the extent to which two or more variables are related. A **correlation coefficient** is the mathematical expression of that relationship and ranges from –1 to +1. A correlation of 0 means that no association exists between two variables; their relationship is totally random. The closer the correlation coefficient is to +1, the stronger the *positive correlation,* or likelihood that the two variables occur together or in parallel fashion. The closer the coefficient is to –1, the stronger the *negative,* or *inverse, correlation,* indicating that the variables do not likely occur together or in parallel fashion. For example, there is a strong inverse correlation between obesity and social class (Goldblatt, Moore, & Stunkard, 1965). The lower the social class, the greater the incidence of obesity (see Figure 10.4). This conclusion has been replicated in more than 30 subsequent studies (Stunkard, 1989).

Researchers use correlational methods extensively in the study of abnormal behavior, particularly in clinical psychology (Cronbach, 1957). Most case studies are limited to single patients, though, whereas correlational research methods typically involve more systematic analyses of the characteristics or performances of entire groups of subjects. Research on personality theory illustrates the systematic nature of the correlational method. For example, suppose an individual scores high on a personality inventory measuring extraversion. According to the trait theory of personality, this extraverted person will behave predictably in different situations. To test the accuracy of these predictions, the personality researcher must measure the individual's behavior in different situations and then determine if these measures correlate significantly with the individual's score for extraversion on the personality inventory. The higher the correlation, the more confidence we can have that the questionnaire is accurately measuring the trait of extraversion.

Correlation and Causality   Correlational methods show only how much two or more events are *associated* with each other. Like case studies, they do not show anything about *causality*—particularly, whether one variable causes the other. For example, patients with eating disorders show high levels of depression, whereas normal dieters do not (Levy, Dixon, & Stern, 1989). In other words, eating disorders are positively correlated with depression: that is, they occur together. Beyond establishing this general finding, the correlation can also identify the nature of the relationship between the two clinical disorders. Three relationships are possible:

1. Depression causes eating disorders.
2. Depression results from eating disorders.
3. Neither causes the other; both depression and eating disorders are products of some third variable or disorder.

For example, an individual may have a genetic predisposition (tendency) to react to stressful life experiences with both depression and an eating disorder, perhaps because of abnormal biochemical functioning. If that's the case, these two disorders—depression and eating disorders—are correlated co-effects of the third variable—the biochemical abnormality.

We can use the "three C's" to help interpret a given correlation: One of the two variables in a correlation will be the *cause,* the *consequence,* or the *correlate* of the other. Sophisticated and powerful research tools are needed to sort out which of the three interpretations is correct and to identify the cause of the eating disorder. Through experimental methods, the depression could be treated and the eating

correlational designs
Research designs in which investigators gather information without altering subjects' experiences and examine relationships between variables; do not permit inferences about cause and effect.

correlation coefficient
Number describing the strength and direction of the relationship between two variables; ranges from +1 to –1.

disorder monitored for change; if the eating disorder changed, it would seem likely that the depression caused the eating disorder. Or the eating disorder could be treated directly and the depression observed; in this case, if the depression changed, it couldn't really be considered a consequence of the eating disorder. (This kind of research is discussed in Chapter 11.)

Epidemiological Research

Epidemiology is a correlational method that studies the prevalence, etiology, and consequences of physical diseases and mental disorders in a population. Epidemiological methods are used in research on how psychological or behavioral factors—such as hostility or cigarette smoking—can influence physical disease—such as heart disease. Epidemiological research studies the social conditions that correlate with specific physical and mental disorders and identifies individuals and groups who are at high risk for developing these disorders.

The famous Framingham Heart Study (Dawber, Meadors, & Moore, 1951) illustrates the value of epidemiological research. Beginning in 1948, a substantial percentage of the adult men and women in Framingham, Massachusetts, have been regularly tested for the development of heart disease. Nearly all these people were healthy when the study began. By continuing to assess their health-related behavior, researchers have shown the effects of high blood cholesterol, high blood pressure, cigarette smoking, obesity, and other risk factors in the development of heart disease. A **risk factor** is a characteristic that predicts illness, even though the reason for the increased risk is unclear. Once identified, the risk factor suggests the type of research needed to uncover the underlying cause or causes of the disease. Identification also encourages interventions to modify the risk factors and thus reduce the occurrence of the disease.

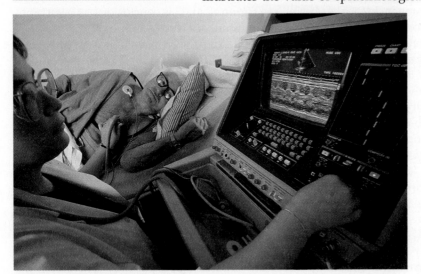

Results from the Framingham study have helped identify risk factors in heart disease.

epidemiology Correlational method that studies the prevalence, etiology, and consequences of physical disease and mental disorders in a population.

risk factor Predicts a clinical disorder and provides a clue to identifying its underlying causes; also encourages interventions to modify the risk and thus reduce the occurrence of the disorder.

Epidemiological research is also crucial in the study of mental health. In Chapter 1, we reviewed the results of epidemiological research showing the prevalence of different forms of abnormal behavior in the United States. Epidemiological family studies have examined the interaction between genetic and environmental factors in the development of abnormal behavior (Weissman, Leaf, Blazer, Boyd, & Florio, 1986). Studies of high-risk subjects focus on the children of parents with clinical disorders. The adult (parent) with the disorder is called the **proband.** The children of probands are at higher risk for developing disorders than comparable children of parents without disorders.

For example, this is true of children of depressed or alcoholic parents. The children are studied using a **longitudinal design,** in which information about them is collected repeatedly over a period of years. By studying changes in these children over time, risk factors that precede development of certain problems can be identified. Researchers can then devise ways to help the children cope with their situations, thereby preventing the development of abnormal behavior. Epidemiological studies can thus form the basis of prevention and treatment programs.

Another epidemiological method, **case-control design,** matches a person who has a clinical disorder with a *control*—namely, someone who doesn't have the disorder but who is similar in age, race, sex, and socioeconomic status. The prevalence

proband Individual who has a particular disorder; the focus of a study of familial transmission of a disorder.

longitudinal design Research design in which one group of subjects is studied repeatedly at different ages.

case-control design Design in which a person with a clinical disorder is matched with a control—namely, someone who does not have the disorder but is similar in age, race, sex, and socioeconomic status.

of the disorder among the family members of the proband (the person who has the disorder) is then compared to that among the family of the control. If the disorder is found more often among family members of the proband, researchers can conclude that the disorder runs in the family.

This evidence of **familial aggregation** does not prove that the disorder is transmitted genetically. Keep in mind that family members also share a common environment, so environmental influences cannot be ruled out. Yet evidence from family epidemiological studies improves our understanding about how disorders are transmitted. If a disorder is transmitted within a family, more powerful experimental designs can be used to separate genetic and environmental determinants of behavior.

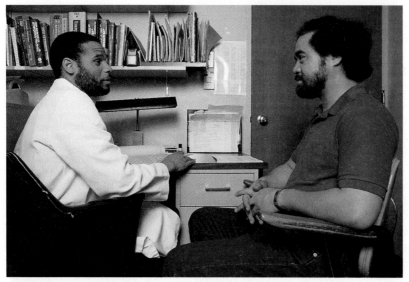

The clinical interview is one of the most important methods psychologists have for gathering detailed information about people's behavior.

Case-control studies also allow researchers to identify risk factors for clinical disorders. Clinicians commonly believe that childhood sexual abuse is a cause of eating disorders, among other things. Chris Fairburn and his colleagues at Oxford University tested this hypothesis in community samples of people with bulimia nervosa, some other clinical disorder, or no disorder at all (Fairburn, 1994). They assessed subjects using a **structured interview,** a method in which the researcher asks each subject the same questions in a standardized way; doing so allows for comparisons among subjects. A typical clinical interview is unstructured, so individual subjects may be asked different questions in a different manner and order; using this method makes it difficult to compare responses among subjects.

The results of the Fairburn study (1994) revealed that a history of sexual abuse was more common among subjects in the two groups with clinical disorders than in the normal controls. But there was no difference between the two groups with clinical disorders. This finding establishes that childhood sexual abuse increases the risk of developing some form of clinical disorder but is not a specific risk factor for bulimia nervosa. Epidemiological studies can never prove that particular risk factors cause particular disorders. They can show only varying degrees of correlation and suggest which risk factors researchers should analyze experimentally.

Recall from the case presented earlier that Laura had told her therapist that "bad things" had happened to her as a child. In response to Dr. Smith's gentle probing, Laura had disclosed that she'd been sexually abused by her stepfather from age 8 through 10. He had threatened to beat her if she said anything to anyone.

The psychotherapist on the TV talk show that Laura had watched had insisted that eating disorders typically result from childhood sexual abuse and that it's essential for treatment to focus on that experience. Laura had thought that she'd overcome her history of sexual abuse. Her mother had eventually left the stepfather and created a new life for Laura. The treatment program she was in made sense to her because it focused specifically on eating disorders. The psychotherapist on TV had been persuasive, though, claiming to have treated numerous cases just like her.

Laura also worried about her conflict with her boyfriend. The psychotherapist had also said that someone who had been sexually abused inevitably would have problems with close personal relationships. Laura's idea about joining a support group for incest survivors was based on this psychotherapist's recommendation.

Dr. Smith reacted with empathy and understanding to Laura's disclosure. But knowing the findings summarized earlier (Fairburn, 1994), she informed Laura that

familial aggregation Finding showing that the relatives of a person with a given disorder are more likely to have the disorder than would be expected by chance.

structured interview Method in which the researcher asks each subject the same questions in the same way.

sexual abuse did not necessarily lead to bulimia nervosa and that the problem could be treated successfully without focusing on her childhood experiences (see Chapter 11). Dr. Smith suggested that Laura stay with her current treatment program; after completing it, they would discuss the prospects of any additional therapy.

Laura responded very well to the treatment. It turned out that she received the combination of cognitive-behavioral therapy and drug treatment with Prozac—which proved to be the most effective approach as we describe later in this chapter.

Imagine what the outcome would have been if Laura had sought treatment from the psychotherapist on TV or someone who shared her views. The primary, if not exclusive, focus of therapy would have been on Laura's experience of childhood sexual abuse. Such a strategy would not be consistent with what's known about the development and treatment of bulimia nervosa (McElroy & Keck, 1995).

This case reminds us of how research findings can inform good clinical practice.

Berkson's Bias Epidemiological research is also necessary to avoid drawing false conclusions from samples of clinical patients. Imagine that you are a psychotherapist with a busy clinical practice, including many patients with eating disorders. Over time, you notice that at least one-third of these patients with eating disorders also report past or present problems of alcohol or drug abuse and dependence. You conclude that the incidence of alcohol and drug problems is unusually high among people with eating disorders. Would you be correct?

One problem in making an inference such as this is that your clinical sample of patients might be an unrepresentative subgroup. People who have two or more medical or psychiatric problems are more likely to seek treatment than those who have only one problem. Accordingly, people with both eating disorders and alcohol or drug use problems would more likely show up in clinical samples than people with only eating disorders. The result is a biased sample, or what is known as **Berkson's bias,** named after the physician who first pointed out this phenomenon (Helzer & Pryzbeck, 1988). A related problem might be that people who have both eating disorders and alcohol or drug use problems are seeking your therapeutic services because you have developed a reputation for treating patients with dual diagnoses.

The only way to test the validity of your inference about eating disorders and alcohol and drug use/dependence is to study how often these two problems occur together in a representative community sample. An important study in England has recently shown that the rate of co-occurrence between these two disorders is much higher in clinical samples than in the community (Fairburn, 1994). From this finding, we would conclude that there is no regular association between the two problems in the population at large, although they do seem to be linked in a subsample of individuals who seek treatment.

Berkson's bias Form of sampling bias in which people who have two or more medical or psychiatric problems are more likely to seek treatment than those who have only one problem; as a result, clinical samples are likely to contain more disturbed people than community samples.

case study Method in which the researcher attempts to understand the unique individual by combining interview data, observations, and sometimes test scores.

Case Studies

In a **case study,** the clinician observes and records the individual's current behavior and gathers information about her past: family, education, employment, crucial social relationships, and general level of psychological adjustment. This information is typically gathered in an interview with the person and may be supplemented by the results of psychological tests and material obtained from family members. The goal of the case study is to describe the patient's problem, relate it to her present and past functioning, and provide a theory about its causes.

The case study has been one of the most influential methods of studying abnormal behavior. All models of abnormal behavior have relied on the case study. For example, a small number of influential case studies established the work of Sigmund Freud (1856–1939). The Freudian, or psychodynamic, model once dominated our understanding and treatment of abnormal behavior and is still one of the most influential approaches. The behavioral model has relied on case studies. Masters and Johnson's (1970) report of a series of case studies on the nature and treatment of sexual dysfunction ushered in the era of sex therapy in the 1970s.

Advantages   Case studies make important contributions to the study of abnormal behavior, serving both scientific and clinical functions. Their scientific function is to provide a useful source of hypotheses that can be tested using powerful experimental methods. Consider, for instance, the radical changes that have recently taken place in our understanding of the anxiety disorders. According to the psychoanalytic model, which dominated American psychiatry until the 1970s (Goodwin, 1986), all anxiety is caused by *intrapsychic conflict,* or the threatened emergence of forbidden or unwanted impulses and feelings into our conscious awareness. In turn, all forms of psychopathology, including schizophrenia, are simply different manifestations of underlying anxiety.

Today, we know differently. In contrast to what was suggested by the psychoanalytic model, Klein (1981) hypothesized that there are qualitatively different types of anxiety and that they have distinctive biological mechanisms. His first evidence for this theory came from clinical case studies of severely anxious psychiatric inpatients. These patients had not responded to traditional therapy, so Klein treated them with imipramine, which was at the time a new drug that had proven effective as an antidepressant. The important finding was that the drug eliminated sudden, acute episodes of intense anxiety, although the patients remained generally apprehensive about the possibility of future episodes. By using the drug, Klein identified a specific type of anxiety reaction—what we call *panic attacks.* Most importantly, his clinical case studies suggested that panic is qualitatively different from other forms of anxiety. Subsequent controlled studies have confirmed Klein's clinical observations (Wolfe & Maser, 1994) (see Chapter 5).

The clinical function of case studies is to allow the report of therapeutic innovations and the description of clinical methods and strategies applied to particular clients. Consider, for example, the following case study:

> A forty-two-year-old housewife erroneously believed she was suffering from cardiac disease. Negative medical tests and reassurance from her physician failed to modify this belief. When asked what evidence she had for the idea that she had cardiac disease, she said that she noticed her heart more frequently than did her husband or colleagues at work and she thought this must indicate that there was something seriously wrong with it. The therapist suggested an alternative interpretation that the problem was her belief that there was something wrong with her heart. This belief then led her to selectively attend to her body, which in turn increased her awareness of her heart. When asked what she thought of this alternative, she said, "You psychologists are very good at thinking of clever explanations, and this would, no doubt, apply to some people, but I don't think that the effects of attention could be strong enough to account for my sensations." Rather than argue with this assertion, the therapist said, "You may be right. But perhaps to get more information it would be good if we did an experiment to see how strong the effects of attention are for you." In this experiment the patient was asked to close her eyes and concentrate on her heart for five minutes. To her great surprise, she found that simply attending to her heart enabled her to detect the pulse in her forehead, neck, arms, chest, and legs without touching these parts of the body. Furthermore, when she was subsequently asked to describe out loud the contents of the room for five minutes, she ceased to be aware of her heart. This demonstration reduced her belief that she had cardiac disease, increased her belief in the alternative explanation, and encouraged her to use distraction as a coping technique when she subsequently felt panicky. (Clark, 1989, p. 85)

This case study not only helps explain the nature of the woman's abnormal fear of heart disease but also provides information about how to treat such a fear. The clinical detail and practical focus of a good case study make it especially appealing to practitioners. Case studies used this way must meet some basic criteria:

1. Treatment methods must be described with sufficient detail and precision to allow replication by other therapists.
2. The methods must be applied to specific problems.
3. Any relevant personal characteristics of the patient must be reported.

Disadvantages Case studies cannot show that one event caused another, which means they cannot prove theories about the etiologies of clinical disorders nor can they establish that certain treatments cure disorders. The problem is that alternative explanations of the results cannot be ruled out. A case study is uncontrolled. The findings may be limited to the particular patient in question, or they may be due to the specific interaction between a particular clinician and patient. Because of these limitations, there is no certainty that the findings from one case study can generalize to other patients with apparently similar problems.

In 1967, Richard Stuart published an account of the behavioral treatment of eight patients who were obese. The results were the best ever reported in the treat-

TABLE 4.1	Advantages and Disadvantages of Common Research Strategies		
Strategy	**Description**	**Advantages**	**Disadvantages**
Controlled Experiment	The investigator manipulates an independent variable and looks at its effects on a dependent variable; requires random assignment of subjects	Permits inferences about causal relationships	Findings may not generalize to the real world
Quasi-Experimental Method	Compares two or more groups of subjects differing on preexisting personal characteristics but matched on other relevant dimensions; a case-control design is an example	Used to study groups of subjects who share a common psychopathology; can show that differences between the groups are attributable to that psychopathology and not other factors	Permits weaker inferences about causal relationships than an experiment, in which subjects are randomly assigned; there is no guarantee that the two groups will be identical, except with respect to the independent variable
Correlational Design	Assesses the degree to which two or more events are associated; uses measures of existing events; does not directly manipulate behavior	Permits study of relationships between variables	Does not permit inferences about causal relationships
Epidemiological Design	Assesses the prevalence, etiology, and consequences of mental disorders in a population	Permits identification of rise for specific disorders	Cannot establish causal relationships between antecedent factors and disorders
Case Study	A detailed analysis of a patient's past and present psychological functioning, using a combination of clinical interviews, observations, and test scores	Provides a clinically rich description of the patient, a source of hypotheses that can be followed up in controlled research, and practical guidelines for treatment	May produce inaccurate information because of the clinician's biases; findings cannot be generalized to other patients; cannot establish causal relationships

ment of obesity: All eight individuals continued to lose 20 pounds or more during the year following therapy. But subsequent research has shown that behavioral treatment of obesity is only modestly effective; it doesn't usually have the dramatic and uniform effects suggested by Stuart's eight cases (Wilson, 1993a). Reliance on case studies alone, then, would falsely inflate the effects of behavioral treatment of obesity, misleading patients about what to expect. For ethical and clinical reasons, individuals who are obese must be alerted to the limited effectiveness of treatment.

Why have case studies been so influential, despite their many limitations? Richard Nisbett and Lee Ross (1980) studied why researchers, including social scientists, assign importance to different data or sources of information. They found that people generally believe that information that's presented dramatically or vividly is more important than information presented in more straightforward ways. Thus, researchers tend to ignore or pay little attention to valid information presented as a summary of well-controlled studies; however, they're willing to base their judgments on less valid information that's more vivid, such as a fascinating case history full of personal details.

Focus on Critical Thinking

Table 4.1 provides a summary of the advantages and disadvantages of the research strategies discussed so far in this chapter. Which of the strategies would be best for studying each of the following (explain your selection in each case):

1. A newly developed antidepressant drug?

2. A known drug for application to a new disorder?

3. The effects of TV on violence on inner-city children?

4. A new virus that caused the death of its only known 10 victims?

EVALUATING THE EFFECTS OF TREATMENT

Single-Case Experimental Designs

The major limitation of the clinical case study, as discussed, is that it is uncontrolled. A significant contribution of the operant conditioning approach of B. F. Skinner (1904–1990) (see Chapter 2) has been the development of **single-case experimental designs** to conduct controlled research and treatment. The clinical adaptation of this type of design shows that behavioral change in an individual patient is the result of specific treatment intervention, not simply the passage of time, a placebo reaction, or some other uncontrolled event.

There are many variations of single-case experimental designs. The principles basic to all of them are illustrated by the two most commonly used variations: the reversal and the multiple-baseline designs.

Reversal Design   In the reversal design, following a period of baseline observation (A), during which no treatment of any kind is attempted, a treatment phase (B) is introduced, while the behavior in question is continuously observed. The behavior will usually show change in the desired direction, after which the treatment is discontinued in a return to the baseline procedure (A). If the treatment itself was responsible for the observed change, then the behavior should generally return almost to the level it was at formerly, during the original (A) period.

A study by Ayllon and Azrin (1965) provides a variation of the reversal design. First, in phase A, investigators increased the level of participation in rehabilitation activities of a group hospitalized with schizophrenia. They did so by making positive reinforcement—in the form of tokens that could later be exchanged for rewards—contingent on participation. Then, in phase B, reinforcement was administered regardless of whether patients participated in activities (see Figure 4.3). That is, all patients received tokens, no matter what their performance.

Giving out tokens in this way broke the contingency (relationship) between the reinforcer (token) and the response (participation), without eliminating the rein-

single-case experimental designs Experimental designs in which individuals serve as their own controls.

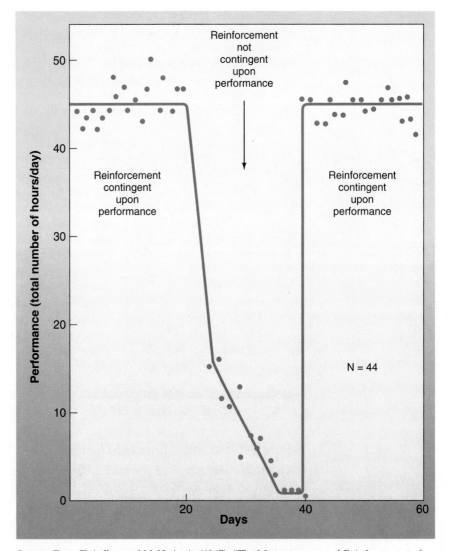

Source: From T. Ayllon and N. H. Azrin (1965), "The Measurement and Reinforcement of Behavior of Psychotics," *Journal of the Experimental Analysis of Behavior, 8,* p. 373.

forcer completely. This had the benefit of ensuring that the amount of social interaction remained unchanged between the attendants and ward staff, who administered the tokens and the patients. If any deterioration in sociability was found, then it could be directly attributed to only one thing: the relationship between behavior and reinforcement.

During phase C, the researchers returned to contingent reinforcement, as in phase A. At this point, it became clear that the treatment had made a difference. The results showed that the specific reinforcing contingency—receiving tokens for group participation—maintained the behavior of the schizophrenics.

The study illustrated in Figure 4.3 demonstrates another characteristic of single-case experimental designs: They typically focus on the behavior of the individual patient. Even so, this methodology is defined by the type of experimental arrangement, not by the number of subjects studied. The number of subjects may vary widely; there were 44 in the Ayllon and Azrin study (1965). The key point is that this group was treated as a single case.

One limitation of reversal design is that the target behavior returns to baseline level once treatment has been withdrawn. It is often ill advised or even unethical to return to a baseline condition after an effective treatment. For example, when a self-destructive child has responded to a particular intervention—such as praise from attendants for positive interactions with other children—it may be detrimental to the child's physical and mental health to ask attendants to withdraw their praise.

A second problem with reversal design is that it requires treatments to be readily reversible. The fact is, certain treatments lead to relatively permanent changes in behavior. For example, if enuretic children (bed-wetters) are given certain toilet training, their bladder size increases and they no longer wet the bed. The withdrawal of treatment does not lead to a return to wetting the bed. This reversibility issue applies especially to learning new skills. After children have learned to read, removing external incentives to read will not make them illiterate. In cases like this, investigators can never reinstate the original baseline. But if the behavior of interest shows no reversal, little of significance can be concluded.

Multiple-Baseline Design   In the multiple-baseline design, several responses are identified and measured over time to provide a baseline to evaluate changes against. Each response is then successively modified, in turn; if each changes greatly only when specifically treated, then a cause-effect relationship can be reliably inferred. Figure 4.4 illustrates the procedure for treating a patient who had the sexual disorder transvestism (that is, a man dressing as a woman for the purposes of sexual arousal) with sadomasochism (deriving pleasure from inflicting pain on oneself or others) (Brownell, Hayes, & Barlow, 1977). First, a specific treatment—known as *orgasmic reconditioning*—was used to increase the patient's heterosexual responsiveness. This intervention left his transvestism and sadomasochism unaffected. Next, a second treatment technique was used to decrease the transvestism, while baseline measures of sadomasochism showed no effect. Finally, sadomasochism was treated and successfully reduced. In sum, the different dimensions of this man's sexual disorder changed only when directly treated. (The details of these sexual disorders and their treatments are discussed in Chapter 8.)

The multiple baseline design is useful if highly specific treatment effects occur, as in Figure 4.4. But what if more than one baseline (that is, more than one type of sexual response) had simultaneously changed? These changes could indicate generalized effects of the specific treatment or nonspecific effects of variables other than the treatment itself (for instance, placebo effects).

Advantages and Disadvantages   Like any type of experimental design, single-case designs have advantages and disadvantages (Kazdin, 1981). One advantage is that they continually assess behavior over time. The target behavior is assessed regularly before, during, and after treatment intervention. This provides researchers with immediate and specific information on treatment progress, making it possible for them to decide whether to continue or modify treatment.

A second advantage of single-case designs is that intervention effects are replicated within the same subject over time. Subjects act as their own controls, and comparisons of their performance are made as different interventions are made. Thus, the treatment of individual patients can be evaluated objectively. The personal quality of the clinical case study is largely preserved without sacrificing experimental rigor. Investigators can therefore study clinical problems that would otherwise be rejected as unsuitable for group methodology.

A limitation of single-case experimental designs is the difficulty of studying the possible interaction of subject variables with the specific treatment technique. Since only a single subject is investigated, the effect of different subject characteristics on the treatment procedure cannot be directly assessed. For example, the treatment might be effective only for a certain type of patient but not for others. Assessing these different patient characteristics requires a group design.

Another disadvantage is that it's hard to generalize findings from single-case designs. A particular patient may respond well to a certain treatment; others may not. One way of avoiding this problem is for the same therapist to apply the same

Sexual arousal in response to
deviant and heterosexual stimuli
was measured using mean penile
circumference changes.

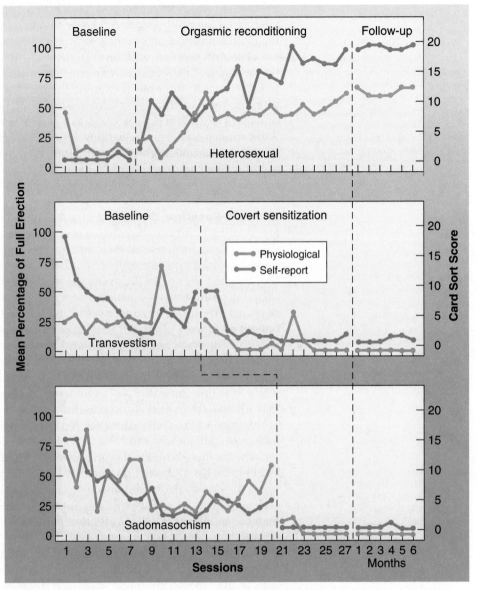

SOURCE: From K. D. Brownell, S. C. Hayes, and D. H. Barlow, "Patterns of Appropriate and Deviant
Sexual Arousal: The Behavioral Treatment of Multiple Sexual Deviations," *Journal of Consulting and
Clinical Psychology, 45,* p. 1149. Copyright © 1977 by the American Psychological Association.
Reprinted by permission.

technique under the same conditions to more than one patient. If the technique is
consistently successful and the results can be replicated in all cases, then interpretation of the results will be clearcut. But if the results are mixed or inconsistent, as
is frequently the case in clinical research, problems in interpretation will arise.

Randomized Group Designs

Evaluating the effects of psychological and drug treatments on abnormal behavior
is a complex task, involving many methodological challenges. Suppose we want to
evaluate the effects of psychotherapy on bulimia nervosa. We could randomly
assign patients to a treatment group and a group that received no treatment at all.
But it would be unethical to withhold therapy from patients in need of it.

Another possibility would be to use what is called a **waiting-list control
group.** Patients in this group would be promised treatment following a certain

waiting-list control group
Control group in which patients
are promised therapy after a
period of time, during which the
experimental group does receive
treatment.

waiting period, which would correspond to the time it takes to administer therapy to the treatment group in the study. A limitation of the waiting-list control group is that treatment can be compared with no treatment only during the period in which treatment is administered. Any follow-up comparison between the treatment and waiting-list groups is impossible because the latter eventually receives treatment.

The most powerful experimental design for evaluating treatment outcome is the **comparative outcome study,** in which two or more treatments are compared without considering either treatment condition as a formal control group. For example, in a landmark study, Paul and Lentz (1977) compared three treatment programs for chronic schizophrenic patients in a mental hospital. The programs involved:

1. *cognitive-behavioral therapy,* using learning principles to modify patients' behavior
2. *milieu therapy,* or creating a therapeutic community in the institution, focusing on the communication of positive expectations and group cohesiveness and group pressure directed toward normal functioning
3. *routine hospital therapy,* emphasizing chemotherapy combined with custodial care and little psychological treatment

On a number of different measures of patient functioning, both cognitive-behavioral therapy and milieu therapy produced greater improvement than routine hospital therapy.

A well-designed study should include independent measures of whether alternative treatments were implemented as planned. In the Paul and Lentz study (1977), for example, continuous assessment of the behavior of the staff of the treatment programs indicated that the social learning therapy and milieu therapy approaches were being faithfully implemented, consistent with their original guidelines. The clear procedural differences between these two programs made it possible to attribute the superior outcome of the subjects in the social learning program to the specific treatment. In other studies, treatment sessions have been audiotaped and later analyzed to ensure that the alternative treatments were correctly administered. Typically, to control for therapist effects the same therapists are trained to administer both treatments being compared. If different therapists conducted different treatments, we wouldn't know what produced the treatment effects: the treatment, the therapist, or some interaction between the two.

With complex clinical disorders, it's unlikely that one treatment will be best for all patients. The ultimate goal of comparative treatment studies is to match treatments to specific patients—namely, to determine which method appears most effective with which patients with a particular disorder. To do this, researchers assess patients on a wide range of pretreatment variables and then see if any of these variables predict outcomes in response to particular treatments.

Evaluation of treatment success must address both short-term and long-term effects. Two treatments may produce equal improvement immediately following therapy. But one may be associated with rapid relapse shortly after posttreatment, whereas the other may have lasting benefits. For example, drug therapy is effective in treating bulimia nervosa, yet once the drug is discontinued, patients rapidly return to binge eating and purging. In contrast, psychological treatment produces comparable short-term effects to drug treatment, but the results are maintained over time (Fairburn, Agras, & Wilson, 1992). Given this pattern of effects, psychological treatment would seem the treatment of choice because it produces durable or long-term improvement. See Table 4.2 for a review of the advantages and disadvantages of the various methods of evaluating treatment outcome.

comparative outcome study Treatment research in which one or more specific treatments are compared with each other.

Focus on
Critical Thinking

1. Refer back to the chapter-opening case of Laura, the young woman with an eating disorder. Explain why the study she participated in required that she postpone additional therapy for dealing with her history of childhood sexual abuse.

TABLE 4.2	Advantages and Disadvantages of Methods of Evaluating Treatment Outcome		
Strategy	**Description**	**Advantages**	**Disadvantages**
Single-Case Experimental Design	Detailed study of treatment effects in the individual patient; unlike the uncontrolled case study, treatment is manipulated experimentally to try to establish causal relationships	The focus on the individual patient is consistent with clinical practice; using patients as their own controls permits detailed analysis of treatment effects; there is continual assessment of the patient's progress over time	The effect of different patient characteristics on the treatment procedure cannot be directly assessed; the treatment might be effective only for a certain type of patient; it is also hard to generalize findings to other patients
Randomized Group Design			
No Treatment Control	Patients are randomly assigned to the treatment group or one that receives no treatment at all	Permits clearcut inference that the treatment intervention is effective	The outcome cannot be attributed to the specific treatment because alternative factors have not been ruled out, such as passage of time
Waiting-List Control	Patients are promised treatment after a delay corresponding to when the treatment would end; patients are assessed in the same way and as often as those in the actual treatment group	Permits researchers to rule out alternative explanations of treatment effects, such as passage of time and repeated assessments	Treatment can be compared with no treatment only during the period in which treatment is administered; follow-up comparison between the treatment and control groups is impossible because the latter eventually receives treatment
Comparative Outcome Studies	A particular treatment is compared with one or more alternative treatments; a control group may or may not be included; typically, the same therapists are trained to provide both treatments, so as to control for the influence of therapist characteristics	Any difference between treatments permits a strong inference that the effect is due to the specific treatment method, rather than some confounding factor—for example, developing a positive relationship with a caring therapist	Alternative treatments must be specified in detailed manuals and differ procedurally; therapists must be trained to administer both treatments with the same skill; taped recordings of sessions must be rated to ensure that different treatments were implemented correctly

Ethics in Psychological Research

informed consent Authorization granted by research subjects based on their understanding of what's involved in the research; all aspects that may affect subjects' willingness to participate must be explained.

The sort of research described in this book is funded mainly by the National Institute of Mental Health (NIMH). This federal agency has strict ethical guidelines that investigators must follow to ensure protecting the people who participate in research studies. Undergraduate students are often research subjects, and many of you reading this book may have participated in research, as well.

To do so, you should have signed an **informed consent** form that stated clearly what you had to do in the experiment, including whether you would be paid for your time. In addition, this form spelled out any risks you might have been exposed to as well as the likely benefits of the research. The informed consent form also asked you to declare that your participation was completely voluntary. It stated that you could withdraw from the study at any time, if you wished, and it ensured that your participation would be kept confidential. No one should have been able to identify you personally after the results of the study were published. After participating in the research, you should also have been given a **debriefing:** a full account of the purpose of the study and any deception that was used.

Laura was asked to sign an informed consent form, which described the details of the study and the research procedures. (She had already been told most of this by the research assistant). She was told that she would be randomly assigned to one of two psychological treatments, each consisting of 19 sessions of individual therapy. All therapy sessions would be tape recorded, so that they could be evaluated by the clinical psychologists and psychiatrists conducting the study.

In addition, she would be given either an antidepressant drug or a pill placebo (an inert, or fake, drug). She was told that this drug had proven effective in other research studies and was now widely used in clinical practice. The possible side effects of the medication were described, as was the purpose of the placebo. (By giving half the subjects real medication and half placebos, researchers could determine whether the drug itself helped patients get better or whether they improved because they believed that they were receiving medication.) Laura would meet periodically with a psychiatrist to assess her progress and check on any side effects from the medication. Neither she nor the psychiatrist administering the medication would know whether she was taking the real drug or the placebo.

Before getting the medication, Laura had to undergo a medical exam, including an electrocardiogram (EKG), which checked the functioning of her heart. She also had a blood test to monitor the levels of her electrolytes, such as potassium, which are often disturbed by the vomiting that is part of bulimia nervosa.

In sum, Laura learned that both therapy and drug treatments were routinely used with patients with her problem and that she was likely to get better as a result of these treatments. All the information gathered in the study would be kept confidential—except in the event that something happened that would make her dangerous to herself or someone else. And when the findings were eventually published, it would be impossible to identify any of the subjects. By signing the informed consent form, Laura indicated that she understood what the study involved and agreed to participate in it.

To ensure that proper procedures are established and followed in conducting research, every university and medical school in the United States has an institutional review board (IRB). An IRB is typically made up of researchers and other individuals who can shed light on ethical concerns, such as lawyers and ethicists. An IRB reviews proposals of all research studies to be conducted at the institution and then decides whether to approve or disapprove them. In particular, IRBs look at whether proposed projects include adequate procedures for obtaining informed consent and for informing subjects of the potential risks and benefits of participation.

Ethical guidelines generally protect both subjects and investigators. Nevertheless, difficult questions often arise and can cause controversy about the ethics of particular studies. For example, is it ethical to allow alcoholics to consume alcohol in a laboratory setting in order to study its effects on behavior? Nathan and O'Brien (1971) were asked this question in conducting pioneering research on alcoholism in the 1960s. Before that, no one had ever carried out experimental analyses of alcoholics when they drank. Although some critics claimed it was unethical to allow alcoholics to drink, Nathan argued that the potential benefits far outweighed the risks. The NIMH and Nathan's university IRB agreed. Ultimately, this study and others like it disproved several myths about alcoholism and led the way to a better understanding of this widespread disorder (see Chapter 9).

debriefing Providing a full account and justification of research activities to subjects who have participated in a study.

Thinking about CONTROVERSIAL ISSUES

The Use of Animals in Experimental Research

ℳost research involving animal subjects uses mice and rats; cats, dogs, and monkeys are used in a small number of cases. Researchers use animal subjects for several reasons. They can conduct experiments on animals that they cannot do with human subjects, for both practical and ethical reasons. Studies of the biological bases of abnormal behavior that require experimental surgery, direct analysis of brain mechanisms, or experimental drug administration must rely on animal subjects. For example, in studies of the process and treatment of drug dependence, animals have been made dependent on heroin and cocaine. The development of new medical or surgical procedures and drugs often begins with animal research, as well.

Animal research also enables researchers to study the developmental conditions that contribute to clinical disorders. Researchers at the University of Wisconsin, for instance, reared monkeys from birth under identical conditions, except for the control the animals were given over environmental events (Mineka, Gunnar, & Champoux, 1986). The experimental group could freely choose access to toys and food treats. The control group had none of these choices. They were yoked to monkeys in the experimental group, which meant they could access these reinforcers (the toys and food) only when one of the experimental group monkeys did. Then, between the ages of seven and nine months, all the monkeys were exposed to anxiety-eliciting situations. Those from the experimental group showed significantly less fear and phobic avoidance than those from the control group. (See Chapter 5 for more discussion of anxiety disorders.)

Animal rights groups vigorously oppose the use of animals in experimental research, objecting to the suffering they sometimes experience. A minority of animal rights activists totally oppose the use of animal subjects, and some have even resorted to violence to show their

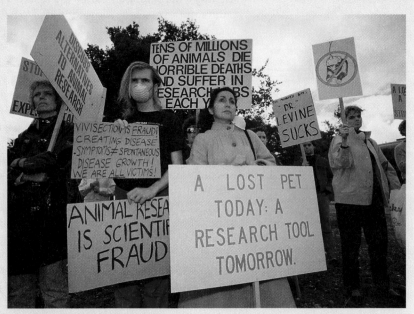

Some animal rights activists oppose all use of animals as subjects in laboratory research.

opposition. The moderate majority, however, have campaigned successfully to reduce the number of animal subjects and to ensure the humane treatment of those that are used.

Many in the biomedical and behavioral research communities share these objectives (Novak & Suomi, 1988). Universities are required to hire veterinarians to monitor the care and treatment of all laboratory animals used in research. And the American Psychological Association (1993) has strict ethical guidelines that are designed to balance the rights of animals with the needs of research.

Think about the following questions:

1. Recall Seligman's research on learned helplessness (described in the Thinking about Research box), in which dogs were given electric shocks. Could he have studied this phenomenon without using animals? Why or why not?

2. Could he have conducted the study without using aversive stimuli (electric shocks)? Why or why not?

Occasionally, ethical guidelines work less well. A study on schizophrenia demonstrates an unfortunate result, despite efforts taken to protect patients. Researchers at the University of California at Los Angeles (UCLA) conducted a study funded by the NIMH to assess the pros and cons of discontinuing drug therapy for schizophrenics. This is the only effective treatment of schizophrenia, but the continued use of these drugs produces serious physical side effects, such as tardive dyskinesia (an irreversible loss of control over movements, such as lip smacking and tongue protrusion). Researchers proceeded to discontinue drug treatment. The results were troubling. One of the patients committed suicide. Another threatened to kill his parents and planned to travel to Washington, DC, to assassinate then-President George Bush on the orders of space aliens ("Editorial," 1994).

The families of these two patients complained to the NIMH, arguing that they had not been sufficiently warned about the possible severity of their sons' being taken off medication. The NIMH issued a report in which they approved the design of the study but criticized researchers for not adequately informing patients about the dangers of stopping the medication. The researchers pointed out that, in addition to the written informed consent they had obtained, they had also orally described the possible risks. The researchers also claimed that the study had allowed immediate reevaluation of patients who began to show psychotic symptoms; medication would have been restored to anyone having serious problems. The parents whose son had threatened their lives disagreed, claiming that they had "practically begged" the researchers to restore drug treatment ("Editorial," 1994).

In response to this episode, UCLA revised its informed consent procedures. Specifically, those procedures now emphasize the possible risks of any clinical research. In addition, the university decided to add a patient representative to its IRB and set up a monitoring system to oversee studies in which researchers are responsible for both research and care of subjects.

The Thinking about Controversial Issues box discusses the controversy surrounding another ethical topic: the use of animals in research on abnormal behavior.

Focus on *Critical Thinking*

Numerous controlled studies have shown that antidepressant drugs (e.g., Prozac) are more effective than a pill placebo in reducing depression. Nevertheless, many clinical researchers still include a pill placebo comparison in ongoing studies of the effects of medication like Prozac.

1. Is it ethical to randomly assign depressed patients to a pill placebo in studies of this sort? Explain your answer.

SUMMARY

The Scientific Study of Abnormal Behavior

▪ To meet scientific standards, a diagnosis or finding must, at a minimum, be consistent and replicable. To ensure reliability, researchers must describe and define the phenomena they study in precise, operational terms.

▪ Validity refers to the accuracy of a test or measure—how well it measures what it was intended to measure. The concept of validity also applies to experimental design and the accuracy and usefulness of the findings they yield.

▪ A scientific theory is a formal statement of propositions designed to explain a phenomenon. To be useful, a theory should integrate known information, be testable, and stimulate new research.

▪ Scientific research has produced several breakthroughs in our understanding of abnormal behavior. It has also corrected several popular and often damaging myths about abnormal behavior—for instance, that childhood autism is caused by cold, emotionally inexpressive parents.

Research Strategies

▪ Controlled experimental methods are needed to show that one event causes another. In a controlled experiment, the independent variable is manipulated, or controlled, by the researcher to measure its effect on the dependent variable.

▪ Hypotheses are ideas that experiments are designed to test.

■ An experiment is internally valid if it allows the researcher to rule out explanations of the observed effects, other than the manipulation of the independent variable. The external validity of a study is the degree to which its findings are generalizable to other subjects in other settings.

■ A control group is the same as the experimental group on all relevant dimensions except the one being manipulated. Control groups are needed to eliminate other explanations of results. Subjects are randomly assigned to experimental and control groups, meaning that each subject has an equal chance of being assigned to either group.

■ In a quasi-experimental design, the nature of the independent variable makes it impossible to randomly assign subjects to the experimental group. A control group is selected by matching the experimental subjects with controls with similar personal characteristics.

■ Correlational design methods assess the degree of relationship between two or more events. The correlation coefficient is a mathematical expression of how strongly two variables are associated. Correlation does not imply causation, however.

■ Epidemiological research is a type of correlational method that examines the prevalence, etiology, and consequences of physical diseases and mental disorders in the population. Epidemiological research identifies risk factors that precede the development of certain diseases and disorders.

■ Using case studies, clinicians gather information about individuals' past and present functioning through interviews and possibly psychological tests. Case studies provide detailed descriptions of clinical methods and generate hypotheses that can be tested by other methods. However, case studies cannot establish that one event caused another, and their findings cannot be generalized to other individuals with the same problem.

Evaluating the Effects of Treatment

■ Single-case experimental designs allow experimental manipulation of the independent variable in an individual patient.

■ Randomized group designs allow the effects of treatments to be evaluated by comparing the treatment condition with no treatment, with a waiting-list control (which receives the treatment after a set period of time), or with alternative treatments. Subjects are randomly assigned to each group.

Ethics in Psychological Research

■ The National Institutes of Mental Health (NIMH), an agency of the federal government, requires that researchers follow strict ethical guidelines in their work.

■ Research subjects must give their informed consent to all procedures, indicating that they understand the nature of the research and any risks or benefits they may experience.

■ Clinical research raises complex and often controversial issues. The likely benefits of research must outweigh any risks to subjects. Researchers must make every effort to protect subjects' well-being.

KEY TERMS

analogue research, **p. 112**
Berkson's bias, **p. 118**
bulimia nervosa, **p. 104**
case-control design, **p. 116**
case study, **p. 118**

comparative outcome study, **p. 125**
confounds, **p. 110**
control group, **p. 110**
correlation coefficient, **p. 115**

correlational designs, **p. 115**
debriefing, **p. 127**
dependent variable, **p. 107**
double-blind strategy, **p. 112**
epidemiology, **p. 116**

CRITICAL THINKING EXERCISE

It has been well known for years that certain chemical substances can trigger anxiety attacks in people. For example, when sodium lactate is infused into the bloodstream of individuals with panic disorder, it frequently triggers a panic attack. The reason for this is unknown, but the chemical does affect important neurotransmitter systems in the body (see Chapter 5).

To test this, Dr. A. conducted an experiment in which he infused sodium lactate into a sample of 20 patients diagnosed with panic disorder and 20 control subjects free from any psychiatric disorder. The experimental and control groups were matched for age, sex (all male), and ethnic identity (all white). Patients in the experimental group were told that "they might experience a panic attack." Subjects in the control group were told that "they might experience an attack with symptoms analogous to those of 'public speaking.'"

The results showed that 75 percent of the panic patients but only 5 percent of the controls experienced panic attacks during the infusion. In general, the panic patients showed significantly more physiological disturbance than the controls. Dr. A. concluded that (a) patients with panic disorder differ from normal individuals in their biological reactivity to an anxiety-inducing chemical, like sodium lactate, and (b) this finding supports the theory that panic disorder is caused by a biological abnormality.

1. What type of validity is necessary if this experiment is to provide a good test of Dr. A.'s theory?
2. Was the control condition appropriate for testing the theory? Why or why not?
3. Was Dr. A. justified in reaching his conclusions? Why or why not?
4. Can you provide an alternative explanation of the findings? If so, what?

Chapter 5
ANXIETY DISORDERS

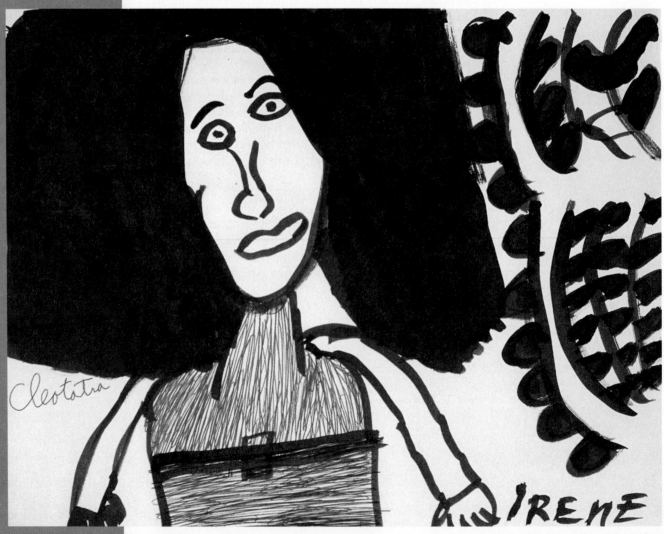

Irene Phillips, **Woman With Big Hair,** HAI

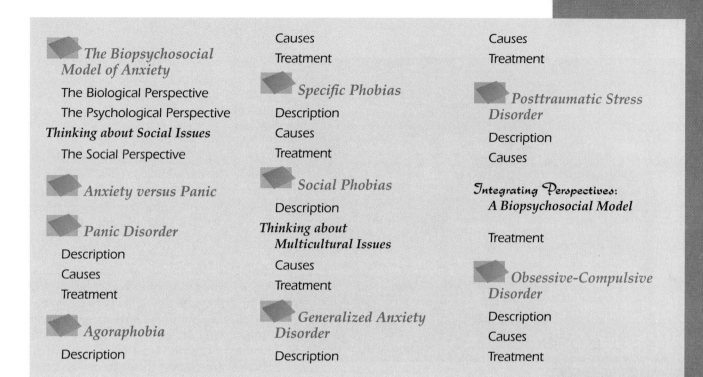

O n this very windy but clear day, Professor Sam Jones was flying home from Denver to San Francisco. After the door closed and the plane began to move away from the gate, he suddenly felt a twinge of terror. He broke out in a cold sweat; his chest felt tight; breathing was difficult and he became dizzy; his legs went weak. Professor Jones felt trapped, wishing he had never boarded the plane. The pilot's announcement that all seat belts should be securely fastened to prepare for a bumpy take-off only heightened his sense of terror.

Eventually turbulence ceased. The professor immediately got up and went to the restroom. The feeling of terror subsided, but he still felt high anxiety. He tried to read but couldn't concentrate. He was fidgety and worried that the passenger next to him would notice that there was something strange about him. At the first available opportunity, he purchased a couple of beers, which he quickly consumed. But the distress persisted. There was no escape from the fear. He resolved never to fly again.

As he struggled to control his anxiety, Professor Jones wondered what was wrong with him. He knew he had never been completely comfortable flying but had been able to distract himself on flights by reading or working. But nothing quite this intense had occurred before. He recalled that he had always disliked small, crowded places. He was typically tense in elevators, and at movies, he would always sit in the aisle seat, near the exit. Yet he was healthy, happily married with a loving family, and a highly regarded professor at a major university in the Bay area. How could this be happening to him?

After this harrowing experience, Professor Jones began to refuse invitations to give lectures in different states if the travel involved flying. He dreaded inventing excuses to explain his sudden change in behavior, which left him feeling humiliated. He had always thought of himself as an adventurous type who was good at handling stress. But anyone can have an anxiety disorder or panic attack.

Professor Jones had **claustrophobia**—the fear of enclosed spaces. This explains why he was distressed when the plane door closed, even before the plane had taken off. The intense fear he experienced on this occasion, characterized by physiological

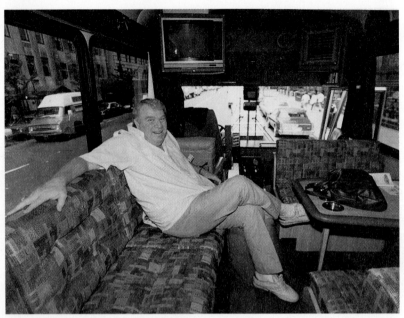

John Madden, the popular TV football analyst, relaxing in his specially outfitted bus, the "Madden mobile." Madden travels around the country in this bus because of his phobia about air travel.

symptoms such as sweating and dizziness, was a panic attack. Panic attacks can occur in all of the anxiety disorders. If frequent enough, they constitute what is called **panic disorder.**

Anxiety disorders are the most common type of psychiatric disorder affecting people in the United States. Structured interviews of a national probability sample found that one in every four of these respondents reported a lifetime history of an anxiety disorder (Kessler et al., 1994). Even "tough guys" suffer from these disorders. One famous person with a fear of flying is John Madden, the former head coach of the Oakland Raiders and current football commentator and commercial spokesman. After a panic attack, he stopped flying and now travels around the country in a specially outfitted bus, the "Madden mobile."

In this chapter, we discuss the nature of anxiety disorders and evaluate the effectiveness of both medication and professional counseling in treating problems like this.

$\mathcal{T}$HE BIOPSYCHOSOCIAL MODEL OF ANXIETY

No concept is more basic in the study of abnormal behavior than **anxiety.** Sigmund Freud (1856–1939) observed that "the problem of anxiety is a nodal point, linking up all kinds of the most important questions; a riddle, of which the solution must cast a flood of light on our whole mental life" (1917/1963, p. 401).

The Biological Perspective

Modern biological models trace the origin of anxiety to the brain. Using sophisticated measures of brain functioning, such as **positron emission tomography (PET scan),** researchers can identify physiological factors that are correlated with the experience of anxiety. For example, PET scans are recorded before and during the experimental induction of anxiety. Researchers can then see which specific areas of the brain become active and can determine if there is any abnormality in brain functioning (Reiman, Fusselman, Fox, & Raichle, 1989).

Brain cells linked to anxiety are located in the portion of the brain stem known as the *locus ceruleus.* Electrical stimulation of these cells triggers fear, whereas destroying them inhibits fear. These cells have specific receptors for **benzodiazepines,** which are anxiety-reducing drugs, such as Librium and Valium. The cell receptors are like locks, and the drugs are like keys. Only these keys fit these locks because they have the right molecular structure. Evidence also points to a genetic predisposition for anxiety and the development of anxiety disorders (Barlow, 1988).

The Psychological Perspective

The Psychodynamic Model   Freud distinguished between reality and **neurotic anxiety.** Individuals who perceive danger in the external world will experience

claustrophobia Fear of being confined in any space.

panic disorder Unexpected, recurrent attacks of intense anxiety occurring in situations that do not normally elicit anxiety.

anxiety A blend of thoughts and feelings characterized by a sense of uncontrollability and unpredictability over potentially aversive life events.

positron emission tomography (PET scan) Brain-imaging technology that permits study of the function of different brain areas.

benzodiazepines Anxiety-reducing drugs, such as Librium and Valium.

neurotic anxiety Anxiety traced to early childhood conflicts, according to psychodynamic theory.

anxiety, a state of painful tension that they seek to reduce. Individuals who experience neurotic anxiety, however, trace their anxiety to early childhood conflicts. Children's aggressive and sexual impulses cannot be directly expressed because they will be met by their parents' punishment or withdrawal of love. As a result, children learn to fear these impulses and develop ways to defend against them.

Repression is the most fundamental **defense mechanism,** allowing the ego to exclude threatening impulses from conscious awareness. However, a weak ego can only partly exclude these impulses, so the repression will not be completely successful. This causes neurotic anxiety as the threatening impulses start to break through the defenses. The impulses are then expressed indirectly or symbolically in ways that are disguised from the individual and others around her.

Before the introduction of the third edition of the *Diagnostic and Statistical Manual of Mental Disorders* (*DSM-III*) in 1980 (American Psychiatric Association), what we now call *anxiety disorders* were known as **neurotic disorders,** or *neuroses.* Based on the psychodynamic model, each of the neuroses was seen as a different, symptomatic expression of underlying neurotic anxiety. That anxiety, in turn, was a product of **intrapsychic conflict.** For example, phobias are the expression of anxiety applied to some external, neutral object.

Freud believed that sexual and aggressive impulses were the basis of neurotic anxiety. Later psychoanalysts expanded this view to include other bases. For instance, Alfred Adler (1870–1937) emphasized power, Karen Horney (1885–1952) emphasized dependency, and Harry Stack Sullivan (1892–1949) emphasized the need for security as the unconscious core of neurotic conflict. According to the psychodynamic model, we must delve into an individual's early childhood conflicts to understand anxiety and the disorders it causes. The overt symptoms that indicate neurotic anxiety provide only clues about the real underlying disorder.

The Cognitive-Behavioral Model   The many competing cognitive and behavioral theories of anxiety share some features. Barlow (1988) has proposed an integrative model that draws not only on cognitive and behavioral research but also on the psychology of emotion. He makes an important distinction between *fear* and *anxiety*. Fear is a primitive, basic emotion that occurs automatically when we are threatened with real or perceived danger. According to emotion theorists, fear is fundamentally an action tendency, defined by the "fight or flight" response that was important to human survival during evolution. Subjectively, we experience this alarm reaction as a strong urge to escape from a threatening situation.

In contrast to fear, anxiety is not a basic emotion but a blend of different emotions, including anger, excitement, and fear itself. Barlow (1988) defines *anxiety* as a fragmented cognitive-affective process in which the individual has a sense of unpredictability or uncontrollability over potentially negative or harmful life events. This concept is similar to Bandura's (1986) theory of self-efficacy, which we will discuss later in this chapter. Our sense of unpredictability and uncontrollability is associated with chronic physiological arousal, such as more rapid breathing and increased heartrate. In terms of feelings, we experience anxiety as apprehension over something bad that's about to happen and concern over our ability to cope with the threat. Anxiety is characterized by self-focused attention that increases arousal, making us more aware of threat-related stimuli.

In his account of the causes of clinical anxiety, Barlow (1988) bases this analysis of how anxiety occurs on a broader biopsychosocial model. Due to heredity, some individuals have a biological (or physical) vulnerability to stress. The exact nature of this vulnerability is still unclear, but it may involve one or more neurobiological systems (for example, a highly reactive or unstable autonomic nervous system). Exposure to stressful life events activates this vulnerability.

Some individuals also have a psychological vulnerability to stress. They may see stressful events as unpredictable—that things happen repeatedly, without reason or warning. Or they may see events as uncontrollable—that they can't do any-

repression Defense mechanism in which the ego excludes threatening impulses from conscious awareness.

defense mechanism Strategy used by the ego to prevent threatening unconscious thoughts or memories from becoming conscious.

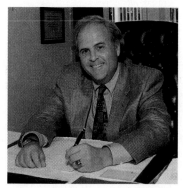

DAVID BARLOW, *Director of the Anxiety Disorders Clinic at the State University of New York at Albany, is one of the country's leading experts on the treatment of anxiety disorders.*

neurotic disorders Describes what the DSM-IV now refers to as anxiety; from the psychodynamic model.

intrapsychic conflict Conflict between the ego and id or the ego and superego.

Thinking about SOCIAL ISSUES   Why Are Anxiety Disorders More Common in Women Than Men?

Research has shown that women are much more likely to suffer from anxiety disorders than men over their lifetime and during the past year. Studies from different parts of the world consistently show that 75 percent or more of agoraphobics are women. And the greater the degree of avoidance behavior among patients with panic disorder, the greater the proportion of women (Reich, Noyes, Hirshfeld, Coryell, & O'Gorman, 1987). Why are women more vulnerable to these disorders?

The usual explanation points to cultural factors. Women supposedly find it easier to cope with anxiety or panic by avoiding fearful situations and staying home. Men may experience the same anxiety or panic as women, but because of societal expectations, they can't avoid difficult situations as easily. Consistent with this view is that the less "masculine" either male or female agoraphobics scored on a measure of sex role, the more avoidance behavior they showed (Chambless & Mason, 1986). It's also been suggested that instead of avoiding fearful situations, men resort to drinking alcohol as a means of self-medicating their anxiety (Barlow, 1988).

One study found that agoraphobics were more dependent and less assertive than nonagoraphobic controls. Women, generally, were more likely to be dependent than men. The passive avoidance behavior shown by women with agoraphobia may be an exaggeration of their stereotypical role (Fodor, 1974). For example, if a young woman feels trapped in her marriage, has no emotional outlet, and cannot be assertive, for fear of losing her husband, she may become fearful and avoidant in an effort to cope. There is no empirical support for this theory, however.

An important but often overlooked finding is that the higher an individual's **socioeconomic status (SES)**, the less likely she will experience a clinical disorder. Data from the National Comorbidity Survey suggest that this is especially true for the anxiety disorders (Kessler et al., 1994). Similarly, Schneier et al. (1992) found that social phobias were more common among lower-SES women in a community sample than those with higher SES. Why would a higher socioeconomic status protect you from anxiety disorders? Once again, perhaps the answer lies in the greater control—and sense of control—that comes with having greater personal resources. Since women are more likely than men to have lower SES, this might help explain the gender gap in vulnerability anxiety disorders.

An alternative interpretation offers a biological explanation: that females are biologically predisposed to be more fearful than males. Research has found that women, in general, are more fearful than men. The same difference has been found in nonhuman primates (Gray, 1987). These findings suggest that a biological predisposition might interact with social influences, leaving women more vulnerable to anxiety disorders.

Think about the following questions:

1. How would you test the theory that women's lower SES makes them more susceptible to anxiety disorders?
2. Women in the United States have become increasingly independent over the years, as social expectations and traditions have changed. Will these changes affect the prevalence of anxiety disorders among women? Explain your prediction and how you would test it.

---

socioeconomic status (SES) Individual's relative standing in society as a function of occupation, income, and education.

Focus on Critical Thinking

1. In 1980, when the American Psychiatric Association replaced the DSM-II (1968) with the DSM-III (1980), it introduced a very different approach to diagnosis (see Chapter 3). Why do you think the DSM-III changed the term neurotic disorders to anxiety disorders?

thing to stop or deal with what happens. Individuals who are both biologically and psychologically vulnerable to stress are likely to develop anxiety disorders.

The Social Perspective

Social and cultural factors are usually provided to explain the greater prevalence of anxiety and its disorders among women than men. In most cultures, when compared to men, women have traditionally been assigned a more dependent role, which may increase their vulnerability to anxiety (as discussed in the Thinking about Social Issues box). Social support from family and friends seems to protect both men and women against the development of anxiety disorders.

ANXIETY VERSUS PANIC

panic Clinical manifestation of fear; usually of sudden onset.

panic attack Sudden feeling of intense fear accompanied by physiological symptoms and thoughts of losing control or dying.

Making a distinction between fear and anxiety helps explain the differences between **panic** and anxiety. The identification and analysis of panic was the most important development in the anxiety disorders of the 1980s and has had a major impact on research and clinical practice, fundamentally altering how anxiety disorders were diagnosed in the *DSM-IV* (American Psychiatric Association, 1994).

A **panic attack** is a sudden feeling of intense fear accompanied by various physiological symptoms, such as those that Professor Jones experienced during his flight from Denver to San Francisco. The diagnostic criteria for a panic attack are listed in the *DSM-IV* table.

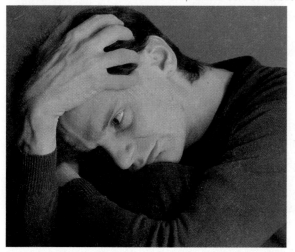

In Barlow's (1988) model, panic is the clinical manifestation of fear. However, it's not a true emotional alarm, triggered by real danger; instead, it's a false alarm because the danger is only perceived. Suppose, for example, you were about to be attacked by a tiger; you would be facing real danger. Out of fear, you would likely have a "fight or flight" response, as described earlier. But suppose that after hurrying to get to class, you're a little out of breath and your heart's beating a bit faster. You mistake these normal sensations as signs of an impending heart attack. This would most likely be panic because unless you had a heart condition or some other medical problem, you wouldn't be facing real danger.

A patient described what it's like to have a panic attack in the following words:

Intense anxiety constitutes both a psychological and physiological burden. What anxiety symptoms are evident in this man's face?

Imagine that you are walking a tightrope between two skyscrapers like the world Trade Center. You are halfway across when a gusty wind starts to blow. You feel your footing go. You look down. It's a long, long drop to the street below. Try to capture the feelings in your body and mind in that situation. The spontaneous panic attack is even worse, and here's why. On the tightrope you know why you're anxious: you can identify things that need to be done to cope. The danger is clear. You are also expecting to feel fear and anxiety. There are no big surprises. On the other hand, with the spontaneous panic attack, it can strike unexpectedly at any time. And worse, you can't identify any good reason for it. You can't pin it on anything. It's a nameless terror. It comes from nowhere and you don't know when it will stop, if ever. Since it can strike any time, anywhere, you are never really safe anywhere. If you invented Hell, you'd have to include this part of the package. (Sheehan, 1983, p. 42)

Like this individual, other patients often report that panic attacks occur unexpectedly and spontaneously. Careful clinical examination, however, usually reveals specific triggering events.

Panic differs from anxiety in two ways: (1) in the specific thoughts associated with the anxiety and (2) in physiological responsive-

Diagnostic Criteria for PANIC ATTACK

A discrete period of fear or discomfort, in which at least four of the following symptoms developed abruptly and reached a peak within 10 minutes:

(1) palpitations, pounding heart, or accelerated heart rate

(2) sweating

(3) trembling or shaking

(4) sensations of shortness of breath or smothering

(5) feeling of choking

(6) chest pain or discomfort

(7) nausea or abdominal distress

(8) feeling dizzy, unsteady, lightheaded, or faint

(9) derealization (feelings of unreality) or depersonalization (being detached from oneself)

(10) fear of losing control or going crazy

(11) fear of dying

(12) paresthesias (numbness or tingling sensations)

(13) chills or hot flashes

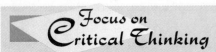

Focus on Critical Thinking

Think of a time when you were very anxious about something and answer the following questions:

1. What thoughts and feelings did you have? What physical symptoms did you experience?
2. Look at the list of symptoms in the DSM-IV table on panic attack (p. 137). How many of them did you have? Do you think you had a panic attack? Explain your answers.

ness. Patients who experience panic report more thoughts about illness, dying, and collapsing than patients with other anxiety disorders (Holt & Andrews, 1989). Panic patients also show greater physiological arousal than other anxiety disorder patients. For example, researchers who monitored patients' heartrates found that panic was associated with a big increase in heartrate (Taylor, Helzer, & Robins, 1986). They did not find the same increase for **anticipatory anxiety,** or anxiety over the prospect of something bad happening.

PANIC DISORDER

Description

The *DSM-IV* distinguishes between panic disorder with and without **agoraphobia.** (*Agoraphobia* is the fear and avoidance of situations that may be difficult to escape from or get help in, should the person experience paniclike symptoms.) The diagnostic criteria for panic disorder without agoraphobia are listed in the *DSM-IV* table. Heart and respiratory symptoms are typical complaints of patients with panic disorder. These individuals frequently consult physicians or go to hospital emergency rooms because they think they're having a heart attack.

Estimates of the lifetime prevalence of strictly defined panic disorder range from 1.5 to 3.5 percent of the population (American Psychiatric Association, 1994), although specific panic attacks occur much more often. Like anxiety disorders, panic disorder is more common in women than men (see Thinking about Social Issues). But it's equally prevalent among whites, African Americans, and Hispanics (Kessler et al., 1994).

Panic disorder with agoraphobia is diagnosed if the patient meets the criteria for agoraphobia in addition to those for panic disorder. (See the *DSM-IV* table on agoraphobia, later in this chapter.) Patients with panic disorder alone or panic disorder with agoraphobia appear identical in terms of descriptive characteristics, such as age of onset and panic frequency (Telch, Brouillard, Telch, Agras, & Taylor, 1989). The prevalence of panic disorder with agoraphobia is as high as 5 percent of the population (American Psychiatric Association, 1994).

Panic disorder is often associated with other clinical disorders, such as depression. An estimated 35 to 91 percent of individuals with panic disorder also report a major depressive episode at some point in their lives (Stein, Tancer, & Uhde, 1990). Research on family genetics has shown that panic disorder and depression are transmitted independently in families (Weissman et al., 1993). In some patients, the disorders occur at the same time, whereas in other patients, panic disorder occurs before depression. Problems with alcohol or other substance abuse also commonly occur with panic disorder. It's commonly believed that individuals with panic disorder try to self-medicate their anxiety by drinking; however, it appears that panic attacks are more likely to *follow* than *precede* alcohol abuse (Kushner, Sher, & Beitman, 1990). Other commonly co-occurring problems include simple and social phobias (Sanderson, DiNardo, Rapee, & Barlow, 1990).

anticipatory anxiety Anxiety over the prospect of something bad happening.

agoraphobia Fear and avoidance of being in places or situations in which help might not be available should some incapacitating or embarrassing event occur.

DSM-IV   Diagnostic Criteria for 300.01 PANIC DISORDER WITHOUT AGORAPHOBIA

A. Both (1) and (2):
  (1) recurrent unexpected Panic Attacks
  (2) at least one of the attacks has been followed by 1 month (or more) of one (or more) of the following:
    (a) persistent concern about having additional attacks
    (b) worry about the implications of the attack or its consequences (e.g., losing control, having a heart attack, "going crazy")
    (c) a significant change in behavior related to the attacks

B. Absence of Agoraphobia

C. The Panic Attacks are not due to the direct physiological effects of a substance (e.g., a drug of abuse, a medication) or a general medical condition (e.g., hyperthyroidism).

D. The panic attacks are not better accounted for by another mental disorder.

In their analysis of data from community samples, Weissman and her colleagues (1989) reported a surprising finding: As many as 20 percent of people with panic disorder had attempted suicide. These individuals were almost three times as likely to attempt suicide as those with other psychological disorders, including major depression. Subsequent research has cast doubt on this finding, however (Beck, Steer, Sanderson, & Skeie, 1991). Clinical studies have found high rates of lifetime suicide attempts in patients with panic disorder, but this association was clearly due to the presence of a third disorder (Friedman, Jones, Chernen, & Barlow, 1992; Lepine, Chignon, & Teherani, 1993). The patients who attempted suicide were those with a borderline personality disorder (see Chapter 12) and those with past or present depression or substance abuse. Among the patients without these disorders, the suicide-attempt rate was very low.

Causes

Currently, the two most promising and influential theories of panic disorder are the biological model and the cognitive-behavioral model. Let's consider each in turn.

The Biological Model   According to this model, *panic* is an unlearned alarm reaction, activated by a biochemical dysfunction, whereas other forms of anxiety are learned. Psychological stress, which might be associated with the onset of panic, is only a nonspecific influence that might worsen but never cause the problem.

Evidence supports the biological model. First, a genetic basis exists for panic disorder that seems independent of other anxiety disorders. About 50 percent of the people with panic disorder have relatives with the same disorder; this is higher than the rate in the general population. Noyes and colleagues (1987) found that the high frequency of panic disorder among the relatives of patients with panic disorder was not seen in the families of people with other anxiety disorders, such as generalized anxiety disorder (GAD). These and other findings indicate that familial risks for panic and GAD are independent. Moreover, **familial transmission** of panic disorder appears to be genetically influenced. Identical twins are more likely to both have the disorder than are fraternal twins (Barlow, 1988).

A second finding is that panic disorder patients have been found to differ physiologically from normal people. A number of pharmacological and physiological reactions (such as hyperventilation and inhalation of carbon dioxide) trigger panic in patients with panic disorder but not in other people. For example, after exercise, the level of lactic acid in the blood rises more in panic patients than in normal individuals. This physiological response can be tested through **sodium lactate infusion,** in which lactic acid is injected directly into the bloodstream. Liebowitz et al. (1984) found that panic patients typically panic, whereas normal controls do not.

A third finding is that specific brain mechanisms have been identified in individuals with panic disorder. PET scans of the brain show differences between patients who panic following lactate infusion and those who do not (Reiman et al., 1989). In the nonpanic state, before lactate infusion, patients who subsequently experienced panic attacks showed an abnormal metabolic rate for oxygen; this was located in a particular region of the brain called the *parahippocampal gyrus.*

A weakness of the biological model is its prediction that panic disorder is treatable only using specific drugs that alter underlying biochemical dysfunction. This is a drawback because based on that prediction, the biological model assumes that psychological methods are incapable of reducing panic (Klein, Ross, & Cohen, 1987).

The Cognitive-Behavioral Model   According to the cognitive-behavioral model, panic disorder results from the individual's catastrophic misinterpretation of normal bodily sensations (Clark, 1988). These misinterpreted sensations may be normal physical sensations—such as heart palpitations or breathlessness—but also

familial transmission
Transmission of a clinical disorder within a family.

sodium lactate infusion
Injection of lactic acid, which tends to trigger panic attacks in people with panic disorder.

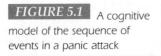

FIGURE 5.1 A cognitive model of the sequence of events in a panic attack

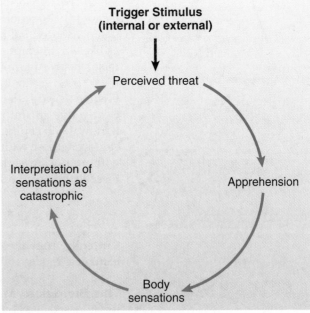

Source: Reprinted from *Behaviour Research and Therapy, 24,* by D. M. Clark, "A Cognitive Approach to Panic," p. 463. Copyright 1986, with kind permission from Elsevier Science, Ltd., The Boulevard, Langford Lane, Kidlington, OX5 1GB, UK.

may include bodily changes in response to excitement or anger. These sensations are perceived as being much more dangerous than they really are. A person with panic disorder might interpret palpitations as evidence of an oncoming heart attack. Stimuli interpreted as threats cause anxiety, which involves different physical sensations. These sensations are then interpreted by the person in a catastrophic way, further increasing anxiety. This response, in turn, causes a further increase in negative physical sensations, perpetuating what becomes a vicious cycle.

In Barlow's (1988) model of anxiety, **catastrophic thinking** is part of the psychological vulnerability—that is, the perceived unpredictability and uncontrollability. This model explains why many people have isolated fear responses or panic attacks that never develop into panic disorder (see Figure 5.1). This disorder develops only when people become anxious about the possibility that a panic attack will reoccur, which then leads them to "catastrophize" about otherwise normal bodily sensations.

Three key, testable predictions follow from the cognitive-behavioral model:

1. Panic patients misinterpret bodily sensations catastrophically more frequently than other anxious patients and normal controls.
2. Eliciting catastrophic cognitions in panic patients leads to panic.
3. Treatment that corrects or changes patients' catastrophic misinterpretations of bodily sensations reduces the incidence of panic attacks.

Research has proven the first two predictions to be true: That is, individuals with panic disorder do misinterpret their bodily functions more often than normal individuals (Rachman & Maser, 1988), and eliciting catastrophic cognitions in panic patients does lead to panic (Clark & Ehlers, 1993).

To test the third prediction about treatment, panic patients were randomly assigned to an experimental or a control group (Clark & Ehlers, 1993). Both groups received sodium lactate infusion, which is supposed to induce panic. The experimental group was given a detailed explanation of all possible sensations attributed to effects of the procedure. This explanation was intended to block patients' naturally occurring tendency to catastrophically interpret the sensations produced by the lactate infusion. The control group received no such explanation.

catastrophic thinking In panic disorder, misinterpretation of normal physical sensations as signs of an impending disaster.

According to the *biological* model, no differences should be found between the two groups, because sodium lactate infusion is supposed to induce panic directly. According to the *cognitive-behavioral* model, the control group should panic, because only they will misinterpret the physical sensations produced by the sodium lactate. The findings were consistent with the cognitive-behavioral model: The subjects who were given no explanation experienced significantly more panic than those whose cognitions had been altered by the explanation (Clark & Ehlers, 1993).

The cognitive-behavioral model is able to accommodate the evidence that biological abnormalities predispose individuals to panic attacks. But it differs from the biological model in suggesting that these abnormalities do not directly cause panic; rather, they have to be misinterpreted in a catastrophic fashion. Again, catastrophic thinking is seen as a necessary condition for panic.

The cognitive model also differs from a related psychological explanation of panic, namely, the **fear of fear hypothesis.** According to this hypothesis, panic patients will panic when they become anxious. But this doesn't always happen. The cognitive-behavioral model explains why: If patients attribute their anxiety to understandable causes, such as a job interview, they don't panic. They panic only when they attribute anxiety to physical sensations that they believe are signs of impending disaster.

Treatment

Pharmacological Therapy   So-called antidepressant drugs are also effective in treating anxiety disorders. Imipramine has proven to be the most effective drug treatment (Telch & Lucas, 1994). Another drug commonly prescribed for treating panic attacks is **Xanax (alprazolam),** a high-potency benzodiazepine. It acts quickly and has few immediate side effects. However, it's unclear whether Xanax is significantly more effective than placebo treatment ("High Anxiety," 1993). Moreover, Xanax is highly addictive. A majority of patients become physically dependent if they take this drug over a period of time. When they discontinue its use, patients develop withdrawal symptoms and their anxiety returns (Otto et al., 1993).

Drug therapy appears to be less effective than psychological treatment. Another important limitation of drug treatment for panic disorder is that many patients are unwilling to take medication for what they consider psychological problems.

Cognitive-Behavioral Therapy   Two treatments that focus on correcting catastrophic thinking have proven highly effective. The first—Clark's (1988) **cognitive therapy**—deliberately activates catastrophic thoughts and teaches patients to reinterpret them so that they no longer trigger panic. For example, patients who respond to normal breathlessness as the sign of an impending heart attack would be instructed to hyperventilate briefly to induce the physical sensations they fear. The therapist would then help these individuals explain the feelings as the normal effects of overbreathing, rather than a heart problem.

A study from Oxford University compared cognitive therapy with drug therapy (imipramine), relaxation training, and no treatment (Clark et al., 1994). Figure 5.2 shows that fully 90 percent of patients treated by cognitive therapy were completely free from panic at the end of treatment and that most continued their recovery after one year. By contrast, only half the patients treated with imipramine or relaxation training were panic free at the end of treatment.

The second treatment has come out of research in the United States that evaluates a broader form of cognitive-behavioral therapy (Craske & Barlow, 1993). This method emphasizes the modification of faulty and catastrophic thinking, as in Clark's (1988) approach. But it also includes other coping techniques, such as relaxation training and systematic exposure to internal cues that trigger panic. In one

fear of fear hypothesis Suggests that patients with panic disorder will panic if they experience anxiety or fear.

Xanax (alprazolam) Potent benzodiazepine often used to treat anxiety and panic.

cognitive therapy In treating anxiety disorders, a form of therapy that focuses on deliberately activating catastrophic thoughts and teaching patients to reinterpret them so that they no longer trigger panic.

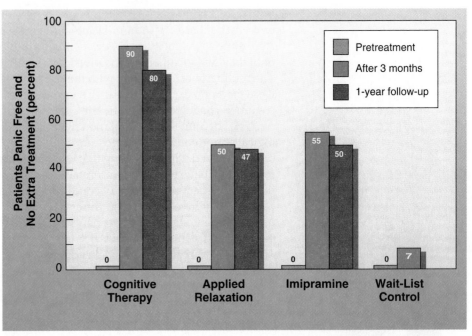

FIGURE 5.2 Success rates of cognitive-behavioral therapy

Source: From D. M. Clark, P. M. Salkovskis, A. Hackmann, H. Middleton, P. Anastasiades, and M. Gelder, "A Comparison of Cognitive Therapy, Applied Relaxation and Imipramine in the Treatment of Panic Disorder," *British Journal of Psychiatry, 6, 759–769,* 1994. Reprinted by permission.

controlled study, 87 percent of the patients were panic free at the end of treatment and were doing well at a two-year follow-up (Craske & Barlow, 1993). In a second study, cognitive-behavioral therapy was superior to Xanax and a pill-placebo condition (Klosko, Barlow, Tassinari, & Cerny, 1990).

Combined Psychological and Pharmacological Treatment The combined treatment method that has been studied most is cognitive-behavioral therapy plus use of the drug imipramine. Several studies have shown that the combined treatment is superior to either psychological or drug treatment alone (Telch & Lucas, 1994).

For example, in one study (Telch, Agras, Taylor, Roth, & Gallen, 1985), patients were randomly assigned to the following three treatments: (1) exposure plus imipramine, (2) exposure plus pill placebo, and (3) imipramine only. To control for the effects of exposure, subjects in the third condition—treatment with imipramine only—were given counterpractice instructions. These instructions emphasized the importance of staying out of phobic situations for the first 8 weeks of treatment, in order for the medication to have time to take effect. In sum, the first treatment—combined exposure plus imipramine—was more effective than the second—exposure plus placebo. But notice what happened to the third/drug-only treatment. In the absence of exposure, this treatment did poorly.

The important question this study raises is: What about imipramine facilitates the effects of exposure? Telch et al. (1985) speculated that the effects of the medication in lowering anxiety made it easier for patients to carry out their exposure tasks. In turn, they were able to derive maximal benefit from exposure.

Focus on Critical Thinking

1. As discussed in the text and the Thinking about Social Issues box, women are more likely than men to suffer from panic disorder. How would the Clark model of panic disorder account for this gender gap?

2. Most people would not hesitate to take medication to cure or reduce the symptoms of a physical ailment. Why do you think that many people are unwilling to take medication for what they consider psychological problems? What does this say about people's attitudes toward psychiatric disorders?

AGORAPHOBIA

Description

Agoraphobia is typically associated with panic disorder. But the *DSM-IV* also includes the diagnosis of "Agoraphobia Without a History of Panic Disorder," although this condition is uncommon (Horwath, Lish, Johnson, Hornig, & Weissman, 1993). In patients with agoraphobia, the anxiety is based on the occurrence of paniclike symptoms such as dizziness or diarrhea. The diagnostic criteria for agoraphobia are listed in the *DSM-IV* table.

Age of onset of agoraphobia is typically in the twenties or thirties, and without treatment, the disorder persists for years. Between 2.7 and 5.8 percent of the adult population in the United States has this disorder. Once more, far more women are affected than men (Barlow, 1988).

Causes

Most of the information we have about this disorder comes from studies of agoraphobics who had panic attacks. We know that agoraphobia runs in families, particularly among female relatives of agoraphobics. The risk for all anxiety disorders was 32 percent among first-degree relatives of agoraphobics (that is, parents and siblings), compared with 15 percent among individuals in the nonanxious control group (Harris, Noyes, Crowe, & Chaundry, 1983). For female relatives of agoraphobic probands (index cases), the risk factor for this disorder was more than twice that for the controls. Male relatives of agoraphobics were also at higher risk for both agoraphobia and alcoholism. Genetic factors account for 30 to 40 percent of the variance in these findings (Kendler, Neale, Kessler, Heath, & Eaves, 1992b).

The family systems model suggests that agoraphobia is the product of a pathological marriage or family system. For example, a wife might develop the disorder as a way of controlling her husband. He would have to spend considerable time with her and maybe take over some of her activities. He couldn't become angry at her without seeming to be uncaring. Alternatively, a husband might unconsciously encourage in his wife the dependency and limited social functioning that are part of agoraphobia as a way of controlling her. Or by focusing on her problems, he might shift attention away from his. Although this family systems approach is popular among clinicians, research evidence to support it is lacking.

The cognitive-behavioral model of panic attacks suggests that once the initial panic or anxiety attack has occurred, the person increasingly avoids the original and related situations. This pattern is maintained by the negative reinforcement of avoiding situations that provoke anxiety. Family members and friends may inadvertently help maintain this pattern of avoidance behavior by taking over the agoraphobic's responsibilities.

Treatment

The most effective psychological treatment of agoraphobia is the cognitive-behavioral therapy technique known as **exposure treatment.** In this technique, patients are encouraged to systematically and gradually confront the situations they fear and avoid. Exposure treatment reliably reduces phobic anxiety and avoidance behavior as well as panic attacks. And the benefits of this treatment usually extend

---

DSM-IV   Diagnostic Criteria for 300.22 AGORAPHOBIA

A. Anxiety about being in places or situations from which escape might be difficult (or embarrassing) or in which help may not be available in the event of having an unexpected or situationally predisposed Panic Attack or panic-like symptoms. Agoraphobic fears typically involve characteristic clusters of situations that include being outside the home alone; being in a crowd or standing in a line; being on a bridge; and traveling in a bus, train, or automobile.

B. The situations are avoided (e.g., travel is restricted) or else are endured with marked distress or with anxiety about having a Panic Attack or panic-like symptoms, or require the presence of a companion.

C. The anxiety or phobic avoidance is not better accounted for by another mental disorder.

---

exposure treatment Behavioral therapy technique in which patients are guided to gradually confront the situations they avoid to help overcome their phobic anxiety.

to other aspects of the patient's life, such as better functioning at home and at work (Klein, Zitrin, Woerner, & Ross, 1983).

Marital factors influence the maintenance of treatment effects. A caring spouse, for instance, may provide emotional support that helps the individual with agoraphobia persist in confronting, rather than avoiding, treatment situations (Arnow, Taylor, Agras, & Telch, 1985). Individuals with agoraphobia who have good marriages at the onset of exposure treatment maintain the reductions they make in phobic anxiety and avoidance better than their counterparts with poor marriages (Bland & Hallam, 1981). Couples training—in which husbands were included in their agoraphobic wives' exposure treatment program—produced superior results to treating wives alone (Barlow, O'Brien, Last, & Holder, 1983).

Focus on Critical Thinking

1. Imagine that you have a close friend who is agoraphobic. List two things that you could do to help him or her.

2. List two actions that would unintentionally help maintain your friend's problem.

3. Many agoraphobics abuse alcohol. Why do you think this is so?

The combination of exposure treatment and antidepressant medication (imipramine) has produced better results than either the drug alone or exposure treatment plus a drug placebo (Telch & Lucas, 1994). A combination of exposure treatment and Xanax seemed better in the short term but significantly less effective at a one-year follow-up (Marks & Swinson, 1993) because patients relapsed after they were withdrawn from the Xanax.

SPECIFIC PHOBIAS

specific phobias Anxiety disorders characterized by the fear and avoidance of particular objects or situations.

Description

Specific phobias were previously called *simple phobias* in the *DSM-III-R* (American Psychiatric Association, 1987). A *phobia* is an excessive fear of a specific object or situation. Professor Jones, in the opening case of this chapter, had a phobia about enclosed spaces—claustrophobia. See the *DSM-IV* table to review the diagnostic criteria for specific phobias.

DSM-IV Diagnostic Criteria for 300.29 SPECIFIC PHOBIA

A. Marked and persistent fear that is excessive or unreasonable, cued by the presence or anticipation of a specific object or situation (e.g., flying, heights, animals, receiving an injection, seeing blood).

B. Exposure to the phobic stimulus almost invariably provokes an immediate anxiety response, which may take the form of a situationally bound or situationally predisposed Panic Attack.

C. The person recognizes that the fear is excessive or unreasonable.

D. The phobic situation(s) is avoided or else is endured with intense anxiety or distress.

E. The avoidance, anxious anticipation, or distress in the feared situation(s) interferes significantly with the person's normal routine, occupational (or academic) functioning, or social activities or relationships, or there is marked distress about having the phobia.

F. In individuals under age 18 years, the duration is at least 6 months.

G. The anxiety, Panic Attacks, or phobic avoidance associated with the specific object or situation are not better accounted for by another mental disorder.

Causes

The Biological Model According to the biological model, genetic factors predispose us to develop phobias (Kendler et al., 1992). Research has shown that in comparison to fraternal twins, identical twins are more alike on measures of emotional expression, shyness, and fear as well as on physiological measures, such as blood pressure (Marks, 1987).

Recall from Chapter 4 the work of psychologist Martin Seligman, who has studied learned helplessness. Seligman has hypothesized that humans, as a

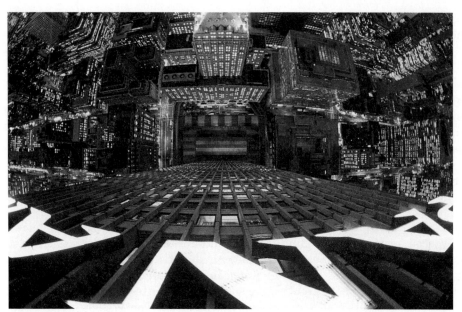

Fear of heights is a common phobia. Do you experience any discomfort when you look down at the street from a tall building, as in this photo?

species, are biologically prepared to develop fears or phobias to certain types of stimuli (Seligman, 1971). Think about what people commonly have phobias about: heights, flying, blood, small animals, and so on. People do not usually have phobias about inanimate objects, such as hammers, electric sockets, or typewriters.

What explains this patterned, nonrandom distribution of phobias? According to the **preparedness hypothesis,** our evolutionary past has prepared us to be afraid of objects or situations that, at one time, were associated with danger. Knowing what to be afraid of— and thus what to avoid or escape from—was essential knowledge in terms of self-preservation and the survival of the species. No doubt, we learn to fear things like snakes and blood more readily than houses and flowers. But is this a legacy of evolution or simply a form of cultural learning?

The Psychodynamic Model   The psychodynamic model takes a different view of phobias. According to this perspective, a phobia is simply one way in which intrapsychic, neurotic anxiety is unconsciously transformed into an external fear of a specific object or situation. In other words, some deep-seated conflict we have is expressed as an irrational fear of something or someone else, without our awareness.

The problems with this model illustrate the general criticisms of the psychodynamic approach. First, the evidence supporting the model is restricted to clinical case studies. Interpreting these case studies is highly subjective; a number of interpretations can be equally plausible—both psychodynamic (Brown, 1965) and nonpsychodynamic (Wolpe & Rachman, 1960). Second, the psychodynamic model predicts that treatment will be ineffective or incomplete if it doesn't unravel the early childhood conflicts that caused the disorder. Through treatment, the overt expression of the disorder may be eliminated, but other symptoms (that is, defense mechanisms) will take their place. Research has shown, however, that this doesn't happen (Barlow, 1988). When phobias are eliminated using exposure treatment, no other problems emerge. If anything, patients report even broader improvements in their lives because of their increased sense of personal mastery.

The Cognitive-Behavioral Model   According to the cognitive-behavioral model, the individual with a specific phobia associates the given object or situation with some threatening event. This fearful association can be learned through classical conditioning, in which an object or situation is paired with a traumatic event. Observing some other person behaving fearfully is another way to acquire phobic anxiety (Mineka, Davidson, Cook, & Keir, 1984). For example, a mother may display intense fear about dogs and pass on this fear to her children through modeling.

A problem with using classical conditioning as an explanation of specific phobias is that most people who are exposed to intense fear-provoking conditions do

preparedness hypothesis
Suggests that our evolutionary history has prepared us biologically to acquire fears of objects or situations that were at one time associated with danger to the species.

not develop phobias. Thus, it seems that some people are predisposed to acquiring phobic reactions, suggesting a biological, not a cognitive-behavioral, origin.

Two central concepts in explaining phobic and other anxiety reactions are predictability and **controllability.** The more we feel capable of predicting and potentially controlling aversive events, the less anxious we become (Bandura, 1986). This type of awareness and confidence about what happens in our lives is called **self-efficacy.** It's a product of what we've learned we can and cannot handle. The greater our feelings of self-efficacy, the less vulnerable we are to developing phobic reactions in response to traumatic experiences.

Research has supported the significance of self-efficacy in developing phobic reactions. An experiment with primates showed that a history of personal control over one's environment has a critical influence on the development of fear (Mineka, Gunnar, & Champoux, 1986). One group of infant monkeys—the "Masters"—were reared in an environment where they controlled when they received food, water, and special treats. A second group—the "Controls"—lived in an identical environment and received the same rewards. The only difference between the groups was that the Controls received their food, water, and treats automatically whenever the Masters chose theirs. Both groups were subjected to fear tests, using a mechanical toy monster to assess fear and exploratory tendencies. The Masters were significantly more willing than the Controls to approach the toy monster, and they were also less fearful in unfamiliar situations. The self-efficacy that the Masters developed in controlling their environment resulted in their having less fearful reactions to life events and situations.

Treatment

Behavior therapy is an effective treatment for specific phobias (O'Leary & Wilson, 1987). As mentioned earlier, the most powerful method is exposure treatment, in which patients confront their phobic situations in a gradual and planned manner (Barlow, 1988). How this treatment helps people overcome their phobias is still debated. Contrary to the predictions of classical conditioning, the amount of exposure during treatment is a poor predictor of outcome. Likewise, neither self-reports of anticipated anxiety nor measures of physiological arousal predict outcome well. Instead, evidence suggests that exposure treatments are effective because they increase patients' perceived self-efficacy. Individuals come to believe that they can cope successfully with the phobic object or situation (Bandura, 1986).

An advantage of self-efficacy theory is that it explains the success of behavioral and other effective nonbehavioral treatments (Klein et al., 1983). Self-efficacy can be increased not only through behavioral performance but also through vicarious experience and verbal persuasion. For instance, we can learn through observing others and how they deal with life events, particularly those we may be afraid of. In effect, individuals with high levels of self-efficacy can model successful behavior. Others can also offer verbal support of our own self-efficacy, encouraging us in situations we might otherwise withdraw from.

After a year of avoiding all air travel, Professor Jones decided to seek professional help. A friend from the psychology department urged him to consult a therapist who specialized in treating phobic and panic disorders.

The therapist planned a graduated series of tasks in which the professor was encouraged to remain in enclosed spaces (such as closets and small rooms) for increasingly longer periods of time until he could control his anxiety. It was then arranged for him to board an airplane together with the therapist—not to take a flight, but to become more comfortable with being in this particular enclosed space. Once the door was closed, the therapist provided emotional support and encouraged the professor to use the relaxation training they had rehearsed as a means of coping with anxiety.

controllability Real or perceived ability to control or influence potentially threatening events.

self-efficacy Attitude that an individual has about her capabilities to exercise control over events affecting her life.

In addition, the therapist used cognitive restructuring to prevent future panic attacks under these conditions. Professor Jones learned to identify specific thoughts that were part of his anxiety. For example, one of his thoughts was that the anxiety he experienced would keep increasing until he would lose control or even go insane. The therapist helped the professor challenge this thought. Using repeated exposure combined with relaxation training, the therapist disconfirmed this thought or expectation, showing the professor that his anxiety would reach a peak and then gradually subside.

After repeated exposures of this kind in a stationary airplane, the therapist arranged for them to take a short flight across the bay from Oakland to San Francisco. After that, increasingly longer flights were arranged. Professor Jones resumed regular air travel. However, his therapist cautioned him that it was possible that he might experience some anxiety at times in the future. Were this to happen, Professor Jones was instructed *not* to avoid but to continue flying while applying the techniques he had learned in treatment.

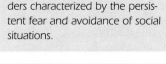

Focus on Critical Thinking

The preparedness hypothesis states that our evolutionary past has prepared us to acquire fears about specific objects or situations that were at one time associated with danger to the species. To test this hypothesis, psychologists paired pictures of either snakes (a biologically "prepared" stimulus) or triangles (a biologically neutral stimulus) with electric shock as an unconditioned stimulus in a classical conditioning study. They measured change in skin conductance, a common measure of fear.

1. What pattern of results does the preparedness hypothesis predict?
2. What should happen during extnction trials when the shock is turned off and the stimulus pictures are presented? Explain your answer.

SOCIAL PHOBIAS

Description

> **social phobias** Anxiety disorders characterized by the persistent fear and avoidance of social situations.

People with **social phobias** dread a variety of social situations because they fear being humiliated or embarrassed—they may even fear being looked at. The phobia may be specific, such as fear of speaking in public, or general, involving virtually all social situations. In extreme cases, social phobics cannot even venture out into the world; just the thought of doing so paralyzes them with fear.

The *DSM-IV* table lists the diagnostic criteria for social phobias. Typical symptoms include tachycardia (elevated heartrate), trembling, blushing, sweating, and shortness of breath—all indicating heightened autonomic nervous system arousal. The anxiety may be enough to provoke a panic attack. In comparison to simple phobics, social phobics also show other psychiatric symptoms, most notably more general anxiety and depression. Alcohol abuse is more often a problem, as well (American Psychiatric Association, 1994).

The distress, anticipation, and avoidance that charac-

DSM-IV Diagnostic Criteria for 300.23 SOCIAL PHOBIA

A. A marked and persistent fear of one or more social or performance situations in which the person is exposed to unfamiliar people or to possible scrutiny by others. The individual fears that he or she will act in a way (or show anxiety symptoms) that will be humiliating or embarrassing.

B. Exposure to the feared social situation almost invariably provokes anxiety, which may take the form of a situationally bound or situationally predisposed Panic Attack.

C. The person recognizes that the fear is excessive or unreasonable.

D. The feared social or performance situations are avoided or else are endured with intense anxiety or distress.

E. The avoidance, anxious anticipation, or distress in the feared social or performance situation(s) interfere significantly with the person's normal routine, occupational (academic) functioning, or social activities or relationships, or there is marked distress about having the phobia.

F. In individuals under age 18 years, the duration is at least 6 months.

G. The fear or avoidance is not due to the direct physiological effects of a substance (e.g., a drug of abuse, a medication) or a general medical condition and is not better accounted for by another mental disorder.

Responses of fear in threatening situations helped our ancestors survive. So it wouldn't be surprising if these responses were passed on through evolution across all species and cultures. Studies have shown that fear and anxiety are determined, in part, by genetic factors; some people have a genetic predisposition to developing anxiety disorders. Given all this, are there ethnic or cultural differences in the occurrence of anxiety?

Certainly, people in all cultures experience fear and anxiety, but how those emotions are expressed differs from culture to culture. Thus, the source of anxiety and how it's understood are culture specific. For example, in some Chinese cultures, there is a focus on sexual symptoms. **Koro,** a paniclike disorder experienced by ethnic Chinese in Singapore, is the fear that the sexual organs will retract into the body, resulting in death (Tan, 1980).

Taijin kyofusho (TKS) is a disorder that's very similar to social phobias that affects Japanese individuals (Kleinknecht, Dinnel, Tanouye-Wilson, & Lonner, 1994). TKS is defined as anxiety about offending others by blushing, emitting offensive odors or being flatulent, staring inappropriately, presenting improper facial expressions, or having physical deformities (Takahashi, 1989). Individuals with TKS are also concerned with being publicly observed and avoiding social situations—characterize

istics that also describe individuals with social phobias (as defined in the *DSM-IV*) (American Psychiatric Association, 1994).

But there is an important difference between the two: Individuals with social phobias are anxious about embarrassing *themselves.* Individuals with TKS are worried about embarrassing or offending *others* (Kleinknecht et al., 1994). This difference reflects the difference between Western and Japanese cultures. Namely, Western culture emphasizes individuality and independence; Japanese culture emphasizes the importance of collectivity and interdependence. Thus, it appears that the same underlying social anxiety is expressed differently according to dominant cultural values.

Are there differences in the expression of disorders among the various ethnic and racial groups in the United States? Although groups differ from each other in terms of some clinical disorders, they do not differ on the anxiety disorders (Kessler et al., 1994).

Think about the following question:

1. In the United States, the rates of prevalence of disorders among African Americans and Hispanics are very similar to those of whites, even when the effects of education and income are eliminated. Why do you think this is true?

---

terize people with social phobias interfere with their jobs or schooling and usual social activities and relationships. Yet social phobics without some associated clinical disorder rarely seek treatment (Schneier, Johnson, Hornig, Liebowitz, & Weissman, 1992).

Social phobias occur in approximately 1.2 to 2.2 percent of the population (Myers et al., 1984). Women are more likely than men to have these disorders, and so are individuals who are single and who are not well educated. The usual age of onset is in early childhood or adolescence (Schneier et al., 1992). Unless treated, this disorder follows a chronic course, becoming worse and worse.

What's the difference between feeling self-conscious or anxious in social situations and actually having a social phobia? After all, most of us experience some anxiety when we have to give a speech or somehow stand out in public. Are these normal reactions totally different from the symptoms of social phobias?

Some investigators suggest that social phobias are simply at the extreme end of a continuum of shyness or social performance anxiety (Barlow, 1988). Others argue that there is a qualitative difference between a social phobia and normal shyness or performance anxiety. Recent research on children's temperament sheds light on this debate. In one study, about 15 percent of 2-year-olds were consistently shy and emotionally inhibited in unfamiliar situations, whereas another 15 percent were sociable and uninhibited (Kagan, 1989a). When studied again at 8 years of age, the children still showed these temperaments: shy versus outgoing. There was no evidence of a continuum between these two extremes; they appeared to be separate categories. However, only children at the extremes of shyness/sociability were followed over time; the lack of evidence was thus built into the study design. It

koro Fear that the sexual organs will retract into the body; experienced by ethnic Chinese in Singapore.

taijin kyofusho (TKS) Japanese social disorder in which people experience social anxiety about the possibility of embarrassing or offending others by their actions or appearance.

remains to be determined, therefore, whether social phobia is more than extreme performance anxiety.

For insight into the effects of cultural differences on social phobias, see Thinking about Multicultural Issues, which looks at variations of these disorders.

Causes

There is some support for a biological model of social phobias. Studies of families of people with social phobias indicate a genetic predisposition for developing these disorders (Torgersen, 1983). Kagan's (1989) research on temperamental differences in young children also supports this model, showing that extreme shyness is inherited, rather than created by early experience.

The psychodynamic view of social phobias is the same as that for simple phobias: Namely, social phobias are caused by a transformation of intrapsychic anxiety into external anxiety, which occurs using the defense mechanism of **displacement.** No empirical evidence is available to test this theory, however.

The cognitive-behavioral model also explains simple and social phobias along the same lines, emphasizing the role of learning processes.

Treatment

Cognitive-behavioral therapy has proven successful in treating social phobias. In one illustrative study, Butler and her colleagues (1984) compared groups receiving one of two forms of treatment with a waiting-list control group. One form of treatment was exposure, in which patients were encouraged to systematically confront situations they had been avoiding. The other form was exposure plus relaxation training and **cognitive restructuring,** a technique in which patients are helped to identify and then challenge and modify dysfunctional thoughts. In the end, both treatment groups improved significantly more than the waiting-list control group.

Drugs are also commonly used to treat social phobias. Benzodiazepines, such as Librium or Valium, provide short-term relief. Antidepressant medication has also proven effective (Levin, Schneier, & Liebowitz, 1989).

A combination of drug and psychological therapy is recommended in treating social phobias. The use of cognitive-behavioral treatment may prevent the return of symptoms that often occurs when drugs are discontinued (Gelernter et al., 1991).

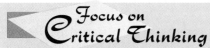

Focus on Critical Thinking

1. Many men are unable to urinate in a public toilet when other men are lining up beside and behind them, waiting for their turn. This has been called a case of the "bashful bladder." Is this anxiety a symptom of social phobia? If it happened repeatedly, would it make someone a social phobic? Explain your answer.

2. In comparison to people with specific phobias, people with social phobias are more likely to have general anxiety and depression, as well. Why do you think this is so?

displacement Defense mechanism in which an unacceptable reaction is shifted unconsciously from the object perceived as threatening to a substitute object that is less threatening.

cognitive restructuring Technique in which patients are helped to identify, challenge, and modify dysfunctional thoughts.

GENERALIZED ANXIETY DISORDER

Description

Consider the following case:

Ray is a thirty-two-year-old rock musician. About five years before his evaluation at the clinic, he had begun to feel very anxious and nervous and found it difficult to sit still. He also found himself worrying constantly about his career, although he had more bookings than ever and had achieved financial independence. Although

Diagnostic Criteria for 300.02 GENERALIZED ANXIETY DISORDER

A. Excessive anxiety and worry (apprehensive expectation), occurring more days than not for at least 6 months, about a number of events or activities (such as work or school performance).

B. The person finds it difficult to control the worry.

C. The anxiety and worry are associated with three (or more) of the following six symptoms (with at least some symptoms present for more days than not for the past 6 months).
  (1) restlessness or feeling keyed up or on edge
  (2) being easily fatigued
  (3) difficulty concentrating or mind going blank
  (4) irritability
  (5) muscle tension
  (6) sleep disturbance (difficulty falling or staying asleep, or restless unsatisfying sleep)

D. The focus of the anxiety and worry is not confined to features of an Axis I. . . .

E. The anxiety, worry, or physical symptoms cause clinically significant distress or impairment in social, occupational, or other important areas of functioning.

F. The disturbance is not due to the direct physiological effects of a substance (e.g., a drug of abuse, a medication) or a general medical condition (e.g., hyperthyroidism) and does not occur exclusively during a Mood Disorder, a Psychotic Disorder, or a Pervasive Development Disorder.

he had previously been a heavy cocaine user, he found that cocaine caused him to be intolerably nervous. Also, he found that marijuana and alcohol, which used to calm him down, no longer did so. He reported symptoms of motor tension, including trembling, twitching or feeling shaky, muscle tension and restlessness, and autonomic hyperactivity; he exhibited extreme vigilance and scanning during the interview. . . . He often felt irritable and had more trouble dealing with frustration than before this episode began. (Taylor & Arnow, 1988, p. 104)

Ray's case illustrates **generalized anxiety disorder (GAD),** a severe disorder that significantly interferes with the routines of daily life. The diagnostic criteria for this disorder are listed in the *DSM-IV* table.

GAD involves what used to be called **free-floating anxiety,** or anxiety that isn't attached to any specific stimulus or situation. Patients with GAD often report a life-long history of generalized anxiety, with no clearcut onset (Brown, O'Leary, & Barlow, 1993). The lifetime prevalence of GAD is 5.1 percent. It occurs twice as often in women than in men (Wittchen et al., 1994).

People with GAD are very likely to have other disorders, too. The National Comorbidity Study found that 90 percent of people with GAD had lifetime **comorbidity** of some other psychiatric disorder (Wittchen et al., 1994). GAD is the most common disorder in patients with a primary diagnosis of another anxiety or mood disorder (Brawman-Mintzer et al., 1993; Brown, O'Leary, & Barlow, 1993).

Although GAD is more common than panic disorder, analyses of patients treated in anxiety clinics indicate that panic disorder is seen far more frequently (Barlow, 1988). GAD patients only seek specialized psychological or psychiatric care when their physical symptoms become too severe. Otherwise, they are likely to put up with their so-called worrying or see a general medical practitioner.

generalized anxiety disorder (GAD) Unrealistic and excessive anxiety about two or more life situations.

free-floating anxiety Old-fashioned term used to describe the pervasive anxiety characteristic of generalized anxiety disorder.

comorbidity Co-occurrence of more than one clinical disorder in the same person.

Causes

Noyes et al. (1987) found a higher frequency of GAD among relatives of people with this disorder than among relatives of individuals with panic disorder or agoraphobia; the same pattern held true in comparing relatives of GAD patients with those of a control group. Research on identical and fraternal twins born to parents with GAD has also shown that familial transmission is genetic. However, because the estimates of heritability of GAD from this research are modest, ranging from 19 to 30 percent, investigators concluded that specific environmental experiences are critical in determining who develops GAD (Kendler et al., 1992a).

Treatment

Medication is the most common treatment for GAD, usually involving the benzo-diazepines, such as Librium, Valium, and Xanax. These drugs are effective in pro-ducing a short-term reduction in anxiety, lasting one to two weeks (Schweizer & Rickels, 1991). Long-term use is discouraged, though. Xanax is highly addictive, and many individuals experience intense anxiety when they try to discontinue use (Barlow, 1988).

Another drawback of medication is that the benzodiazepines tend to make peo-ple drowsy. A newer class of drugs, however, doesn't have these sedative effects. The azapirones, including buspirone, have also been found effective in treating GAD (see Chapter 20). Finally, preliminary findings have indicated that tricyclic antidepressant medication may be effective, as well (Rickels, Downing, Schweizer, & Hassman, 1993).

The most effective and carefully studied psychological treatment has been cognitive-behavioral therapy. CBT combines relaxation training, which directly reduces tension, with cognitive restructuring, which helps patients identify and alter specific anxiety-provoking thoughts. Together, these methods reduce the chronic vigilance characteristic of GAD (Borkovec & Costello, 1993). The cognitive restructuring component of CBT is critical in this treatment approach (Butler, Fennell, Robson, & Gelder, 1991).

Focus on Critical Thinking

1. Think of someone you know who worries a great deal. Does this person display any of the symptoms described in the DSM-IV table on GAD? If so, describe which ones. Could this person be diagnosed with GAD? Why or why not?

2. Why do you think individuals with GAD only seek specialized psychological or psychiatric care when their physical symptoms become severe? Why are they less concerned with their psychological and emotional symptoms? Why might they go to a general medical practitioner instead of a psychological or psychiatric specialist?

POSTTRAUMATIC STRESS DISORDER

Description

Consider the following case:

> Mr. K, a 43-year-old Vietnam combat veteran, was the second-oldest child from a working-class family dominated by a harsh father. His mother died of cancer when he was 13 and his father remarried a year later. Although Mr. K did well in school, he dropped out of school at age 17 to join the Navy for 4 years. During his Navy tour he married the first woman he had ever dated. They produced two children. Following discharge from the Navy he had difficulty finding satisfactory civilian employment and decided to join the Army. . . .
>
> He was sent to Vietnam as a staff sergeant in charge of a vehicle maintenance team. This tour of duty was punctuated with frequent traumatic combat experi-ences, including the death of a close friend, his shooting a Vietcong soldier at close range, . . . finding a burned crew inside a disabled tank, finding the remains of a driver inside a disabled personnel carrier, and witnessing the demolition of a vil-lage. The death of his close friend by sniper fire in a "safe" area was particularly traumatic; Mr. K felt personally responsible for their having been in an avoidable dangerous situation.
>
> When he returned from Vietnam his marriage ended in divorce and he began drinking heavily. He received several Army disciplinary actions, usually for going

absent without leave. After 3 years, Mr. K volunteered for a second tour in Vietnam, which, in contrast to the first tour, was relatively uneventful.

Following his second Vietnam tour he took a discharge from the Army. During the next 15 years, his life seriously deteriorated. He had two short marriages, lived in five different states, and had a long series of various jobs. He began having Vietnam-related nightmares and flashbacks. His abusive drinking became chronic. . . . In addition to numerous alcohol treatments, there were several psychiatric hospitalizations for depression, anxiety, paranoia, and suicide attempts. (Foy, Donahoe, Carroll, Gallers, & Reno, 1987, pp. 369–370)

This case illustrates the diagnostic criteria for **posttraumatic stress disorder (PTSD)** listed in the *DSM-IV* table. Although symptoms of **dissociation**—such as memory loss and identity confusion—are not part of the *DSM-IV* criteria, they are common in PTSD (Bremer, Southwick, Johnson, Yehuda, & Charney, 1993).

PTSD is triggered by a range of life-threatening or personally devastating experiences:

posttraumatic stress disorder (PTSD) Anxiety disorder triggered by a traumatic event and characterized by intrusive thoughts, intense physiological reactivity, and avoidance of the stimuli associated with the trauma.

dissociation Process in which part of mental functioning is split from the rest of consciousness.

 Diagnostic Criteria for 309.81 POSTTRAUMATIC STRESS DISORDER (PTSD)

A. The person has been exposed to a traumatic event in which both of the following were present:
  (1) the person experienced, witnessed, or was confronted with an event or events that involved actual or threatened death or serious injury, or a threat to the physical integrity of self or others.
  (2) the person's response involved intense fear, helplessness, or horror.

B. The traumatic event is persistently reexperienced in one (or more) of the following ways:
  (1) recurrent and intrusive distressing recollections of the event, including images, thoughts, or perceptions.
  (2) recurrent distressing dreams of the event.
  (3) acting or feeling as if the traumatic event were recurring (includes a sense of reliving the experience, illusions, hallucinations, and dissociative flashback episodes, including those that occur on awakening or when intoxicated).
  (4) intense psychological distress at exposure to internal or external cues that symbolize or resemble an aspect of the traumatic event.
  (5) physiological reactivity on exposure to internal or external cues that symbolize or resemble an aspect of the traumatic event.

C. Persistent avoidance of stimuli associated with the trauma and numbing of general responsiveness (not present before the trauma), as indicated by three (or more) of the following:
  (1) efforts to avoid thoughts, feelings, or conversations associated with the trauma
  (2) efforts to avoid activities, places, or people that arouse recollections of the trauma
  (3) inability to recall an important aspect of the trauma
  (4) markedly diminished interest or participation in significant activities
  (5) feeling of detachment or estrangement from others
  (6) restricted range of affect (e.g., unable to have loving feelings)
  (7) sense of a foreshortened future (e.g., does not expect to have a career, marriage, children, or a normal life span)

D. Persistent symptoms of increased arousal (not present before the trauma), as indicated by two (or more) of the following:
  (1) difficulty falling or staying asleep
  (2) irritability or outbursts of anger
  (3) difficulty concentrating
  (4) hypervigilance
  (5) exaggerated startle response

E. Duration of the disturbance (symptoms in Criteria B, C, and D) is more than 1 month.

F. The disturbance causes clinically significant distress or impairment in social, occupational, or other important areas of functioning.

- war, including combat, bombing, and torture
- natural disasters, such as floods, earthquakes, and fires
- human-caused disasters, such as airplane crashes and nuclear accidents
- criminal assaults, such as rape or attempted murder

The symptoms of PTSD may occur immediately after the traumatic event or emerge months, even years, later. The individual may experience mild to total impairment in functioning and biological as well as psychological and behavioral disturbances. Suicide and suicide attempts are not infrequent.

One of the most intensively studied groups of people with PTSD are combat veterans from the Vietnam War. Of the 2.8 million Vietnam-era veterans who served in combat, 0.5 to 1.2 million may suffer from PTSD (Wolfe, Keane, Lyons, & Gerardi, 1987). Diagnosis of PTSD in veterans seeking treatment is as high as 70 percent for those who participated in combat and were wounded. Among those with little combat exposure, the rate of diagnosis is only 25 percent (Foy et al., 1987).

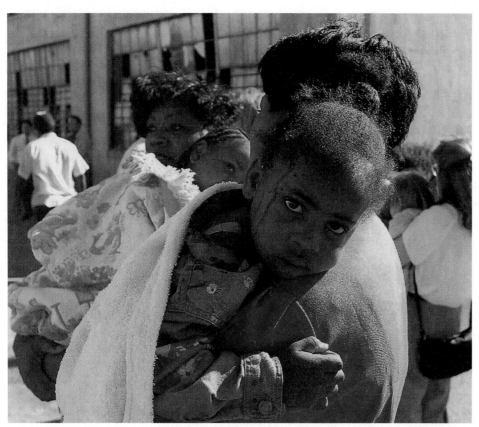

The uncomprehending stare of one of the children who survived the bombing of the federal building in Oklahoma City

Suicide is also common among Vietnam veterans with PTSD. A study of U.S. Army combat veterans found that within five years after returning to civilian life, they had an overall death rate 45 percent higher than veterans who had served elsewhere during the same period (for instance, in Korea, West Germany, or the United States). During the same five-year period, the suicide rate for Vietnam combat veterans was 72 percent higher than that for other veterans of the same era who did not serve in Vietnam (Centers for Disease Control Vietnam Experience Study, 1987).

The prevalence of PTSD among civilians was assessed in a representative national sample of 4,008 women (Resnick, Kilpatrick, Dansky, Saunders, & Best, 1993). The lifetime prevalence rate of PTSD was 12.3 percent, or approximately 11.8 million American women had experienced this disorder at some point in their lives. The current prevalence rate was 4.6 percent. Table 5.1 breaks down lifetime and current prevalence rates according to exposure history. For this sample, physical assault, completed rape, and other sexual assault were the most common causes of PTSD. These findings are consistent with other data, showing that the trauma of rape is a prominent cause of PTSD in women (Breslau, Davis, Andereski, & Peterson, 1991).

TABLE 5.1 Lifetime and Current PTSD Prevalence Rates Associated with Exposure History (in percent)

Event Type	Lifetime PTSD Rate	Current PTSD Rate
Physical assault	38.5	17.8
Completed rape	32.0	12.4
Other sexual assault	30.8	13.0
Any crime victimization	25.8	9.7
Homicide of family or close friend	22.1	8.9
Any trauma	17.9	6.7
Noncrime trauma only (disaster/accident/other)	9.4	3.4
Total Sample	**12.3**	**4.6**

Individuals with PTSD are at heightened risk for all the other anxiety disorders as well as for major depression, suicide, somatization disorder, and substance abuse (American Psychiatric Association, 1994).

Causes

Being exposed to a traumatic event is necessary for the development of PTSD but insufficient by itself. Classical conditioning explains how stimuli associated with a severe trauma elicit stress responses that were part of the original trauma. But not everyone who experiences a traumatic event shows symptoms of the disorder. For example, the majority of Vietnam combat veterans did not develop PTSD. Regardless of the type of trauma experienced, only a minority of those affected develop PTSD (Meichenbaum, 1994). Some combat veterans and survivors of natural disasters have even reported positive effects, saying that the experience increased their sense of being able to cope with crises effectively (Ursano, McCauhey, & Fullerton, 1994).

Genetic factors are strongly related to all the symptoms of PTSD. In a sophisticated genetic analysis of 4,042 identical and fraternal twins of the Vietnam era, genetic influences accounted for at least 30 percent of the variance in PTSD symptoms (True et al., 1993). These findings also applied to cases of PTSD that were unrelated to traumatic experiences in Vietnam. The role of genetic factors applied as much to twins who did not go to Vietnam as to those who served in combat.

Genetic influences predispose people to developing PTSD, creating a critical threshold. If a traumatic event pushes the individual over this threshold, PTSD symptoms result. The lower the threshold, the less traumatic the event needs to be to do damage. A powerful trauma can cause PTSD, even if the threshold is high.

Recent research has indicated that PTSD has a distinctive biological basis. In comparison to patients in other diagnostic groups, patients with PTSD show sustained levels of **catecholamines,** which are stress hormones that prepare the body for an emergency (Kosten, Mason, Giller, Ostroff, & Harkness, 1987). However, PTSD patients showed lower than normal levels of another hormone, **cortisol,** which is important in regulating metabolism (Yehuda et al., 1990). As a result, the ratio of catecholamine to cortisol is twice as high for PTSD patients than it is for patients with other anxiety disorders and from other diagnostic groups. This characteristic imbalance of hormone levels is also consistent with the clinical features of constant vigilance and reactivity, on the one hand (due to high catecholamines), and paranoid-type mechanisms (due to low cortisol), on the other.

What's most intriguing about these biological findings is that the hyperreactivity of the catecholamine system may be due to irreversible changes in brain mechanisms caused by exposure to severe stress (Charney, Deutch, Krystal, Southwick, & Davis, 1993). Traumatic events may cause permanent damage to specific receptors in brain cells (called *alpha 2 receptors*) that regulate the release of catecholamines. Individuals with PTSD have 40 percent fewer alpha 2 receptors than normal control individuals (Southwick et al., 1993).

Severe stress alters three key brain circuits: the locus ceruleus, which regulates brain hormones that prepare for emergencies; the hypothalamus and pituitary gland, which regulate stress-response hormones; and the opioid system, which blunts pain. Thus, a psychosocial event (exposure to trauma) can cause biological changes (in brain neurochemistry) that, in turn, make us more vulnerable to psychological stressors.

Psychological and social factors interact with biological and genetic influences in accounting for different responses to traumatic events. People with preexisting clinical problems are more vulnerable to PTSD when exposed to traumatic events. Helzer, Robins, and McEvoy (1987) found that individuals who had behavioral problems before age 15 (stealing, lying, truancy, fighting, and substance abuse) were

catecholamines Hormones that are part of the stress-response system that prepares us for emergencies.

cortisol Hormone secreted by the adrenal gland that is part of the stress-response system that prepares us for emergencies.

PERSPECTIVE ON POSTTRAUMATIC STRESS DISORDER (PTSD)

BIOLOGICAL FACTORS

Biological mechanisms make certain people more vulnerable to developing PTSD in response to any trauma they might experience:

➤ Genetic factors account for roughly one-third of the variance of all PTSD symptoms.

➤ People with PTSD show abnormal hyperreactivity of the catecholamine and CRF systems, which results in sustained stress responding. This prolonged elevation of neuroendocrine levels can ultimately lead to irreversible changes in brain mechanisms, which in turn impair the brain's ability to regulate catecholamine release and cope with stress.

➤ Excessive release of opioids might explain feelings of emotional numbing.

PSYCHOLOGICAL FACTORS

Psychological factors interact with biological vulnerabilities in producing PTSD symptoms:

➤ The magnitude or perceived severity of the stressor is directly related to the risk of developing PTSD.

➤ Of people exposed to traumatic events, those with a prior history of psychological problems are more likely to be adversely affected by the traumatic experience.

➤ Childhood sexual abuse is a risk factor for developing long-term PTSD.

➤ It is more than the objective traumatic event that results in PTSD. The meaning a person attaches to an event is also important. For example, feeling responsible for an event can be more critical than the event itself.

SOCIAL FACTORS

Both biological and psychological factors operate in specific social contexts:

➤ Social factors increase exposure to trauma (e.g., living in the inner city where personal violence is more common).

➤ Certain conditions produce a higher risk of exposure to traumatic events (e.g., soldiers in combat).

➤ Social factors help determine whether PTSD symptoms are perpetuated or eliminated following exposure to stress. A social network of supportive family and friends can protect against PTSD.

These biological, psychological, and social factors interact to cause problems, as illustrated in the following case:

Greg is a 50-year-old Vietnam veteran currently in treatment for PTSD. He is constantly on edge, moody, irritable, loses his temper easily, and sleeps poorly. He also abuses alcohol. Activities he once enjoyed are no longer fun. Divorced from his wife of ten years, Greg is socially iso-lated and lonely. He is on medication to control high blood pressure.

The biopsychosocial model explains Greg's problems. Greg's father was an alcoholic; his mother was often de-pressed. Greg's childhood psychological problems and repeated trouble at school likely predisposed him to developing PTSD after exposure to combat-related trauma in Vietnam. His sustained stress responding causes his high arousal level, poor sleeping habits, and high blood pres-sure. Heavy drinking perpetuates a nega-tive cycle of stress responding due to the social problems it causes. Alcohol also impairs the sleep cycle, adding to Greg's fatigue and further lowering his threshold for becoming stressed. His behavior has led to divorce and estrangement from friends. The resulting social isolation, in turn, has left him more vulnerable to stress.

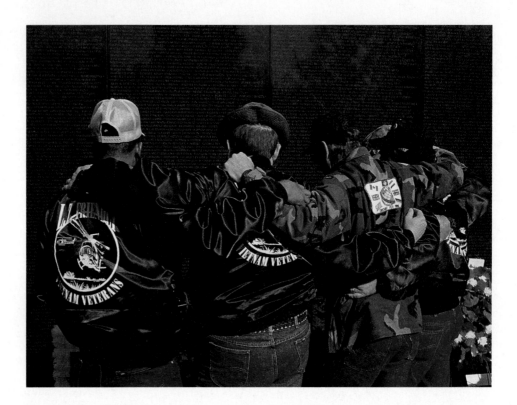

Vietnam veterans share a solemn moment of remembrance at the Vietnam Memorial in Washington, DC.

more likely to develop PTSD or some of its symptoms than those without these childhood problems. Similarly, individuals with family histories of psychiatric problems were more likely to develop PTSD if exposed to military combat than those with no such background (Foy et al., 1987). On the positive side, social support protects against PTSD. The stronger the individual's social network of family and friends, the less the chance of developing this disorder (Barlow, 1988).

Treatment

Given the evidence of biological abnormalities in PTSD, it's not surprising that antidepressant drugs have been used to treat this disorder. Case studies have reported that antidepressant drugs produce a decrease in intensity and frequency of prolonged nightmares, flashbacks, panic attacks, and episodes of anxiety as well as an improvement in mood and the ability to modulate anger. However, evidence from controlled studies about the successful use of these drugs is mixed (Solomon, Gerrity, & Muff, 1992). Pharmacological therapy is usually recommended only as a supplement to other psychological treatment. Antidepressant drugs may be useful, however, in treating associated anxiety and depression in patients with PTSD.

Cognitive-behavioral therapies—particularly *imaginal exposure* methods—have been effective in treating individuals with PTSD, although only a few controlled studies have been completed (Foa, Rothbaum, Riggs, & Murdock, 1991). In these therapies, the patient is asked repeatedly to conjure up detailed images of the events associated with the traumatic experience and to focus on these images until the initial anxiety decreases. Under a therapist's guidance, repeated exposure brings reductions in emotional and physiological arousal and intrusive thoughts.

Both cognitive-behavioral and psychodynamic therapies have shown promise in clinical case studies (Solomon et al., 1992). Horowitz (1989) developed a brief, 12-session psychodynamic treatment that overlaps with cognitive-behavioral therapy. In this treatment, the therapist first establishes a trusting relationship with the

Focus on Critical Thinking

1. Think about someone you know or have heard about who has been raped or experienced some other traumatic event. Did he or she develop any symptoms of PTSD? If so, describe them. What helped this individual cope with his or her problems? Why did this help?

2. The scientific literature on the effects of traumatic events suggests that different types of disasters produce different types of stress reactions. Specifically, disasters that are caused by humans—for example, wars or bombings, such as that of the federal office building in Oklahoma City in 1995—produce more severe stress reactions than natural disasters—for example, hurricanes or floods (Meichenbaum, 1994). What psychological factors might explain these differences?

patient. Within this safe therapeutic relationship, the patient explores self-identity and achieves increasing levels of self-awareness. The goal is for the patient to recognize and accept thoughts about the traumatic event that he had previously warded off.

A form of self-help group treatment for individuals with PTSD are so-called rap groups. These informal discussion groups have been widely adopted to treat Vietnam veterans with PTSD. Because group members have shared the same kinds of experiences, they are able to develop a unique sense of understanding and trust. Disclosing the horrors of a traumatic experience has therapeutic value. Pennebaker (1990) found that victims of the Holocaust, rape, and other traumatic events achieved better physical health if they told others about their secret suffering.

OBSESSIVE-COMPULSIVE DISORDER

Description

Individuals with **obsessive-compulsive disorder (OCD)** are driven to think about certain topics or perform certain behaviors over and over again in an attempt to relieve anxiety. Nearly all individuals with OCD report having both obsessions and compulsions. The diagnostic criteria for OCD are listed in the *DSM-IV* table.

The most common **obsessions** involve themes of aggression, dirt and contamination, sex, religion, and doubt. For example, a highly religious person might be plagued with blasphemous thoughts; a gentle, nonviolent individual might have repeated images of mutilated corpses; or a concerned parent might experience recurring impulses to injure a loved child. Obsessions differ fundamentally from the worries that we all have at one time or another in that they cause marked distress. They are often associated with the fear of losing control. The obsessive person typically tries hard to suppress or neutralize the troubling thought with some other thought or action—although unsuccessfully, in most cases.

Unwanted, unacceptable thoughts are called *ego dystonic.* The person who has such thoughts realizes that they are products of her own mind. The individual's knowing this and actively resisting obsessive thinking is what distinguishes an obsession from a psychotic delusion. As bizarre as some obsessions might seem, they are different from psychotic delusions, for this reason.

The two main types of overt behavioral **compulsions** are cleaning and checking. The classic example of the first type is the compulsive handwasher. A common example of the second type is the person who compulsively checks the security of appliances and entrances to her home. Examples of covert compulsions include mental strategies, such as thinking "good thoughts" or conjuring up particular images to neutralize distressing, obsessional thoughts or images.

Many individuals with OCD realize that their behavior is unreasonable, but some insist that it has a rational basis. For example, a compulsive handwasher might argue that this activity protects against contracting a disease. The *DSM-III-R* described this as an "overvalued idea." Subsequent research has shown that people with OCD vary greatly in how much they recognize that their obsessions or compulsions are senseless (Lelliot, Noshirvani, Basoglu, Marks, & Monterio, 1988). Accordingly, the *DSM-IV* allows clinicians to note how strongly patients believe

obsessive-compulsive disorder (OCD) Anxiety disorder characterized by uncontrollable thoughts or images and behavioral rituals.

obsessions Repetitive thoughts, images, or impulses that cause anxiety the person cannot dismiss.

compulsions Repetitive, stereotyped acts that a person with the disorder feels compelled to carry out, despite some recognition that they are unreasonable.

Diagnostic Criteria for 300.3 OBSESSIVE-COMPULSIVE DISORDER

A. Either obsessions or compulsions:

Obsessions as defined by (1), (2), (3), and (4):

(1) recurrent and persistent thoughts, impulses, or images that are experienced, at some time during the disturbance, as intrusive and inappropriate and that cause marked anxiety or distress

(2) the thoughts, impulses, or images are not simply excessive worries about real-life problems

(3) the person attempts to ignore or suppress such thoughts, impulses, or images, or to neutralize them with some other thought or action

(4) the person recognizes that the obsessional thoughts, impulses, or images are a product of his or her own mind (not imposed from without as in thought insertion)

Compulsions as defined by (1) and (2):

(1) repetitive behaviors (e.g., hand washing, ordering, checking) or mental acts (e.g., praying, counting, repeat-ing words silently) that the person feels driven to perform in response to an obsession, or according to rules that must be applied rigidly

(2) the behaviors or mental acts are aimed at preventing or reducing distress or preventing some dreaded event or situation; however, these behaviors or mental acts either are not connected in a realistic way with what they are designed to neutralize or prevent or are clearly excessive

B. At some point during the course of the disorder, the person has recognized that the obsessions or compulsions are excessive or unreasonable.

C. The obsessions or compulsions cause marked distress, are time consuming (take more than 1 hour a day), or significantly interfere with the person's normal routine, occupational (or academic) functioning, or usual special activities or relationships.

D. If another Axis I disorder is present, the content of the obsessions or compulsions is not restricted to it. . . .

E. The disturbance is not due to the direct physiological effects of a substance (e.g., a drug of abuse, a medication) or a general medical condition.

their symptoms are unreasonable. A patient who believes that he is not unreasonable is described as having "poor insight."

The Epidemiologic Catchment Area (ECA) study of five U.S. communities found prevalence rates of obsessive-compulsive disorder ranging from 1.9 to 3.3 percent of the general population (Karno, Golding, Sorenson, & Burnam, 1988). Unlike the previously discussed anxiety disorders, OCD affects men and women about equally. The average age of onset of OCD ranges from early adolescence to the mid-20s (Rasmussen & Eisen, 1990). The symptoms often begin in childhood.

OCD not only causes severe personal distress but also impairs social, occupational, and sexual functioning. The following case illustrates these devastating effects:

The patient was obsessed with the fear of contamination by germs. As a result she engaged in prolonged and intensive washing and cleaning rituals. Her young child was restrained in one room of the four bedroom house, as it was the only one that she could keep satisfactorily free from germs. Three of the rooms were kept permanently locked because she was incapable of ensuring that they were sufficiently sterile. She used an extraordinarily large amount of disinfectants to clean her house and to wash herself and her child. As is common with many of these patients, she was particularly agitated by contact with doors and doorknobs, and therefore learned how to open a door with her feet in order to avoid contaminating her hands. The large and complicated series of rituals that had to be carried out in preparing food meant that the family was kept on a restricted diet. Meals were seldom complete and rarely ready on time. The patient's fear of contamination made her virtually housebound, and her child was not permitted to leave the house except on a very few essential occasions. On returning from work each day, her husband was obliged to go through a series of decontaminating-cleaning rituals. Their sexual relationship, never satisfactory, had been abandoned because of her fears of contamination. Their social life was damaged beyond repair, and they had lost all but one of their friends; even the members of their families could neither visit them nor be visited by them. Although the patient had been a competent, trained secretary, returning to work was out of the question. (Rachman & Hodgson, 1980, pp. 111–112)

Clearly, this disorder also greatly impacts individuals around the person with OCD. The disorder can be devastating for family members, who find it difficult, if not impossible, to avoid being drawn into the obsessive-compulsive rituals. The preceding case of the woman with the germ obsession shows the effects it had on her husband and child, neither of whom could live normal lives. Many individuals with OCD do not marry, and those who do have a greater than average incidence of marital and sexual problems (Rachman & Hodgson, 1980).

Causes

The Biological Model The first-degree relatives of individuals with OCD often have related psychological and neurological disorders. McKeon and Murray (1987) studied relatives of 50 obsessive-compulsive patients and those of matched control subjects who had no psychiatric disorders. The first-degree relatives of the OCD patients had a significantly higher rate of lifetime psychiatric disorders and much greater rates of depression and generalized anxiety disorder than the relatives of the control patients. The two groups of relatives did not, however, differ in prevalence of OCD, which was very rare. Among the 149 relatives of the obsessive-compulsive patients and the 151 relatives of the controls, only one case of OCD was diagnosed in each group.

These findings indicate that an *anxiety disorder diathesis* (what McKeon and Murray call a *neurotic tendency*) is transmitted within families with OCD. How that tendency is expressed within families, however, is variable. Evidence of a genetic origin of this transmission comes from twin studies that examine the concordance rate (that is, the likelihood of both individuals having the disorder). The concordance rate for anxiety disorders in identical twins is higher than that for fraternal pairs (Andrews, Stewart, Morris-Yates, Holt, & Henderson, 1990). But there is little evidence that this higher concordance applies to OCD itself. This suggests that stressful life events determine how the genetically transmitted diathesis is expressed.

Several other findings also point to OCD having a distinctive biological basis. OCD is often associated with several types of neurological disorders. Over 50 percent of patients with OCD also have *tics*—involuntary motor movements, such as eye blinking and making facial grimaces. From 5 to 15 percent of children and adults with OCD also have **Tourette's syndrome**, which is characterized by a number of distinctive symptoms: displaying intermittent tics, including sudden jerks of the head and other body parts; making sounds, such as barks or yelps; and uttering words, such as obscenities (Leonard et al., 1992). Other examples of neurological disorders that frequently co-occur with OCD are Sydenham's chorea (characterized by rapid, jerky, and involuntary movements), epilepsy, and Parkinson's disease.

The rate of obsessive-compulsive disorder among the first-degree relatives of patients with Tourette's syndrome is significantly higher than estimates from the general population and a control sample of adoptive relatives (Pauls, Towbin, Leckman, Zahner, & Cohen, 1986). This finding suggests that there is some common causal, genetic relationship between the two disorders. All these neurological disorders affect the basal ganglia and particularly the **caudate nucleus** in the brain.

Positron emission tomography (PET) scans have shown that in comparison to controls, patients with OCD metabolize glucose (that is, burn energy) more rapidly in the frontal lobe and cingulate pathway, which connects the frontal lobe to the basal ganglia (Baxter et al., 1987). Moreover, this increased glucose metabolism was correlated with measures of the severity of OCD.

Rapoport (1989) has hypothesized that the basal ganglia and caudate nucleus are "way stations" between sensory input and resulting motor output. In OCD, neural transmission from the frontal lobe to the basal ganglia is disturbed, or "short-circuited," triggering repetitive actions and abnormal motor movements.

We might be able to explain this malfunction, in part, by considering our evolutionary heritage. Obsessions are often dominated by themes of violence, germs or contamination, and checking on things; many phobias are concerned with these issues, as well. During the course of evolution, survival may well have depended on paying attention to these issues. It seems that in OCD, the brain mechanisms responsible for these activities have gone awry.

Tourette's syndrome Disorder characterized by intermittent bodily tics, sounds, and words.

caudate nucleus Cluster of brain cells in the basal ganglia believed to be centrally involved in anxiety disorders such as OCD.

Brain areas showing abnormal activity in OCD depend on **serotonin,** which is a **neurotransmitter.** The most effective drugs for treating obsessive-compulsive disorder increase the amount of serotonin in the brain (Zohar & Insel, 1987).

An alternative biological explanation is that the mechanism of **extinction** is impaired. People with OCD have unusually high levels of vasopressin in their cerebrospinal fluid (Altemus et al., 1992). Vasopressin is a neurohormone that, when injected into the brains of rats, significantly delays the extinction of conditioned avoidance responses that resemble compulsive rituals (Strupp, Weingartner, Goodwin, & Gold, 1983).

The Psychodynamic Model The psychodynamic view is that obsessive-compulsive disorder occurs in people with a particular type of personality—what Freud called **anal-erotic personality.** People with this personality type are characterized by three traits: orderliness, stinginess, and obstinacy. These traits result from fixation of psychosexual development in the anal stage of personality growth. Toilet training occurs during this stage, providing the child with his first experience of imposing external control over an instinctual impulse (that is, defecation). When toilet training is strict or severe, the child takes pleasure in retaining feces. This is expressed symbolically later in life in the traits of orderliness, obstinacy, and stinginess.

These traits identified by Freud are found together in studies of OCD, and there is a loose relationship between the occurrence of OCD and obsessional traits that existed prior to it, as predicted by psychodynamic theory (Fisher & Greenberg, 1977). Yet many people become obsessive-compulsive without ever having displayed preexisting (also called *premorbid*) obsessional traits. A concern with orderliness does not discriminate OCD patients from other patients with nonobsessive anxiety disorder (Rachman & Hodgson, 1980).

Perhaps most critically, the psychodynamic model has failed to produce an effective treatment for obsessive-compulsive disorders.

The Cognitive-Behavioral Model The cognitive-behavioral model suggests that the individual with obsessions has a nonspecific, genetic predisposition to experience anxiety. The model further hypothesizes that the individual grows up in an overcontrolling home environment, leading to rigid standards of personal conduct and vulnerability to self-criticism. These early learning experiences result in a low threshold for regarding certain thoughts and images as being unacceptable; the same thoughts and images would be acceptable to nonobsessive people (Rachman & Hodgson, 1980). For example, sexual thoughts or images often form the content of clinical obsessions because patients find them unacceptable.

The behavioral explanation of the causes of compulsive behavior is similar. In addition to the assumptions mentioned already, additional assumptions are that compulsive cleaners come from overcontrolling and protective environments (which foster a fearful, noncoping disposition) and that checkers come from overcontrolling and overcritical families (which foster obsessional doubt and the need to check "to make sure"). This account of etiology remains speculative, though.

The behavioral model has been more helpful in understanding how compulsive behavior is maintained. It assumes that compulsions constitute a form of escape or avoidance behavior. As they reduce anxiety, the compulsions are reinforced. Preventing obsessive individuals from engaging in or completing compulsive rituals will actually increase their anxiety and will have harmful consequences. This theory is based on the assumption that compulsions are a form of psychic defense, which if removed, would lead to emotional turmoil for the individual.

Rachman and his colleagues (Rachman & Hodgson, 1980), at the Institute of Psychiatry in London, carried out a series of studies to test this anxiety-reduction theory. In the basic experiment, OCD patients agreed to touch an object that was considered to be contaminated. The subjects were allowed to wash their hands

serotonin Neurotransmitter thought to be involved in the causation of different clinical disorders, such as obsessive-compulsive disorder.

neurotransmitter Biochemical substance in the brain that mediates transmission of electrical impulses across the synapses; excesses and deficits are believed to cause psychopathology.

extinction Elimination of the conditioned response when the conditioned stimulus is no longer relevant to or paired with the unconditioned stimulus.

anal-erotic personality Characterized by orderliness, obstinacy, and stinginess.

either immediately after touching the object or after periods of 30 and 60 minutes. Their self-reported anxiety and heartrate were measured before they touched the object, during the time they were waiting to wash their hands, and after they washed their hands. Figure 5.3 summarizes the results. As predicted, touching the contaminated object increased the individuals' urge or discomfort, and completing the compulsive activity (washing their hands) reduced their urge or discomfort. But interrupting the compulsive washing did not increase the urge or discomfort, contrary to predictions of both the behavioral and psychodynamic models.

Although individuals generally perform compulsions to reduce anxiety or discomfort, some individuals may persist in these behaviors even though doing so fails to reduce and may even increase anxiety. These observations are difficult to reconcile with the anxiety-reduction theory. One possibility is that although carrying out some compulsions may produce short-term anxiety, doing so prevents the development of even greater long-term anxiety. For example, a "checker" may be willing to tolerate the discomfort and effort of compulsively making sure that electrical appliances are turned off if doing this eliminates the threat of future disaster, such as fire. The cognitive-behavioral perspective emphasizes that our behavior is influenced more by *anticipated* than by *immediate* consequences (Bandura, 1986).

Obsessions, like phobic stimuli, cause anxiety and discomfort. Why, then, do obsessions persist? They do not extinguish over time, as the learning-based cognitive-behavioral model predicts. While nonobsessional people can control and dismiss their normal obsessions, people with OCD cannot control theirs. Acquiring such control requires more systematic and prolonged exposure to the obsessions than is the case in the naturally occurring disorder.

Treatment

For many years, OCD was difficult to treat and success rates were very poor. Virtually all forms of physical and psychological therapy had been tried. Traditional psychotherapy had been proven ineffective (Goodwin, 1986). In recent years, however, two types of treatment have proven successful, to some degree: cognitive-behavioral therapy and drug therapy. A third treatment—psychosurgery—is sometimes tried in cases in which other methods have failed.

Cognitive-Behavioral Therapy   A significant advance was made in the 1970s with the development of specific cognitive-behavioral methods for treating cleaning and checking compulsions. The most effective treatment is exposure and **response prevention,** as illustrated with compulsive handwashers. First, the different objects or activities that lead the patient to wash his hands are identified. Then, following a thorough explanation of the technique and its rationale, touching the objects that trigger handwashing is systematically encouraged. This is the *exposure* part of treatment. After the patient has touched what is unrealistically viewed as being contaminated, he refrains from washing. This is the *response prevention* part of treatment. In some inpatient treatments using strict response prevention, the therapist may ask the patient to consent to having no opportunity for handwashing. The patient's anxiety typically rises after initially touching the object and then decreases over the course of the session. Focusing the patient's attention on fear of contamination assists the treatment (Steketee & Foa, 1985).

Note that the result of this treatment—reduction in anxiety—is contrary to those theories that would predict a serious increase in anxiety if the individual was prevented from completing the compulsive activity. In this method of treatment, there are three goals:

1. to break the negative reinforcing value of the compulsion
2. to extinguish the anxiety caused by the contaminated object
3. to enhance the patient's self-efficacy in coping with this kind of situation

response prevention
Behavior therapy technique in which phobic or compulsive behavior is prevented so the patient is exposed to anxiety-eliciting stimuli.

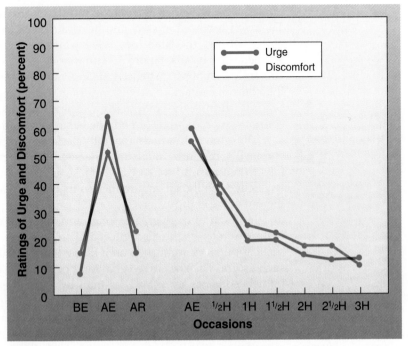

Source: From Rachman/Hodgson, *Obsessions and Compulsions*, © 1980. Reprinted by permission of Prentice-Hall, Inc., Upper Saddle River, N.J.

In cases where in vivo (that is, live) situations are impractical or impossible, imaginal exposure is used. Patients are instructed to conjure up detailed images of compulsive activities and to concentrate on these images until their anxiety decreases.

Roughly 65 to 75 percent of patients with OCD show marked improvement following cognitive-behavioral treatment (Barlow, 1988). This therapeutic success has been maintained during follow-up reviews as long as two years after treatment. Individual improvement typically extends beyond compulsive symptoms to include occupational, social, and sexual functioning (Cobb, McDonald, Marks, & Atern, 1980). Aside from modifying overt behavioral patterns, exposure treatment influences the biological basis of OCD. Successfully treated patients show significant changes in glucose metabolism in the caudate nucleus. These changes are identical to those produced by successful drug treatment (Baxter et al., 1992).

Although in vivo exposure and response prevention seem essential in eliminating compulsive rituals, effective treatment must frequently include supplementary cognitive-behavioral strategies. The clinician usually needs to involve family members in the treatment process, especially if the therapy is intended to help the patient with exposure and response prevention. Getting this participation may prove difficult, however. Marital or family therapy may be necessary to produce treatment effects and to help maintain therapeutic improvement.

Pharmacological Therapy Three drugs have been shown to have specific effects in treating OCD. Of major theoretical significance is the fact that all three increase serotonin in the brain.

The best-studied drug is clomipramine, a tricyclic antidepressant (see Chapter 20), which is superior to other tricyclic drugs (Clomipramine Collaborative Study Group, 1991). Yet only two-thirds of the patients treated with clomipramine respond, and even then, they are not freed from obsessions and compulsions (Zohar, Foa, & Insel, 1989). In addition to having limited effects, clomipramine has negative physical side effects, including the loss of sexual function. The other two drugs used to treat OCD are **Prozac (fluoxetine)** and fluvoxamine. Initial studies

Prozac (fluoxetine) Antidepressant medication that also reduces panic and anxiety by increasing the amount of available serotonin in the brain.

indicate that both are more effective than placebo treatment and also superior to another tricyclic drug, desipramine (Goodman et al., 1990).

A limitation of drug treatment is that patients relapse when it is discontinued. For example, 90 percent of the patients who respond to treatment with clomipramine relapse within weeks after it is withdrawn (Pato, Zohar-Kadouch, Zohar, & Murphy, 1988). Patients treated with a combination of cognitive-behavioral therapy and medication—clomipramine or fluvoxamine—show better maintenance of treatment effects than those treated with medication alone after the drug is withdrawn (Riggs & Foa, 1993).

Psychosurgery   Because OCD has proven so difficult to treat, radical therapies have been tried, including **psychosurgery,** which involves the surgical destruction of certain neural pathways in the brain. One such procedure is **cingulotomy,** which severs the pathway from the frontal lobe to the basal ganglia. As we described earlier, neural transmission from the frontal lobe to the basal ganglia may be abnormal in people with OCD. One of the largest studies of this disorder evaluated 33 OCD patients who underwent cingulotomies at the Massachusetts General Hospital over a 25-year period (Jenike et al., 1991). Researchers concluded that 25 to 30 percent of these individuals reported substantial improvement in OCD symptoms.

The justification offered for such radical treatment as psychosurgery is that it often succeeds where other methods have failed. In the Jenike et al. (1991) study, just mentioned, 8 patients had failed to respond to previous drug (clomipramine) and cognitive-behavioral treatments. Of these, 3 improved moderately or markedly following the cingulotomy. Investigators use these findings to support the continued use of cingulotomy in cases in which all other treatments have failed.

Focus on Critical Thinking

Consider a patient who has the obsession that he will contract AIDS or some other sexually transmitted disease if he uses a toilet seat in a public restroom.

1. How would you differentiate this obsession from a psychotic delusion?
2. What questions might you ask to discover how much insight the patient has about his obsession?

SUMMARY

The Biopsychosocial Model of Anxiety

■ The biological view emphasizes that anxiety originates in the brain, where specific brain cells are activated or inhibited by various chemical substances. Messages from the brain arouse the autonomic nervous system, which is responsible for many of the physiological signs of anxiety, such as increased heartrate.

■ The psychodynamic view traces anxiety to unconscious impulses stemming from conflicts that occurred in early childhood. Anxiety occurs when the impulses break through the defense mechanism of repression. According to the cognitive-behavioral view, anxiety is a learned response to aversive or stressful circumstances that exceed a person's ability to cope.

■ The social view emphasizes the negative effects of exposure to threatening life circumstances and the importance of the positive support of family and friends.

Anxiety versus Panic

■ Fear is a primitive, basic emotion that occurs automatically when we are threatened with real or perceived danger. Anxiety is not a basic emotion but a blend of different emotions, including anger, excitement, and fear itself.

psychosurgery Surgical destruction of certain neural pathways in the brain done in an effort to control a severe mental disorder.

cingulotomy Psychosurgery that severs the pathway from the frontal lobe to the basal ganglia; used to treat OCD.

Panic Disorder

■ Panic disorder, which may be diagnosed with or without agoraphobia, is characterized by repeated attacks of intense anxiety that typically involve symptoms of heart palpitations, shortness of breath, and dizziness.

■ The biological view hypothesizes that panic is a product of biochemical abnormality. The cognitive-behavioral model holds that panic occurs only when patients misinterpret normal physical sensations as signs of illness or disease.

Agoraphobia

■ Agoraphobia is the fear and avoidance of situations that may be difficult to escape from or get help in, should the person experience paniclike symptoms.

Specific Phobias

■ Specific phobias (which used to be called *simple phobias*) involve excessive fear and avoidance of specific situations or objects. Individuals are more vulnerable to becoming phobic if they feel life events are unpredictable and uncontrollable; personal history is a significant factor in creating this feeling.

Social Phobias

■ People with social phobias dread a variety of social situations because they fear being humiliated or embarrassed—they may even fear being looked at. The phobia may be specific, such as fear of speaking in public, or general, involving virtually all social situations.

Generalized Anxiety Disorder

■ GAD involves what used to be called *free-floating anxiety,* or anxiety that isn't attached to any specific stimulus or situation. Patients with GAD often report a lifelong history of generalized anxiety, with no clearcut onset.

Posttraumatic Stress Disorder

■ PTSD can involve a variety of symptoms, including mild to total impairment in functioning and biological as well as psychological and behavioral disturbances. Suicide and suicide attempts are not infrequent.

■ PTSD is caused by exposure to some traumatic event (such as combat or rape), which the individual may reexperience through memories, dreams, and associated images and events.

Obsessive-Compulsive Disorder

■ Obsessions are repetitive thoughts, images, or impulses that cause anxiety the person cannot dismiss. The most common obsessions involve themes of aggression, doubt, sex, and contamination.

■ Compulsions are repeated and stereotyped behaviors, such as handwashing and checking on appliances, locked doors, and so on. Performing the compulsive behavior temporarily reduces anxiety.

■ Obsessions and compulsions typically occur together. Patients usually realize that their behavior is irrational but are unable to stop it.

KEY TERMS

agoraphobia, **p. 138**
anal-erotic personality, **p. 160**
anticipatory anxiety, **p. 138**
anxiety, **p. 134**
benzodiazepines, **p. 134**

catastrophic thinking, **p. 140**
catecholamines, **p. 154**
caudate nucleus, **p. 159**
cingulotomy, **p. 163**
claustrophobia, **pp. 133–134**
cognitive restructuring, **p. 149**

cognitive therapy, **p. 141**
comorbidity, **p. 150**
compulsions, **p. 157**
controllability, **p. 146**
cortisol, **p. 154**
defense mechanism, **p. 135**

CRITICAL THINKING EXERCISE

Dr. Carmen E. was treating Linda, a woman with agoraphobia. After Linda reported increasing marital conflict, Dr. E. arranged a joint session with Linda and her husband, Pat. In the session, Pat seemed frustrated and unsympathetic, and Linda seemed dependent and insecure. Dr. E. noted that this pattern of interpersonal conflict fit the family systems view of agoraphobia. She concluded that Linda's agoraphobia is a symptom of this marital conflict and that treatment needs to focus on the relationship.

1. Is Dr. E. justified in drawing this conclusion? Are there other explanations for Linda's problems? Explain your answer.
2. Design an experiment to test the family systems model of agoraphobia.

Chapter 6
SOMATOFORM AND DISSOCIATIVE DISORDERS

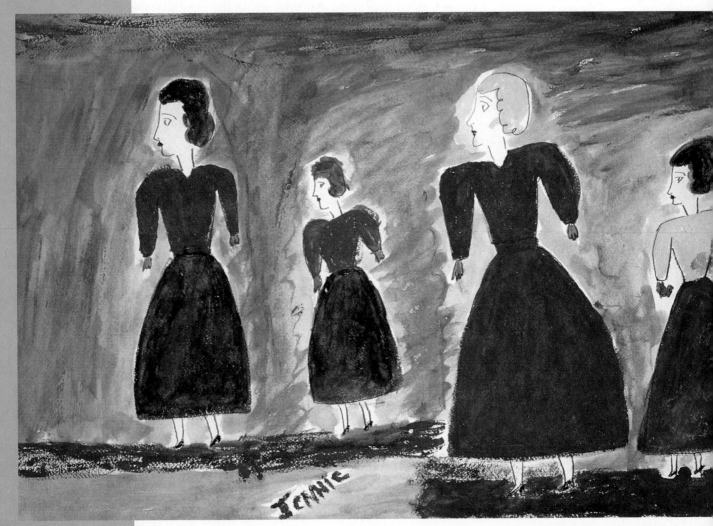

Jennie Maruki, **Four Women,** HAI

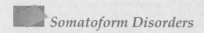
A nna O. was the 21-year-old daughter of a successful Jewish family living in Vienna, Austria. Her father, to whom she was devoted, was dying. She and her mother nursed him constantly, which caused Anna great physical and mental stress. In the fall of 1880, she suddenly developed a number of dramatic symptoms and began to show signs of severe psychological disturbance. These signs included paralysis and loss of sensation in the right side of her body and occasional paralysis in some parts of the left side, as well. Anna complained of not being able to think and worried about becoming blind and deaf. She also had rapid mood changes and terrifying hallucinations of black snakes. She lost her ability to speak German, yet she retained perfect command of English.

Anna O. also suffered from personality alterations. She experienced "absences" that would suddenly interrupt her train of thought. During these times, she would become totally dissociated (separated) from her normal waking self; when she returned to normal, she had no memory of these episodes. Anna alternated between two states of consciousness. During one, she was sad and anxious but relatively normal. During the other—her "naughty self"—she behaved angrily and threw cushions at people. Her mother became alarmed by these symptoms and brought in a physician, Josef Breuer (1842–1925), to treat her daughter.

Breuer treated Anna for 18 months, spending several hours with her each day. He described her as follows:

> This girl, who was bubbling over with intellectual vitality, led an extremely monotonous existence in her puritanically-minded family. She embellished her life in a manner which probably influenced her decisively in the direction of her illness, by indulging in systematic daydreaming, which she described as her "private theater." While everyone thought that she was attending, she was living through fairy tales in her imagination; but she was always on the spot when she was spoken to, so that no one was aware of it. (cited in Dawes, 1994, p. 190)

During therapy, Breuer discovered that Anna's symptoms disappeared if she gave a detailed account of them and the events surrounding their onset. Anna called this her "talking cure" and, jokingly, "chimney sweeping." Breuer called it **catharsis.**

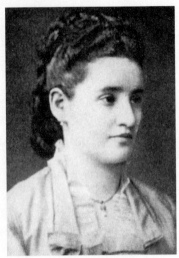

"Anna O.," whose problems allegedly responded to the "talking cure," thereby leading Freud to develop the psychoanalytic technique of free association. Her real name was Bertha Pappenheim, and what really happened to her is one of the ironies of the history of abnormal psychology.

For example, the last of her symptoms—paralysis of the right arm—was eliminated only after she recalled and reported the details of this hallucination: Sitting at her father's bedside, she saw a large black snake. She tried to ward it off with her right arm but was unable to move. She was capable only of reciting an English language prayer. With this final verbal report, her paralysis disappeared and her ability to speak German suddenly returned. Breuer reported his patient cured.

In this chapter, we'll explore the nature of Anna O.'s bizarre symptoms. We'll look into whether people can become functionally blind, even though they are physically able to see. We'll examine whether individuals can have multiple personalities. Are these genuine clinical disorders or intentional attempts to manipulate others? And we'll also describe what finally happened to Anna O. The outcome will surprise you. It's one of the great ironies in the history of abnormal psychology.

SOMATOFORM DISORDERS

We've all experienced an occasional ache, pain, or other unpleasant bodily sensation that come and go without leaving any ill effect. Sometimes, though, they might be more serious and provide signals from our bodies about illnesses or diseases that require medical treatment. Most of us can distinguish between occasional and serious sensations fairly easily. Yet others seem more sensitive to real or perceived bodily sensations; they interpret them as symptoms of undetected physical illness or disease and continually seek medical treatment.

Individuals such as these have **somatoform disorders.** (*Soma* means "body.") They have symptoms typically associated with physical diseases, but no known organic or physiological bases can be demonstrated for their symptoms. By exclusion, then, the symptoms are linked to inferred psychological processes.

To be sure, individuals with somatoform disorders believe their symptoms are serious, despite the absence of any physical disease. These individuals are impulsive and vulnerable to pain. An estimated 30 to 80 percent of patients who visit primary care physicians complain of symptoms not fully explained by any physical problems (Barsky & Klerman, 1983). Patients with somatoform disorders do not initially seek psychological treatment, and only a small fraction come to the attention of clinical psychologists or psychiatrists. Individuals with these disorders are referred for psychological help only after physical causes have been excluded.

The fourth edition of the *Diagnostic and Statistical Manual of Mental Disorders (DSM-IV)* (American Psychiatric Association, 1994) lists five somatoform disorders: conversion disorder, somatization disorder, hypochondriasis, body dysmorphic disorder, and pain disorder. We'll look at each in turn.

Conversion Disorder

The case of Anna O. illustrates **conversion disorder,** the best known of the somatoform disorders. This disorder involves a loss of or change in physical functioning that suggests physical disease but for which no underlying physical problem can be found. The *DSM-IV* table lists the diagnostic criteria for conversion disorder.

Conversion disorder used to be known as *hysterical neurosis.* The term *hysteria* comes from the Greek word meaning "uterus." This reflects the early belief that the uterus of a woman who had no sexual relationship or was childless could dry out and "wander" through the body, symbolizing the desire for procreation. Where the uterus settled determined the specific hysterical symptoms of the woman. For example, if the uterus lodged in her throat, she would feel as if she were choking.

Thus, it was originally believed that hysteria—including conversion disorder—was a women's disorder. Yet evidence suggests that between 20 and 40 percent of

catharsis Psychological relief produced by disclosing emotionally charged thoughts and feelings.

somatoform disorders Disorders characterized by the presence of symptoms typically associated with physical disease for which no known organic basis can be found.

conversion disorder Loss or alteration of physical functioning that suggests a physical disease but for which no underlying physical cause can be found.

DSM-IV   Diagnostic Criteria for 300.11 CONVERSION DISORDER

A. One or more symptoms or deficits affecting voluntary motor or sensory function that suggest a neurological or other general medical condition.

B. Psychological factors are judged to be associated with the symptom or deficit because the initiation or exacerbation of the symptom or deficit is preceded by conflicts or other stressors.

C. The symptom or deficit is not intentionally produced or feigned (as in Factitious Disorder or Malingering).

D. The symptom or deficit cannot, after appropriate investigation, be fully explained by a general medical condition, or by the direct effects of a substance, or as a culturally sanctioned behavior or experience.

E. The symptom or deficit causes clinically significant distress or impairment in social, occupational, or other important areas of functioning or warrants medical evaluation.

F. The symptom or deficit is not limited to pain or sexual dysfunction, does not occur exclusively during the course of Somatization Disorder, and is not better accounted for by another mental disorder.

cases of conversion disorder occur in men (Chodoff, 1974). For both sexes, age of onset is usually in adolescence or early adulthood but can also occur much later in life.

Conversion disorder develops suddenly, usually under severe psychological stress. Often, a prior history of some physical problem provides a model or prototype for the symptom. Remember that Anna O. was physically and mentally stressed by caring for her dying father. Freud coined the term *conversion* when he assumed that anxiety was transformed (converted) into a somatic symptom to prevent it from breaking into the conscious part of the mind.

Individuals with hysterical or dependent personality disorders may be predisposed for developing conversion disorder (see Chapter 12). Patients with conversion disorder are significantly more likely to show a hysterical personality style (Wilson-Barnett & Trimble, 1985). However, no clear link has been shown between hysterical personality and conversion disorder. Conversion symptoms occur in patients with all kinds of different personalities (Wilson-Barnett & Trimble, 1985).

Conversion disorder has declined in prevalence. During the late-nineteenth century, Jean Martin Charcot (1825–1893) in France and Freud in Austria each treated a large number of hysterical patients with conversion symptoms. Today, symptoms such as these are rare—which makes the Cambodian refugees described in the Thinking about Multicultural Issues box all the more intriguing.

The *DSM-IV* distinguishes between conversion disorder and **malingering** (faking). The malingerer shows the same pattern of behavior as characterizes someone with conversion disorder but for a deliberate purpose: to consciously and intentionally obtain some reward or avoid some unpleasant situation. In contrast, the motivation of the patient with real conversion symptoms is unconscious. This distinction is often difficult to make. Common clinical guidelines are based on malingerers voluntarily controlling their symptoms; they can switch back and forth between normal and abnormal behavior more easily and quickly than patients with conversion disorder.

Conversion disorder must also be distinguished from **factitious disorder** with physical symptoms. The individual with factitious disorder intentionally produces symptoms that have an actual physiological basis—for example, accepting a penicillin injection knowing it will cause a toxic reaction. A specific form of this disorder is Munchausen syndrome, in which patients continually attempt to be hospitalized, sometimes even journeying to numerous cities and states to do so.

The concepts of conversion disorder and hysterical neuroses are controversial. In fact, some critics have charged that they do not exist (Slater, 1965). According to this skeptical view, the terms *conversion reaction* and *hysterical neurosis* are merely labels for symptoms that do not have satisfactory physical explanations.

Some support for this radical view comes from a study of 85 patients diagnosed with conversion disorder (Slater & Glithero, 1965). A follow-up study revealed that actual illnesses became evident in all but 21 subjects. In many of them, the physical helplessness they'd developed was demonstrated by symptoms similar to those

malingering Pattern of behavior similar to that seen in a genuine clinical disorder but deliberately and consciously designed to obtain some reward or avoid some unpleasant situation.

factitious disorder Intentional production of symptoms with an actual physiological basis.

ysterical blindness occurs very rarely these days in the United States. It seems to be a disorder from another time and place—perhaps Freud's Vienna at the turn of the century. That's true today with the exception of one place: an area of Long Beach, Los Angeles County, California, where some 85,000 Cambodian refugees live, half of the 170,000 in the United States. Of the Los Angeles County group, about 150 individuals—most of them, women—are functionally blind, even though physically, there's nothing wrong with their eyes. This is perhaps the largest known group of people with this disorder in the world.

These survivors of the so-called killing fields of Cambodia shared a common experience: They witnessed unspeakable atrocities in prison camps. One woman lost her sight shortly after being captured with her brother, his wife, and their three children. The adults were forced to watch as the two older children were beaten to death. Next, the children's parents were killed. Then, one of the Khmer Rouge soldiers "lifted the last child, an infant, by the leg and beat him to death against a tree" (p. 43). Virtually all these Cambodian women—now between the ages of 50 and 70—have seen family members butchered in similar fashion.

The blind refugees were examined by eye specialists using a sophisticated electrophysiological monitoring device, which can check if the brain responds to a visual stimulus. This assessment established that there is no physical reason the Cambodians cannot see.

Do these people suffer from the conversion disorder of hysterical blindness? Did their minds simply shut down their vision as the only way to cope with the horrors they faced? Or are they faking blindness?

We may never know. The investigators admit that they don't know much about these women's histories. But investigators do know the following: The women distrust Western culture and its medicine. They have symptoms of posttraumatic stress disorder (PTSD), such as nightmares and flashbacks. Understandably, they are unwilling to talk about their painful pasts; they would rather avoid cues that remind them of the past.

As these researchers have discovered, it's hard enough to differentiate between conversion disorder and malingering in individuals from our own culture, let alone in those from a foreign culture. And so we are left with the conclusions of the investigators, who are con-

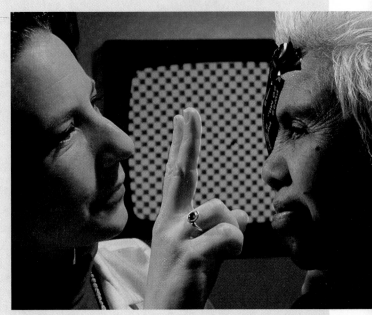

A psychiatrist examining a Cambodian woman in Los Angeles. The woman is one of many refugees from Cambodia who are "blind"—though there seems to be nothing wrong with their eyes.

vinced that the women are not malingering. The researchers argue, "If you're not really blind, you're going to do everything in your power to make me think you are.... People think it's easy. They trip gracefully over the furniture—all this exaggerated motion. But these women behave as the blind really do, which is often in surprisingly normal ways. They rely on sound, air movement; they have a sense of what the room is like" (p. 43).

Think about the following questions:

1. Conversion disorders appear to have declined in Western society. Yet these Cambodian refugees—originally from Eastern society—seem to have developed a conversion disorder (hysterical blindness) in response to trauma. What might account for the difference in prevalence rates between these two cultural groups?

2. It seems that nearly all the refugees who have experienced hysterical blindness are women. Why might this disorder be more common among women than men?

Source: Based on "They Cried Until They Could Not See," by P. Cooke, June 23, 1991, *New York Times Magazine*, pp. 25–43.

originally diagnosed as being hysterical. This suggests that a diagnosis of conversion disorder was mistakenly applied to patients with physical diseases.

Some physical illnesses may also be misdiagnosed as conversion disorder. Nevertheless, the behavior labeled *conversion disorder* cannot be adequately explained by reducing it to underlying physical illnesses.

Causes   Conversion disorder seems to fit well with the psychodynamic model. The key assumption in this view is that the individual derives primary gain from her symptom because it keeps intrapsychic anxiety or conflict out of her awareness. Converting the underlying anxiety into a physical symptom allows the anxiety to be released without being consciously experienced. It works the same way as other means of symbolically coping with anxiety—such as displacing anxiety onto an external object in the form of a phobia. Both mechanisms defend the self against unacceptable anxiety. In addition, the individual with conversion disorder derives secondary gain, allowing her to avoid taking part in unwanted activities and to receive support from others that might otherwise be unavailable.

The psychodynamic model resulted from Freud's early work with Josef Breuer, described in *Studies on Hysteria* (1895/1957). Recall from the opening case in this chapter that Breuer initially reported that his "talking cure" (catharsis) had cured Anna O. Impressed by this success, Freud adapted Breuer's approach in treating his own patients. After confirming the effectiveness of the cathartic method, Freud discarded **hypnosis** completely and asked patients to verbally detail their early life experiences. Under Freud, the "talking cure" became known as **free association,** a fundamental element of contemporary psychoanalytic therapy.

Most textbook accounts of the case of Anna O. (whose real name was Bertha Pappenheim) report the success of therapy. These accounts are incomplete, though. Breuer didn't cure her. She suffered many relapses and was institutionalized in Switzerland for almost two years. She had become addicted to the drug Breuer had prescribed (chloral hydrate) and then later to morphine, which she had received in high doses at the institution (Ellenberger, 1972). Bertha also falsely claimed that she had become pregnant by Breuer, whom she had become very attached to. This ultimately caused Breuer to stop treating her. A year later, he even expressed the hope that Bertha might die so as to be released from her suffering.

Bertha did eventually recover and overcome her addiction. In 1895, she became the director of a Jewish orphanage in Frankfurt, Germany. She traveled widely and campaigned to improve the conditions of women. In 1904, she founded a League of Jewish Women, the first organization of its kind. And in 1907, she began a home for unwed mothers. Committed to the causes of women and children, she can be considered an early feminist. She wrote, "If there is any justice in the next life, women will make the laws and men will bear the children!" (cited in Sulloway, 1979, p. 57). In 1954, the West German government issued a commemorative postage stamp in her honor.

Freud was strongly influenced by Breuer's description of the case of Anna O. Initially, he agreed with Breuer that sexual conflict was not a cause of her symptoms. But after treating other individuals, Freud began to believe that all conversion disorders—indeed, all neuroses—were the product of early, unresolved sexual conflicts. In his discussion of the Anna O. case in later writings, Freud claimed that Breuer had failed to understand Anna O.'s sexual attraction to her therapist—what is known in psychodynamic therapy as **transference.** (Recall that Anna had falsely claimed that she was pregnant by Breuer—what has been called a *hysterical pregnancy.*) Breuer agreed that sexual conflicts were an important cause of hysterical symptoms but rejected Freud's insistence that they were at the root of every case. Disagreement over this issue caused the personal and scientific rift that developed between these two pioneers of abnormal behavior (Sulloway, 1979).

Modern psychodynamic theory is more in accord with Breuer's original position than with Freud's. Any anxiety or conflict—sexual or otherwise—can be repressed and subsequently expressed overtly in the form of symptoms such as those that make up conversion disorder.

Although the psychodynamic model seems to offer a plausible explanation of the etiology of conversion disorder, it has problems. A major prediction of the model is that patients with conversion symptoms should show no anxiety. This absence of anxiety or distress has historically been referred to as **la belle indifference.**

hypnosis Condition in which people behave as if they were in a trance or altered state of consciousness and appear to be highly susceptible to suggestions from a hypnotist.

free association Technique in psychoanalysis in which patients are encouraged to talk in therapy about whatever thoughts or feelings they experience without any effort to censor.

transference Special relationship that develops between patient and therapist in which the patient responds to the therapist as she did toward significant people (usually parents) in her childhood.

la belle indifference Absence of anxiety despite the presence of a somatoform disorder.

To test this psychodynamic assumption, Lader and Sartorius (1968) compared patients with conversion disorder with individuals from two control groups: a matched group of patients with nonhysterical anxiety disorders and nonanxious, normal subjects. The conversion disorder patients showed significantly more physiological arousal and subjective anxiety than the nonhysterical anxiety disorder patients; in turn, the latter group exhibited greater anxiety than the normal control group. Contrary to the notion of la belle indifference, the patients with conversion symptoms reported great concern about their problems. Similarly, an analysis of cases of somatization disorder in the Epidemiological Catchment Area (ECA) study found strong evidence that these individuals showed overt expression of anxiety (Simon & Von Korff, 1991). These findings challenge the psychodynamic model.

In explaining conversion disorder, the psychodynamic model postulates that some mental anxiety or conflict is transformed into a physical symptom. But how does this conversion take place? The theory has been criticized for having no acceptable biological basis that explains this conversion (Chodoff & Lyons, 1958). Psychodynamic treatment follows the classic approach to all anxiety disorders: Exploring and uncovering the childhood trauma or conflict that underlies the hysterical symptoms helps the patient gain insight into these unconscious processes. It's assumed that working through them will eliminate the disorder.

The behavioral model suggests that people with conversion disorder adopt social roles in which their behavior matches that of individuals whose symptoms are caused by physical disease (Ullmann & Krasner, 1969). In other words, people with conversion disorder act like people who are really ill. Two key questions about conversion disorder have guided behavioral research:

1. Are people capable of adopting such social roles?
2. Under what conditions will people act this way?

In answer to the first question, behaviorists have claimed that individuals can mimic hysterical symptoms without being either unconsciously motivated or consciously malingering. To support this assumption, behaviorists point to studies showing that people are responsive to **demand characteristics** in social situations (Orne, 1962). In other words, people are suggestible and will respond in ways that are assumed to be appropriate in specific situations. In answer to the second question, behaviorists suggest that to play these roles, people must have had experience with the symptoms of given disorders and must also be reinforced for such behavior.

According to the behavioral model, conversion symptoms are not unconsciously motivated, although they are functionally the same as malingering. Behaviorists do not differentiate between conscious and unconscious processes and suggest there is no real dichotomy between conversion disorder and malingering. They focus only on observable behavior and its environmental antecedents and consequences.

Although some investigators would agree that it's unproductive to try to distinguish between the so-called real disorder and malingering (Miller, 1987), others maintain that important differences exist between the two. Focusing only on overt behavior fails to address the cognitive processes involved in somatoform disorders. The riddle of **hysterical blindness,** for instance, is that patients behave in ways that prove they are using visual cues yet insist they can't see.

The main shortcoming of the behavioral model in explaining conversion symptoms is that it's more of a *description* than an *explanation* of the disorder (Miller, 1987). Among the questions the model leaves unanswered are: How and why do only some people adopt these social roles in stressful situations? Also, the behavioral model rejects any mention of conscious and unconscious processes.

Somatization Disorder

Somatization disorder is also known as *Briquet's syndrome,* after Paul Briquet (1796–1881), the French physician who first described it in 1859. The key diagnostic

demand characteristics
Cues in a situation people respond to in ways assumed to be socially appropriate.

hysterical blindness Loss of vision that is not due to any physical basis.

somatization disorder
Somatoform disorder characterized by recurrent somatic symptoms, causing the person to consult repeated doctors without finding an organic basis for the problem.

Diagnostic Criteria for 300.81 SOMATIZATION DISORDER

A. A history of many physical complaints beginning before age 30 years that occur over a period of several years and result in treatment being sought or significant impairment in social, occupational, or other important areas of function.

B. Each of the following criteria must have been met, with individual symptoms occurring at any time during the course of the disturbance:

(1) four pain symptoms: a history of pain related to at least four different sites or functions (e.g., head, abdomen, back, joints, extremities, chest, rectum, during menstruation, during sexual intercourse, or during urination)

(2) two gastrointestinal symptoms: a history of at least two gastrointestinal symptoms other than pain (e.g., nausea, bloating, vomiting other than during pregnancy, diarrhea, or intolerance of several different foods)

(3) one sexual symptom: a history of at least one sexual or reproductive symptom other than pain (e.g., sexual indifference, erectile or ejaculatory dysfunction, irregular menses, excessive menstrual bleeding, vomiting throughout pregnancy)

(4) one pseudoneurological symptom: a history of at least one symptom or deficit suggesting a neurological condition not limited to pain (conversion symptoms such as impaired coordination or balance, paralysis or localized weakness, difficulty swallowing or lump in throat, aphonia, urinary retention, hallucinations, loss of touch or pain sensation, double vision, blindness, deafness, seizures; dissociative symptoms such as amnesia; or loss of consciousness other than fainting)

C. Either (1) or (2):

(1) after appropriate investigation, each of the symptoms in Criterion B cannot fully explained by a known general medical condition or the direct effects of a substance (e.g., a drug of abuse, a medication)

(2) when there is a related general medical condition, the physical complaints or resulting social or occupational impairment are in excess of what would be expected from the history, physical examination, or laboratory findings

D. The symptoms are not intentionally produced or feigned (as in Factitious Disorder or Malingering).

feature of this disorder is the pattern of recurrent, long-standing somatic symptoms, which begin before the age of 30 and occur over a period of several years (see the *DSM-IV* table). Patients with these symptoms consult one doctor after another without finding any known medical explanation for their problems.

Patients with somatization disorder often abuse medications and are frequently hospitalized; they might even undergo unnecessary surgery. This disorder is more common among women than men, although the clinical characteristics of the two groups are similar (Golding, Smith, & Kashner, 1991).

Although the *DSM-IV* identifies somatization as a discrete (single) disorder, it can be viewed as a continuum of disturbance, as well. A study of patients who were psychologically distressed and frequently utilized medical services found that those individuals with 9 to 12 symptoms were almost as disturbed as those with 13 or more (Katon et al., 1991). Anxiety and major depressive disorders were comparable in these two groups and far more common in them than in patients with fewer than 6 unexplained somatic symptoms.

Anxiety and depression are commonly associated with somatization disorder, and patients often threaten or attempt suicide. Antisocial behavior and marital and interpersonal difficulties are frequently present, too. We can interpret the association between anxiety and depressive disorders, on the one hand, and somatization, on the other, in at least three ways (Katon et al., 1991):

1. Either anxiety or depression might lower the patient's threshold for being disturbed by perceived physical complaints.

2. Chronic physical symptoms, such as pain, might cause anxiety or depression.

3. Both the anxiety/depressive disorders and the somatization might be a product of some third, underlying disorder.

Causes   The biopsychosocial model provides the most plausible explanation of somatization disorder. Several findings point to a biological predisposition. Family studies, for example, have shown that women with this disorder are more likely to have first-degree female relatives (that is, mothers and sisters) with the same disorder than women in the population at large (American Psychiatric Association, 1994).

There is also a link between somatization disorder and **antisocial personality disorder.** Somatization disorder is more common in women whose biological parents

antisocial personality disorder *Characterized by a consistent pattern of irresponsible and aggressive actions against others.*

PERSPECTIVE ON SOMATIZATION DISORDER

BIOLOGICAL FACTORS

Prominent biological factors contribute to somatization disorder but are not by themselves sufficient causes for this condition:

➤ Women with this disorder are more likely to have first-degree female relatives with the same disorder.

➤ A familial association between somatization disorder and antisocial personality disorder may represent different gender-based expressions of the same underlying biological predisposition. Somatization disorder occurs mainly in women and antisocial personality disorder mainly in men.

➤ Somatization disorder patients score very high on the novelty-seeking dimension of Cloninger's psychobiological personality theory. They tend to be impulsive and vulnerable to pain; behavioral tendencies are linked to a low neurobiological level of dopaminergic activity.

PSYCHOLOGICAL FACTORS

Psychological factors interact with biological vulnerabilities in producing symptoms:

➤ Childhood experiences with pain or serious illness in a family member increases the risk of developing somatization disorder.

➤ Women with somatization disorder are more likely to report a history of childhood sexual and physical abuse than other female psychiatric patients with somatic complaints.

SOCIAL FACTORS

Both biological and psychological factors operate in changing social contexts:

➤ Somatization disorder has been decreasing in prevalence, possibly because it is no longer as socially acceptable. Women are much freer now to express their anger and frustrations more directly.

➤ Rates of female criminality have been increasing, with women committing crimes associated with antisocial personality disorder.

➤ Problems such as borderline personality disorder, which occurs mainly in women, have become prominent in recent years. Somatization disorder covaries with antisocial personality disorder. It may be that cultural changes alter the behavioral expression of underlying predispositions.

These biological, psychological, and social factors interact to cause problems, as illustrated in the following case:

Paula is a 27-year-old single woman who was recently hospitalized for taking an overdose of aspirin and Xanax, an antianxiety drug. At the time, she was taking a variety of other medications, including sleeping pills. Her apparent suicide attempt was in reaction to her boyfriend's decision to end their often-troubled relationship. Paula had been referred by her physician to a psychiatrist, who had prescribed the Xanax in response to her reports of anxiety, dizziness, and shortness of breath.

The biopsychosocial model explains Paula's problems. As a young girl, Paula had been sexually abused by her alcoholic father. Her younger brother drank excessively and had been arrested twice for physically assaulting people while drunk. As a teen-ager, Paula had complained of a variety of somatic symptoms, including frequent headaches and stomach problems. Her mother took her to consult a number of physicians, none of whom could identify a specific medical problem. Paula had a history of failed relationships with men. The conflict with her most recent boyfriend had left her feeling abandoned and depressed.

had antisocial personality disorder (Sigvardsson, Von Knorring, Bohman, & Cloninger, 1984). And conversely, there are high rates of antisocial personality disorder in the first-degree relatives of patients with somatization disorder (Lilienfeld, 1992). Researchers have hypothesized that this familial association between somatization disorder and antisocial personality disorder represents different gender-based expressions of the same underlying biological predisposition (Guze, Cloninger, Martin, & Clayton, 1986). Specifically, somatization disorder occurs mainly in women, and antisocial personality disorder occurs mainly in men.

These two disorders are also linked by several overlapping features. Both somatization disorder and antisocial personality disorder are found mainly among people with low socioeconomic status (SES), begin early in life, follow a chronic course, prove difficult to treat, and are complicated by marital problems, substance abuse, and suicide attempts (Lilienfeld, 1992).

Psychosocial causes of somatization disorder have been inferred from evidence that childhood experience with pain or serious illness in a family member increases the risk of developing this disorder in adulthood (Hartvig & Sterner, 1985). Moreover, women with somatization disorder are much more likely to report a history of childhood sexual and physical abuse than other female psychiatric patients with somatic complaints (Pribor, Yutzy, Dean, & Wetzel, 1993). Given this latter finding, it's tempting to conclude that childhood abuse is a psychological cause of somatization disorder. But how else could we interpret this finding?

One possibility is that women with somatization disorder are more likely to distort their past or simply report childhood abuse. Without independent corroborative evidence, we cannot dismiss this possibility. A second interpretation relies on genetic influences. A daughter with somatization disorder has a greater than normal chance of having a father with antisocial personality disorder. So perhaps the genetic/biological factors they share are the cause of her somatization disorder, rather than the psychological damage caused by child abuse (Pribor et al., 1993).

Social and cultural influences also seem relevant in understanding the link between somatization and antisocial personality disorders. Like conversion disorder, somatization disorder has decreased in prevalence. The usual explanation given for this decrease is that it's no longer as socially acceptable to have this disorder as it was in Freud's time. Consider the role of women, in particular. Today, they are much freer to express their anger and frustrations more directly.

Interestingly, as the prevalence of somatization disorder has declined, rates of female criminality have climbed (Wilson & Herrnstein, 1985). And these crimes tend to be those associated with antisocial personality disorder. In addition, problems such as **borderline personality disorder,** which occur mainly in women, have become prominent (see Chapter 12). This disorder covaries with antisocial personality disorder. Lilienfeld (1992) speculates that as our culture changes, so do our behavioral expressions of underlying predispositions.

Treatment   The per capita cost of health care for patients with somatization disorder is very expensive—up to nine times that of the average person in the United States. Much of this increase in cost is due to excessive and inappropriate hospitalization.

Research has shown that psychiatric consultation with patients with somatization disorder can reduce soaring health costs without affecting the quality of care (Smith, Monson, & Ray, 1986). In one study, patients with somatization disorder were randomly assigned either to a treatment or a control group and then studied for 18 months. The control group received routine medical care; the experimental (treatment) group received more specialized care. The physicians who treated these patients were given detailed information about the nature of somatization disorder and were instructed in how to change their typical management of these patients. For example, these physicians regularly scheduled appointments every four to six weeks to avoid patients' developing new symptoms as a means of getting appointments.

borderline personality disorder Characterized by unstable personal relationships, unpredictable mood swings, and recurrent suicidal gestures.

The physicians were informed that their patients were not consciously making up their symptoms and were instructed not to lightly dismiss a patient's complaints. In treating these patients, the physicians were also encouraged to avoid hospitalization, expensive laboratory tests, and surgery unless clearly indicated.

At the end of the study, researchers found no evidence that the psychiatric consultation had improved patients' mental or physical health. But the results showed the treatment significantly reduced health care costs without affecting patients' self-rated health status or satisfaction with care. The findings demonstrate psychiatric consultation can reduce medical care costs (Smith et al., 1986).

Hypochondriasis

The core feature of **hypochondriasis** is the anxiety of having (or believing that one has) a serious physical illness, despite medical evaluations to the contrary. The diagnostic criteria are listed in the *DSM-IV* table.

The following transcript of a psychologist interviewing a patient with hypochondriasis illustrates the problem:

> **DSM-IV Diagnostic Criteria for 300.7 HYPOCHONDRIASIS**
>
> **A.** Preoccupation with fears of having, or the idea that one has, a serious disease based on the person's misinterpretation of bodily symptoms.
>
> **B.** The preoccupation persists despite appropriate medical evaluation and reassurance.
>
> **C.** The belief in Criterion A is not of delusional intensity (as in Delusional Disorder, Somatic Type) and is not restricted to a circumscribed concern about appearance (as in Body Dysmorphic Disorder).
>
> **D.** The preoccupation causes clinically significant distress or impairment in social, occupational, or other important areas of functioning.
>
> **E.** The duration of the disturbance is at least 6 months.
>
> **F.** The preoccupation is not better accounted for by Generalized Anxiety Disorder, Obsessive-Compulsive Disorder, Panic Disorder, a Major Depressive Episode, Separation Anxiety, or another Somatoform Disorder.

Therapist: So you believe that you have a serious physical problem that the doctors haven't picked up. Is that right?
Patient: Yes that's right.
Therapist: So that thought is very upsetting, and makes you unhappy in a variety of ways. The main ways it affects what you do is it interferes with you being on your own, and it stops you doing things you enjoy, such as tennis. It also has stopped you from eating very much, which might be making eating still more difficult. Is that right?
Patient: Yes. Sometimes I will be on my own, but I won't if I can help it.
Therapist: Right. In general, when people have fears, they usually have reasons for those fears. In your instance, the reasons for your fear about your health are the pains you get, your loss of weight, difficulty eating and swallowing, and bowel problems. These all suggest to you that you are ill, especially as they come every day. Is there any other evidence that makes you think you are ill?
Patient: Yes, it's not a lump, it's a horrible feeling in the throat, tight, when it gets to here it's sore. My doctor checked me, but this has only got worse since I had the X-rays, not before; then it didn't stop me from eating. My waterworks are a problem too. It's very frightening, I can't deal with it. Those are the main things, they make me think I have the same as my mother.
Therapist: Right; so these all make you think the worst; you think you have cancer, like your mother.
Patient: Yes. (Salkovskis, 1989, p. 254)

Hypochondriasis is highly correlated with what Barsky (1992) calls *somatosensory amplification*—namely, the tendency to experience bodily sensations as being unusually intense, aversive, and distressing. Hypochondriasis is strongly associated with other clinical disorders. Of a sample of 42 hypochondriacs from a general medical clinic, 88 percent were diagnosed with one or more Axis I disorders, the most common being anxiety and mood disorders (Barsky, Wyshak, & Klerman, 1992).

hypochondriasis Belief that an individual has a serious physical illness, despite medical judgments to the contrary.

FIGURE 6.1 The Cognitive Model of Hypochondriasis

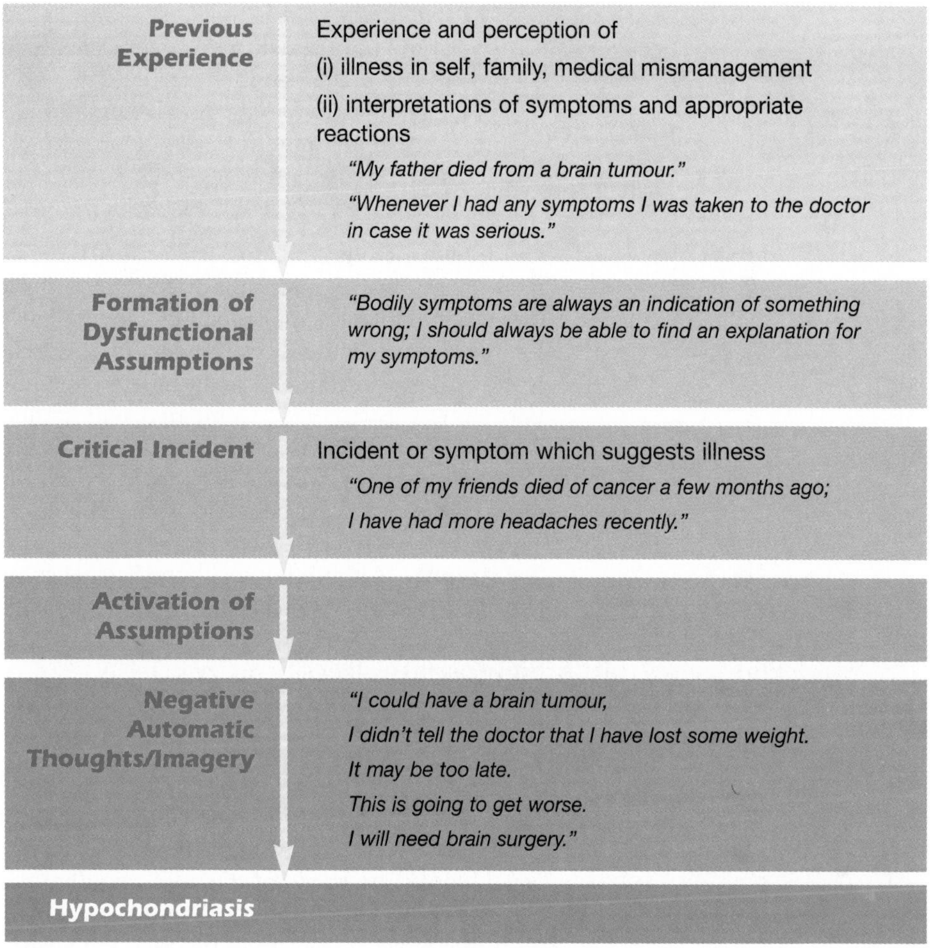

Previous Experience	Experience and perception of (i) illness in self, family, medical mismanagement (ii) interpretations of symptoms and appropriate reactions *"My father died from a brain tumour."* *"Whenever I had any symptoms I was taken to the doctor in case it was serious."*
Formation of Dysfunctional Assumptions	*"Bodily symptoms are always an indication of something wrong; I should always be able to find an explanation for my symptoms."*
Critical Incident	Incident or symptom which suggests illness *"One of my friends died of cancer a few months ago; I have had more headaches recently."*
Activation of Assumptions	
Negative Automatic Thoughts/Imagery	*"I could have a brain tumour,* *I didn't tell the doctor that I have lost some weight.* *It may be too late.* *This is going to get worse.* *I will need brain surgery."*
Hypochondriasis	

Source: Reprinted with permission from: *Advances in Behaviour Research and Therapy,* by P. M. Salkovskis and D. M. Clark, "Panic Disorder and Hypochondriasis," 1993, Elsevier Science, Ltd., Pergamon Imprint, Oxford, England.

Causes   According to the psychodynamic model, hypochondriacs somatize their anxiety to keep it out of conscious awareness. The cognitive model assumes that hypochondriacs have learned to misinterpret bodily sensations as indicating ill health (see Figure 6.1).

There is no direct support for the cognitive model. We don't know whether hypochondriacs have increased rates of medical illness or psychological disorders in their families. Evidence of physical illness in childhood, however, suggests that hypochondriacs may be reinforced for adopting sick roles (Barsky, Wyshak, & Klerman, 1986).

This cognitive model is similar to the discussions about the causes of anxiety in Chapter 5. In explaining panic disorder, the cognitive model also presumes that catastrophic misinterpretation of bodily sensations is the primary cause (Clark, 1989). What, then, are the differences between panic disorder and hypochondriasis?

In first addressing this question, Salkovskis and Clark (1993) predicted three specific differences:

1. *What sensations cause alarm*—Individuals with panic disorder misinterpret sensations involved in acute anxiety reactions (for instance, increased heartrate), whereas hypochondriacs misinterpret a much wider range of sensations as indicating ill health (for instance, a lump in the throat).

2. *Immediacy of effects*—Panic patients misinterpret sensations as causing immediate catastrophe, whereas hypochondriacs perceive their symptoms as eventually leading to irreparable physical harm.

3. *Types of behavior engaged in*—Individuals with panic disorder avoid situations that trigger attacks or immediately escape from threatening situations; hypochondriacs, on the other hand, check their bodies frequently and constantly seek consultation from doctors.

To test these predictions, Salkovskis and Clark (1993) administered a questionnaire to groups of hypochondriacs, panic disorder patients, and patients jointly diagnosed with panic disorder and hypochondriasis. The researchers found support for all three predictions. A second study similarly showed that, despite overlapping features, hypochondriasis can be reliably differentiated from panic disorder (Barsky, Barnett, & Cleary, 1994). Compared with patients with hypochondriasis, patients with panic disorder reported fewer somatic complaints, were less disabled, and were more satisfied with their medical care. Major depression and phobias were more common among panic disorder patients.

Treatment   Although hypochondriasis is commonly alleged, little has been published on treating it. Given the overlap between hypochondriasis and panic disorder, some adaptation of the cognitive-behavioral treatment of panic disorder might prove useful (Salkovskis & Clark, 1993).

Body Dysmorphic Disorder

The diagnosis of **body dysmorphic disorder** describes a preoccupation with an imaginary defect in physical appearance. Common complaints concern excessive facial hair or the shape of the nose, mouth, or jaw. In some cases, an individual's concern about a slight physical anomaly is greatly exaggerated. Being preoccupied with the defect causes great distress, impairing social functioning and work performance. Body dysmorphic disorder should be differentiated from eating disorders, such as anorexia nervosa and bulimia nervosa (see Chapter 11), where the preoccupation is limited to overconcern about body weight.

People with body dysmorphic disorder repeatedly consult physicians such as plastic surgeons and dermatologists. The age of onset of this disorder is in adolescence and early childhood. It's equally common in men and women.

body dysmorphic disorder Pathological preoccupation with an imaginary defect in physical appearance.

pain disorder Somatoform disorder in which the person complains of severe pain that cannot be explained by known physical causes.

Pain Disorder

The diagnosis of **pain disorder** includes both pain disorder associated with psychological factors and pain disorder associated with both psychological factors and a general medical condition. The defining feature of this diagnosis is preoccupation with pain that cannot be accounted for by any known physical abnormality.

Pain symptoms are part of the criteria of somatization disorder, as we have already described, and the two disorders need to be differentiated. Pain disorder is diagnosed only if the pain symptoms occur during periods when the other defining features of somatization disorder do not occur.

Pain disorder causes extreme distress and impairs social and occupational functioning. Some patients may adopt the role of an invalid. The disorder occurs more frequently in women than in men.

Focus on Critical Thinking

1. Many of us know people who are overly and perhaps unrealistically concerned about their health—hypochondriacs. Think of someone you know. Refer to the DSM-IV table on hypochondriasis. Which of the diagnostic criteria does he or she meet? Give examples of behavior.

2. Pop star Michael Jackson has undergone extensive cosmetic surgery, to the extent that his facial features have changed a lot since he was a young boy. Does he meet the DSM-IV criteria for body dysmorphic disorder? Explain your answer.

DISSOCIATIVE DISORDERS

A common theme of **dissociative disorders** is change in the normal, integrated functions of a person's identity, memory, or consciousness. The *DSM-IV* lists four dissociative disorders: dissociative amnesia, dissociative fugue, depersonalization disorder, and dissociative identity disorder. Let's look at each individually.

Dissociative Amnesia

Dissociative amnesia is a sudden loss of memory for important personal information that is not caused by organic deficits. The two most common forms are *localized amnesia* (memory loss of all events in a specific period of time) and *selective amnesia* (failure to remember some but not all events during a period of time). Less common are *generalized amnesia* (memory loss that extends to the person's entire life) and *continuous amnesia* (total memory loss following a specific point in time).

Dissociative amnesia is usually preceded by severe stress. It occurs most frequently in female adolescents and young adults. It has also been reported in young men during war. The disorder disappears as suddenly as it appears, usually with complete recovery and rare instances of recurrence.

The following case report by Kaszniak and colleagues (1988) illustrates the nature of generalized amnesia:

> Mr. M, a twenty-seven-year-old white male, was found lying in a busy road stating he wanted to die. He was admitted to the emergency room of a hospital, not knowing his name or anything else about his past. Neurological and other medical tests revealed no physical abnormality. Mr. M was distressed by his amnesia, alternating between hostility and withdrawal. During psychological testing, he was shown a picture from a projective test depicting one person apparently attacking another from behind. He became so agitated that testing was stopped, and shortly afterward he tried to hang himself in his room. Hypnosis was then used to probe into Mr. M's identity.
>
> In the first three hypnosis sessions, the patient was gradually able to remember his first name and some details about his childhood and recent past. Not until the fourth session did he recall what had happened immediately prior to his admittance to the hospital. He had been lured to an isolated place by two men promising him a job and then raped. During this session, he remembered being overcome with shame and guilt immediately after the attack. When no longer hypnotized he still remembered the rape but refused to discuss it. During a fifth and final session of hypnosis, he recalled his last name and other autobiographical details. When told his name after coming out of his trance, Mr. M reported a sudden "flooding" of memories about his past. For the next ten days his depression increased, and he repeatedly threatened to "kill all faggots." Subsequently, his distress began to subside. Follow-ups at three months and fifteen months after discharge from the hospital showed that he was no longer obsessed with the rape, did not express hostility toward homosexuals, and was successfully employed. But he reported mild depression and increased alcohol consumption. (pp. 100–101)

A study of 110 patients in a state hospital showed that 15 percent met the diagnostic criteria for dissociative amnesia (Saxe et al., 1993). Compared with a control group of patients without any dissociative disorder, the amnesia patients were much more likely to suffer from other disorders, including posttraumatic stress disorder (PTSD), substance abuse, borderline personality, and major depression. Sixty-four percent of the dissociative amnesia patients met criteria for somatization disorder; none of the comparison patients did (Saxe et al., 1994). As with all dissociative disorders, these patients reported histories of severe abuse and neglect.

Child sexual abuse, in particular, has been associated with repressed memories. Several cases have been reported in the news in which adults have remembered

dissociative disorders
Disorders in which the normal, integrated function of a person's identity or consciousness undergoes a sudden change.

dissociative amnesia Disorder in which the person is suddenly unable to recall important personal information to an extent that cannot be explained by ordinary forgetfulness.

Repression is an important but controversial concept in psychodynamic theory. According to this view, the mind copes with a traumatic experience by burying it in some isolated part of the unconscious. The memory lies there, like radioactive waste "in leaky canisters, never losing potency, eternally dangerous" (Hornstein, 1992, p. 260).

Patients with dissociative identity disorder, for example, frequently report having been sexually abused as children. Based on psychodynamic theory, it's widely assumed that the mind deals with such trauma by splitting off and creating a separate personality. Doing so effectively buries the trauma in the unconscious mind, preventing the individual from dealing with it and thus protecting her. Right? Perhaps not.

Recently, we've seen an upsurge of clinical cases in which adults undergoing psychotherapy suddenly recover memories of early childhood sexual abuse. The most sensational case of this nature is that of Eileen Franklin-Lipsker (Terr, 1994). In 1989, while watching her five-year-old daughter playing one day, Eileen had a flashback of witnessing a murder when she was a child. With the help of psychotherapy, she gradually recalled watching her own father first raping and then using a rock to smash the skull of her eight-year-old playmate 20 years earlier.

Eileen told her story to the police, and they eventually charged her 51-year-old father with murder. Impressed by the rich detail of Eileen's story and the testimony of her therapist, who supported the validity of Eileen's account, a jury convicted her father of murder in the first degree.

Was Eileen's recovery of a repressed memory authentic? Most clinicians believe in the concept of repression (Terr, 1994). Critics point out, however, that it's never been validated in experimental research. Its support comes from uncontrolled clinical case studies (Holmes, 1990).

Is it possible that someone could distort or make up such detailed and horrible memories as Eileen's? The answer is yes. Research has clearly established that it's possible for us to create false memories (Loftus, 1993). If you have any doubt, consider the case of Paul Ingram, a deputy in the sheriff's department in Olympia, Washington (Wright, 1994). His two daughters—ages 18 and 22 years—suddenly recalled that he had sexually abused them as children. They recovered this memory after attending a spiritual retreat at which a charismatic preacher had said that someone in the audience had been molested as a child. The daughters' accusations kept changing, as they said they remembered more and more.

Paul Ingram's reaction to his daughters' accusations makes the story even more bizarre. He said that he was shocked and that he didn't remember doing anything bad to his daughters. But he also said that his daughters

would never lie about something like this. He then went into something like a trance, and he did recall abusing his daughters. The harder he tried to remember, the clearer his memories became.

The attorneys prosecuting the case consulted a psychologist who was an expert on cults and mind control. To assess how suggestible Ingram was, the psychologist told him that his son and daughter had reported that he had forced them to have sex with each other. This was known to be false. But within days, Ingram recalled this memory.

Ingram subsequently tried to withdraw his guilty plea, upon deciding that his "memories" were really only fantasies. He also hired a new lawyer. But the legal process was too far along. He was convicted of child sexual abuse and sent to jail; he's appealing the guilty verdict.

Critics of the validity of recovered memories argue that the recent rise in these recoveries is due largely to therapists' making suggestions to impressionable patients, who eventually come to accept these notions as reality (Yapko, 1994). Do some therapists make suggestions that lead patients to recall false memories? Again, the answer is yes. These therapists often assume that abuse must have occurred. They ask leading questions, such as "You seem to have the kind of symptoms that suggest you were abused as a child. What can you tell me about that?" The problem with this approach is that as soon as you begin imagining that something happened, the event becomes increasingly more believable. Research has shown that each time you create a mental image, it becomes more familiar (Loftus, 1993). This is exactly what happened with Paul Ingram.

Are all recovered memories of childhood false or distorted? We can't conclude this. We do know that it's difficult to distinguish true memories from false ones. And we do know that therapists and others should be cautious and adequately informed by research on memory in how they probe for such events. The real tragedy would be if society reacted to the obviously overblown claims about fantastic so-called repressed memories by failing to respond to the many genuine cases of childhood sexual abuse—some of which may well have been buried in memory.

Think about the following questions:

1. Individuals' recovering memories of childhood sexual abuse is a recent development that's confined mainly to the United States. Why might so many people, in such a short period of time, have recovered such memories in psychotherapy? Explain your answer.

2. Imagine that you were on the jury for the trial of either Paul Ingram or Eileen Franklin-Lipsker's father. How might you try to decide the accused's guilt or innocence? How could you judge the authenticity of the claims made by the daughters?

being abused as children. The Thinking about Controversial Issues box explores whether repressed memories are real or imagined.

Dissociative Fugue

The diagnostic criteria for **dissociative fugue** include unexpectedly traveling away from home, taking on a new identity, and failing to recall these actions after recovery. A fugue may last a few hours or days, or it may last months. During a fugue, a person may travel extensively and participate in complex social activities without any sign of psychological disturbance. The new identity the person assumes may be partial or complete. The alteration in identity usually involves an inhibited person becoming more social, with rare episodes of violent behavior.

Dissociative fugue disorder is rare, and the age of onset is variable. Major psychosocial stressors—such as military combat, natural disasters, marital conflict, and personal crises—typically precede a fugue. The effect on the individual depends on the length of the fugue and the acts committed during it. Relatively brief fugues have only minimal impact.

Depersonalization Disorder

dissociative fugue Disorder characterized by sudden and unexpected travel away from home and the adoption of a new identity.

depersonalization disorder Dissociative disorder in which the person feels unreal and disconnected from the self.

dissociative identity disorder Dissociative disorder in which two or more distinctive personalities co-exist within an individual, alternately dominating functioning; previously known as multiple personality disorder.

multiple personality disorder Dissociative disorder now known as dissociative identity disorder.

An individual suffering from **depersonalization disorder** has the sense of being an outside observer of her own thoughts and feelings. In this dreamlike state, the individual's sense of detachment from her body is accompanied by the feeling that she is not in full control of her actions; however, "reality testing" remains intact. This altered sense of self causes personal distress and is chronic or recurrent. Depersonalization disorder is not diagnosed if the depersonalization is a symptom of panic disorder or agoraphobia.

The onset of depersonalization disorder is sudden and usually confined to adolescence or early adulthood. As many as 70 percent of young adults may experience brief spells of depersonalization, but the prevalence of clinically diagnosable cases is unknown.

Dissociative Identity Disorder

Dissociative identity disorder is the new *DSM-IV* label for what has been known as **multiple personality disorder.** An individual with this disorder appears to have two or more distinct personalities or personality states. These personalities take turns in controlling his actions. Because of this, an individual with multiple personalities is unable to recall important personal information—a memory problem that cannot be explained by mere forgetfulness. The diagnostic criteria for dissociative identity disorder are listed in the *DSM-IV* table.

 DSM-IV

Diagnostic Criteria for 300.14 DISSOCIATIVE IDENTITY DISORDER

A. The presence of two or more distinct identities or personality states (each with its own relatively enduring pattern of perceiving, relating to, and thinking about the environment and self).

B. At least two of these identities or personality states recurrently take control of the person's behavior.

C. Inability to recall important personal information that is too extensive to be explained by ordinary forgetfulness.

D. The disturbance is not due to the direct physiological effects of a substance (e.g., blackouts or chaotic behavior during Alcohol Intoxication) or a general medical condition (e.g., complex partial seizures).

Each of the multiple personalities shows distinctive patterns of behavior, attitudes, responses to psychological tests, and even physiological reactivity. One study found that different personalities have distinctive and stable electroencephalograph (EEG) patterns (Putnam, 1984). In that study, a normal group of control subjects who were instructed to fake multiple personalities did not show the same EEG patterns. These findings may reflect neurophysiological differences in perception between personalities. However, the findings may simply reflect the different emotional states that characterize the separate personalities.

In an individual with dissociative identity disorder, the multiple personalities are usually vividly different in behavior and emotional makeup. This sharp contrast among personalities is illustrated by the famous case of Chris Costner Sizemore, described in Thigpen and Cleckley's (1954) classic book *The Three Faces of Eve*. The Oscar-winning movie by the same name starred Joanne Woodward.

One of Sizemore's personalities was named Eve White. She was a sweet, conservatively dressed, and inhibited person, who was a conscientious worker and a devoted mother to her four-year-old daughter. She sought therapy, complaining of severe headaches often followed by blackouts. During a therapy session, another personality emerged—Eve Black—who was the opposite of the original Eve. The second Eve was coarse, seductive, impulsive, and searching for adventure. There were also interesting physiological differences between the two. Eve White had an allergy to nylon, reacting with a skin rash; Eve Black had no allergy. After about eight months of treatment, a third personality emerged—Jane. She was a more self-confident, capable, and spontaneous person than Eve White.

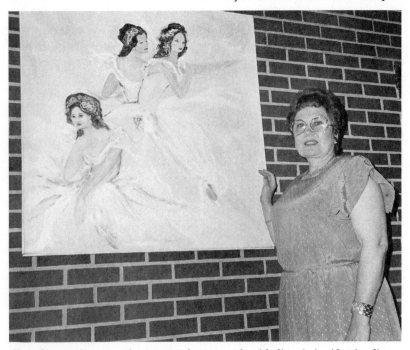

Chris Costner Sizemore, the woman whose struggle with dissociative identity disorder was described in the classic book and movie The Three Faces of Eve

The number of different personalities a dissociative individual may have can vary greatly. According to the *DSM-IV*, roughly half of recently described cases have 10 or more personalities (American Psychiatric Association, 1994). The number may be difficult to determine, as new personalities often emerge over time and during treatment. In autobiographical accounts, Sizemore reported that over 20 new personalities emerged and then disappeared after she had initially been considered cured by Thigpen and Cleckley (Sizemore, 1986; Sizemore & Pittillo, 1977). She describes her last three personalities as the Purple Lady, the Strawberry Girl, and the Retrace Lady. The Purple Lady thought she was 58 years old, needed eyeglasses to read, and wore purple clothes. The Strawberry Girl thought she was 21, read without glasses, wore red, and ate only strawberries. The Retrace Lady was 46 (Sizemore's actual age) and would never repeat anything she did, as though she was trying to avoid previous mistakes. Sizemore reports that she had three personalities at any given time and that they followed a definite pattern.

The diagnosis of dissociative identity disorder requires that at least two personalities repeatedly take full control of the person's behavior. Different personalities can, however, influence behavior, even when they are not dominant. The personality that is in control when the individual seeks treatment usually has no awareness of the other personalities. Yet the separate personalities may be aware of each other and even interact. For example, Eve Black teased Eve White, and after Evelyn White emerged as the dominant personality, she mourned the loss of the two earlier Eves as though they were her sisters (Thigpen & Cleckley, 1954).

Transitions from one personality to another occur suddenly, usually precipitated by stress or some identifiable pattern of social or environmental cues. When Eve White first consulted Thigpen and Cleckley, she was under considerable pressure. One source of pressure was serious marital conflict with a husband she had separated from and divorced. A more dramatic illustration of how a specific set of cues elicit the transition from one personality to another is seen in the case of Sally Beauchamp, the first multiple personality reported in the United States. Her three major personalities appeared on specific, identifiable occasions: after a personal crisis involving a death of someone she felt some responsibility for, when the weather was gloomy and rainy, and on a particular day—June 7 (Rosenzweig, 1988).

The age of onset for dissociative identity disorder is almost always during childhood. But the disorder does not usually come to the attention of professionals until the patient is an adolescent or adult. Sizemore (1986) reports that she knew she was different from other people when she was a child. She experienced frequent headaches, feelings of weakness, and periods of amnesia—all symptoms associated with dissociation. Her case was originally misdiagnosed as amnesia.

Patients with dissociative identity disorder are typically seriously disturbed. Researchers in the Netherlands studied 71 patients who had met the *DSM-III-R* criteria for multiple personality disorder (Boon & Draijer, 1993). The similarities among the patients are quite remarkable. Each had spent an average of 8.2 years receiving one form of treatment or another in the mental health system. Nearly two-thirds (60.6 percent) had been hospitalized at least once, and more than half had, at some time, been treated with antipsychotic, antidepressant, or antianxiety medication. Substance abuse among these individuals was common. All reported suicidal thoughts; two-thirds had made serious suicide attempts. Fully 94.4 percent reported a history of childhood physical or sexual abuse; 80.6 percent met the diagnostic criteria for posttraumatic stress syndrome (PTSD).

Until recently, dissociative identity disorder was thought to be rare and was ignored in the scientific literature. But the number of reported cases has increased dramatically since the early 1970s. In their study of 110 patients consecutively admitted to a state psychiatric hospital in Massachusetts, Saxe and colleagues (1993) found that 4 percent met the diagnostic criteria for dissociative identity disorder.

Some therapists and investigators report seeing far more cases of the disorder than critics allow. What might explain this increase? One argument is that dissociative identity disorder has been misdiagnosed in the past, often as schizophrenia (Kluft, 1987a). Each individual in the Dutch study, described earlier, had received an average of 2.8 different diagnoses prior to being diagnosed as having multiple personality disorder (see Table 6.1). In a U.S. study, Putnam and colleagues (1986) reported that the average patient had been inaccurately diagnosed more than 3 times before being properly diagnosed.

Some symptoms of schizophrenia and dissociative identity disorder do overlap. For example, a common symptom in schizophrenia is the feeling that some external force is withdrawing one's thoughts. Patients with dissociative identity disorder often report their minds going blank, which they explain as other personalities' blocking access to information (Kluft, 1987b). Patients with dissociative identity disorder often report "hearing voices" (Boon & Draijer, 1993). This is not a sign of schizophrenic thought disorder but a symptom of a dissociative disorder.

The difficulty of accurately diagnosing individuals with dissociative identity disorder is compounded because most people try to hide it. Moreover, the different personalities within the individual are often in relative harmony. Only under specific stressful conditions do they conflict with one another and present the classic signs that lead to diagnosis (Kluft, 1987a). The disorder must also be differentiated from malingering, although doing so is often difficult and controversial.

TABLE 6.1	Frequency of Dissociative Symptoms Associated with Multiple Personality Disorder		

		Frequency	
Symptom Cluster		Number	Percent
Amnesia			
Memory gaps		70	98.6
Coming out of blank spell in a strange place		65	91.3
Finding objects that cannot be accounted for		63	88.6
Depersonalization			
Feelings of estrangement		63	90.0
Watching oneself from a point outside the body		69	97.1
Altered perception of the body		55	83.3
Derealization			
Surrounding unreal		53	74.3
Not recognizing one's friends or family		41	57.1
Identity confusion and alteration			
Child part inside		56	78.6
Referred to by strangers by different names		23	32.8
Associated features			
Voices in head talking		64	90.1
Flashbacks/reliving the past as if present		57	83.8

Source: From "Multiple Personality Disorder in The Netherlands: A Clinical Investigation of 71 Patients," by S. Boon and N. Draijer, 1993, *American Journal of Psychiatry, 150,* 489–494. Copyright 1993 by American Journal of Psychiatry. Adapted with permission.

Causes   We'll examine the causes of dissociative identity from four perspectives: (1) psychodynamic, (2) behavioral, (3) cognitive, and (4) biological.

1. *The Psychodynamic Model*—Pierre Janet (1859–1957), working in the early 1900s, was a French pioneer of the study of hypnosis, hysteria, and multiple personality. He first developed the theory of dissociation, describing this disorder as a means of keeping painful events out of consciousness. This view of dissociation is the key element of psychodynamic explanations of all dissociative disorders.

In multiple personality disorder, the dissociated feelings of pain become entrenched as separate selves or personalities. Spiegel (1986) describes a patient's report of the first time a second personality emerged when her father took off his necktie, tied her to the bed, and raped her. "'Come be with me,' this dissociated person said, 'You don't want to be with him, that no good bum!' In this way, she dissociated the pain and fear that she experienced at the time" (p. 125).

Consistent with this model, a strikingly high percentage of individuals with dissociative identity disorder report having experienced serious childhood abuse. Putnam and colleagues (1986) found that of the 100 patients they studied, 83 percent had been sexually abused as children, 63 percent had experienced incest, 75 percent had been physically abused, and 45 percent had witnessed a violent death, often of a parent or sibling. A study by Coons and Milstein (1986) revealed similar results.

The findings of these studies must be viewed cautiously because the studies lacked a control group. Without another group for comparison, we don't know if having a history of childhood sexual abuse is specific to dissociative identity disorder. Individuals who were abused as children are at risk for developing a wide range of mental health problems, including depression, substance abuse, eating disorders, and sexual dysfunction (Finkelhor & Dzulba-Leatherman, 1994).

Patients who develop dissociative identity disorder must have the capacity to dissociate—that is, to split or separate consciousness. For instance, dissociative people have been shown to be highly hypnotizable (Spiegel, 1986). This capacity presumably helps individuals separate themselves from early traumatic experiences. Individuals who cannot dissociate easily may resort to defense mechanisms such as denial or **repression** to protect themselves against intolerably painful experiences.

The psychodynamic model dominates clinical thinking and practice in the dissociative disorders. The model is supported by a wealth of clinical experience, but direct empirical confirmation of its theoretical assumptions is still lacking.

2. *The Behavioral Model*—Behaviorally oriented investigators have largely neglected dissociative disorders. The only behavioral model of these disorders is the same as that for somatoform disorders, which suggests that individuals with dissociative identity disorder—or any other type of dissociative disorder—are playing social roles (Ullmann & Krasner, 1969). That is, they have learned how to play particular roles through prior modeling or exposure to information about given disorders and maintain those roles by reinforcement of their behavior. Playing a specific social role involves paying selective attention to certain stimuli and ignoring others. For the individual with multiple personalities, each personality is defined by a specific behavior in response to a set of restricted situational cues. Behaviorists reject the special states of consciousness and malingering and focus only on observable behavior and its consequences.

To test this model, Kohlenberg (1973) conducted the following study: First, he assessed the baseline rates of occurrence of the behaviors of the three personalities of a hospitalized patient. Then, he selectively reinforced the behaviors of one personality. Predictably, these behaviors increased in frequency and then decreased when reinforcement was withdrawn. This case study shows that reinforcement contingencies can influence the behavior of a multiple personality. We cannot infer anything about etiology, though.

Spanos, Weekes, and Bertrand (1985) have described a social psychological model of dissociative identity disorder that is fundamentally the same as the behavioral model. To demonstrate that normal subjects can adopt the social role of a person with a multiple personality, these researchers conducted a laboratory experiment modeled on the case of the Los Angeles Hillside Strangler. They found that, when given enough coaxing, normal college students would take on the role of a separate personality to cope with a personally threatening situation.

In this study, individuals from three groups of normal college students were each instructed to play the role of an accused murderer claiming innocence. Each subject also agreed to participate in a psychiatric interview, which might involve hypnosis. Each of the three groups was issued different instructions. Subjects in group A each received a brief hypnotic induction and were interviewed. The interviews followed, virtually word for word, the format of that between the Hillside Strangler, Kenneth Bianchi, and the clinical psychologist who interviewed him, Dr. Watkins. As in that interview, subjects were asked, "Pat, are you the same thing as Harry, or are you different in any way?" Subjects of group B were given an explanation of hypnosis that described it as a means of uncovering thoughts and feelings that were "walled off" in a different part of them. The direct question asked of group A was left out, however. Subjects of group C were not hypnotized but told that personality often involved such walled-off thoughts and feelings.

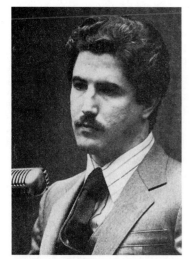

Kenneth Bianchi, the "Hillside Strangler," who tried to fake multiple personality disorder, as he appeared on the witness stand

repression Defense mechanism in which the ego excludes threatening impulses from conscious awareness.

The results of the study showed that more than 80 percent of the subjects in the so-called Bianchi condition (group A) adopted alternative personalities, which was a significantly greater proportion than found among group B or C subjects. Group A subjects showed many of the classic symptoms of dissociative identity disorder. They displayed posthypnotic amnesia—after the interview, they denied awareness of the other personality. Their different personalities were opposite in tastes, emotional expression, and behavior; they even performed differently on psychological tests. Spanos and his colleagues (1985) concluded that subjects who know about multiple personality roles can use this knowledge to achieve their own ends.

The behavioral model fails to provide an adequate account of dissociative identity disorder or the other dissociative disorders because it *describes* rather than *explains* them. Thus, it cannot predict who will adopt such a strange social role as a multiple personality or why anyone would do so. The behavioral model does not account for the remarkably high incidence of childhood trauma in patients with dissociative identity disorder nor does it explain the different forms of psychopathology associated with this disorder. And by rejecting any dichotomy between dissociative identity disorder and malingering, the model fails to address important diagnostic and legal issues.

The behavioral model predicts that using hypnosis to diagnose dissociative identity disorder may encourage patients to show the disorder. Hypnosis may elicit fragments of different personalities, but there is no evidence that hypnosis creates the full clinical disorder (Coons, 1988; Kluft, 1987a). Due to these shortcomings, the behavioral model has had little impact on research or therapy in this area.

3. *The Cognitive Model*—Several research findings in cognitive psychology help us understand dissociative disorders (Bower, 1981). The first finding establishes the significance of *state-dependent memory*, or mood. People remember an event best if, at the time of recall, they can return to the same emotional state they learned it in. For example, college students are hypnotized to feel happy or sad. During their happy moods, they recall happy personal events that occurred during the preceding few weeks; conversely, during their sad moods, they recall events that made them sad. The second finding is about *mood congruity effect*. People learn selectively about material that agrees with their current mood. For example, students are hypnotized to feel happy or sad just before imagining that they're in a number of briefly described situations. Some of these situations are designed to elicit happiness; others, sadness. Students are then returned to a neutral mood and asked to recall the situations. Subjects who were happy during the task learned more about the happy situations; those who were sad learned more about the sad situations.

Bower has proposed an *associative network theory* to explain such results. An emotion—as a unit in our memory system—becomes associated with the events we think cause it to be aroused. When the emotion is aroused again later, even if by another means, it activates the memories we associate with it. Bower (1981, 1986) has speculated that multiple personalities "may be particularly compelling role enactments that have become suffused with distinctly different moods, with the role's behavior perpetuating its mood. . . . A distinctive mood, emotional tone, or set of emotional conflicts associated with a role could easily cause events occurring during enactment of that role to be partially dissociated from, and inaccessible to other states of the person" (pp. 146–147). Consistent with this view is the finding that a single individual's multiple personalities are typically characterized by intense and markedly different emotions.

The speculative nature of this approach must be emphasized. Bower (1987) has reported failures to replicate some of the basic findings on mood and memory. At best, the cognitive model is an incomplete account of dissociative identity disorder. Although these findings do suggest how dissociated memories and feeling states might form and be cognitively organized, they do not address why people might dissociate. The nature of dissociation as an apparent motivational or defensive function is ignored and is the unique feature of the psychodynamic model.

4. *The Biological Model*—In contrast to other disorders discussed in this book, there is no biological model of dissociative identity disorder or other dissociative disorders. This knowledge gap is significant and emphasizes the need for more research on disorders that have been relatively ignored, until recently.

Even the most current research provides only hints of what a biological model might look like. Recent findings show that dissociative symptoms are as marked in PTSD patients as in patients with dissociative disorders (Bremner, Steinberg, Southwick, Johnson, & Charney, 1993). This finding led researchers to hypothesize that dissociative disorders and PTSD share a common etiology. In both, memory and information processing are disturbed following exposure to severe stress. Bremner et al. (1993) speculate that changes in brain mechanisms related to memory might be involved in dissociative disorders.

Treatment   A range of psychological and pharmacological therapies have been used to treat dissociative identity disorder. A survey of over 300 clinicians (Putnam & Loewenstein, 1993), representing a spectrum of mental health professionals, confirmed that the most common treatment methods are hypnosis and psychodynamic therapy. *Hypnosis* is employed to make the primary personality aware of the other personalities. Posthypnotic suggestions encourage the patient's separate personalities to share memories and feelings, eventually fusing them into an integrated whole. *Psychodynamic therapy* focuses on gaining insight into the underlying childhood trauma that caused the dissociation. Making the patient aware of these painful experiences should eliminate the need for a dissociated self and help in personality integration. Pharmacological treatments—using antidepressant and antianxiety drugs—were reported to be adjunctive (supplementary) methods, aimed mainly at dealing with the symptoms of depression and anxiety that accompany this dissociative disorder.

The goals of treatment for all dissociative disorders consist of (1) developing coping strategies so that patients no longer need to rely on dissociation and (2) assisting them in integrating their personality. Spiegel (1986) has identified the following strategies for achieving these therapeutic goals:

1. *Confront the trauma.* To have patients alleviate self-blame, identify the trauma that led to the dissociation. In treating a rape victim, for example, "a therapist who chooses to focus on Oedipal conflicts instead of effects of the rape, reinforces the patient's fantasy that she was somehow responsible for the rape instead of a victim of it, thereby enhancing the need to dissociate the experience of the rape from her view of herself" (p. 128).

2. *Condense the traumatic experience.* Have patients focus on specific images that reflect their traumatic experiences. Hypnosis is especially valuable here. "For example, a combat veteran who suffered a two-day fugue episode in Vietnam after discovering the body of a boy he had adopted, learned to picture an image of the boy's grave next to that of a party he had given him. These two images helped him grieve over the loss by interweaving it with moments of shared pleasure" (p. 128).

3. *Confess.* Help patients disclose their feelings about their traumatic experiences.

4. *Make conscious the dissociated material.* Both hypnosis and psychodynamic therapy share this goal.

5. *Provide therapist support.* Develop a supportive relationship with patients.

6. *Achieve control.* Help patients realize a sense of control in accessing previously repressed memories.

Focus on Critical Thinking

1. In Oshkosh, Wisconsin, a woman consented to have sexual intercourse with her date, Mark Peterson. Upon returning home, she reported that she had been raped. The woman suffered from dissociative identity disorder. She claimed that one of her other personalities was responsible for her behavior (New York Times, 1990). The Wisconsin district attorney prosecuted Mark Peterson for taking sexual advantage of a woman who was mentally ill. What arguments would you make in his defense if you were his lawyer? What position would you take if you were the prosecutor? Explain your answers.

2. Some clinicians have likened multiple personality disorder to posttraumatic stress disorder (which is discussed in Chapter 5). How are the two disorders similar? How are they different?

Controlled evaluations of treatment outcomes in the area of dissociative identity disorder are lacking. Current evidence comes from uncontrolled clinical observations. Coons (1986) followed up 20 patients with dissociative identity disorder for an average of 39 months (range = 3 to 129 months). Only 5 individuals (25 percent) had achieved full personality integration; another 2 had reached partial integration. Those individuals who hadn't improved had experienced significantly more emotional trauma during treatment than those who had achieved integration. Roughly two-thirds of both the patients and their therapists thought that the patients had shown moderate to marked improvement. Antipsychotic medication either had no effect or made patients worse. Antidepressant drugs were rated as being more useful. These modestly successful reports indicate the difficulty of treating this complex disorder.

SUMMARY

Somatoform Disorders

■ Individuals with somatoform disorders report physical symptoms with no identifiable physiological basis and repeatedly seek medical treatment.

■ Individuals with conversion disorder (once known as hysterical neurosis) develop symptoms such as paralysis or loss of sight. Although some physical illnesses may be misdiagnosed as conversion disorder, the problem seems to demand a psychological explanation.

■ Somatization disorder is characterized by recurrent, long-standing somatic symptoms that begin before the age of 30 and occur over a period of several years. These symptoms lead patients to consult one doctor after another, without finding any known medical explanation for them.

■ Hypochondriasis is the anxiety of having or the believing that one has a serious physical illness, despite contrary medical evaluations. This disorder is strongly associated with other problems such as anxiety disorders.

■ Body dysmorphic disorder involves preoccupation with an imaginary defect in physical appearance. This preoccupation causes the individual great distress and impairs social functioning and work performance.

■ Individuals with pain disorder are preoccupied with pain that cannot be accounted for by any known pathophysiology. It causes extreme distress and impairs social and occupational functioning. Pain disorder is diagnosed only if the pain symptoms occur during periods when the other defining features of somatization disorder do not occur.

Dissociative Disorders

■ Dissociative disorders involve serious disruption in the person's identity, memory, or consciousness.

■ Dissociative amnesia is characterized by a sudden loss of memory for important personal information not caused by organic deficits. Symptoms include disorientation and confusion that last several hours or even years.

■ Dissociative fugue involves sudden and unexpected traveling away from home, taking on a new identity, and failing to recall these actions after recovery. Fugues are typically preceded by major psychosocial stressors; they may be as brief as a few hours or days or may last months.

- Individuals with dissociative identity disorder (formerly known as multiple personality disorder) have two or more distinctive and integrated personalities, each with its own pattern of cognitive, emotional, and behavioral responses. The personalities are typically opposite in nature and unaware of each other. Once considered rare, the number of reported cases of dissociative identity disorder has increased dramatically. Critics allege that this increase is not legitimate and due to misdiagnosis. Proponents of the greater prevalence of the disorder argue that it's real and due to improved diagnoses.

KEY TERMS

antisocial personality disorder, **p. 173**
la belle indifference, **p. 171**
body dysmorphic disorder, **p. 178**
borderline personality disorder, **p. 175**
catharsis, **pp. 167–168**
conversion disorder, **p. 168**
demand characteristics, **p. 172**

depersonalization disorder, **p. 181**
dissociative amnesia, **p. 179**
dissociative disorders, **p. 179**
dissociative fugue, **p. 181**
dissociative identity disorder, **p. 181**
factitious disorder, **p. 169**
free association, **p. 171**
hypnosis, **p. 171**
hypochondriasis, **p. 176**

hysterical blindness, **p. 172**
malingering, **p. 169**
multiple personality disorder, **p. 181**
pain disorder, **p. 178**
repression, **p. 185**
somatization disorder, **p. 172**
somatoform disorders, **p. 168**
transference, **p. 171**

*C*RITICAL *T*HINKING *E*XERCISE

Martin, an army veteran, consulted Dr. Susan H., a clinical psychologist, claiming to be totally blind. Dr. H. devised a psychological experiment to investigate Martin's claim. She asked Martin to look at three visual stimuli; two were identical, and one was different. Martin's task was to identify the odd stimulus. The results showed that every time the visual stimuli were presented, Martin identified the wrong one. Dr. H. concluded that Martin was not totally blind. She hypothesized that he was malingering, or faking.

1. What reasoning might support Dr. H's conclusion?
2. To test her hypothesis, Dr. H. used a psychological experiment that's a variation of a strategy for determining whether someone is faking, which is described elsewhere in this chapter. Describe the sort of procedure this experiment would involve.

Chapter 7
MOOD DISORDERS

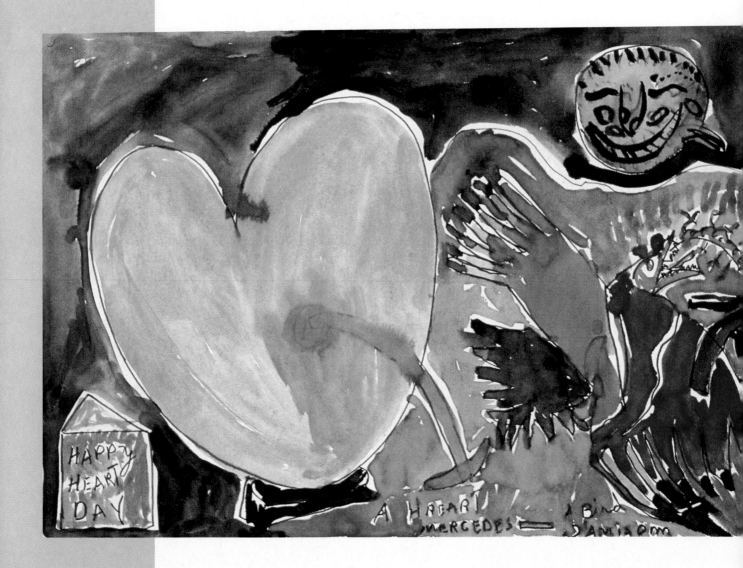

Mercedes Jamison, **Happy Heart Day,** HAI

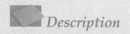
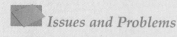

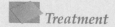
Howard, a 40-year-old high school teacher, felt very depressed after ending his 3-year relationship with Jill. She meant a lot to him. He was scared to leave her, but he felt trapped and controlled in the relationship. So he ended it. And now, he felt guilty and hopeless. He also felt stiffness in his neck, pain in his feet, and tenseness in his groin.

Every so often, the phone would ring late at night or early in the morning, and there would just be a click. Howard thought these were probably hang-ups from Jill. In some ways, the calls made him feel better because he knew that she still must care. Other times, he would awaken early on his own and not be able to get back to sleep. He was afraid to go to work some days for fear that he would cry in front of his class. Sometimes, he cried as he drove to school.

At different times, Howard took various medications for depression. He also had one extremely low time, in which hospitalization was considered. A plan was formulated in which a psychologist saw him and talked with him on the phone. In addition, Howard worked out in a gym and jogged three times a week because he heard that jogging is often associated with reductions in depression.

Howard fought his depression well and ultimately decided not to go into the hospital. He progressed with a considerable amount of his own effort, careful consideration of medications by his psychiatrist, a male support group, and weekly psychotherapy sessions.

We all feel sad at times. But clinical depression is more than occasionally feeling blue. Clinical depression takes over your life. Nothing seems interesting or fun any more. Things that would normally lift your mood—a good meal, an engaging conversation with a close friend, even sex—don't have the same positive effects that they usually do. Your appetite and sleeping patterns may change. You may feel either sluggish and apathetic or agitated and restless. Often, it's extremely difficult to concentrate. Even the smallest decisions become paralyzing.

Major depression strikes people from all racial and ethnic groups and all socioeconomic levels. It's so widespread that it's been called "the common cold of mental illness" (Gelman, 1987). However, unlike the common cold, depression can have serious consequences. Depression is just one of the **mood disorders.** In this chapter, we'll also discuss bipolar disorders (often called *manic depression* or *manic-depressive disorder*) and other forms of both depression and mania. We'll discuss various issues related to the diagnoses, causes, and treatment of mood disorders, as well.

DESCRIPTION

Because most mood disorders are episodic—they come and go over time—the section on mood disorders in the fourth edition of the *Diagnostic and Statistical Manual of Mental Disorders (DSM-IV)* (American Psychiatric Association, 1994) is organized around the different kinds of mood **episodes** that occur.

Types of Mood Episodes

Major Depressive Episodes   Depressive symptoms can occur as a primary problem or in connection with other disorders. Depressive symptoms can also be connected with various problems in life that are not disorders. For instance, an elderly man may develop symptoms of depression following the death of his wife, or a college student may despair over an academic failure or the breakup of a relationship. In each of these cases, the symptoms of depression are secondary to another problem.

In diagnosing depression, the key issue is not whether the symptoms are the primary problem or related to another disorder or problem in life. If enough symptoms occur together for a long enough time, they can be recognized as a mood episode in need of treatment.

Primary Features   What distinguishes a **major depressive episode** from normal distress or a depressed mood that's part of another diagnosis? One major distinguishing factor is the co-occurrence of both somatic (physical) and cognitive symptoms along with the primary mood disturbance. The *DSM-IV* table presents the diagnostic criteria for a major depressive episode.

The core disturbance of a major depressive episode can be shown in one of two ways. First, the person may have a persistent depressed mood. This might be indicated either by her own reports of sadness or emptiness or by similar reports from others—for instance, that she's frequently tearful or doesn't smile or respond to positive events.

A major depressive episode may also be present if the person displays **anhedonia,** which is a marked loss of interest or pleasure in all or nearly all activities. She may stop doing hobbies and have little interest in her work. Even activities that normally would be of special value—for instance, showing affection to her children—may become uninteresting.

Besides these two primary symptoms—persistent depressed mood and anhedonia—a major depressive episode involves at least three or four associated

---

mood disorders Class of mental disorders characterized primarily by disturbances in mood (for example, depression).

episodes Discrete periods of time in which a number of specified symptoms are present and represent a change from previous functioning; the building blocks for mood disorders.

major depressive episode One of two main types of mood episodes; characterized by depressed mood and related changes in behavior and physical and cognitive functioning.

anhedonia Marked lack of pleasure, even in reaction to things that are usually enjoyable; with depressed mood, a core symptom of a major depressive episode.

somatic symptoms Changes in physical functioning, such as sleep and appetite disturbance.

psychomotor agitation Marked increase in physical restlessness; common in major depressive episodes.

 DSM-IV   **Diagnostic Criteria for MAJOR DEPRESSIVE EPISODE**

A. Five (or more) of the following symptoms have been present during the same 2-week period and represent a change from previous functioning; at least one of the symptoms is either (1) depressed mood or (2) loss of interest or pleasure.

1. depressed mood most of the day, nearly every day
2. markedly diminished interest or pleasure in all, or almost all, activities most of the day, nearly every day
3. significant weight loss when not dieting or weight gain, or decrease or increase in appetite nearly every day
4. insomnia or hypersomnia nearly every day
5. psychomotor agitation or retardation nearly every day
6. fatigue or loss of energy nearly every day
7. feelings of worthlessness or excessive or inappropriate guilt nearly every day
8. diminished ability to think or concentrate, or indecisiveness, nearly every day
9. recurrent thoughts of death, recurrent suicidal ideation, or a suicide attempt or specific plan for committing suicide

symptoms. **Somatic symptoms** represent changes in physical functioning, such as a major decrease or increase in appetite or a significant change in weight.

Another common somatic symptom is sleep disturbance. Many depressed people report trouble falling or staying asleep, sometimes because they are worrying about the day's events. Individuals with particularly severe depression may wake two to three hours before they have to get up and be unable to fall back asleep.

Other somatic symptoms of depression have to do with the individual's level of energy and psychomotor arousal. A person who is depressed often feels fatigued. At the same time, the individual may experience **psychomotor agitation,** which results in hand wringing or restless pacing. Or she may have **psychomotor retardation**, which is a great slowing down in motor activity, including simple activities like walking, talking, taking a shower, or preparing a sandwich.

Cognitive symptoms of depression are feelings of worthlessness or excessive inappropriate guilt, greatly increased difficulty in thinking or concentrating, and recurrent thoughts of death or suicide. Depressed individuals tend to be very self-critical. They dwell on their failures, attribute their problems to their lack of skill, and focus on negative events that occur to them and to others. In severe cases, these thoughts can be so extreme that the individual is psychotic (out of touch with reality).

Depressed people often find it particularly hard to concentrate on reading. Thus, depression impairs performance in students and others who need to concentrate for long periods on written materials. If depressed individuals are able to work or attend school, they may have difficulty making decisions, interacting with others, and completing tasks. As a result, they may avoid their real work by filing papers, cleaning equipment, or talking about inconsequential matters.

Suicidal thoughts are also common among depressed people of all ages, including teen-agers. During the 1980s, suicide rose significantly to become the third most common cause of teen-age death; only automobile accidents and homicides take more youths' lives (Berman & Jobes, 1990).

Special Features   To aid clinicians in determining which forms of depression certain individuals have, the *DSM-IV* provides multiple **specifiers** to assist in treatment selection and to improve predictions of the **course** and **outcome** of the disorder. For example, if the depressive episode begins within a month of childbirth, *postpartum onset* can be specified, which may make health care workers more aware of the potential problems in caring for the infant. Clinicians also can specify a range of severity for an episode, from *mild* to *severe with psychotic features.* A severe, psychotic episode may suggest that the individual needs medication, as in the following example:

A 50-year-old widow was transferred to a medical center from her community mental health center, to which she had been admitted 3 weeks previously with severe agitation, pacing, and hand-wringing, depressed mood accompanied by severe self-reproach, insomnia, and a 15-pound weight loss. She believed that her neighbors were against her, had poisoned her coffee, and had bewitched her to punish her because of her wickedness. Seven years previously, after the death of her husband, she had required hospitalization for a similar depression, with extreme guilt, agitation, insomnia, accusatory hallucinations of voices calling her a worthless person, and preoccupation with thoughts of suicide. (Spitzer, Skodol, Gibbon, & Williams, 1981, p. 98)

The specifier **melancholic features** describes a particularly severe type of episode. It's characterized by an almost total loss of pleasure, a lack of reactivity to positive stimuli, and a distinct quality of depressed mood that's quite unlike ordinary sadness. Other symptoms include awakening early in the morning and feelings of depression that are notably worse in the morning. Individuals with melancholic features are less likely to be able to identify particular stressors that triggered

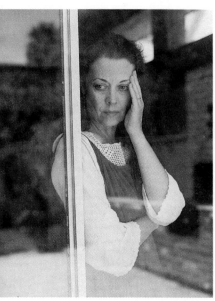

Lethargy, feeling "down" or sad, and loss of interest in daily activities are among the common symptoms of depression.

psychomotor retardation
Significant slowing down of motor activity; common in major depressive episodes.

cognitive symptoms
Changes in content of thought or quality of thought processes, such as poor concentration or suicidal ideation.

specifiers Variety of features describing subtypes of mood disorders; designed to assist in treatment selection and to improve predictions of course and outcome.

course Life history of a disorder; for example, some disorders are chronic (long lasting), whereas others are episodic (come and go).

outcome Eventual result of a disorder; for example, symptoms may go away or persist.

melancholic features
Denote a particularly severe form of major depressive episode; characterized by almost complete loss of pleasure and reactivity to positive stimuli.

Perhaps the most striking and consistent cross-cultural difference in depression is how its symptoms are shown. According to Jenkins, Kleinman, and Good (1991) (who are among the world's foremost researchers of cross-cultural psychiatry), "Most cases of depression world-wide are experienced and expressed in bodily terms of aching backs, headaches, constipation, fatigue, and a wide assortment of other somatic symptoms that lead patients to regard this condition as a physical problem for which they seek out primary case assistance from general practitioners" (p. 73). Of course, we must point out that many people in developed, Western countries also seek treatment for physical problems from their family physicians, who subsequently diagnose them with depression (Katon & Schulberg, 1992). Nonetheless, the professional concept of the disorder places mood disturbance, rather than physical symptoms, at the core of depression.

The particular physical symptoms emphasized vary from culture to culture. For example, in East and South Asia, fatigue is predominant among people with depression, whereas heart distress prevails in Iran; dizziness, in China; and gastrointestinal distress, among Cambodian and Vietnamese refugees (Jenkins et al., 1991). Mumford (1993) has argued, however, that the increased somatic (physical) focus of non-Westerners and the absence of specific words in their languages for *depression* or *anxiety* do not indicate any lack of psychological mindedness and may not represent a true cross-cultural difference. Rather, these issues may simply reflect a greater use of somatic metaphor. For instance, we might express anxiety or fear by saying "I have butterflies in my stomach" or "My heart is in my throat." Similarly, we might object to being called unsophisticated because we designate emotions by colors—"blue" for depression, "green" for envy or jealousy, "black" for anger or upset.

Many of the psychosocial factors that have been causally linked to depression among Americans have similar effects on people from other cultures, too (Jenkins et al., 1991). For example, poor economic conditions were associated with increased depression among rural Kenyans, poor marital relationships characterized depressed women in a South Indian village, negative parenting experiences were reported more often by depressed women of Mexican descent, and traumatic life events increased a variety of psychiatric illnesses among Indochinese refugees. And just as social support was a protective factor among working women in Great Britain, refugees living with families of similar cultural background were less depressed than those who lived in foster or group homes.

We don't mean to say, however, that there are virtually no cross-cultural differences in depression. First, assessment and diagnosis require that judgments be made relative to some normative base, and this base can change significantly across cultures. How emotions are expressed varies greatly from culture to culture; we recognize this when we talk about British people being reserved or Italians being expressive or emotional. Certainly, not all individuals fit the stereotypes of their cultures. On the other hand, stereotypes are not without foundation; they are generalizations about a group based on observations of some of its members. Cultural norms are important, meaningful, and widely varied. Unless we know about them, we might be too ready or too reluctant to diagnose depression in people from other cultures.

Second, we emphasize that the cited findings of cross-cultural researchers have been obtained only after dealing with a large number of methodological difficulties. In many cases, significant cross-cultural differences become hidden within the solutions to these difficulties. For example, we can't simply take a research instrument—say, the Beck Depression Inventory or the Diagnostic Interview Schedule (DIS)—and use it with people in Kenya or South India. Any instrument used cross-culturally must undergo a lengthy and difficult translation process that simultaneously balances the need to be faithful to the original instrument with the need for utility and understandability in the target culture. For example, guilt, shame, and sinfulness are all mentioned together in a single item on the DIS, whereas each term had to be carefully distinguished for use with Hopi Indians (Manson, Shore, & Bloom, 1985).

This translation process reveals that important cultural differences in how depressive symptoms are expressed represent nuisance variables in terms of understanding the basic disorder. However, these cultural differences become hidden in the translation, so researchers who are unaware of the instrument's translation history might draw the mistaken conclusion that there are no cross-cultural differences in how people of different cultures show depression. On the contrary, cultural factors play a profound, if sometimes subtle, role in the development of depression.

Think about the following questions:

1. How many different ways are physical expressions used to designate moods or other psychological states? List as many as you can. What does the existence of these expressions in our language indicate about how we conceptualize these psychological states?

2. If you know another language, think about the different words it uses to describe moods. Do the parallel words in English suggest the same or different feelings to you? If different, what does that tell you about how language shapes our psychological experience?

3. Some causal factors in depression seem common across cultures. Why do you think that might be?

these episodes and are more likely to respond to biological treatments (American Psychiatric Association, 1994).

Some major depressive episodes have **atypical features.** Patients with these features show *mood reactivity*—that is, they respond to positive events with a lightening of their depressed mood. They also experience weight gain or increase in appetite (rather than the classic loss); hypersomnia (sleeping 10 hours or more per day); leaden paralysis (feeling weighted down or very heavy); and extreme sensitivity to interpersonal rejection. This last feature is rather unusual because it's really a personality trait, rather than a symptom. That is, unlike all the other symptoms, it's supposed to be long standing and not just apparent during depressive episodes. Atypical features have been shown to respond best to a particular type of antidepressant medication (Quitkin, Stewart, McGrath, & Tricamo, 1993).

One new specifier allows identifying a **seasonal pattern** to the episodes. People with this subtype—known popularly as *seasonal affective disorder (SAD)*—display symptoms of depression in the winter and then often recover in the spring, even without specific treatment. Interestingly, exposure to bright light is effective in reducing this type of depression (Partonen & Partinen, 1994). The atypical features of weight gain and hypersomnia are more common when a seasonal pattern is present (American Psychiatric Association, 1994). This type of depression is more common among young people and those who live in northern latitudes, where there is a significant decline in sunlight during the winter. Thinking about Multicultural Issues considers other cross-cultural differences, as well.

Manic Episodes   People who are in manic episodes are highly animated and impulsive. For instance, they may be constantly in motion, talk loudly and incessantly, have grandiose ideas, go on wild buying sprees, or engage in unrestrained sexual activity. Sometimes, they're amusing and entertaining, but often, they're irritating and intrude in other people's business.

Primary Features   Like a major depressive episode, a **manic episode** involves a primary mood disturbance plus somatic and cognitive symptoms. However, the symptoms are *bipolar,* or opposite those of a depressive episode. The *DSM-IV* table shows diagnostic criteria for a manic episode. To be diagnosed as manic, an episode must be severe enough to require hospitalization or cause marked impairment in the person's regular functioning.

The elevated mood of a manic episode goes beyond the normal "high" that you might feel after doing really well on a test you studied hard for. A manic mood is unrealistically expansive, accompanied by the feeling that anything is possible—from making a million dollars overnight to writing the perfect novel. For instance, a manic individual who knows how to sew might set out to make blouses for all her friends. In addition, a manic mood is often very **labile,** or changeable. When an individual is in a manic episode, attempts to keep him from carrying out some wild scheme may cause a sudden change of mood to strong anger or irritability.

Like depressed individuals, manic individuals may demonstrate psychomotor agitation. However, manic agitation has a hyperactive, excessive quality often accompanied by reckless behaviors, such as calling friends in the middle of the night, going on

atypical features Denote a subtype of depression; characterized by mood reactivity to positive stimuli.

seasonal pattern Subtype of depression in which symptoms appear in winter and then often go away in the spring, even without specific treatment.

manic episode One of two main types of mood episodes; characterized by extremely elevated mood and related changes in behavior and physical and cognitive functioning.

labile Describes a mood that's very changeable; as in a manic episode, when euphoria quickly changes to anger if the person is provoked.

DSM-IV   Diagnostic Criteria for MANIC EPISODE

A. A distinct period of abnormally and persistently elevated, expansive, or irritable mood, lasting at least 1 week (or any duration if hospitalization is necessary).

B. During the period of mood disturbance, three (or more) of the following symptoms have persisted (four if the mood is only irritable) and have been present to a significant degree:

1. inflated self-esteem or grandiosity
2. decreased need for sleep
3. more talkative than usual or pressure to keep talking
4. flight of ideas or subjective experience that thoughts are racing
5. distractibility
6. increase in goal-directed activity or psychomotor agitation
7. excessive involvement in pleasurable activities that have a high potential for painful consequences

shopping sprees, or starting ill-fated business ventures. Manic speech is loud, rapid, nonstop, often somewhat incoherent, and difficult to direct or interrupt. It may be punctuated by singing, loosely associated plays on words, tangential jokes, and theatrical-type laughter. The following case illustrates these sorts of behaviors:

> B. B., a 39-year-old Hungarian opera singer, was readmitted to a psychiatric hospital after keeping her family awake for several nights with a prayer and song marathon. She was flamboyantly dressed in a floor-length red skirt and peasant blouse and was adorned with heavy earrings, numerous necklaces and bracelets, and medals pinned to her bosom. She spoke very rapidly and was difficult to interrupt as she talked about her intimate relationship with God. She often broke into song, explaining that her beautiful singing voice was a special gift that God had given her to compensate for her insanity. She said that she used it to share the joy she feels with others who are less fortunate. (Spitzer et al., 1981, p. 98)

This case also illustrates another somatic symptom of manic episodes: a much decreased need for sleep. During a manic episode, an individual may sleep only a few hours each night or even stay up for several days at a time.

The cognitive symptoms of a manic episode include lack of control and grandiosity. Manic individuals appear to have inflated self-esteem and may even feel all powerful. Some see themselves as being extremely attractive, which encourages indiscriminate sexual activity. Thoughts come to individuals in manic episodes faster than they can talk. Their **pressured speech** and **flights of ideas** (jumping from topic to topic) may partly reflect a losing attempt to keep up.

Manic individuals are highly distractible. Every little thing around them—such as a bird flitting by, an overheard conversation, or the refrigerator turning on—gets their attention, interrupting any attempt at concentration. Poor judgment during manic episodes seriously interferes with an individual's family and occupational functioning, often to the point that hospitalization is required. In comparison to depressive episodes, manic episodes typically develop more quickly and are briefer. They may start over the period of a day or two and generally last from a week to a few months. Depressive episodes, on the other hand, may come on gradually and last from many months to several years.

pressured speech Loud, fast, nonstop talking that's hard to direct or interrupt; often seen during manic episodes.

flights of ideas Thoughts or speech that jumps from topic to topic with no clear direction or plan; often seen during manic episodes.

hypomanic episode Shorter, milder variant of a manic episode.

mixed episode Mood episode characterized by alteration between full-blown depressive and manic episodes.

major depressive disorders One of the main types of mood disorders; characterized by one or more major depressive episodes but no manic, mixed, or hypomanic episodes.

Hypomanic and Mixed Episodes The characteristics of a **hypomanic episode** are exactly the same as those for a manic episode, with a few important exceptions: Hypomanic episodes are not as long lasting or so severe that they require hospitalization or cause marked impairment in social, interpersonal, and occupational functioning. This type of mood episode was added to the *DSM-IV* after research revealed that many patients had mild maniclike symptoms alternating with depressive episodes or symptoms (Dunner, 1993).

A **mixed episode** is one in which full-blown depressive and manic episodes are *both* present for at least a week, with rapid movement from one extreme to the other. Sleep, appetite, and concentration are all disrupted, and psychomotor agitation and suicidal thoughts are common. Among mood disorder patients, those with mixed episodes may have the poorest prognosis (Keller et al., 1993).

Types of Mood Disorders

Mood disorders represent combinations of episodes and other features. Following this approach, examples of the major types of *DSM-IV* mood disorders are listed in Table 7.1.

Major Depressive Disorders Major depressive disorder, *single episode* is diagnosed when a patient has had a single major depressive episode *without* ever having had any of the other three types of episodes. About 50 to 60 percent of individuals who are diagnosed as such will experience a second episode; their diagnosis

TABLE 7.1 Examples of DSM-IV Mood Disorders		
Disorder	**Type of Episode**	**Features**
Major depressive disorder	Major Depressive	One or more major depressive episodes
		No manic, hypomanic, or mixed episodes
Single episode		One episode only
Recurrent		More than one episode
With melancholic features		Shows particular symptoms associated with this subtype
With seasonal pattern		Seasonal onset and offset (e.g., fall *vs.* spring)
With postpartum onset		Onset follows within 1 month of childbirth
Bipolar I disorder	Manic *or* Mixed	May have experienced major depressive episode in past
With rapid cycling		At least 4 episodes in 1 year
Bipolar II disorder	Hypomanic + Major Depressive	No manic or mixed episodes
With atypical features		Mixed or major depressive episode shows the particular symptoms associated with this subtype

Source: Based on American Psychiatric Association, 1994.

will be major depressive disorder, *recurrent*. Once a second episode has occurred, the likelihood of having a third goes up to 70 percent. And 90 percent of those go on to have a fourth (American Psychiatric Association, 1994). Individuals' degree of recovery between episodes also varies. About two-thirds experience complete **remission** and one-third, only partial remission.

Major depressive episodes without manic or mixed episodes are sometimes referred to as **unipolar disorder** or **unipolar depression.** Whether *unipolar* depression is distinct from *bipolar* depression (for example, whether it's caused by different genetic factors) has been the subject of much research.

The following case is a good illustration of major depression:

Mr. L was to be married on January 1, but never showed up for the wedding. The wedding banquet untouched, his fiancée cried herself to sleep. A biographer described his mood: Where can he be? Has he not looked forward to this, his wedding day? No; to him it is almost his death day. By daybreak [of January 2], after persistent search L's friends find him. The mental strain he has manifested all through the engagement now drives him with restless agitation into a state bordering on melancholia. . . .

After a few days, during which he scarcely eats or sleeps, L appears less agitated, but his thinking is labored and his actions are similarly slow. Periods of silence are broken by lamentations and listlessness. He is indifferent to his surroundings, interrupted by short-lived periods of a pressure of activity as though he were laboring under an intense inner conflict. His thoughts are filled with gloomy forebodings. On the days when he is less perturbed he is able to attend [to his work], yet he is clothed in a constant mood of apathy and gloom. His friends encourage him to attend [to his work], as this activity may take his mind from his recent misfortune, his depression and wedding cancellation.

A few weeks later, he writes, "I have within the last few days been making a most discreditable exhibition of myself in the way of hypochondriasm." And a few days later, in answer to a letter from his partner, he states, "From the deplorable state of my mind at this time, I fear I shall give you but little satisfaction," but he is able to give his partner briefly the news. Yet even this little attention to the issues

remission Lessening or disappearance of symptoms of a disorder.

unipolar disorder or unipolar depression Older name for major depressive disorder.

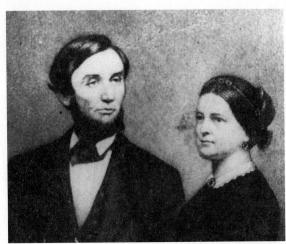

Lincoln's depression was so pronounced that he did not show up for his wedding to Mary Todd. Later in her life, Mary Todd Lincoln was declared insane by a jury, and she then attempted suicide.

at hand fatigues him, and he ends, "I am now the most miserable man living. If what I feel were equally distributed to the whole human family, there would be not one cheerful face on the earth. Whether I shall ever be better, I cannot tell; I awfully forebode I shall not. To remain as I am is impossible; I must die or be better." (L. P. Clark, 1933, pp. 55, 57)

Who was Mr. L? None other than Abraham Lincoln.

Bipolar Disorders   Several diagnoses of **bipolar disorders** are also possible. Bipolar I disorder is diagnosed when a patient is experiencing or has a history of one or more manic or mixed episodes, usually alternating with major depressive episodes. During their "low" times, bipolar patients show the same symptoms as other depressed patients. Most manic episodes—60 to 70 percent—occur immediately before or after a major depressive episode. Individuals who experience only manic episodes are rare, accounting for less than 10 percent of patients with bipolar I disorder (American Psychiatric Association, 1994). The specifier **rapid cycling** can be added to the diagnosis if four or more episodes have occurred within 1 year. Approximately 5 to 15 percent of individuals with bipolar I disorder are rapid cyclers.

As with major depressive disorder, the degree of recovery between episodes is variable. Approximately 20 to 30 percent of individuals with bipolar I disorder continue to display some symptoms and functional difficulties between episodes.

Bipolar II disorder is diagnosed when a patient is experiencing or has a history of one or more major depressive *and* hypomanic episodes but has never experienced a manic or mixed episode. This disorder, which is officially new in the *DSM-IV*, is quite common, can be diagnosed reliably, has clear genetic links to other mood disorders, and is associated with clinically significant problems (Dunner, 1993).

The following case describes a patient with a bipolar II disorder:

A 37-year-old thrice divorced woman was hospitalized in a private psychiatric facility because of an attempt to end her life by putting her head into the oven and turning on the gas. When the acute effects of central nervous system depression had worn off, she complained of hopelessness and uselessness, inordinate fatigue, guilt about having abandoned her 5-year-old daughter, and total anhedonia; she displayed marked psychomotor retardation and slept 12–14 hours a night. This was the patient's sixth episode of this kind. . . .

After 10 days on an antidepressant medication, her mood became elated, flirtatious, and overconfident, and she did not sleep more than 4 to 5 hours a night. This mood receded in 4 days with a downward adjustment of her medication. Review of her history revealed a previous "high period," which had occurred at the tail end of her second depressive episode, when she was on no medication. It had lasted for 2 weeks. She recalled "being on Cloud 9," having an overabundance of energy and a decreased need for sleep, keeping the house immaculate, arranging and rearranging the furniture 2 to 3 times a day, and kissing the children every time they passed by. She denied having racing thoughts and inflated self-esteem, and there was no evidence of poor judgment. (Spitzer et al., 1981, pp. 242–243)

If a patient in a major depressive episode comes for evaluation and if he has *ever* had any distinct periods of abnormally elevated and persistently "high" moods, he should be diagnosed and treated as having a bipolar disorder, even if currently depressed.

Interestingly, there is a documented relationship between bipolar disorder and creativity. A recent study of British artists and writers revealed a much higher rate of mood disorder among these individuals than among the general population. Bipolar disorder was especially common among poets (Jamison, 1993).

bipolar disorders One of the main types of mood disorders; characterized by one or more manic, mixed, or hypomanic episodes.

rapid cycling Subtype of bipolar I disorder, in which 4 or more mood episodes occur per year.

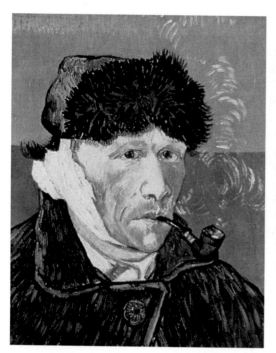
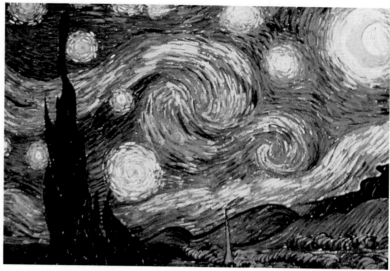

Vincent Van Gogh probably suffered from bipolar disorder. As documented in his self-portrait, he cut off his ear in a fit of despair; his "Starry Night," however, expresses the expansive, creative quality of mania.

dysthymic disorder
Depressive disorder that's less severe but of longer duration than major depression.

double depression
Presence of both dysthymic disorder and a major depressive episode.

Diagnostic Criteria for 300.4 DYSTHYMIC DISORDER

A. Depressed mood for most of the day, for more days than not, for at least two years.

B. Presence, while depressed, of two (or more) of the following:
1. poor appetite or overeating
2. insomnia or hypersomnia
3. low energy or fatigue
4. low self-esteem
5. poor concentration or difficulty making decisions
6. feelings of hopelessness

Specify:
Early onset (before age 21 years)
Late onset (21 years or older)
Atypical features

Specifiers   Table 7.1 also identifies various specifiers. The specifier *with rapid cycling* is limited to bipolar disorders. Other specifiers—*with atypical features* or *seasonal pattern*—can be added to any major depressive episode, whether it appears as a major depressive disorder or as one episode in a bipolar disorder.

Clearly, there are many possible combinations of the different types of episodes and specifiers. This complex system has evolved to characterize the wide variety of mood disorders with as much detail and precision as possible. In this chapter, we'll focus on major depressive disorder and bipolar I disorder, especially in discussing causes and treatments of mood disorders.

Dysthymic Disorder and Cyclothymic Disorder   One important mood disorder that does not entirely fit into the schema just described is **dysthymic disorder**, which is characterized by a relatively chronic mood disturbance, rather than shorter-lived episodes. To diagnose dysthymic disorder, the symptoms must last 2 years or more and be evident most days during this period.

The *DSM-IV* table lists the diagnostic criteria for dysthymic disorder. Like major depression, this disorder is characterized by mood disturbance and loss of energy. Feelings of hopelessness and low self-esteem also are specific criteria. Symptoms do not include psychomotor disturbance or suicidal ideation.

As mentioned earlier, depressive symptoms often occur secondary to other disorders, such as anorexia nervosa (discussed in Chapter 11), anxiety disorders (Chapter 5), and substance abuse (Chapter 9). These symptoms can be diagnosed as dysthymic disorder if they continue for at least 2 years. If an individual with dysthymic disorder is also diagnosed as having a major depressive episode, both diagnoses can be given. Individuals who have **double depression** have a poorer prognosis than those who have only one depressive disorder (Wells, Burnam, Rogers, & Hays, 1992).

The age of onset of dysthymic disorder may be important in predicting its course and outcome. Individuals with early onset are more likely to develop a major depressive disorder later (Klein, Taylor, Dickstein, & Harding, 1988).

Cyclothymic disorder also refers to a chronic mood disturbance that has lasted at least 2 years. In cyclothymic disorder, however, hypomanic symptoms or episodes alternate with depressive symptoms that are less severe than those in a major depressive episode, so a diagnosis of bipolar II cannot be made. Cyclothymic disorder often begins early in life and may represent a risk factor for the development of other mood disorders. For example, 15 to 50 percent of individuals who have cyclothymic disorder eventually develop either bipolar I or bipolar II disorder (American Psychiatric Association, 1994).

Focus on
Critical Thinking

1. According to the DSM-IV, five criteria are required to diagnose an individual as having a major depressive episode. If you were a therapist, what would you do if a patient showed only four symptoms: depressed mood, insomnia, loss of energy, and feelings of worthlessness? Why?

2. Some individuals with dysthymic disorder also experience major depressive episodes. What are the advantages and disadvantages of considering these as separate disorders (that is, as double depression) versus a single depressive disorder with a fluctuating course? Explain your answers.

Issues and Problems

According to a recent community survey, major depression is the single most common psychiatric disorder among people in the United States (Kessler et al., 1994). The fact is, mood disorders affect all people, regardless of race, ethnic group, social class, gender, or age. However, there are demographic patterns to the occurrence of mood disorders, and they often occur with other disorders.

An estimated 15 percent of individuals with mood disorders eventually commit suicide (Kaplan & Sadock, 1991). And as shown in Figure 7.1, 60 percent of suicides are committed by individuals who have depression (Klerman, 1987). In this section, we consider some of the many issues and problems associated with studying mood disorders.

cyclothymic disorder
Mood disorder characterized by frequent alteration between hypomanic and depressive symptoms that don't meet criteria for a major depressive episode.

FIGURE 7.1 Causes of suicide

Sixty percent of suicides are related to depression.

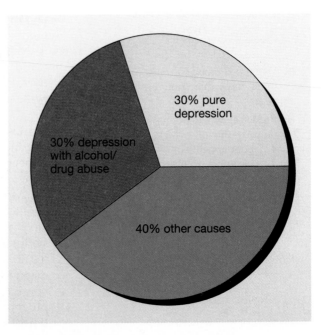

30% pure depression

30% depression with alcohol/drug abuse

40% other causes

Source: From G. Klerman, Dept. of Psychiatry, Cornell University, as reported in *Newsweek,* May 4, 1987. Reprinted by permission of Newsweek.

Prevalence and Risk Factors

Prevalence rates indicate what percentage of a population has a specific disorder. **Point prevalence** indicates the percentage who have the disorder at a particular time or over a given period (such as the past year), whenever the population is sampled.

Figure 7.2 shows prevalence rates for mood disorders among men and women. These data are based on a recent large-scale study (Kessler et al., 1994) of psychiatric disorders in over 8,000 community-dwelling adults in the United States. The 12-month (that is, point) prevalence rates for a major depressive episode were found to be about 8 percent for men and 13 percent for women. Prevalence rates for dysthymia were 2.1 percent and 3 percent for men and women, respectively. For a manic episode, the rates were 1.4 percent for men and 1.3 percent for women.

Lifetime prevalence indicates the percentage of individuals who have ever had a specific disorder at any time. Naturally, lifetime prevalence rates are higher than point prevalence rates. As shown in Figure 7.2, the lifetime prevalence rates for a major depressive episode were 12.7 percent for men and 21.3 percent for women. For dysthymia, the rates for men and women were 4.8 and 8.0 percent, respectively. And for a manic episode, they were 1.6 percent for men and 1.7 percent for women (Kessler et al., 1994).

These figures from Kessler et al. (1994) are considerably higher than those obtained in the Epidemiological Catchment Area (ECA) study, another large-scale study of psychiatric disorders (Regier & Burke, 1987; Regier et al., 1984; Robins et al., 1984) (see Chapter 1). The difference is likely due to the data collection methods

FIGURE 7.2   Gender differences in prevalence of mood disorders

Depression and dysthymia are about twice as common in women as in men, whereas mania appears equally in men and women.

point prevalence
Percentage of individuals with a disorder at a particular point in time.

lifetime prevalence
Percentage of individuals who have had a disorder at any time in their lives.

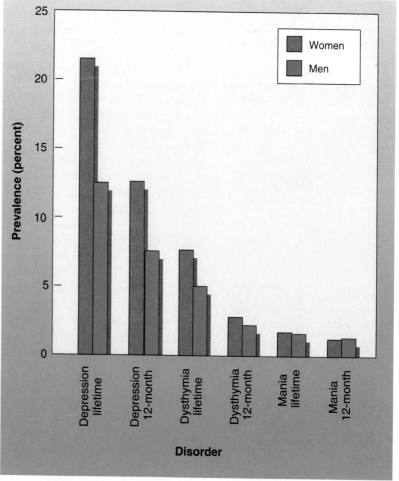

Source: Data from Kessler et al., 1994.

used, but even so, the pattern of prevalence was the same across the two studies. For example, both studies found a greater prevalence of major depressive episodes among women and no difference among men and women in the prevalence of bipolar episodes.

When prevalence rates differ on the basis of a demographic or other factor, that variable is considered a **risk factor** for the disorder. Since the prevalence rate of depressive disorders among women is about twice that of men, sex is a risk factor for depression. But it is not a risk factor for bipolar disorders, because the rates for manic episodes do not differ between the sexes.

These findings (Kessler et al., 1994; Regier & Burke, 1987; Regier et al., 1984) are consistent with those of many other studies and lead to the same conclusion about the different rates of depression for men and women: Those for women are about twice as high as those for men (except in prepubescent youth and the elderly) (Nolen-Hoeksema, 1990; Nolen-Hoeksema & Girgus, 1994). A number of theories have been proposed to account for this finding (see Thinking about Gender Issues).

There are three myths to dispel concerning the relation of mood disorders, especially depression, and the demographic risk factors of age, income, and race/ethnicity. First, major depressive disorder is *not* found frequently among the elderly. One study (Myers et al., 1984) looked at the prevalence of psychiatric disorders in over 9,500 community-dwelling adults over age 18 in the United States. Those 65 and over had the lowest 6-month prevalence rate for all mood disorders, and those from 45 to 64 had generally the next lowest rates. Mood disorders were most common among 18- to 24-year-old men and 25- to 44-year-old women. Ten years later, Kessler et al. (1994) also found higher rates of mood disorders in the 15- to 24-year-old group in their sample. A number of contributing factors might explain this finding: the lack of stable partners, educational and job pressures, and the ambiguity of how to live as an adolescent or young adult.

The second myth is that depression is related to income level. Although rates of mental disorder generally increase with levels of poverty and decrease with levels of education (Bruce, Takeuchi, & Leaf, 1991; Robins, Locke, & Regier, 1991), depression is not strongly related to income across the whole scale. Depressive disorders are more likely to occur in individuals at the extreme low end of the income scale (less than $20,000 per year), but beyond that, there seems to be little relationship between income and mood disorders. By contrast, income is negatively related to anxiety disorders throughout the income range (Kessler et al., 1994). Apparently, a range of income-related stressors relate to anxiety, but only those associated with truly low income (e.g., not being able to pay your bills) increase the likelihood of depression.

The third myth has to do with racial and ethnic groups. Despite some claims that African Americans have higher rates of mood disorders, the status of race/ethnicity as a risk factor in developing these disorders remains unclear. In both of the large survey studies mentioned earlier (Kessler et al., 1994; Weissman, Bruce, Leaf, Florio, & Holzer, 1991), African Americans had slightly (but statistically not significant) lower rates of depressive disorders than Hispanics or non-Hispanic whites. Even when income and education were statistically controlled, the lower rates of mood disorders among African Americans were still evident.

Less research has examined the prevalence of mood disorders among other racial and ethnic groups. However, epidemiological studies of Hispanic populations in Los Angeles (Karno et al., 1987) and Puerto Rico (Canino et al., 1987) found that rates of major depressive disorder were no higher (or even lower) among Hispanics than non-Hispanic whites in these locales.

Comorbidity   Recall the case of Howard, presented at the beginning of this chapter, who experienced repeated bouts of depression throughout his lifetime, along with significant symptoms of anxiety disorders. His pattern of having both anxiety and depression is quite common, and he had to be treated for both problems.

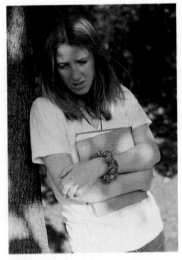

Depression is common among young people, perhaps because the transition from adolescent to adult roles is difficult and stressful. Depression can interfere with the concentration needed for academic success in college.

risk factor Variable that increases a person's tendency to develop a disorder; associated with different prevalence rates of disorders.

matrilineal Describes a society in which family structure and inheritance are based on females' (wives') bloodlines.

artifacts Research findings that result from methodological factors, rather than reflect real differences.

As shown in Figure 7.2, women display nearly twice the rates of unipolar (but not bipolar) depression and dysthymia as do men. These results are consistent across a variety of studies and diverse cultures (Jenkins et al., 1991). Nonetheless, understanding these differences between men and women has proven to be a major challenge. Explanations based on biological, psychological, and social factors all have been offered, but hypothesis after hypothesis has been disproved or only weakly supported by research.

Two general biological explanations have been advanced to account for the gender differences in depression: the genetic hypothesis and the hormonal hypothesis. Neither has received much research support, however. For example, genetic linkage studies provide no evidence that the X chromosome—one of the two chromosomes that determines biological sex—is involved in depression (Nolen-Hoeksema, 1990).

The hormonal hypothesis is partly derived from the observation that some women are at increased risk for depression when their estrogen or progesterone levels change significantly, such as during the premenstrual, postpartum, or menopausal periods. Research findings about this hypothesis have been quite inconsistent (Nolen-Hoeksema, 1990).

Explanations based on social factors also have been proposed. The hypothesis that overall socioeconomic differences between men and women contribute to differences in their rates of depression has not been supported (Nolen-Hoeksema, 1990). Stressful life events by themselves can't account for the observed differences because women don't report having more stressful events than men (Uhlenhuth, Lipman, Balter, & Stern, 1974) nor do they perceive specific events as being more stressful than men do.

Explanations based in differences in gender roles and the expectations that go with them also have been investigated. For example, data suggest that women whose only role is that of the traditional wife and mother may be more vulnerable to depression. These women may be more at risk because they have only one significant source of support and gratification. What's more, their role is undervalued in current Western societies (Nolen-Hoeksema, 1990). In cultures in which both male and female roles are equally valued (for instance, the Old Order Amish community), no gender differences in depression are found. And in some **matrilineal** societies (in which women play dominant roles), men have higher rates of depression (Jenkins et al., 1991).

Finally, a number of psychological explanations also have been offered. It's been proposed, for instance, that gender differences in rates of depression are **artifacts**— that is, they're created artificially by factors basic to the method of data collection. Reporting differences are one such factor. Suppose that women are more willing to report depression and seek treatment; if that's true, then it might appear as if they have higher rates of depression, regardless of whether that's accurate.

Two main lines of evidence argue against this possibility. First of all, research on randomly selected individuals from the community has obtained the same results. This means that the higher rates of depression reported cannot be due to a greater likelihood of women seeking treatment. Second, several studies have examined reporting biases in men versus women. Whether symptoms are reported in face-to-face interviews or anonymously makes no differences in the rates of reporting. Thus, willingness to admit to symptoms cannot account for the gender differences (Nolen-Hoeksema, 1990).

However, Wilhelm and Parker (1994) recently reported on a longitudinal study in which groups of men and women with equal depression rates were studied 10 years later. In sum, men were more likely to have forgotten previous episodes of major depression, whereas women were more likely to recall mild symptoms of depression as full-blown episodes. Differences in depression rates disappeared when these artifacts were controlled for, so the artifact hypothesis cannot be completely dismissed.

A final possible explanation of gender differences that seems promising is differences in the coping strategies of women and men. A body of research by Nolen-Hoeksema and colleagues (Nolen-Hoeksema, 1990, 1991; Nolen-Hoeksema, Parker, & Larson, 1994) suggests that when men are faced with negative emotions aroused by stressful events, they tend to distract themselves from their negative moods through activities such as sports or drinking. Women, on the other hand, tend to focus and maintain attention on the negative mood (that is, they ruminate). If rumination intensifies negative moods, then this response style may make women more likely than men to become clinically depressed.

Still, the rumination hypothesis is not really the final answer to the gender difference puzzle. *Why* women ruminate more than men remains to be explained.

Think about the following questions:

1. Why do you think women ruminate more than men? Develop several hypotheses about this.
2. Gender differences don't show up until adolescence and are not observed among college students. What biopsychosocial factors might lead to the increase in depression in females (but not those who go to college) during adolescence? Explain your answer.
3. What other differences in social behavior between men and women might contribute to higher rates of depression in women? Why?

This co-occurrence of two or more disorders is called **comorbidity.** It presents a difficult challenge to the therapist because selecting the proper treatment may depend on knowing why the disorders are co-occurring. For example, one disorder may be clearly secondary to the other, as when a person with a chronic pain disorder develops opioid (pain medication) dependence. Or the disorders may be entirely independent, as when a person with a sexual disorder experiences a severe, unrelated trauma and develops posttraumatic stress disorder (PTSD). Comorbidity occurs most commonly in mood disorders because the disorders share features ranging from underlying genetic factors to demographic risk factors to environmental stressors.

Mood disorders co-occur with many other disorders, especially anxiety, personality, and substance abuse disorders (L. A. Clark, Watson, & Reynolds, 1995). For example, in a study of depressed outpatients, 74 percent were also diagnosed with a personality disorder (Shea et al., 1990), and in another study, 84 percent of anorexic patients had a current or past mood disorder (Halmi et al., 1991).

The comorbidity of anxiety and depression is a particular problem. Studies have found about a 50 percent overlap between anxiety and depression. This overlap has been consistent regardless of whether the studies examined simply mood (that is, anxious and depressed mood), symptoms associated with anxiety and depression (such as disturbances of sleep, appetite, and concentration), or full-blown anxiety and depressive disorders (L. A. Clark & Watson, 1991b). In some cases, the depression precedes the anxiety problems; in other cases, the reverse is true.

Either way, when anxiety and depression occur together, the combined disorder presents a more serious problem for the individual. In addition, recovery is more difficult. For example, the suicide rate among individuals who have panic disorder with depression is more than three times that for individuals who have panic disorder without depression (Johnson, Weissman, & Klerman, 1990).

Proliferation of Disorders Many more different mood disorders can be described using the *DSM-IV*, given the addition of hypomanic and mixed episodes and all the different specifiers. The section on mood disorders increased in size from 20 pages in the *DSM-III-R* to 75 pages in *DSM-IV* (1987, 1994). Even so, some professionals argue that there still aren't enough mood diagnoses—that there are still other variations of mood disorders not yet included in the *DSM*.

For cases in which this is true, therapists can use the **NOS diagnoses,** which mean "Not Otherwise Specified." An NOS diagnosis is included in every section of the *DSM*. The mood disorder work group who developed this section of the *DSM-IV* attempted to describe more of the common patterns that fall into these groups. Among the mood disorders–NOS, three noteworthy examples are premenstrual dysphoric disorder, minor depressive disorder, and brief recurrent depressive disorder.

Premenstrual dysphoric disorder, commonly known as *PMS,* or *premenstrual syndrome,* was included in the appendix of the *DSM-III-R* (American Psychiatric Association, 1987) as "Late Luteal Phase Dysphoric Disorder." It was studied intensively during the latest revision process, and a set of suggested criteria are listed in the new manual.

Similar decisions were made for **minor depressive disorder** and **brief recurrent depressive disorder.** Both disorders are variants of major depressive disorder. Minor depressive disorder is diagnosed when fewer than the required five symptoms are present, and brief recurrent depressive disorder is diagnosed when the episodes last less than the required 2 weeks. Both diagnoses were found to be very common in community samples and to interfere significantly with individuals' functioning (Angst, 1992).

All these disorders were included in the *DSM-IV* as examples of mood disorder–NOS to encourage further research on them and to help make clinicians aware of their existence. Perhaps in some future *DSM,* these disorders will be listed indi-

comorbidity Co-occurrence of two or more disorders.

NOS diagnoses Not Otherwise Specified diagnoses; used when a patient has a significant clinical problem that doesn't fit any categories in the DSM.

premenstrual dysphoric disorder Commonly known as premenstrual syndrome or PMS; can be diagnosed as a Mood Disorder–NOS.

minor depressive disorder Variant of major depressive disorder with fewer than the required 5 symptoms.

brief recurrent depressive disorder Variant of major depressive disorder that lasts less than the required 2 weeks.

vidually. This is what happened with bipolar II disorder. Previously, patients with bipolar II disorder were diagnosed with mood disorder–NOS.

Suicide

Depression is the most common factor leading to suicide; as such, it is the most lethal mental disorder. Approximately 90 percent of the people who commit suicide have some psychological or psychiatric disorder. Some 45 to 70 percent of those people have a mood disorder, often with another disorder. About 15 percent of individuals with mood disorders eventually commit suicide (Kaplan & Sadock, 1991).

Adolescents and young adults who commit suicide commonly have comorbid alcohol and/or drug dependence and depression (Lesage et al., 1994; Runeson & Rich, 1992). The suicide of rock star Kurt Cobain was related to both depression and substance abuse (Strauss & Foege, 1994). (See Chapters 9 and 14 for more information on substance abuse and disorders of youths, respectively.)

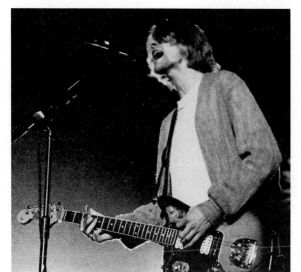

Despite his long history of depression and drug addiction, was rock singer Kurt Cobain's suicide preventable?

Some individuals view suicide as a rational and moral act for the person who is extremely ill or despondent. A recent survey (Cohen, Fihn, Boyko, & Jonsen, 1994) of 938 physicians found that 39 percent thought that physician-assisted suicide was never justified. Fifty-three percent thought that it should be legal in some cases, although only 40 percent said that they'd be willing to assist in a legal suicide. Interestingly, psychiatrists had the most supportive attitudes toward suicide.

Thus, attitudes toward suicide may be changing. Such change will be difficult in Western cultures, though, since suicide has traditionally been condemned by church and state. In some states in the United States, suicide is unlawful. Many religions view it as a sin. Even disregarding the views of church, state, and society, suicide has enormous adverse effects on the family and friends who are left behind; they feel overwhelming guilt, shame, and anger.

Epidemiology   The actual number of people who commit suicide each year is hard to pinpoint. Sometimes, deaths that are reported as being accidental are actually suicides—for instance, single-car accidents, shooting accidents, and even lethal doses of alcohol. About 30,000 individuals commit suicide each year in the United States, and approximately 10 times as many attempt suicide (Andreasen & Black, 1991).

Women make twice as many suicide attempts, which is consistent with the greater prevalence of depression among women. However, men succeed in killing themselves three to four times more often, due to their use of more violent methods, such as guns, hanging, or jumping from high places. Women are more likely to take poison or a drug overdose (Kaplan & Sadock, 1991).

Although suicide *attempts* are most common among young people, *completed* suicide rates increase with age. Particular increases begin at about age 45 for men and 55 for women. People over the age of 65 account for 25 percent of all suicides, although they make up only 10 percent of the population. This may be due partly to physical illness, which increases with age and is a risk factor for suicide. However, the suicide rate among young people—particularly young men—has been rising for the past 25 years. After accidents, suicide is now the second-leading cause of death among individuals in the 15- to 24-year-old group (Kaplan & Sadock, 1991).

There are also trends in suicide rates among racial/ethnic groups and people of different socioeconomic (SES) levels. Although the suicide rate among whites is nearly twice that among nonwhites, "pockets" of increased suicide rates exist among certain Native American, Native Alaskan, and inner-city African American groups. Even though most data show increased psychological problems in lower-income groups, the risk for suicide actually *increases* with SES. Female physicians have one of the highest rates of suicide of any occupational group—about 2.5 to 3 times greater than that of nonprofessional women (Kaplan & Sadock, 1991).

Within the mood disorders group, the risk of suicide is greater for bipolar patients than for patients who experience only depression. Between one-fourth and one-half of bipolar patients attempt suicide at least once (Goodwin & Jamison, 1990), and approximately one-fifth of bipolar patients die by suicide (Jamison, 1993). These high rates may be due to the stress associated with mood cycling.

Reasons for Committing Suicide   The suicides of noted personalities—often, people with beauty, talent, wealth, and fame—draw a lot of publicity. Controversy has surrounded the true causes and motives involved in the deaths of such public figures as Marilyn Monroe, Elvis Presley, Ernest Hemingway, and Kurt Cobain.

Most people commit suicide because they see it as the only solution to an unbearable situation. They are experiencing intense psychological pain, are completely frustrated in their attempts to meet their psychological needs, and have fallen into a state of hopelessness from which they see no other means of escape (Schneidman, 1985). The following suicide note illustrates the overwhelming distress of a father whose wish to die and end his pain stands in marked contrast with his sincere concern for his family (from Schneidman & Farberow, 1957, pp. 206–207):

> To Tom, Betty, John—The stigma I bring upon you cannot be much more than has already been done. Be good to your mother and do all you can to help as she is a wonderful person. Tom—a rather gruesome thought—Remember when we worked in the yard and you asked to see a cadaver at the College? Little did we know that I would be the first deceased for you to encounter. I love you and know you will make a wonderful man. Betty—We have been very close to each other. Please don't think too harshly of my actions. Stabilization takes place in time, and I know you will grow up to be one of the best women in the world. My love, dear. Johnny—You came last in our offspring so couldn't know me as well as your brother and sister. Just follow your brother's example, love your sister and help Mother. Remember, I love you, Johnny. Mary—There is no more or less to say than I have already told you—Truth will triumph eventually.
>
> Bill

A minority of individuals who complete suicide (about 13 percent) do so accidentally, so to speak. For instance, the person who's trying to prevent a lover from leaving or the teen-ager who's had a big fight with his parents and wants to get back at them may die because help is not obtained quickly enough to save the individual. In these cases, the individual is usually ambivalent about wanting to die and, in fact, may not choose to complete the act. About one-third of suicides are thought to involve some combination of truly wanting to die and also trying to manipulate others (Kovacs, Beck, & Weissman, 1975).

Table 7.2 lists the specific problems given as reasons for the suicide attempts of 130 individuals in Oxford, England (Bancroft, Skrimshire, Casson, Harvard-Watts, & Reynolds, 1977). The most common reasons were relationship issues—problems in marriage or with a boyfriend or girlfriend. More recent studies corroborate this. For example, 100 Swedish individuals cited conflict with partners most often as the reason for attempting suicide (Nordentoft & Rubin, 1993). As we discuss later in this chapter, this information is quite consistent with research indicating that marital and interpersonal factors are important in depression.

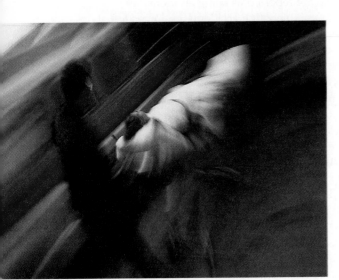

People who have tried to commit suicide commonly require emergency hospital treatment. They are then often admitted to a psychiatric unit for further treatment.

TABLE 7.2	Reasons for Committing Suicide	
Problems	**Females (percent) (N = 91)**	**Males (percent) (N = 39)**
Marital	68	83
Boyfriend/girlfriend	71	77
Sexual	14	15
Children	25	17
Financial	16	26
Work	16	54
Accident/operation	19	3
Alcohol	9	9

Source: From J. Bancroft, A. Skrimshire, J. Casson, O. Harvard-Watts, and F. Reynolds, "People Who Deliberately Poison or Injure Themselves: Their Problems and Contacts with Helping Agencies," *Psychological Medicine, 7,* 289–303. Copyright © 1977 Cambridge University Press. Reprinted by permission of Cambridge University Press.

Warning Signs and Prevention   Sometimes, a person is so successful in hiding his psychological distress from others that his suicide comes as a complete surprise. More typically, however, warning signs provide clues to a potential suicide. Any talk of suicide by a friend or relative should be taken seriously. It's estimated that 80 percent of the people who kill themselves give specific warnings of their intentions. The following are risk factors and warning signs of suicide:

1. previous attempt or fantasized suicide
2. anxiety, depression, exhaustion
3. availability of means of suicide
4. concern for effect of suicide on family members
5. verbalized suicidal ideation
6. preparation of a will, resignation after agitated depression
7. proximal life crisis, such as mourning or impending surgery
8. family history of suicide (Kaplan & Sadock, 1991, p. 556)

Some of these risk factors, such as anxiety and depression, may be reduced with professional intervention. Similarly, if individuals who attempt suicide are referred afterward for psychological or pharmacological treatment, their suicidal thoughts and attempts will decrease. It's difficult to obtain solid empirical data to support the belief that suicide is preventable. Likewise, the effectiveness of suicide prevention centers and hotline services has not been proven (Dew, Bromet, Brent, & Greenhouse, 1987).

Many individuals who commit suicide never seek professional help. Thus, it's especially important that family members and close friends be alert to changes in the person's behavior and respond to her need for love and her lack of hope. These measures are probably the primary suicide preventors.

Focus on Critical Thinking

1. When depression co-occurs with another type of disorder (such as anxiety or substance abuse), the combined disorder seems to be worse than might be expected from simply adding the two sets of symptoms together. What factors might account for these qualitative differences? Explain your answer.

2. Suppose that you were the physician for a severely depressed and suicidal patient. As a professional, how would you feel if your patient wanted to end his pain and distress? Under what circumstances, if any, would you support his desires? Would the patient's age, physical condition, or life situation influence your decision? Again, explain your answers.

CAUSES

Biological models of depression predominated through the 1960s and continue to influence the field greatly. Psychological models of depression became accepted in the 1970s and 1980s. Interpersonal or marital and family models of depression also received significant attention in the 1980s. In the 1990s and as we head into the twenty-first century, researchers are working to integrate these different approaches into a comprehensive biopsychosocial framework.

Biological Factors

Research into biological factors underlying mood disorders continues at a fast pace. We will consider two major areas of investigation: genetic factors and neurobiochemical factors. The latter can be further subdivided into the study of neurotransmitters (chemical messengers in the brain) and neuroendocrine (hormonal) abnormalities.

Genetic Factors   As early as 1621, arguments were made for the genetic transmission of depression. In *The Anatomy of Melancholy*, Robert Burton (1624/1973) asserted that the "inbred cause of melancholia is our temperature, in whole or part, which we receive from our parents" (p. 184). Although no one today thinks body temperature causes depression, the idea that diseases are passed from one generation to the next continues to be supported. Family, twin, and adoption studies all have investigated the role of genetics in causing mood disorders.

Family Studies   Studies of family inheritance patterns provide useful leads in genetic and biochemical research. For example, Lord Byron, the poet, and composer Robert Schumann were both afflicted with bipolar disorder; biographical accounts of their families indicate that many of their relatives were similarly affected (Goodwin & Jamison, 1990).

Katz and McGuffin (1993) found that the relatives of bipolar subjects have a much greater risk of developing bipolar disorder (7.8 percent) than those of unipolar patients (0.6 percent, which is really no different from the population average of about 1.0 percent). Relatives of unipolar patients have a greater risk (9.1 percent) of developing unipolar depression than people in the general population (about 5 percent in the ECA study) (Robins et al., 1984). But relatives of bipolar subjects displayed slightly higher rates of unipolar disorder (11.4 percent).

In other words, family studies suggest that unipolar depression is passed on within families, which is called *familial transmission*. The picture is not as clear cut with bipolar disorders, however. Actually, the relatives of individuals with bipolar disorder have a greater likelihood of developing unipolar than bipolar disorder. These findings suggest that there may be some underlying problem shared by all mood disorders. And perhaps an additional problem is unique to bipolar disorder.

Another finding of family studies is that the risk of relatives' developing a depressive disorder is much greater if the subject was hospitalized for depression (Kendler, Heath, Martin, & Eaves, 1987). This information introduces the notion of a continuum of severity, with mild to moderate unipolar depression at one end, severe unipolar depression (for which people are hospitalized) in the middle, and bipolar disorder at the other (severe) end. As a subject moves from one end to the other, the likelihood of a relative developing a mood disorder increases.

Of course, it's difficult to separate hereditary factors from environmental ones in family inheritance studies. If a daughter, mother, and grandmother were all depressed, for instance, depression could be a genetic trait. But perhaps being raised by a depressed mother causes depression, or maybe all these women lived in a stressful environment. Certainly, the information that a given disorder is transmitted within a family cannot alone settle the question of whether that disorder is genetic.

Twin Studies Recall from Chapter 2 that identical (monozygotic) twins develop from a single egg and are thus genetically identical. Fraternal (dizygotic) twins, on the other hand, develop from separate eggs and are genetically unique.

Twin studies show a clear genetic role in causing major depression. Among identical twins, if one twin is diagnosed with major depression, there's a 40 percent chance of concordance—that the co-twin will also have depression. But among fraternal twins, there's only a 10 percent chance of concordance (Allen, 1976). The role played by genetics is even more apparent in twin studies of bipolar disorders. The concordance rate for identical twins is about 70 to 80 percent, whereas that for fraternal twins is only 10 to 20 percent (Nurnberger & Gershon, 1982).

Research on genetic factors in mood disorders has relied almost solely on using hospitalized patients as subjects. Because the depression of hospitalized patients is likely to be severe, there may be qualitative differences between hospitalized patients and other subjects. Some studies of nonhospitalized twins with major depression have not supported genetic theories (Kendler et al., 1987; Torgersen, 1986).

Adoption Studies Twin studies strongly suggest a predisposition for inheriting depression. It's also possible that twins create similar environments for themselves. For instance, twins reared in the same family spend a great deal of time together as children, which may increase their similarity. Adoption studies assess genetic influences and avoid the similarity of environments of twin studies. Again, recall from Chapter 2 that adoption studies compare people who were adopted with members of both their biological families and adoptive families.

Adoption studies also support the view that genetic factors play an important role in causing mood disorders. Mendlewicz and Rainer (1977) assessed Belgian bipolar patients who had or had not been adopted. The researchers then determined whether the biological and nonbiological (adoptive) parents of the patients had ever had mood disorders. As expected, more mood disorders were found among the biological than nonbiological parents of the patients. Wender et al. (1986) assessed relatives of Danish adoptees with and without depression. Major mood disorders were found more frequently among the biological relatives of depressed adoptees than among the relatives of the adoptees without depression.

The results of these early studies have been confirmed by more recent studies and reviews of the adoption literature for both bipolar (Mitchell, Mackinnon, & Waters, 1993) and unipolar disorder (Maier & Lichtermann, 1993). Moreover, these newer studies have indicated that the severity of disorder is related to the strength of the genetic loading—that is, the extent to which the person has inherited the relevant genes. For example, a person is more likely to develop severe depression if he has many close relatives with mood disorders.

Establishing that a disorder has a genetic basis represents the *beginning* of the larger research enterprise, which involves determining just exactly what's inherited. That is, the fact that even identical twins don't show 100 percent concordance indicates that it's unlikely that *the disorder itself* is inherited. What's more, how mood disorders are transmitted remains unknown (Mitchell et al., 1993). What is inherited is likely to be some kind of vulnerability that's passed on through several, maybe even many, different genes. That vulnerability is probably some complex neurobiochemical predisposition.

Neurobiochemical Factors Early in this century, Kraeplin (1921) proposed that depression was a medical illness with internal causes. However, it was only after the introduction of antidepressant drugs in the 1960s that much research on the biochemistry of depression was conducted. During these years, studies suggested that antidepressant medications worked, at least in part, through effects on **neurotransmitters**: chemicals in the brain that help transmit information in the central nervous system. Study of the reception of these chemical messages followed. In addition, research developed on neuroendocrine abnormalities and sleep disorders in depression.

Neurotransmission   Information is transmitted in the brain via a combination of electrical impulses and neurotransmitters. Within a nerve cell, or *neuron*, information is conveyed by electrical impulses. But for transmission between neurons, neurotransmitters are needed. When an electrical impulse arrives at the end of the neuron, a neurotransmitter is released into a tiny gap—a **synapse**—between it and the beginning of the next neuron. The released neurotransmitter attaches to **postsynaptic receptors** on the next neuron; this action triggers another electrical impulse. Having done its job, the neurotransmitter is then recycled in one of two ways: (1) It may be taken back into the neuron that released it, which is known as **reuptake,** or (2) it may be broken down chemically in the synapse into simpler compounds by **monoamine oxidase (MAO)**. By interfering with this recycling process, the main classes of antidepressants increase how long or how much neurotransmitter remains in the synapse. (This, in turn, increases the frequency or chance of the neurotransmitter attaching to the receptors.) Some antidepressants inhibit reuptake, and others inhibit the chemical breakdown.

Because antidepressants serve to increase the amount or duration of neurotransmitter in the synapse, early investigators (Schildkraut, 1965) reasoned that depression was caused by having too low levels of neurotransmitters. One class of neurotransmitters, in particular—the catecholamines, especially *norepinephrine*—was thought to hold the key to depression. Too much norepinephrine was thought to cause mania and too little, depression. However, researchers quickly found that things were not so simple. A number of neurotransmitters; *serotonin* and *dopamine* soon were shown also to be involved in depression (Goodwin & Jamison, 1990).

Almost immediately after an individual takes antidepressant medication, neural transmissions are increased. Despite this immediate change in biochemical activity at the synapse, the psychological effects of the medication are not seen until 2 or even 8 weeks later. This long delay between the initial biochemical effects and the later psychological effects led researchers to investigate the postsynaptic receptors more closely (Sulser, Gillespie, Mishra, & Manier, 1984).

A tremendous amount of research since then has led to increasingly greater understanding of what has turned out to be an extraordinarily complex process of neural transmission. For example, the brain has a number of **homeostatic mechanisms** that work to keep the system in a steady state, including adjustment of the density and sensitivity of the postsynaptic receptors (Kandel, Schwartz, & Jessell, 1991).

The existence of **presynaptic receptors** has also been discovered. Reuptake by these receptors provides further feedback to the neuron regarding the amount of neurotransmitter in the synapse. It's also been discovered that the various neurotransmitters do not act in isolation. Instead, they interact with each other (Kapur & Mann, 1992) and are further regulated by another class of brain chemicals called **neuropeptides** (Weiss, 1995). Thus, it seems likely that depression is not simply due to the dysfunction of a single neurotransmitter but is caused by an abnormality in how various neurotransmitters interact (Hsiao et al., 1987).

Neuroendocrine Abnormalities   Work in the biochemistry of depression involving the endocrine glands was prompted by the observation that patients with endocrine diseases such as hypothyroidism often have symptoms of depression, as

---

neurotransmitters Complex chemical substances in the brain that are responsible for transmission of information between cells.

synapse Tiny gap between neurons.

postsynaptic receptors Sites on a neuron that receive released neurotransmitters and trigger the next electrical impulse.

reuptake Reabsorption of a neurotransmitter into the neuron it was released from.

monoamine oxidase (MAO) Chemical that breaks down neurotransmitters into simpler compounds.

homeostatic mechanisms Self-regulation processes in the brain that work to maintain a more-or-less steady state.

presynaptic receptors Sites on a neuron that release neurotransmitters that provide feedback regarding the amount of neurotransmitter in the synapse.

neuropeptides Class of brain chemicals that regulate neurotransmitter activity.

well. Development of biochemical tests allowing detection of very small amounts of hormones have also helped the field to expand rapidly.

One endocrine disease associated with depression is Cushing's syndrome, which results in abnormally high levels of the hormone **cortisol** in the blood (Griest & Jefferson, 1992). Initial research (Goodwin & Jamison, 1990) found that over half of patients hospitalized with depression had an excess of blood cortisol. Moreover, severely depressed patients often had high levels of cortisol in their blood throughout the day, rather than only in the morning, as with nondepressed people (Carroll et al., 1981). The test for abnormal cortisol secretion—**dexamethasone suppression test (DST)**—was even used to predict response to treatment. However, it's become evident that other patient groups also have abnormal DSTs (e.g., those with schizophrenia, anorexia, anxiety disorders, and substance abuse), so the DST is no longer used for general diagnosis. Nonetheless, recent progress in neuroendocrine research indicates that a biochemical test for depression may be developed soon.

Sleep Dysfunction   Sleep electroencephalogram (EEG) studies have confirmed that individuals who are depressed usually have disturbed sleep patterns. Specifically, they have less deep (slow-wave) sleep, earlier onset of **rapid eye movement (REM) sleep** (the stage associated with dreams and nightmares), and increased amounts of REM sleep (Sandor & Shapiro, 1994). The EEG sleep abnormalities of people with depression can be distinguished from those of people with insomnia, anxiety disorders, and panic disorder. Interestingly, the neurotransmitters serotonin and norepinephrine are involved in initiating and maintaining non-REM sleep. Thus, the dysfunction of these neurotransmitters may be responsible for the sleep problems of people who are depressed (Thase, Frank, & Kupfer, 1985).

Psychosocial Factors

Psychodynamic Factors   Psychodynamic ideas often seem strange in their original form, yet it's noteworthy that this approach continues to develop and influence thinking in the field. There are two major areas of importance in psychodynamic thinking about mood disorders: interpersonal relationships and self-esteem.

Interpersonal Relationships   Psychoanalytic views of depression originally emphasized the loss of love and emotional security as key variables in depression. In his classic paper *Mourning and Melancholia* (1917/1950), Sigmund Freud (1856–1939) hypothesized that the individual who lost a lover or spouse became angry at that person. Because anger at a loved one is an uncomfortable feeling, it's redirected toward the self. In sum, it's experienced first as self-hate and ultimately as depression.

Although research has confirmed the association of interpersonal loss with depression, Freud's specific hypothesis has not been supported. For example, early dream analyses found incompetence and failure—not internalized anger—to be the most common themes in the dreams of depressed individuals (Beck, 1963). Moreover, individuals who are depressed may be openly hostile with others; they do not simply internalize their negative feelings (Gotlib & Whiffen, 1991).

Revised psychodynamic hypotheses continue to link depression and anger in various ways and some have received research support. For instance, Blatt (1974) hypothesized that difficulty expressing anger was not a feature of all types of depression but only of a particular subtype characterized by excessive dependency. Moreover, data support Blatt's idea that excessive interpersonal dependency constitutes a vulnerability to depression that becomes apparent when the individual faces significant interpersonal loss or rejection (Blatt & Zuroff, 1992; Hirschfeld & Shea, 1992). In turn, dependency is associated with difficulty expressing anger and aggression (Blatt & Zuroff, 1992; L. A. Clark, Watson, & Mineka, 1994).

cortisol Hormone related to depressive symptoms.

dexamethasone suppression test (DST) Test for abnormal secretion of cortisol; formerly used in diagnosis of depression.

rapid eye movement (REM) sleep Stage of sleep characterized by rapid eye movements and associated with dreaming.

Self-Esteem   Many psychodynamic theorists have placed greater emphasis on the loss of self-esteem, rather than the loss of a beloved object or person. Especially important is the idea that vulnerability to depression is particularly strong in people who depend either on other people's love and approval or on their own achievement and success to maintain self-esteem (Butler, Hokanson, & Flynn, 1994).

Roberts and Monroe (1994) recently reviewed the literature associating self-esteem and depression and found similarities among the psychodynamic, cognitive, and social-environmental perspectives. They noted that according to all three models, low self-esteem alone was not sufficient to cause depression. Rather, other factors also contributed to vulnerability, such as having few or externally based sources of self-worth, experiencing stressful events, or having an unstable sense of self.

In addition to dependency-based depression, Blatt (1974) also hypothesized about another subtype of depression that's seen in people who are focused on achievement concerns and are highly self-critical. When faced with failure—say, losing a job or getting a bad grade—these people are more likely to develop depression. Some studies have supported this idea, including Segal, Shaw, Vella, and Katz (1992), who studied self-critical patients who had recovered from depression. These researchers found that those patients who had a negative experience that was achievement related were more likely to relapse than those who experienced a negative experience that was not achievement related. Similarly, Hewitt and Flett (1993) found that patients with self-oriented perfectionism were more depressed when they experienced achievement-related stressors. Other studies, however, have not found this pattern to hold true (Blatt & Zuroff, 1992; Neitzel & Harris, 1990), perhaps because various studies have used different (sometimes completely unrelated) measures of self-criticism, achievement orientation, and perfectionism (L. A. Clark et al., 1994).

In short, the psychoanalytic notions that depression is caused by disturbances in close relationships and self-esteem continue to be refined by research. Modern explanations emphasize the interaction between personality factors (such as dependency and self-criticism) and stressful experiences (such as loss and failure).

Psychodynamic theorists have also hypothesized about self-esteem in bipolar disorder. They see mania as a defense against the underlying, repressed, low self-esteem that accompanies severe depression. Winters and Neale (1985) reported that on a self-report measure, bipolar patients obtained higher self-esteem scores than unipolar depressives. Yet when these individuals' self-esteem was measured in a manner not obvious to them, the bipolar subjects had lower self-esteem scores than the unipolar depressive subjects. The researchers concluded that bipolar subjects' overt self-esteem was a defense against an underlying low level of self-esteem.

Cognitive Factors   The role of cognition in mood disorders has probably been the subject of more research in the past decade than any other factor. In the following sections, we'll discuss several intertwined yet separable lines of inquiry, including the cognitive distortion model, attributional models, self-focus and rumination, and the importance of positive thinking.

The Cognitive Distortion Model   Beck's (1967, 1976) cognitive theory of depression has been enormously influential in the study of depression over the past 25 years. His original hypothesis was that the cognitions of individuals with depression are distortions of reality and **depressogenic**—that is, they *cause* depression. This proved to be too simple a view, and Beck's theory continues to be modified by research. There is little doubt, however, that cognitive factors play an important role in the maintenance—if not the cause—of depression.

According to Beck (1967, 1976), the distorted cognitions that cause depression are **automatic thoughts**. They simply pop into our minds or, more often, flit through our minds on the edges of consciousness. The depressed person accepts these thoughts without questioning their accuracy. There are several common types of automatic thoughts:

depressogenic Causing depression.

automatic thoughts Cognitions that pop into our minds without effort; negative automatic thoughts are associated with emotional distress, like depression and anxiety.

1. *arbitrary inferences*—drawing conclusions despite having little, no, or contrary evidence; for example, a man concludes "She *hates* me" when his boss fails to make a positive remark about his report
2. *overgeneralization*—drawing sweeping conclusions about your ability or self-worth based on a single incident; for example, a woman concludes "I'm worthless" because she's having trouble finding a particular address
3. *magnification and minimization*—exaggerating the frequency or importance of negative events and devaluating positive events; for example, a student thinks "I was just lucky that the test was easy" when she gets an A on an exam

Beck also hypothesized that our beliefs and knowledge about ourselves are organized into **schema** (Kovacs & Beck, 1978). These belief systems help us make sense of our experiences by processing and organizing information, selectively focusing on information that fits our schemas and ignoring or distorting that which doesn't.

According to Beck, depressed people have a **cognitive triad** of negative schema—that is, they have characteristically negative ways of thinking about the self, the world, and the future. Beck further hypothesized that the automatic thoughts of depressed individuals would show **content specificity** (Beck, Brown, Steer, & Eidelson, 1987) by focusing on experiences of loss and failure. This hypothesis fits with the psychodynamic notions that experiences of loss and failure cause depression.

Many studies have confirmed Beck's hypothesis that people who are depressed have more distorted, automatic cognitions than people who are not depressed (Gotlib, 1992; Haaga, Dyck, & Ernst, 1991). And as hypothesized, the content of the automatic cognitions of depressed patients has been shown to focus on themes of loss or failure; in contrast, the automatic cognitions of anxious patients are more oriented toward future threats (D. A. Clark, Beck, & Stewart, 1990; Haaga et al., 1991; Jolly, Dyck, Kramer, & Wherry, 1994).

Beck's idea that negative cognitions *cause* depression has not been confirmed, however. Although there are contrary findings (Giles, Etzel, & Biggs, 1989), most studies find that when people have recovered from depression, their negative thinking disappears, as well (Barnett & Gotlib, 1988). One likely explanation of these inconsistent findings is that many individuals do not fully recover between depressive episodes; instead, they have some residual symptoms, including negative cognitions.

Attributional Models   A second major cognitive model of depression is the **learned helplessness** model, originally proposed by Seligman (1975). He found that animals who were exposed to repeated, unavoidable shocks acted helpless and looked visibly upset and depressed when they were later given the chance to escape the shock. Seligman extended this finding of learned helplessness to people. Specifically, he argued that individuals who were exposed to uncontrollable aversive situations would develop depression that was rooted in feelings of helplessness. This view has also been modified over the years, first by Abramson, Seligman, and Teasdale (1978) and later by Abramson, Metalsky, and Alloy (1989).

Abramson and colleagues (1978) focused on how people who are depressed interpret the causes of events that happen in their lives. This outlook on life events and what causes them is called **attributional style**. The researchers hypothesized that depressed people have an internal, stable, and global attributional style:

■ *Internal* refers to the tendency to attribute negative events to your own failings or incompetence; for example, "I got a D on that exam because I'm stupid."
■ *Stable* refers to the belief that the causes of negative events remain consistent across time; for example, "I *never* get good grades because I've *always* been stupid."
■ *Global* refers to believing that the causes of negative events have a very broad and general effect in your life; for example, "My stupidity causes me

schema Underlying belief system about yourself or the world that filters and organizes your experiences.

cognitive triad Negative beliefs about yourself, the world, and the future; said to characterize depression, according to Beck's cognitive theory.

content specificity Hypothesis that the focus of negative thoughts is specific to a disorder; for instance, depressive cognitions are characterized by themes of loss and failure.

learned helplessness Theory that experiencing uncontrollable stress leads to depression.

attributional style Cognitive style regarding beliefs about the causes of events; a particular style is characteristic of depression.

all sorts of problems, from not doing well in school, to losing jobs, to not being able to find a girlfriend."

Reviews of research on depression and attributional style support the basic hypothesis that people who are depressed show the so-called depressive attributional style (Sweeney, Anderson, & Bailey, 1986). However, many patients with other psychological disorders also show this attributional style (L. A. Clark & Watson, 1991a), so it's not specific to depression, as was hypothesized.

Data regarding the important question of whether this attribution style *causes* depression are again largely negative (Barnett & Gotlib, 1988). For example, attribution style isn't very consistent over time, isn't necessarily seen in individuals before they become depressed, doesn't predict increases in depression over time, and doesn't remain after the depression disappears.

Partly in response to these negative findings, Abramson and colleagues (1989) proposed a further revision of the model, termed the **hopelessness theory** of depression. Like the original learned helplessness model, this is a **diathesis-stress model**. According to this theory, hopelessness is the immediate cause of a subtype of depression called *hopelessness depression*. Hopelessness develops when a person with a cognitive vulnerability (the diathesis) experiences a negative life event (the stress) and so makes negative, stable, global attributions about its cause.

Research-based evaluations of the hopelessness model are beginning to appear in the literature, and support is mixed. Depression seems most likely to develop when there's a match between the person's personality or value orientation (interpersonal versus achievement) and the type of stressful life event (L. A. Clark et al., 1994). However, contrary to the model, hopelessness expectancies may develop independently of the depressive attributional style (DeVellis & Blalock, 1992). Thus, the helplessness/hopelessness model of depression seems to be a fairly accurate *description* of selected aspects of depression. But it is less successful as an *explanation* of how and why depression develops and is maintained.

hopelessness theory Revision of the learned helplessness theory; suggests that expectancies of hopelessness are the immediate cause of depression.

diathesis-stress model Causal model for pathology in which two elements are necessary: a vulnerability (diathesis) and a negative event (stress).

Self-Focus and Rumination In the early 1970s, social psychologists Duval and Wickland (1972) postulated that by focusing attention on ourselves, we initiate a self-evaluative process. If this process leads us to conclude that we haven't met our goals, then self-focus can produce negative emotions. Extensive clinical experience has shown that individuals who are depressed may engage in a negative cycle, beginning with self-focus and ending in self-criticism.

Reviewing the self-focus literature, Pyszczynski and Greenberg (1987) found support for this idea. Not only do elevated levels of self-focus characterize people with mild depression (Ingram, Lumrey, Cruet, & Seiber, 1987), but individuals self-focus more when they experience a loss in the personal, social, or work sphere.

Nolen-Hoeksema (1990) noted that women self-focus more than men. Given this observation, she hypothesized that persistent self-focusing in women was one possible explanation for the 2 to 1 ratio of depression in women versus men. She further theorized that persistent self-focus could maintain depression in additional ways, besides leading to negative self-evaluation (Nolen-Hoeksema, Morrow, & Fredrickson,

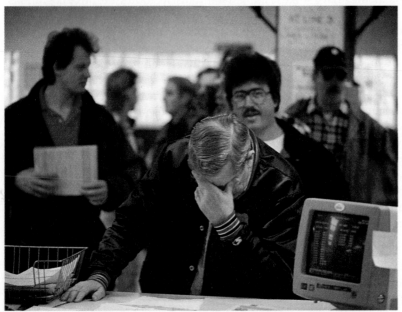

Stressors such as unemployment often precede the onset of depression. What type of person might be most affected by losing a job?

1993). For example, in a depressed person, persistent self-focus—termed a **ruminative response style** (or more simply, *rumination*)—could enhance a memory bias for negative experiences that occurs in depression. Rumination may also interfere with concentration, so that things that need to be done (such as appointments or assignments) don't get done, causing social, school, or work problems. Similarly, rumination may interfere with complex thinking and problem solving, which makes it less likely that people who are depressed will come up with creative solutions to their difficulties.

The Importance of Positive Thinking   A number of studies have yielded a variety of results that support the idea that lack of positivity is a specific characteristic of depression. McCabe and Gotlib (1995) found that attentional differences between individuals who were clinically depressed and nondepressed were not due to a depressive negative bias. Rather, these attentional differences stemmed from the fact that the depressed individuals didn't show the positive bias seen in the nondepressed individuals. Needles and Abramson (1990) had similar findings. They reported that depressed students who experienced more positive events and who also had an enhanced attributional style for positive events became more hopeful and recovered from depression. Ingram, Slater, Atkinson, and Scott (1990) reported that lower scores on a measure of positive automatic thoughts differentiated depressed patients from nondepressed pain patients and healthy control subjects. Dyck, Jolly, and Kramer (1994) found that lack of positive emotions and positive cognitions together predicted patients' depression but not their anxiety.

These findings are all congruent with L. A. Clark and Watson's (1991b) **tripartite model**, which was proposed to explain similarities and differences between depression and anxiety. The tripartite model suggests that anxiety and depression overlap because they share an important personality factor called **negative affectivity,** *negative emotionality,* or *neuroticism.* The core characteristic of negative affectivity is a temperamental sensitivity to negative stimuli; that is, people who have high negative affectivity react frequently and strongly to every little thing that happens to them. They often feel nervous, angry, distressed, fearful, or similarly negative in terms of emotions. Someone who's temperamental and sensitive in this way could be prone to developing an anxiety disorder, a mood disorder, or both.

Negative affectivity has long been linked to anxiety, but only recently has it been connected to depression. A **meta-analysis** (a method of statistically combining the results of multiple studies) revealed that nondepressed individuals who later developed depression scored higher on negative affectivity than those who never developed depression (Clark, Watson, & Mineka, 1994).

According to the tripartite model, however, anxiety and depression can be distinguished because each is characterized by its own specific factor, too. In anxiety, the specific factor consists of the physical symptoms (such as heart palpitations, sweating, and feelings of choking) that accompany an anxious mood (see Chapter 5). The specific factor in depression is disturbances in another personality dimension called **positive affectivity,** or *positive emotionality, extraversion,* or *behavioral engagement.* Individuals with high levels of positive affectivity are temperamentally cheerful and energetic. They are more sensitive to the rewarding aspects of their environments, so they often feel joyful, enthusiastic, proud, confident, and so on. By contrast, individuals low in positive affectivity are less sensitive to rewards, so they are less likely to experience positive emotions. They are often anhedonic (unable to feel pleasure) and feel flat and dull, drowsy and sluggish. Note that the two extremes of this dimension resemble the opposite poles of mania and depression.

Putting the cognitive and tripartite models together, both depressed and anxious patients have high negativity—that is, they feel nervous and distressed and have negative thoughts. This common factor explains their co-occurrence. In addition, individuals with depression have specifically depressive thoughts (focused

ruminative response style
Persistent focus on negative experiences that serves to maintain depression.

tripartite model Theory that explains the overlap and distinction of anxiety and depression by hypothesizing the interaction of three factors: one shared factor and one unique factor for each type of problem.

negative affectivity
Temperamental sensitivity to negative stimuli; one of the three factors of the tripartite model.

meta-analysis Method of statistically combining the results of more than one study.

positive affectivity
Temperamental sensitivity to positive stimuli; one of the three factors of the tripartite model.

on loss) and low positive affectivity (anhedonic, dull and sluggish) (Jolly et al., 1994). These unique dimensions help distinguish depression from anxiety.

One of the exciting things about this research area is that connections are being made between the surface temperament dimensions and the underlying biological systems. For some years, Jeffrey Gray (1982, 1987) has been investigating a motivational model that he proposes involves three biological systems: the **behavioral inhibition system (BIS),** the **behavioral activation system (BAS),** and the fight-or-flight system (which relates to the feeling of fear or panic discussed in Chapter 5).

The BIS is the "stop, look, and listen" system that alerts the organism to potential dangers. Individuals with an overactive BIS are oversensitive to negative stimuli and thus come to anticipate danger; they are hypervigilant and behaviorally inhibited. In short, they resemble anxious individuals or those high in negative affectivity. Indeed, research suggests that the BIS may be the biological system underlying generalized anxiety and negative affectivity (Fowles, 1993a).

The BAS, on the other hand, is an approach system. It activates the organism to seek rewards by exploring the environment. Individuals with an active BAS are energetic, curious, alert, and confident; those with an inactive BAS are lethargic, disinterested, inattentive, and pessimistic. Mounting evidence suggests that dysfunction of the BAS (which principally involves the dopamine system) underlies mood disorders (Depue & Iacono, 1988). Thus, research is beginning to weave threads from cognitive theory and personality/temperament theory with those of biological models of motivation.

Interpersonal Factors   Several trends—beginning with such influential neo-Freudians as Harry Stack Sullivan (1892–1949) and Erik Erikson (1902–1994)—have led to a greater focus on interpersonal factors in depression. One such trend was the increased popularity and use of marital, family systems, and social therapies in the 1960s and 1970s, which highlighted the importance of interpersonal relationships in a variety of psychological disorders. This trend was followed by critical attention from researchers in the 1980s. Three interrelated aspects have received special notice: lack of social support; marital discord, in particular; and disturbance in interpersonal relationships, in general.

Lack of Social Support   *Social support* refers to the social network that's available to meet an individual's interpersonal needs and to provide support during stressful times. Psychological problems can arise if the individual has too few contacts, is not close enough to confide in other people, or has negative interactions with support group members that interfere with developing positive relationships (Henderson, Byrne, & Duncan-Jones, 1981). One study (Beach, Arias, & O'Leary, 1986) found that the risk for depression was 13 times greater in community members who were socially isolated than in those who were not.

Although there is clearly an association between poor social support and depression, it's difficult to establish exactly what that association means. In many studies, the measures of support and depression are obtained simultaneously, so it's impossible to determine what is causing what. This is especially true in studies that use self-reports of subjects' support levels, which may be distorted by their depression (Paykel & Cooper, 1992). When that's the case, the lower level of social support may be either a cause or result of the mental state or both.

Longitudinal studies, however, suggest that lack of social support may be a causal factor in depression and that the presence of social support may provide a buffer against the negative effects of stressful events (Brown & Harris, 1978; Paykel & Cooper, 1992). It follows that receiving more social support during episodes of depression will help bring about a better outcome—that is, recovery will occur more quickly and completely. It's still unknown, though, exactly *how* levels of social support cause or reduce depression.

behavioral inhibition system (BIS) Biological motivation system proposed to underlie anxiety; acts to inhibit activity in response to potential threat.

behavioral activation system (BAS) Biological motivation system proposed to regulate the seeking of positive stimuli; dysregulation of the BAS may underlie mood disorder.

Marital Discord Marital discord and depressive symptoms often occur together. In a community sample of 328 married couples, the odds of one partner showing significant depressive symptoms was 10 times greater if the couple was having marital troubles (O'Leary, Christian, & Mendell, 1994).

As with social support, the causal link between marital discord and depression appears to go both ways—that is, each can lead to the other. The influence of significant marital problems on depression is seen quite clearly in the following study (Christian-Herman, Avery-Leaf, & O'Leary, 1994).

Fifty women were each assessed just after experiencing a significant negative marital event, such as discovering that her husband was having an affair or learning that he was planning to leave the relationship. In order to be selected for the assessment, the negative events reported by each woman had to be judged by three experienced clinicians to be highly stressful for any individual. The 50 women were screened from a larger pool of women in order to assure that they had never been clinically depressed before. They were assessed with clinical interviews using standard diagnostic criteria for major depressive disorder and 38 percent of them proved to be clinically depressed. All of them reported that their depressive feelings were caused by the significant marital problem.

It's also been shown that depression can lead to marital discord. This is particularly true if the depression is long standing (dysthymia). Beach and O'Leary (1993) assessed 264 couples at two times: before marriage and 6 to 18 months later. They found that premarital depressive mood was tied to later marital dissatisfaction.

In looking at the relationship between marital satisfaction and depression, it's interesting to consider whether there are different issues for men and women. The effects that being married has on mental health—especially that of women—is addressed in the Thinking about Social Issues box.

Disturbance in Interpersonal Relationships It's likely that at least some of the factors linking depression with marital discord (and perhaps also poor social support) are the same as or similar to those linking depression with more general disturbances in interpersonal relationships. In 1976, Coyne (1976a, 1976b) proposed an **interactional perspective** on depression. He hypothesized that the needs and demands of people who are depressed place a strain on their interpersonal relationships. Being around or living with someone who is constantly uninterested in socializing with others, who mopes around, and who is down on life can lead a friend or partner to become dissatisfied with the relationship.

Evidence is mounting that people who are depressed are not simply victims of interpersonal stress; rather, behavior associated with their depression contributes to causing relationship stress. For example, Hammen (1991) followed samples of women who were unipolar depressed, bipolar depressed, medically ill, and healthy (controls) over the period of 1 year. The unipolar depressed women were significantly more likely to have "negative interpersonal events to which they had contributed" (p. 559).

A review by Gotlib and Whiffen (1991) found evidence for a negative interactive cycle in the interpersonal behavior of depressed individuals. They appear to have social skills deficits, which are characterized by a pattern of low involvement and responsiveness (Segrin & Abramson, 1994). In comparison to nondepressed individuals, they maintain less eye contact, are less verbal, speak more softly and monotonously, make more negative statements about things, and take longer to respond to others' verbalizations (Gotlib & Robinson, 1982).

Individuals with depression also show more difficulty "reading" photographed facial expressions and more discomfort when presented with negative or ambiguous facial expressions (Persad & Polivy, 1993). Since facial cues are important in social interactions, this finding suggests one possible reason as to why depressed individuals have difficulty responding appropriately in social situations.

interactional perspective
View that depression is developed and maintained, in part, by negative interpersonal cycles.

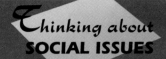
The role of marriage in mental illness has been hotly debated for decades. Sociologists such as Bernard (1972) have concluded that men like to be married because it benefits them: Marriage provides child care, household maintenance, and often cooked meals. In contrast, Bernard has argued that traditional marriage could be mentally harmful to women because of their service to their husbands and the lack of emotional and financial support they could receive from employment. In support of this view, Weissman and Klerman (1977) found lower rates of mental illness and depression among single, divorced, and widowed women compared to men in these same categories. This did not hold true, however, in a comparison of married women and men.

Note that these findings were reported in the 1970s. Have things changed since then? A number of studies from the 1980s and early 1990s examined how spousal, parental, and work-related roles interact in relation to mental health. Although some research supported the view that marriage is better for men's mental health than women's (Fowers, 1991; McRae & Brody, 1989), other studies found the opposite effect, at least for some groups (Menaghan, 1989; Pugliesi, 1989). On closer examination, a more complex picture began to emerge, in which employment played a major role.

A study of over 1,800 men and women revealed that having multiple-role identities—that is, husband/wife, worker, parent—significantly reduced distress for both men and women (Thoits, 1986). In fact, much of the gender difference in depression was accounted for by the greater likelihood of employment among men. Pugliesi (1989) further found that employment enhanced well-being through its effect on self-esteem. In his book *Marriage and Mental Illness: A Sex Role Perspective*, Julian Hafner (1986) also concluded that the combination of marriage and lack of employment outside the home was a critical ingredient in causing depression in young wives.

We should not jump to the conclusion, however, that being married and not working outside the home is unequivocally bad for all women. In fact, if their marriages are close and confiding, then women who either want to work (and feel supported in that decision) or who feel they must work (for economic reasons) are at reduced risk for marital problems and depression (Barling, 1990). Similarly, Ross, Mirowsky, and Huber (1983) found that both spouses were less depressed when the wife's employment status was consistent with their preferences.

Neither should we jump to the conclusion that employment or other roles protect women against depression. McRae and Brody (1989) found that having multiple roles did not diminish the effect of marital discord on women's mental health. That is, marriage itself may not be bad for the mental health of women. Rather, bad marriages are bad for the mental health of men as well as women, presumably.

One consistent finding is that women, compared to men, spend more than twice the amount of time working in the home and providing child care. Even with the increased participation of women in the workforce, the number of hours they spend doing these chores hasn't varied much for decades. Arlie Hochschild (1989) documented the extent of this inequity in her book *The Second Shift*. She reported that most men (61 percent) in dual-career households contributed less than one-third of the effort needed to complete household tasks, including car repair and lawn work as well as laundry and sewing. Only 18 percent of the men shared these tasks equally with their partners, and not a single man in the survey did more than 55 percent of the work. One study found that employed mothers averaged 65 hours per week of paid and unpaid work (Schor, 1991); another reported a figure of 87 hours per week (Hochschild, 1989). Comparable figures for men ranged from 17 to 30 hours a week *less*.

Not surprisingly, this gender gap in work burden versus leisure time contributes to depression. Wearing (1989) found a significant relation in first-time mothers between general mental health and leisure time plus time for oneself. And Ross et al. (1983) reported that wives were less depressed "if their husbands helped with the housework, and husbands were not more depressed as a result of helping" (p. 809). (It's interesting to note that even the wording of this professional report implies that the work is the women's and that the men simply "help.")

What conclusions can we draw from this research? It seems that men do benefit more from marriage than women, given that women typically do the greater share of caretaking, which has a negative impact on leisure time and mental health. However, this blanket statement must be modified by considering the quality of the marriage (including egalitarianism in task sharing) and the opportunities that women have for obtaining gratification from outside employment.

Think about the following questions:

1. From one point of view, men have no reason to change the current system, in which women do most of the domestic caretaking. What arguments could be made that men's *own* mental health would benefit from changes in the current system?

2. Data generally indicate that women are less satisfied with marriage than men and that being married (especially unhappily) can contribute to depression in women. Knowing these facts, how would you counsel a young woman contemplating marriage? Explain your answer.

People who are depressed may be in a vicious cycle, in which their own social skills deficits, negativity, and interpersonal distance result in less positive attention from others. This, in turn, may make them feel more rejected and depressed. How do these negative cycles get started in the first place? Drawing from Bowlby's (1973) work on attachment, researchers have looked to early parent/child relations as a possible origin. Much of this research is based on the memories that depressed and nondepressed individuals have of their parental relationships. An association between recall of poor maternal care and later depression has been confirmed by several studies (Birtchnell, 1993; Mackinnon, Henderson, & Andrews, 1993; Parker & Hadzi-Pavlovic, 1992). The recollection of extremely disturbed parental relationships, however (for example, abusive relations), may be more characteristic of personality disorders than depression (Nigg, Lohr, Westen, Gold, & Silk, 1992; Rose, Abramson, Hodulik, Halberstadt, & Leff, 1994).

Biopsychosocial Approach

Some form of diathesis-stress model of depression is clearly needed to account for all the factors that have been shown to be causally related to depression. In this section on causes, we have discussed a number of models in which the diathesis is a psychological variable. But often the term *diathesis* refers to a biological predisposition—in particular, a family or genetic background that makes developing the disorder more likely. Having such a family history (and therefore a genetic vulnerability to mood disorders) does not inevitably lead to development of such disorders, though. Some other factors such as stressful life events may be responsible.

In an early study evaluating the role of stressors in developing depression, Paykel et al. (1969) compared the histories of 185 depressed patients and 185 community control subjects who were matched with the patients for age, sex, and education. The depressed subjects reported having almost three times as many undesirable life events as the control subjects. The groups didn't differ, however, on desirable life events, such as promotion, engagement, or marriage. Even *endogenous* depression—a type of depression often thought to be strongly influenced by biological factors—has been shown to be associated with stressful life events, both in the United States (Frank, Anderson, Reynolds, Ritenour, & Kupfer, 1994) and Great Britain (Brown, Harris, & Hepworth, 1994).

The question remains of *how* stressors interact with a biological vulnerability to cause depression. One hypothesis is that stress causes depressogenic changes in brain functioning. For example, in one study, both patients who were depressed and people undergoing severe life stressors showed reductions of about 50 percent in certain natural immune functions (Irwin et al., 1990). The particular immune functions that are associated with depression vary somewhat from study to study. Moreover, depression does not affect immune functions consistently. Nevertheless, when depression has a biological effect, it lowers immune functions (A. O'Leary, 1990; Schleifer & Keller, 1989; Stein, Miller, & Trestman, 1991).

Beginning with the learned helplessness studies, animal research has also documented that uncontrollable physical stress affects neurotransmitter functioning. In an exciting research program extending over 20 years, Jay Weiss (1995) has provided solid evidence for the diathesis-stress model of depression based on work with laboratory rats. Rats exposed to uncontrollable stress (electric shock) were more likely to give up and stop struggling when placed in a bucket of water than rats who were able to control the shock. (Weiss kept the rats from drowning by putting little "water wings" on them.)

Weiss made the important observation that there were large individual differences in how much the stressed rats struggled before they gave up (because giving up was associated with abnormal norepinephrine functioning). He hypothesized that the rats who gave up more quickly had a genetic predisposition to depression.

PERSPECTIVE ON MAJOR DEPRESSION

BIOLOGICAL FACTORS

Biological factors play key roles in the development of major depression:

➤ Genetic predisposition to major depression has been indicated through family, twin, and adoption studies. The genetic vulnerability probably includes a neurochemical oversensitivity to negative experiences. It may also include a dysfunction of the mechanisms that restore the brain's neurochemistry to normal when it has been disrupted by stress.

➤ Life traumas may lead to changes in neurochemistry that create the same effect as genetic predisposition.

PSYCHOLOGICAL FACTORS

Psychological factors, particularly developing a sense of self, interact with biological vulnerabilities in the development of major depression:

➤ Self-worth is based on internal reactions to experience as well as the feedback received from interacting with the environment, including other people.

➤ A person with too many stressors, failures, and poor interpersonal experiences may develop a *negative schema*, including lack of confidence in ability to cope, no expectations of support from others, and little hope that things will improve in the future.

SOCIAL FACTORS

Both biological and psychological factors operate in specific social contexts:

➤ Childhood traumas such as death or divorce of caretaker(s)

➤ Physical traumas such as accidents, abuse, or serious illness

➤ Environmental factors such as extreme poverty

These biological, psychological, and social factors interact to cause problems, as illustrated in the following case:

Emily's early childhood was fairly routine, although her mother was rather anxious and overprotective. She was faintly aware that her aunt had been hospitalized for a major depression. Her parents' divorce was particularly traumatic, as she had been close to her father. She became quiet and withdrawn but recovered in a few years.

At college Emily was acutely homesick and intimidated by all the decisions she had to make living on her own. By spring semester, she found it increasingly hard to concentrate and often missed class due to lack of energy or minor illnesses. When she got her first D on a midterm, she became very depressed, certain that she was incapable of college-level work.

The biopsychosocial model helps explain Emily's problems. Emily may have inherited a vulnerability to depression (remember her aunt) in the form of a neurochemical oversensitivity to negative experiences. Thus, the childhood trauma of divorce may have affected her more deeply than it would the average child, especially since she was so attached to her father. This early loss further sensitized her, both neurochemically and psychologically, and led to Emily's developing a negative schema about herself and her world. These negative expectations were then activated by the social stressors of living away from home at college, resulting in a major depressive episode.

To test that hypothesis, he bred those rats to produce a strain that might be strongly biologically predisposed to depression. These genetically vulnerable rats were then exposed to the uncontrollable shock and their norepinephrine functioning was examined. Weiss (1995) found that their brains didn't return to normal until up to 6 weeks later, compared with the 3 days normally observed.

Bipolar Disorder   The manic phases of a patient with bipolar disorder are so unusual and powerful that, for many years, researchers have looked for their origins almost exclusively in biochemistry and genetics. The appearance of mania is sudden, and the individual's energy and racing thoughts seem endlessly driven. Sleep appears totally unnecessary. Since a manic episode can develop within an hour and often without an apparent precipitating event, searches for biochemical causes seem reasonable. Indeed, as discussed earlier, genetic models of bipolar disorder have definite support. A great deal of research in recent years (Diehl & Gershon, 1992; Young, Warsh, Kish, & Shannak, 1994) on patients with bipolar disorder has documented abnormalities in neurotransmitter (particularly dopamine) functioning.

Psychological factors may also be important, although they haven't been studied as much until recently. Based on a review of 14 studies, Goodwin and Jamison (1990) concluded that stressful events were important in the initial onset of manic episodes but not in their recurrence. Three recent studies document the importance of life stressors for some aspects of bipolar disorder. Ellicott et al. (1990) examined the impact of life stressors on the course of bipolar disorder in 61 outpatients. They found a significant association between life events and recurrence of the disorder over a 2-year period. Later, this same group of researchers (Hammen, Ellicott, & Gitlin, 1992) followed 49 other bipolar patients for an average of 18 months after recovery from their current episode. Symptom severity—but not episode recurrence—was significantly associated with interpersonal life stressors, especially if the person showed dependent personality traits. Finally, Marks, Wieck, Checkley, and Kumar (1992) studied women after they'd given birth. These researchers reported that the recurrence of mania seemed to reflect a physiological or psychological vulnerability made worse by marital difficulties.

Because bipolar individuals often spend large sums of money, act promiscuously, and indulge in other impetuous behavior during their manic phases, they often have very unsatisfactory marriages. The clinical impression is that spouses who have a clear understanding of bipolar disorder are better able to support their troubled partners. Indeed, research has found that bipolar patients whose families were not very critical were less likely to relapse after being discharged from the hospital (Miklowitz, Goldstein, Neuchterlein, Snyder, & Mintz, 1988). This research on family environment underscores the role of psychological variables, even in situations in which disorders have clear genetic components.

Focus on Critical Thinking

1. Most psychosocial theories of mood disorder have focused on depression; for example, depressed patients are said to have negative self-schema, which makes them more vulnerable to depression. How might these theories need to be modified to explain depression in bipolar patients who also have manic episodes?

2. It seems likely that some type of diathesis-stress model of mood disorders will be needed to account for all the research data. Devise such a model, working in as many of the variables that we've discussed as possible.

TREATMENT

A variety of factors have been suggested or shown to cause mood disorders. So it's not surprising that there are also many types of treatment available, including both biological and psychological therapies. Increasingly, different types of therapies are being used in combination to treat these complex and multifaceted disorders.

Biological Therapies

Several key biological therapies are used in treating mood disorders: medications for unipolar and bipolar disorders, electroconvulsive treatment for major depressive disorder, and light therapy for major depressions with a seasonal pattern.

Medications   Since their advent around 1960, many different types of drugs have been used to treat mood disorder. In this section, we'll discuss the major classes of these medications. (See Chapter 20 on biological therapies.)

Tricyclic Antidepressants   The oldest type of antidepressant medication is a group of drugs called **tricyclic antidepressants** (which get their name from their 3-ring molecular structure). Tricyclics remain one of the most commonly prescribed treatments for depression. They include such medications as imipramine (sold under the brand name Tofranil), amitriptyline (Elavil), and clomipramine (Anafranil).

Tricyclics successfully reduce or alleviate the symptoms of about 50 to 65 percent of the patients with major depression who take them. We must compare these figures, though, to the 25 to 30 percent of patients who respond positively to a **placebo**, or so-called sugar pill, which looks just like the real medication but contains no active substance (Depression Guideline Panel, 1993a). In other words, about twice as many patients respond positively to tricyclics as do so to a placebo.

Tricyclics have some nonserious unpleasant side effects, such as dryness of the mouth, constipation, blurred vision, and difficulty urinating. They tend to be the worst at the beginning of treatment, when patients start taking the medication. Some patients even experience side effects when taking a placebo, which again indicates that the power of suggestion is very strong.

Exactly how tricyclic antidepressants work is not entirely understood. Their initial effect is to increase the amount of available neurotransmitter by blocking reuptake into the synapse that it was released from. It usually takes several weeks of taking daily medication before the depressive symptoms begin to decrease. So other processes must also be affected by the drug, including adjustment of the density and sensitivity of the postsynaptic receptors (Kandel et al., 1991).

Partly because the mechanisms of action are not fully known, there's still debate over what is the appropriate length of time for patients to take tricyclic antidepressants. Traditionally, patients were phased off the drugs after 6 to 8 months, but recent research suggests that continuing the medication helps prevent relapse (Kupfer, 1993). This information is important because, as discussed earlier, once a person has had a depressive episode, he is at significant risk of becoming depressed again (American Psychiatric Association, 1994).

tricyclic antidepressants Class of medications used in treating depression that interfere with reabsorbing various neurotransmitters back into the neuron.

placebo So-called sugar pill that looks just like real medication but contains no active substance.

selective serotonin reuptake inhibitors (SSRIs) Class of medications used in treating depression that interfere with reabsorbing the neurotransmitter serotonin back into the neuron.

Selective Serotonin Reuptake Inhibitors (SSRIs)   In the 1980s, a class of drugs was developed called **selective serotonin reuptake inhibitors (SSRIs).** They selectively inhibit the reuptake of the neurotransmitter serotonin and, unlike tricyclic antidepressants, do not affect other neurotransmitters, such as norepinephrine. Fluoxetine (Prozac) was the first widely known drug of this class, although other similar drugs exist, such as paroxetine.

In the mid-1980s, Prozac proved very successful in treating people with mood disorders, and its use increased greatly. Many thought it would be the wonder drug of the 1990s (Cowley, 1990). Others expressed concern about its widespread use, however, due to a small number of cases of increased violence or suicide that were attributed to its use.

The research done on the SSRIs clearly documents the following:

1. They are about equally effective as the tricyclics in reducing depression (Depression Guideline Panel, 1993a).
2. They have fewer side effects than the tricyclics (Kupfer, 1993), so more patients are willing to take them long enough to have an effect.

3. They are not associated with increased violence, suicide, or suicide attempts (Beasley, Dornseif, Bosomworth, & Sayler, 1992; Tollefson, Fawcett, Winokur, & Beasley, 1993).

4. They have a lower risk of fatal overdose (Henry, 1992).

5. They may be effective for treating dysthymic disorder that has not responded to psychotherapy (Kaplan & Sadock, 1991).

Thus, although the SSRIs are not wonder drugs, they do have some distinct advantages over the older tricyclics. We should note, however, that the SSRIs are much more expensive than tricyclics, which may be a factor in treatment decisions in this age of health care cost containment. What's more, some SSRI and tricyclic medications make individuals unable to have orgasms (Long & Rybacki, 1994).

Monoamine Oxidase Inhibitors (MAOIs)   When depressed patients do not respond to the tricyclics or SSRIs, another option is to use **monoamine oxidase inhibitors (MAOIs).** The drugs in this group slow down the rate of chemical breakdown of neurotransmitters in the synapse. They appear to work best for patients with atypical depressive features (including mood reactivity, increased sleep and appetite, leaden paralysis, and rejection sensitivity) and those with features of personality disorder (see Chapter 12). MAOIs also may be useful in treating dysthymic disorder, particularly if atypical features or features of personality disorder are present (Kaplan & Sadock, 1991).

According to the Depression Guideline Panel (1993a), MAOIs are about as effective as the other antidepressant medications. However, when MAOIs are taken with food or drink that contains the amino acid tyramine—such as cheese, alcohol, or chocolate—severe hypertension and occasionally death can result. Therefore, patients taking MAOIs must adhere to special dietary restrictions. Overall, the MAOIs are superior to placebos in alleviating depression, but they obviously are not the first choice of medication for most depressed individuals.

Let's take another look at Howard, from the chapter-opening case. Like many individuals with depression, he'd taken a number of medications to treat his disorder at various points in his life. First, he took Prozac, the "wonder drug," but it made him lose weight and have trouble sleeping. He took a second antidepressant medication—another SSRI—and initially responded very well to it. His appetite improved, he slept well, and his hopelessness lessened considerably. Unfortunately, he became very concerned about his inability to have an orgasm, which is a common problem with this medication. So, he switched to yet another antidepressant medication—a tricyclic—which made him feel quite good. While on this third medication, he also took a benzodiazepine to reduce his anxiety. Howard's experience with multiple medications is typical of many individuals with depression.

Lithium   In contrast to the medications already discussed, **lithium** (lithium carbonate) has proven effective in the treatment of bipolar disorder, including bipolar I, bipolar II, and severe cyclothymia. Approximately 50 to 80 percent of individuals with bipolar I disorder report full or partial alleviation of both manic and depressive episodes (Kaplan & Sadock, 1991). However, a naturalistic (that is, not experimentally controlled) follow-up evaluation of 73 manic patients, done approximately 2 years after their hospitalization, concluded that those who had initially been treated with lithium had no better outcome than those who had not (Harrow, Goldberg, Grossman, & Meltzer, 1990). If the medication is discontinued shortly after the episode has cleared, there is a 50 percent chance of relapse within 3 months (Goodwin, 1994). It appears that long-term treatment with lithium is required, lasting approximately 2 years.

Lithium also has been shown to be effective in treating recurrent unipolar illness—again, whether used alone (Souza & Goodwin, 1991) or with other antidepressant medication (Katona, Robertson, Abou-Saleh, & Nairac, 1993). As when treating bipolar disorder, continued use seems to be required to prevent relapse.

monoamine oxidase inhibitors (MAOIs) Type of medication used primarily in treating depression; slows down the rate of chemical breakdown of neurotransmitters in the synapse.

lithium Medication used primarily in treating bipolar disorder.

Common side effects of lithium include gastric distress (such as nausea and abdominal pain), weight gain, tremor, and fatigue. Moreover, lithium is toxic at high levels, and the difference between effective and toxic doses is relatively small. At toxic levels, lithium may impair kidney and thyroid functioning.

Electroconvulsive Therapy   Perhaps the most controversial biological treatment for the mood disorders in widespread use is **electroconvulsive therapy (ECT).** It involves sending electrical charges through a person's brain to induce a generalized seizure, similar to that which occurs in some forms of epilepsy. ECT is most often used for the following types of patients:

1. those who are seriously depressed (for example, highly suicidal patients) and need a quicker treatment than antidepressant medications, which require several weeks to take effect
2. those with psychotic features to their depression that do not respond well to medication alone
3. those in acute manic episodes

Approximately 80 percent of depressed patients show significant improvement after ECT. And the decreases in depressive symptoms following ECT are comparable to those of other treatments for depression (Piper, 1993). Moreover, in treating bipolar disorder, ECT has been shown to be as effective as lithium and may act more quickly (Kaplan & Sadock, 1991).

Much of the misunderstanding regarding ECT and its effects may stem from problems associated with how it was used in the 1930s, when it was first introduced. In those early years, patients were awake during ECT, so the procedure was both fearful and unpleasant. Worse yet, patients often suffered bone fractures from the seizures' motor activity. Today, however, these problems have been eliminated through the use of general anesthetics and muscle relaxants. Patient fear still remains an important clinical issue, however (Fox, 1993).

Currently, ECT is provided by a medical team, who monitors the induction of electrical current as well as the patient's brain functioning. Electrodes are placed on the patient's head, and an electric shock is administered for 0.1 to 0.5 seconds. Previously, the electrodes were placed on both sides of the head, but unilateral placement is as effective or only slightly less so and is associated with fewer negative cognitive effects (such as memory impairment). Shortly after receiving the shock, the patient has a seizure lasting 30 to 60 seconds.

A course of ECT for depression usually involves between 4 and 12 sessions, administered 2 to 3 times a week over several weeks. Most individuals who are depressed show improvement after the first few treatments. Those who are manic may require more frequent treatments (even daily) and a greater number of treatments (up to 25) (Kaplan & Sadock, 1991). It's important to note that ECT is best used as a treatment for a depressive or manic *episode*; that is, it is not a long-term solution for either unipolar or bipolar disorder. Further treatment with drugs and psychotherapy is needed to prevent relapse.

Memory impairment is common with ECT, but almost all patients recover normal memory functions within 6 months. Heart problems also occur in patients with cardiac disease. However rare, these problems are of concern and have led to recommendations for using less electrical charge and few treatments (American Psychiatric Association, 1990).

The mechanism by which ECT reduces mood-related symptoms remains unclear, although this topic has received more research attention recently. Most likely, effects on neurotransmitter, peptide, and neuroendocrine functioning all need to be considered (Cooper, Scott, & Whalley, 1990; Smith, 1994).

Light Therapy and Related Therapies   As discussed earlier, for some individuals, depression follows a seasonal pattern. These cases are more common in

electroconvulsive therapy (ECT) *Treatment for depression in which electrical charges are sent through the brain to induce a generalized seizure.*

northern latitudes, which have markedly decreased winter light (American Psychiatric Association, 1994). It stands to reason, therefore, that increased exposure to light might be used to treat depressions of this type.

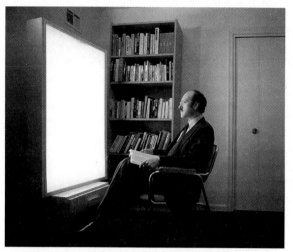

Exposure to very bright light for 2–3 hours a day appears to be an effective treatment for major depression with a seasonal pattern.

More than 25 controlled studies have confirmed this hypothesis (Kaplan & Sadock, 1991). The most effective treatment appears to be exposure to very bright light of 2,500 lux (which is about 200 times greater than typical indoor light) for 2 to 3 hours, early each morning (Terman, Terman, Quitkin, & McGrath, 1989). Response to this treatment is usually quite rapid—2 to 4 days. But if the treatment is stopped, relapse is just as rapid (Kaplan & Sadock, 1991).

Research into how light therapy works suggests that it may shift the body's biological **circadian rhythms**. These bodily rhythms regulate a host of functions, including the daily sleep/wake cycle and body temperature variation. For individuals with seasonal depressive episodes, their circadian rhythms are dysregulated (that is, out of sync) during even nonseasonal episodes (Healy & Williams, 1988). There is also growing evidence that the disruption of sleep and appetite during mood episodes is also related to the dysregulation of biological circadian rhythms (Bunney, Goodwin, & Murphy, 1992).

It's interesting to note that one complete night of sleep deprivation brings about dramatic short-term reductions in depressive symptoms (Kaplan & Sadock, 1991). Another treatment approach is to advance the sleep cycle methodically—for instance, ignoring the clock and going to bed earlier and earlier each day until coming around full circle to nighttime again. Phase advancing also has antidepressant effects that last up to a week or so, in some patients (Bunney et al., 1992).

Psychological Therapies

Psychotherapy has been established most clearly as an effective treatment only for unipolar depression. Psychotherapy can be used either in addition to or as an alternative to medication because individuals may refuse to continue medication due to adverse side effects. Furthermore, many mental health professionals and consumers of mental health services recognize that medication only directly addresses the "bio" portion of this complex disorder; it does not address life stress, negative cognitions, or interpersonal problems related to depression. In addition, many individuals want to have a nonmedical way of coping with depression.

Two major types of psychological therapies for depression have been most widely investigated: cognitive (or cognitive-behavioral) therapy (Beck, 1976) and interpersonal psychotherapy (Klerman, Weissman, Rounsaville, & Chevron, 1984). A third treatment is marital therapy, which is effective in treating individuals with unipolar depression who also have marital discord (Beach, Smith, & Fincham, 1994; O'Leary & Beach, 1990).

circadian rhythms Daily biological cycles of various bodily functions, such as the sleep/wake or body temperature cycles.

collaborative empiricism Process in cognitive therapy through which the therapist and patient together identify, analyze, and test the validity of the patient's dysfunctional cognitions.

Cognitive and Cognitive-Behavioral Approaches Although cognitive therapy for depression has many variations, it's still quite closely identified with its originator, Aaron Beck (1967). He recommends that therapists teach the cognitive model of depression to patients in a straightforward manner. Patients learn how cognitions, moods and emotions, and behavior are interrelated by analyzing the associations among them in their own lives. They are taught to view depression as the product of dysfunctional thoughts. Then, with the therapist, they work to uncover their own maladaptive cognitions and beliefs and to explore the connection between them and their negative emotions. Through a process called **collaborative empiricism**, therapist/patient teams design personal experiments to test the validity of patients' dysfunctional beliefs against their own real life data. By the end of treatment, typically 20 sessions, patients learn specific techniques for changing their faulty beliefs and thought processes, thereby relieving their depressed mood.

The following dialogue shows how a therapist may ask specific questions to help a patient discover the negative consequences of assuming that a person should always work up to her potential:

> **Patient:** I guess I believe I should always work up to my potential.
> **Therapist:** Why is that?
> **Patient:** Otherwise, I'd be wasting time.
> **Therapist:** But what is the long-range goal in working up to your potential?
> **Patient:** (Long pause) I've never really thought about that. I've just assumed that I should.
> **Therapist:** Are there any positive things you give up by always having to work up to your potential?
> **Patient:** I suppose it makes it hard to relax or take a vacation.
> **Therapist:** What about "living up to your potential" to enjoy yourself and relax? Is that important at all?
> **Patient:** I've never really thought of it that way.
> **Therapist:** Maybe we can work on giving yourself permission not to work up to your potential at all times. (Young & Beck, 1982, p. 201)

This patient/therapist team might go on to list and evaluate the long- and short-term advantages and disadvantages of changing the assumption that she should always work up to her potential. They might also explore the patient's automatic thoughts about what would happen if she didn't work up to her potential all the time; they could then design an experiment to test this belief. For example, the patient might believe that she will lose her job. To test this belief, she might agree to take a weekend at the beach and see whether it affects her job standing.

In addition to using cognitive strategies to change dysfunctional thoughts, cognitive-behavioral therapists also use behavioral techniques, such as scheduling activities and giving concrete homework assignments. It's important to avoid having patients who are depressed not meet (or even feel that they have not met) their goals. To help ensure that this won't happen, therapists encourage patients to set realistic schedules and to be flexible in following their activity plans. Therapy can help individuals who are depressed learn how to talk to themselves in ways that enhance their coping efforts and reduce the impact of experiences of failure or perceived failure.

Evaluation Cognitive therapy was originally evaluated by Rush, Beck, Kovacs, and Hollon (1977). On both self-ratings and clinicians' ratings of depression, these researchers found cognitive therapy superior to treatment involving the antidepressant medication imipramine. The dropout rate for the cognitive therapy group was also much lower than that for the medication group. The meaning of these findings was debated for methodological reasons, so the study stimulated a great deal of cognitive therapy research on depression and served as a springboard for a large government study comparing various therapies. (See discussion of the National Institute of Mental Health study later in this chapter.)

Recently, two major reviews of this research have appeared. The first (Hollon, Shelton, & Davis, 1993) considered the literature of **therapy outcome studies**, which asks two questions: Does therapy X work? and Does therapy X work better than therapy Y? Hollon et al. concluded that cognitive therapy was certainly better than a minimal treatment condition and generally fared quite well in comparison to other treatments. In addition, these researchers indicated that cognitive therapy was helpful in preventing relapse, even after therapy had been terminated. This finding is particularly important in light of research that shows a high relapse rate

therapy outcome studies
Research to determine how effective a therapy is in comparison to placebo or minimal treatment controls or to other treatments.

upon discontinuing drug use for depressed individuals treated with medication alone (Evans et al., 1992; Hollon, 1990).

The second review (Whisman, 1993) considered the question of whether cognitive therapy works the way it's supposed to work—that is, by changing patients' dysfunctional cognitions. Whisman concluded that there was strong research support for the idea that changes in cognition and depression occurred together but limited support for the hypothesis that the changes in cognition *caused* the changes in depression. Another difficulty was that there were many methodological problems and ambiguities in the research. Thus, this review concluded that cognitive change does seem to play an important role in reducing depression. Exactly how cognitive therapy works, however, was not conclusively determined.

Interpersonal Psychotherapy   An approach called **interpersonal pscyhotherapy (IPT)** was developed in the early 1980s by the husband/wife team of Gerald Klerman and Myrna Weissman (Klerman et al., 1984). IPT has been perceived positively because it's been used successfully with a wide variety of disorders, including bulimia, dysthymia, and major depression (Weissman & Markowitz, 1994). IPT is also attractive to many therapists because it's the most widely researched treatment to have evolved from a psychodynamic framework—particularly through the influence of neo-Freudian theorist Harry Stack Sullivan. IPT was also influenced by John Bowlby's studies of attachment; it stresses the importance of how disrupting bonds with a parent can initiate depression (Klerman et al., 1984).

In contrast to classic psychodynamic therapy, interpersonal psychotherapy is directive and limited to a particular timeframe, lasting from 12 to 16 weeks. IPT addresses childhood, family background, and developmental issues only in terms of how they are directly relevant to current problems. It emphasizes coping with the loss of relationships, interpersonal disputes, interpersonal skill deficits, and interpersonal challenges related to role changes—for instance, interacting with coworkers upon entering a full-time job outside the home after full-time parenting. As discussed earlier, individuals who are depressed often engage in negative cycles of interaction with the important people in their lives.

The ultimate goals of IPT are to reduce depressive symptoms and improve self-esteem. To do so, the overall therapeutic emphases are:

1. to help patients identify the interpersonal conflicts in their lives
2. to develop strategies for more successful communication and conflict negotiation
3. to cope more effectively with interpersonal stressors

Evaluation   Interpersonal psychotherapy has been evaluated in several independent studies and in one large collaborative study on the treatment of depression (Elkin, Shea, Watkins, & Imber, 1989). Reviews of this literature (Jarrett & Rush, 1992; Stravynski & Greenberg, 1992) indicate that IPT is effective in treating depression (Weissman & Markowitz, 1994). In fact, the effects of IPT have been successful enough that it is included in the 1993 American Psychiatric Association "Practice Guidelines for Major Depressive Disorder in Adults" (Karasu et al., 1993). The IPT standard therapy has been adapted by professionals dealing with a range of problems—from depression in alcoholics who are trying to remain abstinent to posttraumatic stress disorder in young women with breast cancer.

Marital Therapy   The relationship between marital discord and depression is quite strong, but it's unclear whether depression causes marital problems or vice versa (Beach et al., 1994). Marital difficulties are the most frequently associated problem of women seeking treatment for depression—approximately half of all depressed women have serious marital problems (Beach, Sandeen, & O'Leary,

interpersonal psychotherapy (IPT) Directive and time-limited treatment for depression that focuses on identifying and coping with current interpersonal problems; derived from psychodynamic therapy.

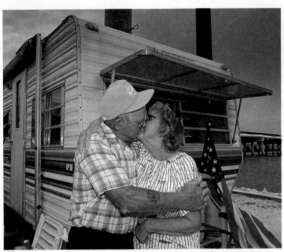

How might a close, supportive relationship be a buffer against depression?

1990; Weissman, 1987). Marital problems also may minimize the therapeutic value of antidepressant medication (Coyne, 1986).

Beach and O'Leary (1986) developed a **marital therapy** program that emphasized increased feelings of closeness, open sharing of thoughts and feelings, positive interchanges, and effective problem solving for marital disputes. The researchers compared it with another program using individual cognitive therapy for depressed women who were unhappily married. Individual cognitive therapy led to reductions in depression but did not impact marital discord (Beach & O'Leary, 1990). By contrast, the marital therapy program led to reductions in depression as well as to increases in marital satisfaction.

The effectiveness of marital therapy highlights the social or interpersonal context of depression. Given that, marital therapy should be seriously considered for depressed women who want to remain in their troubled marriages. Like IPT, marital therapy has been included in the list of treatments for major depression in the 1993 American Psychiatric Association's practice guidelines (Karasu et al., 1993).

Comparative Outcome Research

As mentioned earlier, both cognitive therapy and IPT have been found more effective than minimal treatment conditions. The review by Hollon et al. (1993) concluded that, overall, cognitive therapy also fared quite well in comparison to treatment with either antidepressant medications or other psychological therapies. Moreover, Frank et al. (1990) provided evidence that continued IPT reduces the likelihood of relapse for patients who have recovered from depression.

The National Institute of Mental Health (NIMH) conducted a major study comparing different treatment therapies for depression called the "Treatment of Depression Collaborative Research Program" (Elkin et al., 1989). It compared cognitive therapy, interpersonal psychotherapy, antidepressant medication, and placebos. Both of the medication conditions (real and placebo) also involved 20 minutes per week of "clinical management" with a psychiatrist. The therapies were conducted at three different universities with 239 depressed persons treated by 28 therapists. Patient outcomes on several different measures were assessed after 4 months of treatment.

Patients in all four conditions—including the placebo/control—showed improvement. Regardless of the outcome measure, the rank order of the results was almost always the same: Patients improved the most on medication and the least on the placebo, with the two psychotherapies falling in between (see Figure 7.3A). However, statistical analyses indicated that many of the differences were not significant. In sum, the treatments didn't clearly help patients more than spending 20 minutes a week with a supportive professional.

Further analyses revealed a great deal of variation within each treatment group, and the overall conclusion appeared limited to patients with less severe depression. That is, more severely depressed patients clearly benefited more from active medication compared to placebo. IPT also showed statistically significant effects, but cognitive therapy did not. These results are shown in Figure 7.3B.

These results are still generating comment and controversy over 5 years later. For example, some professionals have criticized the methods or interpreted the study's results differently. Hollon et al. (1993) noted that cognitive therapy fared poorly with severely depressed patients at only *one* of the three study sites. They also expressed concern that there were important differences in the cognitive therapy training across sites. Klein and Ross (1993), on the other hand, questioned the

marital therapy Treatment for couples experiencing marital discord that's also effective in reducing depression.

FIGURE 7.3 Treatment responses of depressed patients

Part A: Both medication and placebo groups received 20 minutes per week of clinical management. Controversy raged over whether cognitive therapy was more effective than the placebo. **Part B:** No differences in recovery rate were found for mildly depressed patients. Again, there was controversy over the cognitive therapy results.

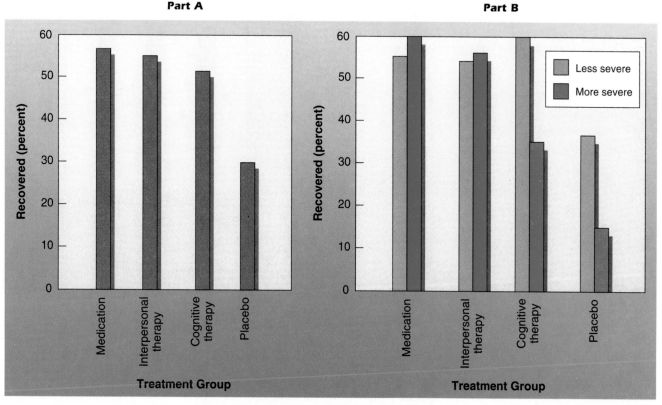

Source: Data from Elkin, Shea, Watkins, & Imber, 1989.

statistical analyses used in the original report. Their reanalysis indicated that medication was superior to both psychotherapies and both psychotherapies were somewhat superior to placebo, with again the most marked differences among the more severely depressed patients.

One and one-half years after the treatment portion of the study ended, follow-up data showed that only 24 percent of the patients who had started the study had recovered and never relapsed (Shea et al., 1992). These data also suggested that psychotherapy—especially cognitive therapy—might help maintain recovery. But statistically, there was no difference among the types of treatments received (see Figure 7.4). The NIMH researchers concluded that 16 weeks of treatment was too short for most patients to achieve a full and lasting recovery. In addition, these data underscore the fact that depression is a cyclic disorder and that maintenance therapy is important in managing it.

Biopsychosocial Approach

Because mood disorders are caused by a number of factors, combinations of treatments might be more effective than single treatments. For instance, medications do not (at least not directly) affect patients' interpersonal relations, social support or skills, negative schema, attributional or ruminative style, and so forth, and psychosocial treatments do not directly change neurochemistry.

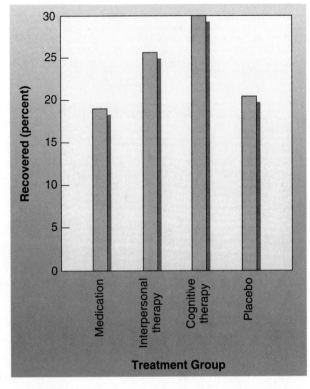

FIGURE 7.4 Recovery from depression

Psychological therapies may be more successful in preventing relapse following recovery from depression. This figure shows the percentages of patients who recovered from depression and were still well 1.5 years later.

SOURCE: Data from Shea et al., 1992.

Surprisingly few studies have examined combined treatments (Muñoz et al., 1994). What few research data are available suggest three main conclusions:

1. Combined treatment may help keep patients from dropping out of therapy, perhaps because it achieves a faster response than single treatments (Simons, Levine, Lustman, & Murphy, 1984).
2. The overall response rate for a typical course of treatment (that is, 3 to 4 months) isn't different for single versus combined treatments (Hollon, Shelton, & Loosen, 1991).
3. Psychological treatment—either with or without medication—appears to be effective in preventing relapse or recurrence (Fava & Kaji, 1994; Muñoz et al., 1994).

The next step is to research the mechanisms behind therapeutic change. Psychosocial stressors, for instance, seem to change neurochemistry for the worse. So does psychosocial treatment change it for the better? Are patients' interpersonal behaviors indirectly affected by taking medications because of the effects they have on mood?

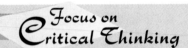

Focus on Critical Thinking

1. Suppose that you or someone close to you were severely depressed or manic and a psychiatrist suggested treatment involving either medication or electroconvulsive therapy. Which would you choose? Why?
2. Some manic patients discontinue taking lithium because taking it brings them down off a "high" that feels good. Think about what kind of psychotherapy might encourage bipolar patients to continue taking their medication.

SUMMARY

Description

■ There are two major types of mood episodes—major depressive and manic—and two variants, or subtypes, of these—mixed and hypomanic. These types and subtypes form the basis for the wide variety of mood disorders.

- Symptoms of a major depressive episode include affective symptoms (depressed mood and loss of interest in activities), cognitive symptoms (difficulty concentrating, excessive guilt), and somatic symptoms (disturbances in sleep and appetite).
- Manic episodes are characterized by elevated or irritable mood, grandiosity, high levels of energy and activity, decreased need for sleep, racing thoughts, and distractibility. A hypomanic episode is a milder version of a manic episode.
- Mood episodes form the basis of mood disorders. For example, major depressive disorder is characterized solely by depressive episodes, bipolar I disorder is characterized by both major depressive and manic (or mixed) episodes, and bipolar II disorder is characterized by major depressive plus hypomanic episodes.
- Specifiers such as seasonal pattern and postpartum onset in depression and rapid cycling in bipolar disorder are used to describe the full variety of major mood disorders.
- Dysthymic disorder and cyclothymic disorder have milder symptoms than the major mood disorders but are chronic (long lasting) in nature.

Issues and Problems
- Major depression is a very common disorder, with a lifetime prevalence as high as 13 percent for men and 21 percent for women. Mood disorders are more common among young people and those with very low incomes but are not consistently related to race/ethnicity.
- Mood disorders are comorbid (co-occur) with many other disorders, especially anxiety, personality, and substance abuse disorders. Comorbidity complicates treatment and interferes with recovery.
- Depression is the most common precipitant of suicide. About two-thirds of suicide attempts are made by persons who are depressed.
- Women make twice as many suicide attempts as men, but men actually kill themselves three to four times more often. Completed suicide increases with age and socioeconomic status and is higher among whites than other races and ethnic groups.
- Suicide can be reduced by paying attention to its warning signs, such as talking about and having the means to commit suicide.

Causes
- Family, twin, and adoption studies all indicate that mood disorders have a genetic basis. What is inherited, most likely, is not the disorder itself but a predisposition to developing it. Some complex neurobiochemical dysfunction is probably passed on through several, maybe even many, different genes.
- The psychodynamic view is that loss in close relationships and disturbances in self-esteem cause depression. That these factors are associated with depression has received research support, but psychodynamic theories about *how* these factors cause depression have not.
- Cognitive factors are certainly correlates of depression, but it's unclear whether they are a cause, an effect, or both. Recent theories have focused on biased negative schema, a depressogenic outlook on the causes of life events, a ruminative style, and the absence of positive thinking.
- Interpersonal problems—particularly social stressors, lack of social support, and marital difficulties—can contribute to the development and maintenance of depression. The interactional perspective emphasizes that the behavior of individuals who are depressed contributes to negative interpersonal cycles. This behavior reflects poor social skills and difficulties with interpersonal attachment that may stem from early childhood.
- Given that many factors have been shown to contribute to the development of mood disorders, it seems clear that depression is a biopsychosocial disorder.

Treatment

■ Several different types of medications have been developed to treat depression: tricyclic antidepressants, selective serotonin reuptake inhibitors (SSRIs), and monoamine oxidase inhibitors (MAOIs). Overall, these drugs are equally effective, but the newer SSRIs (such as Prozac) have fewer side effects. Lithium is largely successful in treating individuals with bipolar disorder and may also help in treating some with nonbipolar depression.

■ Electroconvulsive therapy (ECT) is a quick, safe, and effective method for treating severe depressive and manic episodes. It is not a good long-term treatment for mood disorders, however.

■ Light therapy can be effective in treating mood disorders with seasonal patterns.

■ Cognitive treatment of depression tries to relieve the disorder by changing the patient's maladaptive thought processes. It's been proven as effective as other treatments and may be more effective in preventing relapse.

■ Marital therapy and interpersonal treatment for depression are based on the assumption that dysfunctional relationships contribute to depression. Both types of treatment have been shown effective in a number of studies and are included in the list of treatments for major depression in the 1993 American Psychiatric Association's practice guidelines. Marital therapy is also considered an important adjunct to medication in the treatment of bipolar disorder.

■ The biopsychosocial approach suggests that a combination of biological therapy and psychotherapy might be best for treating mood disorders. Existing research shows that medication may lead more reliably to initial recovery, whereas psychotherapy may play a more important role in preventing relapse or recurrence.

KEY TERMS

anhedonia, **p. 192**
artifacts, **pp. 202–203**
attributional style, **p. 213**
atypical features, **p. 195**
automatic thoughts, **p. 212**
behavioral activation
   system (BAS), **p. 216**
behavioral inhibition
   system (BIS), **p. 216**
bipolar disorders, **p. 198**
brief recurrent depressive
   disorder, **p. 204**
circadian rhythms, **p. 225**
cognitive symptoms, **p. 193**
cognitive triad, **p. 213**
collaborative empiricism,
   p. 225
comorbidity, **p. 204**
content specificity, **p. 213**
cortisol, **p. 211**
course, **p. 193**
cyclothymic
   disorder, **p. 200**
depressogenic, **p. 212**
dexamethasone
   suppression test
   (DST), **p. 211**

diathesis-stress
   model, **p. 214**
double depression, **p. 199**
dysthymic disorder, **p. 199**
electroconvulsive therapy
   (ECT), **p. 224**
episodes, **p. 192**
flights of ideas, **p. 196**
homeostatic
   mechanisms, **p. 210**
hopelessness theory, **p. 214**
hypomanic episode, **p. 196**
interactional
   perspective, **p. 217**
interpersonal psycho-
   therapy (IPT), **p. 227**
labile, **p. 195**
learned helplessness,
   p. 213
lifetime prevalence, **p. 201**
lithium, **p. 223**
major depressive
   disorders, **p. 196**
major depressive
   episode, **p. 192**
manic episode, **p. 195**
marital therapy, **p. 228**

matrilineal, **pp. 202–203**
melancholic features, **p. 193**
meta-analysis, **p. 215**
minor depressive
   disorder, **p. 204**
mixed episode, **p. 196**
monoamine oxidase
   (MAO), **p. 210**
monoamine oxidase
   inhibitors
   (MAOIs), **p. 223**
mood disorders, **pp. 191–192**
negative affectivity, **p. 215**
neuropeptides, **p. 210**
neurotransmitters, **p. 210**
NOS diagnoses, **p. 204**
outcome, **p. 193**
placebo, **p. 222**
point prevalence, **p. 201**
positive affectivity, **p. 215**
postsynaptic receptors,
   p. 210
premenstrual dysphoric
   disorder, **p. 204**
pressured speech, **p. 196**
presynaptic
   receptors, **p. 210**

ℭRITICAL ThINKING EXERCISE

It was reported widely in the media that the suicide of rock star Kurt Cobain in 1994 was due to problems with both depression and substance abuse. But beyond that, what do we really know about him? Consider the following details of his life and death:

In 1979 and 5 years later, in 1984, two of Cobain's great uncles fatally shot themselves. It was rumored that other relatives had also committed suicide—some, way back in the family's history (Gilmore, 1994).

When Cobain was 8, his parents went through a bitter divorce. After that, he was shuttled around between his parents' and other relatives' homes. There are unconfirmed reports that he was physically abused and exposed to drug abuse during this period. He even had to live with one of his high school teachers for a year.

His high school teachers said that he never let anyone get close. "Around Kurt there was an aura of 'Back off,'" one of them said (Gilmore, 1994, p. 46). By high school, he already had been diagnosed with depression. In addition, he was suffering from the severe stomach pain that plagued him all his life, which may have been the result of chronic anxiety. His friends also confirmed that Cobain had rapid mood swings—that he'd go from being funny and outgoing to moody and uncommunicative in a matter of hours.

The suicide attempt that killed him was not Cobain's first. He had overdosed before at least twice and had once left a suicide note (although he later insisted it wasn't intended to be that). For some weeks before his death, his friends and family had been trying to talk him into getting treatment for his drug use and depression (Strauss & Foege, 1994). He finally checked into a drug rehabilitation program but left after 2 days. A few days later, he was dead.

Cobain had repeated domestic disputes with his wife that, from time to time, were so violent that the police were called in. On at least one occasion, they confiscated his guns to keep him from harming himself or someone else. He eventually killed himself with a 20-gauge shotgun, which he'd talked a friend into buying for him. He was reportedly afraid that if the police found out he'd bought a gun for himself, they'd take it away (Strauss & Foege, 1994).

Cobain left a suicide note that contained elements of guilt (that he faked enjoying his music), anger, and frustration. Ironically, these are the same emotions felt by those he left behind.

1. Think about the warning signs of suicide. Could anything have been done to prevent this suicide? If so, what? If not, why not?

2. How much did Cobain's genetics, early childhood experience, introverted personality, stressful lifestyle, marital discord, and drug use contribute to his death? Can the influence of each of these factors be separated? Explain your answers.

Chapter 8
SEXUAL DISORDERS

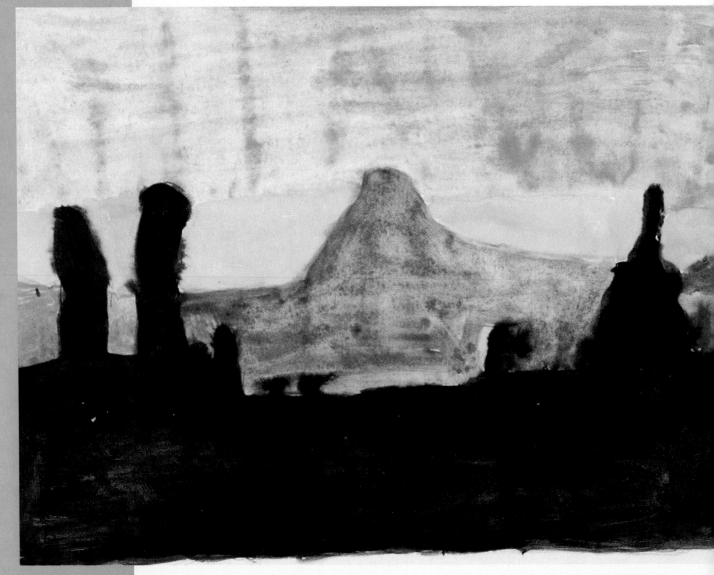

James Prendergast, **Untitled,** HAI

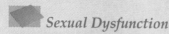
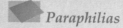
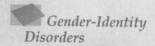
H enry X. was a big man—more than 6 feet tall and overweight. His physical presence was imposing, so it was immediately apparent why women would easily be threatened by his actions. Henry had been referred to Dr. Rogers for evaluation and treatment for exhibitionism. At the time, Henry was under grand jury indictment for exposing himself and was facing the possibility of receiving a lengthy prison term—even a life sentence. Treatment was the last resort. This time, if he was unsuccessful in changing his behavior, he would go to prison.

It's unusual for an exhibitionist to be sentenced to such a severe prison term. But Henry X. was a most unusual patient.

Henry was 35 years old. He was married and had two sons, ages 8 and 5 years. He came from a successful, middle-class family. For the last 20 years, he had been exposing his genitals to unsuspecting adult women—often, as many as five or six times a week. He would also occasionally engage in **frotteurism,** an act in which he would rub up against a woman in a crowd, usually with his penis partly out of his pants. He had never physically assaulted anyone, nor did he expect to have sex with any of the women he exposed himself to. He became sexually aroused just by fantasizing about exposing himself and even more excited during the exposure. Henry reported that he hoped the women he exposed himself to would express some form of approval, either by smiling or making some sexual comment. But most of them simply ignored him; some called the police.

Typically, Henry would masturbate to orgasm following the exposure. It wasn't uncommon for him to have mutually satisfactory sexual intercourse with his wife, either before or after exposing himself to some anonymous woman.

Although Henry regarded what he did as harmless, his exhibitionism had serious consequences in his life. He had spent 15 years in intermittent outpatient psychoanalytic treatment and had been hospitalized at psychiatric institutions. These efforts had failed to change his unwanted but apparently uncontrollable behavior.

What's more, Henry X. had been apprehended by the police on numerous occasions. He was usually able to escape serious consequence by paying a fine. But a number of years ago, his behavior had landed him in jail for a time in another state. He recalled being in prison with fear and distress. The other inmates had mocked and humiliated him. Another sexual offender had tried to rape him. As much as he had suffered in this harsh environment, though, the experience did little to control his behavior. In fact, on one occasion, while he was serving his sentence, he had tried to expose himself to a woman who was one of a group of visitors to the prison. The prison psychiatrist had diagnosed Henry X. as untreatable and had advocated his removal from free society.

When Henry X. came to Dr. Rogers, the immediate cause of his legal problems was being caught exposing himself. As always, he had targeted an adult woman. But this time, unbeknownst to him, he had also been seen by a group of Girl Scouts, whose leader had called the police. Henry was now charged with a sexual offense against a juvenile. This charge—combined with his chronic history of repeated exhibitionism, a failure to respond to treatment, and a prior jail term—explained the prosecutor's request for a lengthy jail sentence. Henry's lawyer had bargained for another attempt at treatment before the sentence was pronounced.

The case of Henry X. illustrates some of the issues we will cover in this chapter. It also raises a number of challenging questions: Why would someone who has a satisfactory sexual relationship with a caring wife engage in acts such as exhibitionism? Is this type of behavior merely a social nuisance, or is it part of a more ominous pattern of sexual violence against women and children? Should Henry be jailed for committing a sexual offense or treated for having a sexual disorder? Can sexual disorders be treated successfully? Why do so many more men than women seem to commit sexual offenses?

Sexual Dysfunction

The formal, scientific study of sexual pathology can be traced to late-nineteenth-century Europe. Richard von Krafft-Ebing (1840–1902), professor of psychiatry at the University of Vienna, Austria, helped found the scientific study of sexual disorders as an independent field of inquiry. His great work—*Psychopathica Sexualis* (1886/1965)—is generally credited with ushering in the scientific analysis of sexual disorders as an important yet controversial branch of medical psychology. During the first half of the twentieth century, the field was dominated by the pioneering clinical observations and concepts of Sigmund Freud (1856–1939), Krafft-Ebing's colleague in Vienna. Freud and his followers' continuing emphasis on human sexuality in the study of clinical disorders has been a major emphasis of psychoanalysis.

frotteurism Paraphilia involving touching or rubbing against a nonconsenting and unsuspecting person.

After Freud, the next great name in sex research was that of an American biologist, Alfred Kinsey (1894–1956). Kinsey was a revolutionary. His famous surveys (Kinsey, Pomeroy, & Martin, 1948; Kinsey, Pomeroy, Martin, & Gebhard, 1953) of the sexual preferences and practices of American men and women broke through the social taboos about investigating sexual behavior. His work also produced the first reliable information about Americans' sexual behavior and paved the way for the objective study of sexual activity.

Kinsey's surveys were based on self-reports given by people during interviews. Self-reports—particularly those divulging sensitive information—are always open to the criticism that they may be biased. People may not be accurate in what they report, whether deliberately or otherwise. Thus, it's one thing

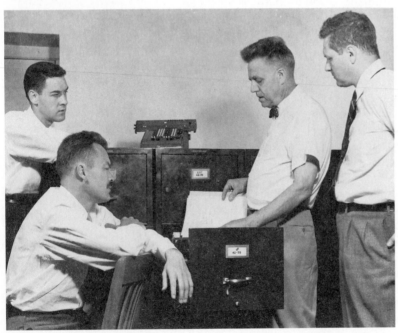

Alfred Kinsey, pioneering sex researcher (standing second from the right), with some of his staff at Indiana University

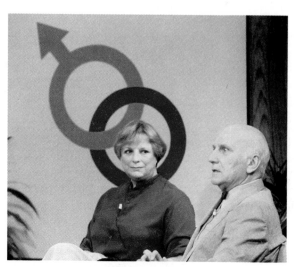

William Masters and Virginia Johnson, whose laboratory studies of sexual behavior led the way to a greater understanding and more effective therapy for sexual dysfunction

to ask people to describe their sexual behavior but quite another to observe such behavior directly.

Observation was the source of the next major advance in our knowledge about sexual behavior. In 1966, William Masters and Virginia Johnson published the results of their detailed observations and recordings of a variety of explicit sexual acts, such as masturbation, intercourse, and oral sex. Their book, *Human Sexual Response* (1966), and its sequel on therapy, *Human Sexual Inadequacy* (1970), fundamentally changed the field. Masters and Johnson added significantly to our knowledge about sex and its disorders. Moreover, they shattered some of the myths about sexual functioning and helped make the study of sexual behavior a legitimate scientific subject.

It's not uncommon for both men and women to experience transitory sexual difficulties at some point in their lives. For example, in a survey of 100 well-educated, happily married couples (who had not sought therapy), 36 percent of the men reported difficulties with ejaculating too quickly and 16 percent reported problems with obtaining or maintaining erections (Frank, Anderson, & Rubinstein, 1978). Most men manage to cope with such problems. Yet when these difficulties persist and cause distress, they become clinical dysfunctions requiring treatment.

The fourth edition of the *Diagnostic and Statistical Manual of Mental Disorders (DSM-IV)* (American Psychiatric Association, 1994) divides sexual dysfunctions into four major categories:

1. desire disorders
2. arousal disorders
3. orgasmic disorders
4. pain disorders

These categories correspond to different phases of the normal cycle of sexual response. *Desire* refers to how often or strongly a person wants sex, *arousal* to how excited someone becomes once sex is initiated, and **orgasm** to the male's ability to ejaculate and the female's capacity to reach climax after arousal. For men and women, orgasm is an intensely satisfying physiological reflex, releasing sexual tension. Sexual *pain* refers to any genital discomfort felt during sexual intercourse.

Sexual dysfunction is diagnosed only if it's not the result of some other disorder, such as major depression. Any sexual dysfunction may be lifelong or acquired following a particular life event. Sexual dysfunction may be generalized to all sources of sex or specific to a particular person or situation. If the dysfunction is the result of a medical condition—which is often the case, as discussed later—the diagnosis is *sexual dysfunction due to a general medical condition.*

orgasm Intensely satisfying physiological reflex, releasing sexual tension.

hypoactive sexual desire (HSD) Absence of sexual fantasies and wish for sexual activity.

sexual aversion disorder Paraphilia in which an individual avoids all or almost all genital sexual contact with a partner.

Desire Disorders

Description   There are two major sexual desire disorders. The first—**hypoactive sexual desire (HSD)**—is marked by the absence of sexual fantasies and the wish for sexual activity (see the *DSM-IV* table). The second type of desire disorder—**sexual aversion disorder**—involves avoiding all or almost all genital sexual contact with a partner and causes definite personal or interpersonal distress.

HSD is the most controversial and least understood sexual disorder (Rosen & Leiblum, in press). Defining *low sexual desire* is difficult because there are no objective standards of what is normal or healthy interest in sex.

For instance, how often do couples have sex in good marriages? A study involving 100 couples (Frank et al., 1978) found the following:

DSM-IV   **Diagnostic Criteria for 302.71 HYPOACTIVE SEXUAL DESIRE DISORDER**

A. Persistently or recurrently deficient (or absent) sexual fantasies and desire for sexual activity. The judgment of deficiency or absence is made by the clinician, taking into account factors that affect sexual functioning, such as age and the context of the person's life.

B. The disturbance causes marked distress or interpersonal difficulty.

C. The sexual dysfunction is not better accounted for by another Axis I disorder (except another Sexual Dysfunction) and is not due exclusively to the direct physiological effects of a substance (e.g., a drug of abuse, a medication) or a general medical condition.

- 8 percent reported having intercourse less than once a month
- 23 percent, two to three times a month
- 24 percent, once a week
- 31 percent, two to three times a week
- 12 percent, four to five times a week
- 1 percent, daily
- 2 percent, never

Some people with low levels of sexual desire may not view this as a dysfunction. It's their partners' dissatisfaction that leads them to seek help. So when a couple complains about low desire, the problem may be desire discrepancy, in which one partner wants sex more often than the other (Zilbergeld & Ellison, 1980). For example, suppose a man prefers to have sex only once or twice a month, but his wife would like to have sex almost daily. Is the man suffering from a sexual disorder?

Before the 1960s sexual revolution, the answer to this question would have been a clear no. Since then, however, the answer has become less obvious. Partner dissatisfaction is often the reason people seek treatment.

Prevalence rates of HSD vary, but the problem is common. The rates are higher among women than men (Rosen & Leiblum, in press). Findings from a large, multicenter study of the treatment of sexual disorders indicated that 65 percent of all patients seeking treatment met the criteria for HSD (Segraves & Segraves, 1991). Clinical studies show that the number of patients seeking treatment for HSD has increased during the past 20 years (LoPiccolo & Friedman, 1989).

Causes   Sexual function and desire are complex products of biological, psychological, and sociocultural influences. Illness, disease, and surgery may all lower sexual desire. Sexual desire seems linked to hormones. In one study, the level of **testosterone**—often called the "sex hormone"—was lower in physically healthy men with HSD than in men from an age-matched control group (Schiavi, Schreiner-Engel, White, & Mandeli, 1988). But the same study failed to find differences in levels of testosterone or other hormones between women with HSD and normal controls.

Depression and severe stress may also cause low sexual desire. Both involve physiological as well as psychological determinants. A person's sexual desire often returns to normal when a depression lifts or stressful life circumstances change. But occasionally, negative sexual consequences of these conditions persist. Both men and women with HSD report greater lifetime histories of depression than normal controls (Schreiner-Engel & Schiavi, 1986).

There are several psychological causes of lowered sexual desire. One such cause is negative early experiences in learning about sex—for instance, being taught that sex is sinful or dangerous. Lowered sexual desire can also be caused by traumatic experiences, such as **child sexual abuse** or rape (Becker, Skinner, & Abel, 1983). Men's and women's sexual problems are frequently caused by or become enmeshed with feelings of anxiety, anger, jealousy, and guilt. Intrapsychic conflicts can trigger what Kaplan (1979) calls the "turn-off" mechanism. Based on her clinical experience, she believes that people may unconsciously and involuntarily suppress sexual desire by focusing selectively on the negative characteristics of their partners or the situation. The motivation behind this sexual turn-off is an unconscious fear of sexual intimacy. In psychodynamic terms, the fear that originates in unresolved childhood conflicts is transferred to the person's sexual partner. For example, a woman may see her husband as her father, with whom sex is forbidden.

Interpersonal problems—particularly underlying hostility and conflict—often cause sexual disorders. The following case illustrates how relationship problems may cause sexual desire disorder:

testosterone Hormone that's critical in regulating sexual arousal in men.

child sexual abuse Use of a child for sexual gratification of an adult.

Max and Carol, a couple in their mid-twenties, had been living together for three years. Max, a third-year medical student, felt frustrated by Carol's growing lack of interest in sex. Although Carol was able to become aroused and have orgasms, she was seldom in the mood for sex and rarely initiated it. Carol, a laboratory assistant, felt equally frustrated by Max's preoccupation with his medical-school training. His school pressures had become so great that the couple spent little time together. Carol also complained that when they had sex, Max was usually impatient and rushed through foreplay. Max agreed that during the week, they saw too little of each other but usually planned to make it up on the weekends. By the time the weekend began, he said, he'd been bottling up his desire all week and generally felt very horny. When Carol showed no interest in his advances, he became angry because of the tension, and the couple often found themselves arguing about something. Max saw Carol's low level of sexual desire as a major problem for them. (Rosen & Hall, 1984, p. 373)

male erectile disorder
Persistent or recurrent failure to attain or maintain an adequate erection until completion of sexual activity.

female sexual arousal disorder Persistent or recurrent failure to be physiologically aroused until completion of sexual activity.

DSM-IV   **Diagnostic Criteria for 302.72 MALE ERECTILE DISORDER**

A. Persistent or recurrent inability to attain, or to maintain until completion of the sexual activity, an adequate erection.

B. The disturbance causes marked distress or interpersonal difficulty.

C. The erectile dysfunction is not better accounted for by another Axis I disorder (other than a Sexual Dysfunction) and is not due exclusively to the direct physiological effects of a substance (e.g., a drug of abuse, a medication) or a general medical condition.

DSM-IV   **Diagnostic Criteria for 302.72 FEMALE SEXUAL AROUSAL DISORDER**

A. Persistent or recurrent inability to attain, or to maintain until completion of the sexual activity, an adequate lubrication-swelling response of sexual excitement.

B. The disturbance causes marked distress or interpersonal difficulty.

C. The sexual dysfunction is not better accounted for by another Axis I disorder (except another Sexual Dysfunction) and is not due exclusively to the direct physiological effects of a substance (e.g., a drug of abuse, a medication) or a general medical condition.

Arousal Disorders

Description   Male erectile disorder is the persistent or recurrent failure to attain or maintain an adequate erection until completion of sexual activity. The *DSM-IV* table lists the diagnostic criteria for this disorder.

Male erectile disorder causes a good deal of personal or interpersonal distress. One noted authority on male sexuality summarized the psychological impact as follows:

A man without an erection feels that he has failed as a man. His partner may be sympathetic and supportive, but he may be so consumed with self-loathing that he cannot accept what she offers. Many men distance themselves from their partners after such "failures" and engage in orgies of self-flagellation. The result is usually a miserable time for everyone concerned. (Zilbergeld, 1992, p. 37)

The *DSM-IV*, like the *DSM-III* (American Psychiatric Association, 1994, 1980), identifies this disorder using the term *erectile disorder*, but the more common word is *impotence*. Many sex therapists avoid this term because it tends to stigmatize men. The negative implications of being impotent go beyond the inability to complete a sexual action. The presumption is that if a man is impotent, he has lost power; he is supposedly "less of a man." Nevertheless, Kinsey and Masters and Johnson used the term in their work, and it's standard usage in current medical literature (Feldman, Goldstein, Hatzichristou, Krane, & McKinlay, 1994). In this chapter, we will use the term used by the investigator whose work is being described.

The man with *lifelong erectile disorder* (previously called *primary erectile dysfunction*) has never been able to achieve a sufficient erection to have intercourse with a partner. Cases of this severity seem relatively rare. In *acquired erectile disorder* (previously called *secondary erectile dysfunction*), the man is currently unable to achieve a sufficient erection to engage in sexual intercourse but was able to do so at least once in the past.

Female sexual arousal disorder is characterized by a woman's persistent or recurrent failure to be physiologically aroused until completion of sexual activity (see the *DSM-IV* table). As with males, this may be a *lifelong* or *acquired* problem.

Causes   For a time, it was believed that roughly 95 percent of all cases of male sexual arousal disorder were caused by psychological problems (for example, see Masters & Johnson, 1970). Over the past 15 years, however, the view has shifted to the other extreme—namely, that 50 percent or more of cases are due to physical causes (Blakeslee, 1993b). Much of the research on impotence is now conducted by urologists and other medical specialists (Krane, Goldstein, & DeTejada, 1989).

An erection begins in the mind. The brain sends a signal that travels down the spinal cord and along specific nerves that connect to the blood vessels and smooth muscle cells in the penis. Erection is produced by the inflow of oxygen-rich blood into the spaces in the penile tissue. When the smooth muscle cells around the spaces are constricted, very little blood flows in and the penis is flaccid. When the muscle cells are relaxed, blood flows in and the penis becomes erect.

Erectile dysfunction is caused by factors that impair the hormones, nerve pathways, or bloodflow that form the physiological basis of erection. Examples include illness (such as diabetes), surgery (such as prostatectomy), chronic alcohol abuse, and commonly prescribed medications (such as antihypertensive or antidepressant drugs). The drug Prozac, for instance—widely prescribed for depression and other clinical disorders—often produces decreased sexual desire (Jacobsen, 1992).

A recent study by Feldman and colleagues (1994)—the largest and most comprehensive evaluation of male sexuality and health since that done by Kinsey and colleagues (1948)—found that the ability to have an erection declines with age. In this study, almost half the men over 40 years of age had experienced problems with impotence. At age 40, 5 percent of the men reported total impotence. By age 70, three times as many (or 15 percent) reported impotence (see Figure 8.1). Other factors that correlated positively with impotence were heart disease, high blood pressure, and low levels of high-density lipoprotein (so-called good cholesterol).

Men with erectile problems should be checked for organic causes. Sophisticated medical diagnostic tests are now available to assess the role of hormonal, vascular, and neurological factors. For example, ultrasonographic techniques can be used to measure bloodflow in the penile arteries before and after the injection of a chemical that relaxes smooth muscle tissue.

While sleeping, the average healthy adult male may experience an average of about 1 erection every 90 minutes. This increase in penile tumescence (or swelling)

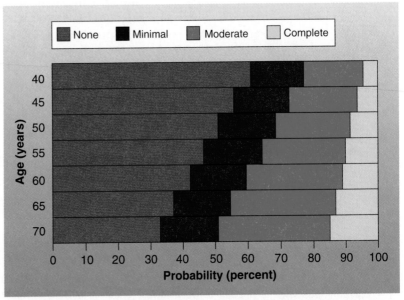

FIGURE 8.1   Impotence and age

The ability to have an erection declines with age. In this study, almost half the men over 40 years of age had experienced problems with impotence. Other factors that correlated positively with impotence were heart disease, high blood pressure, and low levels of high-density lipoprotein (so-called good cholesterol).

Source: From H. A. Feldman, I. Goldstein, D. G. Hatzichristou, R. J. Krane, and J. B. McKinlay, "Impotence and Its Medical and Psychosocial Correlates: Results of the Massachusetts Male Aging Study," *The Journal of Urology, 151*, p. 56. Copyright © 1994 by Williams & Wilkins. Reprinted by permission of Williams & Wilkins.

usually occurs during the rapid eye movement (REM) stage of sleep. The term **nocturnal penile tumescence (NPT)** describes these erections. During sleep, this naturally occurring physiological process is assumed to be unimpaired by the inhibitions, fears, and anxieties that affect erection during the waking state. Therefore, if the man has erections while sleeping, it's concluded that his sexual problem is caused by psychological factors; otherwise, it's assumed that organic factors are responsible.

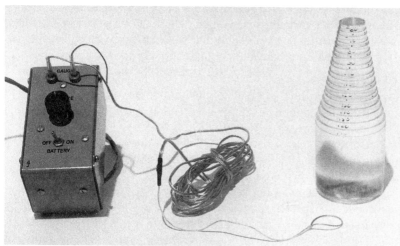

Left *A mercury-in-rubber strain gauge, attached to an electronic recording device, which fits over the penis and measures penile erection* **Right** *A cone for calibrating the strain gauge so as to provide accurate measurement*

Penile erection—during either the waking or sleeping state—is measured using a penile plethysmograph. This instrument has a thin rubber gauge filled with mercury. A very weak electrical current runs from an attached wire and flows through the mercury. The man places the rubber gauge over his flaccid penis. When his penis becomes erect, the rubber gauge expands, thereby changing the flow of electric current. A polygraph then records these alterations.

Despite the importance of organic causes of impotence, the influence of psychological factors is quite real. The sudden onset of impotence, typically associated with life stresses, clearly points to psychological causes. Even the medical tests in which chemicals are injected into the penis to assess bloodflow are influenced by the man's current psychological state. Many cases of erectile disorder involve both organic and psychological causes, and psychological treatment is often effective, despite some degree of physical impairment (Buvat, Buvat-Herbaut, Lemaire, Marcolin, & Quittelier, 1990; Carey, Wincze, & Meisler, 1993).

It's useful to divide psychological causes into two groups: (1) historical influences and (2) those currently maintaining the sexual problem (Masters & Johnson, 1970). Rigid adherence to orthodox religious beliefs and practices is a common factor in the backgrounds of men and women with different forms of sexual dysfunction. Strict religious teaching—regardless of the particular religion—often results in negative attitudes toward sexuality. Individuals come to believe that sex is sinful.

Of course, deeply religious people don't necessarily develop sexual dysfunctions. But the findings of Masters and Johnson (1970) have been corroborated by other sex therapists, indicating that strong religious beliefs and other background factors increase the probability of a person having sexual difficulties. Other underlying causes of lifelong erectile dysfunction include the following:

- having a dominating, overcontrolling parent who undermines self-esteem
- having a traumatic initial sexual encounter, such as a humiliating failure to perform that destroys self-confidence and heightens fears of inadequacy
- experiencing homosexual leanings that compete with heterosexual arousal

Acquired erectile disorder is caused by a broader range of factors than lifelong erectile dysfunction. Religious orthodoxy, traumatic sexual experiences, conflicts about sexual identity, and premature ejaculation have been identified as common antecedents of acquired erectile dysfunction. Alcohol abuse and a variety of nonsexual causes, such as inhibited emotional development, can also lead to erectile failure.

Masters and Johnson (1970) concluded that, irrespective of antecedent causes, an individual's current anxiety about sexual performance is responsible for most forms of sexual dysfunction. Such performance anxiety leads to what Masters and Johnson called **spectatoring.** That is, the man grows self-conscious and becomes an observer of his sexual response—a "third person"—looking for signs of failure. Instead of

nocturnal penile tumescence (NPT) Erection that occurs in healthy males during the rapid eye movement (REM) stage of sleep.

spectatoring Individual's self-conscious role during sexual activity, in which he becomes an observer of his sexual response and looks for signs of failure.

being open and responsive to erotic stimulation and enhanced sensory input, he is distracted by critical self-evaluation. The result is to generate even more anxiety and undermine the body's natural psychophysiological response to erotic cues.

Research by Barlow and his colleagues has clarified the psychological mechanisms that cause erectile problems (Cranston-Cuebas & Barlow, 1990). These researchers compared the typical sexual response of sexually dysfunctional men with that of normally functioning men. In a series of laboratory studies, these two groups viewed erotic movies under various anxiety-eliciting conditions—namely, the threat of receiving an electric shock. The men's subjective sexual arousal, erectile responses (measured by the penile plethysmograph), and attentional processes were assessed. The following differences were revealed between the two groups of men:

1. The experimental induction of anxiety usually increased sexual arousal in normally functioning men but impaired erection in sexually dysfunctional men.
2. When performance demand was induced in the laboratory setting by instructing men to become sexually aroused, erection was impaired in dysfunctional men but improved in functional men.
3. Exposure to erotic cues brought on negative feelings in dysfunctional men but positive feelings in functional men.
4. Distraction—for instance, being asked to notice a nonsexual stimulus while attending to an erotic cue—impaired erection in functional but not dysfunctional men. The explanation given for this finding was that men with erectile problems were already attending to nonsexual cues.

clitoris Female organ that's the main site of sexual responsiveness in women.

female orgasmic disorder Persistent or recurrent delay in or absence of orgasm following adequate sexual arousal

male orgasmic disorder Persistent delay in or absence of orgasm following normal arousal during sexual activity; typically means the inability to ejaculate in the vagina.

FIGURE 8.2 Current causes of sexual dysfunction

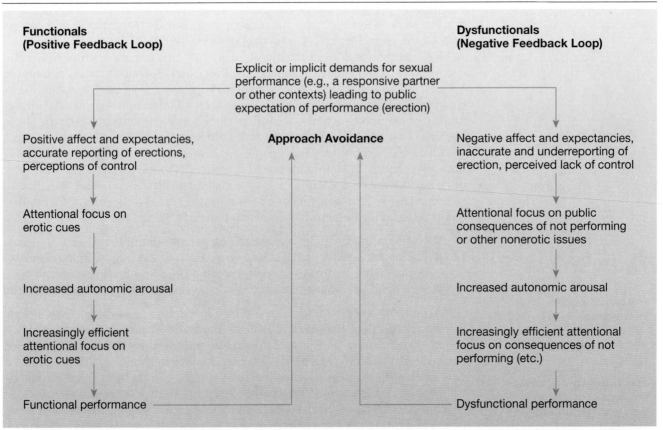

SOURCE: From D. H. Barlow, "Causes of Sexual Dysfunction," *Journal of Consulting and Clinical Psychology,* 54, p. 146. Copyright © 1986 by the American Psychological Association. Reprinted by permission.

5. Dysfunctional men reported less subjective arousal than functional men, even when their ability to have an erection did not differ.

Based on these research findings, Barlow (1986) proposed a psychological model of sexual arousal disorder (see Figure 8.2). This model assumes that any demand for sexual performance brings on anxiety and feelings of inadequacy. Instead of attending to normal erotic cues, the person is distracted and worries about his perceived inability to perform. The resulting cognitive distraction or interference leads to erectile failure. This negative cognitive-affective response to sexual performance is rooted in the historical factors summarized previously.

Much less is known about the causes of female sexual arousal disorder. For the female, the **clitoris** is the organ that's sensitive to sexual stimulation. Anything that reduces the flow of oxygen-rich blood to it may impair sexual arousal and orgasm. In this respect, the clitoris and penis are highly similar. Preliminary evidence suggests that the sexual arousal disorder model in Figure 8.2 (which was based on research involving men) may also apply to women. Women with normal sexual responses (like the functioning men) showed increases in sexual arousal with both the induction of anxiety (Palace & Gorzalka, 1990) and performance demand (Laan, Everaerd, Van Aanhold, & Rebel, 1993).

Orgasmic Disorders

Description   **Female orgasmic disorder** is the persistent or recurrent delay in or absence of orgasm following adequate sexual arousal (see the *DSM-IV* table). **Male orgasmic disorder** refers to the persistent delay in or absence of orgasm following normal arousal during sexual activity (see the *DSM-IV* table). This problem typically means the inability to ejaculate in the vagina. Male orgasmic disorder causes distress and a variety of interpersonal problems.

As with the arousal disorders, female and male orgasmic disorders can be divided into three subtypes, based on whether they are (1) *lifelong* or *acquired,* (2) *generalized* or confined to a *specific* situation (for example, orgasm is reached with masturbation but not intercourse), or (3) due primarily to psychological or combined psychological and medical factors.

Causes   Among the most common causes of orgasmic disorders identified by Masters and Johnson (1970) were the same negative influences responsible for male sexual disorders: restrictive religious prohibitions, homosexual commitments, and negative family influences. According to Masters and Johnson, "cold, formal, and controlled" childhood conditions can result in female sexual difficulties.

The most frequent source of sexual orgasmic difficulty is the woman's emotional dissatisfaction with her partner. These negative emotional reactions might include shame, resentment, jealousy, boredom, disappointment, and even disgust. At various times, sexual difficulties may also reflect unhappiness over financial failure, physical appearance, social shortcomings, lack of affection, and the man's relationships with other women. Sexual problems in women can also result from experiencing specific traumas (such as rape or attempted rape), being molested as a child, or feeling severe pain or panic during the first sexual encounter.

Women are also vulnerable to the negative influences of sexual inadequacy in their partners. A man may not concern himself with his

DSM-IV   Diagnostic Criteria for 302.73 FEMALE ORGASMIC DISORDER

A. Persistent or recurrent delay in, or absence of, orgasm following a normal sexual excitement phase. Women exhibit wide variability in the type or intensity of stimulation that triggers orgasm. The diagnosis of Female Orgasmic Disorder should be based on the clinician's judgment that the woman's orgasmic capacity is less than would be reasonable for her age, sexual experience, and the adequacy of sexual stimulation she receives.

B. The disturbance causes marked distress or interpersonal difficulty.

C. The orgasmic dysfunction is not better accounted for by another Axis I disorder (except another Sexual Dysfunction) and is not due exclusively to the direct physiological effects of a substance (e.g., a drug of abuse, a medication) or a general medical condition.

DSM-IV   Diagnostic Criteria for 302.74 MALE ORGASMIC DISORDER

A. Persistent or recurrent delay in, or absence of, orgasm following a normal sexual excitement phase during sexual activity that the clinician, taking into account the person's age, judges to be adequate in focus, intensity, and duration.

B. The disturbance causes marked distress or interpersonal difficulty.

C. The orgasmic dysfunction is not better accounted for by another Axis I disorder (except another Sexual Dysfunction) and is not due exclusively to the direct physiological effects of a substance (e.g., a drug of abuse, a medication) or a general medical condition.

Integrating Perspectives
A Biopsychosocial Model

PERSPECTIVE ON ERECTILE DISORDER

BIOLOGICAL FACTORS

Biological factors contribute to erectile disorder:

➤ Erection occurs when oxygen-rich blood flows into the spaces in penile tissue. Anything that interferes with this process can cause erectile problems. Examples include nerve damage (e.g., from diabetes) and vascular damage (e.g., atherosclerosis).

➤ Acute and chronic effects of alcohol and drugs impair erectile function.

➤ Erectile problems reliably increase with age.

PSYCHOLOGICAL FACTORS

Psychological factors interact with biological vulnerabilities in causing erectile disorder:

➤ Performance demand—the pressure to get and maintain an erection adequate for mutually satisfying intercourse—can cause erectile failure.

➤ Negative psychological states (e.g., depression or low self-esteem) and critical attitudes about sex (e.g., guilt or "sex is sinful") can cause erectile problems.

SOCIAL FACTORS

Both biological and psychological factors operate in specific social contexts:

➤ Relationship problems with a partner contribute significantly to erectile problems, even when the primary cause is biological. Examples include lack of trust, poor communication of feelings, and interpersonal conflict.

➤ Social pressures may overemphasize the importance of sexual performance to the exclusion of caring and mutual pleasure.

➤ Rigid religious contexts regard most sex as sinful.

These biological, psychological, and social factors interact to cause problems, as illustrated in the following case:

Joe had a date on Friday night. He was up late the night before studying for an exam the next morning. He worked hard all of Friday and then took Karen out to dinner, after which they went to a party. By the time they went home to his apartment, it was 1 A.M. He was dead tired. On top of that, he had drunk at least six beers and a few glasses of wine. When they tried to have sex, he was unable to get an erection.

The biopsychosocial model explains what happened. Joe's first failure was due to fatigue and too much alcohol—biological factors. The failure caused him to worry and doubt his sexual capacity. He became a victim of performance demand ("I have to prove to Karen that I can do it next Saturday night"). Once in bed, he became a "spectator," attending to nonerotic cues. The original biological causes had triggered psychological factors, which, combined with more drinking, caused the problem.

If Joe understands that the failures were due to fatigue and alcohol, he will probably shrug them off. Karen's reaction, a social relationship factor, is also critical. If she remains patient and supportive, she can help Joe overcome the problem. But if she dumps him or withdraws from sex because she begins to doubt her own ability to arouse Joe, the problem might worsen.

partner's sexual satisfaction; he is physically able to have orgasm through sexual intercourse, regardless of his mate's sexual responsiveness. For a woman to achieve orgasm during sexual intercourse, however, her partner must maintain an erection and control his ejaculation for a sufficient period of time. Even then, a clumsy or insensitive lover may interfere with a woman's orgasmic response (assuming the presence of the necessary sexual mechanics of erection and ejaculatory control). The woman also frequently worries about her partner's inability to control ejaculation or maintain an erection, thereby impairing her own sexual response. She might even feel guilty about his erectile failure, doubting her own sexual allure. Of the couples that Masters and Johnson (1970) treated in which both partners showed sexual dysfunction, premature ejaculation and orgasmic dysfunction was the most common combination.

Based on their work, Masters and Johnson concluded that most forms of sexual dysfunction in women are rooted in society's double-standard of sexual values: Male sexuality is culturally sanctioned, if not implicitly encouraged, while women's sexual nature has been ignored, even denied (except when it involves satisfying men). This topic is examined further in Thinking about Social Issues.

Sexual responsiveness is not simply an innate drive that automatically unfolds as men and women mature physically. Our biological potential for sexual responsiveness is elaborated on and probably channeled into different directions, depending on our subsequent psychosocial experiences. In short, as Gagnon (1977) has argued, we have to *learn* to be sexual. If the social opportunities necessary for this learning are unavailable or if the response to sexual stimulation is systematically punished, the individual will not develop into a healthy sexual being. The woman who has lived up to social expectations for "female virtue" and thus has little or no sexual experience, will have difficulty in suddenly becoming orgasmic upon taking a marriage vow or accepting her first invitation to go to bed with a man.

Related to American society's double-standard of sexual values is the assumption that the man—as the sexual expert—must initiate and orchestrate sex. A U.S. study of college students who were seriously dating found that, despite the recent easing of the double-standard, the male was still expected to make the first move in sexual encounters (Peplau, Rubin, & Hill, 1977). The overwhelming majority of women waited for men to make sexual overtures, although 95 percent of both men and women advocated identical moral standards for sex. What explains the women's hesitancy to initiate sex? They were afraid of threatening their partners' egos.

In their research, Masters and Johnson (1970) observed the typical script of the man taking the lead, with usually brief, stereotyped foreplay, followed by the ultimate objective of vaginal intercourse. This relatively unvarying pattern among heterosexual couples often places the woman at a sexual disadvantage because the timing may not align with her pattern of sexual responsiveness. This single-minded emphasis on sexual intercourse as the end goal also places unnecessary pressure on the man to perform, which can result in erectile problems.

As with male sexual dysfunction, organic factors can play a role in female orgasmic dysfunction. However, the biological basis of sexual dysfunction in women has received less direct research attention than disorders in men.

Premature Ejaculation   The sexual disorder **premature ejaculation** occurs when the male ejaculates too soon. But what's "too soon"? Any attempt to specify arbitrary time periods seems misguided. Sexually functional women vary greatly in the amount of stimulation they require for orgasm. Even the same woman will vary from time to time, depending on a number of factors—some, changeable, physiological factors and others, psychosocial factors specific to the situation.

The *DSM-IV* defines *premature ejaculation* as that occurring with "minimal sexual stimulation before, on, or shortly after penetration and before the person wishes it" (p. 509). The clinician making the diagnosis must take into account fac-

premature ejaculation
Disorder in which the male is unable to prevent reaching orgasm before he wants to during vaginal intercourse.

Thinking about SOCIAL ISSUES

The Sexual Double-Standard for Men and Women

American society has always had a double-standard regarding sexuality for men and women. You are probably aware of this—perhaps you have even experienced it. In sum, men are expected to be more sexual and allowed to be more permissive than women. For instance, society generally tolerates men having premarital sex and even extramarital affairs but frowns on women doing so.

You may not have thought about how this double-standard has constrained women's sexuality and contributed directly to sexual dysfunction. One of the important contributions of Masters and Johnson's (1966) research was that it helped prove that women are no less sexual than men. Women have been shown to be at least as sexually responsive as men. For example, they are capable of having multiple orgasms in response to effective sexual stimulation.

Women have suffered from false assumptions about the development of female sexuality. Until Masters and Johnson (1966) proved otherwise, it was widely believed by psychotherapists that there was a difference between clitoral and vaginal orgasms. Freud (1917/1963c) declared that in childhood, the clitoris was the focus of the little girl's sexuality. He felt it had a "special excitability" that enabled her to gain sexual satisfaction through masturbation (p. 318). For the girl to become a woman and achieve psychosexual maturity, the clitoris had to "hand over its sensitivity, and at the same time its importance, to the vagina" (Freud, 1933/1964a, p. 118). Allegedly, this development allowed the woman to experience mature sexual satisfaction through vaginal intercourse, rather than masturbation. By doing so, she reached the hallmark of psychosexual maturity. Freud predicted that sexual dysfunction would result if the clitoris retained its sensitivity (Freud, 1917/1963c, p. 318).

Through their research, Masters and Johnson (1966) showed that the physiological basis of all orgasms is stimulation of the clitoris, either directly during masturbation or indirectly during vaginal intercourse. The sensitivity of the clitoris is vital to healthy sexuality. With hindsight, the Freudian view can be seen as sexist. It's sobering to reflect on the possibly harmful consequences this view brought the many women who underwent unnecessary psychotherapy to overcome their supposed "arrested psychosexual development."

In the last 20 or 30 years, dramatic changes have occurred in how we view sexual dysfunction. This change in mindset highlights the importance of cultural values in defining and treating sexual disorders. Masters and Johnson's early research appeared during the 1960s, a period of intense social unrest and change in the United States. People talked of a sexual revolution, in which sexual attitudes became more liberal. Behaviors that were previously prohibited—such as premarital and extramarital sex—became more acceptable to many people. Women, in particular, were freed from the fear of unwanted pregnancy by the development of "the pill" and other birth-control methods. As a result, they became increasingly independent in their career choices and social roles and began to demand sexual equality.

These heightened expectations increased the pressure for sexual performance in women and in their partners, too. And with that pressure can come sexual dysfunction. Consider the increase in hypoactive sexual desire (HSD) disorder that's occurred in the United States over the last 20 years. It has been attributed, in part, to the newfound freedom of women to initiate sexual activity (Rosen & Leiblum, in press).

The societal double-standard may have changed, but female sexuality still seems underemphasized. The focus in scientific research has been on male impotence. For example, nothing like the Feldman et al. (1994) study of Massachusetts men exists for women. Great strides have been made in understanding the basic physiology of erections (Blakeslee, 1993b) but not in understanding the mechanisms of female sexual arousal.

John Bancroft, a leading sex researcher in Great Britain, points out another significant gender bias: For men, the explanation and treatment of erectile problems has been medicalized. For women, psychological explanations are still favored. Bancroft (1992) noted:

> When colleagues of mine in the United States sought official approval for the investigation of a new drug in the treatment of sexual problems of women, they were told that what a sexually troubled woman required was not a drug, but a new or better sexual partner. Elsewhere, we are told that what the sexually troubled, impotent man requires is not a new partner, but a new or more effective penis, kicked into action by its injection with drugs, or reinforced with plastic rods. From this viewpoint, male sexuality is the key to human sexuality. The crucial issue is to get that right; female sexuality will then follow. (p. viii)

Think about the following questions:

1. Do you think that a societal double-standard still exists when it comes to male and female sexuality? Explain your answer.
2. Why do you think the medical investigation of sexual dysfunction has focused almost exclusively on men?

tors that affect duration of the excitement phase, such as age, novelty of the sexual partner, and frequency of sexual activity.

Many sex therapists now emphasize the importance of *both* sexual partners feeling satisfied with the male's ejaculatory control during intercourse. Previously, a man with premature ejaculation might not have thought that he had a problem. This change in thinking reflects the modern trend toward equality between the sexes and the recognition of the sexual needs and wishes of women.

Masters and Johnson's (1970) study of almost 200 men with premature ejaculation revealed a correlation between a man's educational level and his concern about his partner's sexual satisfaction. The better educated the man, the more likely he was to be troubled by his inability to satisfy his partner sexually. Men who had not completed high school rarely complained about premature ejaculation. Also, premature ejaculation seems related to unusually hurried early sexual experiences.

We can't make too much of these preliminary findings, since they're based on a relatively small and nonrandom sample of sexually dysfunctional men.

Pain Disorders

Women who experience **dyspareunia,** or painful intercourse—involving aching, burning or itching sensations—often lack adequate vaginal lubrication. In women, lubrication is, roughly speaking, the functional equivalent of erection in men. Thus, inadequate lubrication usually means the woman is insufficiently aroused. Some emotional or interpersonal factor is usually responsible for this problem.

However, physical factors may be at work. Deep pelvic pain felt during intercourse may be caused by vaginal infections, which damage the ligaments supporting the uterus. Such damage may be the result of childbirth or brutal physical assault. Dyspareunia may also be caused by endometriosis, a disease affecting the vaginal lining. These types of physical conditions require diagnosis by a gynecologist.

Vaginismus refers to involuntary tightening in the outer one-third of the vagina. These spasms can make it difficult, if not impossible, for the woman to have intercourse. Diagnosis of this disorder is made on the basis of a physical examination, in which the presence of the muscle contractions are established by one-finger insertion. In addition to some of the psychosocial causes of sexual dysfunction (such as punitive religious prohibitions), vaginismus can result from being raped.

Treatment of Male Sexual Dysfunction

Psychological Therapies   Current psychological treatment methods of male sexual dysfunction are largely derived from Masters and Johnson's (1970) sex therapy. The core assumption of this therapy is that sexual dysfunction stems mainly from the fear of failure to perform. Accordingly, treatment techniques are designed to overcome this fear through a desensitization procedure. The following key concepts form the basis of the typical therapy program for most men's sexual problems:

1. *Desensitization*—The objective is to reduce the performance anxiety that leads to spectatoring. The first step is to prohibit any sexual activity that's not specifically sanctioned by the therapist. Thus, sexual intercourse is initially forbidden, thereby removing the pressure on the man to perform. Thereafter, the couple is instructed in how to start a carefully graduated program of mutually pleasurable sensual and sexual involvement. This program is conducted at the couple's own pace and involves no explicit goals, so performance pressure is effectively undercut.

2. *Sensate focus*—The mutual, non–goal oriented sensual interaction between partners is known as **sensate focus,** involving the physical or sensory stimulation of each other's body. The couple is taught to think and feel sensuously by giving and receiving bodily pleasure—first, by nongenital contact and then, by specific genital stimulation. The fundamental goals of sensate focus exercises are (a) to

dyspareunia Condition in which burning or itching sensations are felt during vaginal intercourse.

vaginismus Involuntary tightening or spasms in the outer layer of the vagina.

sensate focus Therapeutic technique involving mutual, non-performance-oriented sensual interaction between partners.

increase the partners' verbal and nonverbal communication and (b) to teach them that sexual gratification does not necessarily depend on intercourse. As sexual arousal occurs spontaneously in these "homework" assignments, the treatment is oriented toward the specific form of sexual dysfunction in question.

3. *Focus on couples*—It's recommended that both partners participate in treatment, even if only one of them is clearly dysfunctional. Emphasis on treating the sexually dysfunctional couple reflects the significance given to improving effective interpersonal communication. Treating the couple also prevents the possibility that the partner who is not being seen in therapy will conduct "sexual sabotage"— namely, accidentally or purposefully interfering with treatment because of other emotional or interpersonal conflicts.

Variations of this basic treatment program can be tailored to treat different sexual problems. The consensus among therapists is that hypoactive sexual desire (HSD) is the most difficult disorder to treat. A national survey of sex therapists in the 1980s revealed that patients with HSD required a greater number of therapy sessions than individuals with other sexual disorders. What's more, the therapeutic success rate was less than 50 percent (Kilmann, Boland, Norton, Davidson, & Caird, 1986).

The treatment of erectile problems is similarly based on the Masters and Johnson program. Couples are instructed to continue with sensate focus exercises until erection occurs spontaneously. Thereafter, the woman uses a "teasing technique" in which she manipulates the penis to erection and then relaxes with her partner until the erection disappears. She repeats this procedure several times, gradually reducing the man's fear of losing an erection and not regaining it during sexual interaction. The therapy continues with the woman making it easy for the man to insert his penis into her vagina without any pressure. This stage is followed by progressively more vigorous thrusting until the man's orgasm occurs.

Like any other sexual problem, erectile dysfunction is often embedded in a troubled relationship. Because of this, treatment methods have to extend beyond specific sexual techniques. In addition, therapy must address the role of marital difficulties in maintaining sexual dysfunction. The following case study, reported by Brady (1976), illustrates the role of relationship factors in therapy:

> The patient was a twenty-seven-year-old man with acquired erectile dysfunction. Standard sex therapy failed completely. The patient disobeyed the therapist's explicit instructions and drank before a session of sensate focus. (Alcohol consumption can significantly suppress erectile capacity.) His wife also ignored instructions by engaging almost immediately in direct genital stimulation and urging her husband to attempt intercourse. Mutual recriminations inevitably followed these interactions. As soon as this self-defeating pattern of behavior became apparent, the therapist delved more deeply into the nature of the couple's marital relationship. This showed the client plagued by self-doubt and a lack of assertiveness; his wife, while expressing occasional warmth and support, was predominantly critical and aggressive in manner. Therapy was redirected to changing the couple's relationship, and as a result, it improved greatly over the following five months of treatment. The client's erectile problem persisted, however, and he naturally still felt anxiety about his sexual performance. At this stage, the original desensitization program was reintroduced, and the sexual dysfunction eliminated within a few weeks. (p. 898)

This clinical case underscores an important point: Effective treatment of specific sexual disorders will sometimes require therapy for other nonsexual aspects of the couple's functioning, such as competitive tendencies and lack of communication.

Premature ejaculation has been successfully treated using the "squeeze technique." The woman manually stimulates her partner's penis to full erection. Then, just prior to ejaculation, she firmly squeezes the penis for 3 or 4 seconds, using her thumb and first two fingers of the same hand. This pressure stops the man's urge to ejaculate. The same procedure is repeated after about 30 seconds. By using this technique, the man is gradually able to maintain increasingly longer erections. Next, the progression moves from the woman straddling the man and inserting his penis into her vagina (while otherwise remaining motionless) to slowly building up to vigorous pelvis thrusting. If at any time the man feels that he's going to ejaculate too quickly, the woman—who is in the superior coital position, on top of the man—raises her body, repeats the squeeze technique, and then reinserts the penis.

It's vitally important that the man be able to recognize when he's close to ejaculation and that he communicate this to his partner. If he waits too long, he will reach the point of ejaculatory inevitability and will be unable to restrain ejaculation.

Lifestyle factors are also important in treating male sexual dysfunction. The Feldman study (Feldman et al., 1994) of Massachusetts men (mentioned earlier in this chapter) found that a number of lifestyle choices can improve erectile functioning: improving diet, quitting cigarette smoking, moderating alcohol consumption, and overcoming stress.

Surgical and Pharmacological Treatments   A range of possible treatments has come from the recent "medicalization" of impotence, in which the approach is exclusively physiological. Several surgical techniques have been developed. The most common is the penile implant, involving insertion of a semirigid rod or hydraulic device that can be pumped up to produce an erection (see Figure 8.3). The implant produces an erection hard enough for intercourse, and ejaculation is possible.

A study of 52 men who received penile implants showed that the surgery was technically successful. When surveyed, 90 percent of the subjects would choose the surgery again, if confronted with the same problem (Steege, Stout, & Carson, 1986). Yet 25 percent of the men reported significant dissatisfaction with the outcome. They were troubled by the size and stiffness of their erections and decreased sensations during ejaculation. In addition to these problems, little is known about the long-term effects of implants and their psychological effects on the sexual experiences of both men and their partners (Melman & Tiefer, 1992).

FIGURE 8.3 Penile prosthesis with pump for inflation

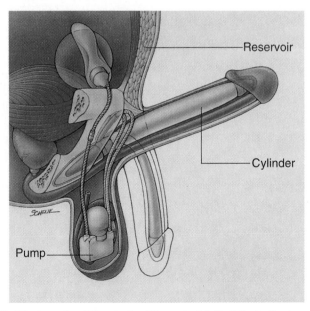

Source: Courtesy of American Medical Systems, Inc., Minnetonka, Minnesota. Medical illustration by Michael Schenk.

The most widely used medical technique for treating male sexual dysfunction is pharmacological, or drug, therapy. Men inject themselves with drugs such as papaverine, which relax the smooth muscles and allow blood to flow into the penis. Within 15 minutes following injection, these drugs produce partially or completely stiff erections that last 1 to 4 hours. They are often used in combination with standard sex therapy, even in cases in which erectile problems are caused by psychological factors.

A one-year study (Althof et al., 1991) examined the effects of self-injection of papaverine and phentolamine on 42 men. It showed that 83 percent of the men experienced satisfactory erections. They injected themselves an average of five times a month. After they started using injections, the men reported having intercourse more often, more frequent orgasm, greater sexual satisfaction, less depression and anxiety, and enhanced self-esteem.

The following case study illustrates the positive effects of drug therapy:

A 30-year-old financial analyst hoped to save a few dollars by climbing up a 30-foot ladder to clean the gutters on his house. He fell, sustaining a spinal cord injury. Upon being told he would never walk again, he and his wife, a registered nurse, sought additional consultation. Their persistence paid off when they found a surgical team with considerable expertise. Although he never really regained control over bowel and bladder functions, he was eventually able to walk with a limp. Despite his partial response to spinal cord decompression surgery, he had unreliable, short-lived erections, decreased penile sensation, and rare ejaculations. The couple was eager to have children and was pursuing artificial insemination when first seen in our clinic.

Injections of papaverine and phentolamine induced good erections. The patient's ejaculation frequency increased to two-thirds of the time. He reported, "The injection treatment is working wonderfully. I still don't get good erections without the injections, but our reaction is different; we don't get so frustrated. What surprises us, though, is all the other effects. I feel more normal, more like there's a real place in the world for me. I am more assertive and less depressed. Our relationship is more comfortable and more loving, and the idea that we can get pregnant like everybody else and be normal parents is wonderful." His wife confirmed these changes and added, "I even feel more self-confident. It's funny; even though I knew his problems were physical, I hadn't realized how inadequate I felt and how much I thought things were my fault. You really have turned our lives around." (Althof & Turner, 1992, p. 290)

Self-injections also have significant limitations, though. They are accepted by only 40 to 50 percent of the men referred for such treatment (Althof et al., 1991). Drug treatment also has negative side effects, such as scarring of the penis, liver problems, and occasional experiences of priapism (or prolonged erection in the absence of sexual stimulation).

Hormone replacement therapy—involving, for instance, testosterone—is helpful in treating erectile disorder when the failure is due to a hormonal deficiency. This approach is of little value if the man is within the normal range or hormone levels (Rosen & Leiblum, 1992).

Treatment of Female Sexual Dysfunction

Many of the basic treatment concepts and procedures just described for dysfunctional men are appropriate for dysfunctional women, as well. Like men, women benefit from reducing performance pressure and developing improved verbal and nonverbal communication. In addition, sensate focus exercises encourage the woman to show her partner what she does and does not find sexually arousing, rather than passively allowing him to do what he thinks she wants. The therapist instructs the couple in the details of specific sexual positions for stimulation and intercourse, stressing the importance of timing.

For example, Masters and Johnson's (1970) observations of heterosexual couples having sex revealed that the man typically begins to stimulate his partner's clitoris as soon as sex is initiated. But this immediate stimulation may be ineffective, if not unpleasant, for the woman, unless she is psychologically ready for it. Instead, the man is taught how to stimulate nongenital areas of his partner's body to build up arousal gradually before moving to more direct genital play. This more varied or imaginative pattern of sexual stimulation—carried out with explicit concern for the woman's sensual and sexual pleasure—is very different from the more typical sexual script between man and woman. This latter pattern involves only minimal foreplay, followed by a rapid, male-initiated move to have sexual intercourse. Following sensate focus exercises, the couple proceeds gradually to nondemanding penile insertion, with the woman in the superior coital position, controlling the pace.

As sex therapy has developed, several additional treatment procedures have proved effective in enhancing female sexual responsiveness. A widely used approach with women who have never experienced orgasm is a systematic program of directed masturbation (Heiman, LoPiccolo, & LoPiccolo, 1976). The woman is first taught to familiarize herself with her body—particularly the genital area—and to identify pleasurable sensations. A female therapist then instructs the woman in the intricacies of masturbation, including the use of electric vibrators. Once the woman reaches orgasm through masturbation, her partner is introduced to the procedure by observing her masturbate. This step not only desensitizes the woman to being sexually aroused in his presence. It also provides a learning experience for her partner, who, in the next step of the program, will masturbate her to orgasm. Although most women become orgasmic in response to direct genital stimulation, far fewer achieve orgasm during intercourse with their partners.

In women, sexual dysfunction may also be caused by the decreased production of estrogen, which occurs after menopause or having a hysterectomy. Lower levels of this hormone result in the reduction of lubrication, which may, in turn, result in painful intercourse. This problem may be alleviated through hormone replacement therapy, in which women take estrogen supplements.

Summarizing Treatment Effectiveness

Masters and Johnson (1970) originally claimed that only 19 percent of their patients failed to respond to their sex therapy. But their study has subsequently been criticized as lacking good outcome measures and necessary scientific controls (Zilbergeld & Evans, 1980). Modern sex therapists make more modest claims about the success of their treatments.

Simple sexual problems, uncomplicated by other personal or interpersonal difficulties, are relatively easy to treat—often, without therapy. Women can become orgasmic and men can overcome premature ejaculation using self-help manuals and receiving minimal instruction from therapists (Morokoff & LoPiccolo, 1986). Clinical experience, though, shows that relationship problems tend to complicate sex therapy and hinder its success.

Successful sex therapy for both men and women usually involves more than applying specific methods, such as sensate focus, the squeeze technique, or desensitization. Sex may be part of the balance of politics and power in the marriage. For example, the resolution of a man's erectile failure might drastically alter this balance, threatening an insecure partner for whom the dysfunction served a controlling purpose. Should a man with erectile dysfunction become functional, his partner will be faced with the prospect of greatly increased sexual contact, which she may not want or may even fear. Conversely, improvement in a woman's orgasmic responsiveness might produce erectile problems in her male partner, whose own problems were masked by her sexual inhibitions.

Most sexual disorders require a multimodal approach, including many components: education, desensitization of performance anxiety, changing negative attitudes and dysfunctional beliefs about sex, and improving communication between partners (Rosen, Leiblum, & Spector, 1994). Combinations of psychological and medical treatment are often required.

The special issues involved in treating sexual dysfunctions in gay and lesbian individuals are addressed in Thinking about Multicultural Issues. In sum, Masters and Johnson (1979) carried out the same studies with homosexual couples as they had done with heterosexual couples. The results were surprisingly similar, including those with implications for treatment.

Focus on Critical Thinking

Masters and Johnson (1970) claimed that a couple in sex therapy had to be treated by male and female co-therapists. Their reasoning was that only a female therapist could fully understand a woman's problems and only a male therapist could fully understand a man's difficulties.

1. Do you agree with Masters and Johnson about the need for male and female co-therapists? Why or why not?

2. If you had a sexual problem, would you have any preference for a female or male sex therapist? Explain your answer.

PARAPHILIAS

The study of sex blends modern science with social issues, such as morality and politics. Not unexpectedly, this mix often creates controversy. Any analysis of sexual behavior, then, requires us to think seriously about ethics, law, lifestyles, cultural influences, and the psychological and biological bases of behavior.

Most of us engage in sexual activities that fall within the conventions of the particular society we live in. Some individuals, however, are stimulated by unconventional acts or odd objects. In the *DSM-IV*, these types of sexual activities are labeled **paraphilias.** The term comes from combining two Greek words: *para*, meaning "beyond" or "amiss," and *philia*, meaning "love." Thus, *paraphilias* are sexual disorders in which bizarre or unusual acts, imagery, or objects are required for sexual stimulation. A clinical diagnosis of paraphilia is made only if the individual acts on these unconventional urges or is distressed by them. Most of these acts—such as exhibitionism and voyeurism—are also against the law in the United States. (We will discuss specific types of paraphilias later in this section.)

Previously, paraphilias were labeled using the term *sexual deviance*. The problem with using this label is that it's difficult, if not impossible, to define what is deviant or abnormal. Considerable diversity exists across cultures as to what forms of sexual expression are deviant. Few patterns have universally been disapproved of as being abnormal. Another problem with the term *sexual deviance* is that it implies a judgment. The term *paraphilia* seems more descriptive and less judgmental.

The question of defining what is abnormal remains, nonetheless. Perhaps the most useful approach is to define as abnormal those acts that people feel compelled to do that make them unhappy or that cause distress or harm for other individuals. This definition acknowledges that something that might be considered normal in one context might be considered abnormal in another.

Description

Researchers face unusual difficulties when they try to obtain accurate information on paraphilias. Arrest records of individuals who have committed paraphilias are inadequate sources of data because most paraphiliacs are not caught. Moreover, those who are caught have usually committed a number of offenses—many more than the one they've been arrested for. Thus, researchers must rely on information provided by paraphiliacs. But because their actions are, in most cases, criminal offenses, paraphiliacs remain understandably reluctant to disclose their behavior.

paraphilias Sexual disorders in which bizarre or unusual acts, imagery, or objects are required for sexual stimulation.

Thinking about MULTICULTURAL ISSUES   Sexual Dysfunction in Gays and Lesbians

ntil recently, any discussion of homosexuality in books on abnormal psychology would center on efforts to change homosexuals into heterosexuals. The gay rights movement and an increasing acceptance of alternative lifestyles has changed that. Now, the clinical focus has shifted to helping homosexuals overcome problems that impair their sexual functioning as homosexuals.

Masters and Johnson (1979) carried out the same laboratory studies with homosexual couples as they had done with heterosexual couples. The results were clearcut: Despite their differences in sexual orientation, homosexuals exhibited the same physiological pattern of sexual response as heterosexuals. Homosexuals also experienced the same sexual dysfunctions as heterosexuals. It follows, then, that dysfunctional homosexuals may overcome their sexual difficulties by the same methods used successfully to treat heterosexuals.

Masters and Johnson (1979) treated male and female homosexuals in the same two-week rapid treatment program used to treat heterosexuals. All patients were required to find a same-sex partner willing to participate in the therapy. Masters and Johnson developed definitions of homosexual dysfunctions similar to those of heterosexual dysfunctions. For example, a lesbian with *lifelong (primary) orgasmic dysfunction* was defined as "a person who had never experienced orgasm in response to one of three primary sources of sexual stimulation: masturbation, manual stimulation by partner, or oral sex (cunnilingus)." A gay male with *lifelong (primary) erectile dysfunction* was defined as "someone who had never been able to achieve an erection in response to masturbation (either by self or partner or oral sex)." In sum, the results that Masters and Johnson achieved in treating homosexual couples were as good as those for heterosexual couples.

Modern sex therapists who treat gay men emphasize the importance of confronting negative attitudes about homosexuality. These therapists argue that gay men need to accept their homosexuality, both emotionally and sexually (McCarthy, 1992). Not surprisingly, the devastating impact of AIDS (acquired immune deficiency syndrome) among gay men has had a major impact on sexual behavior and dysfunction. The risk of contracting this deadly disease has increased anxiety about sexual encounters. In one large study of gay men seeking treatment for sexual dysfunction, almost half reported erectile problems (Paff, 1985).

As with heterosexuals, there are gender differences among sexually dysfunctional homosexuals. Masters and Johnson (1979) pointed out that sexually dysfunctional lesbians and their partners were more cooperative and communicated more openly during sex therapy than gay couples with erectile problems.

There is also gender bias regarding research on gays and lesbians. Again, as with heterosexuals, the focus of clinical research is almost entirely on problems in men. If anything, we know even less about sexual dysfunction in homosexual women than in their heterosexual counterparts.

Think about the following questions:

1. Clinical reports suggest that anxiety about contracting AIDS might contribute to erectile problems in some gay men. How would you treat someone who consulted you with such a problem?

2. Imagine that you're a psychotherapist who has been consulted by a young woman. She thinks she's bisexual, since she has had sexual relationships with both men and women. She's unhappy and reports that she is not orgasmic with either men or women. How would you treat her for sexual dysfunction? Explain your answer.

Virtually all the information available on paraphilias comes from men who have been imprisoned for their deviant sexual behavior. But even these individuals may be reluctant to talk to researchers. In the culture of prison, individuals who have committed sexual crimes—such as rape and child sexual abuse—are considered the dregs of the criminal population. These incarcerated men risk violence from fellow prisoners if the nature of their crimes becomes known. Most textbook accounts of the nature of paraphilias, consequently, rely on very limited, if not inaccurate, information.

Research by Abel and his colleagues has overcome the problem of obtaining more accurate information (Abel et al., 1987; Abel, Becker, Cunningham-Rathner, Mittelman, & Rouleau, 1988). Using a certificate of confidentiality from the federal government, these researchers guaranteed privacy to 56 nonincarcerated paraphiliacs seeking voluntary evaluation or treatment at centers in Tennessee and New York City. With this guarantee, these men had little reason to withhold relevant information.

The results of Abel's research have challenged many long-held assumptions about paraphiliacs. Three findings, in particular, stand out:

1. Previous research had suggested that the average paraphiliac commits fewer than two crimes. Abel et al. (1987) found that the number is much higher.
2. Paraphiliacs were previously thought to engage in only one type of deviant behavior. Abel and colleagues (1988) found that these individuals participate in as many as 10 different forms of paraphilia, on average. In fact, it seems rare to find a paraphiliac with a history of having committed only 1 paraphilia.
3. Paraphiliacs often have normal sexual involvements with adult partners that do not involve paraphilic fantasies or activities. Recall from the beginning of this chapter the case of Henry X., who often exposed himself shortly after having satisfactory intercourse with his wife. As with Henry, deviant and nondeviant sexual behaviors coexist in most paraphiliacs.

Given this general description of paraphilias and the individuals who engage in them, we'll look at specific disorders in the following sections.

Exhibitionism   The **exhibitionist**—or "flasher," as he is often called—either exposes his genitals to unsuspecting individuals or has strong and persistent urges and sexually arousing fantasies concerning such exposure. His victims may be adults or children. The exhibitionist's average age at conviction is 30 years. Approximately one-third of these men are married; one-third are separated, divorced, or widowed; and the remaining one-third have never been married.

The exhibitionist acts compulsively in exposing himself and is obsessed with his immediate feelings and intentions. As a result, he becomes oblivious to the consequences of his actions and the danger he may be in. This is what happened to Henry X. He became caught up in a pattern—as most paraphiliacs do—one step leading to another. And with each step, it becomes harder to stop. Here's an analysis of the typical series of events that led up to Henry X. exposing himself:

1. *The trigger*—Different events triggered Henry's acts of exposure. Negative emotions were common precursors. For example, after a heated argument with his father, Henry's anger would often lead him to consider exposure as a means of dealing with his emotion. Even if he were not emotionally upset, particular situations would trigger the urge to expose himself—for example, the sight of a woman standing alone at a bus stop as he drove past in his car.
2. *The fantasy*—Triggers elicited fantasies of exposing himself. He would begin to imagine the details of the woman and how he would feel during the situation. He would develop the image and think about masturbating, either during or shortly after the exposure. The more he fantasized, the stronger the urge became.
3. *Dysfunctional thoughts*—Henry X. would rationalize the act by thinking that he wasn't harming anyone. He even thought that women might actually like it.
4. *The plan*—Once the fantasy had been fully developed, Henry would begin to plan the act. In the case of the solitary woman standing at the bus stop, he would drive around the block several times, trying to ensure that he would not be detected. Then he would drive up, stop the car in front of the woman, open the door, and expose himself.
5. *Acting out*—Once committed to his plan, Henry X. could not seem to turn back. He tuned out everything except his immediate feelings and intentions. He had entered a trancelike state, becoming oblivious to the consequences of his actions. This explains why he didn't realize that he'd been

exhibitionist Man who exposes his genitals to unsuspecting women and has strong and persistent urges and sexually arousing fantasies concerning such exposure.

Thinking about CONTROVERSIAL ISSUES   Pee-Wee's Punishment

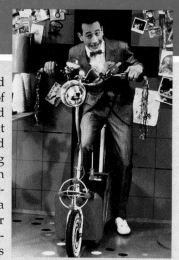

Paul Reubens in his TV role as Pee-Wee Herman

You probably know of Pee-Wee Herman—the movie and TV actor with the goofy grin and weird voice. He made a movie called *Pee-Wee's Big Adventure* and had a Saturday morning TV show on CBS called *Pee-Wee's Playhouse*. The TV show, which started in 1986, was a smash hit and received an Emmy Award. Its audience was primarily young children who were entertained by the dumb but funny things Pee-Wee said and did.

Then, in 1991, everything changed. Paul Reubens—the 39-year-old actor who created and played the role of Pee-Wee Herman—was arrested by the police and charged with "exposure of sexual organs." He had been caught masturbating in a pornographic movie theater in Sarasota, Florida.

Massive publicity followed as soon as the media got hold of this story, and the consequences were swift in coming. CBS immediately canceled Reubens's TV show. The Disney-MGM studio in Orlando withdrew a 2-minute film clip that featured Pee-Wee and was shown as part of a stage tour of the theme park in Florida. Well-known psychologists appeared on TV and radio to advise parents about how to explain this event to their children. Pee-Wee Herman jokes abounded.

Not everyone joined in the public trashing of Reubens. Some raised questions about what he'd been arrested for and criticized CBS for rushing to dismiss him. The truth is, he'd been masturbating—by himself—in a darkened movie theater while watching pornography. Technically, this counts as public exposure, which is illegal.

Think about the following questions:

1. Based on the information presented here, does Reubens have a sexual disorder? Is he a paraphiliac? Why or why not?
2. Should Reubens have been arrested? Was CBS justified in firing him and canceling his TV show? Explain your answers.

seen by the troop of Girl Scouts, whose leader reported him. (Recall from earlier in the chapter that this event landed him in jail, charged with a sexual offense against juveniles.) Henry's attention had been focused on an adult woman. He'd become so engrossed in thinking about and looking at her that he'd failed to see the Girl Scouts arrive on the scene.

The traditional textbook view is that most exhibitionists tend to be inhibited, show no associated psychopathology, and otherwise conform to society's customs. These individuals feel guilty about their problem, are motivated to regain control of their behavior, and often respond well to treatment. Henry X. was a patient like this.

In contrast to this group of so-called pure exhibitionists, a much smaller number have antisocial behavior histories, show personality disturbances, and engage in other illegal activities (Forgac & Michaels, 1982). Abel and colleagues (1988) found that the exhibitionists in their sample frequently engaged in other paraphilias. For example, as many as 46 percent had molested young girls, which is *pedophilia* (discussed in a later section). Several in Abel's sample reported acts of sexual aggression, and 25 percent said that they had raped someone. These findings are clearly contrary to the traditional view of exhibitionists as being harmless nuisances.

The debate about whether exhibitionists are indeed harmless was brought into the public arena in 1991 with the arrest of TV star Paul Reubens—known to millions of children as Pee-Wee Herman. The details of his arrest for exhibitionism and the severe consequences it brought are discussed in Thinking about Controversial Issues.

Voyeurism   The voyeur—or "peeping Tom," as he is often called—is a male whose preferred or exclusive means of gaining sexual excitement is observing unsuspecting women undressing or engaging in sexual activity. The voyeur may masturbate to orgasm while watching the activity or afterward in response to his memory of it. The element of risk seems crucial for the voyeur; his victim must be unaware of being observed.

The majority of voyeurs are young, single, timid men, who are fearful about having direct sexual contact with women. Yet a subcategory of voyeurs who have been arrested are aggressive and may go on to commit sexual assault.

Masochism and Sadism   Although separate paraphilias, **masochism** and **sadism** are closely related. The *masochist* is sexually aroused by fantasizing about or engaging in the act of being dominated, humiliated, or even beaten. The *sadist* is aroused by fantasies or actions involving the domination or beating of another person. The *sadomasochist* responds to both sources of stimulation.

Sadists and masochists get their stimulation from a range of activities, including whipping, biting, burning, and cutting. These rituals may result in injury and even death. For example, a sadomasochist who administers electric shock to his genitals may inadvertently electrocute himself.

Sadism and masochism occur in heterosexual and homosexual individuals. Unlike other paraphilias, sexual masochism occurs in women as well as men. However, the sex ratio is 20 males for every 1 female (American Psychiatric Association, 1994). Clubs and bars labeled "S & M" establishments cater to this clientele. Abel et al. (1988) found that 46 percent of the sadists in their sample of nonincarcerated men reported having committed rape—the highest percentage of rape reported for any category of paraphiliac.

Fetishism   The disorder **fetishism** involves becoming sexually aroused by persistent fantasies about or actual use of nonliving objects, such as women's panties. Often, the fetishist fondles or smells the object while masturbating. Many men are turned on by female partners wearing sexy lingerie; for example, a woman wearing only a garter belt and net stockings is a common pornographic image. This excitement does not constitute a fetish, however, unless the man cannot function sexually without having or thinking about the object. Fetishists tend to be lonely, withdrawn people and lack appropriate social skills.

Transvestic Fetishism   A **transvestite** is a man who becomes sexually aroused by dressing as a woman, which is also known as *cross-dressing*. This behavior is usually done in limited circumstances. The transvestite cross-dresses in secrecy, often with the knowledge of and occasionally the cooperation of his wife. For the most part, though, these men are masculine in appearance and activities. Most are heterosexual and married.

> Jack M.—a married, 31-year-old police officer—suffered from uncontrollable urges to appear in public dressed as a woman. In addition to his transvestism, Jack had a history of sadomasochism. During sexual intercourse with his wife, he tied her to the bed, handcuffed her, and had her wear an animal collar and leash. When he cross-dressed, he also tied himself with ropes, chains, handcuffs, and wires. He was concerned that he would injure himself seriously. His wife had threatened divorce because of his cross-dressing, yet she frequently purchased women's clothing for him and was compassionate while he wore it. This collusion by the wife in the patient's deviant sexual behavior is not unusual (Brownell, Hayes, & Barlow, 1977).

Pedophilia   The unnatural desire to have sexual contact with a prepubescent child (age 13 or younger) is called **pedophilia**. The nature of the sexual contact may vary from genital fondling to sex-

masochism Paraphilia in which an individual becomes sexually aroused by fantasizing about or engaging in being dominated, humiliated, or beaten.

sadism Paraphilia in which an individual is aroused by fantasies or actions involving dominating or beating another person.

fetishism Paraphilia in which an individual becomes sexually aroused by persistent fantasies about or actual use of nonliving objects, such as women's panties.

transvestite Man who become sexually aroused by dressing as a woman.

pedophilia Paraphilia characterized by the unnatural desire to have sexual contact with a prepubescent child (age 13 or younger).

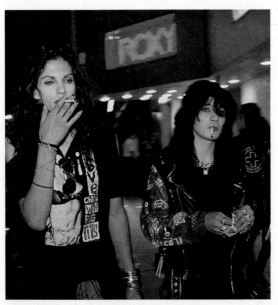
Transvestites are men who dress as women.

ual intercourse. Pedophiles, or *child molesters,* may be males or females. Their targets may be boys or girls of any age—even toddlers.

Pedophilia has been in the news. Within the last few years, celebrities such as singer Michael Jackson and filmmaker Woody Allen were accused of molesting children in highly publicized scandals. And over the last decade, the Catholic Church has reportedly paid millions of dollars to cover legal costs and settlements arising out of numerous charges against priests for molesting young boys and girls (Sleek, 1994).

In July 1985, the *Los Angeles Times* conducted a telephone poll of a random sample of 2,627 men and women from every state in the United States. The results made front page news: 27 percent of the women and 16 percent of the men reported having been sexually abused as children (*Los Angeles Times*, 1985). Most cases of abuse involved physical contact. Fully one-third of the individuals polled had never disclosed their history of abuse to anyone; only 3 percent had contacted the police.

These numbers indicate how widespread but hidden child sexual abuse is. Children may be too frightened to tell their parents what's happened. Pedophiles are usually very effective in manipulating their victims to participate and then keep quiet about it. Even if parents find out their children have been sexually abused, they might be unwilling to go to the police or child protective services for fear of negative publicity and unwanted attention.

Public and professional awareness of the alarming incidence of child sexual abuse—both within and outside the family—may appear to be a recent phenomenon. But the problem was identified professionally almost 100 years ago by none other than Freud. Virtually all his female patients who suffered from what Freud called "hysterical illness" reported having been sexually abused as children. In most cases, the women had been abused by their fathers, which is called *incest* (discussed later in this section). Freud hypothesized that child sexual abuse was the main cause of adult neurotic behavior.

This idea—the **seduction theory of neurosis**—was widely rejected by Freud's colleagues. Within two years, Freud changed his mind about the source of his patients' neuroses. He decided that his patients had not really experienced incest; rather, they unconsciously wished to have sex with their fathers (Masson, 1984). This new theory was called the **theory of infantile sexuality** and became a cornerstone of psychoanalysis.

Freud's abandonment of the seduction theory was unfortunate, for several reasons. We know today that Freud was more correct with the first theory: that being sexually abused as a child contributes significantly to the risk of developing mental disorders later in life (Burnam et al., 1988). We also know that in the past, female patients' reports of sexual abuse to their therapists were misinterpreted as unconscious fantasies. Consequently, the women who were molested were often held responsible for their own abusive experiences (Crewdson, 1988).

A study of 453 male pedophiles by Abel (1989) has cast new light on the dimensions of pedophilia. Of these men, more had assaulted girls than boys. But those who had assaulted boys had done so more frequently. Sixty-three percent of all reported victims were males. Many pedophiles abuse both boys and girls—children within and outside the family.

Pedophiles and the children they abuse are drawn from all socioeconomic and educational levels (Abel et al., 1987). There are no differences between blacks and whites (Crewdson, 1988). Pedophiles often try to justify their behavior. For instance, they may claim that children who do not physically resist really want to have sex with them or that they are performing a service by teaching the children about sex. Like other paraphiliacs, pedophiles may engage in other forms of paraphilia, including rape (Abel et al., 1988). When the pedophile and his or her victim are related, the offense is **incest.**

Textbooks have traditionally differentiated between nonincestuous and incestuous child molesters. The former were said to be attracted to younger victims than the latter. A common stereotype of the incestuous child molester is the man under

seduction theory of neurosis Early Freudian theory that neurotic disorders in women were caused primarily by having been sexually abused as children.

theory of infantile sexuality Freud's revised theory, in which he assumed that patients' reports of child sexual abuse were not real, instead reflecting their unconscious desire for sex with their fathers.

incest Sexual relations between family members; typically, sex between fathers and daughters or between siblings.

stress, turning to his daughter for the emotional support or sexual expression not available from his wife. But if this scenario were realistic, why wouldn't the man have extramarital affairs with other adult women? What makes him turn to a child? Abel et al. (1988) reject this traditional view and conclude that the incestuous pedophile turns to a child because he's generally attracted to young girls or young boys. A large proportion of pedophiles who molest their own sons or daughters molest children from outside the family, as well (Abel et al., 1988).

Other Paraphilias   Although we won't discuss them in detail, you should be familiar with several other paraphilias:

- *frotteurism*—sexual urges involving touching or rubbing against a nonconsenting and unsuspecting person
- *necrophilia*—sexual obsession with corpses, perhaps including intercourse
- *klismaphilia*—sexual excitement that results from having enemas
- *coprophilia*—sexual interest in feces
- *zoophilia*—sexual gratification from having sexual activity with animals

Causes

Psychodynamic Theory   According to psychodynamic theory, all paraphilias are expressions of a common underlying psychopathology—namely, a form of personality disturbance. Thus, a pathological sexuality derives from unconscious, intrapsychic conflicts originating in early childhood. For example, the exhibitionist defends himself against underlying castration fears. The observer's reaction to the sight of his genitals supposedly reassures him that he has not been castrated. For the transvestite, cross-dressing as a female serves as his symbolical protection against castration.

Robert Stoller, a prominent psychoanalytic authority on sexual disorders, has argued that sexual aggression (for example, sadomasochism) is simply a more extreme form of the same sexual drive that arouses people who engage in conventional sexual activities. According to this view, the difference between giving someone a "love bite" and committing rape is only one of degree. Stoller asserts, "It is hostility—the desire, overt or hidden, to harm another person—that generates sexual excitement" (1979, p. 6). Thus, it follows that sadomasochists and other sexual aggressives act out their unconscious hostilities, whereas normal individuals restrict this drive to the fantasy level or subordinate it to positive feelings of affection.

Abel (1989) rejects this theory of specific paraphilias being the products of particular psychological conflicts. Instead, he points to evidence that shows that paraphiliacs suffer from a generalized lack of control over their sexual arousal and behavior.

Cognitive-Behavioral Theory   A behavioral, or social learning, analysis of what causes paraphilias emphasizes the importance of interpersonal and environmental factors. Kinsey originally outlined this view:

> Learning and conditioning in connection with human sexual behavior involve the same sorts of processes as learning and conditioning in other types of behavior. . . . From its parents, from other adults, from other children, and from the community at large, the child begins to acquire its attitudes toward such things as nudity, the anatomic differences between males and females and the reproductive functions; and these attitudes may have considerable significance in determining its subsequent acceptance or avoidance of particular types of overt sexual activity. (Kinsey et al., 1953, pp. 644–645)

Masturbation may be the key. Males masturbate frequently and early in their psychological development. And when they do, they fantasize about a variety of specific sexual stimuli—sometimes, deviant or unconventional stimuli. Each time a fantasy is associated with masturbation, a trial of classical conditioning occurs (see Chapter 2). Orgasm is a very powerful form of reinforcement. Research has shown that repeatedly pairing sexual arousal with a formerly neutral stimulus can experimentally induce a mild fetish. Rachman and Hodgson (1968) showed that penile erection in response to pornographic stimuli could be classically conditioned using a previously neutral stimulus—for example, a boot.

Parents may model and maintain deviant sexuality patterns through direct and vicarious reinforcement. Stoller's (1967) study of transvestites, for example, revealed that wives and mothers could initiate men into transvestism by providing strong reinforcement for dressing in feminine clothes. The following adult transvestite's narrative illustrates the influence of social learning in developing this behavior:

> The highlights of my life as a girl came when I was between the ages of ten and seventeen. I had an aunt who was childless and wanted to take me through the steps from childhood to young womanhood. She knew of my desires to be a girl. I would spend every summer at her ranch. The first thing she would do was to give me a pixie haircut, which always turned out pretty good since I would avoid getting a haircut for two months before I went to her ranch. She then would take me into the bedroom and show me all my pretty new things she had bought me. The next day, dressed as a girl, I would accompany her to town and we would shop for a new dress for me. To everyone she met, she would introduce me as her "niece." This went on every year until I was thirteen years old. Then she decided I should start my womanhood. I will never forget that summer. When I arrived I got the same pixie haircut as usual but when we went into the bedroom there laid out on the bed was a girdle, a garter belt and bra, size 32AA, and my first pair of nylons. She then took me over to the new dressing table she had bought me and slid back the top to reveal my very own makeup kit. I was thrilled to death. She said she wanted her "niece" to start off right and it was time I started to develop a bust. The next morning I was up early to ready myself for the usual shopping trip to town, only this time it was for a pair of high heels and a new dress. I remember I stuffed my bra with cotton, put on my garter belt, and slipped on my nylons with no effort. After all, I became an expert from practice the night before. My aunt applied my lipstick because I was so excited I couldn't get it on straight. Then off to town we went, aunt and "niece." What a wonderful day. I shall never forget it. (Stoller, 1967, p. 335)

A Psychobiological Model   John Money is arguably the world's leading expert on how the complex links among anatomy, hormones, and life experience determine a person's sexuality. Together with colleague Margaret Lamacz, he has proposed a novel theory of the early development of paraphilias (Money & Lamacz, 1989).

The core concept is that paraphilias result when the natural link between romantic love and sexual lust is blocked or distorted in some way. In the natural psychobiology of sexual development, a pattern of brain functioning is established that determines what the person will find sexually arousing. Money and Lamacz (1989) call this brain program a **lovemap.** They believe that it's developed between the ages of 5 and 8 years. Traumatic childhood experiences, such as sexual abuse or emotional neglect, can disrupt the patterning of the lovemap. Errors may be programmed into the map that involve either the displacement or distortion of elements within the sequence of behaviors that normally lead to sexual activity for that species. These sorts of behaviors, which are characteristic of a species, are called *phyletic* behaviors. For example, fondling a sexual partner is normal for humans. Doing so becomes abnormal, though (a paraphilia), when the behavior is displaced—as when someone like Henry X. becomes aroused by rubbing against an unsuspecting stranger (frotteurism). Money and Lamacz believe that having a strict upbringing, in a family with

lovemap Hypothesized pattern of brain functioning that determines what sexual imagery and actions an individual will find stimulating.

repressive attitudes toward sex, puts individuals at risk for the development of paraphilias. These researchers discount the influence of pornography, asserting that men with abnormal lovemaps seek deviant pornography.

Although it's original, Money and Lamacz's (1989) lovemap theory fails to address some important questions. For instance, only a small subset of children who experience traumatic life experiences go on to develop paraphilias. What is special about this subset? Money and Lamacz answer that these individuals have some inherent vulnerability to acquiring a lovemap that's programmed with errors. But there is no evidence to suggest what this vulnerability might be.

The Cycle of Abuse   It's widely believed that children who are sexually abused are at increased risk for becoming abusers themselves (Crewdson, 1988). The common assumption is that the experience of being sexually abused steers the individual in the direction of becoming an offender.

Seligman (1994) has proposed an alternative explanation. He correctly points out that abused children—especially those who have experienced incest—very often come from dysfunctional families. The members of these families have higher rates of psychopathology than people in the population at large. For example, the father or older brother who abuses the younger child likely has other clinical disorders in addition to pedophilia. These associated problems might be responsible for the child who's been abused eventually becoming an offender.

Moreover, it's likely that some of this pattern of family disturbance is passed on genetically. It follows, then, that genetics might also influence the development of pedophilia. Based on their detailed review of the literature, Abel and colleagues (1992) point out that there is no satisfactory evidence to support the hypothesis that abused individuals become abusers.

Paraphilias are confined almost exclusively to men. Nonetheless, recent reports have identified females who have molested young boys and girls (Sleek, 1994). The evidence suggests that these female pedophiles suffer from associated clinical disorders (O'Connor, 1987). For instance, they share a history of acting out sexually before adolescence and report high rates of depression, posttraumatic stress disorder (PTSD), and suicidal thinking. They often use force or the threat of force to overcome their victims, and they frequently carry out their offenses while babysitting young children. As with male paraphiliacs, these women are believed to have been sexually abused as children (Sleek, 1994).

To explain this gender gap, Money and Lamacz (1989) propose that something goes wrong with development of the lovemap. The prenatal, structural differentiation of the male fetus is more complex than that of the female. It follows that sexual development is more complex in the male and thus more subject to errors. These errors involve either the displacement or distortion of elements within the sequence of behaviors leading to sexual activity.

The social learning explanation of the male/female difference in paraphilia emphasizes the greater role that visual cues and fantasy play in male as opposed to female sexual arousal. In comparison with heterosexual women, both heterosexual and homosexual men were found more responsive to visual sexual stimuli (Bailey, Gaulin, Agyei, & Gladue, 1994). Moreover, as noted earlier, males masturbate more often and earlier in development, employing vivid fantasies about specific sexual stimuli.

Treatment

Psychological Therapies   Paraphilias may be treated using psychodynamic, cognitive-behavioral, and drug therapies. Lengthy psychodynamic treatment has not proven effective with these problems, but alternative therapies have been successful (Abel, Osborn, Anthony, & Gardos, 1992).

Cognitive-behavioral treatments focus on five major areas:

1. suppression or elimination of the individual's unwanted or undesirable sexual arousal
2. substitution of a more acceptable source of sexual arousal and behavior
3. development of self-control or coping skills to resist the problem behavior
4. cognitive restructuring
5. relapse prevention training

Let's look at each area in turn. To address the first area, aversion therapy is used to suppress unwanted sexual arousal. Although different methods have been used, the most common employs aversive imagery. In this technique of **covert sensitization,** the patient first imagines engaging in the deviant behavior and then imagines an aversive consequence occurring. For example, as part of Henry X.'s therapy, he was instructed to imagine that just as he approached a woman and planned to expose himself to her, a police car with flashing red lights and blaring siren pulled up and he was apprehended.

One advantage of this technique is that it teaches the patient to use a self-control method any time he feels the urge to expose himself. For the technique to be effective, the patient must repeatedly and actively rehearse this association between his deviant activities and realistic aversive consequences. Based on his clinical practice, Maletzky (1980) reported a success rate of roughly 90 percent in treating exhibitionists with aversive imagery. This success rate held up in follow-up evaluations for up to 2.5 years. In the absence of controlled research, however, we should interpret this estimate of success with caution.

In addressing the second area, orgasmic reconditioning helps paraphiliacs develop sexual arousal to more conventional heterosexual activities. Consider, for example, the treatment of Jack M., the transvestite police officer described earlier. In therapy, he was instructed to continue to masturbate in his usual fashion to deviant fantasies of cross-dressing and sadomasochism. Then, just prior to ejaculatory inevitability (the point at which the male ejaculates involuntarily), he was to switch to an erotic fantasy of more conventional heterosexual behavior. To ease this switch to heterosexual arousal, Jack was given pictures of nude women from magazines. Gradually, he made the switch earlier and earlier in the sequence, until he could initiate masturbation and reach orgasm exclusively using heterosexual fantasies. Prior to treatment, Jack had shown virtually no arousal to conventional heterosexual stimuli. Following approximately 20 sessions of orgasmic reconditioning, he displayed strong erections to it.

Next, self-control training begins with assessing the thoughts, feelings, and events preceding exposure. The patient is shown how he actively contributes to his problem by focusing on inappropriate thoughts and feelings. He learns to recognize early warning signs of the temptation to expose himself and then to institute self-control procedures at that point. If he waits too long and the temptation becomes too strong, his chances of self-control greatly diminish. If tension or anxiety lead to exposure, the patient is taught relaxation procedures as an alternative means of control. Social-skills training helps the individual learn how to relate better to adult partners.

The fourth area of treatment—cognitive restructuring—is designed to alter distorted thinking. Many men with paraphilias deny wrongdoing. They try to rationalize their behavior and to minimize its impact on others. For example, Henry X. always referred to the women he exposed himself to as "the other party." He tried to make it sound as if these women were somehow active participants. Therapy focused on helping Henry accept that the women were unwilling victims and on getting him to take personal responsibility for his behavior. Current treatment programs train patients to develop empathy for their victims—in other words, to put themselves in their victims' places and to try to feel how threatening and abusive the experience is. Henry X., for example, was asked to play the role of the woman in an exposure episode.

covert sensitization
Behavior therapy technique used to decrease a patient's desire for negative sexual activity; patient is taught to use imagery that links a negative consequence with the activity.

Finally, treatment emphasizes relapse prevention (Laws, 1989). The risk of relapse following initially successful therapy is high in paraphilic disorders. The first step in **relapse prevention training** is to educate patients about the probability of relapse. Next, patients are taught to identify and anticipate the early warning signs of the return of their deviant behavior. The third step is to help patients rehearse cognitive and behavioral methods for coping with high-risk triggers that increase the likelihood of relapse. Finally, patients are coached to deal with a lapse in behavior—whether having a strong paraphilic fantasy or committing a sexual act. Instead of giving up and experiencing a full-blown relapse, patients are prepared to get back on track by implementing self-control strategies or seeking therapeutic help immediately.

The lack of well-controlled outcome studies makes it difficult to evaluate the effectiveness of cognitive-behavioral treatment programs. The relapse rate has ranged from 3 percent to 31 percent in different studies, depending on the type of patient population and the length of follow-up (Abel et al., 1992). A study at the Vermont State Corrections program revealed that of 147 pedophiles, only 3 percent had relapses during a 6-year follow-up (Pithers, Martin, & Cumming, 1989). The relapse rate for rapists in the same program was much higher (see Chapter 17).

An important study in California (Goleman, 1992b) compared the outcome of men treated with cognitive-behavioral therapy with that of a control group matched for type of paraphilia. Among the pedophiles, 5 percent of those from the treatment group committed a new offense within 3 years of being released from prison, compared with 9 percent of the control group. In general, treatment cuts the relapse rate by roughly half. Nonetheless, the overall results of treatment are modest, at best.

Pharmacological Therapies In the past decade, we have seen a dramatic increase in the use of chemical treatments to reduce paraphilic behavior. One class of drugs used in such therapy are hormonal agents. Cyproterone acetate (CPA) is an **antiandrogen drug** that reduces testosterone level. The drug virtually eliminates relapse among paraphiliacs, provided they continue to take sufficiently high doses that reduce their testosterone levels by at least 30 percent (Bradford, 1989). A related antiandrogen drug is medroxyprogesterone acetate (MPA), more commonly known as Depo-Provera or Provera. This is the most frequently used drug treatment for paraphilias in the United States; CPA is unavailable here but is used in Europe.

A second class of drugs involves nonhormonal agents. Preliminary research has shown that the antidepressant drug Prozac significantly decreases deviant fantasies and behavior without interfering with conventional heterosexual functioning (Kafka & Prentky, 1991). The promising results obtained with drugs such as this encourage therapists to search for safe and more effective chemical treatments that could be combined with psychological methods of treating paraphilias.

relapse prevention training Therapeutic strategy that prepares patients to cope with threats to self-control and thus to prevent relapse.

antiandrogen drug Used to reduce testosterone level in treating males with sexual disorders.

Focus on Critical Thinking

1. Recall from the chapter-opening case that Henry X. had never been violent toward anyone; he had been arrested for exposing himself before, however. His latest arrest was for exposing himself to some adolescent girls, a more serious offense than the others. The public prosecutor wants to send Henry X. to jail for a long time. Do you think this would be an appropriate course of action? Explain your answer.

2. Imagine that you are a counselor at a local high school. An exhibitionist has been caught exposing himself to students as they leave school one day. You are asked to talk to the youths about this experience. What would you say to them? What would you say about the exhibitionist?

Administration of Therapies Treatment doesn't work for all sex offenders—especially the most violent and the most dangerous. And of those who are helped initially, many subsequently relapse, posing a growing problem for public safety.

A far bigger threat to society, though, is this reality: Only a minority of individuals who are imprisoned for sexual offenses such as pedophilia receive effective treatment before eventually being released. Estimates are that at least 75 percent of all jailed sex offenders get no treatment at all (Goleman, 1992b). So once they're released from prison, these individuals will very likely repeat their crimes (see Chapter 17).

GENDER-IDENTITY DISORDERS

Gender-Identity Disorder

Description   An individual's *sexual identity* is his or her biological designation—namely, male or female. **Gender-role identity** is the individual's perception of himself or herself as consistently male or female. Individuals with **gender-identity disorder** want to be members of the opposite sex. They identify completely with members of that sex. For example, a man might insist that he's "a woman trapped in a man's body." The *DSM-IV* table summarizes the diagnostic criteria for gender-identity disorder.

Before the *DSM-IV* (American Psychiatric Association, 1994) was issued, the term used to describe an individual with gender-identity disorder was **transsexual.** His or her usual goal was to obtain a sex-change operation—that is, surgery that would alter his or her body to become that of the opposite sex. This is a very rare disorder. Based on data from European studies, roughly 1 per 30,000 adult males and 1 per 100,000 adult females seek sex-change surgery (American Psychiatric Association, 1994).

We shouldn't confuse *transsexuals* with *transvestites* or *homosexuals*. As discussed in the previous section, transvestites are almost always heterosexuals who achieve

Diagnostic Criteria for 302.6 GENDER-IDENTITY DISORDER

A. A strong and persistent cross-gender identification (not merely a desire for any perceived cultural advantages of being the other sex).

In children, the disturbance is manifested by four (or more) of the following:

(1) repeatedly stated desire to be, or insistence that he or she is, the other sex

(2) in boys, preference for cross-dressing or simulating female attire; in girls, insistence on wearing only stereotypical masculine clothing

(3) strong and persistent preferences for cross-sex roles in make-believe play or persistent fantasies of being the other sex

(4) intense desire to participate in the stereotypical games and pastimes of the other sex

(5) strong preference for playmates of the other sex

In adolescents and adults, the disturbance is manifested by symptoms such as a stated desire to be the other sex, frequent passing as the other sex, desire to live or be treated as the other sex, or the conviction that he or she has the typical feelings and reactions of the other sex.

B. Persistent discomfort with his or her sex or sense of inappropriateness in the gender role of that sex.

In children, the disturbance is manifested by any of the following: in boys, assertion that his penis or testes are disgusting or will disappear or assertion that it would be better not to have a penis, or aversion toward rough-and-tumble play and rejection of male stereotypical toys, games, and activities; in girls, rejection of urinating in a sitting position, assertion that she has or will grow a penis, or assertion that she does not want to grow breasts or menstruate, or marked aversion toward normative feminine clothing.

In adolescents and adults, the disturbance is manifested by symptoms such as preoccupation with getting rid of primary and secondary sex characteristics (e.g., request for hormones, surgery, or other procedures to physically alter sexual characteristics to simulate the other sex) or belief that he or she was born the wrong sex.

C. The disturbance is not concurrent with a physical intersex condition.*

D. The disturbance causes clinically significant distress or impairment in social, occupational, or other important areas of functioning.

*For example, androgen insensitivity syndrome

gender-role identity
Individual's self-perception as consistently masculine or feminine in characteristics and behavior.

gender-identity disorder
Paraphilia in which an individual wants to be a member of the opposite sex.

transsexual Individual with gender-identity disorder; wishes to be a member of the opposite sex.

specific sexual satisfaction by cross-dressing. They don't fundamentally and consistently identify with the opposite sex, like transsexuals do. Gender-role identity, defined earlier, distinguishes transsexuals from transvestites.

Sexual orientation—whether heterosexual or homosexual—is yet another matter. A transsexual man is usually sexually attracted to other men. For the man who's had a sex-change operation—biologically becoming a woman—*her* sexual orientation is heterosexual. She relates to men as a woman does. But transsexuals may also have a homosexual orientation. *Gender role* is a behavioral characteristic that differs from both gender-role identity and sexual orientation. Gender role refers to what men and women do—what activities they prefer and how masculine or feminine they appear.

Gender-identity disorder can occur in young children as well as adolescents and adults. A boy with this disorder will find his genitals disgusting. His behavior will go well beyond the fairly typical tendency of some young boys, for example, to dress up occasionally in their mother's clothes or assume the role of a girl in play. The boy with gender-identity disorder does so persistently, rejecting typical boys' games. Behavior such as cross-dressing is not an isolated act but part of a consistent pattern or syndrome. For girls, gender-identity disorder is marked by a comparable unhappiness about their anatomy and the desire to possess a penis and be a boy.

In the following excerpt, a mother describes her 8-year-old son, who seems to have gender-identity disorder:

> **Mother:** He acts like a sissy. He has expressed the wish to be a girl. He doesn't play with boys. He's afraid of boys, because he's afraid to play boys' games. He used to like to dress in girls' clothing. He would still like to, only we have absolutely put our foot down. And he talks like a girl, sometimes walks like a girl, acts like a girl.
>
> **Therapist:** How long have you had these concerns?
>
> **Mother:** For about three years.
>
> **Therapist:** What was the very earliest thing that you noticed?
>
> **Mother:** Wanting to put on a blouse of mine, a pink and white blouse which if he'd put it on would fit him like a dress. And he was very excited about the whole thing, and leaped around and danced around the room. I didn't like it and I just told him to take it off and I put it away. He kept asking for it. He wanted to wear that blouse again. And I said, "No, I'm sorry that belongs to me, not to you. You wear your clothes and I wear mine." But he asked many times for it.
>
> **Therapist:** You mentioned that he's expressed the wish to be a girl.
>
> **Mother:** I remember distinctly his making this remark. And it's such a dramatic remark that you don't forget it. He'd make it many times.
>
> **Therapist:** What does he say, exactly?
>
> **Mother:** "I would like to be a girl. I don't like to be a boy. Boys are too rough. When I play boys' games the ball hurts my legs. I don't want to go to school today because I'll have to play baseball." So he goes and plays gently with the girls.
>
> **Therapist:** Has he ever said, "I am a girl"?
>
> **Mother:** Playing in front of the mirror, he'll undress for bed, and he's standing in front of the mirror and he took his penis and he folded it under, and he said, "Look, Mommy, I'm a girl." (Green, 1987, pp. 2–3)

Causes   Researchers don't know what causes gender-identity disorder. Among the possible biological influences are the effects of prenatal hormones. Some findings indicate that young boys whose mothers took female hormones during pregnancy may show fewer so-called masculine behaviors (Yalom, Green, & Fisk, 1973). But there's no evidence that mothers' taking hormones caused their children to have gender-identity disorder or adult transsexualism. It's not unusual for young boys to engage in some stereotypically feminine activities and for young girls to participate in some masculine activities. By themselves, these activities do not indicate or cause any abnormal gender development.

Both psychodynamic and behavioral theories emphasize the importance of early childhood experiences in psychosexual development. Psychodynamic theorists believe that for normal sexual development to occur, the child must identify successfully with the parent of the opposite sex. Behavioral theorists also focus on parents as role models and sources of social reinforcement (Rosen & Hall, 1984). Yet the family environment seems to have surprisingly little effect on the development of gender disorders. Green (1978) studied 16 children reared by transsexual parents. Most of the children knew about their parents' sex changes. All became heterosexual, and none developed gender-identity problems.

Researchers cannot even predict with any certainty that children with gender-identity disorder will become transsexuals as adults. Many become heterosexual

(Zucker, Finegan, Deering, & Bradley, 1984), and others become homosexual or bisexual, as discussed later (Green, 1987).

Treatment   In the 1960s, **sex reassignment surgery** became an established form of treating transsexuals. In the male-to-female reassignment, the man first takes estrogens to develop breasts and other female characteristics. Next, he is castrated, and an artificial clitoris and vagina are constructed. In the female-to-male reassignment, the woman initially takes androgens to reduce her breasts, develop male characteristics, and stop menstruation. A surgeon then removes her uterus and remaining breast tissue and constructs a penis; this organ is unsatisfactory for intercourse, however, and cannot be stimulated to orgasm.

The merits of sex reassignment surgery have been vigorously debated. One influential study found that transsexuals who had undergone surgery were no better adjusted subsequently than those who had not (Meyer & Reter, 1979). This study has been criticized for various methodological inadequacies, however, including the failure to assess patients' psychological adaptation (Lothstein, 1982). The best estimate is that roughly two-thirds of patients show improved adjustment following sex reassignment surgery, with female-to-male subjects faring better (Abramowitz, 1986). The negative outcome rate of this surgery is significant, as well: About 7 percent of subjects request surgical reversal, require psychiatric hospitalization, or commit suicide.

Psychological treatment of gender-identity disorder has been limited primarily to behavioral methods. Although some successful case studies have been reported (Barlow, Abel, & Blanchard, 1979; Khanna, Desai, & Channabasavanna, 1987), controlled studies are lacking and few therapists have adopted these methods. The treatment of gender-identity disorder in young boys has been highly controversial, as illustrated in the following case study by Rekers and Lovaas (1974):

> Kraig was a physically normal 5-year-old boy who was referred for treatment by the family physician. He had cross-dressed since the age of 2, played with cosmetic items belonging to his mother and grandmother, displayed exaggerated feminine mannerisms, preferred to play with little girls, and emphasized his desire to be a girl. The two therapists, Rekers and Lovaas, helped Kraig's mother alter her behavior to reinforce more masculine activities and decrease gender-inappropriate behavior. The result was that Kraig's gender disorder decreased dramatically, and he began to act in a more masculine manner. Using sophisticated methodological control procedures, Rekers and Lovaas were able to show that this behavioral change was due directly to the reinforcement procedures that formed the basis of the treatment program. At a follow-up over two years later, Kraig looked and acted like any other boy his age.
>
> The therapists justified their treatment program on the following grounds: This sort of exaggerated feminine behavior in boys makes them subject to social isolation and ridicule by their peers. Cross-gender preferences predict severe adjustment problems in adulthood. (Most adult transsexuals and transvestites report a history of childhood gender disturbances.) Altering cross-gender preferences is most likely to be successful during early development. The treatment program was consistent with the parents' wishes, social mores and cultural expectations of the community the family lived in, local laws, and views of other professionals. The child also cooperated throughout the program.

Critics of this sort of treatment program have argued that adult pathology, such as transsexualism, cannot be reliably predicted from highly effeminate behavior displayed in early childhood. They have also noted the emphasis placed on the masculine gender role in programs such as the one described. As an alternative, they advocate the idea of androgyny (Winkler, 1977). *Androgyny* is the state of being neither masculine nor feminine, in the stereotypical sense. It includes supposedly desirable attributes from each gender—for example, strength and independence

sex reassignment surgery
Surgery performed to physically change an individual's sexual identity from male to female or vice versa; an established means of treating transsexuals.

from the masculine role; affection and compassion from the feminine role. Supporters of this view assert that androgynous behavior is more likely to lead to better adjustment than extreme sex-role typing as masculine or feminine.

In addition to the ethical issues raised by this type of operant conditioning program, there are questions about its efficacy, as well. In comparison to the outcomes reported by Rekers (1982), Green (1987) reported far less success in trying to change the sexual identity of these boys.

Sexual Disorders Not Otherwise Specified

The *DSM-IV* (American Psychiatric Association, 1994) diagnosis of "Sexual Disorders Not Otherwise Specified" is reserved for problems that are neither sexual dysfunctions nor paraphilias. One example of a disorder in this category is "Persistent and Marked Distress about Sexual Orientation" (p. 538). The story behind the development of this seemingly innocuous description has been one of the major controversies in the study of abnormal psychology. It's the debate about the nature of homosexuality.

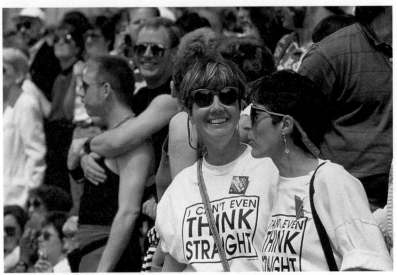

Protests by gays and lesbians have helped change how homosexuality is perceived by mental health professionals.

In the second edition of the *Diagnostic and Statistical Manual of Mental Disorders (DSM-II)*, published in 1968, the American Psychiatric Association officially listed homosexuality as a major clinical disorder. In response to pressure from gay activist groups and concerned professionals, this designation was changed in the *DSM-III*, published in 1980. Homosexuality was no longer inevitably seen as a form of psychopathology. The *DSM-III* recognized homosexuality as a possible nonpathological, alternative lifestyle. The category "Ego-Dystonic Homosexuality" was, nevertheless, included as a diagnosis for those homosexuals who were distressed by their sexual orientation and wanted to become heterosexuals. The word *homosexuality* cannot be found in the *DSM-IV* (1994). But the category mentioned earlier— "Persistent and Marked Distress about Sexual Orientation"—seems to refer to anxiety over being homosexual, not heterosexual.

Homosexuality: Fact and Fiction Psychodynamic theory was very influential in shaping clinicians' views of homosexuality. In this view, homosexuality is caused by having an overprotective, close-binding mother and a distant, ineffectual father. As a result of these negative parental influences, the person is believed to get stuck at an immature level of psychosexual development (Bieber et al., 1962). There is no evidence to support this view, though.

A study by Green (1987) followed 44 extremely feminine boys for 15 years— from early childhood to adolescence or young adulthood. Three-fourths of these boys later became homosexuals or bisexuals (that is, individuals who are attracted to both sexes). The results from this group are greatly different than those from a comparison group of typically masculine boys, in which only 1 boy became a homosexual. In cases in which parents tried to discourage feminine behavior, their sons' homosexual tendencies were lessened but not reversed. Similarly, treatment by professionals designed to alter this pattern of behavior did not prevent later homosexuality, although the boys did show more typical masculine behavior. No consistent evidence was found to indicate that parents shaped their feminine sons, causing them to be homosexuals. In fact, some parents had other typically masculine sons. These findings support the view that some individuals have a biological predisposition to homosexuality.

Several major research findings in the past few years have established the biological basis of homosexuality. The first finding points to anatomical differences between the brains of heterosexual and homosexual men. One difference is in the anterior commissure, which is a bundle of nerve fibers that allows the two halves of the brain to communicate with each other. It's larger in gay men than in heterosexual men or women (Allen & Gorski, 1992). A second difference is that the hypothalamus is smaller in gay men than in heterosexual men (LeVay, 1991). Some critics have pointed out that these differences in brain structure might be a *consequence* rather than a *cause* of sexual orientation (Byne & Parsons, 1993). However, animal studies have shown that sexual differences in brain structure occur early during prenatal development (Hooper, 1991). This determination makes it unlikely that the differences in brain structure that have been identified are the results of a gay lifestyle.

A second major finding points to the genetic basis of male homosexuality. Twin studies of both gay men and lesbians show significantly higher concordance rates for homosexuality between identical (monozygotic) twins than fraternal (dizygotic) twins (Bailey, Pillard, Neale, & Agyei, 1993). In other words, it was more likely among identical twins that both individuals were homosexual. This supports the genetic basis of homosexuality because identical twins develop from a single fertilized egg and thus have the same genetic makeup. (Fraternal twins develop from separate eggs and are genetically different.)

Other evidence comes from a study using DNA linkage analysis of the families of gay men (Hamer, Hu, Magnuson, Hu, & Pattatucci, 1993). The rates of homosexuality among the brothers, maternal uncles, and maternal male cousins of these gay men were much higher than rates among the general population. DNA analysis traced this pattern of inheritance to a gene that lies within a small stretch of the X chromosome. This gene is inherited by men from their mothers.

The third major finding in support of the biological basis of homosexuality is that gay and heterosexual men differ in specific cognitive abilities that reflect differences in brain architecture. On tests of visual/spatial ability, the scores of gay men fell between those of heterosexual men, at one extreme, and heterosexual women, at the other (Witelson, 1991). This and related findings have led to the view that gay men represent a "third sex" at the neurological level.

Collectively, these findings strongly support the view that heredity plays an important role in homosexuality. The traditional view that homosexuality is simply a product of childhood learning has no scientific basis. Likewise, the claim seems groundless that gays and lesbians choose their sexual lifestyle—something people who oppose gay rights have long argued.

Treatment   A critical implication of this biologically based view is that changing an adult's sexual orientation should be difficult, if not impossible. Research has shown that it is. Psychotherapies aimed at changing sexual orientation—including hundreds of hours of intensive psychoanalytic therapy—have proven ineffective (Bancroft, 1974). Behavior therapy has not fared much better, particularly with homosexuals who have no history of heterosexual interest (O'Leary & Wilson, 1987).

Instead of trying to convert homosexuals into heterosexuals, current therapies are designed to help gays and lesbians lead more fulfilling lives as homosexuals. Specific treatments for sexual dysfunction among gays and lesbians were discussed in the Thinking about Multicultural Issues box.

Focus on Critical Thinking

In a controversial paper, Davison (1976) argued that no therapist should try to help a homosexual patient become heterosexual, even if doing so seemed to be what the patient wanted. To try to bring about this change, Davison insisted, would be to support society's bias and prejudice against homosexuality.

1. Do you agree with Davison? Explain your answer.
2. Might there be certain circumstances in which a therapist should try to help a homosexual patient convert to heterosexuality? Explain your answer.

SUMMARY

Sexual Dysfunction

- The general category of sexual dysfunction is divided into disorders of desire, arousal, orgasm, and pain.

- Hypoactive sexual desire is the absence of sexual fantasies and wish for sexual activity.

- Male arousal disorders involve impaired erections, a condition also known as *impotence*. Female disorders involve the absence of vaginal lubrication.

- Orgasmic disorders refer to a man or woman's inability to reach orgasm following sexual arousal.

- Painful intercourse (also called *dyspareunia*) and vaginismus are the most common pain disorders.

- A variety of psychological, social, and biological factors can cause sexual dysfunctions. Biological causes, which are more common than once believed, include the normal aging process, illness, certain medications, and alcohol and drug abuse. Psychological causes are divided into historical influences (for instance, a strict religious upbringing that equates sex with sin) and current causes (such as negative self-evaluation and anxiety about sexual performance).

- Modern sex therapy derives mainly from the methods of Masters and Johnson. Core components include desensitization of performance anxiety, mutual pleasuring, improved communication between sexual partners, and elimination of interpersonal conflict.

- A variety of surgical and pharmacological treatments are used to alleviate erectile problems, including penile implants and self-injections with drugs that produce erections.

Paraphilias

- Paraphilias are sexual activities defined as deviant by a given society.

- In the past, most knowledge about paraphilias was obtained from men who were imprisoned because of their deviant behavior. More recent research is based on paraphiliacs in the community who voluntarily seek treatment and are guaranteed confidentiality; these findings show a broader extent of deviant sexual activities than previously thought. Paraphiliacs often commit numerous offenses, engage in several different kinds of paraphilia, and have normal sexual involvements with adult partners.

- Primary types of paraphilias include exhibitionism, voyeurism, masochism and sadism, fetishism, transvestic fetishism, and pedophilia.

- Pedophilia is the unnatural desire to have sexual contact with a prepubescent child (age 13 or younger). The incidence of pedophilia—or *child molesting*—is difficult to establish due to underreporting. However, the incidence seems to be increasing.

- Incest occurs when the pedophile abuses a relative—usually, a sibling or daughter. Many pedophiles who molest their own children also abuse children from outside the family.

- Paraphilias occur when the natural link between romantic love and sexual lust is blocked or distorted in some way. In the natural psychobiology of sexual development, a pattern of brain functioning—called a *lovemap*—is established that determines what the person will find sexually arousing. It's hypothesized that traumatic childhood experiences, such as sexual abuse or emotional neglect, can disrupt the patterning of the lovemap.

- Psychological treatment is effective in reducing the relapse rate of paraphiliacs who have been released from prison. Drug treatments that lower the testosterone level show promise in helping these men control their deviant behavior. A major problem is that only a fraction of jailed sex offenders ever receive systematic treatment.

Gender-Identity Disorders

■ People with gender-identity disorder (formerly known as *transsexualism*) believe they are members of the opposite sex and are intensely dissatisfied with their own sex. Psychological treatment appears ineffective; sex reassignment surgery is often used to treat these individuals.

■ Gender-identity disorder can occur in early childhood as well as adolescence and adulthood. Young boys with this disorder have the strong desire to be girls; they typically cross-dress and reject their male anatomy. Girls with this disorder show comparable unhappiness with their anatomy and the desire to have penises.

■ Under the category "Sexual Disorders Not Otherwise Specified," the *DSM-IV* includes dissatisfaction with sexual orientation, which is a reference to homosexuality. Simply being gay or lesbian is no longer considered a clinical disorder.

■ Homosexuality seems to be biologically determined. There is no evidence that even prolonged treatment can alter this sexual orientation.

KEY TERMS

antiandrogen drug, **p. 262**
child sexual abuse, **p. 238**
clitoris, **pp. 242–243**
covert sensitization, **p. 261**
dyspareunia, **p. 247**
exhibitionist, **p. 254**
female orgasmic disorder,
    pp. 242–243
female sexual arousal disorder, **p. 239**
fetishism, **p. 256**
frotteurism, **pp. 235–236**
gender-identity disorder,
    p. 263
gender-role identity, **p. 263**
hypoactive sexual desire
    (HSD), **p. 237**

incest, **p. 257**
lovemap, **p. 259**
male erectile disorder,
    p. 239
male orgasmic disorder,
    pp. 242–243
masochism, **p. 256**
nocturnal penile
    tumescence (NPT),
    p. 241
orgasm, **p. 237**
paraphilias, **p. 252**
pedophilia, **p. 256**
premature ejaculation,
    p. 245
relapse prevention training,
    p. 262

sadism, **p. 256**
seduction theory of neuro-
    sis, **p. 257**
sensate focus, **p. 247**
sex reassignment surgery,
    p. 265
sexual aversion disorder,
    p. 237
spectatoring, **p. 241**
testosterone, **p. 238**
theory of infantile sexuality,
    p. 257
transsexual, **p. 263**
transvestite, **p. 256**
vaginismus, **p. 247**

ℭRITICAL THINKING EXERCISE

A young woman—23 years of age—entered psychological treatment, claiming to be a man in a woman's body. She wanted to physically become a man. After successfully completing psychotherapy, she had sex reassignment surgery. She now leads life as a man. But sexually, she/he is attracted only to other men. Explain your answer to each of the following questions:

1. What is this person's *DSM-IV* diagnosis?
2. What is this person's gender-role identity?
3. What is this person's sexual orientation?
4. What is this person's gender role?
5. Which of these three characteristics—gender-role identity, sexual orientation, and gender role—is hardest to change? Which is easiest to change?

Chapter 9
SUBSTANCE-RELATED DISORDERS

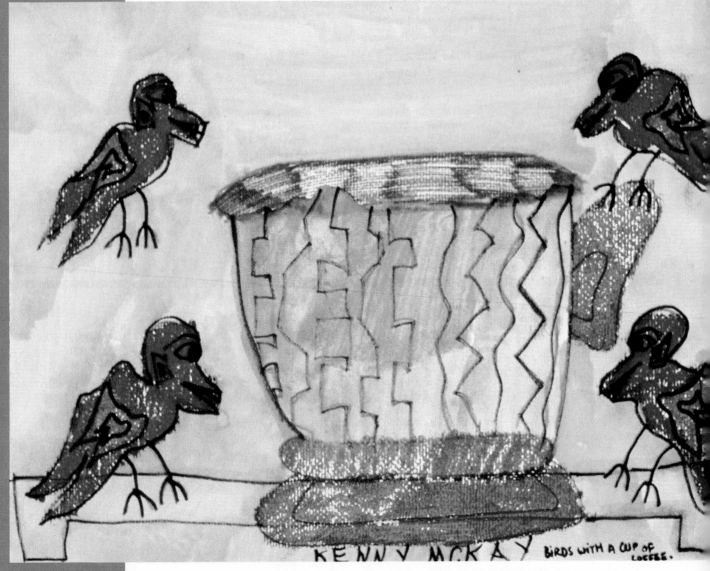

Kenny McKay, **Birds with a Cup of Coffee**, HAI

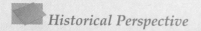
I'll always regret missing J. P.'s funeral, because it means that his death—like so much of his life—will remain a mystery to me.

I'm a clinical psychologist. I met J. P. during the early days of my first job. I had started working in a large city hospital, where one of my responsibilities was to be the psychologist in an outpatient clinic for alcoholics. Like most public alcoholism clinics, its patients couldn't pay for treatment but badly needed it. Perhaps one-third of the patients on any given Tuesday night were drunk, half were on welfare, and almost all had lost jobs, families, and self-respect because of their drinking over the years. After a while, the hopelessness of this place affected even the therapists—most of them, psychologists and psychiatrists fresh out of training.

John Paul Hennessey (J. P.'s real name, although almost no one ever used it) was one of the first patients I saw in the clinic. He was a distinguished-looking, white-haired man who looked 20 years older than his age of 40. When we first met, J. P. expressed polite skepticism about whether I could be of much help to him. He'd been drinking for all but a dozen years of his life. His drinking had cost him a marriage, his relationship with his son, countless jobs, and his ambition, health, and youth. How was I, this young psychologist, barely out of graduate school and knowing just about nothing about substance abuse, going to help? To be honest, I had my doubts (which I kept to myself).

Yet, somehow, I did help J. P.—or rather, I helped him help himself. From the beginning of our relationship, I respected him, and I guess I showed it. That wasn't very hard. J. P. was bright, sincere, and self-reflective, despite what his alcoholism had done to him through the years. As sometimes happens, the respect I gave J. P. gradually enabled him to regain it for himself. And in the process, he was able to take better advantage of treatment opportunities, including both a local Alcoholics Anonymous group and our treatment relationship at the clinic.

I also helped J. P. find something else to do with his life, besides drinking. He had a dismal work history—mostly odd jobs and low-paying restaurant work. After getting sober, he went to work as an attendant on the research unit I directed. After staying sober and being on the job a few years, he worked his way up to managing the unit. These were the best years of his life: He enjoyed the respect of his co-workers; spent an interesting, challenging day with research subjects who, like himself, were recovering alcoholics; looked forward to a steady paycheck; and even developed a regular relationship with a woman, after years of solitary living.

Unfortunately, J. P.'s job ended when the research unit closed. He wasn't able to find another job because of his age and work history, so he had to go back on welfare. But he remained sober—that is, until the cancer was diagnosed. Then, J. P. returned to the bottle. He spent the last painful months of his life drunk (whenever he could afford it), isolated by an alcoholic haze from the world he'd never come to terms with, sober or drunk.

J. P. died of stomach cancer at age 52. He was buried in the Hennessey family plot. The gravesite service was attended by his two sisters and a handful of the people he'd worked with at the city hospital. His brothers—the successful ones, who'd long since written him off—were too busy to be there.

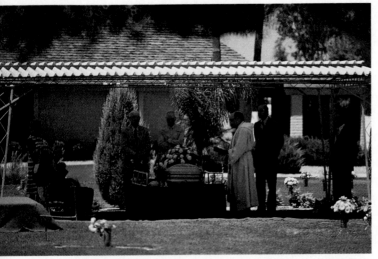

Stomach cancer is one of several diseases common among alcoholics.

Because I knew J. P. so well, I learned firsthand about alcohol dependence, which is remarkably cruel and unforgiving. I've applied that knowledge in writing this chapter. The case of J. P. may have special relevance for some of you, too. As you'll learn, J. P. had a son named Tim. They only lived in the same home for the first four years of Tim's life. Nonetheless, as J. P.'s son, Tim is the child of an alcoholic. Moreover, because Tim's mother broke off contact with J. P. shortly after they were divorced, Tim only knew of his father's abusive drinking. He knew nothing of J. P.'s strengths, achievements, and love for his son.

Like Tim Hennessey, some of you may be the children of alcoholic parents. We consider the significance of that status later in the chapter. A few of you may even be the children of alcoholic parents you never knew. That was Tim's lot, as well, and we can be sure that it shaped his life in a multitude of ways.

$\mathcal{H}$ISTORICAL PERSPECTIVE

Alcohol and drug abuse have long been part of human history. The Hebrew Bible, written 2,500 years ago, accurately describes such essential diagnostic features of alcoholism as the symptoms of physical and psychological dependence, alcohol-induced memory deficits, and withdrawal. The authors of both the Old and New Testaments warn against drunkenness, link it with sinful behavior, and severely admonish those who lack the strength to resist the temptation to imbibe. Reflecting this strongly judgmental view of substance abuse, chronic alcohol abusers were stoned to death during the Old and New Testament eras. Through the Middle Ages, alcoholics could be tortured or burned at the stake for demonic possession, alongside people who were psychotic and mentally retarded. Those who escaped torture or death could still be confined indefinitely to prison or the almshouse, since it was believed that alcohol abusers and psychotics had made sinful behavioral choices.

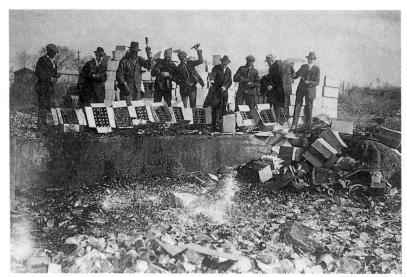

This photo chronicles the destruction of 749 cases of beer, which were confiscated by federal authorities from a Prohibition-era bootlegger.

It was not until the mid-eighteenth century that a few individuals began to advocate another view, which was radical for the time: namely, that excessive alcohol use was a disease, rather than a sinful, conscious choice. Among the first of these individuals was Benjamin Rush (1745–1813), a signer of the Declaration of Independence and a founder of American psychiatry. Since heavy drinking and drug use were common in both American and English society at the time, this view was controversial. So was the view of physicians in both the United States and Great Britain, who, later in the nineteenth century, concluded that the habitual use of drugs like the opiates, tobacco, and coffee stemmed from inherited or acquired biological vulnerability. These views of addiction as a disease helped promote the establishment of the first few publicly funded treatment programs, including what came to be called *inebriate asylums.*

The worldwide temperance movement, which peaked at the beginning of the twentieth century, viewed alcohol, not drunkenness, as the cause of alcoholism. Accordingly, the movement advocated control and, where possible, prohibition of the sale of alcoholic products. Prohibition—"the noble experiment that failed"— became law in the United States with the passage of the Eighteenth Amendment in 1919, shortly after the end of World War I. Even though the ban on alcohol succeeded in reducing rates of alcoholism, it dramatically increased rates of crime, much of which was associated with the illegal sale and distribution of alcohol. Prohibition was repealed with the Twenty-First Amendment in 1933.

A more enlightened view of alcohol and other drug abuse has emerged over the last 40 or 50 years. Americans became convinced that alcoholism was not simply a moral issue during World War II, when countless numbers of soldiers engaged in substance abuse. A self-help group called Alcoholics Anonymous (AA), which was established shortly before World War II, also helped change public attitudes toward alcoholism. The philosophy of AA persuaded many Americans that alcoholism is more a medical and social problem than a moral one. Today, AA has members worldwide.

Continuing advances have also been made in the scientific understanding of what causes alcoholism—many of them achieved during the past 25 years. This knowledge has also moved the addictions from the moral to the medical and social realms.

Until relatively recently, alcohol had few rivals as the principal drug of abuse in Western society. Opium—"the flower of happiness"—had been cultivated in the Fertile Crescent of the Middle East some 2,000 years before the birth of Christ, and its use had become well established in India and China by A.D. 800. However, opium was essentially unknown in the Western world before Swiss physician and alchemist Philippus Aureolus Paracelsus (1493–1541) formulated *laudanum* (tincture of opium) in the fifteenth century.

Until the end of the eighteenth century, most Western opium addicts were either survivors of battlefield trauma or victims of chronic pain. Both groups of individuals had become dependent on the pain-killing properties of the opium family of drugs. Opium, morphine, and heroin were all available without restriction in the United States until the Pure Food and Drug Act and the Harrison Narcotic Act were passed in the early twentieth century. In the absence of research on their long-term effects, these drugs were not believed to be dangerous.

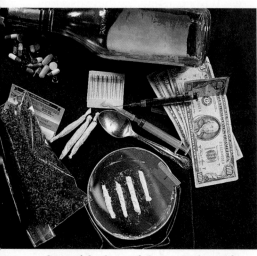

Some of the drugs of abuse, together with implements for their use and the means to purchase them

The abuse of drugs other than alcohol and the opiates in Western countries increased sharply in the early nineteenth century, for two reasons: (1) The veterans of Napoleon's Egyptian campaign brought back marijuana and hashish to French society and (2) cocaine, the potent alkaloid of the coca leaf, was introduced in Europe and the United States at about the same time. Sigmund Freud (1856–1939) contributed a great deal to the drug's appeal with his rave review of cocaine's magical analgesic and sedative properties in the late 1800s. Popular fictional detective Sherlock Holmes also promoted cocaine as a mental stimulant. At the time, it was widely believed that the use of cocaine and opium had virtually no harmful consequences. As a result of all this, by the end of the nineteenth century, alcohol had become only one of the drugs that Americans abused.

Focus on Critical Thinking

1. Why has the use of alcohol and drugs been linked through the ages with immorality and sin?
2. What are some of the factors responsible for the recent change in our views of the substance-related disorders as largely medical and social problems, rather than moral ones?

DIAGNOSIS OF SUBSTANCE-RELATED DISORDERS

Early Diagnostic Conceptions

Alcohol and drug addiction were included in both the *DSM-I* and *DSM-II* (American Psychiatric Association, 1952, 1968). However, they were not included as independent diagnostic conditions in either manual. Instead, they were listed as varieties of **sociopathic personality disturbance**, a catchall diagnostic category that also covered antisocial behavior and the sexual disorders. The implication of this classification was that people diagnosed with alcoholism, drug addiction, antisocial behavior, or one of the sexual disorders threatened society's moral fabric as a result of their intemperate or immoral behavioral choices.

The *DSM-III* (American Psychiatric Association, 1980) gave the alcohol- and drug-related disorders their own separate identity: the *substance-use disorders.* This classification eliminated the moralistic, "guilt by association" stigma of the previous diagnostic manuals. The *DSM-III* highlighted new research findings that pointed to sociocultural and genetic factors in the etiology (causation) of the conditions. Based on this research, the symptoms of *tolerance* and *withdrawal* were assigned key diagnostic roles. The *DSM-III* also established a separate diagnosis for **substance abuse.** The purpose of this diagnosis was to identify persons whose substance use was problematic but had not yet reached the proportions of **substance dependence.** The *DSM-III-R* (American Psychiatric Association, 1987) retained many of the diagnostic advances achieved by the *DSM-III.*

The **DSM-IV** *Substance-Related Disorders*

In preparing the *DSM-IV* (American Psychiatric Association, 1994), the Substance Disorders Work Group undertook a very extensive series of field trials and data analyses. This research was designed to establish the criteria for substance abuse and dependence on the firmest possible empirical base (Cottler et al., 1995; Schuckit, 1994b). These efforts led the work group to retain many of the criteria developed for the *DSM-III* and *DSM-III-R* (American Psychiatric Association, 1980, 1987) because of their sound predictive validity (Helzer, 1994; Nathan, 1994b). The work group also reaffirmed the *DSM-III*'s diagnostic emphasis on tolerance and withdrawal symptoms; these symptoms frequently accompanied substance dependence in the field trials. Finally, the work group reemphasized the valuable role of substance abuse as a diagnosis separate from substance dependence. This sepa-

sociopathic personality disturbance Catchall diagnostic category in the DSM-I and DSM-II that included antisocial behavior and the sexual deviations as well as alcoholism and drug addiction.

substance abuse Maladaptive pattern of substance use, characterized by recurrent and significant adverse consequences related to the repeated use of substances.

substance dependence Cluster of cognitive, behavioral, and physiological symptoms that indicate that the individual continues use of a substance despite significant substance-related problems.

Operational Criteria for SUBSTANCE DEPENDENCE

A maladaptive pattern of substance use, leading to clinically significant impairment or distress, as manifested by three (or more) of the following, occurring at any time in the same 12-month period:

(1) tolerance, as defined by either of the following:
   (a) a need for markedly increased amounts of the substance to achieve intoxication or desired effect
   (b) markedly diminished effect with continued use of the same amount of the substance

(2) withdrawal, as manifested by either of the following:
   (a) the characteristic withdrawal syndrome for the substance
   (b) the same (or a closely related) substance is taken to relieve or avoid withdrawal symptoms

(3) the substance is often taken in larger amounts or over a longer period than was intended

(4) there is a persistent desire or unsuccessful efforts to cut down or control substance use

(5) a great deal of time is spent in activities necessary to obtain the substance (e.g., visiting multiple doctors or driving long distances), use the substance (e.g., chain-smoking), or recover from its effects

(6) important social, occupational, or recreational activities are given up or reduced because of substance use

(7) the substance use is continued despite knowledge of having a persistent or recurrent physical or psychological problem that is likely to have been caused or exacerbated by the substance (e.g., current cocaine use despite recognition of cocaine-induced depression, or continued drinking despite recognition that an ulcer was made worse by alcohol consumption)

Specify if:

With Physiological Dependence: evidence of tolerance or withdrawal (i.e., either item 1 or 2 is present)

Without Physiological Dependence: no evidence of tolerance or withdrawal (i.e., neither item 1 nor 2 is present)

rate diagnosis allows identification of a unique group of persons who benefit from the clinical attention they subsequently receive (Widiger et al., 1994).

The *DSM-IV* (American Psychiatric Association, 1994) operational criteria for substance dependence and substance abuse, shown in the tables, illustrate the range of behaviors linked to these diagnoses. In reviewing these tables, you may recognize familiar alcohol- or drug-related behaviors that you have observed in friends or family members.

You may also recall the case of J. P., presented at the beginning of this chapter. He met the *DSM-IV* criteria for both alcohol and nicotine dependence before he was 14. At the time—1933—there was no *DSM*. The *DSM-I* lay almost 20 years in the future (American Psychiatric Association, 1952), and the *DSM-IV* would not appear for more than 60 years (1994). Rather than try to guess at the symptoms that J. P.'s family doctor used to diagnose his condition so many years ago, we'll describe J. P.'s symptoms in current terms—those of the *DSM-IV*.

J. P. had his first taste of alcohol at the age of 6. The setting was the bedroom of his best friend, who was the son of the proprietor of the neighborhood tavern. That's where J. P.'s father and uncles spent most weekend nights. Since J. P.'s friend lived above the tavern, it wasn't much of a challenge for the two boys to go downstairs and, when no one was looking, draw a glass of beer from the tap.

J. P. didn't remember having any particular reaction to that first drink. The next time he tried alcohol, though, three years later, things were quite different. He and the same friend split a six-pack one Saturday afternoon—this time, at J. P.'s house. After finishing his three beers plus two of his friend's, J. P. felt better than he had ever felt in

Operational Criteria for SUBSTANCE ABUSE

A. A maladaptive pattern of substance use leading to clinically significant impairment or distress, as manifested by one (or more) of the following, occurring within a 12-month period:

   (1) recurrent substance use resulting in a failure to fulfill major role obligations at work, school, or home (e.g., repeated absences or poor work performance related to substance use; substance-related absences, suspensions, or expulsions from school; neglect of children or household)

   (2) recurrent substance use in situations in which it is physically hazardous (e.g., driving an automobile or operating a machine when impaired by substance use)

   (3) recurrent substance-related legal problems (e.g., arrests for substance-related disorderly conduct)

   (4) continued substance use despite having persistent or recurrent social or interpersonal problems caused or exacerbated by the effects of the substance (e.g., arguments with spouse about consequences of intoxication, physical fights)

B. The symptoms have never met the criteria for Substance Dependence for this class of substance.

his whole life. It was as though a new world had opened before him, a world more full of promise and pleasure than he ever could have imagined. He had to have more!

By the time he was 14, alcohol had become the center of J. P.'s life. Unlike his brothers and sisters, he spent little time on homework or sports. For J. P., the perfect afternoon was spent with a few like-minded friends in a quiet spot in a shady park (or a vacant building, when winter came on)—drinking beer or wine, smoking hand-rolled cigarettes, and talking.

Even at the age of 14, J. P. easily met the *DSM-IV* standard for alcohol dependence. For more than a year before that, he'd been gradually adjusting his consumption upward to maintain the marvelous feeling of tranquillity alcohol had provided him virtually from the start. J. P. had developed tolerance. On those few occasions when he hadn't had enough money to drink and had had to stop for a day or two, he had begun to experience the nausea, restlessness, agitation, and sleeplessness associated with withdrawal. Though he seldom tried to cut down his drinking, on the rare occasions when he did—for instance, when he planned to try out for the junior high football team—he had been unable to do so. And ever since alcohol had taken the central role in his life, he had had to spend a great deal of his time figuring out how to earn the money he needed to buy it. Schoolwork, athletics, dances and dating, evenings with parents and siblings—J. P. gradually gave them all up in favor of the opportunity to acquire and consume the substance that made him feel incomparably better than he had ever felt before.

Tolerance and withdrawal are important symptoms of substance dependence (Nathan, 1994b). For that reason, the diagnosis of substance dependence in the *DSM-III* (American Psychiatric Association, 1980) required the presence of one or both symptoms. This requirement was based on the belief that dependence could not develop in the absence of these symptoms. The drafters of the *DSM-III-R* (1987) did not hold this view; they concluded that a person could be dependent without demonstrating either symptom. The *DSM-IV* (1994) work group, however, thought that the presence of these symptoms was important enough to distinguish between two types of addicted persons: those with tolerance or withdrawal symptoms (diagnosed as **with physiological dependence**) and those without either symptom (diagnosed as **without physiological dependence**). This diagnostic distinction implies that the two varieties of dependence may differ in etiology, in the course of the disease, or in response to treatment.

Tolerance occurs at both the cellular and the psychological levels (Chiu et al., 1994; Nathan, 1994b). Cells adjust to the long-term presence of alcohol and other drugs in the bloodstream; they do so by altering certain biochemical processes to achieve physiological balance with the substances. This response is comparable to how long-term, substance-abusing humans learn to adjust to certain psychological and behavioral consequences of using alcohol or drugs on a regular basis. (We'll discuss learned tolerance later in this chapter.) Tolerance requires the individual to use more of the substance to maintain its original reinforcing effects. The individual who's achieved tolerance will also feel a gradual decline in those effects if the dosage of the substance isn't increased over time.

Withdrawal refers to the physical and psychological symptoms that occur when the individual stops drug or alcohol intake after a period of use long enough to induce dependence (Hughes, 1994a, 1994b). Symptoms include nausea, vomiting, restlessness and agitation, and sleeplessness. In severe withdrawal states, such as delirium tremens (described in Chapter 16), withdrawal may actually be life threatening. The symptoms of withdrawal, like those of tolerance, are influenced by both psychological and cellular factors (Crowley, 1994).

---

with physiological dependence Substance dependence that includes tolerance or withdrawal symptoms or both.

without physiological dependence Substance dependence that does not include tolerance or withdrawal symptoms.

tolerance Consequence of addiction to a substance; over time, requires that increasing amounts be ingested in order to achieve the same subjective effects.

withdrawal Physical and psychological consequences that result when use of an addicting substance is stopped.

Focus on Critical Thinking

1. Do you think the diagnostic distinction between substance abuse and substance dependence is useful in understanding these problems? For instance, does it help you understand the behavior of family members or friends who have experienced substance-related problems? Explain your answers.

2. Which of the criteria for substance abuse/dependence are most relevant for someone your age? Which are relevant regardless of age? Again, explain your answers.

*A*MERICANS *WITH* *S*UBSTANCE-*R*ELATED *D*ISORDERS

Between 5 and 7 percent of the U.S. population—or between 14 million and 16 million people—meet the *DSM-IV* (American Psychiatric Association, 1994) criteria for alcohol abuse or dependence (NIAAA, 1993; Regier & Burke, 1987). Between 4 and 6 million Americans—many of whom are alcohol dependent, as well—abuse illicit drugs. More than 45 million Americans are dependent on the nicotine in cigarettes (NIDA, 1991). As Figure 9.1 indicates, the economic costs of substance abuse to Americans are substantial, totaling well over $200 billion in 1990.

As Figure 9.2 indicates (see pages 278–279), the average annual alcohol consumption of an individual in the United States has remained steady over the past 140 years, with two exceptions (Horgan, 1993). Alcohol consumption declined during the Prohibition years, 1919–1933. And since about 1960, alcohol consumption first increased and then decreased. Rates of alcohol abuse and dependence have probably remained steady over the same timespan.

Rates of alcohol and drug abuse and dependence vary with age, sex, and ethnicity (NIAAA, 1993; NIDA, 1991). Among men between the ages of 18 and 44, rates of abuse and dependence are more than double the overall rates; women's rates for the same age groups are about one-quarter those of men. Between the ages of 45 and 64—and especially from 65 years and beyond—rates of abuse and dependence for both men and women plummet to half the overall rates. At most ages, African Americans and Hispanics of both sexes demonstrate slightly higher rates of abuse and dependence than whites.

FIGURE 9.1   Economic costs of substance abuse: 1990

Associated medical, illness, death, and other costs of drug abuse, alcohol abuse, and smoking in the United States (in billions of dollars).

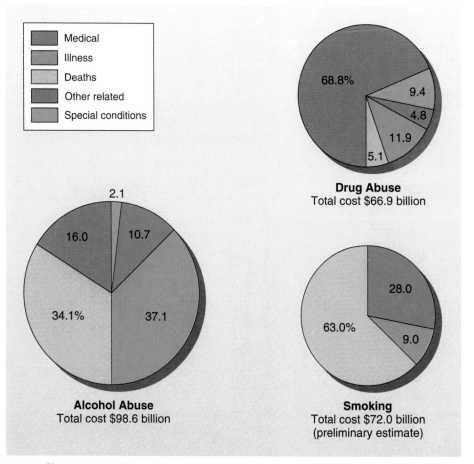

Source: Chart 4, p. 16, *Substance Abuse: The Nation's Number One Health Problem,* Robert Wood Johnson Foundation. Reprinted by permission.

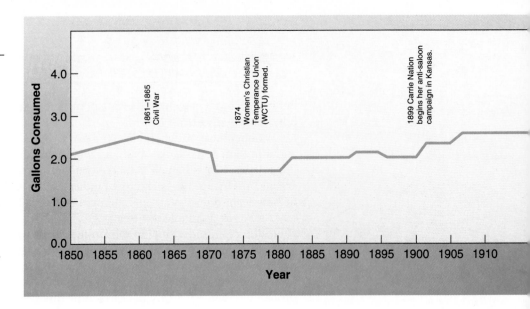

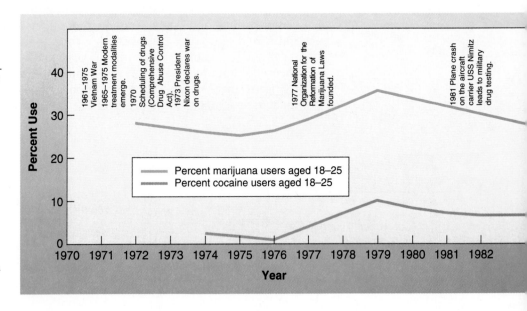

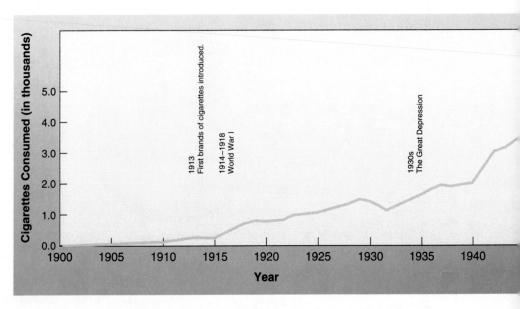

278

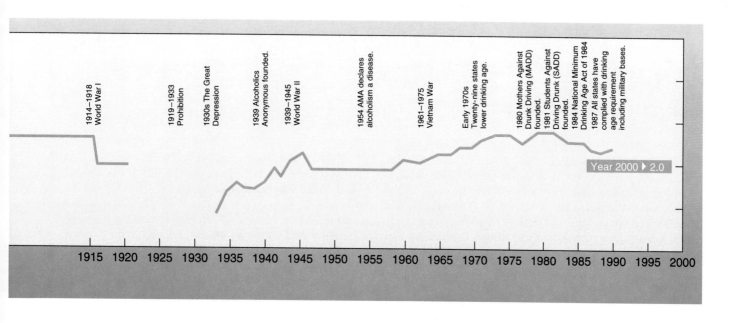

1914–1918
World War I

1919–1933
Prohibition

1930s The Great
Depression

1939 Alcoholics
Anonymous founded.

1939–1945
World War II

1954 AMA declares
alcoholism a disease.

1961–1975
Vietnam War

Early 1970s
Twenty-nine states
lower drinking age.

1980 Mothers Against
Drunk Driving (MADD)
founded.

1981 Students Against
Driving Drunk (SADD)
founded.

1984 National Minimum
Drinking Age Act of 1984

1987 All states have
complied with drinking
age requirement
including military bases.

Year 2000 ▶ 2.0

1915 1920 1925 1930 1935 1940 1945 1950 1955 1960 1965 1970 1975 1980 1985 1990 1995 2000

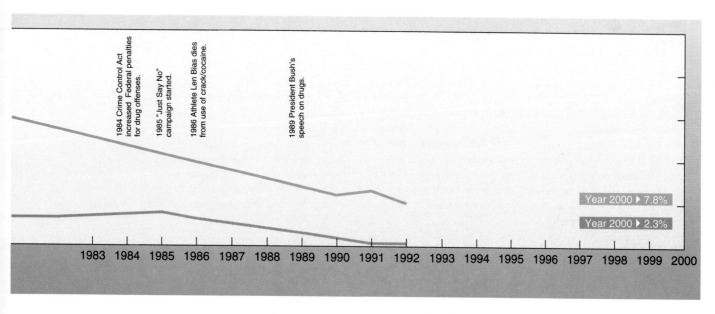

1984 Crime Control Act
increased Federal penalties
for drug offenses.

1985 "Just Say No"
campaign started.

1986 Athlete Len Bias dies
from use of crack/cocaine.

1989 President Bush's
speech on drugs.

Year 2000 ▶ 7.8%

Year 2000 ▶ 2.3%

1983 1984 1985 1986 1987 1988 1989 1990 1991 1992 1993 1994 1995 1996 1997 1998 1999 2000

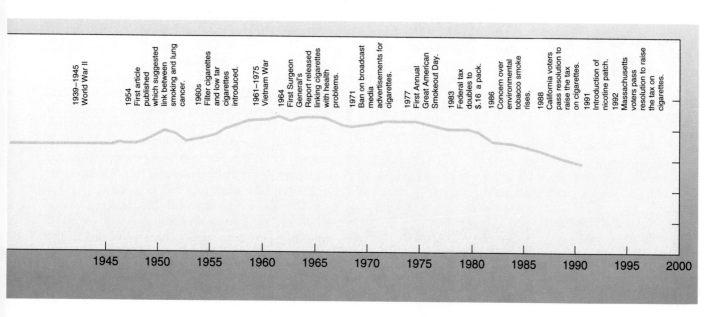

1939–1945
World War II

1954
First article
published
which suggested
link between
smoking and lung
cancer.

1960s
Filter cigarettes
and low tar
cigarettes
introduced.

1961–1975
Vietnam War

1964
First Surgeon
General's
Report released
linking cigarettes
with health
problems.

1971
Ban on broadcast
media
advertisements for
cigarettes.

1977
First Annual
Great American
Smokeout Day.

1983
Federal tax
doubles to
$.16 a pack.

1986
Concern over
environmental
tobacco smoke
rises.

1988
California voters
pass resolution to
raise the tax
on cigarettes.

1991
Introduction of
nicotine patch.

1992
Massachusetts
voters pass
resolution to raise
the tax on
cigarettes.

1945 1950 1955 1960 1965 1970 1975 1980 1985 1990 1995 2000

Thinking about MULTICULTURAL ISSUES

A Life on the Streets with "Crack"

Derek was 11 years old when he first tried "crack." At the time, he was an impressionable African American youth who spent most of his free time on the streets of the urban ghetto where he, his four siblings, and his mother lived. Most of Derek's older friends regularly used drugs. The person he most admired, Jonathan, had been dealing drugs off and on for as long as Derek could remember. Jonathan wore expensive clothing, always seemed to have spending money, was clearly well liked by the girls, drove an expensive car, and was always smiling and laughing. Derek had decided long ago that he wanted to be like Jonathan when he grew older, even though his mother told him that Jonathan was bound to get into serious trouble with the law.

Derek first tried crack a few months after having his first drink of alcohol and his first "joint." An older boy in the neighborhood shared a small bag of the delicate white powder. When Derek inhaled the crack smoke into his lungs, an intense euphoria overcame him and he felt completely free from the pressures of his life on the streets. Crack made Derek forget the three roach-infested rooms that he and his family lived in; the constant struggle that his overburdened mother had, trying to stretch her paycheck from one week to the next; and his persistent worry that she wouldn't be able to continue to care for five active children by herself.

Crack had a powerful effect on Derek. He knew that he had to experience it again, and he did. It quickly led him to make everything else in his life secondary to the effort to get the money to buy it. And when he couldn't earn the money, he stole it—from other children on the street, from old people in the neighborhood, and finally, from the proprietors of stores. Derek and his friends held up local stores at gunpoint.

During one of these armed robberies, Derek was caught by the police, who were on stakeout. He was tried and convicted and is now serving an indeterminate juvenile sentence, which is likely to stretch to his eighteenth birthday. Although he has completed a drug program in the juvenile detention center, Derek isn't sure he can withstand the allure of crack when he returns to the streets. He sure would like to, though.

Think about the following questions:

1. Does Derek meet the operational criteria for crack cocaine dependence or abuse? Why or why not?
2. How does this story illuminate the possible role played by social factors in the development of Derek's substance use? Explain your answer.
3. Does Derek's story suggest reasons as to why urban minority youth are at heightened risk to abuse illicit drugs? Why or why not?

polysubstance abuse
Concurrent abuse of or dependence on more than one substance.

Focus on Critical Thinking

1. Figures 9.2, 9.3, and 9.4 show trends in substance use over a number of years. Examine the trends over your lifetime. What do you think were the most important environmental and social influences on alcohol, illicit drug, and cigarette use over that time? Why?
2. What factors help explain the greater prevalence of substance abuse among men than women?

Polysubstance abuse—most often involving alcohol and one or more additional substances—is more the rule than the exception these days. This trend makes it even more difficult to get an accurate picture of the numbers of drug abusers in the United States.

Figure 9.3 (on pages 278–279) illustrates the trends in regular marijuana and cocaine use from 1972 to 1992 among Americans between the ages of 18 and 25. Use of both drugs has decreased sharply since peaking in 1979. Cigarette smoking has also decreased in recent years among people of all ages, as Figure 9.4 (on pages 278–279) shows (Horgan, 1993). The decline has been especially sharp since the 1964 U.S. Surgeon General's report linking cigarettes with health problems (U.S. Department of Health, Education, and Welfare, 1964).

Derek's story—detailed in Thinking about Multicultural Issues—illustrates one of the most troubling substance dependence problems in the United States: the abuse of "crack" cocaine by urban minority youngsters.

THE NATURE OF SUBSTANCE ABUSE AND DEPENDENCE

Alcohol Abuse and Dependence

After it's ingested, alcohol enters the stomach and small intestine, where it's quickly absorbed into the bloodstream. Then it's carried to the brain, where it affects the central nervous system and thus behavior. In moderate doses, alcoholic beverages initially produce a mild sense of stimulation and enhanced well-being, followed by relaxation and calm. In larger doses, alcohol interferes with cognitive functioning, balance and coordination, judgment, memory, and perception. In extremely high doses, the sedative effects of alcohol can impair respiration and breathing and lead to death from respiratory failure.

The concentration of alcohol in the body is usually measured by taking a blood sample. The amount of alcohol in the bloodstream is called the *blood-alcohol level*. Table 9.1 summarizes the most common behavioral effects at various blood-alcohol levels. These data help explain why the acute effects of alcohol in the blood not only cause direct negative effects but also lead to a variety of indirect negative outcomes (Klatsky & Armstrong, 1993).

For instance, the effects of alcohol intoxication include a heightened risk of having an automobile accident; in 1991, nearly half (47.9 percent) of traffic-related deaths involved the use of alcohol (National Highway Safety Administration, 1992). Likewise, intoxication causes substantially more alcohol-related accidents and

TABLE 9.1	Behavioral Effects of Blood-Alcohol Levels
Blood-Alcohol Level (percent)	**Behavioral Effects**
0.05	Lowered alertness; usually good feeling; release of inhibitions; impaired judgment
0.10	Slowed reaction times; impaired motor function; less caution
0.15	Large, consistent increases in reaction time
0.20	Marked depression in sensory and motor capability; decidedly intoxicated
0.25	Severe motor disturbance; staggering; sensory perceptions greatly impaired; smashed!
0.30	Stuporous but conscious; no comprehension of the world around them
0.35	Surgical anesthesia; minimal level causing death
0.40	About half of those at this level die

NOTE: A 160-pound man will achieve a blood-alcohol level of 0.05 in the course of an hour by consuming about two beers or two 5-ounce glasses of wine or two highballs, each containing an ounce of Scotch, bourbon, vodka, or gin. A blood-alcohol level of 0.10 will be achieved by consuming roughly twice that amount of beverage alcohol during an hour, or 25 percent more during two hours (because alcohol metabolizes or disappears from the system at the constant rate of about 0.015/hour).

SOURCE: From O. Ray and C. Ksir (1990), "Behavioral Effects of Blood Alcohol Levels," *Drugs, Society, and Human Behavior,* 5th ed. Reprinted by permission of Mosby-Year Book, Inc.

injuries on the job and at home (Trice, 1992). High blood-alcohol levels are also associated with crime of all kinds. In 1991, between 40 and 60 percent of violent crimes in the United States were alcohol related (Martin, 1992), and in 1992, almost 80 percent of crimes involving the possession or sale of drugs also involved the use of alcohol or drugs (U.S. Department of Justice, 1993). Being intoxicated causes high-risk sexual behavior (Leigh, 1990) and increased levels of family violence, such as spouse and child abuse. Overall, women who are battered report that approximately 50 percent of their husbands have long-term alcohol problems (Leonard, 1993).

In terms of individual health, the long-term effects of alcohol are equally devastating, if not worse. Chronic alcohol abuse is associated with permanent, disabling changes in brain function, reflecting alcohol's toxic effects on brain tissue (Hunt & Nixon, 1993) (also see Chapter 16). The chronic abuse of alcohol has also been linked to a variety of specific birth defects (Michaelis & Michaelis, 1994; Streissguth, 1994). In addition, long-term alcohol abuse is responsible for life-threatening physical disorders affecting the brain, heart, liver, and gastrointestinal system. As a result, chronic abuse of alcohol is a major cause of premature death in the United States. On average, people who die from alcohol-related causes lose 26 years from their normal life expectancies (Horgan, 1993).

You may recall from the chapter-opening case that J. P. died prematurely at the age of 52 from stomach cancer, an alcohol-related disorder. But the cancer that killed him was not the only grievous consequence of J. P.'s lifelong pattern of abusive drinking.

J. P. was certainly smart enough to make his way in life; his formal IQ measured in the "superior" range. Yet, until he worked at the hospital, he had never held a job for more than a year or two. Typically, after an initial period of sobriety and excellent performance on the job, J. P. would start drinking again, coming to work late, and eventually missing work altogether. After a few weeks of this, he would get fired—again.

J. P. had four serious automobile accidents in his lifetime, all of them alcohol related. In the first accident, J. P., his wife, and 3-year-old son were injured when he swerved to avoid an oncoming car and slid on an icy road into a tree. Both he and the other driver had blood-alcohol levels in excess of the legal limit. J. P.'s other auto accidents were also alcohol related. He spent several months in jail following the third accident and permanently lost his license to drive after the fourth. As a result, toward the end of his life, J. P. didn't drive at all, both because he couldn't afford a car (let alone the insurance) and because his driver's license had been permanently revoked.

Perhaps J. P.'s greatest alcohol-related loss was that of his family—in particular, his only child. J. P. married a neighborhood girl, Maureen, when he was 22. He was drinking heavily then and continued to do so for the 7 years they were married. Three years into the marriage, the Hennesseys had a son, Tim. Bright, energetic, affectionate, and adventurous, he quickly became the apple of his father's eye. Tim loved being with his father, who was a lot of fun, even after he'd been drinking. Tim's mother, on the other hand, became increasingly disheartened at her husband's inability to stay sober and hold a job. The auto accident in which they had all been injured was the final straw. Shortly after Maureen and Tim recovered from their injuries, they moved out. Tragically, J. P. spent the last 20 years of his life totally out of touch with both his ex-wife and son.

The stomach cancer that killed J. P. was only the latest and most serious of the many alcohol-related physical disorders he had experienced through the years. He had been hospitalized at the city hospital a number of times for a range of digestive and cardiac problems that were either caused or made worse by his drinking. In fact, by the time he came to the clinic for treatment of alcohol abuse, J. P. had become one of the hospital's best-known figures.

Nicotine Dependence

The number-one public health problem in the United States is not the use of cocaine, "crack," or heroin. It's not even the abuse of alcohol, which is clearly a major problem in American society, given the number of deaths it causes annually. By that criterion, the most serious public health problem in the United States is the use of tobacco.

Tobacco contains nicotine, a substance that induces dependence (Abrams, Emmons, Niaura, Goldstein, & Sherman, 1991). Nicotine is found in all tobacco products, including cigarettes and cigars, pipe tobacco, and different types of so-called smokeless tobacco. The use of smokeless products, such as chewing tobacco and snuff, has increased in recent years, especially among young males. In contrast, the average annual per capita consumption of cigarettes has fallen from more than 4,000 in 1965 to 2,700 in 1992. Nonetheless, in 1990, cigarettes still cost the United States $72 billion and over 400,000 lives—more than 100,000 of them from lung cancer. Even though alcohol abuse cost the country about $25 billion more in the same year, it took less than half as many lives (Horgan, 1993).

As mentioned earlier, cigarette smoking has declined markedly in the United States since 1964, when the U.S. Surgeon General issued his initial report on the catastrophic health consequences of smoking (U.S. Department of Health, Education, and Welfare, 1964). However, as Figure 9.5 shows, the decline in cigarette use has been very uneven among young people. Among high school seniors, whites are

FIGURE 9.5 Trends in alcohol and cigarette use among youth: 1976–1992

High school seniors in the United States who are heavy users of alcohol and cigarettes, by racial/ethnic group (in percent).

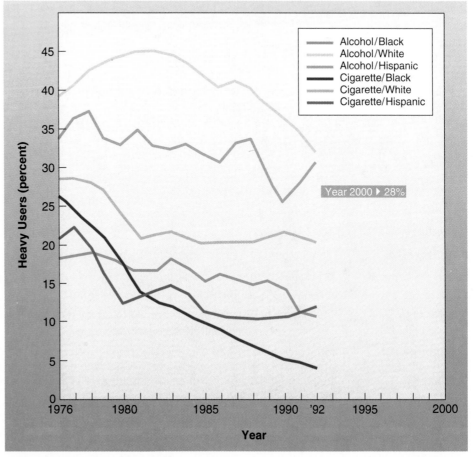

Source: Chart 6, p. 27, *Substance Abuse: The Nation's Number One Health Problem,* Robert Wood Johnson Foundation. Reprinted by permission.

now most likely and blacks least likely to be heavy smokers and drinkers. Rates for Hispanic youths fall in between (Horgan, 1993).

Nicotine is a central nervous system (CNS) stimulant that's chemically related to the amphetamines (which are discussed in the next section). Like the amphetamines, nicotine causes withdrawal symptoms and tolerance and induces dependence. In low doses, nicotine acts as a mild CNS stimulant. But at higher doses, it can cause agitation and irritability, interfere with thinking and problem solving, and bring on dramatic alterations in mood.

Whereas the tars and other toxic components of cigarette smoke represent substantial health risks, it's the nicotine that ensures people will become dependent and continue to smoke. Two experts on substance abuse have concluded that the dependence produced by nicotine is greater than that produced by any of five other commonly abused substances, including heroin and cocaine (Hilts, 1994d). These experts' ratings of substances are shown in Table 9.2. So, contrary to widespread belief, nicotine is an extremely potent compound. Fortunately, its potency is diminished somewhat because it's not ingested in purified form. Once inhaled, though, up to 90 percent of the nicotine in cigarettes is absorbed through the lungs.

The health hazards caused by cigarette smoking have been known for some 30 years now, yet cigarette manufacturers continue to deny that their products bring

---

TABLE 9.2 Experts' Ratings of the Addictive Properties of Problem Substances

Dr. Jack E. Henningfield of the National Institute on Drug Abuse and Dr. Neal L. Benowitz of the University of California at San Francisco ranked six substances based on five problem areas.

1 = Most serious   6 = Least serious

Henningfield Ratings   Benowitz Ratings

Substance	Withdrawal		Reinforcement		Tolerance		Dependence		Intoxication	
Nicotine	3	3*	4	4	2	4	1	1	5	6
Heroin	2	2	2	2	1	2	2	2	2	2
Cocaine	4	3*	1	1	4	1	3	3	3	3
Alcohol	1	1	3	3	3	4	4	4	1	1
Caffeine	5	4	6	5	5	3	5	5	6	5
Marijuana	6	5	5	6	6	5	6	6	4	4

Withdrawal	Presence and severity of characteristic withdrawal symptoms.
Reinforcement	A measure of the substance's ability, in human and animal tests, to get users to take it again and again, and in preference to other substances.
Tolerance	How much of the substance is needed to satisfy increasing cravings for it, and the level of stable need that is eventually reached.
Dependence	How difficult it is for the user to quit, the relapse rate, the percentage of people who eventually become dependent, the rating users give their own need for the substance and the degree to which the substance will be used in the face of evidence that it causes harm.
Intoxication	Though not usually counted as a measure of addiction in itself, the level of intoxication is associated with addiction and increases the personal and social damage a substance may do.

*Equal ratings

Source: From Philip J. Hilts, "Is Nicotine Addictive? It Depends on Whose Criteria You Use," *The New York Times*, August 2, 1994, p. B6. Copyright © 1994 by The New York Times Company. Reprinted with permission.

In a three-part series of articles, published on the front pages of the *New York Times* in June 1994, Philip J. Hilts describes the complex interplay of social, economic, and moral issues that cigarette manufacturers had to confront when, in the late 1950s and early 1960s, they first began to suspect the health hazards their products posed. The first of Hilts's three articles—"Cigarette Makers Debated the Risks They Denied" (Hilts, 1994a)—captures the executives' dilemma. In sum:

> For more than 40 years, American tobacco executives followed a two-track approach to the health dangers of cigarettes, saying in public that there was no proven risk, while privately debating how to deal with the very risk they were denying. (p. 1)

Hilts's writing is based, in part, on more than 4,000 pages of documents from the archives of one of the nation's largest cigarette manufacturers. In his articles, he portrays the struggles of company executives to find a way to deal with the medical and moral issues their products raised while also working to protect their company's profits.

In the second article in the series—"Tobacco Maker Studied Risk but Did Little about Results" (Hilts, 1994b)—Hilts tells of the company's initial hopes that technology would solve their problems by enabling them to develop a safer cigarette. However, as Hilts notes:

> The business side of the company was less optimistic about the prospects for making smoking a safer endeavor than company researchers were. Even if such products were available, the businessmen in the companies asked, could they ever be palatable in a competitive market? . . . Behind these concerns lurked the legal issues: Would the companies be sued over the effects of their products? Could they afford to be honest about the hazards? Could they afford not to be? (p. C16)

The cigarette manufacturer eventually concluded that making a safer cigarette was not technically feasible.

So it closed its research laboratories in the 1970s and began denying publicly the nature and extent of the health risk—even while executives continued internal debates on the best course of action. The third article in the series—"Grim Findings Scuttle Hope for 'Safer' Cigarette" (Hilts, 1994c)—brings the reader to the present. It quotes extensively from a presentation by the company's directors of public relations and marketing research, which epitomize the stance that cigarette manufacturers have taken for the past decade:

> Doubt is our product, since it is the best means of competing with the "body of fact" that exists in the mind of the general public. With the general public, the consensus is that cigarettes are in some way harmful to the health. . . . If we are successful in establishing a controversy at the public level, then there is an opportunity to put across the real facts about smoking and health. Doubt is also the limit of our "product." Unfortunately, we cannot take a position directly opposing the anti-cigarette forces and say that cigarettes are a contributor to good health. No information that we have supports such a claim. (p. 10)

To put this in perspective, keep in mind that cigarette smoking is the leading public health problem in the United States. Smoking is responsible for more than 400,000 deaths a year. Also keep in mind that this company debate was probably not limited to just one cigarette manufacturer; it was no doubt replicated in the executive suites of every other cigarette manufacturer across the country. So, if this debate had had a different outcome, how many millions of lives might have been saved over the 40 years that have elapsed since the first research findings on the health consequences of smoking appeared?

Think about the following questions:

1. Why do you think this cigarette manufacturer adopted the strategy described to deal with the health risks of smoking?
2. Will this strategy ultimately be judged to have been a good business decision? Why or why not?

serious harm. The Thinking about Social Issues box examines the complicated mix of social, economic, and moral factors that the tobacco industry has had to face in defending their products.

Amphetamine Abuse and Dependence

The amphetamines are also CNS stimulants. Methamphetamine—commonly called "speed"—is the best-known and most commonly used member of this drug class. It's also the most potent. When a very pure form of methamphetamine—

called "ice"—is smoked, it produces a powerful stimulant effect. Most drugs in this class are usually taken orally or intravenously. Substances that are structurally different but also have amphetaminelike actions—for instance, methylphenidate and other appetite suppressants (so-called diet pills)—are also included in this class. All these drugs increase the brain's activity level, especially that of the reticular activating system (RAS). The RAS, located in the mid- and hindbrain, plays a key role in the sleep/wake cycle.

For many years, the amphetamines were commonly used to help control appetite. That use is now illegal because the drugs were abused so often by dieters. The amphetamines were also taken to reduce fatigue and heighten concentration by military personnel, long-distance truck drivers, and others who needed to maintain alertness. Again, because of the drugs' abuse potential, that use is also uncommon today. One drug from this class—Ritalin—is still widely used, however. It's prescribed to control the agitated behavior of children with attention-deficit hyperactivity disorder. Ritalin calms many of these children, even though it's a stimulant for adults.

Caffeine—the sympathetic nervous system stimulant that gives coffee its "kick"—is related to this family of stimulant drugs. Some scientists also consider several of the antidepressant drugs to be stimulants, since their behavioral actions mimic those of the amphetamines and other CNS stimulants. In fact, as discussed in Chapter 7, part of the controversy surrounding the new antidepressant Prozac stems from the profound stimulating effects it has on some patients.

Low to moderate doses of a stimulant lead to elevated mood and increased mental alertness and energy. In higher doses, stimulants produce hyperactivity and restlessness, insomnia, anxiety, impaired judgment, and even anger and fighting, at times. Stimulant intoxication also induces marked physiological changes, including changes in heartrate, blood pressure, gastrointestinal functioning, and respiration. Confusion, seizures, and coma can also occur at high concentrations. Chronic stimulant intoxication is associated with emotional blunting (that is, numbness or apathy), fatigue, sadness, and social withdrawal. Agitation, concentration difficulties, and paranoid delusions can occur upon taking increasing doses of these drugs repeatedly for an extended period of time. Such behaviors may ultimately produce a psychoti-clike state—called *toxic psychosis*—which resembles paranoid schizophrenia.

Let's look at how taking amphetamines affected Mary Beth:

> Mary Beth was a 20-year-old college student when she began using amphetamines to stay awake during the final exam period in the spring of her sophomore year. Although her exams didn't turn out very well (in part, because the drugs interfered with her ability to concentrate and remember), she continued to use them on and off over the next few months. Because tolerance gradually reduced the effects of the drug, she began taking more and more of it. Increasingly, the feelings of euphoria that had first accompanied use of the drug were replaced by restlessness, irritability, and anger. People learned to stay away from her when she was studying late at night, because they knew she could lash out at them for the slightest provocation. Worse, though, were the profound feelings of depression that Mary Beth had begun to experience when the acute drug effect wore off. At those times, the best she could do (if she had no more drug to take) was go to bed and try to fall asleep. The depression she experienced when she "crashed" was worse than anything she'd ever experienced before.

Stimulant withdrawal typically involves a "crash": a period of profound despair and depression, accompanied by a variety of CNS and gastrointestinal abnormalities, which can last for several days or more. A crash can be especially severe when a substantial amount of drug has been ingested. Tolerance also develops to the stimulant's ability to induce euphoria and energy. This explains why very high doses of the drug—capable of inducing serious behavioral and physical consequences—are taken.

Cocaine and "Crack" Abuse and Dependence

Cocaine is a short-acting, powerful stimulant. Its effects are very much like those of the amphetamines, only shorter lived and more intense. The only therapeutic use for cocaine is as a topical anesthetic for minor operations.

Cocaine is a natural substance that's refined from the coca plant. As such, it's long been used by South American natives to induce euphoria and counteract fatigue. The chewing of coca leaves by Andean people is still very common.

When taken by mouth, cocaine's potency is significantly reduced. As a result, it's generally inhaled ("snorted"), smoked, or injected. When inhaled, the peak effects of cocaine occur in about 20 minutes; they diminish within about an hour. An intense, though short-lived, feeling of well-being—the "rush"—is what makes cocaine so sought after.

"Crack"—the source of a recent epidemic of stimulant use in many U.S. cities—is the dried mixture of the powdered hydrochloride salt of cocaine, water, and baking soda. It's smoked ("free-based") to yield a very intense, 20- to 30-minute "high." Arnold Washton, a psychologist with long experience treating drug dependence, calls crack "the most addictive drug known to man right now. It is almost instantaneous addiction. . . . There is no such thing as the 'recreational use' of crack" (Morganthau, 1986, p. E1).

Cocaine and crack cause dependence rapidly, for two reasons: (1) The euphoria they produce is profoundly reinforcing and (2) the effect is so short lived and so often followed by depression that the abuser ingests repeated doses, one after another, in an attempt to regain the high and postpone the low. When cocaine and crack are involved, the vicious cycle of abuse and dependence so often associated with psychoactive drugs is established with unparalleled swiftness:

> While alcoholism takes its toll over the course of years, coke, free-basing, and crack are causing people to bottom out within months. "It's very simple," says Paul, a 45-year-old real-estate broker with a large investment firm, who became a born-again Christian when he kicked his coke habit. "There's a line you cross when it becomes impossible. It usually takes twenty years with alcohol, ten to fifteen years with pot, five years with snorting cocaine, six months for shooting it, and a matter of weeks for crack." (Hoban, 1989, p. 40)

In addition to the catastrophic psychological effects of cocaine and crack addiction, free-basing cocaine and crack can lead to significant cardiovascular and lung damage. Cocaine has also been linked to pregnancy complications and birth defects. And the obvious financial incentives of the cocaine/crack trade have led to drug wars, murders of rival drug suppliers, and the virtual siege of drug-infested areas of some cities. The problem of drug dependence in U.S. cities is no longer solely one of heroin. Crack and cocaine have become equally destructive contributors.

Wider public recognition of cocaine's harmful effects is reflected in the data shown in Figure 9.6 on page 288. In sum, the number of occasional cocaine users in the United States declined by about 50 percent between 1985 and 1991. Unfortunately, the number of heavy users (that is, individuals who use cocaine once a week or more) has remained essentially unchanged (Horgan, 1993).

Sedative-Hypnotic Abuse and Dependence

The sedative-hypnotic drugs reduce brain activity, especially the activity of the reticular activating system (RAS). As a result, these drugs are commonly used to sedate and calm (in low doses) and to induce sleep (in higher doses). The drugs that belong to this class include the barbiturates (e.g., secobarbital), the benzodiazepines (e.g., Librium and Valium), the carbamates (e.g., meprobamate), and the barbituratelike hypnotics (e.g., methaqualone). In addition to the barbiturates,

FIGURE 9.6 Trends in cocaine use: 1985–1991

Even though the number of cocaine users in the United States decreased by more than 50 percent, the number of heavy users remained essentially constant.

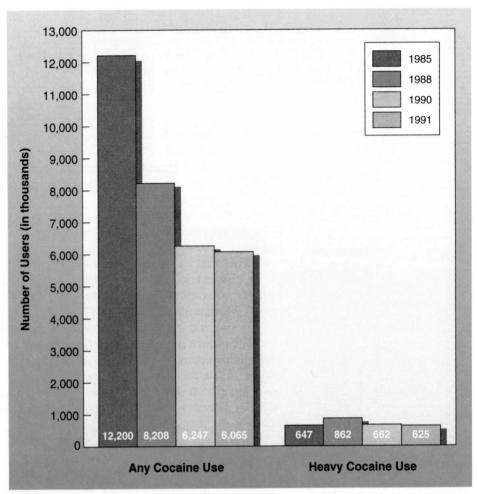

Source: Chart 5, p. 25, *Substance Abuse: The Nation's Number One Health Problem*, Robert Wood Johnson Foundation. Reprinted by permission.

other sedative-hypnotics that require a prescription include such common sleeping medications as Quaalude, Doriden, and Noludar. Like the barbiturates, they are most commonly used to sedate or induce sleep. The minor tranquilizers, including Librium and Valium, are also classified as sedative-hypnotics; they are prescribed as muscle relaxants and to induce relaxation.

The abuse potential of the sedative-hypnotic drugs is very high. In lower doses, they induce mild sedation, relaxation, and a sense of well-being—the feelings for which they are abused. Most of these drugs also cause strong physical dependence and tolerance, so users must take higher and higher doses in order to maintain their reinforcing effects. However, higher doses of these drugs induce behavioral and CNS depression and respiratory failure. Because the sedative-hypnotics produce profound tolerance, stopping use abruptly can cause a variety of life-threatening consequences, including convulsions, coma, and death.

The sedative-hypnotic drugs are *additive:* that is, combining them with another drug yields a greater effect than would be obtained with either substance alone. A popular combination is taking barbiturates with alcohol, which is also a sedative. Combinations of sedative-hypnotics have been fatal in many instances when the effects included severely depressed respiration and CNS functioning. Perhaps the most famous victim of the synergistic (combined) effects of sedative drugs and alcohol was Elvis Presley.

Opioid Abuse and Dependence

Three groups of powerfully addicting drugs are included in this drug class:

1. *the natural opiates*—refined from the opium poppy; for example, morphine and codeine
2. *the semisynthetic opiates*—chemical derivatives of morphine or codeine; for example, heroin
3. *the synthetic opiates*—manufactured drugs whose actions mimic those of the opiates; for example, methadone, Darvon, and Demerol

People have known for millennia about the effects produced by the dried matter that comes from the cut seedpod of the opium poppy. Almost 6,000 years ago, the Sumerians described a "joy plant," which was almost certainly the opium poppy. The opiates produce euphoria and a profound sense of well-being, passivity, and warmth. They also give the individual a striking subjective sense of being removed from physical reality and put into a dreamlike state. In addition, they are very effective in dampening pain.

The principal therapeutic use of the opiates centers on the last effect: controlling pain. Morphine, in particular, has been used as a premier analgesic (painkiller) for two centuries. It continues to be used for that purpose today, especially for managing the extreme pain of orthopedic surgery and some varieties of cancer.

Heroin is the most commonly abused opiate, in part, because it's several times stronger than morphine. Heroin is a white, odorless, bitter-tasting powder. Users prefer to mix the drug with water and inject it because this route of action produces a rapid effect. Heroin produces a powerful rush of relaxation, dreaminess, and well-being. Many users have compared the heroin high to orgasm. It's a very expensive habit, however.

Another frequently abused opiate is the codeine contained in cough syrup, which is available only by prescription. The high from codeine is not nearly as dramatic as that from heroin. But codeine is also less dangerous and less expensive.

Both the natural and synthetic opiates are profoundly addicting. They induce rapid tolerance, physical dependence, and a disagreeable period of physical withdrawal that is characterized by nausea, vomiting, psychomotor irritability, and insomnia. Opiate overdose can cause respiratory depression and sedation.

Many addicts die when they unknowingly use heroin that is more pure than they are used to. The result is an overdose that effectively shuts down breathing and causes death from asphyxiation. Another hazard is the use of adulterants, such as bleach and talc, to "cut" the drug. These materials are used, in effect, to dilute the heroin, reducing its potency and also making the amount of drug go further. The trouble is, some of these substances are toxic in their own right. Even more hazardous is the practice of injecting heroin with dirty needles. As you likely know, intravenous (IV) drug abusers—most of them heroin addicts—are one of the groups at highest risk for contracting HIV (human immunodeficiency virus), which causes AIDS.

Hallucinogen Abuse and Dependence

The hallucinogens include LSD, psilocybin, morning glory seeds, mescaline, and phencyclidine (PCP). They are ingested to induce hallucinations—visual and auditory distortions of the environment—which distance the user from her surroundings and sometimes force a rethinking of relationships. Reaching this so-called altered state of consciousness is reinforcing to some people. In fact, in certain cases, doing so is important enough to cause individuals to structure their lives around taking hallucinogens, rather than on home, school, family, and friends.

Hallucinogens have been used throughout history. Religious leaders have often used these drugs as "mind-expanding" agents that seem to bring them into closer contact with the "cosmic forces" of the universe. For example, a number of tribes of Native Americans used natural hallucinogens for religious purposes. When taken on a very occasional basis, these substances are unlikely to cause irreversible damage. But when taken frequently, they can cut the user off from the real world, further alienating a person who may be estranged from society to begin with. Hallucinogens also have the potential to permanently alter neurotransmitter functioning in the brain and cause prolonged paranoid and delusional psychoses that are difficult to treat.

Cannabis (Marijuana and Hashish) Abuse and Dependence

Cannabis products—namely, marijuana and hashish—are related chemically and by the effects they produce to the hallucinogens. The psychoactive ingredient in cannabis—**tetrahydrocannabinol (THC)**—is concentrated in the resin of the hemp plant, *Cannabis sativa*. Marijuana is the dried mixture of the leaves and seeds of this plant. Hashish, a more potent form of THC, is the highly resinous mixture of the flowering tops of the plant.

In sufficient amounts, both marijuana and hashish can induce hallucinations and paranoid delusions. In moderate doses, individuals experience subjective effects such as a sense of relaxation and well-being. On occasion, individuals become disinhibited, such that things are seen in a new light—for instance, humorous, silly, or offbeat. These drug effects may enhance a party or celebratory atmosphere, which is one reason marijuana is often ingested in group settings. Moderate doses of marijuana produce behavioral effects similar to those of moderate doses of alcohol. The physical effects of marijuana include increased respiration and heartrate and a dry mouth and throat.

The most troublesome consequence of chronic use of marijuana is called the **amotivational syndrome.** It's characterized by the individual having great difficulty rousing himself from profound self-absorption to become reinvolved with friends, work, family, and school. There is considerable scientific dispute over whether long-term marijuana use is associated with other damaging psychological or physical consequences (Ray & Ksir, 1990).

CAUSES OF SUBSTANCE ABUSE AND DEPENDENCE

Genetic/Biological Factors

It has long been recognized that alcoholism and drug abuse/dependence run in families. It is not as clear, however, why. Is it because a genetic predisposition (tendency) to substance abuse or dependence is transmitted from parent to child? Does an alcoholic or drug-using parent create an environment conveying psychological and behavioral factors that lead to similar behavior in their children? Or are both hypotheses valid? In the following sections, we review the substantial data supporting the former view—that of a genetic predisposition to abuse and dependence.

Concordance Rates for Alcoholism in Twins   If there is a genetic component in the risk for developing alcoholism or drug dependence, then identical twins (who share identical genes) should have similar histories of use and abuse (that is, high rates of concordance). Fraternal twins (who are genetically different, though born at the same time) would be more likely to differ in their tendencies to develop problems with abuse and dependence. In general, researchers using twin studies to examine the genetics of alcoholism have confirmed these expectations. (Note that twin studies have not been used extensively to study the genetics of other types of substance abuse and dependence.)

tetrahydrocannabinol (THC) Psychoactive ingredient in cannabis products, such as marijuana and hashish.

amotivational syndrome Condition associated with heavy use of marijuana; the individual loses motivation for virtually everything in life except continuation of heavy use of marijuana.

In an early, influential study, Kaij (1960) reported that the concordance rate for alcohol abuse among Swedish monozygotic (identical) twins was 54 percent and among dizygotic (fraternal) twins, 28 percent. A study by Leohlin (1977) involved 850 pairs of American same-sex twins who were high school juniors at the time. In comparing data from identical versus fraternal twins, it was observed that both individuals in sets of identical twins were more likely to be heavy drinkers.

A recent study (Kendler, Heath, Neale, Kessler, & Eaves, 1992) of 1,030 female/female twins in Virginia had similar findings: Concordance for alcoholism was consistently higher in identical than in fraternal twins. Overall, 58 percent of the identical twins were concordant for alcoholism, compared to only 29 percent of the fraternal twins. Commenting on these findings, Kendler cautioned, "Women with relatives who have been alcoholic should be warned early in life to watch for early signs of alcohol dependence, like repeatedly finding yourself drinking more than you want to" (Goleman, 1992c).

Despite the consistency of these findings, twin studies of alcoholism have been criticized. Even though most of us assume that identical and fraternal twins share their environments equally and differ only in the amount of shared genetic material, that's not necessarily so. Identical twins may actually share more features of the environment than fraternal twins because their parents and the world may treat them as being more alike. In other words, the environment side of the environment/heredity equation for identical twins may differ significantly from that for fraternal twins.

Adoption Studies of Children of Alcoholics   Adoption studies hold environmental influences constant—which twin studies may not—while systematically varying genetic factors. As a consequence, many behavioral scientists believe these studies provide the best perspective on the role of genetic factors in mental disorders.

The most influential adoption studies of alcoholism are a series of Danish studies by Goodwin (1976, 1979, 1985) that compared four groups of young adult children of alcoholics (ACOAs). The groups included (1) sons of alcoholics raised by nonalcoholic foster parents, (2) sons of alcoholics raised by their biological parents, and daughters of alcoholics raised, respectively, by (3) nonalcoholic foster parents and (4) their biological parents. Paired with each group was a control group matched for age and adoption status. All adoptees had been separated from their biological parents during the first few weeks of life and then adopted by nonrelatives.

These extensive studies yielded two principal findings about ACOAs:

1. Sons of alcoholics were about four times more likely than sons of nonalcoholics to become alcoholic adults, regardless of whether they had been raised by their own alcoholic biological parents or by nonalcoholic adoptive parents.
2. The influence of genetics on the daughters of alcoholics was not as strong as that on the sons of alcoholics.

Subsequent Swedish research on adopted children has confirmed Goodwin's initial conclusions on the role of genetic factors in male alcoholism (Bohman, Cloninger, von Knorring, & Sigvardsson, 1984). What's more, this research has shown that genetic factors significantly affect female alcoholism, as well—a finding much stronger than that of Goodwin's research. The Swedish research also suggested that there are at least two forms of inherited alcoholism. By analyzing data from 2,000 Swedish adoptees, these researchers (Bohman, Sigvardsson, & Cloninger, 1981; Cloninger, Bohman, & Sigvardsson, 1981) identified two groups of alcoholics differing in alcoholism heritability.

The more common, lower-heritability, Type I alcoholics begin drinking in their midtwenties to thirties; however, they typically don't develop alcohol problems until middle age. These individuals have a high risk of developing liver disease and show little antisocial behavior and relatively few social and occupational problems. Children of Type I alcoholics are twice as likely to become alcoholics as children without family histories of alcoholism. Sons of Type I alcoholics, raised in troubled adoptive homes, are at even greater risk to develop alcoholism.

In contrast are the higher-heritability Type II alcoholics. Their alcoholism begins very early, and they experience profound social and occupational problems but relatively few medical difficulties. The biological sons (but not the biological daughters) of Type II alcoholics are nine times more likely to become alcoholics, regardless of environmental influences.

Heritability Studies of Children of Drug Addicts and of Cigarette Smokers   In one of the few empirical studies of the role played by genetic factors in the development of drug abuse, Cadoret, Troughton, O'Gorman, and Heywood (1986) reported significant relationships among parental alcoholism, antisocial behavior, and drug problems in adults who were adopted as children. These findings suggest that at least some forms of drug abuse—like some forms of alcoholism—have a genetic component. Since antisocial personality and parental alcoholism have both been associated with the development of drug abuse (Helzer et al., 1990), these data suggest a genetic link between drug abuse in biological parents and drug abuse in their children.

A recent series of reports on the role of genetic factors in smoking (Heath & Martin, 1993; Heath et al., 1993) strongly suggests that two smoking behaviors are heavily influenced by genetics: (1) initiation (whether a nonsmoker becomes a smoker) and (2) persistence (whether a smoker quits smoking). Heath and his colleagues obtained self-report data on smoking initiation from three large samples of adult twins, totaling almost 10,000 pairs. (The first two samples were gathered in Australia and Virginia; the third was a national survey sponsored by the American Association of Retired Persons.) In their study on smoking persistence, Heath and Martin (1993) examined questionnaire responses from Australian twin pairs who were over 30 years of age. Differences in concordance rates for smoking initiation between identical and fraternal twins were substantial—so much so that these researchers estimated the genetic contribution to the risk of becoming a smoker in the U.S. sample to be 60 percent in men and 51 percent in women. Heritability estimates in the Australian sample were also substantial: 33 percent in men and 51 percent in women. For smoking persistence, the combined heritability estimate for men and women was 53 percent.

Electrophysiological Studies of Children of Alcoholics   Two electroencephalographic (EEG) techniques commonly used to study the brain's electrical activity—**evoked potential (EP)** and **event-related potential (ERP)**—have been employed to study genetic influences on alcoholism. EP techniques measure the brain's electrical response to external stimuli, like flashes of light or loud sounds. ERP techniques measure electrical events that arise during the brain's processing of information.

There is substantial evidence (Hill, 1995) that EP and ERP waveforms are genetically determined. Noting this, Begleiter, Porjesz, Bihari, and Kissin (1984) hypothesized that a specific ERP response—the P300 wave deficit—may be a genetically determined antecedent of alcoholism, rather than a consequence, as previously believed. Begleiter and his colleagues tested this hypothesis by comparing the ERPs of 25 12-year-old boys who had alcoholic fathers with those of 25 same-aged boys who had no histories of paternal alcoholism.

Significant differences in P300 voltage were found between the two groups (see Figure 9.7). Interestingly, the boys who had paternal histories of alcoholism showed a pattern of significantly reduced P300 voltage. This pattern was similar to one previously seen in chronic alcoholics who were no longer drinking (Porjesz &

evoked potential (EP)
Brain's electrical response to external stimuli.

event-related potential (ERP)   Electrical events that arise during information processing in the brain.

FIGURE 9.7   Event-related response

There are marked differences in event-related responses shown by a normal control subject and a high-risk subject.

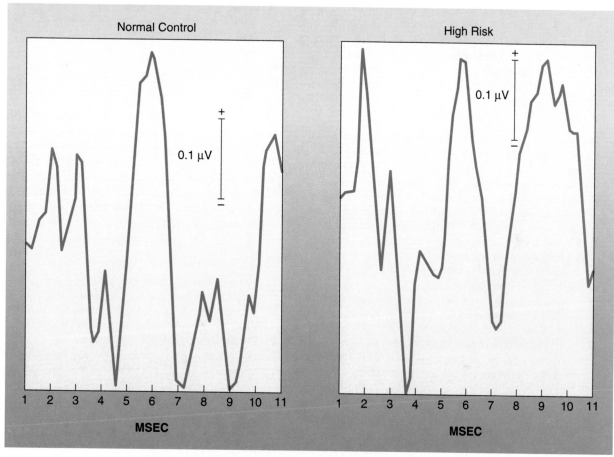

Source: From H. Begleiter, B. Porjesz, and B. Bihari, "Auditory Brainstem Potentials in Sons of Alcoholic Fathers," *Alcoholism: Clinical and Experimental Research, 11*, p. 478. Copyright © 1987 Williams & Wilkins. Reprinted by permission of Williams & Wilkins.

Begleiter, 1983). The similarity between these two groups supported the notion that reduced P300 voltage is a factor in developing alcoholism. Two recent reports of reduced P300 voltage in groups of boys and girls who had family histories of alcoholism (Hill & Steinhauer, 1993; Steinhauer & Hill, 1993) further strengthen the likelihood that ERP may reflect a genetic predisposition to alcoholism that is based in the central nervous system.

A Biological/Genetic Basis for Substance Abuse and Dependence   Do these findings prove that the children of alcoholics and drug addicts are doomed to follow in their parents' footsteps? Absolutely not. Certainly, some researchers believe that the adult children of alcoholics bear extra burdens in life (as reviewed in Thinking about Research). But the fact is, most children of substance abusers do not become substance abusers, and most substance abusers are not the children of substance abusers. These realities prove how important environmental factors are in the development of substance abuse (Prescott et al., 1994; Schuckit, 1994a).

Instead, when we discuss a genetic basis for alcoholism and drug dependence, we simply imply that there's a heightened predisposition to developing the disorder. That is, if your father or mother was or is a substance abuser, you have a greater chance of developing a problem.

Some authorities believe that adult children of alcoholics (ACOAs) bear an additional burden beyond their heightened risk for developing alcoholism. Namely, they claim that ACOAs suffer lifelong psychological consequences of their parents' alcoholism, even if they never develop the disorder. Dr. Timmen L. Cermak, who is the adult child of an alcoholic, lists the following burdens that ACOAs must bear (1988):

■ Hard-driving; workaholic; always preoccupied by projects and things that "have to be done"; rarely satisfied with accomplishments; in denial of feelings, relationships take a back seat.

■ Defensive; fearful of closeness to others; plays cards close to the vest; unable to deal honestly on an emotional level; longing for relationships; chronic anger.

■ Overwhelmed by feelings; buffeted by emotional storms; desperately trying to get other people to behave properly; often unable to work effectively.

■ Alcohol and drug addiction.

■ Depressed, with a chronic sense of emptiness within; lacking a sense of direction in life; apathetic; low self-esteem; may be self-destructive.

■ Victim identity; constant sense of being attacked, misunderstood, ignored, and betrayed—all of which justifies an angry, demanding attitude toward others.

■ Martyr identity; long-suffering; unwilling to take care of oneself; constantly excusing the faults of others; willingness to submit oneself to painful situations for others' sake.

■ Generous, helpful, and thoughtful—to a fault.

■ Constantly searching for answers, rules and guidelines for finding happiness and social/emotional success.

Researchers who have surveyed the existing literature on ACOAs question whether a specific set of psychological consequences results from parental alcoholism. They suggest, instead, that most ACOAs do not differ from other people and that if there is a lasting effect of parental alcoholism in some individuals, it's not distinguishable from the effects of living with a parent who suffered from any other chronic, recurrent illness (Goleman, 1992a; Sher, 1991).

Think about the following questions:

1. What factors might explain how the belief developed that ACOAs bear a special burden as adults, even though the adult children of parents with other serious disorders haven't been implicated in this way?

2. Do you know any ACOAs? Are you one, perhaps? Do any of Cermak's characteristics describe your friends or yourself? If so, discuss them.

So, if you are the child of an alcoholic, you owe it to yourself to be aware of your increased risk of developing alcoholism. How? You should be more careful than friends who do not share your heightened risk in how you use alcohol. Logically, you will be more likely to develop an abusive drinking problem if you drink heavily. Everyone should use alcohol responsibly. But remember that you have an obligation to treat alcohol with even greater care and respect than persons without your family history.

Sociocultural Factors

Think about the groups you belong to: racial/ethnic, religious, and national groups as well as those defined by your sex, profession, education, and age. All these groups influence who you are, including how you behave. This is hardly surprising, since your parents' group memberships influenced the childrearing patterns that, in turn, affected you. Group identification also directly affected your behavior in the past, during childhood, and will continue to do so now and in the future. We all try to behave like our elders or others we admire.

Given all this, you may not be surprised to learn that group membership influences behaviors of alcohol and drug use and abuse. You may be surprised, however, to learn just how much (Johnson, Nagoshi, Danko, Honbo, & Chau, 1990; Kandel, Davies, Karns, & Yamaguchi, 1986).

Table 9.3 summarizes the widely differing rates of alcohol consumption across the nine census regions of the United States, illustrating the effects of group membership on alcohol consumption (Midanik & Room, 1992, p. 185). These differences in per capita consumption reflect regional population differences in the religious, ethnic, and

| TABLE 9.3 | Per Capita Consumption of Alcohol in Nine Census Regions of the Coterminous United States: 1940, 1964, 1979, and 1988 (in gallons of pure alcohol, rather than beverage alcohol) | | | | | | | |

	Per Capita Consumption				Rank Order on Per Capita Consumption			
Region	1940	1964	1979	1988	1940	1964	1979	1988
Pacific	1.9	2.6	3.4	2.8	1	1	1	2
Middle Atlantic	1.8	2.4	2.7	2.4	2	3	5	6
East North Central	1.8	2.3	2.7	2.4	3	4	5	5
New England	1.7	2.5	3.1	2.9	4	2	3	1
Mountain	1.3	2.1	3.3	2.8	5	5	2	3
West North Central	1.2	1.8	2.5	2.2	6	7	8	8
South Atlantic	1.1	1.9	2.8	2.5	7	6	4	4
West South Central	0.9	1.7	2.6	2.3	8	8	7	7
East South Central	0.6	1.0	2.0	1.9	9	9	9	9

Source: From "The Epidemiology of Alcohol Consumption," by L. T. Midanik and R. Room, 1992, *Alcohol Health & Research World, 16*(3), Table 1, p. 185.

racial makeup of the American "melting pot." In turn, we can observe regional differences in rates of alcoholism, which are closely related to rates of consumption.

For example, New England is populated with large numbers of Northern Europeans, whose parents and grandparents came from countries with high alcoholism rates. Per capita consumption in this region is much higher than in the three southern census regions, which are populated with a substantial number of Southern Baptists, for whom drinking is forbidden. Moreover, periodic shifts in the rank order of per capita consumption shown in the table likely reflect geographic shifts in population groups. For instance, since 1940, more individuals from groups with lower rates of drinking have moved north to the Middle Atlantic region in search of employment. Likewise, more persons from groups with higher rates of drinking have moved to the South Atlantic region for the same reason (Midanik & Room, 1992, p. 185). You may have observed regional differences in drinking patterns if you have lived in several census regions, perhaps to go to school or work.

Earlier in this chapter, we reviewed data indicating that age, ethnicity, and sex all affect rates of alcohol and drug consumption. How does membership in groups like these exert such strong effects on rates of alcohol use and abuse? It's not simply that one group discourages consumption of alcohol and another especially encourages it. In fact, ethnic groups in the United States with low rates of alcoholism—including Italian Americans, Jewish Americans, and Chinese Americans—generally show low rates of abstinence, as well. The opposite is also true: High rates of alcoholism and abstinence characterize Americans with Irish, African, and Eastern European heritage (Lex, 1985).

These puzzling findings (which are similar to those of Harford, Parker, Grant, & Dawson [1992]) point to the importance of cultural patterns. Specifically, it seems that cultural groups that stress the moderate use of alcohol, especially in a family or religious context, produce large numbers of members who use alcohol but few alcoholics. By contrast, cultural groups that focus on both the dangers and the pleasures of alcohol use tend to produce more members who abstain from alcohol as well as more who drink to excess (Lex, 1985).

FIGURE 9.8 Lifetime prevalence rates of alcoholism for men and women

In a worldwide study involving subjects from five regions, striking differences were found between men and women. Prevalence rates for alcoholism were most disparate among Korean subjects.

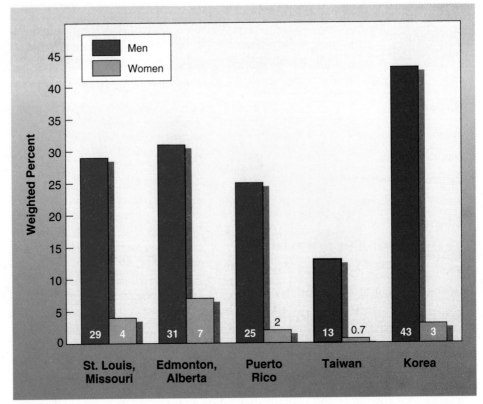

Source: From J. E. Helzer, G. J. Canino, E.-K. Yeh, C. K. Lee, H.-G. Hwu, and S. Newman, "Alcoholism—North America and Asia," *Archives of General Psychiatry, 47,* p. 315. Copyright 1990 American Medical Association. Reprinted by permission.

In the late 1980s, a population survey (Helzer et al., 1990) examined alcohol abuse and addiction in five sites around the globe: St. Louis, Missouri; Edmonton, Alberta, Canada; Puerto Rico; Seoul, South Korea; and Taipei City, Taiwan. Researchers confirmed that sex is a major risk factor for alcoholism, just as it is for drug abuse and disorders like depression and antisocial personality disorder. The marked disparity in lifetime prevalence for alcoholism between men and women in all five geographically diverse sites is illustrated in Figure 9.8. (*Lifetime prevalence* means, for example, that 29 percent of the men and only 4 percent of the women interviewed in St. Louis had been diagnosed as being alcoholic at some point in their lives.) In sum, men are at much higher risk for alcoholism than women. These data confirm studies reviewed earlier, which also reported differences in alcoholism rates between men and women in the United States.

What explains these significant differences between men and women in alcohol abuse and dependence? Two theories are most widely accepted. First, many observers point to the lower tolerance shown in most societies for heavy alcohol use by women, due to their traditional role in caring for children. Second, researchers have examined the different rates at which men and women metabolize alcohol (Frezza et al., 1990). Recent empirical data suggest that women possess smaller amounts of a crucial enzyme that detoxifies alcohol in the stomach and small intestine. Such a sex-based metabolic difference would explain why alcohol consumed in equivalent doses by men and women has greater behavioral and physiological effects on women (Gallant, 1987; Jacobsen, 1986). Simply put, fewer women than men may drink to excess because when drunk in large quantities, alcohol produces more aversive behavioral and physical consequences for women.

The abuse of illicit and prescription drugs among Americans has long been related to ethnic and racial identity (Schuckit, 1995). Even today, heroin use is largely (though by no means entirely) confined to people who are poor, largely

African American or Hispanic, and living in urban ghettos. By contrast, the abuse of prescription drugs is largely a phenomenon of middle-class women, whose physicians originally prescribe these drugs to alleviate depression, anxiety, and insomnia.

Learning-Based Factors

Classical Conditioning   Mechanisms of classical conditioning have been implicated in such common symptoms of dependence as craving and tolerance. A series of experiments with alcohol (Crowell, Hinson, & Siegel, 1981) and morphine (Siegel, 1978) demonstrated that drug-dependent rats that had developed drug tolerance maintained tolerance only when tested under the environmental conditions originally associated with drug or alcohol administration. Tolerance was not observed when the drugs were given in new environments.

These experiments led Siegel (1978) to propose the **conditioned compensatory response model,** a classical conditioning model of drug tolerance. Siegel (1978) argued that environmental stimuli associated with drug intake become linked with the drug's effects on the body to produce a conditioned response opposite to the drug's effect. This is a compensating response, designed to maintain bodily homeostasis (balance). As this conditioned homeostatic response increases in magnitude with continued drug intake, the drug's effects continue to decrease and tolerance increases.

The **conditioned appetitive motivational model** is a classical conditioning model of craving (Stewart, deWit, & Eikelboom, 1984). According to this model, the conditioned stimuli associated with the positive reinforcing effects of drugs—for example, the smells, sounds, and lighting of the place where heroin is most often injected—become capable of bringing about a positive motivational state, similar to the one elicited by the drug itself. This state, in turn, creates strong, continuing urges to seek and use the drug. This model explains why former abusers have such great difficulty staying off drugs when they return to the environments where they developed their addictions.

Operant Conditioning   One of the first studies of the operant conditioning mechanisms involved in alcohol self-administration by humans was reported by Nathan and O'Brien (1971). They examined alcoholic subjects living in an experimental environment on a Boston City Hospital ward during 33-day studies. The social behaviors, moods, and drinking behaviors of matched groups of alcoholics and nonalcoholics were compared over these prolonged periods. Operant procedures were used to assess the differing reward values of alcohol and social interaction, both of which are extremely powerful reinforcers for these subjects. All subjects had to repeatedly press a button on an operant panel at a high rate. By doing so, they earned points to "purchase" alcohol, time out of their rooms in a social area, or both.

Comparisons of the operant behavior of the alcoholic and nonalcoholic groups revealed the following:

- The alcoholics worked much longer and harder to earn points to purchase alcohol. As a result, even though both alcoholics and nonalcoholics reached the same high blood-alcohol levels early in drinking, the alcoholics remained at these levels longer and returned to them more frequently. The alcoholics drank almost twice as much as the nonalcoholics.
- The nonalcoholics worked much longer and harder to earn points that permitted them to leave their rooms and spend time with each other in a social area. By contrast, the alcoholics remained social isolates before, during, and after drinking.
- Once the drinking began, the alcoholics became significantly more depressed and less active than the nonalcoholics. The alcoholics also demonstrated significantly more psychopathology, including anxiety, manic behavior, depression, paranoia, and phobic and compulsive behavior.

conditioned compensatory response model   Siegel's classical conditioning theory of acquired behavioral tolerance to dependency-inducing drugs.

conditioned appetitive motivational model   Classical conditioning theory explaining the craving addicted individuals experience for the substances they're dependent on.

This research program (Nathan & O'Brien, 1971) ultimately led a number of other clinical researchers to explore operant programs that are designed to reinforce alcoholics for reducing or stopping their drinking. Bigelow and his colleagues (Bigelow, Cohen, Liebson, & Faillace, 1972; Bigelow, Liebson, & Griffiths, 1974), for example, reported a major reduction in alcoholics' drinking when subjects were reinforced with money and other rewards for maintaining limited periods of abstinence in laboratory settings.

Modeling and Vicarious Reinforcement   As we have already observed, we tend to drink the way our parents and others in our environment drink. During the early 1970s, Bandura (1969, 1977) studied the learning-based mechanism that helps explain this phenomenon. Bandura's research—much of it with children—demonstrated that we can acquire new knowledge and behaviors and modify existing knowledge and behaviors simply by watching other people and events. It isn't necessary for us to engage in these behaviors ourselves, and the consequences of these behaviors don't have to affect us. Vicarious reinforcement and modeling provide learning-based explanations for the impact that social and peer group memberships have on drinking rates and patterns. These explanations also address why the children of alcoholics sometimes drink abusively.

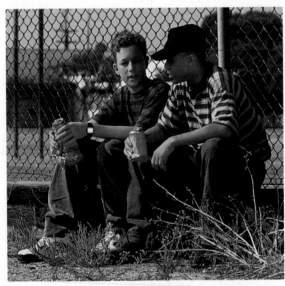

As adolescents get older, many become increasingly convinced of the positive benefits of alcohol consumption. These expectations play an important role in inducing youths to become regular drinkers. What are some of the roots of alcohol expectancies?

Alcohol Expectancies   In a 1985 study of adolescent **alcohol expectancies,** Christiansen, Goldman, and Brown found that as adolescents age, they become increasingly convinced that alcohol improves social behavior, increases sexual arousal, and decreases tension. Subsequently, the same investigators (Goldman, Brown, & Christiansen, 1987) reported that adolescent alcohol abusers differ from nonabusers in terms of what each group expects alcohol to do for it. A group of 116 adolescents was split into four groups: alcohol abusers and nonabusers with and without family histories of alcoholism. All the youths completed the *Alcohol Expectancy Questionnaire* (Christiansen, Goldman, & Inn, 1982).

A review of the results found that the four groups had striking differences in expectancies. Adolescent alcohol abusers anticipated significantly more pleasure from drinking than their nonabusing peers. Moreover, adolescents who had alcohol-abusing parents expected more cognitive and motor enhancement from alcohol than did those without family histories of alcoholism. These findings confirm that adolescents' alcohol use patterns and family histories of alcoholism affect their attitudes toward drinking. In addition, these findings suggest that alcohol expectancies may affect adolescents' chances of developing more serious drinking problems as adults (Goldman, Brown, & Christiansen, 1987).

Psychopathological and Personality Factors

alcohol expectancies
Expectations of the effects of alcohol on behavior.

comorbidity Presence of two or more psychiatric disorders in an individual.

Comorbidity   Psychopathological explanations of substance abuse assume that it occurs, at least partially, because of **comorbidity**—the presence of two or more psychiatric disorders in a single person. Individuals who are alcohol dependent are more likely than those with other *DSM* disorders to suffer from other psychiatric conditions (Neighbors, Kempton, & Forehand, 1992; Sher & Trull, 1994). More specifically, the conditions that most often accompany alcohol dependence are depression and antisocial personality disorder, followed by schizophrenia, anxiety disorders, and sleep disorders (Schuckit, 1994c).

FIGURE 9.9 The biochemistry of cocaine

Blocking Normal Restraints

Cocaine, in effect, prevents the brain from calming itself down.

Normally, in response to certain external stimuli, specific neurons release a chemical called dopamine that helps trigger good feelings, or euphoria. The dopamine enters the junction, or synapse, between the first neuron and its neighbor. It stimulates the neighboring cell and thereby acts as a messenger (or neurotransmitter), sending information along so-called dopamine pathways.

Normally, the dopamine is then reabsorbed by the sending neuron. But cocaine somehow blocks the reabsorption. The neighboring nerves thus become overexcited and the euphoria intensifies greatly. Not for long, however. The brain's supply of dopamine becomes depleted, and once that happens, the crack user crashes into profound depression.

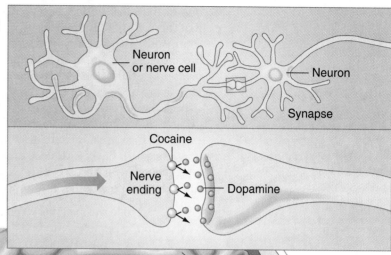

Pathway to Euphoria

One dopamine pathway goes through the major emotional centers of the brain, in the limbic system. When crack brings about an oversupply of dopamine, these centers are rapidly overstimulated and many changes occur: Heartbeat quickens, the stomach churns, sexual desire is enhanced, mood is greatly elevated.

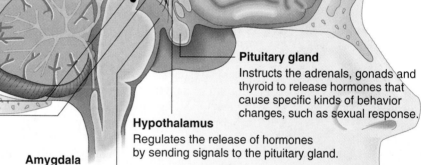

Centers of Stimulation

Ventral tegmental area
Nucleous accumbens
Thought to be learning and reinforcing centers. An animal will repeat an activity that stimulates these areas.

Amygdala
Strongly implicated in originating emotional behavior. Regulates the hypothalamus.

Hypothalamus
Regulates the release of hormones by sending signals to the pituitary gland.

Pituitary gland
Instructs the adrenals, gonads and thyroid to release hormones that cause specific kinds of behavior changes, such as sexual response.

SOURCE: From *The New York Times*, August 24, 1989, p. B7. Copyright © 1989 by The New York Times Company. Reprinted by permission.

Some researchers have speculated that the heavy use of marijuana leads to other psychiatric disorders. If strong evidence were provided to support this hypothesis, it would make a convincing argument against heavy use of this drug. In fact, though, the evidence for this link is mixed. When 100 regular marijuana users were followed for 6 to 7 years, researchers failed to observe a higher incidence of psychopathology in the users than in a comparison group of 50 young men and women who were not users (Weller & Halikas, 1985). On the other hand, as we noted earlier, marijuana is associated with an amotivational syndrome in some chronic users, which interferes significantly with their ability to function. Although this syndrome is not a formal diagnosis in the *DSM-IV* (American Psychiatric Association, 1994), it might someday be recognized as a distinct disorder, worthy of diagnosis and treatment.

More and more data in recent years support the view that substance use disorders are partly due to central nervous system dysfunction. Figure 9.9 illustrates one of the most widely accepted current theories of cocaine addiction—namely, that the drug blocks the reabsorption of dopamine, one of the most important neurotransmitters. In doing so, cocaine simultaneously induces euphoria and lays the groundwork for one of its principal effects, the "crash" on withdrawal that leads to profound depression. A key unanswered question in this theory is whether some people are more susceptible than others to the allure of cocaine's euphoria, to the depression accompanying withdrawal, or to both. Presumably, an individual with one or both of these vulnerabilities would likely have an inborn abnormality in metabolizing neurotransmitters.

To explain the coincidence of substance abuse and other psychiatric disorders, researchers must resolve the "chicken-and-egg" problem. In other words, they must determine whether the symptoms of the other disorder or disorders:

1. precede the substance abuse, in which case the abuse may have developed in the person's effort to dampen the symptoms of the other disorder
2. are the consequences of the troubled life of the substance abuser
3. follow the development of substance abuse and result from it, since substance abuse often produces symptoms that mimic other disorders
4. or some combination of the above

The empirical data available to resolve this problem have been inconsistent. The weight of the evidence seems to suggest two things, however: (1) that antisocial behavior frequently precedes substance abuse and may help trigger its onset (Sher & Trull, 1994) and (2) that depression as often follows as precedes substance abuse, leaving its causal role uncertain (Gawin & Ellinwood, 1988). It remains even more unclear whether schizophrenia, anxiety disorders, and sleep disorders contribute to developing substance abuse and, if they do, how. As Schuckit (1994c) observes, "There is no simple and perfect way to use multiple diagnoses in the context of substance use and abuse to indicate prognosis and treatment. Even with the amount of data that have accrued on the high prevalence of multiple labels among patients meeting criteria for alcohol- or drug-related problems, no single theoretical approach . . . appears to accomplish the goals clearly" (p. 61).

Personality Factors   The psychodynamic model of alcoholism and drug dependence portrays these disorders as ultimately unsuccessful efforts to satisfy in adulthood strong dependency needs that were unmet in infancy and early childhood. According to this view, the individual has substituted substance abuse for the satisfaction of oral dependency needs that went unsatisfied much earlier (Khantzian, 1985). The psychodynamic explanation for substance dependence is less influential than it was several decades ago because efforts to confirm it empirically have not been successful.

But what about the so-called *addictive personality?* Is it true that alcoholics and drug addicts—not to mention compulsive gamblers and maybe even compulsive eaters—share a set of personality characteristics that make them different from others? Put another way, have behavioral scientists been able to identify a particular personality pattern that predicts substance abuse?

Supporters of this position point to indications that many alcoholics share certain behaviors and personality characteristics (like antisocial and depressive tendencies) that differentiate them from nonalcoholics (Morey & Skinner, 1986; Sutker & Allain, 1988). Nathan (1988), however, claims that the personality factors that appear to distinguish substance abusers from others (again, like antisocial and depressive traits) are consequences, rather than causes, of these disorders, so they do not play a role in the development of the substance abuse. Sher and Trull (1994), who also reject the idea of the addictive personality, nonetheless believe that personality factors play a role in the etiologies of both alcoholism and antisocial personality disorder. What's more, these authors believe that the same factors might be responsible for both conditions. They refer to *broad-band personality trait dimensions* that mediate disinhibitory behavior.

Cloninger's (1987) theory of *neurogenetic adaptive mechanisms* is one of the most interesting developments in this dialogue (see Chapter 2). According to Cloninger, genetic and neurobiological factors, personality factors, and environmental factors interact to produce persons who are at substantially higher risk to develop alcohol dependence than persons without these predisposing factors. This theory, if confirmed empirically, would give strong support to the role that personality factors play in alcoholism.

A Biopsychosocial Model

The biopsychosocial model best fits what we know about substance abuse. Data on the role of genetic factors in substance abuse and dependence are strong. They suggest that individuals with family histories of substance-related disorders are at heightened risk to develop abuse and dependence—in part, because they share genetic material with substance-abusing parents or other family members. These data don't explain, however, why most individuals with such family histories never develop substance-related disorders. Likewise, further explanation is needed as to why most of the people who do develop substance abuse disorders do not have family histories of these problems.

These issues are explained somewhat by the contemporary social learning model, which has recently been supported by empirical findings (summarized in NIAAA, 1993). This support has come from long-accepted findings that point to the impact of sociocultural factors on drinking and also from the literature on the role of comorbidity and personality disorders in substance abuse.

In sum, we've examined a number of explanations for what causes substance-related disorders: genetic/biological factors, sociocultural factors, learning-based factors, and psychiatric or personality factors. Alone, none of these views explains the onset and course of substance abuse and dependence as convincingly as they all do when considered together. The addictions field is getting closer than ever to integrating the separate findings on etiology and thus creating a coherent understanding. Although it's not the final word on etiology, Cloninger's theory of neurogenetic adaptive mechanisms serves as a model of the kind of integration of complex mechanisms and divergent findings that will likely emerge at some point.

> ### Focus on
> ### Critical Thinking
>
> **1.** Think about your own drinking or that of someone close to you. Can you identify any biological factors responsible for the consumption pattern you observe? What about social or psychological factors? Explain your answer.
> **2.** Have you known enough heavy or abusive drinkers to be able to categorize them, based on consumption pattern and perhaps family history and abuse consequences? Again, explain your answer.

TREATMENT OF SUBSTANCE ABUSE AND DEPENDENCE

Many of the treatments reviewed in this section are used with both alcohol and drug abusers. That's because most patients today are polydrug abusers, who combine alcohol abuse with the abuse of one or more additional drugs.

Group and Family Therapy

group therapy Approach to therapy that brings a therapist and several patients together; after a time, the patients begin to play a therapeutic role that complements that of the therapist.

Group Therapy   Group and family therapy have become treatments of choice for many substance abusers during the past 25 years. **Group therapy** first gained popularity because it offered therapists a way to confront their patients' denial of

PERSPECTIVE ON SUBSTANCE-RELATED DISORDERS

BIOLOGICAL FACTORS

Biological factors contribute substantially to but are not, by themselves, sufficient to cause the substance-related disorders:

➤ Children of substance abusers are at increased risk to abuse substances. Studies of twins and adults adopted as children indicate genetic predisposition.

➤ Substance intoxication, tolerance, and withdrawal are cardinal features of the substance-related disorders; each results from the effects of the abused substance on the central nervous system. Long-term substance abuse is associated with marked damage to the cardiovascular, gastrointestinal, and central nervous systems—which can lead to premature death.

➤ The impact of alcohol and drugs on specific brain neurotransmitter systems, which determine the individual's unique intoxication, withdrawal, and craving experiences, may be the prime means by which genetic transmission of these disorders take place.

PSYCHOLOGICAL FACTORS

Psychological factors interact with biological vulnerabilities in the substance-related disorders:

➤ Depression, antisocial personality disorder, anxiety disorder, and schizophrenia may precede, accompany, and follow substance abuse. Substances may be used excessively to alleviate the symptoms of these disorders.

➤ The physical and social consequences of substance abuse are often negative. This may influence the development of additional psychological symptoms which, in turn, can lead to further abuse.

➤ Expectancies of the effects of substance use on behavior, both positive and negative, influence use patterns and the ultimate risk of abuse and dependence.

SOCIAL FACTORS

Both biological and psychological factors operate in specific social contexts to determine substance abuse patterns:

➤ Gender, age, ethnicity, education, social class, societal norms, and geography all play important roles in determining both initial substance use patterns and the ultimate risk of substance abuse.

➤ Group pressures, especially during adolescence, establish use patterns that may last a lifetime.

➤ Living conditions and the impact of racial and ethnic discrimination are thought to play a central role in the epidemic of illicit drug abuse in our inner cities.

These biological, psychological, and social factors interact to cause problems, as illustrated in the following case:

Tom never knew his alcoholic father. His parents had divorced when Tom was a baby. Tom began drinking with high school buddies several afternoons a week before their parents got home. In college, Tom continued drinking regularly. One Saturday night, he and his friends spent most of the evening drinking at an off-campus bar. Tom agreed to drive back, even though he knew he'd drunk too much. A state trooper pulled him over. Aware of the likely consequences of a DWI conviction, Tom immediately started arguing with the trooper. One thing led to another, harsh words were exchanged, and Tom took a swing at the trooper.

The biopsychosocial model helps explain Tom's behavior. Fatigue and intoxication—biological factors—impaired Tom's judgment about driving and his physical ability to control the car. Social pressure from friends also influenced his decision to drive. Finally, psychological factors—his reaction to feelings of powerlessness and panic when he was stopped by the trooper—influenced still another unwise decision: to confront the trooper rather than accept the inevitable.

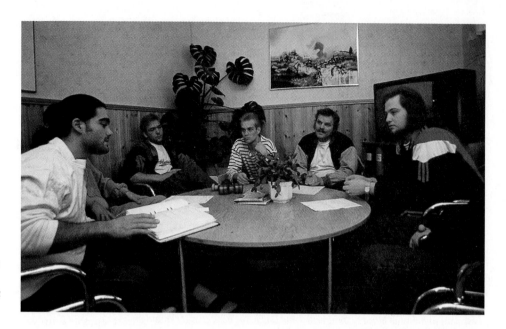

Participants in group therapy have many therapists—their fellow group members—all trying to help them confront the denial that is so much a part of the abuse syndrome.

the seriousness of their abuse problems. Fellow substance abusers can often confront one another about denying their abuse with greater effectiveness than therapists can. The following dialogue illustrates such a confrontation during a group therapy session attended by eight young men, all of them convicted of drunken driving and most of them abusers of both alcohol and drugs:

> **Roy:** You guys have got it all wrong. Sure, I drink. In fact, I had a few beers the night of the accident. But it was raining. The roads were slick and my old Buick wasn't too good going around curves even under the best conditions. But for you to say—
>
> **Thomas:** Roy, you're giving us a bunch of crap.
>
> **Roy:** —that I'm an alcoholic just because I had an accident is ridiculous. I can control my drinking whenever I want. I always drink with friends and never alone, I've never had a blackout—
>
> **Thomas:** Why won't you take responsibility for anything, for the accident, for being an addict, for beating up on your wife when you're high, for anything?
>
> **William:** Roy, we've all been where you are. It took losing my child and wife and the best job I ever had for me to face up to my part in my troubles, that maybe it was my drinking and drugging—
>
> **Roy:** Why are all of you after me, what'd I do to deserve this? Why don't you pick on somebody else?
>
> **Thomas:** Because if we don't call you on this, you're going to do it again. And when you do, you might kill somebody in that old car of yours!

Family Therapy During the past decade, **family therapy** has also become a popular treatment for individuals with alcohol and drug dependence disorders (Bowers & Al-Redha, 1990; McCrady, Stout, Noel, Abrams, & Nelson, 1991). One appealing feature of family therapy is that it assumes that substance abuse is not the abuser's problem alone. Because it affects every member of the family, family therapists are convinced that substance abuse is everyone's problem and that all family members must participate in treatment.

Family therapy enables family members to share with the substance abuser the negative impact that his behavior has on them. The supportive atmosphere of the family therapy session makes it easier for family members to share these feelings with the abuser, thereby confirming deeply felt, long-hidden truths. This difficult

family therapy *Therapeutic method that involves assessment and treatment of all immediate family members; emphasizes treating the family as a system.*

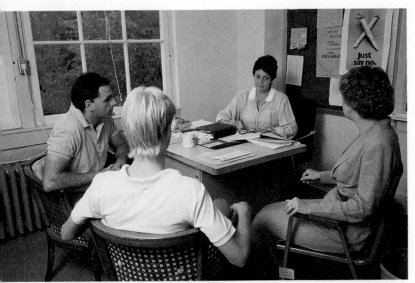

Family therapy involving a substance abuser and her family is often the best way to help the abuser comprehend the impact of her behavior on other family members.

exchange is as important for the abuser as for the family. Once all these feelings are out in the open, it becomes more difficult for the abuser to later deny the impact his behavior has had on those he claims to love.

Family therapists are convinced that alcohol and drug abuse is a family disorder, created and maintained by disordered family relationships. Therapists look for family patterns that lead to substance abuse—for instance, the wife who drinks so she can forget her husband's infidelity, the husband who uses sedatives to dampen the stress of his job, and the adolescent who smokes marijuana to deal with his parents' constant bickering.

The following is an excerpt from a long, intimate statement written by a recovering alcoholic who traces her sobriety to understandings she achieved in family therapy:

In the four years that I've been sober, one of the changes that has taken place is my attitude toward my childhood and family. I am now 35 and have a brother, 39, and a half sister from my father's second marriage who is 28; we are just getting to know each other. My mother is still living, but my father died about 15 years ago. While I was drinking I laid the blame for my failures squarely at my mother's feet and tried in various ways to scare or coerce her into showing love. It was convenient to use her, my parents' divorce, and my brother's hostility when we were children as an excuse for my insanities. I did not seem capable of seeing my mother as a separate person who also happened to be my mother and who had a life and problems of her own. This attitude of self-pity and blame has changed to a better evaluation of where my own sickness lay; I have been able to extract from the past just where my confusions were and find out how to begin to sort them out. Whatever anger I have is confined to the present; I do not see my family as the villains I once did, nor myself as the victim. (Kaufmann & Lilly, 1979, p. 245)

Behavior Therapy

Behavioral approaches to understanding and treating substance abuse have become well accepted over the past two decades. In essence, they assume that some of the substance abuser's behavior is learned and thus can be unlearned.

Aversive Procedures   Chemical aversion, which is based on the principles of classical conditioning, was developed in the late 1930s (Voegtlin, 1940). Today, it's an accepted, though still controversial, form of treatment. When used in treating alcoholism, chemical aversion conditioning involves repeatedly pairing the sight, smell, and taste of the patient's preferred alcoholic beverage with drug-induced nausea and vomiting. Doing so establishes a conditioned aversion to alcohol. After this has been accomplished, the patient will reexperience strong feelings of nausea and disgust at the sight, taste, or smell of alcohol. As long as the aversion persists (generally, a few months), she can enjoy a craving-free interval. Also during this time, she can work toward a more lasting solution to her substance abuse problem.

The data on outcomes of **chemical aversion treatment** have consistently been among the most promising of all approaches to treating alcoholism (Smith, Frawler, & Polissar, 1991). This success can be explained, at least in part, by the fact that chemical aversion conditioning requires patients to be strongly motivated. Keep in mind that it's an extremely unpleasant and demanding treatment, requiring repeated experiences of nausea and vomiting during conditioning sessions.

chemical aversion treatment   Treatment for alcoholism; involves pairing the sight, smell, and taste of alcoholic beverages with the onset of chemically induced nausea and vomiting, producing a conditioned aversion to alcohol.

The patients' high level of motivation alone probably accounts for a substantial part of the success rate of this treatment (Nathan & Skinstad, 1987).

Aversion techniques were also among the first formal treatments for smoking (Lichtenstein & Glasgow, 1992). When aversive stimuli such as painful electric shocks, nausea-inducing drugs, and negative images are paired with lighting up cigarettes, individuals are induced to stop smoking. But when that association no longer exists, individuals' smoking tends to return quickly to pretreatment levels. Cigarette smoke has also been used therapeutically. In rapid smoking treatment programs, individuals smoke several cigarettes in rapid succession, drawing deeply and repeatedly on each. This induces an aversion to the highly concentrated dose of nicotine and tars they are ingesting. Although rapid smoking has achieved some success in inducing short-term abstinence, its long-term consequences have been disappointing.

Broad-Spectrum Behavioral Treatment with Nonabstinent Treatment Goals

Several behavioral treatment programs developed over the past 25 years have focused simultaneously on the abusive drinking of alcoholics and the negative vocational, interpersonal, and emotional consequences it brings. The ambitious focus of these programs explains why they have been termed *broad-spectrum treatments*. Several of these programs have also tested a revolutionary concept: **nonabstinent treatment goals** (Alden, 1988; Miller, Leckman, Delaney, & Tinkcom, 1992; Pomerleau, Pertschuk, Adkins, & D'Aquili, 1978; Sobell & Sobell, 1973, 1976).

Individualized behavior therapy for alcoholics (IBTA) was one of the first and best-known of these programs (Sobell & Sobell, 1973, 1976). At the time of the IBTA study, most alcoholism treatment programs tended to emphasize nonspecific treatment goals—for instance, personality change or increased psychological maturity. It was hoped that these nonspecific changes would somehow lead to positive change in the drinking problem, too. The IBTA program, however, was targeted. Its interventions were designed specifically (1) to modify subjects' abusive drinking by providing them with controlled social drinking skills and (2) to redress abuse-related deficits in social, interpersonal, and emotional skills. This approach assumed that addressing only the abusive drinking or its consequences constituted incomplete treatment.

The success of the IBTA program was evaluated by determining which group of patients drank less at the follow-up intervals: those receiving IBTA or those receiving standard treatment. At 6-month and 2-year follow-up periods, patients receiving IBTA treatment did drink less—in terms of both quantity and frequency—than patients receiving standard treatment. The patients who did best of all at follow-up turned out to be those who had received both IBTA treatment and the assigned treatment goal of controlled social drinking—a nonabstinent treatment goal—rather than the traditional goal of abstinence.

Most clinicians today reject the use of **controlled drinking goals** for chronic alcoholics, due to lack of supportive research findings. There is more support, though, for the use of nonabstinent drinking goals for drinkers who have just begun to have problems with their drinking. You may fall into this category if, after having a few drinks, you've experienced a drunken-driving arrest, episodes in which you've blacked out, or a few angry or violent encounters. Individuals in the early stages of problem drinking tend to be unwilling to stop drinking altogether. Yet if they can be guided to see that they have a problem, they might be willing to participate in a program designed to help them develop a pattern of moderate drinking and avoid future drinking-related problems.

It seems that the use of controlled drinking goals is feasible for **early stage problem drinkers,** in contrast to chronic alcoholics. Studies of early stage problem drinkers testing nonabstinent treatment have shown promising results (Kivlahan, Marlatt, Fromme, Coppel, & Williams, 1990; Taylor, Helzer, & Robins, 1986).

nonabstinent treatment goals Synonym for controlled drinking goals for alcoholism treatment.

controlled drinking goals Goals for alcoholism treatment that do not aim for abstinence, which is traditional, but for nonabusive drinking.

early stage problem drinker Person who has not developed alcohol dependence but has experienced one or more problems because of drinking.

Behavioral treatment for these drinkers typically includes several components, such as self-control training to help set limits on drinking and concentrated efforts to identify rewarding alternatives to heavy drinking. Cognitive restructuring is also used to alter the frequently held mindset that it's not possible for someone who's already had a problem with alcohol to become a moderate drinker.

Relapse Prevention Marlatt, Gordon, and their colleagues (Larimer & Marlatt, 1994; Marlatt & Gordon, 1985) argue that treatment for substance abuse should not end when formal treatment ends for the newly sober patient. At that point, she is in the midst of confronting the many risky situations that can prompt a return to substance abuse. These risks are maximized when the newly abstinent person returns to her job, neighborhood, friends, and family—all of which may have been associated with abusive drinking before treatment.

Marlatt and Gordon's **relapse prevention model** addresses this phase of treatment. The model stresses the importance of identifying the cues in the recovering person's environment that are associated with relapse—for example, situations that elicit the anger, depression, and anxiety that typically precede relapse in recovering persons. The model also aims to develop and strengthen coping strategies that the recovering person can use to deal with these high-risk situations. Such strategies typically involve cognitive restructuring, such as having the individual redefine herself as being strong enough to cope with the risk of relapse. Frequent rehearsal of coping skills is also needed to strengthen the individual's ability to confront risky situations without relapsing. Several clinicians (Annis, 1986; Rankin, 1986) have developed relapse prevention programs that are designed to extend alcoholism treatment beyond the period of an inpatient program.

The following recounts an effort to maintain smoking cessation by the use of relapse prevention techniques:

> Mr. L, who had been ordered by his doctor to stop smoking, was a veteran of several smoking cessation programs. Each time he applied himself vigorously to quitting, but was not able to maintain abstinence for very long. He complained that, after a while, not smoking so interfered with his ability to work that he was "forced" to start smoking again. A discussion of Mr. L's self-monitoring data was a stimulus for a discussion of his lifestyle. Mr. L was a classic "workaholic." He typically worked 12-hour days 6 days a week and found little time for anything else. He reported that he nearly always felt rushed and . . . agreed that his two-pack-a-day habit helped him maintain this lifestyle.
>
> A "want-should" analysis of Mr. L's life showed a nearly total absence of wants (i.e., reinforcers). While Mr. L easily identified several behaviors that might become wants for him (gym workouts and tennis were high on the list), he claimed that all were too time consuming given his busy schedule. Mr. L's therapist forcefully pointed out that this issue was critical to Mr. L's success in quitting smoking, and that he had been willing to commit substantial time and energy to this project. Mr. L contracted to work out three times a week on a trial basis. With Mr. L's permission, the therapist contacted Mrs. L and encouraged her to engage Mr. L in positive conversation about his workouts. Mr. L reported a slight decrease in tension on the workout days. When the clinic ended, Mr. L was unwilling to commit firmly to continuing his workouts. However, his wife reported that he seemed to be enjoying them and thought he would continue. (Shiffman, Read, Maltese, Rapkin, & Jarvik, 1985, p. 515)

relapse prevention model
Attempts to identify the cues associated with relapse and to strengthen strategies to cope with the high-risk situations these cues refer to.

A recent review of smoking cessation treatments (Lichtenstein & Glasgow, 1992) has concluded that "a particular disappointment has been the mediocre showing of relapse prevention" (p. 521). Despite the enthusiasm these authors had for the relapse prevention approach shortly after it was proposed (Glasgow & Lichtenstein, 1987), they concluded that research on its effectiveness for smoking cessation has not proven its superiority over other methods of treatment.

Motivational Interviewing   William Miller, a well-known behavior therapist, has developed a **motivational interview** to be administered to alcoholic patients just after they enter treatment. The interview provides patients direct feedback on 44 measures of past and present alcohol consumption, abuse, and dependence. It was developed from individual questionnaire items taken from three well-established alcohol screening questionnaires. Miller created the interview because the treatment literature suggested that straightforward feedback on the status and severity of drinking-related problems sometimes increases patients' motivation to change their drinking patterns for the better (Brown & Miller, 1993).

In an initial test of the impact of the motivational interview, 14 chronic alcoholic inpatients completed it early in their hospitalization (Brown & Miller, 1993). As a consequence, they participated more fully in their treatment. What's more, they showed significantly lower alcohol consumption at a 3-month follow-up interview than 14 patients who did not complete the motivational interview but did participate in all other treatments in the same setting. While much more research on the usefulness of the motivational interview is clearly called for, this initial finding is nonetheless promising.

Detoxification

Before treatment for substance abuse of any kind can get under way, the patient should be detoxified—that is, completely withdrawn from the substance or substances he is dependent on. Besides preserving the patient's physical health, **detoxification** increases his chances for treatment success. Alcohol- or drug-dependent persons cannot cooperate with their treatment if they continue to be intoxicated during much of the day. In fact, even after alcohol-dependent persons have been detoxified, it takes 2 to 3 months before their thinking processes return to normal (Hitzemann et al., 1992). For that matter, some older, chronic alcoholics never fully recover their cognitive abilities upon regaining sobriety after a lengthy period of heavy alcohol abuse (Roehrich & Goldman, 1993) (see also Chapter 16).

Detoxification from some substances can safely take place outside a hospital, whereas withdrawal from others requires resources available only to inpatients (Gold, 1991; NIAAA, 1993). Several groups of abusers are at particular risk in attempting withdrawal outside a hospital: namely, persons with long histories of heavy drinking who are still consuming substantial quantities of alcohol daily, people dependent on barbiturates, individuals who have acquired tolerance to the synthetic sedatives (including Valium and Librium), and persons dependent on more than one substance (including sedatives).

In order to be safe, withdrawal in these high-risk situations requires a gradual daily-dose reduction, spread over a week or more. Otherwise, life-threatening withdrawal symptoms may develop. The individual who abruptly stops abusing barbiturates and other sedative-hypnotic drugs, for example, may have withdrawal seizures, which can cause brain damage, coma, and death. Although withdrawal from other drugs of abuse is highly unpleasant, it's not usually associated with life-threatening withdrawal symptoms. The individual's physician is the best judge of where and how detoxification should take place.

Pharmacological Interventions

Alcohol- and Drug-Sensitizing Agents   The drug **Antabuse (disulfiram)** blocks the chemical breakdown of alcohol. Individuals who have ingested Antabuse cannot metabolize alcohol beyond the point at which it has been broken down in the bloodstream to a chemical called *acetaldehyde*. Acetaldehyde is toxic to the body in very small quantities. When even the smallest amount of alcohol has been consumed by someone with Antabuse in his bloodstream, an **acetaldehyde reaction** takes place

motivational interview Interview with an alcohol- or drug-dependent person, designed to heighten motivation for change in drinking by providing direct feedback on the status and severity of his substance-related problem.

detoxification Process of withdrawing an alcohol- or drug-dependent person from the substance or substances she is addicted to.

Antabuse (disulfiram) Chemical that blocks the breakdown of alcohol and permits acetaldehyde to accumulate in the bloodstream whenever alcohol is consumed.

acetaldehyde reaction Aversive treatment for alcoholism; takes place when sufficient acetaldehyde has accumulated in the bloodstream to precipitate nausea, vomiting, and other bodily reactions.

(Christensen, Moller, Ronsted, Angelo, & Johansson, 1991). At that point, the individual quickly begins to experience nausea, vomiting, profuse sweating, and markedly increased respiration and heartrate. Alcoholics who have had an acetaldehyde reaction say it's an experience they would do almost anything to avoid.

It's precisely because of the acetaldehyde reaction that Antabuse has been used for several decades to treat alcoholism. Alcoholics who take an Antabuse tablet every day generally cannot consume alcohol without experiencing an acetaldehyde reaction. Thus, they are protected from the impulse to drink, even if they are tempted by alcohol-related cues. Because of the dangers of the acetaldehyde reaction, however, physicians only prescribe Antabuse to patients who are physically fit, motivated to stop drinking, and fully able to appreciate the consequences if they drink while taking the drug.

Nan Robertson's firsthand account of her recovery from alcoholism (1988) contains the following endorsement of Antabuse:

> Antabuse meant that I made one decision a day not to drink, instead of dozens. Some people call it a crutch, but I call it blessed insurance that strengthened my determination to stay sober a day at a time. . . . [My doctor] told me that when you are saturated with Antabuse, you know you cannot drink safely after the last dose for the next four or five days, or even longer. . . . She called it "a time bomb that will never go off unless you trigger it with alcohol." (Robertson, 1988, p. 255)

Some experienced clinicians swear by Antabuse; others find it ineffective. Data on the drug's effectiveness are ambiguous (Wright & Moore, 1989), largely because it works well for some patients and not at all for others. Patient differences in sensitivity to the effects of the drug may explain its inconsistent usefulness. In general, clinicians prescribe Antabuse to give alcoholics a recovery "window" or grace period that reduces their risk of succumbing to craving. During this time, the alcoholic can make psychological and behavioral gains that will allow him to discontinue use of the drug at some point.

Narcotic antagonists such as **naloxone** are also quite controversial. They bring on immediate withdrawal from narcotic drugs. When an addict who is on a maintenance dose of naloxone slips and ingests or injects an opiate like heroin, he will not experience its reinforcing effects because the heroin will be rapidly dissipated from the body. Narcotic antagonists abolish or greatly diminish all the effects that heroin addicts find pleasurable. As is the case with Antabuse, narcotic antagonists should be given only to patients who are determined to end their dependence on these drugs. Otherwise, these patients might ingest their drug of choice despite being on the narcotic antagonist, which will produce effects almost as unpleasant and sometimes as dangerous as those of an Antabuse reaction.

Like Antabuse, naloxone has its supporters and detractors. Empirical data have not yet answered the all-important question of the therapeutic utility of either drug (Gold, 1991).

narcotic antagonist Drug that precipitates immediate withdrawal from narcotics.

naloxone Narcotic antagonist; used to treat narcotic addiction.

methadone Synthetic opiate drug that replaces heroin in the addict's CNS opiate receptors, thereby markedly reducing heroin's reinforcing effects.

Methadone   A drug used to treat heroin addiction—**methadone**—is even more controversial than Antabuse and naloxone. As a synthetic opiate, methadone essentially replaces heroin in the addict's central nervous system opiate receptors when it's ingested on a regular basis. As a result, the reinforcing effects of heroin are greatly reduced. For most users, methadone produces a less powerful high than heroin. Addicts who have chosen to undergo methadone maintenance therapy have agreed to give up heroin's powerfully reinforcing effects in order to live a life free from the extraordinary requirements of maintaining a heroin habit (Ball & Ross, 1991).

Critics of methadone maintenance point out, however, that the drug does produce a moderate high, so that it creates an active and illegal drug market. Consequently, the usual methadone maintenance procedure requires the addict to report to a treatment center for her daily oral dose of the drug, which is consumed in the staff's presence. Critics also complain that even though the treatment may ease heroin abuse, it leaves the addict free to abuse a wide range of other substances.

One striking feature of contemporary heroin addicts is their tendency to abuse multiple substances, including alcohol, cocaine, and benzodiazepines. In treating a group of urban heroin addicts through methadone maintenance, Stitzer, Iguchi, and Felch (1992) were able to significantly reduce the incidence of polydrug abuse in their patients. They achieved this by giving the patients the privilege of taking their methadone doses home, so they would not have to make daily trips to the clinic. This privilege was offered only when a patient showed two consecutive weeks of urine samples free from drugs other than methadone.

Agents for Managing Withdrawal and Maintaining Sobriety   Twenty years ago, clinicians routinely gave alcoholics the minor tranquilizers Librium and Valium during withdrawal. It was widely assumed that these drugs eased the physical and psychological pains of detoxification and prevented development of more serious withdrawal phenomena, like delirium tremens. But today, many clinicians recognize that relatively few alcoholics have severe enough withdrawal symptoms to warrant pharmacological intervention (Wartenburg et al., 1990). As a result, many more patients are routinely detoxified without the use of drugs.

In years past, antianxiety agents were given to alcoholics in the hope that these drugs would help individuals stop drinking by treating the anxiety that many of them try to self-medicate. Instead, many alcohol abusers simply added the abuse of Librium or Valium to their abuse of alcohol and other drugs. Both Librium and Valium induce dependency; addiction to them tremendously complicates withdrawal from alcohol. As a result, antianxiety drugs are now rarely given to persons dependent on alcohol or other drugs.

Nicotine gum or tablets and lobeline (a drug related to nicotine) reduce nicotine-induced withdrawal symptoms and help prevent a return to smoking by the newly abstinent individual. These drugs have had moderately positive results (Hughes, 1993) but only with smokers who are highly motivated to change their behavior (Cepeda-Benito, 1993). Nicotine "fading"—in which the individual smokes cigarettes that contain successively lower concentrations of nicotine—has also been tried with mixed results. This technique has generally been used in conjunction with behavioral self-control programs (Burling, Lovett, Frederiksen, Jerome, & Jonske-Gubosh, 1989).

Nicotine gum successfully confronts another common consequence of continued abstention from cigarettes: weight gain (Perkins, 1993). Women—especially young women—have been particularly resistant in recent years to efforts at smoking cessation. One reason may be that smoking diminishes appetite and inhibits weight gain (Perkins, 1993). As a result, young women who continue to smoke can successfully maintain diets and avoid gaining weight. It's true that smoking cessation often results in increased food intake and changes in food preferences to favor sweet, high-carbohydrate foods (Perkins, Epstein, & Pastor, 1990). But as the period of smoking cessation lengthens beyond several months, the evidence of increased eating becomes much less clear (Moffatt & Owens, 1991; Perkins, 1993).

Anticraving Agents   Over the past decade, researchers have investigated several drug classes that act on neurotransmitters in the brain, including serotonin reuptake inhibitors, dopamine agonists, and opioid antagonists. This research has led to the development of drugs that have the exciting potential to decrease the craving and reinforcing effects of alcohol. These drugs are promising because they might be able to prevent alcohol abuse and dependence, rather than simply treat its effects.

Serotonin reuptake inhibitors increase quantities of the neurotransmitter serotonin in the brain. They have produced modest decreases in alcohol consumption in males who are heavy drinkers with mild to moderate alcohol dependence (Naranjo, Kadlec, Sanhueza, Woodley-Remus, & Sellers, 1990), probably because serotonin exerts an anticraving effect. *Dopamine agonists* also decrease alcohol consumption and self-reported craving because they affect the concentration of the neurotransmitter dopamine in the brain (Dongier, Vachon, & Schwartz, 1991); dopamine appears to increase craving. Finally, the opioid antagonist **naltrexone**—originally developed to treat opioid dependence by inducing withdrawal in opioid addicts—also appears to have a marked impact on alcohol consumption by alcoholics. O'Malley and her colleagues (1992), for example, reported that naltrexone led to a marked decrease in alcohol consumption by outpatient alcoholics. This probably resulted because the drug appeared to reduce the pleasurable feelings that alcohol induces.

Self-Help Groups

Alcoholics Anonymous

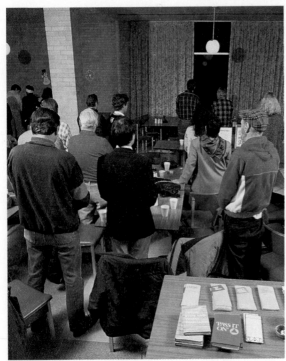

Alcoholics Anonymous meetings provide a protected, alcohol-free social environment, especially during the crucial first months of abstinence from alcohol.

This is not the story of my life. It is the story of how I got drunk, and how I got sober. I have told it before, many times: at A.A. meetings, and to my A.A. sponsor, and to other close A.A. friends gathered in coffee shops—what we in A.A. call "the meeting after the meeting." But I have never before told it in full. . . .

My name is Nan, and I am an alcoholic. (Robertson, 1988, p. 238)

This excerpt was written by Nan Robertson, who was, at the time, a reporter for the *New York Times.* It's from a compelling, first-hand account of the workings of Alcoholics Anonymous called *A.A.: Inside Alcoholics Anonymous* (1988). In it, the author describes her struggles with alcohol and her ultimate recovery, which came about with the help of the fellowship of Alcoholics Anonymous.

Alcoholics Anonymous (AA) is the best-known, largest, and most influential of the addiction self-help groups. In 1992, AA reportedly served more than 850,000 alcoholics in the United States; worldwide, the figure was more than 1.7 million (Alcoholics Anonymous, 1993). The organization has grown dramatically since it was founded in 1935 in Akron, Ohio, by Doctor Bob and Bill W., two alcoholics who came together to share their problems and try to solve them.

AA seems to work best when people who are determined to do something about their abusive drinking commit as much time as possible to attending meetings, embrace AA's 12-step program, and "put their trust in a higher power." In fact, the prescribed goal for newly sober alcoholics is "90 meetings in 90 days." Members believe that attending a meeting every night during the crucial initial recovery period is the best way to prevent a return to drinking, partly because AA meetings represent a protected, alcohol-free social environment. The program's commitment to being nonjudgmental is particularly helpful for individuals whose drinking has caused family, friends, and themselves to make harsh judgments about their behavior—and their self-worth.

Nan Robertson put it this way:

Soon, I began to see why A.A. members kept going to meetings. . . . The people in them steadied and supported me in ways as small but crucial as an arm around my shoulder. Sometimes my attention wandered for stretches of time while I retreated into my own thoughts. . . . But a speaker, or even a sentence uttered from the floor,

naltrexone Opioid antagonist; originally developed to treat opioid dependence by inducing withdrawal in opioid addicts; also appears to have a strong impact on alcoholics by reducing craving.

would get through to me. At one meeting, a man said, "I began coming to these basements and I discovered that I was right about myself—I am a decent person." I thought with surprise, "So am I." (Robertson, 1988, p. 250)

A typical AA meeting is preceded and followed by socializing periods, involving vast quantities of coffee. When the meeting begins, members who have been abstinent for periods ranging from 3 months to 30 years and more tell their stories: what alcohol did to them; how they lost their families, jobs, friends, and self-respect; how they've become sober with the help of the fellowship; and what sobriety means to them. New members quickly realize that they're not alone, that what has happened to them has happened to others (which is a surprise to many). They also realize that by being sober, they can look forward to a very different kind of life. AA warns, however, of looking beyond the next 24 hours of sobriety, believing that no one is ever fully cured of alcoholism.

Similar self-help groups are available to people with alcoholics in their lives. Al-Anon provides support for the spouses, relatives, and friends of alcoholics, and Al-Ateen offers help to their adolescent children. Both groups are rooted in the same sort of philosophy as AA and function similarly.

Although AA has been a major factor in alcoholism treatment for some 60 years, its impact has been hard to quantify (McCrady & Miller, 1993). This difficulty is due, in part, to the organization's decentralized nature. While broadly conforming to the traditions of AA, each group develops its own focus, traditions, and helping procedures. Although this philosophy has maintained AA as a vital organization, capable of continuous renewal, it has also made the coordinated study of treatment outcomes across individual groups extremely difficult.

The modest amount of research on AA's effectiveness that is available suggests an abstinence rate of between 25 and 50 percent at the 1-year mark. This rate is within the range of outcomes for other treatments (NIAAA, 1993). A recent membership survey (Alcoholics Anonymous, 1993) reports an average sobriety length of 50 months for those individuals who attend meetings regularly. (*Regularly* is defined as an average of 4 meetings a week by the typical member.) The survey also found that about half of those individuals who attend 3 or 4 AA meetings a week don't continue to do so for longer than 3 months.

Walsh and colleagues (1991) undertook one of the most important treatment outcome studies involving Alcoholics Anonymous. Industrial workers with newly identified alcohol problems were assigned to one of three treatment groups: (1) compulsory inpatient treatment for alcoholism followed by compulsory AA attendance; (2) compulsory AA attendance only; and (3) free choice of what treatment program, if any, to enter. Of the subjects in the third, free-choice condition, 46 percent chose to attend AA and 41 percent chose inpatient treatment.

Following treatment, all three groups showed comparable improvement on measures of job performance. But subjects in the first group—who were compelled to enter inpatient treatment and attend AA meetings—did better than those in either of the other two groups on measures of drinking. This finding led the authors to conclude that inpatient treatment was more often associated with long-term abstinence than was AA membership. However, AA membership seemed to have contributed substantially to positive outcomes, as well (Walsh et al., 1991).

Synanon and Narcotics Anonymous   Two self-help treatment programs for drug addiction include **Narcotics Anonymous** and **Synanon**. The programs are drastically different, however.

Narcotics Anonymous was modeled after Alcoholics Anonymous. In slightly modified form, Narcotics Anonymous follows the AA path to recovery. It involves heroin abusers in daily meetings and urges them to trust a "higher being," to shed their overwhelming guilt, and to take responsibility for restarting their lives as

Narcotics Anonymous Self-help group for narcotics addicts modeled after Alcoholics Anonymous.

Synanon Self-help group for heroin and cocaine addicts, requiring a lengthy residential stay and involving successive group confrontations to break through addicts' denial.

drug-free persons. Even though data on the treatment outcomes of Narcotics Anonymous are difficult to obtain, many believe it's a viable approach to the difficult task of getting narcotics and cocaine abusers to give up drugs.

In comparison, Synanon offers a very different approach to treatment, though its goal—permanent abstinence from drugs, primarily heroin and cocaine—is the same. A lengthy period of residence in a Synanon House is required; during it, members confront each other in a constant effort to break down defenses and denial. Synanon's basic assumption is that the addict's denial of personal responsibility for and the negative consequences of substance abuse are key factors in his decision to maintain the addiction. Alcoholics construct much the same denial system. However, AA seeks to break through the denial in a much less confrontational way than is typical of Synanon programs.

Virtually every day of a resident's stay at a Synanon House includes a group therapy session that everyone attends. Although the focus of the session shifts from person to person, it always emphasizes taking more responsibility for individual behavior (especially drug-using behavior) and confronting realistically what impact that behavior has on others. Again, group confrontation is the touchstone of Synanon treatment. It's assumed that abusers will continue their drug abuse until or unless their denial is broken and they face up to the consequences of their drug abuse—for themselves and others.

As with Alcoholics Anonymous, reliable data on the success rates of Synanon treatment are generally unavailable, so we cannot compare outcomes to those of other treatment approaches. Nonetheless, the dramatic growth shown by this program attests to its acceptance by those people who are most concerned: the abusers it seeks to help.

Stages of Change in Addictions Treatment

During the past 15 years, psychologist James O. Prochaska and his co-workers (Prochaska & DiClemente, 1983, 1986) have intensively studied how people intentionally change addictive behaviors. These researchers have concluded that modifying addictive behaviors progresses through five **stages of change:**

1. precontemplation
2. contemplation
3. preparation
4. action
5. maintenance

Persons who are substance dependent typically recycle through these stages several times before they achieve stable abstinence (Prochaska, DiClemente, & Norcross, 1992). Moreover, different specific treatments seem to be most effective at each stage (Prochaska & DiClemente, 1992).

The first of the stages of change is **precontemplation.** During this stage, the individual has no intention to change behavior in the foreseeable future; in fact, she may not be aware of having an addiction problem. **Contemplation** is the next stage; in it, the individual is aware that she has an addiction problem, is seriously thinking about doing something about it, but has not yet made a commitment to do so. **Preparation** is the stage that brings together the intention to change with preparations for doing so; small changes may even have been initiated, like reducing drinking by a few beers a week or smoking three or four fewer cigarettes a day. During the **action** stage, the individual confronts her addiction most directly by changing her behavior or environment; abstinence is the most meaningful of these behavior changes. During **maintenance,** the final stage, the individual's principal task is to prevent relapse and consolidate the gains she made in the action stage.

stages of change Research program on the process of behavioral change in treating addictions; has led to development of an assessment technique that places an individual at one of five stages of change.

precontemplation stage First stage of change; the person has no intention of changing behavior any time soon.

contemplation stage Second stage of change; the person is aware a problem exists, is seriously thinking of confronting it, but has not made a commitment to do so.

preparation stage Third stage of change; the person intends to take action within a month.

action stage Fourth stage of change; the person modifies behavior, experiences, or environment in order to overcome problems.

maintenance stage Final stage of change; the person works to prevent relapse and consolidate gains made in the action stage.

Although most of Prochaska's research program has focused on stages of change in people who are trying to quit smoking, it has also investigated stages of change in those trying to quit drinking. In a recent study (Snow, Prochaska, & Rossi, 1992), for example, researchers assessed the readiness to stop smoking of current smokers who were also former problem drinkers. Since so many recovering problem drinkers are or have been regular smokers, understanding how these two common addictions interact during recovery is important.

A group of 191 adults was recruited who admitted to once having a drinking problem but who were no longer drinking (Snow, Prochaska, & Rossi, 1992). Of the group, 41 percent were current smokers; 81 percent had smoked regularly in the past. The average length of alcohol sobriety was slightly less than 6 years. Of the 79 current smokers in the sample, 52 percent were in the precontemplation stage, 34 percent were in the contemplation stage, and 14 percent were in the preparation stage of change. These stage distributions were comparable to the stages of change found in smokers in other studies. The only difference was that women smokers in this sample were at an earlier stage of change. (Sixty-seven percent of women and 38 percent of men were in the precontemplation stage.)

Focus on Critical Thinking

1. What components of the Alcoholics Anonymous/Narcotics Anonymous experience seem most important to their effectiveness? Explain your choices.

2. What do you think about the controversial issue of controlled drinking treatment for alcoholics? Consider the alcohol abusers you have known. Could any of them have maintained a controlled drinking pattern for an extended period of time? Why or why not?

3. Think of someone you know who has a problem with alcohol or drug dependence. Try to place him or her at one of the stages of change in addictions treatment. Explain what your placement is based on.

EFFECTIVENESS OF PREVENTION AND TREATMENT PROGRAMS

Preventing Substance Abuse

Many alcohol and drug prevention efforts in the United States focus on the schools (Hansen, in press). School-based programs are tailored to the ages of the students involved. They describe the metabolism and physiology of alcohol and drugs and provide detailed information on the range of potentially dangerous effects of abuse. These programs may also go into the causes of substance abuse, the impact of parental alcoholism and drug dependence, and the kinds of treatments available. Some combine information on the effects of alcohol and drugs with ways to resist peer pressure to use and abuse them (Botvin, Baker, Filazzola, & Botvin, 1990). Parents are sometimes invited to join their children in these discussions (Hawkins, Catalano, & Kent, 1991).

All these prevention programs share the same goal: to convince children and adolescents to seriously consider the negative consequences they will face if they decide to drink or use drugs. In doing so, these programs attempt to change the attitudes that youthful users have about alcohol and drugs. Instead of seeing these substances as symbols of emerging adulthood and sophistication, educators want youths to see them as agents of injury, disease, and death.

Most available data (Hansen, in press; Nathan, 1983) on the outcomes of preventive education and attitude-change programs in secondary schools and colleges show that they are successful in increasing information level and changing attitudes on use from positive to less positive. However, such programs are only modestly successful in changing consumption levels in young people who are already using alcohol and drugs.

In contrast, efforts over the past 30 years to change public attitudes toward smoking have been very successful; efforts to prevent alcoholism and other drug dependencies have been less so. Since 1964—the time of the U.S. Surgeon General's *Report on Smoking and Health*—a variety of public figures (including a more recent Surgeon General, Dr. C. Everett Koop) have led an ultimately successful campaign to alter public attitudes toward smoking. This campaign has been especially effective in reducing smoking in public settings, as shown by several efforts:

- involvement of entire communities in programs for smoking cessation (LeFebvre, Cobb, Goreczny, & Carleton, 1990)
- increased public concern about the health effects of passive smoking (that is, inhaling someone else's cigarette smoke)
- society's willingness to support imposing health warning labels on cigarette packages; restrictions on smoking in public places, including restaurants and airplanes; and prohibitions on advertising tobacco products

A significant reduction in smoking has taken place in the United States. Only 29 percent of adults smoke today, compared to 40 percent in 1965. Men have stopped smoking at the highest rates: Half of all men smoked in 1965; fewer than one-third do today.

Preventing the Consequences of Substance Abuse

Strategies for reducing certain negative consequences of alcohol use have been much more successful than efforts to prevent use in the first place. For instance, the number of fatal automobile accidents involving youthful drinkers has been reduced substantially over the years. This has been achieved primarily through two measures: (1) by limiting the availability of alcohol to youthful drivers through raising the legal age for purchase of alcoholic beverages to 21 and (2) by increasing the effective enforcement of laws pertaining to alcohol sales to underage individuals (Hingson, 1993; Klitzner, Stewart, & Fisher, 1993). In addition, the frequency of fetal alcohol syndrome (FAS) has been reduced significantly by programs designed to educate women on the risks of drinking during pregnancy (NIAAA, 1993). (FAS afflicts the children of mothers who drink heavily during pregnancy, causing physical, cognitive, and emotional defects.) Finally, programs to prevent problems in the workplace due to alcohol and drug use (Ames, 1993) have shown promising results, as have those aimed at preventing alcohol- and drug-related HIV infection (Strunin & Hingson, 1993).

Drunken driving and FAS are major public health problems in the United States. Drunken drivers kill and injure thousands of Americans and cause millions of dollars of property damage each year. Similarly, victims of FAS number in the thousands; the loss of their full productivity and the costs of caring for and educating these individuals are enormous. Hence, the success of efforts to reduce drunken driving and the incidence of fetal alcohol syndrome represents an important public health advance. Although more difficult to determine, the costs of alcohol and drug problems in the workplace and those due to alcohol-related HIV infection are also very substantial. So increased success in preventing these problems has also had substantial positive consequences for the country.

Treating Substance Abuse

Let's return to the case of J. P., introduced at the beginning of the chapter. Over the years, he'd become quite an authority on treatment. Dr. N., the young psychologist who treated J. P., thought that he knew something about how to treat alcoholics. After all, Dr. N. had read the most current books and articles on the subject and had been supervised by senior clinicians while treating more than 10 alcoholic patients during his years of training. But the doctor's "overconfidence bubble" burst 10 minutes into his first therapy session with J. P.

In that session, J. P. recounted the diverse treatments he had received during his three decades of chronic alcoholism: AA; Antabuse; individual, group, and marital therapy; behavioral therapy; even a course of Gestalt treatment and one session of primal therapy; eight inpatient stays; and countless outpatient treatments. J. P. was a walking encyclopedia of information on the latest fads and fancies in alcoholism treatment. That he continued to abuse alcohol, despite all the treatments he had gone through, was testimony to their failure to help him.

Given this history, Dr. N. decided to focus on the basics with J. P. During the first few months, they spent most of their time together on the laborious process of relationship building. When Dr. N. first started seeing J. P., he was completely out of touch with his ex-wife, son, and family. He was living on welfare in a small room near the hospital, eating at a soup kitchen. His self-esteem couldn't have been lower. He was convinced that he had nothing to offer and couldn't imagine why anyone could want to have a relationship with him. For Dr. N.'s part, he hoped that as the relationship grew, J. P. would realize that he did have something to offer. That realization would lay the groundwork for small but significant changes in his feelings about his worth as a person. To the extent that J. P. would begin to feel better about himself, his motivation to do something about his drinking might increase.

And that's about the way things worked out. From small beginnings, J. P.'s interest in the world gradually reawakened. Cognitive restructuring helped correct J. P.'s chronically negative view of himself and his ability to remain sober and contribute to society. So did behavior rehearsal; J. P. and Dr. N. anticipated high-risk situations for relapse and role-played successful efforts to deal with them without drinking. J. P.'s brief periods of sobriety grew longer, and his occasional unskilled jobs were replaced by steadier, more demanding ones.

After more than 2 years of treatment, J. P. felt much better about himself. He started attending a church singles group, where he met a woman with a history only slightly less formidable than his own. But he was making progress, and it continued through and beyond the 8 years that Dr. N. worked at the city hospital. Some of those years were J. P.'s best.

As you know, however, J. P. didn't stay sober. After years of success, he started drinking again upon learning that he had stomach cancer. And he spent the last painful months of his life drunk. He died at age 52.

Many substance abusers have personal stories as devastating as J. P.'s. Most have been in and out of treatment their entire lives, with little or no success. A review of treatment statistics paints a gloomy picture.

First of all, no more than 10 percent of all alcohol-dependent people enter treatment in any given year in the United States (NIAAA, 1993). The comparable figure for drug-dependent individuals is almost certainly lower, given that the use of most abused drugs is illegal. If we adopt the most widely accepted prevalence estimate, we can say that between 7 and 9 percent of the U.S. population—around 18 million people—suffers from a significant alcohol or drug problem. And a substantial number of these people are polysubstance abusers. These data suggest that between 1.6 and 2 million alcohol and drug abusers enter treatment during any given year.

Next, let's look at treatment outcomes for alcoholism and drug dependence. Again, if we adopt the most widely accepted figure, only 30 percent of those individuals who begin treatment programs remain abstinent for a year after treatment has ended (Nathan & Skinstad, 1987; NIAAA, 1993; NIDA, 1991). Over 50 percent of patients entering treatment drop out before its conclusion, and a substantial number who complete treatment fail to benefit from it. As we'll discuss later in this section, patients in some programs are better than average prospects for successful outcomes; these programs do better than 30 percent. On the other hand, programs that treat more difficult patients do worse than 30 percent.

In order to determine how many substance abusers are helped out of dependence in any single year, we can multiply this 30 percent average positive outcome figure by 10 percent, which represents the group of alcoholics and drug addicts treated in a year in the United States. In doing so, we get a product of 3 percent. That means that only 3 of 100 substance abusers successfully end dependence in the United States each year.

Judging from these figures, we treat alcoholism and drug dependence with very modest effectiveness. However, the situation is not as bad as it seems, and it will likely become even better in years to come. Substantial research on treatment outcomes for substance abuse that was undertaken in the past 20 years has begun to yield important results. For example, data reported in recent years suggests that patient variables and perhaps even therapist variables play important roles in the success of both alcoholism and drug treatment. In fact, these variables may be more important than the specifics of the treatment itself (McLellan et al., 1994).

Patient variables that influence treatment success include marital status (married people do better), education (more educated people do better), and employment status (employed people do better). Even more important is the patient's drinking and drug use history. Predictably, patients whose abusive drinking or drug use has not progressed to dependence or led to physical disease are better treatment prospects than patients whose drug or alcohol abuse is of long duration and has long been out of control (Langenbucher, McCrady, Brick, & Esterly, 1993). Likewise, patients who have shown that they're able to abstain from using substances or control their intake for significant periods in the past as well as those who have minimal polydrug use are better treatment prospects.

Abusers' motivation to change their abusive drinking or drug use pattern is an especially important determinant of treatment success (Brown & Miller, 1993; Miller, Benefield, & Tonigan, 1993). For this reason, clinicians have begun to make specific efforts to increase their patients' treatment motivation and to select individuals for treatment who are clearly motivated to benefit from rigorous treatments.

Another promising effort to improve treatment success involves matching patients both to treatments and to therapists. This strategy is based on research suggesting that particular patients may be motivated to work hardest in particular treatment settings, with particular kinds of therapists (Litt, Babor, DelBoca, Kadden, & Cooney, 1992; Mattson & Allen, 1991). Two of the nation's leading researchers on treatment matching, however, caution against believing that significant breakthroughs are imminent (Moos, Finney, & Cronkite, 1990). As you can imagine, the conceptual and methodological problems associated with treatment matching are quite complicated.

Research on new alcohol- and drug-sensitizing agents and anticraving agents has also been encouraging. By themselves, these drugs are unlikely to affect substantial numbers of alcoholics and drug addicts. But when used in combination with psychological and behavioral interventions, they hold great promise. Both classes of drugs can provide alcohol- and drug-dependent persons an interval of freedom from their addiction that's long enough to help them reorganize and reorder their lives more permanently.

Focus on **Critical Thinking**

1. Based on what you've read thus far, compare the rate of successful treatment for substance-related disorders with those for other psychopathologic disorders. What might explain these differences in success?

2. What are some of the reasons that treatment for substance-related disorders has not been more successful?

3. In general, efforts to prevent some of the consequences of substance-related disorders (such as drunken driving and fetal alcohol syndrome) have been more successful than efforts to treat these disorders. What might explain this?

SUMMARY

Historical Perspective

■ Alcoholism was recognized in the Old Testament and for centuries thereafter as evidence of sinfulness.

■ Benjamin Rush was among the first medical professionals to view alcoholism as a physical disorder, rather than a moral condition.

■ The addiction problems of soldiers during World War II convinced many Americans that alcoholism is a medical and psychological problem.

■ In the Western world, the abuse potential of drugs such as the opiates, cocaine, and marijuana was recognized in the late 1800s, when these drugs were introduced to these societies.

Diagnosis of Substance-Related Disorders

■ The *DSM-I* and *DSM-II* included substance abuse as a category of sociopathic personality disturbance.

■ The *DSM-III* provided a separate category for the substance-related disorders, assigned tolerance and withdrawal key diagnostic roles, and distinguished between substance abuse and substance dependence.

■ The *DSM-III-R* based diagnosis on the substance dependence syndrome, deemphasized the diagnostic importance of tolerance and withdrawal, and made substance abuse a residual category.

■ The *DSM-IV* drew on an extensive research base and combined the strongest diagnostic features of the *DSM-III* and *DSM-III-R;* it also strengthened the criteria for substance abuse.

Americans with Substance-Related Disorders

■ Between 14 and 16 million Americans meet the criteria for alcohol abuse or dependence. Rates vary with age, sex, and ethnicity. African Americans and Hispanics show slightly higher rates of abuse and dependence than their Caucasian counterparts.

■ Polydrug abuse—involving alcohol and one or more additional substances—is very common today, making it difficult to estimate the number of drug abusers in the United States.

The Nature of Substance Abuse and Dependence

■ Alcohol and drug intoxication are associated with heightened risk of automobile accidents, accidents and injuries on the job and at home, crimes of all kinds, high-risk sexual behavior, and family violence, such as spouse and child abuse.

■ Chronic alcohol and drug abuse are associated with disabling changes in brain function and life-threatening physical disorders affecting the brain, heart, liver, and gastrointestinal system.

Causes of Substance Abuse and Dependence

■ The etiology of substance abuse and dependence includes genetic/biological, sociocultural and group membership, sex, learning-based, and psychiatric and personality factors.

■ The causes of substance abuse and dependence can best be explained by a biopsychosocial perspective.

Treatment of Substance Abuse and Dependence

■ Treatments for alcohol and drug abuse and dependence include group, family, and marital therapy; behavior therapy; detoxification and inpatient treatment; pharmacological intervention; and self-help groups.

■ The stages of change model has helped improve the success of smoking cessation efforts.

Effectiveness of Prevention and Treatment Programs

■ Efforts to prevent substance-related disorders have achieved only modest success.

■ Efforts to reduce the incidence of drunken driving, fetal alcohol syndrome, workplace alcohol problems, and alcohol-related HIV infection have been more successful.

■ Treatment reaches only about 10 percent of alcohol and drug abusers in any given year, and of that group, only about one-third benefit from treatment.

KEY TERMS

acetaldehyde reaction, **p. 307**
action stage, **p. 312**
alcohol expectancies, **p. 298**
amotivational syndrome, **p. 290**
Antabuse (disulfiram), **p. 307**
chemical aversion treatment, **p. 304**
comorbidity, **p. 298**
conditioned appetitive motivational model, **p. 297**
conditioned compensatory response model, **p. 297**
contemplation stage, **p. 312**
controlled drinking goals, **p. 305**
detoxification, **p. 307**

early stage problem drinker, **p. 305**
event-related potential (ERP), **p. 292**
evoked potential (EP), **p. 292**
family therapy, **p. 303**
group therapy, **p. 301**
maintenance stage, **p. 312**
methadone, **p. 308**
motivational interview, **p. 307**
naloxone, **p. 308**
naltrexone, **p. 310**
narcotic antagonist, **p. 308**
Narcotics Anonymous, **p. 311**
nonabstinent treatment goals, **p. 305**
polysubstance abuse, **p. 280**

precontemplation stage, **p. 312**
preparation stage, **p. 312**
relapse prevention model, **p. 306**
sociopathic personality disturbance, **p. 274**
stages of change, **p. 312**
substance abuse, **p. 274**
substance dependence, **p. 274**
Synanon, **p. 311**
tetrahydrocannabinol (THC), **p. 290**
tolerance, **p. 276**
with physiological dependence, **p. 276**
withdrawal, **p. 276**
without physiological dependence, **p. 276**

CRITICAL THINKING EXERCISE

Suppose that you have recently become worried about your roommate Sarah's drinking and drug use. Both of you are juniors in college. You have roomed together for three years, so you know each other pretty well. Although Sarah has always liked to party, her use of alcohol and marijuana was more or less recreational—something to look forward to after an intense week of classes and studying. During the past 6 months, however, that's begun to change.

After breaking up with her boyfriend, Sarah became consumed with depression and self-blame. She started to bring wine back to the apartment and would drink it alone while watching television, sometimes instead of eating. Then, after having a few glasses of wine, she'd sometimes bring out marijuana and roll herself a hefty joint. At first, this was just on the weekends, maybe two or three nights a week. But now, she spends most nights this way: alone at home, in front of the television, drinking and smoking.

Your relationship has also changed. Before, Sarah shared almost all her thoughts and feelings with you; now, she doesn't tell you anything. Her school-work has suffered, as well. Understandably, she gets little studying done when she's drinking and smoking.

What has you worried most is that Sarah complains now of needing more of the substances to experience the feelings she first enjoyed. Not surprisingly, you've become very concerned about your roommate.

1. Refer to the *DSM-IV* tables of operational criteria for substance abuse and dependence (see page 275). Can you make a diagnosis of substance abuse or dependence on the basis of what you know about Sarah's drinking and drug use and their consequences? If so, make a diagnosis. If not, explain what else you need to know.

2. What are some of the things you might do to help your roommate deal with her substance abuse problems?

3. Do you think this behavioral pattern is common or unusual among college students? Explain your answer.

Chapter 10

PSYCHOLOGICAL FACTORS AFFECTING HEALTH

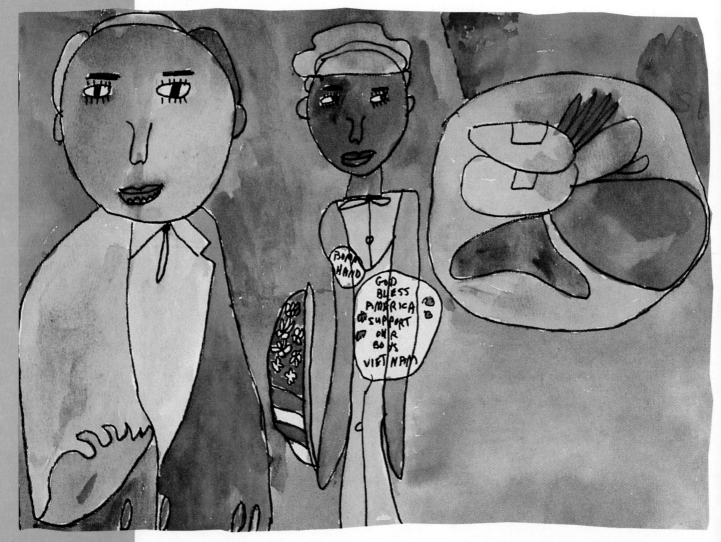

Helen Kossoff, **God Bless America,** HAI

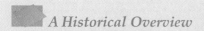
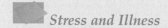
Barbara Boggs Sigmund died of cancer on October 10, 1990. She was the mayor of Princeton, New Jersey, and a member of one of the most prominent political families in the United States. One of her daughters, Cokie Roberts, is a well-known journalist.

Less than a year before she died, Barbara Boggs Sigmund wrote an article for the *New York Times,* in which she reflected on cancer and personal responsibility:

In late October, a medical exam revealed that my eye cancer—an ocular melanoma—had spread to various parts of my body. Very soon thereafter, the self-help books started arriving. I had caused my own cancer, they told me, so it was up to me to cure it.

"Bull ----," exclaimed my husband, when I informed him of having this interesting new fact to face so soon on the heels of the news itself. "What about babies? Do they cause their own cancer?"

Clearly, babies do not "cause" their own cancer through "stress" in their young lives or "lack of self-love" or a "need to be ill" or a "wish to die." And so it is with most of us with cancer. I did not cause my own disease. Overexposure to the sun is the only known suspect in melanoma, but the sun hasn't glimpsed my head unhatted nor my skin unoiled for decades. Only people who deliberately use or expose themselves to proved carcinogens can justly be accused of self-inflicted cancer.

But, say the gentle proponents of the self-cure books, what you are objecting to is merely "the dark side" of these theories. Don't forget, I'm reminded, these books also tell you how to heal yourself.

Yes. And everywhere I turn I see evidence that the last frontier of rugged individualism in America is relentless self-belief. Even in the beauty parlor, I run across a book excerpt trumpeting, once again, that the only limit on the success and happiness we can achieve is the belief in limits themselves. No racism, sexism, sickness, poverty or just plain lack of talent need apply.

But, alas, there is more to fear than fear itself. Evil, illness, accident, injustice and bad luck strike the self-improved and unimproved alike.

Does this mean I don't believe there is any merit to theories that positive and more loving attitudes can't help us bear and possibly cure our sicknesses, even

321

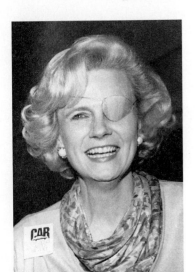

Barbara Boggs Sigmund, former mayor of Princeton, New Jersey, died of eye cancer in 1990, not long after she reflected on the role of personal responsibility in having cancer.

cancer? Or that changes in ourselves and the way we live can't influence these things? Of course not.

But seven years ago, I lost my eye to cancer. This time, the odds are better than even that I will lose my life. And it simply doesn't help to tell me that, rah-rah-sis-boom-bah, I can beat the odds if I only learn to love myself enough. Of course, I want to live. I'm at the top of my form, happy, useful, looking forward to new challenges. My boys are in their early 20's now, and I want to see their lives unfold.

But if I die, I don't want to feel like a failure.

It isn't through lack of love in return that I report that picturing white blood cells as so many little men of war against the cancer cells, "imaging" techniques, or a no-nonsense all-American determination to redirect their lives may be fine and life-giving for others, but not for me. I'm sticking with the medal of Jesus and Mary around my neck and novenas to St. Jude. It's strictly a utilitarian decision: The data base of success stories is larger by far. (Sigmund, 1989)

It's easy to see what Barbara Boggs Sigmund was referring to. You have only to look at popular magazines and best-selling books on self-help to discover that people see a link between psychological factors, such as an individual's personality or level of life stress, and the development of different physical diseases (Siegel, 1986). This belief goes back to ancient times, but is it only folklore? Does solid scientific evidence connect stress and illness?

A HISTORICAL OVERVIEW

The physical disorders discussed in this chapter are significantly influenced by psychological factors. Before publication of the third and fourth editions of the *Diagnostic and Statistical Manual of Mental Disorders* (*DSM-III-R* and *DSM-IV*) (American Psychiatric Association, 1987, 1994), these disorders were known as *psychosomatic* or *psychophysiological* disorders. Some common examples are heart disease, hypertension, headaches, arthritis, diabetes, and obesity. The *DSM-IV* describes problems of this sort as "Psychological Factors Affecting Medical Condition." The diagnostic criteria for these disorders are summarized in the *DSM-IV* table. These disorders must be distinguished from the somatoform disorders discussed in Chapter 6, which have no known physiological basis.

In this chapter, we discuss the scientific evidence relating to the concerns shared by Barbara Boggs Sigmund. Can psychological factors cause or contribute to health and illness? And if so, how do mental processes alter biological mechanisms? This question of how the mind and body interact has been the focus of philosophical debate over many centuries.

Psychosomatic Medicine

Tracing the origins of the systematic investigation of the links between psychological factors and physical illness takes us back to the development of psychoanalysis. In his pioneering book *Psychosomatic Medicine* (1950), Franz Alexander argued that specific unconscious emotional conflicts cause certain diseases. For instance, consider the diagnosis of gastrointestinal disorders, such as peptic ulcer, diarrhea, and colitis. Alexander suggested that these disorders are caused by an emotional conflict between the unconscious wish to remain passive and dependent (loved and cared for, like an infant), on the one hand, and the need to be independent and achieving, on the other (like an adult). Ulcer patients overcompensate for their unconscious need for dependence by acting aggressively and being independent in real life; these behaviors contribute to development of an ulcer. By contrast, patients with diarrhea and colitis compensate for their need to be dependent through the unconscious

Diagnostic Criteria for 316 PSYCHOLOGICAL FACTORS AFFECTING MEDICAL CONDITION

A. A general medical condition is present.

B. Psychological factors adversely affect the general medical condition in one of the following ways:

(1) the factors have influenced the course of the general medical condition as shown by a close temporal association between the psychological factors and the development or exacerbation of, or delayed recovery from, the general medical condition

(2) the factors interfere with the treatment of the general medical condition

(3) the factors constitute additional health risks for the individual

(4) stress-related physiological responses precipitate or exacerbate symptoms of the general medical condition

Choose name based on the nature of the psychological factors (if more than one factor is present, indicate the most prominent):

Mental Disorder Affecting . . . [Indicate the General Medical Condition]

(e.g., an Axis I disorder such as Major Depressive Disorder delaying recovery from a myocardial infarction)

Psychological Symptoms Affecting . . . [Indicate the General Medical Condition]

(e.g., depressive symptoms delaying recovery from surgery; anxiety exacerbating asthma)

Personality Traits or Coping Style Affecting . . . [Indicate the General Medical Condition]

(e.g., pathological denial of the need for surgery in a patient with cancer; hostile, pressured behavior contributing to cardiovascular disease)

Maladaptive Health Behaviors Affecting . . . [Indicate the General Medical Condition]

(e.g., overeating; lack of exercise; unsafe sex)

Stress-Related Physiological Response Affecting . . . [Indicate the General Medical Condition]

(e.g., stress-related exacerbations of ulcer, hypertension, arrhythmia, or tension headache)

Other or Unspecified Psychological Factors Affecting . . . [Indicate the General Medical Condition]

(e.g., interpersonal, cultural, or religious factors)

symbolism of excrement. According to psychoanalytic theory, defecation is an infantile form of gift giving or meeting obligations. Thus, this behavior is an emotional substitute for performance and accomplishment.

Psychosomatic medicine suggests similar explanations for the cardiovascular disorders, such as hypertension and migraine headaches. For example, specific emotional conflict in these disorders is attributed to repressed hostility. Alexander (1950) also linked coronary heart disease to excessive responsibility and mental stress. This clinical observation anticipated development of the theory of a Type A behavior pattern, discussed later.

Consistent with the general psychodynamic view of abnormal behavior, the early approach taken by psychosomatic medicine resulted from clinical observations, not empirical investigation. It explained why different people with various types of personalities and emotional conflicts developed particular physical disorders. But in fact, this approach to psychosomatic medicine had relatively little influence on either general medicine or the behavioral sciences (Agras, 1982). This was due partly to the lack of evidence linking specific diseases to particular personalities as well as the failure to develop effective methods for changing behavior related to medical problems. The emergence of behavioral medicine and health psychology in the 1970s changed this, however, and dramatically altered the study and treatment of health and disease.

Behavioral Medicine and Health Psychology

Behavioral medicine is the term used to describe the integration of behavioral and biomedical sciences in order to better understand, prevent, and treat physical illness (Schwartz & Weiss, 1978). Behavioral medicine emerged as a field of interdisciplinary study in the 1970s, in large part due to the impact of behavior therapy. Investigators had already demonstrated the effectiveness of behavioral principles and procedures in modifying many traditional psychiatric disorders (such as phobias), so they turned to problems associated with illness and disease (Blanchard, 1982). Biofeedback (discussed later in this chapter) lent itself to the assessment and treatment of different physical problems. Similarly, self-control strategies could be

psychosomatic medicine
Study of clinical disorders in which emotional conflicts are said to cause physical damage or symptoms such as hypertension, headaches, and ulcers.

behavioral medicine
Integration of behavioral and biomedical science to better understand, prevent, and treat physical illness.

directly applied to preventing and coping with chronic diseases (such as coronary heart disease). The medical community quickly accepted the availability of effective methods for changing a wide range of behaviors related to physical conditions, together with strategies for evaluating the effects that resulted.

Health psychology largely overlaps with behavioral medicine, since both focus on the influence that psychological factors have on health and illness. Yet there are differences:

1. Behavioral medicine is more closely identified with the modification of specific diseases. In contrast, health psychology is concerned not only with specific interventions but also with a number of other issues, including socioenvironmental factors and individual differences affecting health and illness as well as the analysis of health policy and the health care system.
2. Behavioral medicine tends to be interdisciplinary—medical specialists working with behavioral scientists. In contrast, health psychology is based solely on the discipline of psychology, representing the activities of both basic and applied psychologists.

The development of behavioral medicine and health psychology reflects a significant change in our health and illness models. A biopsychosocial perspective (Engel, 1977), which emphasizes the interactive influences of psychosocial and biological factors, is replacing the traditional biomedical model, which has a more limited emphasis on biology and disease. To a large extent, current health concerns focus on chronic diseases, such as cardiovascular problems, and identify behavior and lifestyle as the main risk factors, including stress, diet, substance abuse, physical inactivity, and unsafe sexual behavior. Each successive generation is living longer. And to maximize our health as we get older, we must avoid health-damaging behaviors and adopt health-enhancing habits.

> ## Focus on Critical Thinking
>
> The biopsychosocial model emphasizes that behavior plays an important role in influencing health.
>
> 1. Does this mean that people are responsible for their own health? Explain your answer.
> 2. How might the biopsychosocial model affect public health policy in the United States?

THE RELATIONSHIP BETWEEN MENTAL HEALTH AND PHYSICAL HEALTH

It's easy to show that emotional problems such as anxiety and depression are frequently associated with physical illnesses such as cancer. It's much more difficult, though, to determine which came first. That is, are the emotional problems the cause or the consequence of the physical illness?

To answer this challenging question, we need longitudinal data that show whether emotional problems preceded development of physical illness. If they did, we could infer that such problems caused or contributed to the illness. Vaillant (1979) conducted such a study and provided evidence that people's mental health has a direct influence on their physical health. The subjects in this study were 204 male Harvard University sophomores. All were physically healthy and free from any emotional problems. The men were first assessed between 1942 and 1944 and then followed up every year or two, when they would complete either questionnaires or interviews.

Based on these measures, the men's mental health status at the 1967 assessment was compared to their physical health at the 1975 examination. The relationship was highly significant. For example, between the ages of 21 and 46, only 2 of the 59 men rated with the best mental health became chronically ill or died. Yet 18 of the 48 men with the worst mental health became chronically ill or died.

health psychology
Application of psychology as a discipline to promote health and prevent and treat illness.

TABLE 10.1   *Association between Psychological Factors and Poor Health in Men 53 Years Old*

Predictor Variables Assess: 1940–1967	Health: 1975	
	Excellent Health (N = 100 men) (percent)	Ill, Disabled, or Dead (N = 34 men) (percent)
Psychiatric visits	12	56
Heavy use of mood-altering drugs	10	44
Little occupational progress	15	44
Job dissatisfaction	21	44
Little recreation with others	39	76
Marriage unhappy or terminated	31	50
Little vacation	26	50
College psychologic soundness rated poor ("C")	11	29
More than 5 days sick leave/year	14	32
Low income (less than $20,000/year)	14	26
Total adult adjustment score		
Best scores (10–12)	43	6
Worst scores (16–23)	14	59

Source: Adapted from G. E. Vaillant, "Natural History of Male Psychological Health," *New England Journal of Medicine*, 1979, *301*, p. 1251. Reprinted by permission.

Table 10.1 lists the factors that defined "poor" mental health in the men in the 1967 assessment. The corresponding data show that these qualities were found significantly more often in the men who later became ill or died (Vaillant, 1979). The effect of mental health on subsequent physical health held true even when statistical analyses controlled for the influence of other factors that might confound the results, such as cigarette smoking, obesity, and parents' longevity. This finding is important because many studies linking psychological stress with disease have not taken these factors into account.

The subjects in Vaillant's study were a homogeneous sample of white, economically advantaged men. We can't say whether these results generalize to women or people from other racial, ethnic, or socioeconomic groups. The data, nevertheless, strongly suggest that poor mental health predicts premature aging and deterioration of physical health.

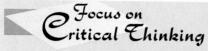
Focus on Critical Thinking

Research has often shown that people who have psychological problems also have existing physical illnesses.

1. Does this correlation allow us to infer that mental disorders contribute to physical illness? Explain your answer.

2. Based on Vaillant's study, can you infer a causal effect of mental health on physical health? Again, explain your answer.

STRESS AND ILLNESS

risk factor Characteristic that increases the likelihood that an individual will get an illness, even though the reason for the increased risk may be unclear.

Individuals who are exposed to severe psychological stress are, on average, less healthy and develop more physical illnesses than their less stressed peers. Evidence from several different sources has demonstrated that stress is a risk factor for disease (McEwen & Stellar, 1993). A **risk factor** is a characteristic that increases the likelihood that an individual will get an illness, even though the reason for the increased risk may be unclear. Once identified, a risk factor suggests the types of studies needed to uncover the underlying causes of the disease. Identification also encourages intervention to modify the risk factor and thus reduce occurrence of the disease.

A Response Model

Stress has been defined in terms of a complex physiological response by Hans Selye (1956), a pioneering biological researcher in this field. He conceptualized stress as a nonspecific body response that follows three predictable stages:

1. *Alarm and mobilization reaction*—The autonomic nervous system is aroused.
2. *Resistance*—The body tries to adapt to the physiological demands placed on it.
3. *Exhaustion*—Following prolonged exposure to the harmful stimulation, the body dies or suffers irreversible damage.

Subsequent research has demonstrated that Selye's complex series of physiological responses occur in response to psychological states as well as to physical stimulation (Weiner, 1977).

The Biological Basis of Stress   The human nervous system is organized as a hierarchy of different components. The brain is at the top of this hierarchy. Two parts of the brain—the hypothalamus and the limbic system—exert primary control over our emotions and motivation. Let's look at the role played by each.

The hypothalamus influences the autonomic nervous system and the endocrine system. The sympathetic division of the autonomic nervous system activates key organs such as the heart, blood vessels, stomach, and various glands (such as the adrenal glands) (see Chapter 2). In response to emotion or stress, the autonomic nervous system mobilizes the body's resources for emergencies—for instance, by increasing heartrate.

The **endocrine system** consists of glands that secrete hormones into the bloodstream. These hormones allow the brain to send chemical messages to different parts of the body in addition to direct neural transmission. The hypothalamus is a gland as well as a center of nerve cells. The chain of influence on the endocrine system, initiated by the hypothalamus, is shown in Figure 10.1. The secretion of corticotropin-releasing hormone (CRH) by the hypothalamus stimulates the pituitary gland. Together, the hypothalamus and pituitary control emotional responses, hunger and thirst, digestion, and sexual behavior. The pituitary gland, in turn, activates the adrenal gland by releasing adrenocorticotrophic hormone (ACTH).

The **adrenal gland,** which is also stimulated by the autonomic nervous system, consists of two parts—the inner portion (the *adrenal medulla*) and the outer portion (the *adrenal cortex*). In response to stress, the adrenal cortex secretes **corticosteroids** and the adrenal medulla secretes **catecholamines** (epinephrine and norepinephrine). The effects of these secretions are summarized at the bottom of Figure 10.1. These hormones also influence the brain in a complex feedback loop.

The second part of the brain critically involved in regulating emotion and motivation is the **limbic system,** a neural structure at the base of the forebrain. One part of the limbic system is the **hippocampus,** which plays a major role in memory. The hippocampus seems particularly responsive to corticosteroids released by the adrenal cortex. This feedback action of corticosteroids on the hippocampus helps turn off the stress response.

A Stimulus Model

Stress has also been defined in terms of stimuli, events, or environmental conditions that are assumed to influence all or most of us in the same way. Cohen et al. (1982) have classified these stimuli, or *stressors,* into four broad categories:

---

stress   State of physical and psychological tension caused by pressure or strain; a complex physiological response, according to Selye.

endocrine system   Physiological system that consists of glands secreting hormones into the bloodstream; these hormones allow the brain to send chemical messages to different parts of the body in addition to direct neural transmission.

adrenal gland   Located just above the kidneys; consists of two parts—the inner portion (the adrenal medulla) and the outer portion (the adrenal cortex); in response to stress, the adrenal cortex secretes corticosteroids and the adrenal medulla secretes catecholamines (epinephrine and norepinephrine).

corticosteroids   Hormones secreted by the adrenal cortex in response to stress.

catecholamines   Hormones (epinephrine and norepinephrine) secreted by the adrenal medulla in response to stress.

limbic system   Neural structure at the base of the forebrain; regulates emotion and motivation.

hippocampus   Part of the limbic system that plays a major role in memory.

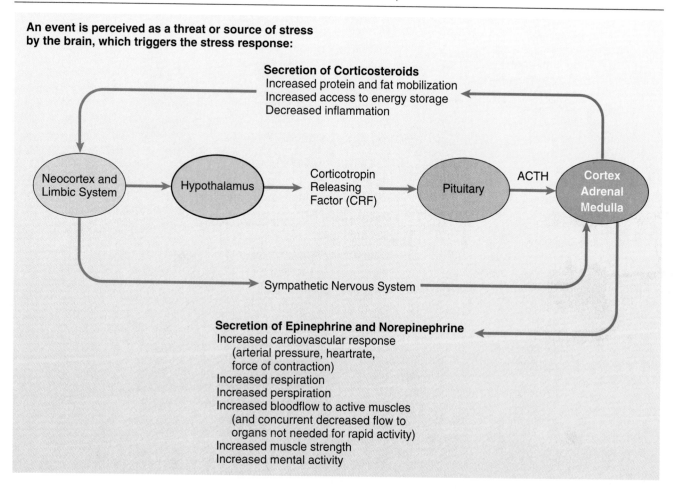

**An event is perceived as a threat or source of stress
by the brain, which triggers the stress response:**

Secretion of Corticosteroids
Increased protein and fat mobilization
Increased access to energy storage
Decreased inflammation

Neocortex and Limbic System → Hypothalamus → Corticotropin Releasing Factor (CRF) → Pituitary → ACTH → Cortex Adrenal Medulla

Sympathetic Nervous System

Secretion of Epinephrine and Norepinephrine
Increased cardiovascular response
(arterial pressure, heartrate,
force of contraction)
Increased respiration
Increased perspiration
Increased bloodflow to active muscles
(and concurrent decreased flow to
organs not needed for rapid activity)
Increased muscle strength
Increased mental activity

1. *acute stressors*—for example, awaiting surgery
2. *stressor sequences triggered by particular events*—for example, divorce or death of a spouse
3. *chronic stressors*—for example, unemployment
4. *chronic but intermittent stressors*—for example, weekly contact with family members that reliably produces conflict

Researchers have tried to measure stress by identifying stressful life events (Holmes & Rahe, 1967). In studies designed for this purpose, people are asked to recall major life events that occurred within a specified period of time (typically, 1 year). Each life event is given a weight—that is, decisions are made about how stressful events are in comparison to one another (see Table 10.2). The sum of the weighted scores is then taken as the degree of stress that person was exposed to. Positive life events, such as marriage, as well as negative events have been assumed to cause stress. In sum, any change from our normal routine is considered stressful.

Measuring major life events in this way has increased our knowledge of the association between stress and disease. But it's often difficult to interpret the association, due to several problems. One is that not all possible stressors are included in the different life event scales. For example, chronic conditions such as gender-role conflict are not assessed in the life event approach, although they are certainly related to health. Additionally, many minor everyday stressors, or "hassles," have been linked to health outcomes (Kanner, Coyne, Schaefer, & Lazarus, 1981). A second problem is that it's difficult to know if the occurrence of common stressors

TABLE 10.2 The Holmes and Rahe Life Events Stress Scale

Rank	Life Event	Mean Value
1	Death of spouse	100
2	Divorce	73
3	Marital separation	65
4	Jail term	63
5	Death of close family member	63
6	Personal injury or illness	53
7	Marriage	50
8	Fired at work	47
9	Marital reconciliation	45
10	Retirement	45
11	Change in health of family member	44
12	Pregnancy	40
13	Sex difficulties	39
14	Gain of new family member	39
15	Business readjustment	39
16	Change in financial state	38
17	Death of close friend	37
18	Change to different line of work	36
19	Change in number of arguments with spouse	35
20	Mortgage over $10,000	31
21	Foreclosure of mortgage or loan	30
22	Change in responsibilities at work	29
23	Son or daughter leaving home	29
24	Trouble with in-laws	29
25	Outstanding personal achievement	28
26	Wife begin or stop work	26
27	Begin or end school	26
28	Change in living conditions	25
29	Revision of personal habits	24
30	Trouble with boss	23
31	Change in work hours or conditions	20
32	Change in residence	20
33	Change in schools	20
34	Change in recreation	19
35	Change in church activities	19
36	Change in social activities	18
37	Mortgage or loan less than $10,000	17
38	Change in sleeping habits	16
39	Change in number of family get-togethers	15
40	Change in eating habits	15
41	Vacation	13
42	Christmas	12
43	Minor violations of the law	11

Source: Reprinted with permission from *Journal of Psychosomatic Research, 11,* by T. H. Holmes and R. H. Rahe, 1967, Elsevier Science Ltd., Pergamon Imprint, Oxford, England.

(such as divorce) preceded or resulted from the illness. A third problem is that not everyone responds similarly to the same stressful event. People feel differently about divorce, for instance; it may be more traumatic for some than for others. Finally, many people experience negative life events without becoming ill; this finding requires a different approach to the assessment of stress.

A Biopsychosocial Model

Selye's (1956) view of stress as a unitary response to varied stimuli is no longer useful. For example, in comparison to positive events, negative life events may have different psychological and physiological consequences. Negative life events also appear to be better predictors of illness than positive events (Cohen et al., 1982). The evidence clearly shows that different people respond differently to the same negative stimulus or stressful life event. It is now well accepted that a number of different biological and psychosocial processes and conditions determine or influence how a particular person will respond to a stressor.

Cognitive Appraisal   The emotional and physiological impact that a potentially stressful event will have can be determined somewhat through **cognitive appraisal** (Lazarus, 1991). A stressful event can be appraised according to three criteria:

1. *harm*—damage already done
2. *threat*—future or anticipated consequences
3. *challenge*—future events that might involve personal gain

For instance, the student who is threatened by a pending exam worries about failure. In contrast, the student who is challenged by the same exam anticipates the opportunity to perform well.

Cognitive appraisals are not necessarily rational or conscious; instead, they are often automatic, unconscious, and irrational. An example of cognitive appraisal is Bandura's (1986) self-efficacy theory (see Chapter 5). As you may recall, this theory suggests that it's not so much actually being exposed to stressful (phobic) stimuli that evokes psychological distress and biological measures of stress; rather, it's how confident individuals are perceived to be about coping with the stimuli.

Another cognitive variable that seems linked to physical illness is **explanatory style,** which is the way in which we each habitually explain the negative life events we experience (Peterson, 1988). These explanations are coded as causes that are stable versus unstable, global versus specific, and internal (due to ourselves) versus external (due to our environment). Explanatory style can be assessed using either a questionnaire or an analysis of an individual's written or spoken material. A pessimistic explanatory style reflects the belief that bad events are caused by stable, global, and internal factors.

In an illustrative study, Peterson, Seligman, and Vaillant (1988) analyzed the explanatory styles of 99 randomly chosen men from Vaillant's (1979) sample of Harvard University graduates, described earlier. The following statement is an example of pessimistic explanatory style: "I have symptoms of fear and nervousness . . . similar to those my mother had. She is still very nervous" (p. 25). Notice that this statement refers to internal causes (fear) and stability or permanence (that his mother has always had this problem). The study found that pessimistic explanatory style predicted poor health in these Harvard men from ages 45 through 60, even when physical and mental health at age 25 were controlled.

We don't know exactly how pessimistic explanatory style is linked to poor health, although both direct and indirect influences have been suggested. People who explain bad events in terms of stable, global, and internal attributions reportedly showed suppression of the immune system later. People with this explanatory style might also neglect health care because they have negative, passive views. For

cognitive appraisal Individual's judgment as to whether a potentially stressful event poses a personal threat.

explanatory style Habitual manner in which people explain the negative life events they experience.

PERSPECTIVE ON HOW STRESS CAN LEAD TO DISEASE

BIOLOGICAL FACTORS

Biological responses to stress provide the mechanisms whereby stressful events lead to disease:
➤ Genetic factors strongly influence response to stress.
➤ Biological aspects of gender help determine response to stress. For example, premenopausal women are protected by estrogen.
➤ Relative reactivity of the autonomic nervous system influences the impact of stressors.

PSYCHOLOGICAL FACTORS

Psychological factors influence whether an individual responds to life events with stress:
➤ How a person appraises a stimulus determines whether it's perceived as a threat or stressor.
➤ Good coping responses minimize the impact of stress; poor coping responses result in stress.
➤ Perceived control over life events protects against stress.
➤ Psychological stress affects the autonomic nervous system and neuroendocrine system. These neuroendocrine changes can ultimately cause neuron damage in the brain and subsequently impair the body's ability to cope effectively with stressful stimuli. Prolonged stress leads to the excessive release of glucocorticoids, which can seriously damage or even kill neurons in the hippocampus.

SOCIAL FACTORS

Biological and psychological factors interact with social elements in causing stress:
➤ Social stress produces an increase in the hormone cortisol, resulting in increased insulin secretion. Elevated levels of cortisol and insulin combine to increase the risk of heart disease.
➤ Social stress may also lead to maladaptive coping responses, such as eating a high-fat diet or excessive amounts of food. Social stress is more likely to produce heart disease when combined with a high-fat diet than a low-fat diet.
➤ Availability of social support and a person's socioeconomic status can protect against stress.

These biological, psychological, and social factors interact to cause problems, as illustrated in the following case:

Bill was 55 years old when he had a heart attack. He was at the airport when he collapsed, running to catch a flight home from a hectic business trip. Fortunately for him, airport security responded immediately. He was taken to a nearby hospital, where he received prompt medical attention that stabilized his condition.

The biopsychosocial model helps explain Bill's problems. He was genetically at risk for cardiovascular disease. His father had died of heart disease at age 40 and his uncle, at age 48. Both Bill and his younger brother had hypertension. In addition, Bill's health habits were poor: He was somewhat overweight, had a high cholesterol level, ate a high-fat diet, and didn't exercise. Bill failed to follow his doctor's advice to reduce fat intake and lose weight. He frequently neglected to take his antihypertensive medication, despite his doctor's repeated warnings.

As an executive in a major pharmaceutical company, Bill's job was often very stressful, requiring long hours of work. His fellow workers referred to him as a Type A personality. The demands of his job kept his time for family and friends at a minimum. So socially, Bill had little support. He lived alone, after divorcing his wife of 25 years, and he rarely saw his children.

example, pessimistic college students who contract colds or influenza may be less likely than their optimistic peers to take steps to ease their recovery, such as sleeping more and drinking more liquids.

Coping   Understanding the nature and effects of stress is linked to the concept of coping. The availability and use of specific coping mechanisms strongly influences our psychological and physiological responses to stressors. Coping can be how we think about events or how we behave in response to stressors. Both cognitive and behavioral coping strategies can be effective in modifying the effects of stress.

Lazarus (1991) has distinguished between two major forms of coping. In *active,* or *problem-focused,* coping, people work to change the situation directly. For example, a college student might be upset by her roommate's inconsiderate behavior, such as entertaining friends in the apartment until late at night when she's trying to study for a test the next day. The student might speak to the roommate, explaining how she needs time to study for tests and suggesting that the roommate check with her first before inviting friends over. In *passive,* or *emotion-focused,* coping, people try to accept and manage their feelings. This form of coping is helpful in situations that are beyond an individual's control and thus cannot be changed by appropriate problem solving. For example, coping with terminal illness might be emotion focused, such as trying to accept death.

The effects of different coping styles partly depend on variables such as the specific social and cultural context. Active coping or personal control may occasionally have negative, rather than positive, effects on health. For example, Dressler (1985) studied the relationships among coping styles, chronic economic stress, and psychosomatic distress symptoms among residents of a rural, southern, black community. Having an active coping style reduced the effects of stress on women but increased the effects on men. According to Dressler, the social norms within the conservative community where the study was conducted explain this gender-linked difference.

Specifically, in this community, active coping by black men was more likely to conflict with the barriers put up by institutionalized racism. The more the men tried to change their economic conditions, the more frustration and failure they met with. In response, they learned to suppress their resentment—but at the cost of increased psychosomatic distress. In contrast, the women's attempts at active coping were confined mainly to improving conditions for their children. As Dressler (1985) observed, these efforts were more acceptable within the community. What's more, in comparison to the men, the women felt they had more personal control over their behavior.

Interestingly, women are sick more often than men, but men die younger than women. This issue and other differences in men's and women's health and mortality are considered in Thinking about Gender Issues.

Social Support   The environmental factor of **social support** mediates the relationship between stress and illness (Cohen & Syme, 1985). Social support is the network of people that provides a foundation for an individual, showing concern and caring, communicating acceptance and group inclusion, giving tangible help when needed, and offering advice about coping with problems. Epidemiological research has consistently linked social relationships with mortality rates. For example, death rates (from all causes) are higher among unmarried than married individuals. Measures of social relationships—for example, marriage, contacts with extended family and friends, church membership, and other formal and informal social connections—predict subsequent death rates.

Thus, in a study conducted in Tecumseh, Michigan, House, Robbins, and Metzner (1982) found measures of social relationships and activities strongly related to death rates during the following 10 to 12 years. The relative risk for men

social support Network of people that provides a foundation for an individual, showing concern and caring, communicating acceptance and group inclusion, giving tangible help, and offering advice.

Thinking about GENDER ISSUES

Sex Differences in Health and Mortality

There is an intriguing gender difference in health: Women are sick more often than men, but men die younger than women (Rodin & Ickovics, 1990). Health surveys in the United States and Europe reveal that compared to men, women have higher rates of visits to physicians, disability days, and uses of prescription and nonprescription medication. The explanation given for these gender differences is that women suffer from transient, nonfatal illnesses (such as arthritis, digestive conditions, and migraines) to a much greater extent than men. However, men are more likely to die from their illnesses (such as heart disease).

Based on statistical analyses of health data, Verbrugge (1989) concluded that women's higher rate of sickness is due primarily to their social role and attitudes toward health. The psychosocial risk factors that predict greater morbidity in women include their lower level of paid employment, higher level of emotional stress, feeling of greater vulnerability to illness, and less strenuous physical activity. When these risk factors are statistically controlled, the difference in morbidity between men and women disappears. If anything, men are more likely to get sick and seek medical care. A crucial implication of these findings is that women's health can be significantly improved by psychosocial interventions, such as better employment opportunities, reducing stress, and encouraging aerobic activity.

The mortality data tell a different story: Men die younger than women. This finding transcends racial differences; black women live longer than both black and white men. In fact, this finding holds true even when lifestyle risk factors are controlled for, such as heavier cigarette smoking, alcohol consumption, and greater job hazards among men (Verbrugge, 1989).

Part of the explanation for this trend is that women are biologically more advantaged than men. Women's more resilient biology could be due to genetic or hormonal differences. Women have estrogen, which clearly protects against cardiovascular disease. After menopause, when women no longer produce estrogen, their rates of heart disease match those of men. It's likely that these biological differences interact with psychosocial factors to account for women's lower death rates (Matthews, 1989).

Think about the following question:

1. The social role of women in the United States has been steadily changing. More and more women are entering the workforce and pursuing professional careers. They have become increasingly independent in other ways, too. Do you think that this changing social role will affect gender differences in health? Explain your answer.

---

was 3.0 and for women, 1.5. (A relative risk for death of 3.0 means that someone who scores low on the measure of interest—in this case, the extent of social relationships and activities—is three times as likely to die as individuals who score high on the measure.) These results were obtained even though investigators controlled for the effects of known risk factors, such as high blood pressure and blood cholesterol levels. Prospective studies overall have shown that the apparent protective effect of social relationships holds for men and women across different populations. But data suggest the effect is greater for men than women and possibly for whites more than blacks (House et al., 1982).

The link between social support and health has been well established. But how does social support influence biological functioning? One view is that social support (such as emotional support or practical assistance with challenging tasks) gives us a buffer against the negative biological effects of stress. Several correlational studies back up this view. For example, among college students experiencing the stress of final exams, those individuals with more social support had superior immune function (Jemmott & Magliore, 1988).

In the first experimental study of this question, Cohen, Kaplan, Cunnick, Manuck, and Rabin (1992) randomly assigned nonhuman primates to experiencing 26 months of stable or unstable social conditions. Among the unstable conditions group, each monkey was housed with a different group of monkeys every month, which is known to produce severe and chronic stress. Among the stable conditions group, the animals remained with the same three or four monkeys for the full 26 months.

During this period, the researchers systematically observed the monkeys' affiliative behavior (how they related to others in the group) and their immune response. It was found that stress—the unstable social conditions—significantly impaired the monkeys' immune function. The animals in the unstable conditions were more affiliative than those in the stable conditions, and those who were the most affiliative showed the least impairment in immune response. In other words, the monkeys with the most social support were protected against the negative biological effects of chronic stress (Cohen et al., 1992).

Another view is that social support enhances health directly in ways unrelated to any buffering effect against stress. Among the hypotheses about social support is that it fosters a sense of meaning or coherence about life, thereby enhancing health. Another theory is that social support encourages health-promoting behaviors, such as getting enough sleep, following a beneficial diet, being physically active, getting good medical care, and avoiding alcohol and drug abuse (Umberson, 1987).

The *quantity* of social support we each enjoy is a function of life experience. But how we perceive the *quality* of that social support is strongly influenced by genetic factors (Bergeman, Plomin, Pederson, McClearn, & Nesselroade, 1990). This intriguing finding suggests that the positive effect of social support on health is not only a product of environmental events; it's also the result of genetic factors that influence what social environments we select and how we interpret those environments.

Focus on Critical Thinking

1. Assume that stable social conditions and support promote good health. Given that, suggest which subgroups of people in the United States are most exposed to stress and should show more physical illness. Explain your answers.

2. A high school girl feels stressed because a boy in her class makes unwanted sexual comments about her and often touches her body. Should she respond with an active or passive coping style? Explain your answer.

PSYCHOLOGICAL EFFECTS ON BIOLOGICAL MECHANISMS

Available evidence consistently shows that factors such as mental health and psychological stress significantly affect our physical health. So the key question is: How do psychological factors cause the physiological changes that define physical illness and disease?

Psychological factors influence health in two major ways. First, they affect the basic biological mechanisms and functions that mediate illness and disease. And second, they determine specific health-promoting and health-damaging behaviors, such as coping better with stress, quitting cigarette smoking, following a healthy diet, and adopting safe-sex practices.

To illustrate the direct influence of psychological factors on medical conditions, we will focus on diseases related to the immune system (such as cancer), cardiovascular disorders (such as heart disease), and metabolic diseases (such as diabetes). These medical conditions not only afflict large numbers of people but also provide excellent examples of current research in the complex interactions between psychological processes and biological functioning.

Immune System Function and Disease

immune system Physiological system that protects the body against viral and bacterial disease.

The **immune system** protects the body against viral and bacterial disease. Although immune function is highly complex and not yet fully understood, you should be aware of some of its basic workings.

Immune function is measured by drawing blood and analyzing the number and specialized functions of various subgroups of white blood cells (*leukocytes*) and their biochemical mediators. The immune system has two main components—the humoral and the cellular. *Humoral immunity* involves the release of antibodies into the blood and other body fluids, which defend against bacteria and viruses. B-cells and their immediate derivatives, plasma cells, are primarily involved in humoral immunity. *Cellular immunity* protects against viruses, cancer cells, and foreign tissue (as in organ transplants). T-cells, or lymphocytes, from the thymus gland are primarily responsible for cellular immunity.

Besides T- and B-cells, several other cell types and plasma components are involved in immunological processes. **Natural killer (NK) cells,** for example, which are derived from bone marrow and related to T-cells, destroy viruses and some tumor cells. In a well-functioning immune system, these complex, interdependent components precisely balance each other. When their delicate balance is disrupted, disease may result. Autoimmune disease occurs when the immune cells mistakenly attack the body's normal tissue, as if it were foreign matter.

Impairment Due to Stress   Animal studies have consistently shown that stress reduces resistance to infection and enhances the incidence and development of tumors (Ben-Eliyahu, Yirmiya, Liebeskind, Taylor, & Gayle, 1991). Stress reduces both humoral and cellular immune responses. How much control the individual has over the stressor, in relative terms, seems especially likely to make a difference. For example, two groups of rats each received stressors in the form of electric shocks. One group could terminate these shocks by making an escape response; in other words, they could control the stressors. The other group received the same number and duration of electric shocks but could not terminate them; that is, they had no control. Only the inescapable shock had the effects of suppressing NK cell activity and enhancing tumor growth in the rats (Laudenslager, Ryan, Drugan, Hyson, & Maier, 1979). Even receiving the same amount of shock had very different outcomes, depending on the degree of control available to the rat.

Research with people has shown that a variety of stressful events can influence immune function. In one series of studies, Kiecolt-Glaser and Glaser (1987) assessed immune function in medical students one month before and then during final exams. These researchers found significant reductions in a number of immune functions due to the stress of examinations, including decreased helper T-cell and NK cell activity. Students taking exams, of course, typically change their behavior in several ways—for instance, they sleep fewer hours and eat less well than normal. So immune function may be influenced by either sleep loss or inadequate nutrition, rather than stress. The researchers controlled for these potentially confounding factors and concluded that the observed immunological changes resulted directly from the stress of taking exams.

Although many students may disagree, the stress of taking examinations is relatively mild. What about more severe stress? Bereavement over the death of a spouse or immediate family member is usually considered the most powerful of all stressful events, and it does affect immune function. For example, husbands of women with advanced breast cancer showed significant immune system suppression in the months following their wives' deaths compared to the months prior to bereavement (Stein, Keller, & Schleifer, 1985). Marital separation and divorce are also reliably associated with increased rates of illness and mortality. Compared with married controls, separated or divorced women show poorer immune function (Kiecolt-Glaser & Glaser, 1987).

People who perceive that they have control over exposure to stressors seem to be protected against the immunosuppressive effects of stress (Sieber et al., 1992). For example, perceived self-efficacy directly affects responses of the autonomic nervous system and the immune system. To demonstrate this, Wiedenfeld and her col-

natural killer (NK) cells
Part of the immune system; destroy viruses and some tumor cells; derived from bone marrow.

leagues (1989) used an experimental methodology previously described in the treatment of phobic disorders (see Chapter 5). Using modeling and guided exposure treatments, researchers systematically increased self-efficacy in subjects who had snake phobias. The researchers measured immunological responses to the phobic stressor (the snake) before, during, and after the subjects acquired self-efficacy about coping with the snake. The development of self-efficacy enhanced the subjects' immunological responses to the stressor.

The research we've summarized here establishes that psychological stress can alter immune function. But are these effects of stress clinically significant? Do they lead to or delay recovery from infectious diseases? Increasing evidence suggests that for some diseases, the answer to both questions is yes.

The Common Cold   You've surely heard the old saying that if you're run down, you're more likely to get sick. Catching a cold, for example, is often attributed to being tired and stressed out. Now we know that this age-old belief is correct.

Stress increases our susceptibility to viral infections, like colds. Researchers in England administered nasal drops containing one of five different cold viruses or saline as a control to 394 healthy subjects (Cohen, Tyrrell, & Smith, 1991). The subjects were then quarantined so that they did not come into contact with any other infectious agents. Detailed measures were obtained of the life stress that the subjects had been experiencing. Subjects were assessed for cold symptoms and clinical colds—namely, symptoms in addition to the infection verified by isolation of the responsible virus.

Both symptoms and clinical colds increased significantly among subjects who were exposed to a cold virus and who reported the most stress. A particularly strong finding was that the more stress the subjects experienced, the more likely they were to develop colds. This held true with all the cold viruses tested, suggesting that stress has a general impact on lowering resistance to various viral infections.

Cancer   Some investigators have dismissed the relevance of psychosocial factors in the cause and course of cancer (Cassileth, Lusk, Miller, Brown, & Miller, 1985). However, data show that psychological factors may influence at least some forms of cancer in some patients. A study of women with breast cancer (Spiegel, Bloom, Kraemer, & Gottheil, 1989) has provided some of the most provocative and potentially important evidence to date. Researchers found that women who participated in a psychotherapy group and used self-hypnosis to control pain lived almost twice as long as those in a control group. Both groups received normal medical treatment. Women in the therapy group also reported less anxiety, depression, and pain than the controls.

Colorectal cancer has been linked to stress, as well. A recent Swedish study found that people who reported a history of workplace problems over the past 10 years faced 5.5 times the risk of colorectal cancer of adults who reported no such problems (Courtney, Longnecker, Theorell, & de Verdier, 1993). The association held even after researchers accounted for diet and other factors that had previously been linked to these cancers.

Stress can contribute to cancer by impairing the immune system. A similar result can occur from lesions in DNA, which are caused by stress. Japanese scientists have shown that chronically stressed rats develop oxidative damage (lesions) in liver DNA (Adachi, Kawamura, & Takemoto, 1993). This damage can lead to cell mutation and the growth of cancers.

The chapter-opening case of Barbara Boggs Sigmund illustrates some of the controversy that surrounds the role of psychological factors in cancer. For example, in his best-selling book *Love, Medicine, and Miracles* (1986), Bernie Siegel—a surgeon at Yale Medical School—argued that self-love is as important in surviving cancer as receiving an accurate medical diagnosis and treatment. Siegel believes that cancer is despair experienced at the cellular level. According to him, "If we ignore our despair, the body receives a die message. If we deal with our pain and seek help, then the message is 'Living is difficult but desirable' and the immune system works to keep us alive" (p. 29). (An earlier version of this notion was proposed by Wilhelm Reich, who attributed Sigmund Freud's dying of cancer to his sexually unfulfilling and unhappy marriage [Sontag, 1977].) Siegel also contends that when we fail to face psychic conflict, we get cancer in the organs in which those conflicts are focused (or somatized). Thus, "Women who have unhappy love relationships are especially vulnerable to breast or cervical diseases" (Siegel, 1986, p. 29).

Barbara Boggs Sigmund talked about assertions made by people like Siegel. She rejected his view, based on her own experience (Sigmund, 1989).

As described in this chapter, some physical states are significantly influenced by psychological factors and may even be altered using psychological treatments. But statements about how love can cure cancer only invite skeptical reactions and premature rejection of the possible influence that psychological factors might actually have on cancer and other diseases. Perhaps more important is the unintended impact that these much publicized pronouncements have on people with diseases. Susan Sontag, in her book *Illness as Metaphor* (1977), argued that simplistic psychological theories of this sort blame the patient for having the disease. As you may remember, Barbara Boggs Sigmund wrote poignantly about not wanting to die feeling "like a failure."

AIDS **Acquired immune deficiency syndrome (AIDS)** is a particularly deadly disease in which the cells of the immune system are attacked. The cause is infection with the human immunodeficiency virus, or HIV. Infection with HIV is believed to inevitably lead to the full clinical disease, AIDS. However, a small but possibly growing number of people with AIDS live 5 or more years after diagnosis. This is remarkable, considering that the average life expectancy of someone with AIDS ranges from 2 to 18 months after diagnosis. Some investigators have speculated that psychosocial factors may influence the onset and the course of the disease through their effects on the immune system.

Psychosocial factors might influence the course of AIDS by reducing the negative effects of stress on immune function (Solomon, 1989). One way to test this would be to compare patients who died rapidly following onset of the disease with those who survived for 2 years or longer. Some research has indicated that patients who lived longer were more likely to use active coping strategies and reach out for help in solving problems (Solomon, Temoshok, O'Leary, & Zich, 1987). Autonomic arousal was also correlated with greater NK cell activity. Moreover, autonomic arousal measures predicted patients' survival at a 3-year follow-up (O'Leary, Temoshok, Jenkins, & Sweet, 1989). Researchers hypothesized that increased autonomic arousal is associated with the release of catecholamines, enhancing NK activity. This view is consistent with other research that correlates minimal expression of emotion with bad outcomes in cancer patients.

Other findings call into question the role of psychological factors on the progression of AIDS. Severe stress is commonly believed to speed the deadly progression of AIDS. Yet gay men bereaving the deaths of lovers and friends from AIDS do not show different immunological responses than gay men who are not bereaving (Kemeny, Cohen, Zegans, & Conant, 1989). A detailed epidemiological analysis of the impact of stressful life events on the onset of symptoms in gay men showed no effect (Kessler et al., 1991). The researchers concluded that gay men with HIV infection do not need to reduce exposure to stressful events in their lives.

For people with HIV, depression does not speed the onset of AIDS or eventual death. Those who develop HIV-related symptoms are more likely to become depressed, but depression does not influence progression of the disease. An 8-year study of 365 depressed and 1,858 nondepressed patients with HIV showed that

acquired immune deficiency syndrome (AIDS)
Fatal disease caused by the human immunodeficiency virus (HIV), in which cells of the immune system are attacked.

depression was not associated with any measurable impairment of immune function in these patients. Moreover, no difference was found in the amount of time before death (Lyketsos et al., 1993). Even in people who do not have HIV, depression has not been shown to have consistent effects on the immune system or on the development of disease states (Stein, Miller, & Trestman, 1991).

Cardiovascular Disease

The cardiovascular system consists of the heart and blood vessels. To illustrate the role of psychological factors in cardiovascular disease, we will focus on the problems of hypertension and coronary heart disease.

Hypertension The condition of having chronic, abnormally high blood pressure is called **hypertension.** A blood pressure measure of 140/90 is defined as borderline hypertension; a measure of 160/95 characterizes definite hypertension. (Note that in a measure of blood pressure, the first number is the *systolic* reading, which is when the heart is actively pumping blood, and the second number is the *diastolic* reading, which is when the heart is resting.) Sometimes, hypertension is called the "silent killer" because it is *asymptomatic,* which means that you're unaware of this condition unless you have your blood pressure checked. Hypertension affects roughly 30 million people in the United States. It can cause stroke, heart disease, and kidney damage. It is more prevalent in men than women and twice as common among blacks as among whites, as discussed later in this section.

Hypertension has multiple causes, including genetic, dietary, and sociocultural factors. As a result, understanding and treating hypertension requires a biopsychosocial perspective, taking into account the separate and interactive effects of different risk factors.

Genetic factors predispose some people to develop the problem, in that hypertension runs in families. White children who have at least one parent with hypertension respond to stress with greater increases in blood pressure than those without such family histories—even if the children themselves have normal blood pressure. A likely explanation for the greater prevalence of hypertension among blacks is that black children and adults show greater **autonomic reactivity** than whites (Anderson, McNeilly, & Myers, 1991). Reactivity refers to changes in arousal of the autonomic nervous system in response to stressors. Autonomic reactivity is significantly associated with risk for hypertension. One prospective study with white male medical students found that a change in systolic blood pressure in response to a physical stressor predicted the development of hypertension more than 20 years later (Menkes et al., 1989).

In addition to genetic factors, psychological factors are linked to hypertension. A recent study has shown that highly anxious men are twice as likely to develop hypertension as less anxious men (Markovitz et al., 1993). Diet affects blood pressure, too. Reducing sodium intake is a major means of preventing and treating hypertension. Similarly, excessive alcohol consumption is positively correlated with increased blood pressure (Altura, 1986).

Sociocultural factors also play a role in hypertension. Cross-cultural research has shown a strong association between rates of hypertension and industrialization. It remains uncertain whether this association is due to increased levels of stress being placed on people in modern, industrialized societies or is a function of other variables, such as changed dietary practices. Norman Anderson—a leading hypertension researcher—has proposed that the heightened autonomic reactivity in African Americans is a function of the chronic social and environmental stress that they encounter in U.S. society (Anderson et al., 1991). This chronic stress increases autonomic arousal, sodium retention, and the release of stress hormones like norepinephrine, which leads to vasoconstriction (constriction of the blood vessels).

hypertension Chronic, abnormally high blood pressure; measure of 140/90 is borderline hypertension and one of 160/95 is definite hypertension.

autonomic reactivity Arousal of the autonomic nervous system in response to stress.

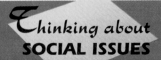

Thinking about SOCIAL ISSUES   Socioeconomic Inequalities in Health

Socioeconomic status (SES) is a strong predictor of disease and death. The lower people are in the SES hierarchy, the more likely they are to contract virtually all diseases and to die at a younger age (Adler, Boyce, Chesney, Folkman, & Syme, 1993). This inverse relationship between SES and health holds true whether SES is defined in terms of income, education, or occupation. In the United States, differences in mortality rates between whites and blacks seem more attributable to differences in SES than race. Blacks tend to have lower SES and so have worse health outcomes than whites.

An obvious explanation for the inverse relationship between SES and health is that people of low SES are burdened with poverty and lack of access to adequate health care, as is the case for many people in the United States. But this alone cannot explain the phenomenon (Adler et al., 1993), for several reasons:

1. People of low SES are more likely to have health problems even in countries where there is universal health care, such as Sweden and England.
2. SES differences occur not only at the bottom of the hierarchy but also at the top, where all people have access to health care.
3. The differences occur in diseases that respond to treatment as well as those that are not. If it were simply a matter of access to health care, there should be a greater difference in treatable diseases, which is not the case.
4. SES differences occur even within single treatment settings. A study of patients recovering from heart attacks revealed that those with higher levels of education died less often even after age, race, sex, and severity of heart disease were taken into account (Tofler et al., 1993).

This pattern of findings certainly does not mean that access to medical care is unimportant. But it does suggest that other broad psychosocial factors might play significant roles in determining health. Nancy Adler and her colleagues (1993) have suggested what these factors might be. Behaviors such as cigarette smoking, poor nutrition, and lack of exercise have all been shown to impair health, as we've described in this chapter. These behaviors are also inversely related to SES, as are the related risk factors of hypertension, high cholesterol, and obesity. When these behaviors and risk factors are controlled for, the SES differences are reduced but not eliminated. So other factors must be at work.

Considering various physical and psychological sources of stress provides a plausible explanation. People with low SES are exposed to more adverse physical and social conditions—for instance, cancer-causing materials and violence. These people experience more stressful life events and social isolation (Ruberman et al., 1984), and they have fewer material and psychological resources to cope with these problems. For people with low SES, life is less controllable and more unpredictable than for those with higher SES. And as noted in several chapters of this book, controllability and predictability are reliably linked to anxiety, stress, and biological harm.

In 1994, President Clinton proposed legislation to ensure that every American would have health insurance. Estimates were that roughly 30 million Americans had no health coverage. Opposition to Clinton's proposal came from many sources and for different reasons, and it was defeated in Congress. But even if universal health insurance were achieved, Adler and her colleagues (1993) point out that it would not eliminate SES inequalities in health. Medical coverage is necessary but not sufficient to overcome the SES differences.

Think about the following question:

1. What can be done to reduce SES inequalities in health? If you were in charge of public health policy in the United States, what would you do to improve this situation?

Over time, this stress-induced reactivity results in structural damage to the system of blood vessels and thus the development of hypertension.

Several lines of evidence support this model. Compared to whites, blacks are exposed to greater levels of psychosocial stress due to unemployment, poverty, crime, and crowded housing conditions. These chronic stressors are associated with higher blood pressure and hypertension within the black population. For example, there is a strong inverse relationship between **socioeconomic status (SES)** and hypertension among blacks. In fact, SES is a strong predictor of health problems and even death; see Thinking about Social Issues for more on this topic.

socioeconomic status (SES) Person's relative status in society as a function of income and education.

coronary heart disease (CHD) Partial or total obstruction of one or more of the coronary arteries due to atherosclerosis.

Coronary Heart Disease   The etiology of **coronary heart disease (CHD)** is complex. Like hypertension, heart disease runs in families. Vulnerable individuals inherit a biological tendency that may then interact with different physiological, nutritional, and environmental factors to produce heart disease.

For some time, researchers have considered a number of psychological factors that may contribute to heart disease. To be sure, no personality trait has received more publicity as a possible cause than the Type A behavior pattern. Beginning in the 1950s, San Francisco cardiologists Meyer Friedman and Ray Rosenman suggested that people with a particular behavior pattern—Type A—are at greater risk for coronary heart disease than people without such a behavioral style—Type B. In general, the Type A person responds to stress with hostility or aggression, feels a sense of time pressure (always has deadlines to meet), and is competitive and ambitious. By contrast, the Type B person is less aggressive, more relaxed, and sets fewer deadlines (Friedman & Rosenman, 1974).

Friedman and Rosenman illustrated the Type A pattern in the case of Paul, a 52-year-old company manager in California:

> Paul is not merely an impatient man; he is also a harried man. A very disproportionate amount of his emotional energy is consumed in struggling against the normal constraints of time. "How can I move faster, and do more and more things in less and less time?" is the question that never ceases to torment him.
>
> Paul hurries his thinking, his speech, and his movements. He also strives to hurry the thinking, speech, and movements of those about him; they must communicate rapidly and relevantly if they wish to avoid creating impatience in him. Planes must arrive and depart precisely on time for Paul, cars ahead of him on the highway must maintain a speed he approves of, and there must never be a queue of persons standing between him and a bank clerk, a restaurant table, or the interior of a theater. In fact, he is infuriated whenever people talk slowly or circuitously, when planes are late, cars dawdle on the highway, and queues form.
>
> He also strives as often as he can to do several things at once. While driving his car to work, he sometimes dictates letters into his portable tape recorder, or he shaves himself with an electric razor. He also keeps his car radio on in order to hear the news. (1974, pp. 108–109)

One of Friedman and Rosenman's (1974) early studies showed that stress directly affects cholesterol level in the blood (serum cholesterol), which is an established risk factor for heart disease. Using a sample of accountants, the cardiologists measured the individuals' serum cholesterol levels from January to June of one year. Cholesterol levels rose sharply as April 15 approached, reflecting the intense pressure that accountants are under to complete income tax returns by this deadline. Cholesterol levels then declined significantly during May and June, when the stress had subsided. These results could not be attributed to changes in the accountants' diet, cigarette smoking, or exercise habits, which remained stable during this period.

The first prospective epidemiological study seemed to confirm the importance of the Type A behavior pattern. The Western Collaborative Group Study (WCGS) followed 3,154 healthy men, ages 39 to 59, for $8\frac{1}{2}$ years. Men with Type A behavior pattern were twice as likely to develop coronary heart disease as their Type B counterparts (Rosenman et al., 1975).

Even stronger support came from studies of patients undergoing a medical procedure known as coronary **angiography.** This procedure involves inserting a catheter (or fine needle) to inject a special dye into the coronary arteries to examine them under X-ray and determine the extent of plaque buildup, or **atherosclerosis.** Initial studies found that Type A patients had more extensive coronary artery disease at the time of catheterization than other patients, even when other risk factors were held constant (Blumenthal, Williams, Kong, Schanberg, & Thompson, 1978).

But soon after these early studies, contradictory findings began to appear. That was the case with a 25-year follow-up of the original WCGS subjects (Matthews & Haynes, 1986). This study showed that patients with Type A behavior pattern who had recovered from heart attacks were significantly less likely than Type B patients to die of subsequent coronary heart disease (Ragland & Brand, 1988). In other

angiography Medical procedure that involves inserting a catheter (fine needle) to inject a special dye into the coronary arteries; done to examine them under X-ray and determine the extent of plaque buildup.

atherosclerosis Condition in which plaque of cholesterol, fat, and calcium has built up in the coronary arteries; obstructs bloodflow and causes chest pain (angina) and heart attack (myocardial infarction).

words, in subjects who survived their first heart attacks, having a Type A behavior pattern appeared to be a protective factor, not a risk factor. Studies using angiography have been even more damaging to the Type A behavior pattern hypothesis. After the three initial supportive studies, subsequent investigations failed to show a significant association between Type A behavior pattern and degree of coronary heart disease at the time of catheterization.

The inconsistency among these findings shows that the association between personality and heart disease is more complex than Friedman and Rosenman had thought. The current consensus is that not all components of the complex set of reactions labeled Type A behavior pattern are related to coronary heart disease. Only some components may be harmful or toxic; others may be neutral or even protective. In the WCGS data, the hostility component of Type A behavior pattern was the strongest predictor of heart disease (Matthews, Glass, Rosenman, & Bortner, 1977). Other studies have linked a questionnaire measure of hostility to subsequent heart disease and death. For example, 255 physicians who had completed the Minnesota Multiphasic Personality Inventory (MMPI) in medical school were assessed 25 years later (Barefoot, Dahlstrom, & Williams, 1983). Those with high hostility scores on the MMPI's Ho scale had a cumulative heart disease rate four or five times higher than those with low scores. (See Chapter 3 for more information about the MMPI.)

Stress and Heart Disease   Stress can contribute to heart problems through two mechanisms. In the first, stress accelerates the buildup of plaques in the arteries. Kaplan, Adams, Clarkson, Manuck, and Shively (1991) subjected monkeys to chronic social stress by changing their cagemates on a regular basis. These monkeys developed more atherosclerosis than those who lived in stable conditions. When the stressed monkeys were put on the drug propranolol, they did not develop atherosclerosis. This drug blocks the effect of sympathetic arousal of the autonomic nervous system, which suggests that this arousal is responsible for plaque buildup.

In the second mechanism, an acute stressful event triggers a heart attack by causing a rupture of the atherosclerotic plaque. The rupture leads to formation of a thrombus (bloodclot) that blocks bloodflow and can cause sudden death (Fuster, Badimon, Badimon, & Chesebro, 1992). The acute event may be a physical stressor, such as excessive exercise, or a psychological stressor.

Depression and Heart Disease   Depression doesn't seem to impair the immune system, as we've already noted. But results from a study of risk factors for heart disease in a study of 1,225 men in Finland indicate that depression can contribute to heart problems (Bower, 1992). It appears that depression increases the effect of two well-known risk factors: cigarette smoking and higher than normal levels of fibrinogen (a blood-clotting protein that facilitates plaque formation in the arteries). The amount of plaque buildup in the carotid artery was three times greater in depressed men who smoked than in nondepressed men who smoked, with years of smoking and cigarettes smoked per day held constant. Depressed men with elevated fibrinogen levels had nearly four times as much carotid atherosclerosis as nondepressed men with the same levels of the protein.

People's general outlook on life was one of the factors considered by a group of researchers studying mortality rates among Chinese Americans. Thinking about Multicultural Issues presents their findings on the link between psychological states and illness and disease.

Metabolic Disease

Diabetes is a disorder of carbohydrate metabolism in which individuals have trouble regulating their blood-sugar levels. It afflicts roughly 11 million Americans.

diabetes Disorder of carbohydrate metabolism in which individuals have trouble regulating blood-sugar levels.

Thinking about
MULTICULTURAL ISSUES

Chinese American Traditions and Mortality Rates

According to Chinese astrology and medicine, a person's fate is influenced by the year of his birth. Each birthyear is associated with one of five phases: fire, earth, metal, water, or wood. In turn, each phase is associated with an organ or symptom—for instance, fire with the heart and earth with lumps and tumors. So a person born in a fire year would be especially susceptible to heart disease.

Researchers at the University of California at San Diego have hypothesized that these beliefs might influence health (Phillips, Ruth, & Wagner, 1993). People who share these cultural beliefs and who contract diseases associated with the phases of their birthyears might feel hopeless and helpless—psychological states that have often been linked to illness and disease. Given this reasoning, people with heart disease who were born in fire years and people with cancer who were born in earth years should have lower average ages at death than those born in other years.

To verify this, researchers reviewed the deaths of 28,169 Chinese American adults and 412,632 randomly selected, matched controls coded as being "white" on their death certificates in California. The results showed that Chinese Americans, but not whites, died at earlier ages if they contracted diseases that Chinese medicine linked to their own birthyears. Moreover, the more strongly the Chinese Americans believed in Chinese traditions, the earlier they died. This association held for all causes of death. Chinese American females died sooner than their male counterparts. Phillips and his colleagues explained this gender gap by noting that the women were less exposed to Western influences and thus more likely to believe in Chinese medical traditions.

It's important to note the limitations of this study. Its correlational design makes it impossible to rule out other explanations of the early death rate among Chinese Americans. The researchers considered possible explanations—such as changes in the behavior of the Chinese American patients or their doctors—but concluded that other explanations could not completely account for the data. The researchers were left with the conclusion that their findings were due, at least in part, to some form of psychological influence. Although no definitive conclusion can be drawn, the findings are consistent with other evidence presented in this chapter that psychological factors can influence the development of illness and disease in some individuals.

Think about the following questions:

1. You may have heard about so-called voodoo death in some subcultures in countries like Haiti, in which a person is put under a spell by someone endowed with a special status and alleged mystical powers (like a witch doctor) and then dies. How feasible is the notion of voodoo death? How might beliefs in special powers and people contribute to death?

2. How might information that cultural traditions influence health affect the ways in which physicians treat their patients?

Uncontrolled diabetes can have a number of serious effects on health: a significantly increased risk of heart disease and stroke; blindness (the second-leading cause of blindness in the United States); susceptibility to infection, increasing the risk of gangrene (thus resulting in an amputation rate 20 times greater than in nondiabetics); and loss of sexual function in both men and women.

The body of the diabetic loses its capacity to produce or use the hormone **insulin.** Without insulin, the body cannot convert sugar, or glucose, into energy to store in cells. High levels of glucose collect instead in the bloodstream, serving as an ineffective energy source. In Type I diabetes—also known as insulin-dependent or juvenile-onset diabetes—the body lacks sufficient insulin because insulin-producing cells in the pancreas degenerate. Thus, the person with Type I diabetes depends on daily injections of the hormone. The onset of this disease is related to some form of infection, so Type I diabetes is currently viewed as a form of autoimmune disease.

Roughly 80 percent of all diabetics have the Type II form, which is characterized by a sufficient level of insulin that is metabolically ineffective. Type II diabetes typically occurs among adults and is closely associated with obesity. Figure 10.2

insulin *Hormone that converts glucose into energy to store in cells.*

FIGURE 10.2 Rates of diabetes and obesity among people of different sexes and races

Diabetes is closely correlated with obesity.

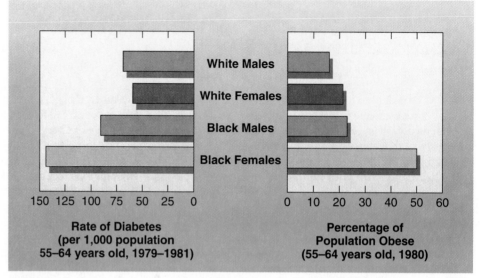

SOURCE: From "Closing the Gap," 1990. Office of Minority Health, USDHHS. Reprinted with permission.

shows the correlation between diabetes and obesity. Researchers speculate that the fat cells of people who are obese undermine the ability of insulin to regulate blood glucose. Obesity is most likely to lead to Type II diabetes in people with family histories of the disease. Weight reduction is an effective way for people who are genetically at risk for the disease to avoid getting it. Rates of Type II diabetes are significantly higher among black Americans (particularly women) than whites (see Figure 10.2). More blacks than whites die from diabetes, as well (Berg, 1991).

Diabetes and Stress Stress affects diabetes in two ways. As an indirect influence, stress affects how well people adhere to a behavioral treatment program (Fisher, Delamater, Bertelson, & Kirkley, 1982). For example, when under stress, diabetics may eat too much or eat the wrong foods. The other influence of stress on blood glucose is direct and mediated by the autonomic nervous system (Surwit, Ross, & Feingloss, 1991). In response to perceived stress, **cortisol** and the catecholamines are released into the bloodstream. They prompt the pancreas to release glycogen, which is then converted into glucose by the liver; they also block the release of insulin from the pancreas, which increases levels of circulating glucose still more.

In one study, Type II diabetics showed increased blood glucose in response to stressful imagery and the threat of electric shock (Goetsch, 1989). Increased blood glucose has also been found in Type I diabetics during the stress of a competitive video game (Cox, Goner-Frederick, Clarke, & Carter, 1988). A Swedish study of Type I diabetes in children found that stressful life events significantly increased the relative risk of developing the disease (Haggloff, Blom, Dahlquist, Lonnberg, & Sahlin, 1991). Clinical treatment studies provide additional evidence of a causal link between stress and blood glucose. Type II diabetics who were treated with progressive relaxation (discussed later in this chapter) showed reductions in blood glucose, probably as a function of lowered cortisol levels (Goetsch, 1989).

cortisol Hormone released by the adrenal gland in response to stimulation from the pituitary gland.

Focus on Critical Thinking

1. Research has shown that the death rate among Jewish people decreases by 31 percent just before Passover and then rises sharply by the same amount just after the holiday (Phillips & King, 1988). There are no corresponding patterns in death rates for people of other religious and ethnic groups. What psychological factors might explain this mortality pattern among Jewish people?

2. Recall the case of Paul, the company manager with a Type A behavior pattern (see p. 339). Do you or someone you know exhibit any of the behavioral characteristics he showed? Explain your answer.

*P*SYCHOLOGICAL *D*ETERMINANTS OF *H*EALTH-*P*ROMOTING AND *H*EALTH-*D*AMAGING *B*EHAVIORS

Adherence

Most of us know that we would be healthier if we exercised, reduced fat intake, refrained from smoking, avoided unprotected sex, and took medicine when our doctors prescribed it. But frequently, we don't follow this good advice. Our **adherence** to health-promoting behavior—or *compliance,* as it is often called—is poor.

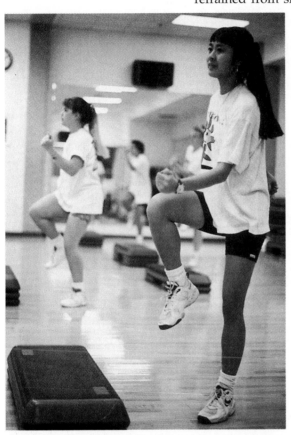

Studies have shown that only about half of all patients follow their doctors' advice (Ley, 1977). For instance, hypertension can be controlled by the appropriate use of medication. Yet 50 percent of patients fail to follow referral advice, over 50 percent drop out of care within 1 year, and only two-thirds of those remaining under care use enough medication to control their blood pressure adequately (Vetter, Ramsey, Luscher, Schrey, & Vetter, 1985). Similarly, diabetics frequently do not take their insulin as prescribed, and only 30 to 40 percent of people with epilepsy adhere to their medication schedules. Adherence is also poor among patients who survive heart attacks; half drop out of rehabilitative exercise programs within the following year (Meichenbaum & Turk, 1988).

Adherence to medical interventions may be linked to health in still another way. Simply *taking* medication faithfully seems to improve health—even if the medication is a placebo. In one study, patients who had survived heart attacks were given either medication (propranolol) to prevent another attack or a placebo. Unexpectedly, those patients who adhered to the medication were more likely to be alive at a 1-year follow-up than those patients who did not. What is of particular interest here, however, is that the same pattern was found among patients receiving the placebo. Patients with poor adherence had an increased risk of death, regardless of whether they received the active medication or placebo (Horwitz & Horwitz, 1993).

Do you exercise regularly? Physical activity is associated with positive health effects, including lower blood pressure and cholesterol levels.

The most obvious explanation of this result is *selection bias*—namely, that the poor adherers had more severe disease than the good adherers to begin with. But the same result was obtained even when the initial clinical severity of the patients was controlled. Horwitz and Horwitz (1993) explained this finding by suggesting that the act of adhering activates patient self-efficacy and related coping responses that lead to improved health outcomes. This result raises the possibility that adherence can enhance health in a number of ways—certainly beyond ensuring that individuals take their medication.

Obesity

adherence Extent to which a patient follows professional advice to take certain medications or change behavior patterns.

Americans seem to talk a lot about the need to exercise and maintain a healthy diet, but for many, that's as far as it goes—talk. The most recent data show that 1 in 3 American adults is overweight, which is a dramatic increase over past years. In fact, from 1960 through 1980, the number of overweight adults remained stable at about 1 in 4. That figure rose sharply between 1980 and 1991 to the present level (Kuczmarski, Flegal, Campbell, & Johnson, 1994). See Table 10.3, which presents more specific data on trends in weight among men and women and people of different races and ethnic groups.

TABLE 10.3	The Fattening of America (percent of population that is obese)				
	1962	**1974**	**1980**	**1991**	**Increase from 1980–1991**
Both sexes	24.4	24.9	25.4	33.3	31.1
Men	22.9	23.6	24.0	31.6	31.7
Women	25.6	25.9	26.5	35.0	32.1
White men	23.1	23.8	24.2	32.0	32.2
White women	23.5	24.0	24.4	33.5	37.3
Black men	22.2	24.3	25.7	31.5	22.6
Black women	41.7	42.9	44.3	49.6	12.0
White, non-Hispanic men			24.1	32.1	33.2
White, non-Hispanic women			23.9	32.4	35.6
Black, non-Hispanic men			25.6	31.5	23.1
Black, non-Hispanic women			44.1	49.5	12.2
Mexican American men			31.0	39.5	27.4
Mexican American women			41.4	47.9	15.7

By age group	20–34 years old	35–44 years old	45–54 years old	55–64 years old	65–74 years old	75 years and over
Men	22.2	35.3	35.6	40.1	42.9	26.4
Women	25.1	36.9	41.6	48.5	39.8	30.9

Source: Data from *The New York Times*, July 17, 1994, p. 18.

obesity Body weight 20 percent or more than a person's desirable weight.

abdominal obesity Pattern of obesity in which more body fat is carried above than below the waist; typically shown in men.

femoral obesity Pattern of obesity in which more fat is carried below than above the waist; typically shown by women.

Obesity is defined as being 20 percent or more above your desirable weight. That's about 25 pounds for an average woman (height 5′4″) and 30 pounds for an average man (height 5′10″). As shown in the table, in 1991, the groups with the highest proportions of overweight people were black non-Hispanic women (49.5 percent) and Mexican American women (47.9 percent).

This "fattening of America" is disturbing, considering the health consequences it causes. Obesity is linked to hypertension, diabetes, pulmonary and kidney problems, osteoarthritis, some types of cancer, and complications in recovery from surgery (NIH, 1992). Moreover, obesity is an independent risk factor for cardiovascular disease in men and women. A prospective study of 115,886 U.S. women between ages 30 and 55 showed that being even mildly to moderately overweight increased their risk of heart disease (Manson et al., 1990). More recent research has shown that obesity increases the risk of esophageal cancer in men (Raloff, 1995) and retards recovery from breast cancer in women (Bastarrachea, Hortobagyi, Smith, Kau, & Buzdar, 1994). Even modest weight loss has significant benefits for health, such as reduction in blood pressure (Wadden & VanItallie, 1992).

Interestingly, where on their bodies people carry their extra pounds affects the general risk of being overweight. Irrespective of overall obesity, people whose extra weight is stored mainly above the waist are at a significantly higher risk for disease and death than those whose extra pounds are stored predominantly below the waist (Greenwood, 1989). The pattern where fat storage is greater above than below the waist is called **abdominal obesity**. Obese men typically show this pattern—the so-called "beer belly." The pattern where fat storage is greater below than above the waist is known as **femoral obesity.** Women typically show this pattern. In more common terms, people with the abdominal pattern are sometimes called "apples" and those with the femoral pattern, "pears."

Causes   Obesity runs in families. Both twin and adoption studies have established a strong genetic predisposition toward obesity. Research has shown that identical

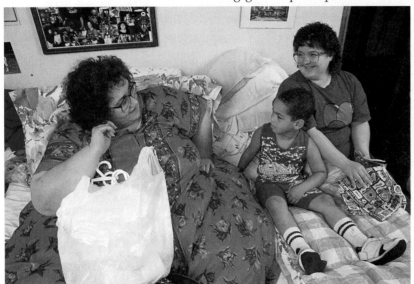

(monozygotic) twins have significantly greater concordance for being overweight than fraternal (dizygotic) twins (Stunkard, Harris, Pedersen, & McClearn, 1990). Similarly, adopted children are more likely to weigh the same as their biological parents than their adoptive parents (Stunkard, Foch, & Hrubec, 1986).

The **set-point theory** of body weight assumes that all individuals have a biologically programmed weight range. Whereas some individuals are naturally lean, others are naturally fat because of the biological settings in their bodies. Accordingly, our bodies defend particular weight ranges (Stallone & Stunkard, 1991). Most individuals of normal weight biologically resist significant weight loss or gain over the long term (Keys, Brozek, Henschel, Mickelsen, & Taylor, 1950; Sims et al., 1968).

Obesity runs in families. Some people have a genetic predisposition to become overweight.

The mechanisms responsible for this biological regulation of weight are still unknown. However, an individual's genetically determined metabolic rate is a determinant of body weight. Having a low metabolic rate puts an individual at risk for obesity (Ravussin et al., 1988). Once obesity has been established, it's maintained by several potent biological mechanisms, including the irreversible formation of fat cells (Bjorntorp, 1986) and an increase in metabolic efficiency (Shah & Jeffery, 1991).

As discussed in Chapter 4, obesity is related to socioeconomic status (SES), which describes a person's relative status in society as a function of income and education. To be specific, obesity is about six times more common among women of low SES than high SES (Goldblatt, Moore, & Stunkard, 1965). To reiterate, this correlation does not allow us to infer a causal relationship between obesity and social class. But we can attempt to explain what's behind this pattern.

Look at Figure 10.3 on page 346. Notice that the SES of origin—in other words, the status a woman was born into—is almost as strong a correlate of obesity as her own SES. This suggests that the influence of SES on obesity is stronger than the effect of obesity on SES (Stunkard, 1989). Since blacks have lower SES than whites, on average, this finding might help explain the greater rate of obesity among blacks. In addition to environmental influences, biological factors are also likely involved. Some data suggest that blacks might be more efficient in storing fat and expending energy (Kumanyika, 1987).

Treatment   Even though there's evidence of genetic and biological influences on obesity, this does not mean that psychological factors are insignificant or that obese individuals cannot lose weight. The most effective treatments for obesity consist of multiple components:

set-point theory Suggests that each individual has a biologically programmed weight range that the body defends against change.

- behavior modification to alter eating habits
- nutritional counseling to increase knowledge about diet and health
- self-control strategies to achieve lifestyle change
- cognitive restructuring to change unhealthy attitudes about body weight and shape
- increased physical exercise to promote fitness (Brownell & Wadden, 1992)

FIGURE 10.3 The relationship between obesity and socioeconomic status (SES)

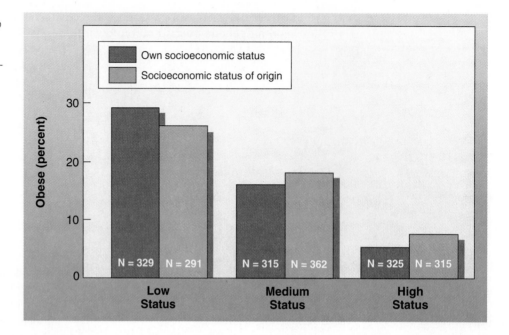

Treatments that include these elements help individuals achieve an average weight loss of 30 to 40 pounds over a 6-month period. Health benefits from such treatments include reductions in blood pressure and cholesterol level, decreased depression, and enhanced self-esteem.

Although dietary and behavioral weight-loss treatments are successful in the short term, they are ineffective in the long term (NIH, 1992; G. T. Wilson, 1993a). Roughly two-thirds of obese adult patients who lost weight during dietary and behavioral treatment had maintained their weight loss at a 1-year follow-up. However, 90 to 95 percent of these patients returned to their baseline weight after 5 years (Wadden, Sternberg, Letizia, Stunkard, & Foster, 1989). Relapse can be delayed for periods as long as 1 to 3 years (Ohno et al., 1991), but it cannot be denied. The reason for relapse is that patients eventually abandon the nutrition and behavioral strategies they learned in treatment. This occurs even with extended maintenance sessions designed to prevent relapse (G. T. Wilson, 1993a).

But there is some good news. Children who are obese can be treated effectively. In another study, 10 years after treatment, 34 percent of obese children had maintained some weight loss; 30 percent were no longer obese. These are the best results ever achieved in research on behavioral treatment of obesity (Epstein, Valoski, Wing, & McCurley, 1994). Note that the obese parents (who were treated in the same program as their children) showed the familiar pattern of initial weight loss followed by relapse. At a 5-year follow-up, virtually all the parents had returned to their baseline weights, and after 10 years, parents in all groups were even more overweight. These results underscore once again the problems that adults have in maintaining long-term weight loss.

Why do children succeed where adults fail? One reason is that it's easier to teach healthy eating and activity habits to children than to adults. A second possibility is that parents can exert external control—including social support and food management—on children and even adolescents living at home. Adults don't usually have that oversight. Obese adults who lose weight regain it because their self-control gradually falters.

AIDS

AIDS is a fatal, infectious disease for which there is no cure. It is now the second-leading cause of death among American men between ages 18 and 44 (Kelly, Mur-

Greg Louganis, a gold medal winner in diving in the 1992 Olympics, recently disclosed that he is HIV positive.

phy, Sikkema, & Kalichman, 1993). It's estimated that as many as 20 to 50 percent of gay men in cities such as San Francisco and New York have the HIV infection. The prevalence among intravenous (IV) drug abusers is similarly high. But AIDS is not confined to these two high-risk groups. Increasingly, it's spreading to heterosexuals and women—particularly those who live in the inner cities and already have high rates of other sexually transmitted diseases (O'Leary, Raffaelli, &

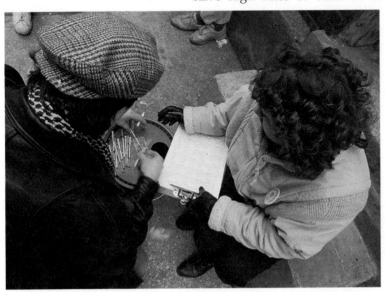

AIDS is transmitted by IV drug abusers' sharing needles to inject themselves. Needle exchange programs are used to try to prevent the spread of AIDS.

Allende-Ramos, in press). Heterosexual contact is the main source of transmission of AIDS in most developing countries (World Development Report, 1993).

Initially, the AIDS epidemic prompted significant behavioral changes in the gay male population. In New York City, for example, Martin (1987) interviewed a sample of 745 gay men, ages 20 to 65, to assess the impact of AIDS on their sexual behavior. Their sexual activity with different partners had declined by 78 percent; the frequency of sexual contacts involving the exchange of bodily fluids (blood and semen) had decreased an average of 70 percent; and condom use during anal intercourse had increased from 1.5 to 20 percent.

The success of efforts to change behavior among homosexual men is generally attributed to community-based activism. The gay communities in big cities such as New York City and San Francisco are stable and cohesive. In response to the AIDS epidemic, members educated themselves about the spread of the disease, devised instructional programs, and were able to spread this knowledge throughout the community. Social norms and support were enlisted to cope with despair, encourage safer sex, and reward individuals for making prudent lifestyle changes (Coates, 1993). The social learning principles of modeling and social reinforcement of behavior change are clearly illustrated in these programs. Education alone does not change behavior.

IV drug users are at risk for contracting HIV mainly because they share contaminated needles. Efforts to change the behavior of this high-risk group have been less successful (Des Jarlais, 1988). Most IV drug users know about AIDS and how it is transmitted. But they don't have the means for behavior change, including more effective treatment designed to stop drug use and sterile needles for safer injections. The psychosocial factors that facilitated behavior change by gay men are typically absent among IV drug users. Namely, they lack educational and financial resources, are caught up in illegal activities, and have little social support.

Even when IV drug users have increased the use of safer injections (for instance, sterilizing needles with bleach), they have not made similar changes in their sexual behavior. This lack of change puts their sexual partners at risk, too. Studies have found that introducing condoms is an obstacle to behavior change because their use is often associated with the breakup of heterosexual relationships. Condoms not only signal that one partner has the HIV infection but also raise concerns about sexual infidelity. The majority of IV drug users are heterosexual males, who may infect female partners, who may transmit the infection to their infants during pregnancy. Minority groups living in poor communities with widespread drug use are at particularly high risk for AIDS (O'Leary et al., in press).

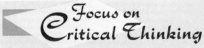

Focus on Critical Thinking

Imagine that you are a consultant to a national task force that is responsible for reversing the steadily increasing rate of obesity in the United States.

1. What advice would you give? Why?
2. What sort of public health policy should the United States adopt in order to control obesity and reduce its serious health consequences? Explain your answer.

PREVENTION AND TREATMENT OF HEALTH-DAMAGING BEHAVIORS

Clinicians have used a broad range of psychological approaches to prevent and treat stress-related medical conditions. The psychosomatic medicine of the 1940s and 1950s was a direct application of the psychodynamic model to medical conditions. It followed that some form of psychodynamic therapy was the treatment of choice. Despite the decline of the early psychosomatic medicine approach, psychodynamic therapies continue to be widely used. The basic assumption is that helping patients resolve unconscious psychological conflicts improves what are presumed to be associated conditions, such as diabetes, obesity, and so forth.

Pennebaker, Kiecolt-Glaser, and Glaser (1988) provided an intriguing example of how this psychotherapeutic approach might enhance health. College students were asked to write about the most traumatic experiences in their lives over four consecutive days. Consistent with the psychodynamic model, this expression of subjects' feelings was designed to relieve pent-up emotional conflict and reduce the psychological cost of inhibiting behavior. Researchers found that subjects who wrote about their experiences showed enhanced immune function and subsequently made fewer visits to the health center than subjects in a control group.

Cognitive-behavioral methods are frequently used to prevent and treat a variety of stress-related medical conditions. Among the most commonly employed are biofeedback and relaxation techniques. Let's look at each.

Biofeedback

Until the late 1960s, it was believed that physiological functions regulated by the autonomic nervous system—for example, heartrate and blood pressure—could be classically conditioned but not brought under direct instrumental or operant control. Then, in a series of dramatic studies, Miller (1969) reported how operant conditioning directly modified autonomic nervous system responses.

biofeedback Direct modification of physiological responses such as blood pressure by feedback that makes the person aware of the process.

The typical experiment to show this in rats involved spontaneous fluctuations in an autonomic response (such as heartrate) that can be shaped or followed by reinforcing consequences. Under these conditions, the rat learned to increase or decrease heartrate—a physiological function previously considered involuntary. In these experiments (Miller, 1969), the rat received an injection of curare (a drug that paralyzes the skeletal muscles) and was kept alive on artificial respiration. By paralyzing the rat's muscles, researchers were able to rule out alternative explanations of the observed changes in heartrate by the indirect effects of skeletal activity or altered respiratory patterns. The rats were rewarded by direct electrical stimulation of pleasure centers in the brain.

Subsequent studies failed to replicate these animal findings and raised questions about the reality of direct operant control of autonomic responses. Nonetheless, Miller's ground-breaking research led to the development of operant conditioning methods that could be used to modify a wide range of human physiological responses: skin temperature; heartrate speeding, slowing, and stabilizing; electrodermal activity; systolic and diastolic blood pressure; and peripheral vasomotor responses (Schwartz & Beatty, 1977). These methods became known as biofeedback.

Biofeedback is the direct modification of physiological responses such as blood pressure by feedback that makes the person aware of the process. Biofeedback equipment continuously monitors physiological responses and converts them into signals such as lights

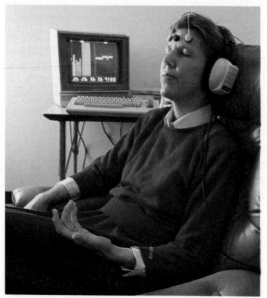

A patient receiving biofeedback treatment

or sounds that the person can easily perceive. Because it is more difficult to rule out explanations of results (such as changes in heartrate) in terms of indirect mediating influences (like breathing and other skeletal responses), it is unclear if autonomic responses in humans are modified directly. From a practical viewpoint, however, the specific mechanism of change is less important than the fact that different autonomic responses involved in medical disorders can, in fact, be changed.

The therapeutic use of biofeedback can be illustrated by one of its most common and successful applications: **tension headache.** Among the general population, 31 percent of males and 44 percent of females report severe headaches. A study of college students revealed that over 50 percent suffered from headaches at least once or twice a week (Andrasik, Holroyd, & Abell, 1979).

What causes tension headaches is unclear. They may result from sustained contraction of skeletal muscles of the face, scalp, neck, and shoulders in response to psychological stress. Biofeedback treatment involves auditory or visual feedback regarding muscle tension, called electromyographic (EMG) feedback. The typical procedure is to attach an electrode to the forehead and provide the patient with continuous visual or auditory information signaling a reduction in muscle tension. This electronic feedback is then phased out as progress is made. Experimental studies have shown that the effectiveness of EMG feedback is no greater than that of alternative psychological treatments, such as progressive relaxation training or cognitive coping strategies (Blanchard, 1992).

EMG biofeedback effectively reduces tension headaches, but its mechanism of action is still debated. The original explanation was that this feedback reduced the muscle tension that caused the headache. Yet the successful treatment of tension headaches is often unrelated to changes in forehead muscle tension. Biofeedback may work not because it directly changes physiological responsiveness, which was the original rationale of this form of treatment. Instead, it may work because it causes changes in cognitive mechanisms—such as self-efficacy for coping with stress—which then reduce headaches (Holroyd et al., 1984).

Relaxation Training

Progressive relaxation is the most widely used relaxation method in treating stress-related disorders. Adapted from a technique originally described by Jacobson (1938), it consists of teaching an individual to systematically tense and relax different muscle groups of the body. These tensing/relaxing procedures help the person learn to become especially attentive to her feelings of tension and to substitute for them feelings of relaxation. The typical brief method—taught in 4 to 10 sessions—emphasizes the suggestion of relaxation. (It therefore has a cognitive thrust.) In contrast, Jacobson's technique takes months, even years, to master and is exclusively somatic (physical), based on acquiring the skill of muscle relaxation. Progressive relaxation is used as an active coping skill, in which patients are taught to identify early warning signs of stress and to respond by using their relaxation skills.

Transcendental meditation (TM) is another form of relaxation training. Benson (1975) developed a simplified form of TM in which the person becomes comfortable in a quiet environment, assumes a passive attitude, and repeats a word or mantra (a special message or chant) with each exhaled breath. Benson called this simple method the *relaxation response,* and it has typically been used in behavioral medicine.

Progressive relaxation training has been used successfully to treat a remarkable range of different disorders, including some of the anxiety disorders (described in Chapter 5) as well as asthma, tension headaches, migraines, hypertension, Type A behavior pattern, chronic pain, and insomnia (Lehrer & Woolfolk, 1984; O'Leary & Wilson, 1987). Relaxation training has also helped ease the distress of people with cancer.

As many as 25 percent of cancer patients who undergo chemotherapy have conditioned aversive reactions to this treatment. That is, these individuals experi-

tension headache Painful contraction of skeletal muscles of the face, scalp, neck, and shoulders in response to psychological stress.

progressive relaxation Form of relaxation training widely used to treat different stress-related disorders; involves alternate tensing and relaxing of different muscle groups.

transcendental meditation (TM) Form of relaxation training in which the person adopts a passive attitude and focuses on a single object.

ence profound nausea and vomiting before drug administration, often in response to approaching the hospital, seeing the nurse who gives the injection, or even talking about their chemotherapy. Antiemetic drugs, which are used to control this anticipatory or conditioned nausea, are often ineffective. So consequently, psychological procedures have been used, including hypnosis and variations of relaxation training and guided imagery. Relaxation, as the primary component of these procedures, reliably reduces distress (Redd & Andrykowski, 1982).

Interventions for Multiple Risk Factors

Thus far, we have described how to treat individual risk factors for illnesses and disease. But it seems obvious that the most effective treatments—say, for reducing the occurrence of coronary heart disease—would involve targeting multiple risk factors at the same time. Moreover, for optimal effectiveness, these interventions should be aimed at the whole community, not just specific individuals.

One of the best known and most successful interventions of this kind is the Stanford Three-Community Study. In this pioneering work, researchers evaluated the effects of a broad intervention program for reducing the risk of coronary heart disease (CHD) in two small communities in northern California (Meyer, Nash, McAlister, Maccoby, & Farquhar, 1980). One community (Gilroy) received a media-based intervention. A second (Watsonville) received the media-based intervention supplemented by an intensive program of face-to-face instruction in behavior change for participants who were judged to be at high risk for CHD. A third community (Tracy) served as the control and thus received no intervention. The study involved a quasi-experimental design because constraints on selecting the communities meant that they could not be randomly assigned to experimental conditions. (See Chapter 4 for information on research designs.)

To evaluate the impact of the interventions, sample surveys gathered baseline and yearly follow-up data from a random sample of adults ages 35 to 59 in all three communities. Each survey included a behavioral interview and a medical examination of each subject. The behavioral interview assessed the subject's knowledge and self-reported change in risk factors; the medical examination included measures of plasma cholesterol and triglyceride concentrations, blood pressure, relative weight, and an electrocardiogram. Both behavioral and medical data were combined into a single risk factor estimate, based on one developed in the Framingham Heart Study (Dawber, Meadors, & Moore, 1951) that predicts a person's probability of developing CHD within the next 12 years.

The content of the intervention programs was based on social-cognitive theory and behavioral self-control principles such as self-monitoring, modeling, and reinforcement. Media campaigns were presented in both English and Spanish, using a variety of media materials. Over 2 years, about 3 hours of television programs and over 50 television commercials were produced, as well as about 100 radio spots, several hours of radio programming, weekly newspaper columns, and newspaper advertisements and stories. Printed materials of many kinds were sent via direct mail to participants, and posters were placed in buses, stores, and worksites. The face-to-face intensive instruction intervention—conducted with 107 high-risk individuals and their spouses in the Watsonville community—consisted of a 10-week program of weekly and then semimonthly sessions. The therapists who carried out this instruction were mainly college graduates who received 4 weeks of training in the counseling methods.

Results of the Stanford study showed that subjects in both intervention communities (Gilroy and Watsonville) gained a good deal of knowledge about risk factors for CHD. The media-based intervention in Gilroy also produced changes in individuals' self-reported consumption of cholesterol and fats. The intensive instruction plus media program in Watsonville achieved the best results after 3 years; the risk for CHD was lowered significantly, predominantly through reducing cigarette smoking (Meyer et al., 1980). Compared with the control community, the treated communities showed significant reductions in systolic blood pressure and dietary cholesterol. The Watsonville community also had significantly lowered plasma cholesterol.

The more recent Stanford Five-City Project was designed to replicate and extend the findings from the Three-Community Study (Farquhar et al., 1990). The Five-City Project included a longer intervention period (5 to 6 years versus 2 years), reached a more diverse population, and focused more intensively on using grass-root community organizations to promote healthy behavior. Two cities (Monterey and Salinas) received continual education about cardiovascular risk factors. The focus was on reducing cholesterol level, blood pressure, body weight, and cigarette smoking and on increasing physical activity. Educational efforts—based on the same social learning principles used in the previous study—included the use of television and radio, newspapers, direct mail, community meetings and workshops, and changes in school curricula. Three cities (Modesto, San Luis Obispo, and Santa Maria) received no intervention and served as controls.

The results of the Five-City Study confirmed the general success of the Three-Community Study in altering risk factors for heart disease. Residents of the two cities that received the communitywide education campaign showed greater reductions in plasma cholesterol, blood pressure, and rate of cigarette smoking than did residents of the control cities (Farquhar et al., 1990). Combined, these changes reduced the overall risk of heart disease by an impressive 16 percent. The effect on weight loss was negligible, however (Taylor et al., 1990), indicating once again how difficult it is to change this risk factor for disease.

The value of an intensive intervention program involving multiple risk factors was dramatically illustrated in a recent study by Haskell and his associates (1994). Three hundred men and women with coronary artery disease were randomly assigned to participate in a multiple risk factor reduction program or to receive usual care from their physicians. The reduction program consisted of training individuals to lower fat intake, lose weight, increase exercise, stop cigarette smoking, and reduce cholesterol through diet and medication. Over a 4-year period, the patients enjoyed highly significant improvements in all risk factors, with weight loss being the smallest (–4 percent). Patients receiving routine medical care, on the other hand, failed to show changes in risk factors. Compared with routine care, the risk factor reduction program greatly decreased the narrowing of coronary arteries due to atherosclerotic plaque buildup. The reduction program also reduced the number of hospitalizations due to heart problems.

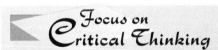

Focus on Critical Thinking

1. Raynaud's disease is a serious disorder in which bloodflow to the fingers and toes is restricted because of spasms in the peripheral blood vessels. Patients complain of pain and coldness. How could biofeedback be used to help these individuals? Explain your answer.

2. Both biofeedback and progressive relaxation training have been used to treat hypertension (high blood pressure). Explain how these treatments might help lower high blood pressure.

SUMMARY

A Historical Overview

■ As psychosomatic medicine developed in the 1940s and 1950s, psychoanalytic clinicians linked psychological factors to physical illness. Different medical disorders were seen as expressions of specific personality types.

■ In the 1970s, development of the fields of behavioral medicine and health psychology went beyond the psychoanalytic approach in emphasizing the use of behavioral science methods for assessing, preventing, and treating medical conditions.

■ Instead of the traditional biomedical model (with its limited emphasis on biology and disease), we now have a broader biopsychosocial perspective, emphasizing the interactive influences of psychological and biological factors in health and illness.

The Relationship between Mental Health and Physical Health

■ Serious emotional problems, such as anxiety or depression, increase people's risk of developing diseases and dying.

■ Individuals who are exposed to severe stress in their lives are, on average, less healthy than those who are not severely stressed.

Stress and Illness

■ According to the response model, stress is a complex physiological response that follows three predictable stages: alarm and mobilization reaction; resistance; and exhaustion.

■ The stimulus model defines stress in terms of stimuli, events, or environmental conditions that are assumed to influence all or most people in the same way. There are four kinds of stressors: acute stressors; stressor sequences triggered by particular events; chronic stressors; and chronic but intermittent stressors.

■ According to the biopsychosocial model, stress involves more than mere exposure to stressful life events, such as bereavement. It also includes how people cognitively appraise such events, what coping mechanisms they use, and how much social support they have. These factors all determine whether a specific life event elicits stress. Different people respond very differently to the same life stressors.

Psychological Effects on Biological Mechanisms

■ Psychological factors influence physical health in two major ways: by affecting basic biological mechanisms and functions that control illness and disease and by determining specific health-promoting and -damaging behaviors.

■ Psychological factors have a direct affect on health and illness by influencing the immune system, which protects the body against infection and disease. Psychological stress impairs immune function and enhances the risk for diseases such as cancer and AIDS.

■ Stress is directly linked to cardiovascular diseases such as hypertension and coronary heart disease (CHD). Blacks have higher rates of hypertension than whites. This difference has been attributed to the greater levels of chronic psychosocial stress that many blacks experience.

■ The Type A behavior pattern—characterized by aggressiveness, time urgency, and the need to control—has been linked to CHD. The evidence on this relationship, however, is inconsistent.

■ Stress can contribute to heart problems through two mechanisms: by accelerating the buildup of atherosclerotic plaque and by triggering a heart attack due to a rupture of the atherosclerotic plaque.

■ Psychological factors also influence metabolic diseases, such as diabetes. Direct influences include mediation of blood glucose by the autonomic nervous system; indirect influences include reduced adherence to behavioral treatment programs.

Psychological Determinants of Health-Promoting and Health-Damaging Behaviors

■ An important element in health-promoting behaviors is adherence, or the extent to which medical advice is followed (for instance, taking medication to control high blood pressure).

■ Obesity is defined as being 20 percent or more above an individual's desirable weight. It is a genetically predisposed, chronic disease linked to numerous medical problems and higher rates of mortality. Although obesity is resistant to change, individuals can reduce their weight and manage their condition in ways that either promote or damage health. It is easier to produce lasting weight loss in children than in adults.

■ AIDS is a fatal disease for which there is still no cure. The emphasis must be on prevention, namely, lifestyle change. Organized communities of gay men have made dramatic changes in adopting safer sex habits. Efforts to change the behavior of IV drug users have been less successful, however.

Prevention and Treatment of Health-Damaging Behaviors

■ Clinicians have used a broad range of different psychological methods to prevent and treat health-damaging behaviors: from individual therapy for specific problems (such as biofeedback for tension headaches) to community-based programs targeted at lifestyle change (changes in diet, physical exercise, cigarette smoking, and alcohol use).

KEY TERMS

abdominal obesity, **p. 344**
acquired immune
    deficiency syndrome
    (AIDS), **p. 336**
adherence, **p. 343**
adrenal gland, **p. 326**
angiography, **p. 339**
atherosclerosis, **p. 339**
autonomic reactivity, **p. 337**
behavioral medicine, **p. 323**
biofeedback, **p. 348**
catecholamines, **p. 326**
cognitive appraisal, **p. 329**
coronary heart disease
    (CHD), **p. 338**

corticosteroids, **p. 326**
cortisol, **p. 342**
diabetes, **p. 340**
endocrine system, **p. 326**
explanatory style, **p. 329**
femoral obesity, **p. 344**
health psychology, **p. 324**
hippocampus, **p. 326**
hypertension, **p. 337**
immune system, **p. 333**
insulin, **p. 341**
limbic system, **p. 326**
natural killer (NK) cells,
    p. 334

obesity, **p. 344**
progressive relaxation,
    p. 349
psychosomatic medicine,
    p. 323
risk factor, **p. 325**
set-point theory, **p. 345**
social support, **p. 331**
socioeconomic status (SES),
    p. 338
stress, **p. 326**
tension headache, **p. 349**
transcendental meditation,
    p. 349

CRITICAL THINKING EXERCISE

Recall from the chapter-opening case that Barbara Boggs Sigmund preferred to pray for recovery from cancer, rather than use psychological techniques such as imagery. She wrote that the "data base of success stories" of religious belief justified this faith (Sigmund, 1989). People of all religious faiths believe in the value of prayer or meditation. But can its effectiveness in treating disease or sickness be studied scientifically?

1. Do you think it's appropriate to try to study the effects of prayer on health? Why or why not?

2. Design a research study that would evaluate the effects of prayer on health or sickness.

Chapter 11
EATING DISORDERS

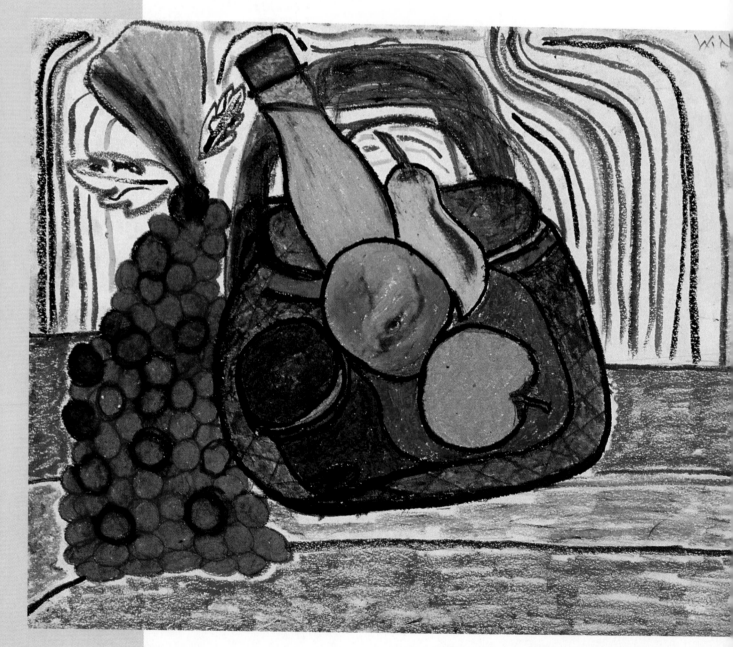

Wally C. Nicholson, **Untitled,** HAI

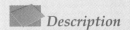 *Description*

Anorexia Nervosa

Bulimia Nervosa

Integrating Perspectives:
A Biopsychosocial Model

Binge-Eating Disorder

Thinking about
Controversial Issues

 Causes

Genetic Factors

Biological Factors

Dieting

Psychological Factors

Thinking about Social Issues

Social/Cultural Factors

Thinking about
Multicultural Issues

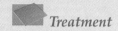 *Treatment*

Anorexia Nervosa

Bulimia Nervosa

Binge-Eating Disorder

Julie is an attractive 18-year-old college student. But she looks pale and tired. Her eyes are bloodshot; her cheeks, puffy. She has been crying recently and is close to tears again. She's just had her first session with a clinical psychologist at an eating disorders clinic, in which she described her problems.

Every day, Julie tries hard to restrict the amount of food she eats. She has rigid rules about when and what she can eat. She skips meals—especially breakfast—because she wants to eat no more than 1,000 calories a day. And she avoids a wide range of foods that she thinks are high in fat content, including cake, cookies, ice cream, pizza, and many others. In fact, Julie is preoccupied with food and its potential effect on her weight.

Although she severely restricts her eating, Julie ends up binge eating three or four days a week. The binges typically consist of the foods she tries to avoid and are characterized by a sense of lost control. Julie feels powerless to resist eating or to stop once she's started. Terrified of gaining weight, Julie vomits after each binge. She used to stick her finger down her throat to stimulate the gag reflex, but now she can simply bend over the toilet and throw up. Vomiting relieves her immediate anxiety about gaining weight. But it's a draining experience. What's more, Julie has begun to notice that she gets headaches after vomiting. And last week, she became very frightened when she saw some blood in her vomit. She feels scared, ashamed, and angry about losing control again. The cycle of binge eating and vomiting makes her hate herself.

Julie weighs 126 pounds, which is normal for a young woman of her height (5'4"). But she wants to lose the 10 pounds she gained during her freshman year in college. She wants to be thinner—the way she was as a cheerleader in high school. She weighs herself constantly. Her greatest fear is that she will keep gaining weight. She is especially self-conscious about her thighs and stomach. She freely admits that nothing is more important to her sense of well-being than having what she feels is an acceptable body weight and shape.

Julie's concerns about her eating and body weight have begun to interfere with her social life and personal relationships, too. She has become self-conscious about eating in public, which makes any social occasion difficult, including those with her friends or family. She thinks her mother knows that she has an eating problem. Visits home are tense because Julie increasingly senses that her mother is watching what she eats. Even her relationship with her boyfriend has been affected. Julie doesn't like him to touch her when she feels fat. His reassurances that she is physically attractive do little to ease her anxiety.

Julie has an eating disorder known as *bulimia nervosa.* It causes significant emotional and physical distress and is a chronic condition that is unlikely to go away without treatment. In this chapter, we discuss why today, young women like Julie are particularly vulnerable to this disorder. We also discuss how to assess bulimia nervosa and other eating disorders, according to several criteria. Finally, we look at how to treat eating disorders. There's good news about effective treatments for problems such as Julie's, but treating the more severe, life-threatening disorder of anorexia nervosa remains difficult.

$\mathcal{D}$ESCRIPTION

Eating disorders are characterized by severe disturbances in eating behavior, maladaptive and unhealthy efforts to control body weight, and abnormal attitudes about body weight and shape. The two most thoroughly studied eating disorders are anorexia nervosa and bulimia nervosa. Other disorders are closely related to these two but do not meet all the formal diagnostic criteria. The fourth edition of the *Diagnostic and Statistical Manual of Mental Disorders (DSM-IV)* (American Psychiatric Association, 1994) classifies these other disorders as **eating disorder not otherwise specified (EDNOS).** A large number of the patients seen in clinical practice receive this diagnosis (see Figure 11.1). However, the different variations of eating disorders included within this category are not well specified and have been relatively ignored in the clinical and research literature.

The single exception and perhaps most common example of disorders in this category is what the *DSM-IV* identifies as binge-eating disorder (BED). This disorder is characterized by recurrent binge eating but without the inappropriate weight-control behaviors that are part of bulimia nervosa. In this chapter, we will focus on three disorders: anorexia nervosa, bulimia nervosa, and binge-eating disorder.

You may be surprised to learn that obesity is *not* considered a psychiatric disorder or an eating disorder. Nonetheless, many mental health professionals lump obesity (or what is sometimes called a "weight disorder") together with the eating disorders. Doing so only serves to stigmatize people who are obese. Their condition is

eating disorder not otherwise specified (EDNOS) DSM-IV designation of disorders that are closely related to anorexia nervosa and bulimia nervosa but do not meet all the formal diagnostic criteria.

FIGURE 11.1 A schematic representation of the relationship among types of eating disorders

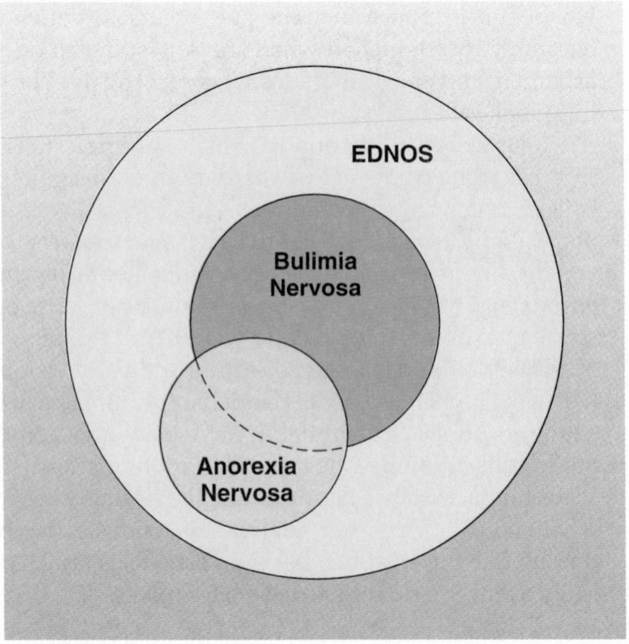

Source: From C. G. Fairburn and G. T. Wilson, "Binge Eating: Definition and Clarification," in *Binge Eating: Nature, Assessment, and Treatment* (pp. 3–14). Copyright © 1993 Guilford Publications, Inc. Reprinted by permission.

better viewed as a complex metabolic disorder, rather than as a behavioral problem (Garner & Wooley, 1991; G. T. Wilson, 1993a). Some obese people may develop eating disorders. A small fraction of patients with bulimia nervosa are obese. And still more obese patients engage in binge eating and receive the diagnosis of BED.

The best way to determine whether your weight is reasonable is to calculate your **body mass index (BMI).** BMI is calculated as follows:

$$BMI = \frac{\text{Weight (in kilograms)}}{\text{Height}^2 \text{ (in meters)}}$$

You can calculate your BMI easily:

1. Multiply your weight in pounds by 700.
2. Divide that number by your height in inches.
3. Divide that number once more by your height in inches.

Empirical research has shown that a BMI between 20 and 25 is optimal for health and long life. The ranges 18–20 and 25–27 are marginal areas that represent being slightly underweight and slightly overweight, respectively. People with BMIs in these areas run a slightly higher risk of having health problems. Individuals with BMIs of 30 or more are obese and at significant risk for health problems (Bray & Gray, 1988). And those with BMIs under 18 are significantly underweight. One of the diagnostic criteria for anorexia nervosa is a BMI of less than 17.5 (American Psychiatric Association, 1994).

Binge eating has two defining features. One is the consumption of amounts of food that are definitely larger than most people would eat during similar periods of time and under similar circumstances. The second feature is a sense of loss of control over eating—namely, the feeling that you cannot stop. People often describe an episode of binge eating as something like an altered state of consciousness, in which they "space out." One patient described it like this:

> It all starts with the way I feel when I wake up. If I am unhappy or someone has said something to upset me, I feel a strong urge to eat. When this urge comes, I feel hot and clammy. My mind goes blank, and I automatically move toward food. I eat really quickly, as if I'm afraid that by eating slowly I will have too much time to think about what I am doing. I eat standing up or walking around. I often eat watching television or reading a magazine. This is all to prevent me from thinking, because thinking would mean facing up to what I am doing. (Fairburn, 1995, p. 8)

body mass index (BMI) Value used to assess healthy and unhealthy body weights; calculated as weight in kilograms divided by height in meters.

binge eating Uncontrolled consumption of unusually large amounts of food.

anorexia nervosa Eating disorder characterized by serious weight loss (more than 15 percent of normal body weight) and distorted body image.

Anorexia Nervosa

Anorexia nervosa has been identified as a psychiatric disorder for more than a century (Gull, 1873). It's defined by a serious loss of weight and disturbed body image; the diagnostic criteria are listed in the *DSM-IV* table. In contrast to previous diagnostic schemes, the *DSM-IV* (American Psychiatric Association, 1994) divides anorexia nervosa into subtypes

DSM-IV   Diagnostic Criteria for 307.1 ANOREXIA NERVOSA

A. Refusal to maintain body weight at or above a minimally normal weight for age and height (e.g., weight loss leading to maintenance of body weight less than 85% of that expected; or failure to make expected weight gain during period of growth, leading to body weight less than 85% of that expected).

B. Intense fear of gaining weight or becoming fat, even though underweight.

C. Disturbance in the way in which one's body weight or shape is experienced, undue influence of body weight or shape on self-evaluation, or denial of the seriousness of the current low body weight.

D. In postmenarcheal females, amenorrhea, i.e., the absence of at least three consecutive menstrual cycles. (A woman is considered to have amenorrhea if her periods occur only following hormone, e.g., estrogen, administration.)

Specify Type

Restricting Type: during the current episode of Anorexia Nervosa, the person has regularly engaged in binge-eating or purging behavior (i.e., self-induced vomiting or the misuse of laxatives, diuretics, or enemas)

Binge-Eating/Purging Type: during the current episode of Anorexia Nervosa, the person has regularly engaged in binge-eating or purging behavior (i.e., self-induced vomiting or the misuse of laxatives, diuretics, or enemas)

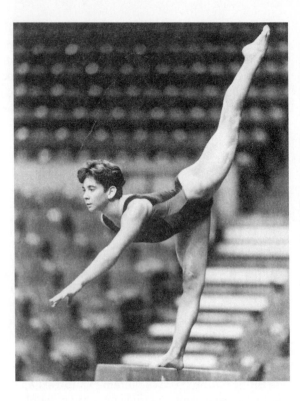

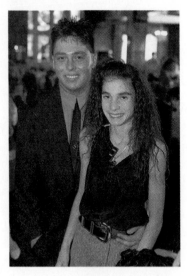

Left *Christy Henrich as a nationally ranked gymnast in the late 1980s* **Right** *Christy Henrich, with her fiancé, a year before she died of anorexia nervosa in 1994*

based on the nature of binge eating and purging. (**Purging** refers to self-induced vomiting or laxative misuse designed to influence body weight and shape.) Namely, there is a *binge-eating/purging type,* which involves regular episodes of binge eating or purging, and there is a *restricting type,* in which binge eating and purging do not occur regularly. The basis for this distinction is the evidence that, compared with the restricting group, those who regularly binge or purge tend to have stronger personal and family histories of obesity and higher rates of so-called impulsive behaviors, including stealing, drug misuse, deliberate self-harm, and moodiness (Garner, 1993).

The tragedy of anorexia nervosa is illustrated by the fate of world-class gymnast Christy Henrich. When she died of liver and kidney failure at the age of 22, the 4'10" Christy weighed 64 pounds. At one point, she had weighed as little as 47 pounds; a few years earlier, at the peak of her career, she had weighed 95 pounds. Christy had been in and out of hospitals for treatment; her medical bills totaled over $100,000. Before one hospitalization, her parents found that her suitcase had a false bottom, which she was hiding laxatives in. And in a treatment center, she had to be confined to a wheelchair to prevent her from running everywhere in a desperate effort to lose weight through excessive exercise (Noden, 1994).

Unfortunately, it's more common for patients to come to professional attention because of the concerns of family members over their extreme weight loss than it is for them to seek help themselves. Patients with anorexia nervosa actively resist change because they do not want to gain weight. Unless physical or psychological symptoms resulting from starvation cause sufficient distress, these patients cannot be persuaded that their intense fears of weight gain and dangerously low weights are unreasonable.

The two subtypes of anorexia nervosa have significantly different clinical characteristics. Individuals with the restricting subtype are highly controlled, rigid, and often obsessive. Those with the binge-eating/purging subtype alternate between periods of rigid control and impulsive behavior. Individuals in the second subtype

purging Self-induced vomiting or laxative misuse designed to control weight.

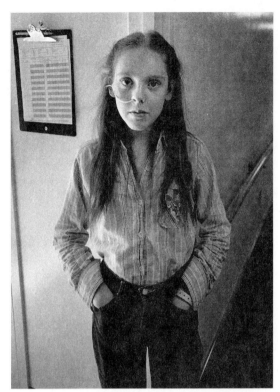

An adolescent girl with anorexia nervosa. Notice the loose-fitting shirt, which is often used to hide the extreme thinness that characterizes this disorder.

display significantly more psychopathology and are more likely to attempt suicide than those in the restrictive subtype (Hsu, 1990; Strober, 1995).

The prevalence of anorexia nervosa ranges from 0.2 to 0.8 percent (Hoek, 1993). The disorder typically develops in adolescence; evidence indicates that the average ages of onset are 14 and 18 (American Psychiatric Association, 1994). The course and outcome of the disorder are highly variable. Some individuals recover after a single episode. Others continue to fluctuate between restoring normal weight and relapsing. This fluctuating course is often marked by periods of hospitalization, which become necessary when an individual's weight sinks to a dangerously low level. Still other individuals gain weight but continue to experience bulimia nervosa or EDNOS. A significant minority never recover. Between 5 and 18 percent of individuals with anorexia nervosa die as a result of this disorder.

Associated Psychopathology   The most common form of psychopathology associated with anorexia nervosa is depression. Rates of co-occurrence range from 21 to 91 percent (Kaye, Weltzin, & Hsu, 1993). However, these findings must be interpreted cautiously because many of the symptoms associated with starvation closely resemble those of depression. One way to clarify this issue is to study patients who have gained weight after successful treatment for anorexia nervosa. To do so, researchers compared the rates of affective disorders between patients who were still symptomatic and those who had improved and no longer experienced symptoms for the year prior to assessment. It was found that the relationship between anorexia nervosa and affective disorders did extend beyond the secondary effects of starvation (Toner, Garfinkel, & Garner, 1988). (See Chapter 7 for more information on mood disorders.)

Anorexia nervosa also co-occurs with anxiety disorders (Halmi et al., 1991)—in particular, obsessive-compulsive disorder (OCD) (see Chapter 5). Obsessional tendencies in anorexia nervosa have been noticed by numerous observers. Specifically, obsessive behaviors have been reported to predate the development of anorexia nervosa and to exist after weight restoration, as well (Kaye et al., 1993). In their long-term follow-up study of patients with anorexia nervosa, Toner et al. (1988) reported that 26.7 percent of symptomatic anorexics, 38.5 percent of improved anorexics, and 36.8 percent of asymptomatic anorexics showed evidence of lifetime OCD.

Substance abuse is common in patients with anorexia nervosa. Rates of co-occurrence range from 6.7 to 23 percent (G. T. Wilson, 1993b). Levels of substance abuse are higher among individuals in the binge-eating/purging subtype compared with those in the restricting subtype. (See Chapter 9 for further discussion of substance-related disorders.) Personality disorders are also associated with anorexia nervosa. Rates range from 27 to 93 percent, depending on the particular study (Skodol et al., 1993). Anorexia nervosa appears to be most strongly associated with what's called the *cluster C personality,* which is avoidant, dependent, and obsessive-compulsive. (See Chapter 12 for more on this and other personality disorders.)

Medical Complications   Serious complications can emerge in anorexia nervosa as a result of starvation and malnutrition. Common physical signs include dry, sometimes yellowish skin and lanugo (fine, downy hair) on the trunk, face, and extremities. Individuals with anorexia nervosa are also sensitive to cold and experience a number of cardiovascular problems, including hypotension (chronically low blood pressure) and bradycardia (slow heartbeat) (Hsu, 1990). Self-induced vomiting may cause the salivary glands to become enlarged and dental enamel to erode. The most dangerous complications of anorexia nervosa are chronic dehydration and electrolyte imbalance, which are also due to excessive vomiting. In particular, depletion of serum potassium may lead to hypokalemia, increasing the risk of both renal (kidney) failure and cardiac arrhythmia (irregular heartbeat).

As many as 10 percent of individuals with anorexia nervosa die from medical complications such as these or from committing suicide (American Psychiatric Association, 1994). Christy Henrich, described earlier, was one such case. These potentially serious conditions make thorough medical assessment an essential part of treatment for anorexia nervosa.

Bulimia Nervosa

Recall the case of Julie, from the beginning of this chapter. Her symptoms illustrate **bulimia nervosa.** As described earlier, she rigidly tries to restrict her food intake, even skipping meals. But periodically, she loses control and binge eats. After these episodes, she purges to prevent weight gain—and so the cycle goes. Julie's problem is not that she eats too much; rather, she eats too little. Her rigid dieting and subsequent binge eating and purging are driven by an overconcern with the importance of body shape and weight. The diagnostic criteria for bulimia nervosa are listed in the *DSM-IV* table.

The real-life impact of having bulimia nervosa is illustrated by looking at the life of another world-class gymnast: Nadia Comaneci. She is the Romanian gymnast who, at the age of 15, captivated the world with her perfection in winning the gold medal at the 1976 Olympics. Within two years, she had grown 4 inches and gained 21 pounds. This signaled the beginning of her struggle with a weight and eating disorder. At age 28, she described herself as "fat and ugly," even though she was a size 6 (Noden, 1994). In a story on Nadia in *Life* magazine, Barbara Grizzuti Harrison described having dinner with the former gymnast:

> Her appetite for food is voracious. She eats her own food and [her companion] Constantin's too. After each course, she goes to the bathroom. She is gone for a long time. She comes back, her eyes watery, picks her teeth and eats some more. She eats mountains of raspberries and my creme brulee. She makes her way to the bathroom again. When she returns, she is wreathed in that rank sweet smell. (quoted in Noden, 1994, p. 56)

Happily, Nadia seems to have been able to deal with her eating disorder and a series of other problems that contributed to it. She has

bulimia nervosa Eating disorder characterized by binge eating, extreme methods of weight control, and abnormal attitudes about the importance of body weight and shape.

DSM-IV   Diagnostic Criteria for 307.51 BULIMIA NERVOSA

A. Recurrent episodes of binge eating. An episode of binge eating is characterized by both of the following:

(1) eating, in a discrete period of time (e.g., within any 2-hour period), an amount of food that is definitely larger than most people would eat during a similar period of time and under similar circumstances

(2) a sense of lack of control over eating during the episode (e.g., a feeling that one cannot stop eating or control what or how much one is eating)

B. Recurrent inappropriate compensatory behavior in order to prevent weight gain, such as self-induced vomiting; misuse of laxatives, diuretics, enemas, or other medications; fasting; or excessive exercise.

C. The binge eating and inappropriate compensatory behaviors both occur, on average, at least twice a week for 3 months.

D. Self-evaluation is unduly influenced by body shape and weight.

E. The disturbance does not occur exclusively during episodes of Anorexia Nervosa.

Specify Type

Purging Type: during the current episode of Bulimia Nervosa, the person has regularly engaged in self-induced vomiting or the misuse of laxatives, diuretics, or enemas

Nonpurging Type: during the current episode of Bulimia Nervosa, the person has used other inappropriate compensatory behaviors, such as fasting or excessive exercise, but has not regularly engaged in self-induced vomiting or the misuse of laxatives, diuretics, or enemas

Integrating Perspectives
A Biopsychosocial Model

PERSPECTIVE ON BULIMIA NERVOSA

BIOLOGICAL FACTORS

Biological factors contribute to the onset of eating disorders, but are not by themselves sufficient causes of such behavior:

➤ Family studies show that anorexia nervosa and bulimia nervosa are more common among biological relatives of patients with bulimia nervosa than in the general population. Twin studies indicate that this familial aggregation is due to genetic influences. The concordance rate is much higher for identical twins than for fraternal twins.

➤ Disturbances in both the noradrenergic and serotonergic systems have also been observed in anorexia nervosa and bulimia nervosa, although it is unclear whether these abnormalities are the cause or consequence of disordered eating.

PSYCHOLOGICAL FACTORS

Psychological factors interact with biological vulnerabilities in producing symptoms:

➤ Negative self-evaluation and low self-esteem result in an increased focus on the importance of body shape and weight.

➤ Abnormal attitudes about the importance of body shape and weight drive young women to rigid and unhealthy dieting.

➤ Patients with bulimia nervosa show a cognitive style marked by rigid rules and all-or-nothing thinking. This tendency to think in terms of extremes contributes to binge eating following a perceived transgression of a dietary rule.

➤ Women are more vulnerable to eating disorders than men because their self-images are more interpersonally oriented. Interpersonal success is closely linked to physical attractiveness, hence body weight and shape become critical determinants of self-acceptance and self-esteem.

SOCIAL FACTORS

Both biological and psychological factors operate in specific social contexts:

➤ Current cultural norms in the United States and other Western countries place great value on an ideal body shape that is biologically impossible for many women to attain.

➤ The desire to achieve the ideal body shape and weight drives women to unhealthy dieting. Dieting interacts with other psychological or biological vulnerabilities in a minority of women to produce bulimia nervosa.

➤ These cultural norms are shared most strongly by middle- and upper-class white women, among whom the rate of eating disorders is the highest. Black women are less likely to accept and internalize these norms, and they show correspondingly lower rates of eating disorders.

➤ Certain sports—such as gymnastics, dance, and track—that often equate body size with ability to succeed may create a higher prevalence of eating disorders.

These biological, psychological, and social factors interact to cause problems, as illustrated in the following case:

Lisa, a college sophomore, suffers from bulimia nervosa. Obsessed with her body weight and shape, Lisa constantly diets, works out in the gym nearly every day, and weighs herself several times each day. But almost daily she loses control of her eating, binges on the foods she denies herself, and then forces herself to vomit. She feels gross and shameful about her behavior and has increasingly withdrawn from social contact.

The biopsychosocial model explains Lisa's eating disorder. As a child, Lisa was slightly overweight. Most members of her father's side of the family were overweight, suggesting a genetic predisposition to gaining weight. Her younger sister is normal weight but has begun to vomit as a means of controlling her weight. Lisa's mother, who has a history of depression, is very concerned with her own weight and shape and with that of her daughters. In high school, Lisa lost weight. Athletic and good looking, she became a cheerleader. But when she went to college, she found it harder to control her weight. There was the pressure of studying and less time to exercise. She began to diet and binge. She learned about vomiting from a college friend who also had an eating disorder.

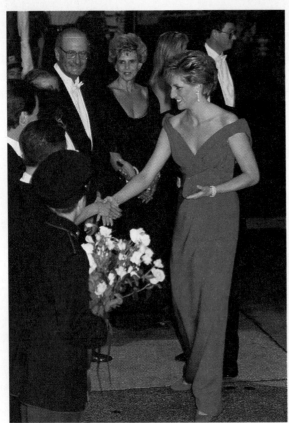

Diana, the Princess of Wales, has publicly disclosed her struggle with bulimia nervosa.

returned to professional competition and helps train young gymnasts.

In contrast to previous diagnostic systems, the *DSM-IV* (American Psychiatric Association, 1994) identifies two subtypes of bulimia nervosa: purging and nonpurging (see the table). Evidence suggests that the purging type is a more severe and chronic form of the disorder (Hay et al., 1995). Notice also that the *DSM-IV* specifies that a person with bulimia nervosa does not currently meet diagnostic criteria for anorexia nervosa. This specification restricts the diagnosis of bulimia nervosa to individuals who are of average or above-average weight.

The main reason for allowing the diagnosis of anorexia nervosa to override that of bulimia nervosa concerns therapeutic implications. In anorexia nervosa (but not bulimia nervosa), there is the need for weight gain. Furthermore, the therapeutic outlook is quite different. Bulimia nervosa can be effectively treated in the majority of cases, with good prospects for a full and lasting recovery (Fairburn et al., 1995). Again, that was the case with Nadia Comaneci. Anorexia nervosa, however, is more resistant to successful long-term treatment (Hsu, 1990), as illustrated by the case of Christy Henrich.

The eating behaviors of patients with bulimia nervosa have been studied directly under controlled laboratory conditions (Walsh, 1993). Patients were instructed either to overeat or to eat normally on different occasions. Their eating behaviors were then compared with those of control subjects (free of any eating disorders), who were tested under the same instructions. The results showed that patients with bulimia nervosa ate significantly larger amounts of food than normal control subjects when instructed to overeat. However, the bulimia nervosa patients did not differ from the normal controls in terms of the relative amounts of nutrients they consumed. In an average binge-eating episode, the bulimic patients got 47 percent of their calories from carbohydrates, whereas the controls got 46 percent. The comparable figures for fat calories were 40 percent for the bulimics and 39 percent for the controls (Walsh, 1993).

As is true of patients with anorexia nervosa, those with bulimia nervosa show a cognitive style marked by rigid rules and all-or-nothing thinking (Butow, Beumont, & Touyz, 1993). Patients view themselves in absolute terms—as being either completely in control or out of control, virtuous or indulgent. Likewise, food is either good or bad.

Bulimia nervosa usually begins in adolescence or early adulthood. Binge eating develops during or after a period of restrictive dieting, which is followed closely by purging (Hsu, 1990). The lifetime prevalence of bulimia nervosa ranges from 1 to 2 percent among adolescent and young adult women in the general population (Fairburn, Hay, & Welch, 1993). This prevalence rate reflects only those cases that meet the full diagnostic criteria. It does not provide a full picture of the extent of subclinical eating problems in the population.

Bulimia nervosa was originally described in 1979 by Gerald Russell in England. It is now widely accepted that bulimia nervosa emerged as a clinical disorder during the 1970s. This development can be seen by analyzing referrals to prominent centers in different countries that have been created to treat eating disorders (Fairburn, Hay, & Welch, 1993). In Toronto, Canada, for instance, the referral rate for anorexia nervosa was relatively stable between 1975 and 1986, but there was a noticeable increase in the referral rate for bulimia nervosa. The same trends occurred in Wellington, New Zealand (Hall & Hay, 1991), and in England (Lacey, 1992).

Associated Psychopathology Bulimia nervosa is strongly associated with other forms of psychopathology in clinical samples. It co-occurs so frequently with depression that some researchers have hypothesized that the two disorders share a common etiology. Therapy outcome studies, however, have shown that depression usually disappears following successful treatment of the eating disorder (Strober & Katz, 1987). This and other evidence suggests that depression is a consequence or correlate of bulimia nervosa, not a cause.

Anxiety disorders also frequently co-occur with bulimia nervosa. Schwalberg and colleagues (1992) examined 20 bulimia nervosa patients, 20 social phobics, and 20 individuals with panic disorder for comorbidity between eating and anxiety disorders. Seventy-five percent of the bulimia nervosa patients met the *DSM-III-R* (American Psychiatric Association, 1987) criteria for an additional diagnosis of one or more anxiety disorders. The most commonly diagnosed anxiety disorders in this population were generalized anxiety disorder and social phobia. Elevated levels of eating disorders among subjects with anxiety disorder were not found, which argues against a simple relationship between eating disorders and anxiety disorders (Schwalberg et al., 1992).

Substance abuse is associated with bulimia nervosa, as well. The lifetime prevalence rate of substance abuse in patients with bulimia nervosa ranges from 9 to 55 percent (Wilson, 1993b). This apparent relationship between the disorders might simply reflect an increased tendency for persons with more than one problem to find their way into treatment. However, Kendler et al. (1991)—in their examination of over 1,000 female twin pairs in Virginia—found that of the 123 subjects with bulimia nervosa, 15.5 percent had a lifetime diagnosis of alcoholism. These results indicate that bulimia nervosa and alcohol abuse co-occur even in the general population. Thus, earlier reports of co-occurrence are not simply the results of sample bias.

If eating disorders and substance abuse do co-occur, then there should be a higher than normal frequency of eating problems among individuals with substance abuse problems. This association has been found to hold true (G. T. Wilson, 1993b). The largest study, conducted in Japan, examined a sample of 3,592 patients who were admitted for alcohol abuse or dependence. Researchers found that 11 percent of the females and 0.2 percent of the males also had eating disorders—most commonly, bulimia nervosa (Higuchi, Suzuki, Yamada, Parrish, & Kono, 1993).

The similarities between eating and substance-related disorders is addressed further in Thinking about Controversial Issues. Can we become addicted to food?

Medical Complications   As with anorexia nervosa, the purging that is part of bulimia nervosa can produce serious negative health effects. Recall from the chapter-opening case that Julie had physical complaints, such as fatigue, headaches, and puffy cheeks. This puffiness is due to enlargement of the salivary glands, a result of repeated vomiting. The most serious medical complications are probably posed by electrolyte abnormalities, such as low potassium, which can disrupt heartrate and cause kidney failure. To force vomiting, some patients ingest ipecac, a drug that may lead to heart damage. Excessive laxative abuse entails the risks of becoming dependent on these medications and suffering severe constipation on withdrawal or even permanent damage to the colon. Given these possible effects, it's important that any individual who purges be medically screened and have blood tests to assess electrolyte status and fluid imbalances.

binge-eating disorder (BED) Eating disorder characterized by recurrent binge eating but not inappropriate weight-control behaviors.

Binge-Eating Disorder

Individuals with **binge-eating disorder (BED)** engage in recurrent binge eating but do not meet the criteria for bulimia nervosa. Binge-eating disorder is not an official disorder in the *DSM-IV* (American Psychiatric Association, 1994); the proposed diagnostic criteria are listed in the *DSM-IV* table. For example, individuals with

Thinking about CONTROVERSIAL ISSUES   Are Eating Disorders a Form of Addiction?

How many times have you heard someone say "I'm addicted to chocolate" or "I can't stop eating cookies, once I start"? Comments such as these encourage the view that eating can become an addiction. Actually, it's true that binge eating and bulimia nervosa share many similarities with alcohol and drug abuse. Common experiences among individuals with these problems include:

- the urge or craving to consume the substance
- a sense of lost self-control—the substance takes control of the individual
- use of the substance to cope with negative feelings or stress
- preoccupation with the substance and repeated attempts to stop consuming it
- denying the magnitude of the problem or attempting to keep it secret
- adverse psychological and social consequences because of the problem behavior

Many people experience both eating and alcohol or drug problems—sometimes simultaneously. Because of these similarities, certain forms of overeating and eating disorders have been viewed as types of chemical dependency or addictive behavior. Can we become addicted to food?

The answer to this question is important. If food is addictive, then the treatment used for other addictive behaviors (such as alcohol and drug abuse) may be effective in treating certain eating disorders. If food is not addictive, however, using traditional approaches to treating addictions may not be effective. In fact, they might even be harmful.

Use of the addiction approach to treating overeating is exemplified by the 12-step program Overeaters Anonymous (OA), which has been modeled after Alcoholics Anonymous (AA) (see Chapter 9). Among the assumptions of this approach are:

- that some individuals are biologically vulnerable to certain foods (such as sugar) that can cause chemical dependence
- that treatment is based on abstinence from these toxic foods (chemicals)

- that the eating problem is a progressive illness that can never be eliminated but only managed as a life-long problem

Despite the similarities between overeating and alcohol and drug abuse, there are important differences. Chemical dependency or addiction is distinguished by characteristics that include tolerance, physical dependence and withdrawal, craving, and loss of control over the substance. These characteristics do not seem to define eating disorders (G. T. Wilson, 1993b).

There is no scientific evidence that people with eating problems experience craving after eating particular nutrients. Moreover, studies have not shown that individuals with bulimia nervosa crave sugar or even prefer foods with simple sugars during overeating episodes. In laboratory studies, when the eating patterns of persons with eating disorders were compared with the eating patterns of normal persons, the types of foods selected from the major food groups (such as carbohydrates, proteins, and fats) were similar for both groups. The most striking difference found between the binge meals and regular (nonbinge) meals of people with bulimia nervosa was the amount of food they eat, not its nutrient composition (Walsh, 1993). The finding that patients with bulimia nervosa don't consume abnormally large amounts of carbohydrates during binges discredits the widespread myth that binge eating is caused by carbohydrate craving. Typical binge foods (desserts and snacks) tend to be sweet with high fat content. For example, do you know what percentage of the calories in Häagen-Dazs vanilla ice cream are from fat versus carbohydrate? (The answer is 57 percent fat and 36 percent carbohydrate.)

Think about the following question:

1. Julie, the young woman described in the chapter-opening case, severely restricts how much and what she eats. She claims that whenever she eats a sweet dessert, she can't stop eating and goes on to binge. She wonders whether she is addicted to sweets. Explain Julie's problem with sweets without relying on the addiction model.

BED do not regularly engage in purging (Marcus, 1993). The BED criteria do not specify any weight range; however, in contrast to findings about bulimia nervosa, preliminary data clearly indicate that BED occurs predominantly in individuals who are obese (Spitzer et al., 1992). Such individuals who binge are often referred to as "compulsive overeaters" in the clinical and popular literature.

DSM-IV   Proposed Diagnostic Criteria for BINGE-EATING DISORDER

A. Recurrent episodes of binge eating. An episode of binge eating is characterized by both of the following:

   (1) eating, in a discrete period of time (e.g., within any 2-hour period), an amount of food that is definitely larger than most people would eat in a similar period of time under similar circumstances

   (2) a sense of lack of control over eating during the episode (e.g., a feeling that one cannot stop eating or control what or how much one is eating)

B. The binge-eating episodes are associated with three (or more) of the following:

   (1) eating much more rapidly than normal

   (2) eating until feeling uncomfortably full

   (3) eating large amounts of food when not feeling physically hungry

   (4) eating alone because of being embarrassed by how much one is eating

   (5) feeling disgusted with oneself, depressed, or very guilty after overeating

C. Marked distress regarding binge eating is present.

D. The binge eating occurs, on average, at least 2 days a week for 6 months.

E. The binge eating is not associated with the regular use of inappropriate compensatory behaviors (e.g., purging, fasting, excessive exercise) and does not occur exclusively during the course of Anorexia Nervosa or Bulimia Nervosa.

Laboratory studies have shown that obese patients with BED consume significantly more food than obese nonbingers when instructed to binge or to eat normally (Yanovski et al., 1992). The two groups do not differ in terms of what they eat. For example, obese patients with BED do not consume more carbohydrates than obese nonbingers. In fact, compared with bulimia nervosa patients of normal weight, binge eaters who are obese diet much less. They typically consume a lot of food between binges (Yanovski & Sebring, 1994).

People with BED not only consume a lot of food but also report disorganized and even chaotic eating habits (Marcus, 1993). For example, an early morning breakfast might consist of pizza left over from the previous night's dinner, followed by a more conventional bowl of cereal. Dinner might begin with a piece of pie, followed by takeout from a fast-food restaurant and then more pie. This disorganization contributes significantly to the individual's sense of loss of control. What's more, eating many of these so-called meals turns into a binge.

Spitzer and his colleagues conducted two large multisite studies based on a self-report questionnaire (Spitzer et al., 1992). They reported a 30 percent rate of BED among obese patients who were seeking weight-control treatment and a 2 percent rate among community samples. In another study in England, Fairburn, Hay, and Welch (1993) examined a sample of 243 women from their community-based study. They found that 4.1 percent of the women reported having objective bulimic episodes (binges) once a week, on average, and 1.7 percent reported having such episodes twice a week. These researchers concluded that "binge eating, as defined in *DSM-IV*, does not appear to be a common behavior even among the group thought to be most at risk (i.e., young women)" (Fairburn, Hay, & Welch, 1993, p. 134).

One of the strengths of this English study was that the subjects were a representative sample from the population. Another advantage was that binge eating was assessed using a semistructured clinical interview—the Eating Disorder Examination (EDE) (Fairburn & Cooper, 1993)—which is the best available means of assessment. The data from the Fairburn, Hay, and Welch (1993) study also confirm earlier reports that recurrent binge eating (or BED) is more common among individuals who are obese.

The proposal to identify BED as a new diagnosis has been controversial. Critics contend that it's premature to single out this particular subgroup of EDNOS patients. As more research is conducted, more useful or valid ways of classifying different subgroups of individuals with recurrent binge eating might emerge (Fairburn, Jones, Peveler, Hope, & O'Connor, 1993). In addition, critics find fault with the two main studies on which the case for including BED as a new diagnosis were based (Spitzer et al., 1992; Spitzer et al., 1993). That is, both studies used self-report questionnaires, which could have yielded unreliable estimates of binge eating.

In response to critics, Spitzer et al. (1993) suggest that more attention needs to be devoted to specifying the nature of EDNOS. They contend, however, that working out the diagnosis of BED is an important step in this direction.

Focus on Critical Thinking

1. As you've read about the eating disorders, have you been reminded of anyone you know? If so, what symptoms did that person have? Would he or she have met any of the diagnoses described here? Explain your answer.

2. Self-induced vomiting is the most common way of purging food by individuals with eating disorders. What about vomiting causes these individuals to continue such behavior?

Associated Psychopathology Obese individuals who binge show significantly greater levels of psychopathology than obese nonbingers (de Zwaan et al., 1994). For example, Schwalberg et al. (1992) found a 60 percent lifetime prevalence of affective disorder and a 70 percent lifetime rate of anxiety disorders in their sample of obese binge eaters. Unlike bulimia nervosa, however, BED does not seem to be significantly associated with alcohol abuse (G. T. Wilson, 1993b).

CAUSES

Biological, psychological, and social factors combine to cause eating disorders. As with the other clinical disorders we've looked at throughout this book, a biopsychosocial model is required to understand how these problems are caused and maintained.

Genetic Factors

Family studies show that anorexia nervosa and bulimia nervosa are more common among biological relatives of patients with eating disorders than among the general population (Strober, 1995). Twin studies indicate that this **familial transmission** is due to genetic influences. For example, Holland, Sicotte, and Treasure (1988) found that the concordance rate for anorexia nervosa in identical twins was 55 percent compared with only 7 percent in fraternal twins.

Strober (1995) has hypothesized that the genetic predisposition in anorexia nervosa may be expressed through certain types of personality structures. Research and clinical observations have revealed that certain personality traits seem to cluster in patients with anorexia nervosa, including obsessional tendencies, rigidity, emotional restraint, preference for the familiar, and poor adaptability to change. According to Strober, individuals with these anorexic personality traits are at a disadvantage when dealing with the issues typical of adolescence and puberty. The disorder that results is seen as a maladaptive way of coping with the conflict between adolescence and the individual's need for order and predictability.

Recent twin studies similarly suggest a hereditary influence in bulimia nervosa. In a well-controlled study of 1,033 female twin pairs, Walters et al. (1992) found a significantly higher concordance for identical versus fraternal twins. This finding suggests that genetics help determine who develops eating disorders.

Biological Factors

Changes in eating behavior can have significant effects on how the nervous system works. This poses a problem for researchers examining the biological bases of eating disorders. Do the biological abnormalities seen in patients with eating disorders result from or cause their disturbed eating behaviors?

Individuals with bulimia nervosa exhibit abnormalities in the function of **serotonin,** a neurotransmitter in the brain that plays a key role in regulating mood and

familial transmission
Pattern in which a disorder occurs at a higher than expected rate among family members.

serotonin Neurotransmitter that plays a key role in regulating mood and eating behavior.

eating behaviors. How serotonin regulates feelings of hunger and fullness or satisfaction has led researchers to hypothesize that binge eating is influenced by abnormally low serotonin function (Kaye & Weltzin, 1991). The available evidence is mixed. A number of studies support the hypothesis that people with bulimia nervosa have decreased serotonin activity (Jimerson, Lesem, Kaye, Hegg, & Brewerton, 1990). But other studies have found no significant difference in serotonin levels between individuals with bulimia nervosa and controls (Jimerson, Lesem, Kaye, & Brewerton, 1992).

Family History of Psychopathology   As we noted in the section on genetic influences, the familial transmission of anorexia nervosa and bulimia nervosa is well documented (Strober, 1995). Evidence from clinical samples of patients has suggested that a family history of depression or substance abuse is a risk factor for bulimia nervosa. Parental alcohol or drug abuse has also emerged as a specific risk factor in a community-based sample of women with bulimia nervosa (Fairburn, 1994). This conclusion has been strengthened by Strober's (1995) data comparing relatives of patients with bulimia nervosa or the binge-eating/purging subtype of anorexia nervosa with relatives of both normal controls and the restricting subtype. Relatives of the former group of patients had a three- to fourfold increase in their lifetime risk of acquiring substance-related disorders.

Personal and Family Weight History   A history of being overweight and parental obesity are both specific risk factors for bulimia nervosa that pose sizable attributable risks (Fairburn, 1994). **Attributable risk** is the proportion of cases in the population that are due to the risk factor. In this case, 10 percent of individuals with bulimia nervosa have this sort of personal and family weight history. Moreover, the greater the severity of the obesity, the stronger the risk factor.

The significance of this association is strengthened by two additional findings. The first is that the only two predictors of outcome from a 6-year follow-up of the psychological treatment of bulimia nervosa were the patients' own and parental obesity (Fairburn et al., 1995). The second finding is that a 10-year follow-up of the behavioral treatment of childhood obesity (children between the ages of 6 and 12) noted what seems to be an unusually high rate of occurrence of bulimia nervosa: 6 percent in girls (Epstein, Klein, & Wisniewski, 1994; Wilson, 1994). A likely explanation of this finding is that a tendency toward being overweight makes it more difficult for women to achieve or maintain the thinness that is culturally valued. They are therefore driven to take more extreme weight-control measures (such as rigid dieting), which puts them at greater risk for bulimia nervosa, as we discuss next.

Dieting

Dieting is closely linked to the onset and maintenance of eating disorders. Clinical reports indicate that virtually all patients with these disorders have histories of dieting prior to the onset of binge eating (Pyle et al., 1990). Two studies verify this link. One consisted of a representative sample of 15-year-old schoolgirls in London. Compared with nondieters, dieters were significantly at risk for developing eating disorders within 1 year. Only a small portion of the girls who were dieting at the beginning of the study (21 percent) subsequently were diagnosed as having eating disorders. However, dieters were eight times more likely than nondieters to develop eating disorders (Patton, Johnson-Sabine, Wood, Mann, & Wakeling, 1990). The second prospective study was an analysis of more than 1,000 female twins located through the Virginia Twin Registry. Self-reported weight fluctuation and current dieting status predicted the diagnosis of bulimia nervosa during interviews conducted 1 to 3 years later (Kendler et al., 1991).

attributable risk Proportion of cases in the population that are due to a particular risk factor.

Dieting has various biological, cognitive, and affective consequences that may predispose persons to binge eating. Among the biological effects, short-term dieting in normal female subjects has produced evidence of reduced serotonin function in the brain (Cowen, Anderson, & Fairburn, 1992). Disturbances in levels of serotonin in the brain have been linked to eating disorders, as noted earlier in this chapter.

Dieting also has a number of cognitive effects. Many dieters have unrealistically rigid standards of their control over food intake. On a cognitive level, this leaves them with feelings of deprivation. Under these strict conditions, dieters are vulnerable to loss of control if they break their diets. And dietary lapses lead to all-or-nothing cognitive reactions. According to this phenomenon—called the **abstinence violation effect**—individuals attribute their lapses to a complete inability to maintain control. Thus, they abandon all attempts to regulate food intake and overeat.

It's now widely accepted that dieting plays a significant role in the development of eating disorders. Some clinicians have gone so far as to suggest that we should refer to *dieting* disorders, rather than *eating* disorders (Beumont, Garner, & Touyz, 1994). But dieting is not a sufficient cause of eating disorders. A majority of young women in North America diet in order to influence body weight and shape. Yet only a small minority develop eating disorders. Dieting is certainly a risk factor but a relatively weak one. Clearly, it must interact with other biological or psychological vulnerabilities in precipitating an eating disorder. Nor is dieting a necessary causal condition for development of an eating disorder. Data show that the disorder can develop in the absence of dieting (Fairburn, 1994).

The role of dieting among obese individuals with BED is unclear. In contrast to individuals with bulimia nervosa, binge eating often precedes dieting in individuals with BED (Berkowitz, Stunkard, & Stallings, in press). Obese binge eaters show significantly less dietary restraint than people with bulimia nervosa (Marcus, 1993). Yanovski and Sebring (1994) found that obese binge eaters reported greater average food intake than nonbingers on both total caloric (2,707 versus 1,869 kcal/day) and weight-adjusted bases. What's more, obese individuals with BED had higher intake on nonbinge days, which strongly contrasts the pattern among individuals with bulimia nervosa.

Psychological Factors

A variety of personal and familial factors have been suggested as causes of eating disorders, but until recently, none has received much empirical support. Speculation about etiological factors has been based mainly on clinical samples. This is an important limitation, because as we have emphasized throughout this book, patients seeking treatment may not be representative of the majority of people with a given disorder.

Recent research from Oxford University in England has remedied this and other methodological deficiencies in the study of what causes bulimia nervosa (Fairburn, 1994). Using a **case-control design,** investigators recruited a representative, community-based sample of 102 people with bulimia nervosa. Each of these individuals was matched with a normal control and a psychiatric control subject. This psychiatric control group—comprised mainly of cases of depression—was needed to identify risk factors that are specific to the eating disorder and not to psychopathology in general.

The Oxford study (Fairburn, 1994) revealed that roughly 75 percent of the sample had never received treatment for bulimia nervosa. This finding underscores the importance of basing etiological analyses on community-based, rather than clinical, samples. Research that is based on individuals who seek treatment clearly represents only a small subset of the population with eating disorders. Another distinguishing feature of this well-designed study was the use of state-of-the-art

abstinence violation effect Occurs when someone on a strict diet breaks a dietary rule; she attributes the lapse to a complete inability to maintain control, abandons all attempts to regulate food intake, and overeats.

case-control design Experimental design in which a person with an identified clinical disorder is matched with a control subject of the same sex, age, and socioeconomic status.

clinical interviews for screening and assessing the prevalence of bulimia nervosa and its possible risk factors.

Several important findings have emerged from this research. It is popularly believed that early sexual abuse is a cause of bulimia nervosa, although empirical support for this belief has been lacking. The Oxford study found that childhood sexual abuse occurred more frequently in both the bulimia nervosa and psychiatric control subjects than in the normal controls. In other words, childhood sexual abuse is a *general* risk factor for psychopathology but not a *specific* risk factor for bulimia nervosa. Negative self-evaluation, perfectionism, and shyness were identified as specific risk factors with attributable risks of 11, 13, and 15 percent, respectively.

The Stress of Adolescence   Both anorexia nervosa and bulimia nervosa typically develop among girls during adolescence. Why might this be a period of heightened risk for young women?

The answer seems to be that adolescence is a period during which females have lower self-esteem and are more vulnerable to affective disturbance than males. Postpubertal changes in body weight and shape are more stressful for females than males. In contrast to males, the self-images of female adolescents are more interpersonally oriented. Adolescent girls are also more concerned with their appearance and their relationships with others. Consequently, for females far more than males, any emotional problem is likely to involve body image and attempts to influence it.

The Role of the Family   Families of daughters with anorexia nervosa have been portrayed as being concerned with external appearances. They are said to be anxious to maintain a show of harmony and solidarity at the expense of open communication and expression of negative feelings. And they supposedly often speak for one another, as if they could read each other's minds (Bruch, 1978). Although this family systems approach has had considerable clinical appeal, there is little empirical support for it.

In an early observational study, Minuchin, Rosman, and Baker (1978) identified the following characteristic patterns of interaction in families of adolescents with anorexia nervosa:

1. Enmeshment characterizes families where members are overinvolved with one another and personal boundaries are easily crossed.
2. Overprotectiveness hinders children's development of autonomous functioning.
3. Rigidity causes families to feel threatened by changes that come with puberty and adolescence in their daughters.
4. Conflict avoidance and poor conflict resolution hinder effective communication.

Minuchin and colleagues (1978) portrayed the daughter with anorexia nervosa as a regulator in the family system. She is overinvolved in parental conflict in one of two ways: as the object of diverted conflict or after being drawn into coalition with one parent against the other.

A study that attempted to operationalize these patterns found high levels of enmeshment in families of both anorexia nervosa and bulimia nervosa patients, but evidence for the other patterns was weak (Kog, Vandereycken, & Vertommen, 1985). Further research, based on coding videotaped family discussions, has shown systematic differences between the families of individuals with eating disorders and controls (Humphrey, 1989). In comparison with the controls, the eating disorder families revealed more criticism and contradictory communication and less trusting, helping, and nurturing.

Thinking about SOCIAL ISSUES   Why Are Eating Disorders Mainly Confined to Women?

At the sociocultural level, it's clear that physical attractiveness is more important for women than men. This societal double-standard has been demonstrated in numerous studies (Rodin, 1993). The cultural pressure to be thin influences the developmental psychology of women. Ruth Striegel-Moore (1993) has argued that two aspects of the contemporary female gender-role stereotype have particular relevance to women's risk for eating disorders.

First, beauty is a central aspect of femininity. Girls learn early in life that being pretty is what draws attention and praise from others. Consider how often girls in books and on television focus on their appearance while boys are playing and doing. As early as fourth grade, body build and self-esteem are positively correlated for girls but not for boys (Striegel-Moore, Silberstein, & Rodin, 1986).

A second aspect is women's interpersonal orientation. Theorists about the psychology of women argue that self-worth is closely tied to establishing and maintaining close relationships (Gilligan, 1978). Thus, women's self-concepts are interpersonally constructed. In comparison to boys, girls' self-descriptions at age 7 have been found to be more based on the perceptions of others (Striegel-Moore et al., 1986). Consequently, women are said to derive significant self-worth from other's opinions and approval of them. And in U.S. culture, social approval is significantly related to physical attractiveness. Research has consistently shown a significant correlation between self-esteem and feelings about one's body—especially in women, whose self-esteem is significantly related to how they are evaluated by others (Hsu, 1990). Even lesbians—who generally take a more critical stance toward sociocultural norms regarding women and female gender-role stereotypes—are not significantly different from heterosexual women in their attitudes about weight. In one study, self-esteem was strongly related to feelings about one's body, and the prevalence of bulimia nervosa among lesbians was similar to that among heterosexual women (Heffernan, 1994).

The ideal standard of physical attractiveness has become thinner over the past few decades. This trend has made it harder for women to meet the standard, so they resort to such extreme methods of weight control as rigid dieting and purging. Some men also diet to lose weight and achieve leaner bodies. Examples include jockeys and wrestlers (Brownell & Rodin, 1992). Both groups report some features of eating disorders when their sport is in season, but these features disappear during the off-season (King & Mezey, 1987).

There is a crucial difference between these male athletes and women, however: The men want to lose weight to improve their athletic performance. Their concern with body weight is secondary to their goal of performing well. For women, dieting to achieve an ideal weight has more profound psychological meaning. Namely, it's related to their self-identity and self-evaluation. Consistent with this explanation are several clinical reports that among men, gays are most likely to develop eating disorders (Heffernan, 1994).

Biological factors might also help explain the gender gap. Women not only diet more than men but might also suffer more serious effects of dieting than men. Studies of dieting in normal, healthy male and female college students showed a differential effect on brain serotonin function. The women showed reduced serotonin activity, whereas the men were unaffected (Cowen et al., 1992).

Think about the following questions:

1. In comparison to heterosexual males, why might gay men be more likely to develop eating disorders?
2. In recent years, women have become more independent and strived to attain sexual and social equality with men. At the same time, women appear to have become more vulnerable to eating disorders. Is there any connection between these trends? Explain your answer.

The problem in interpreting these findings is a familiar one in correlational research of this kind. That is, the disturbed relationship is identified only after an eating disorder has become serious and treatment has been sought. So again, we ask the question: Are these family characteristics the cause or consequence of the eating disorder? In the absence of controlled, prospective studies, this question cannot be answered.

A family focus on the importance of body shape and weight may also contribute to the development of eating disorders. Teen-age girls whose mothers were

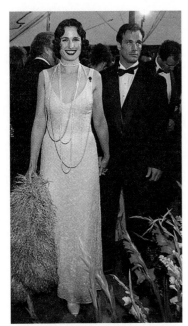

Andie MacDowell, former super-model and star of movies such as Four Weddings and a Funeral, *has confessed to using diet pills and cocaine to lose weight.*

critical of their weight reported higher rates of disordered eating than girls whose mothers were more accepting of their appearance (Pike & Rodin, 1991). The Oxford epidemiological study showed that family dieting and critical comments by parents of their daughters' weight or eating were specific risk factors for bulimia nervosa (Fairburn, 1994). This study also revealed that a number of more general aspects of parenting were surprisingly specific risk factors, including frequent parental absence, underinvolvement, high expectations, criticism, and discord between parents.

Social/Cultural Factors

We cannot explain the causes of eating disorders without understanding the social forces women experience. (A number of these forces are addressed in Thinking about Social Issues.) In sum, the current cultural context defines the ideal female body shape as thin and lithe. This trend started with the model Twiggy at the end of the 1960s, coinciding roughly with the emergence of bulimia nervosa. Before that time, the ideal female shape had more body fat, wider hips, and more curves.

Evidence of the increasing preference for thinness may be observed in the declining average weights of *Playboy* centerfolds (see Figure 11.2) and Miss America contestants from the late 1950s to the late 1970s (Garner, Garfinkel, Schwartz, & Thompson, 1980). Notice that the average weight of women in the general population under 30 years old actually *increased* by 5 pounds over the same 20-year period. This clash between biological reality and psychosocial pressure is the key to understanding eating disorders.

Studies have consistently shown that a majority of young women in the United States are dissatisfied with their body shapes and weights. And most consider themselves overweight, even though many are statistically at normal or below-normal

Left *Marilyn Monroe, the sex symbol of the 1950s, would not conform to today's norms of the perfect female body.* **Right** *Twiggy, the British model of the late 1960s, helped create Western society's emphasis on thinness in the ideal female body. What factors influenced this shift in ideals?*

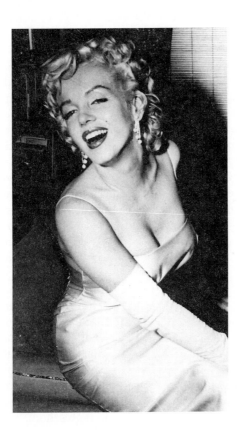

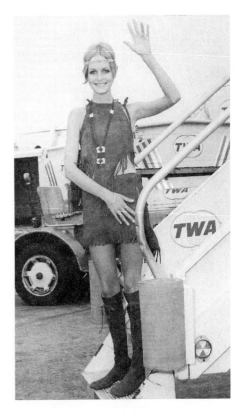

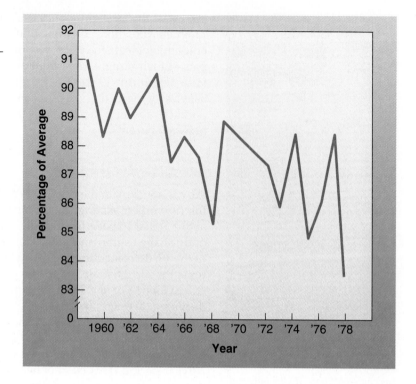

Source: Reprinted with permission from the authors and publisher from: D. M. Garner, P. E. Garfinkel, D. Schwartz, and M. Thompson, "Cultural Expectations of Thinness in Women," *Psychological Reports*, 1980, *47*, 483–491. © Psychological Reports 1980.

FIGURE 11.2 Weight changes of *Playboy* centerfolds: 1960–1978

The average weight of a *Playboy* centerfold decreased to the point that in 1978, she weighed only 83 percent of the weight of an average woman.

weights (Rodin, 1993). Judy Rodin and her colleagues (1985) coined the term *normative discontent* to describe women's pervasive dissatisfaction with their bodies. To try to improve their looks, women diet. Over 60 percent of adolescent females in the United States diet (Rosen & Gross, 1987). In a minority of women who have additional biological or psychological vulnerabilities, dieting causes eating disorders.

Being thin is particularly important among white, middle- and upper-class women. Obesity is strongly and inversely correlated with socioeconomic status, and the desire to be thin is positively correlated with socioeconomic status for women but not men. White adolescent girls from higher-income families become leaner during adolescence than black females and their peers from lower-income families, presumably because they deliberately restrict food intake. Eating disorders are most common among the very population that is most concerned with dieting to achieve thinness: white, upper-socioeconomic-level females.

Overall, there is a positive correlation between the cultural pressure to be thin and the prevalence of eating disorders both across and within different ethnic groups (Hsu, 1990). The link between ethnic identity and eating disorders is looked at more closely in Thinking about Multicultural Issues.

Eating disorders also occur more frequently among individuals in specific occupations and activities that place pressure on females to be thin—for instance, modeling and ballet dancing. The same pressure can be seen in sports that demand that women be thin, such as gymnastics and cheerleading. Cheerleaders and majorettes must often attain unrealistically low weight goals in order to participate in sporting events (Humphries & Gruber, 1986). Remember from the case at the beginning of the chapter that Julie had been a cheerleader in high school.

Focus on *Critical Thinking*

1. Jane and Sarah are both 18-year-old ballet dancers. After doing well in a national competition, Jane has been accepted into an elite ballet school in New York City. Sarah continues to take lessons in her hometown. All things being equal, which of these young women is more likely to develop an eating disorder? Why?

2. Dieting typically precedes the development of bulimia nervosa in young women. Does this mean that all forms of dieting are bad for your health? Explain your answer.

Thinking about MULTICULTURAL ISSUES

Ethnic Identity and Eating Disorders

In the United States, eating disorders are less prevalent among blacks than whites (Dolan, 1991). The reason seems to be that young black females do not experience the same pressure to be thin as their white counterparts. Surveys have shown that black females wish to lose less weight than whites (Rosen & Gross, 1987), report significantly fewer negative thoughts about their body shapes, and voice less concern about dieting and weight fluctuation (Rucker & Cash, 1992). Moreover, as has been discussed in other chapters, the rate of obesity in the United States is significantly higher among black than white women.

These cultural factors have protected black women against the development of eating disorders. But what happens as blacks become increasingly acculturated and integrated into mainstream U.S. culture? Recent findings indicate that as black women become assimilated, they increasingly value thinness and resort to dieting (Abrams, Allen, & Gray, 1993). Accordingly, we can expect that the rate of eating disorders will increase in the black population.

Similar trends have been observed among other ethnic groups as they become assimilated to Western cultural ideals of female beauty. For example, a study of female high school students at English-medium schools in Pakistan found only one case of bulimia nervosa (Mumford, Whitehouse, & Choudry, 1992). Yet when the same investigators studied 204 Indian and Pakistani high school students living in England, they found seven cases, or a prevalence rate of 3.4 percent (Mumford, Whitehouse & Platts, 1991).

Eating disorders also occur in non-Western cultures, such as those of Japan and Malaysia, showing the same concentration among females of upper-socioeconomic status (Hsu, 1990). The prevalence of bulimia nervosa in Japan seems similar to that in the United States—that is, roughly 2 percent (Higuchi et al., 1993). And in China, a prevalence rate of 1.1 percent for bulimia nervosa was reported among 509 college freshmen (male and female) (Chun et al., 1992).

Thus, there is a consistent pattern of findings showing that assimilation to Western values is associated with increased dieting, concern about shape and weight, and the rate of eating disorders. This pattern provides strong support for the importance of sociocultural forces in the etiology of eating disorders.

Think about the following question:

1. Consider a woman you know who is from a different country or a different ethnic group than yours. What are her attitudes about body shape and weight? Do they differ from your own? Explain your answer.

TREATMENT

A variety of therapies have been used to treat eating disorders: drug therapies, individual psychological therapies, and family therapy. Let's consider how these therapies are used in treating the specific disorders.

Anorexia Nervosa

For individuals with anorexia nervosa, the medical complications brought about by reaching dangerously low weights often require hospitalization. The first goal of treatment is to restore individuals to something near normal body weight. This can usually be achieved with therapeutic support and carefully planned nutritional treatment. More drastic interventions, such as tube feeding, are not necessary except in the most resistant patients whose lives are at risk.

Behavior modification has proven effective in increasing the rate of weight gain during hospitalization (Halmi, 1993). Such treatment consists of providing the individual with positive reinforcements for gradual weight gain. Typical rewards would be increased visiting privileges and physical and social activities. Inpatient treatment of this kind is effective in restoring weight. The problem, however, is that short-term improvements do not predict long-term outcomes (Hsu, 1990). Patients tend to relapse and lose weight, often necessitating readmission to the hospital.

Several psychological treatments have been used to produce more enduring improvements in weight and psychosocial functioning. **Family therapy** is one of the most commonly employed approaches. It's rooted in the assumption that the overall functioning of the anorexic patient's family is disturbed and serves to maintain her eating disorder (Minuchin et al., 1978). So if the family system is the problem, then the entire family needs to be the focus of therapy.

Despite clinical reports of the success of family therapy, empirical research on its effectiveness is lacking. The only controlled outcome study completed to date compared family therapy with individual supportive psychotherapy (Russell, Szmukler, Dare, & Eisler, 1987). At the end of a 1-year treatment period, the outcomes achieved by family therapy were superior to those of individual psychotherapy for patients with a young age of onset (under 18 years) and short duration of the disorder (less than 3 years). The results as a whole were discouraging, however; only 23 percent of patients were classified as having good clinical outcomes.

Individual psychotherapy has typically consisted of some form of psychodynamic treatment (Johnson, 1991). The most promising approach to date has been that described by Crisp and his colleagues in London (Gowers, Norton, Halek, & Crisp, 1994). It involved offering female patients mainly psychodynamic therapy with some cognitive-behavioral elements. This approach is based on the assumption that anorexia nervosa is a phobia about normal weight gain caused by conflict over becoming a mature woman, which means gaining weight and body fat. The eating disorder is a maladaptive means of coping with this emotional conflict. Therapy is therefore aimed at resolving the underlying conflict and helping patients develop more constructive ways of coping with their psychosexual development.

The Crisp group compared their treatment approach with a no-treatment control group that received only the intensive pretreatment assessment (Gowers et al., 1994). Twenty young female patients were randomly assigned to each condition. Therapy consisted of 12 sessions of 60 to 90 minutes, spread out over a 10-month period. Some of the sessions included family members of patients in an effort to improve communication and end any interactions that maintained the young women's problems.

The results at both 1- and 2-year follow-up evaluations indicated that the treatment group was significantly more improved than the control group, even though many of the women in the latter group had received treatment elsewhere (Gowers et al., 1994). The treatment group had gained more weight and showed improved social and psychosexual functioning. For example, after 2 years, the mean weight of the treatment group was 94.5 percent of what would normally be expected, compared with 83 percent in the control group. Before treatment, both groups were at 75 percent of normal weight. What is unusual about this study is how well both groups of patients fared over follow-up. In contrast, both treatment groups in the Russell et al. (1987) study did relatively poorly.

Drug therapy for eating disorders has included both neuroleptic (antipsychotic) and antidepressant drugs. At best, they have had only marginal effects in promoting weight gain (Hsu, 1990). Whether some type of medication can help reduce relapse among anorexic individuals remains to be studied.

family therapy Treatment approach involving the entire family; based on the assumption that the functioning of a patient's family is disturbed and serves to maintain her eating disorder.

Bulimia Nervosa

Medication   Antidepressant drugs have proven effective in treating bulimia nervosa (Mitchell & de Zwaan, 1993). Research has found that drugs such as imipramine and desipramine (tricyclics) and fluoxetine (Prozac) are reliably more effective than a pill placebo. One of the advantages of using antidepressant medication is that it effectively treats the depression that is commonly associated with bulimia nervosa (Mitchell et al., 1990).

There are several problems with using these drugs, though (Wilson, 1995):

1. Many individuals with bulimia nervosa are reluctant to take medication for their problem.
2. More patients drop out of pharmacotherapy than psychological treatment because of the side effects caused by the drugs.
3. Individuals tend to relapse rapidly when the drugs are withdrawn.

In sum, no study has yet demonstrated that drug treatment can produce long-term improvement (Fairburn, Agras, & Wilson, 1992).

Psychological Treatment   Cognitive-behavioral therapy (CBT) has been the most intensively studied treatment of bulimia nervosa. It typically consists of 16 to 20 sessions administered over a 4- to 5-month period. CBT is aimed at normalizing the chaotic eating patterns of patients, modifying their abnormal attitudes about shape and weight, and equipping them with more constructive coping skills for handling stressful life events. This treatment approach produces an average reduction in binge eating and purging that ranges from 73 to 93 percent. Roughly 50 percent of all patients stop these behaviors (Wilson, 1995). In addition, CBT reduces unhealthy dietary restraints and helps patients become more accepting of their body shapes and weights. Improvement is usually maintained for up to 1 year; one study found up to 6 years' maintenance (Fairburn et al., 1995).

CBT is superior to antidepressant medication. A combination of CBT and antidepressant drugs has been found no more effective than CBT plus a placebo but more effective than the medication alone in treating binge eating and purging (Agras et al., 1992).

CBT has also been shown to be significantly more effective than alternative psychological treatments, with the exception of **interpersonal psychotherapy (IPT)**. This time-limited treatment has been shown effective in treating depression (see Chapter 7). It focuses on the individual's current social functioning, interpersonal conflicts, and role transitions (for instance, an adolescent leaving home to attend college). The success of IPT is not as great as that of CBT immediately after treatment, but that changes over time. The two have been found equally effective at 1- and 6-year follow-ups (Fairburn et al., 1995).

cognitive-behavioral therapy (CBT) *Psychological treatment approach designed to restore normal eating patterns, help patients cope with stressful situations, and alter abnormal attitudes toward body weight and shape.*

interpersonal psychotherapy (IPT) *Time-limited treatment approach that focuses on the individual's current social functioning, interpersonal conflicts, and role transitions.*

Focus on Critical Thinking

1. Interpersonal psychotherapy seems effective in treating bulimia nervosa. However, IPT focuses only on the patient's current social functioning, not on eating habits or attitudes about body weight. What does this tell us about the factors that cause or maintain bulimia nervosa?

2. One theory about antidepressant medication is that it reduces binge eating by decreasing hunger, thereby making it easier for patients to restrict food intake. If this theory is correct, should this medication be used to treat bulimia nervosa? Why or why not?

Binge-Eating Disorder

Preliminary studies have shown that both antidepressant medication and psychological treatments can significantly reduce binge eating in patients with BED (Agras, 1993; Yanovski & Sebring, 1994). As with treating bulimia nervosa, the two most promising psychological approaches are CBT (Marcus, 1993) and IPT (Wilfley et al., 1993). Although these treatments reduce, if not eliminate, binge eating, it is important to note that they do not appear to promote weight loss. (Remember that most BED patients are obese.)

SUMMARY

Description

■ Anorexia nervosa is characterized by medically serious weight loss of 15 percent or more of normal body weight; intense fear of weight gain; and abnormal attitudes about body shape and weight, including denial of the seriousness of the current low body weight.

■ Bulimia nervosa is characterized by binge eating; extreme methods of weight control, such as purging, starvation, or excessive exercise; and abnormal attitudes about the importance of body shape and weight.

■ Binge-eating disorder (BED) is characterized by binge eating but not extreme methods of weight control, as in bulimia nervosa. The majority of BED patients are obese.

Causes

■ Both anorexia and bulimia nervosa run in families. This familial transmission is genetically influenced.

■ It's difficult to determine whether the biological abnormalities seen in patients with eating disorders result from or cause the disturbed behavior.

■ Dieting typically precedes the onset of binge eating and is a risk factor for the development of eating disorders.

■ A personal or family history of obesity, parental substance abuse, and traits of negative self-evaluation and perfectionism are risk factors for bulimia nervosa.

■ Current cultural norms about the ideal female body drive women to diet and hence increase their risk for eating disorders. Women, far more than men, feel societal pressure to be thin. Also, women's sense of self-identity is influenced more by physical attractiveness than men's.

Treatment

■ The first goal of treatment for patients with anorexia nervosa is to restore weight. Hospitalization is often required. Family therapy, individual psychotherapy, and drug therapy have all been used with limited success.

■ Both psychological and drug therapies are effective in treating bulimia nervosa and BED. Cognitive-behavioral and interpersonal therapies result in broad and lasting improvement.

KEY TERMS

abstinence violation effect, **p. 368**
anorexia nervosa, **p. 357**
attributable risk, **p. 367**
binge eating, **p. 357**
binge-eating disorder (BED), **p. 363**
body mass index (BMI), **p. 357**

bulimia nervosa, **p. 360**
case-control design, **p. 368**
cognitive-behavioral therapy (CBT), **p. 375**
eating disorder not otherwise specified (EDNOS), **p. 356**

familial transmission, **p. 366**
family therapy, **p. 374**
interpersonal psychotherapy (IPT), **p. 375**
purging, **p. 358**
serotonin, **p. 366**

CRITICAL THINKING EXERCISE

Paula is a 20-year-old college student. Her current BMI is 20. However, the weight she really wants to be would give her a BMI of 16. She talks about her frustration that she's stopped losing weight over the past month. She has not had her period in the last 3 months.

Paula wishes fervently that she could live without ever eating. Her daily food intake is highly restricted, rarely exceeding 800 calories. Occasionally, she's tempted to eat such "forbidden" foods as cookies, but she never consumes more than two or three. She experiences enormous guilt and discomfort when she does this. She claims that she can "feel the fat cells in her thighs expanding" after eating chocolate chip cookies. She always vomits after eating what she regards to be fattening food. She also consistently purges what most people would regard as a normal meal. As a result, she vomits several times every week.

The reason Paula has given for seeking treatment is to help control her eating. She says that she is doing well in her studies and is generally happy in school. She is close to her family but reports more and more conflict with her mother when she goes home from college.

1. If you were the therapist, what diagnosis would you give Paula? Why?

Chapter 12

PERSONALITY DISORDERS

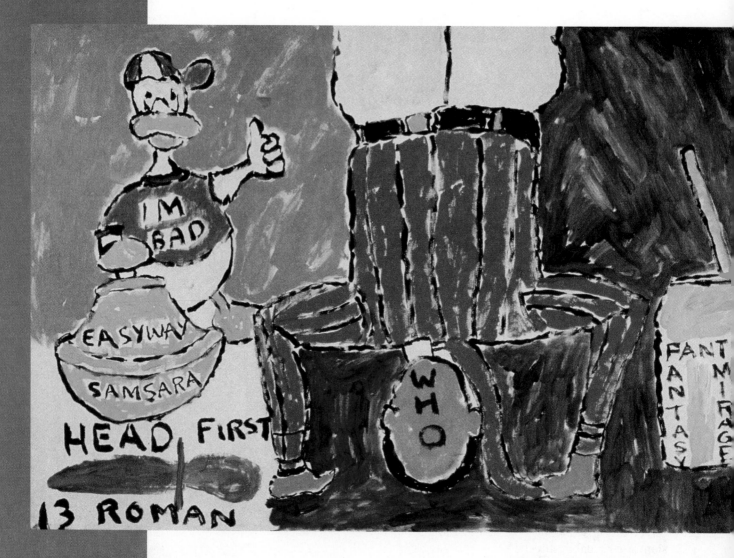

William Gonzalez, **Head First,** HAI

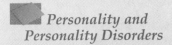
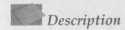
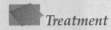

L uanne['s] . . . first symptoms began when she went away to college. She became increasingly withdrawn and preoccupied and was unable to finish the year. She was employed twice briefly but quit each job because she was convinced she could not succeed. She began psychotherapy and soon vacillated between hating her therapist one day and refusing to leave his office the next. She was hospitalized psychiatrically twice for a total of 8 months. Few details were given of her treatment or her mental state except a note about her being very hot tempered.

On admission to Chestnut Lodge, [20-year-old] Luanne was hostile, assaultive at times, and "impulsive." She devalued her therapist, constantly telling him he was insignificant. She did not appear to be motivated for therapy but nevertheless settled into a long-term stay as an inpatient and day patient. Luanne was discharged [on the advice of her psychiatrist] in the late 1950s.

While still a day patient at Chestnut Lodge, Luanne met and married . . . a former patient from another psychiatric hospital. She became pregnant twice and had a son each time. She described these pregnancies as the greatest times in her life. She was physically well and felt that having children gave her a reason to live. Her marriage, however, was quite unstable, as her husband was frequently psychotic and hospitalized. After 5 years, Luanne left her husband and moved to another city to be near her parents. At this time she was depressed, anxious, panicky, and occasionally suicidal. She screamed at and hit her children. She drank three to four beers per night and went on heavier "drinking binges" periodically. She entered psychotherapy, felt that her doctor was a "lousy therapist," and became more disturbed instead of less. Her therapist eventually refused to treat her anymore, sending her for consultation elsewhere (McGlashan, 1993, pp. 248–249).

Luanne's case is one example of the personality disorders—a very diverse group of disorders. For some individuals, having a personality disorder severely affects every aspect of their lives for decades. But for other people, these disorders have a shorter-term, moderate impact. How personality disorders develop is a complex process that is still not well understood, but we know that these disorders are typically difficult to change. We'll discuss in this chapter how personality disorders can be diagnosed along with other clinical syndromes, such as alcoholism, depression, and sexual dysfunction.

PERSONALITY AND PERSONALITY DISORDERS

Have you ever known people who had trouble talking about anything other than themselves? People who, no matter what the topic, quickly find a way of making themselves the center of conversation? You probably thought that they were extremely self-centered or conceited. Or maybe you've known people who seem extremely well organized but never quite manage to finish anything. They spend hours getting ready to work or study—arranging their desks, books, and papers—but then don't have enough time left to complete what actually needs to be done. You might have thought of such people as being obsessive. Or perhaps you've known people who can't ever make decisions on their own. They constantly ask for advice on what to wear, what to order at a restaurant, whether to apply for a certain job, or even whether they should marry a certain person. You might consider these people to be insecure or dependent.

All these kinds of behaviors are commonly thought to reflect **personality**—the more or less stable, characteristic way a person feels and behaves in a wide variety of situations. For the most part, we enjoy the personality differences among the people we know. Moreover, people are typically able to adapt their behavior to different situations in their lives. For example, even very talkative people usually manage to keep quiet while attending lectures, religious services, or plays.

But some people exhibit personality traits that are so exaggerated and inflexible that they distress them or cause problems in their school, work, or interpersonal relationships. According to the fourth edition of the *Diagnostic and Statistical Manual of Mental Disorders* (*DSM-IV*), such individuals have **personality disorder** (American Psychiatric Association, 1994).

Recall from Chapter 3 that in the multiaxial system of the *DSM-IV*, the personality disorders (together with mental retardation) form a second level: Axis II. The symptoms of Axis I disorders tend to come and go, whereas those of Axis II disorders are longer lasting; they are part of a person's fundamental makeup. The general diagnostic criteria for personality disorder are listed in the *DSM-IV* table.

DSM-IV   **General Diagnostic Criteria for PERSONALITY DISORDER**

A. An enduring pattern of inner experience and behavior that deviates markedly from the expectations of the individual's culture. This pattern is manifested in two (or more) of the following areas:
   (1) cognition (i.e., ways of perceiving and interpreting self, other people, and events)
   (2) affectivity (i.e., the range, intensity, lability, and appropriateness of emotional response)
   (3) interpersonal functioning
   (4) impulse control

B. The enduring pattern is inflexible and pervasive across a broad range of personal and social situations.

C. The enduring pattern leads to clinically significant distress or impairment in social, occupational, or other important areas of functioning.

D. The pattern is stable and of long duration and its onset can be traced back at least to adolescence or early adulthood.

E. The enduring pattern is not better accounted for as a manifestation or consequence of another mental disorder.

F. The enduring pattern is not due to the direct physiological effects of a substance . . . or a general medical condition.

personality More or less stable, characteristic way a person feels and behaves in a wide variety of situations.

personality disorder Extreme and inflexible personality traits that are distressing to the person or that cause problems in school, work, or interpersonal relationships.

Background

The modern history of the study of personality disorders is usually traced to the concepts of *manie sans delire* ("insanity without delirium") (Pinel, 1801/1962) and *moral insanity* (Prichard, 1835). These terms describe the occurrence of wildly inappropriate behaviors in persons whose intellect was otherwise intact—for example, extreme, irrational outbursts of temper or apparently uncontrollable stealing and lying. Sigmund Freud (1856–1939) and other early psychoanalysts also described a number of character disorders (Frances & Widiger, 1986), including melancholic, masochistic, hysterical, narcissistic, phobic, and obsessive-compulsive characters. Similarly, Kurt Schneider (1934/1958) identified 10 personality types, such as the insecure, attention-seeking, or labile (emotionally unstable) personalities. Although the system for categorizing personality disorders continues to evolve, many of the disorders recognized today were identified long ago.

Classification of Personality Disorders

So far, we've been talking about both personality *traits* and personality *types* without distinguishing between them. *Traits* are dimensional; they're characteristics that people have some quantity of. Some people, for example, are very aggressive or insecure, whereas others are not at all that way; most people fall somewhere between these two extremes. Personality *types*, by contrast, are categorical; they're descriptions that center on a few striking features. If we say that someone has an "obsessive personality," for instance, we are characterizing that person according to a single, strong feature of his behavior. But if we say that someone has many "obsessive traits," we are mentioning one aspect of his whole personality.

The *DSM-IV* classifies personality disorders using a **categorical system** based on personality types. In the *DSM-IV*, 10 personality disorders are each described using a few prominent characteristics; for example, *antisocial personality disorder* is described as reflecting "a pervasive pattern of disregard for and violation of the rights of others" (p. 649). In addition, a more detailed set of criteria is given for each personality disorder; for example, criterion 5 for antisocial personality disorder is "reckless disregard for safety of self or others" (p. 650).

To be diagnosed with a personality disorder, a person must show 4 or 5 of these specific criteria. This method is used because it's recognized that a person may exhibit a general behavioral pattern (such as disregard for the rights of others) through any number of different specific behaviors. In the next section, we'll describe each of the 10 personality disorders included in the *DSM-IV*. Then, we'll consider some major problems with this categorical system and discuss alternative ways of thinking about personality disorder. Finally, we'll discuss the causes and treatments of these disorders.

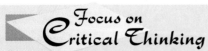

Focus on Critical Thinking

1. What differentiates ordinary inappropriate or obnoxious behavior from a personality disorder? What criteria can we use to decide if someone has a personality disorder?

2. Think about a few people you know well and a few you know only in one particular context. How well can you capture each of his or her personalities with a few choice words versus a longer list of descriptors? Do your descriptions differ, depending on how well you know each person? Explain your answer.

DESCRIPTION

The *DSM-IV* groups the personality disorders into three *clusters*, based on certain descriptive similarities. Table 12.1 lists the diagnoses forming each cluster and the features shared by the disorders in it. The *DSM-IV* acknowledges that "the clustering system . . . has serious limitations and has not been consistently validated" (p. 630). Nonetheless, this method of organization is helpful in understanding the personality disorders.

Cluster A: Odd and Eccentric Personality Disorders

The first cluster, Cluster A, includes disorders characterized as odd and eccentric personality disorders. Table 12.2 lists the essential features that are specific to each of the three Cluster A diagnoses: paranoid, schizoid, and schizotypal.

Paranoid Personality Disorder   The essential feature of **paranoid personality disorder** is "a pervasive distrust and suspiciousness of others such that their motives are interpreted as malevolent" (American Psychiatric Association, 1994, p. 637). By early adulthood, these individuals begin to believe that others are tak-

categorical system Method of classification that separates things into distinct types; in terms of personality disorder, individuals are diagnosed according to specific disorders.

paranoid personality disorder Characterized by ongoing feelings of distrust and suspicion of others, whose motives are seen as harmful.

TABLE 12.1	DSM-IV Personality Disorder Clusters	
Cluster	**Common Feature**	**Diagnoses**
Cluster A	Odd, eccentric	Paranoid; Schizoid; Schizotypal
Cluster B	Dramatic, emotional, erratic	Antisocial; Borderline; Histrionic; Narcissistic
Cluster C	Anxious, fearful	Avoidant; Dependent; Obsessive-Compulsive

Source: American Psychiatric Association, 1994.

ing advantage of them; they even harbor doubts about the loyalties of friends and associates. People with paranoid personality disorder feel slighted by little things and are easily angered by perceived insults that are not apparent to others. They tend to be secretive, jealous, rigid, unforgiving, argumentative, sarcastic, cold, and frequently hostile. Individuals with this disorder tend to think that they're fault-less, so they attribute their mistakes to others, going so far as to assign devious motives to others. People with paranoid personality disorders are supersensitive to rank, class, and power issues; they resent others who have things that they don't, and experience obvious problems in the workplace.

Schizoid Personality Disorder The essential features of **schizoid personality disorder** are "a pervasive pattern of detachment from social relationships and a restricted range of emotions in interpersonal settings" (American Psychiatric Asso-ciation, 1994, p. 641). Individuals with schizoid personality disorder are reclusive, engaging in solitary activities, choosing work with minimal social interactions. Because of this they often appear cold and detached. These individuals can form *stable* relationships, but they don't form *close* relationships, even with family mem-bers. They take pleasure in few, if any, activities and express very little desire for sexual experiences. Individuals with this condition seldom date or marry and often work in low-level jobs that require little interpersonal contact.

Schizotypal Personality Disorder **Schizotypal personality disorder** has one of the shortest histories of any personality disorder. It evolved out of clarifying the

schizoid personality dis-order Characterized by being detached from social relationships and showing a restricted range of emotions in interpersonal exchanges.

schizotypal personality disorder Characterized by social and interpersonal deficits that are shown primarily by intense discomfort in inter-personal relationships and impaired ability to form close relationships as well as cognitive or perceptual distortions and eccentric behavior.

TABLE 12.2	Essential Features of Cluster A, "Odd and Eccentric," Personality Disorders
Diagnosis	**Pervasive Pattern**
Paranoid	Distrust and suspiciousness of others
	Interpretation of others' motives as malevolent
Schizoid	Detachment from social relationships
	Restricted range of expression of emotions in interpersonal settings
Schizotypal	Social and interpersonal deficits marked by:
	■ acute discomfort with close relationships
	■ reduced capacity for close relationships
	Cognitive or perceptual distortions
	Eccentricities of behavior

Source: American Psychiatric Association, 1994.

boundary between schizophrenia and borderline personality disorder. Evidence suggests that this personality disorder is related to schizophrenia in a number of important ways (Siever, Bernstein, & Silverman, 1991), leading some to argue that it should be considered a schizophrenia-related disorder and placed on Axis I.

A schizotypal personality exhibits two sets of qualities: (1) intense discomfort in interpersonal relationships and impaired ability to form close relationships and (2) cognitive or perceptual distortions and eccentric behavior. For example, people with schizotypal personality disorder may dress in mismatched clothing or clothing that's out of fashion or out of season—for instance, wearing a sweater on a hot summer day. These individuals' speech and perception of the world may also be unusual; they may claim to be clairvoyant or believe that they can feel the presence of "a force" in the room. Unlike schizophrenic individuals, however, people with schizotypal personality disorder have not totally lost contact with reality. They are likely to be superstitious and believe in astrology, crystal power, megavitamin therapy—whatever fringe fad is popular at the time.

Schizotypal personalities are loners. Like those with paranoid personality disorder, they are suspicious of others, but their affect is more likely to be anxious than hostile. This anxiety does not diminish with increased familiarity, so individuals with schizotypal personalities tend to remain socially isolated. Because this isolation limits their opportunities to learn the subtleties of appropriate social behavior, conversations with these individuals are often awkward and constrained.

Cluster B: Dramatic, Emotional, and Erratic Personality Disorders

The second group of personality disorders identified by the *DSM-IV,* Cluster B, includes dramatic, emotional, and erratic personalities. Table 12.3 lists the core features of the four diagnoses: antisocial, borderline, histrionic, and narcissistic.

Antisocial Personality Disorder   Because of its impact on society, **antisocial personality disorder** has been the subject of more research than any other personality disorder. Severe antisocial behavior (criminal behavior) is addressed by the law enforcement and legal systems. In addition, antisocial behavior causes a variety of other major problems for families and friends.

antisocial personality disorder Characterized by frequent disregard for and violation of others' rights occurring since age 15 with evidence of conduct disorder beginning before age 15.

TABLE 12.3	**Essential Features of Cluster B, "Dramatic, Emotional, and Erratic," Personality Disorders**
Diagnosis	**Pervasive Pattern**
Antisocial	Disregard for the rights of others
	Violation of the rights of others
Borderline	Instability of interpersonal relationships
	Instability of self-image
	Instability of affects (emotions)
	Marked impulsivity
Histrionic	Excessive emotionality
	Attention seeking
Narcissistic	Grandiosity in fantasy or behavior
	Need for admiration
	Lack of empathy

Source: American Psychiatric Association, 1994.

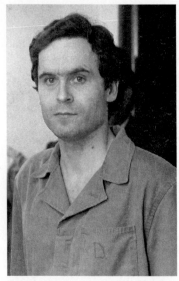

Ted Bundy epitomized the aggressive nature of antisocial personality disorder. Just before he was electrocuted, he confessed to the murders of 16 women from coast to coast. He described himself as "the most cold-blooded son-of-a-bitch that you will ever meet."

psychopathy Conceptualization of a personality disorder similar to the DSM-IV antisocial personality disorder; emphasizes such traits as lack of empathy, glib and superficial charm, egocentricity and inflated self-worth, emotional unresponsiveness and irresponsibility, poor judgment, deceitfulness, and impulsive behavior.

borderline personality disorder Characterized by pervasive instability in interpersonal relationships, self-image, and emotions as well as marked impulsivity.

The essential features of antisocial personality disorder are "a pervasive pattern of disregard for and violation of the rights of others occurring since age 15," with evidence of conduct disorder before age 15 (American Psychiatric Association, 1994, p. 649). This pattern must include at least three of the following:

1. Failure to conform to social norms
2. Deceitfulness
3. Impulsivity or failure to plan ahead
4. Irritability and aggressiveness
5. Reckless disregard for the safety of self or others
6. Irresponsibility
7. Lack of remorse (p. 649)

Antisocial personality disorder is much more common among males than females. In community populations, approximately 3 percent of men and 1 percent of women display characteristics of antisocial personality (American Psychiatric Association, 1994). The *DSM* has been criticized for overemphasizing criminal behavior and underemphasizing psychological factors in establishing the diagnostic criteria for antisocial personality disorder (Frances, 1980).

For 25 years, Hare (1991) has been researching an alternative set of criteria, based on Cleckley's (1941/1982) classic criteria for **psychopathy.** These criteria emphasize such traits as lack of empathy, glib and superficial charm, egocentricity and inflated sense of self-worth, emotional unresponsiveness and irresponsibility in interpersonal relationships, poor judgment and failure to learn from experience, deceitfulness, and impulsive behavior. Hare (1991) reported that about half of incarcerated criminals meet the *DSM* criteria for antisocial personality disorder; however, consistently fewer (about one-third) are diagnosed with psychopathy.

Robins, Tipp, and Przybeck (1991) also looked at criminal behavior among people with antisocial behavior as part of the Epidemiologic Catchment Area (ECA) study (see Chapter 1). About half of those diagnosed with antisocial personality disorder did not have significant arrest records. More common features were job troubles (94 percent), violence (85 percent), multiple moving traffic violations (72 percent), and severe marital difficulties (67 percent). These data led Robins and colleagues to suggest that the actual degree of overlap found between criminality and antisocial personality disorder is consistent with theoretical and clinical expectations—that is, they are related but not the same thing.

The puzzle of the overlap between psychopathy and antisocial personality disorder is not resolved by these data. The *DSM* criteria may identify small-time swindlers, who have conned, duped, or charmed their way through life yet somehow were never arrested for a major offense. But these data also suggest that the *DSM* might not identify other individuals who would meet the criteria for psychopathy—for example, politicians who proclaim their ethics while being "on the take" from various illegal ventures, Wall Street investors who engage in insider trading, or television evangelists who amass personal fortunes and engage prostitutes while preaching "the good, clean life."

Borderline Personality Disorder   Now recognized as a specific diagnostic category, **borderline personality disorder** is the least distinct of all the personality disorders. In a review of 10 studies, only 3 to 10 percent of individuals with borderline personality disorder didn't have some other personality disorder, too (Gunderson, Zanarini, & Kisiel, 1991). A study of over 18,000 patients seeking evaluation at a psychiatric clinic reported that 70 percent of those diagnosed with borderline personality disorder also had an Axis I disorder, such as major depression (Fabrega, Ulrich, Pilkonis, & Mezzich, 1991).

Borderline personality disorder was not widely researched until it appeared in the *DSM-III* in 1980. But since then, research on this personality disorder has surpassed that on any other and has also come to be one of the most frequently

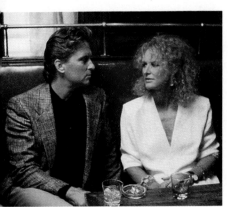

Glenn Close ("Alex Forrest") in Fatal Attraction *portrayed the extreme variability of individuals with borderline personality disorder.*

diagnosed personality disorders: About 10 percent of psychiatric outpatients and 20 percent of inpatients receive this diagnosis (American Psychiatric Association, 1994). Moreover, a review of four studies found that among patients with personality disorders, borderline personality disorder was the most common at 38 percent (Widiger & Rogers, 1989). Approximately 3 out of 4 individuals diagnosed with borderline personality disorder are women. This phenomenon may be related to the fact that childhood physical and sexual abuse are possible risk factors in the development of this disorder.

The essential features of the *DSM-IV* borderline personality disorder are "a pervasive pattern of instability in interpersonal relationships, self-image, and affects [emotions], and marked impulsivity" (American Psychiatric Association, 1994, p. 654). Recent research suggests that poor impulse control may be a more central feature of this disorder than unstable self-image or mood (Gunderson et al., 1991). Characterized by marked uncertainty about major life issues (for instance, goals and values, sexual orientation, career choice, and types of friends), such uncertainty proved common among people with a number of other disorders and among normal adolescents, as well. Emotional instability—another traditional hallmark of people with borderline personality disorder—was especially common among people with mood disorders.

What seems distinctive about mood in borderline personality disorder is its reactivity—that is, the fluctuation of intense dysphoria (unhappiness), anxiety, and rage within a matter of hours or days in response to seemingly trivial events. Individuals with this disorder also tend to have intense and unstable interpersonal relationships. Supposedly best friends become enemies on the basis of ordinary disagreements. Consequently, people with borderline personality disorder fear abandonment and often make desperate efforts to maintain relationships.

Mood reactivity also may be related to poor impulse control. Individuals with borderline personality disorder often act impulsively in self-destructive ways, such as driving recklessly or bingeing on food, alcohol, drugs, or sex. In one study (Soloff, Lis, Kelly, & Cornelius, 1994), 72 percent of individuals with borderline personality made suicide attempts or suicidal gestures, such as cutting themselves with razors or burning themselves with cigarettes. Completed suicide occurs in 8 to 10 percent

TABLE 12.4	**Self-Destructive Acts by 57 Hospitalized Patients with Borderline Personality Disorder**	
Variable	**Number of Patients**	**Noteworthy Patterns**
Suicide threats	42	To get attention
		To cause trouble
		In rage
Overdose	40	No usual pattern
		Barbiturates most frequent
Self-mutilation	36	Wrist slashing, body banging, burning, puncturing, hair removal
Drug abuse	38	Polydrug abuse, amphetamines, alcohol binges, marijuana
Promiscuity or alcohol	36	Usually under the influence of drugs
Accidents	14	Reckless driving

Source: From J. G. Gunderson (1984), *Borderline personality disorder.* Washington, DC: American Psychiatric Association, p. 86.

of such cases. Table 12.4 on page 385 shows the variety of self-destructive acts of borderline hospital patients (Gunderson, 1984).

A final characteristic of borderline personality disorder, in about 75 percent of cases (Gunderson et al., 1991), is stress-related paranoid ideation or severe dissociative symptoms that are quite transient, lasting only a few minutes or no more than a few hours. Often, the stressor is the threat or fear of abandonment; in these cases, the symptoms disappear when the relationship is no longer perceived to be in danger of breaking up. This feature is one of the most discriminating of the diagnostic criteria for this disorder.

Histrionic Personality Disorder   As its name suggests, **histrionic personality disorder** evolved out of the ancient concepts of hysteria (see Chapter 6) and later, hysterical personality. A number of older studies documented the overlap between somatization disorder and either histrionic features or histrionic personality disorder (Lilienfeld, Van Valkenburg, Larntz, & Akiskal, 1986). Recent research reveals that histrionic personality disorder overlaps even more with other personality disorders (Rost, Akins, Brown, & Smith, 1992). This finding calls into question any special relationship among these disorders. Nevertheless, research has shown that women are more likely to be diagnosed with histrionic personality disorder than men (Maier, Lichterman, Klingler, Heun, & Hallmayer, 1992).

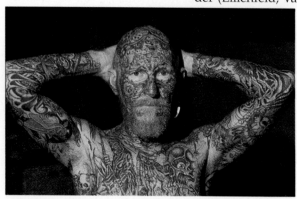

People with histrionic personalities seek attention in unusual many ways. This man may be seeking attention through his tattoos. Does this mean he has a personality disorder?

The essential feature of this disorder is "a pervasive pattern of excessive emotionality and attention seeking" (American Psychiatric Association, 1994, p. 657) in which individuals attempt to gain attention in unusual ways. They may dress in brightly colored clothing and have strikingly different hairstyles. Their behavioral style itself is dramatic—the word *histrionic* means "dramatic or theatrical." These individuals are often provocative or sexually seductive, and they overreact behaviorally and emotionally to many situations.

Individuals with histrionic personality disorder are highly impressionable, so they often become enthusiastic about the latest fad. These individuals develop convictions based on little evidence; they defend these views passionately but not consistently over time. There's a shallowness about the speech and emotional expression of people with histrionic personality disorder. They may refer to a person they hardly know as "a very special friend," yet be unable to describe someone they actually know well. Individuals with this disorder may be in the throes of anxiety one moment—say, over a minor error they made at work—and be gushing with gratitude the next—perhaps when their supervisor brushes off the mistake as being unimportant.

Narcissistic Personality Disorder   The word *narcissist* is derived from the Greek myth about Narcissus, a handsome young man who was told by his mother that he would have a long life if he never looked at his features. Despite her warning, Narcissus gazed into a spring at his reflection and fell in love with his own image. Accordingly, people who adore themselves are described as being *narcissistic*.

The essential features of **narcissistic personality disorder** are "a pervasive pattern of grandiosity (in fantasy or behavior), need for admiration, and lack of empathy" (American Psychiatric Association, 1994, p. 661). This grandiosity is often seen in arrogant, boastful behavior, such as making unwarranted claims of achievement or intimacy with famous people. In others with this disorder, the grandiosity is expressed only in fantasy. They have a rich "inner life," dreaming of how their next business scheme will lead to wealth or of owning a big house, driving an expensive car, attracting the ideal mate, and so on.

histrionic personality disorder Characterized by excessive expression of emotion and attention seeking.

narcissistic personality disorder Characterized by grandiose fantasies or behavior, constant need for admiration, and lack of empathy.

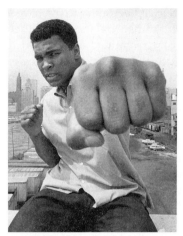

The word narcissism *derives from the figure Narcissus in Greek mythology, who fell in love with his own reflection. Muhammed Ali was as well known for his narcissistic style as for his athletic prowess. He frequently exclaimed, "I am the greatest!"*

Narcissists have a strong sense of superiority, which leads naturally to expectations of special treatment, callous use of other people to further their own ends, and blindness to others' needs and feelings. One narcissistic patient felt that she deserved special privileges; when asked why she deserved them, she looked surprised and stated, "Because I want them!" People with narcissistic personality disorder expect admiration and become very upset, even enraged, when they don't receive it. Although not part of the *DSM-IV* criteria, beneath the narcissist's grandiosity and need for admiration lies a very vulnerable and fragile self-esteem (Cooper & Ronningstam, 1992). Individuals with this disorder often become anxious and/or depressed when their sense of self-worth is threatened. When a friend, lover, or therapist begins to give honest feedback and refuses to feed the exaggerated sense of self-importance, the narcissist will be threatened and withdraw.

As in the myth, data suggest that more men have narcissistic traits than women. But the full disorder is rarely found among community samples (less than 1 percent) (Weissman, 1993) and hardly more common (approximately 6 percent) in researched clinical samples (Widiger, 1993).

Cluster C: Anxious and Fearful Personality Disorders

Table 12.5 lists the features of the diagnoses in Cluster C personality disorders, which share the feature of anxiety or fearfulness. The diagnoses in this cluster include avoidant, dependent, and obsessive-compulsive personality disorders.

Avoidant Personality Disorder   The *DSM-III* (American Psychiatric Association, 1980) was the first to include **avoidant personality disorder.** In the *DSM-IV*, this disorder is characterized by "a pervasive pattern of social inhibition, feelings of inadequacy, and hypersensitivity to negative evaluation" (1994, p. 664).

These three characteristics are highly intertwined in avoidant people. For example, due to their fears of criticism or disapproval, people with this personality disorder avoid occupational situations that involve any significant contact with other people. Similarly, because they view themselves as being socially inept and inferior to others, they have excessive worries about rejection and so refrain from becoming involved in relationships until they receive clear signs that they'll be accepted. Individuals with avoidant personality disorder also worry about embarrassing themselves and so do not attempt anything new. When they are in

avoidant personality disorder *Characterized by social inhibition, feelings of inadequacy, and extreme sensitivity to negative remarks.*

TABLE 12.5	Essential Features of Cluster C, "Anxious and Fearful," Personality Disorders	
Diagnosis	**Pervasive Pattern**
Avoidant	Social inhibition
	Feelings of inadequacy
	Hypersensitivity to negative evaluation
Dependent	Excessive need to be taken care of
	Submissive and clinging behaviors
	Fears of separation
Obsessive-Compulsive	Preoccupation with orderliness and perfectionism
	Preoccupation with mental and interpersonal control
	Restricted flexibility, openness, and efficiency

Source: American Psychiatric Association, 1994.

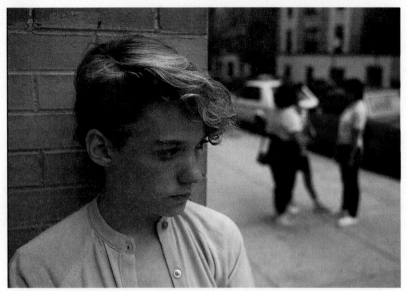

Extreme social anxiety may reflect avoidant personality disorder. What biological and psychosocial factors can contribute to its development?

a social situation or beginning to develop a friendship or intimate relationship, they behave in a very restrained and inhibited manner because they believe that they're personally unappealing and fear being criticized, shamed, or ridiculed. In contrast to individuals with schizoid personality disorder, those with avoidant personality disorder desire contact with others. So, they live lives of continual conflict—wanting relationships yet avoiding the risk of becoming involved.

The behavior of individuals with avoidant personality disorder can set up a vicious cycle: They appear aloof and distant to co-workers and other peers, who may then keep their distance, too. As a result, avoidant persons never receive the signals of acceptance we all look for and end up feeling more sure than ever of their inadequacy. They have a similar problem with intimacy, which develops through mutual self-disclosure. Because avoidant individuals' interpersonal restraint interferes with this process, it contributes to the very outcome that they fear: rejection (Meleshko & Alden, 1993). The same pattern can be seen in social skills, which are learned behaviors (Turner, Beidel, Cooley, & Woody, 1994). By following an avoidant behavior pattern, the individual limits how much interpersonal experience she gets and the more she avoids such experiences, the less socially skilled she is likely to be (Herbert, Hope, & Bellack, 1992). Thus, there may be some factual basis for the self-view of the person with avoidant personality disorder, who sees herself as socially inept. Regardless, the vicious cycle continues.

Dependent Personality Disorder   The concept of dependency has multiple historical roots, including psychoanalytic theory, social and developmental psychology, and ethology (Hirschfeld, Shea, & Weise, 1991). The *DSM-IV* description of **dependent personality disorder** represents a blend of these various traditions. It focuses on two interrelated essential features: (1) "a pervasive and excessive need to be taken care of" and (2) the "submissive and clinging behavior and fears of separation" that this need causes (American Psychiatric Association, 1994, p. 668).

Individuals with dependent personality disorder rely on others to make most of their decisions. They passively allow others to take responsibility for their lives; for example, they may never move out of their parents' homes, make no friends other than those of their roommates, or accept jobs that their spouses obtain for them.

To gain approval and to assure the support of those they depend on, these individuals may voluntarily make unreasonable sacrifices or do mundane and thankless tasks for others. One patient with dependent personality disorder gave her possessions away to anyone who complimented or admired them. On the other hand, out of fear of losing support and approval, these individuals are very reluctant to disagree with others. When close relationships end, they may take up with the first available person to avoid having to depend on themselves.

dependent personality disorder Characterized by a pervasive and excessive need to be taken care of, which causes submissive, clinging behavior and fears of separation.

Obsessive-Compulsive Personality Disorder   In 1908, Freud described the anal character as "orderly, parsimonious and obstinate" (1908/1959, p. 169) and elaborated that these traits incorporated being fastidious, conscientious, trustworthy, miserly, and argumentative. This concept has gone through various transfor-

PERSPECTIVE ON OBSESSIVE-COMPULSIVE PERSONALITY DISORDER

BIOLOGICAL FACTORS

Biological factors may make certain people more vulnerable to developing obsessive-compulsive personality disorder:

➤ Sensitive temperament—which research has shown to be under genetic influence—appears to be an important element in the development of many types of psychopathology, including personality disorders.

➤ Children with sensitive temperaments react quickly and strongly to everything. They may appear to be very anxious or to overreact to minor negative events.

➤ Children with less sensitive temperaments react less easily and less strongly; therefore, they may fail to be affected by negative events when it would be appropriate to become anxious.

PSYCHOLOGICAL FACTORS

Psychological factors interact with biological vulnerabilities in producing personality problems:

➤ Interpersonal dysfunction is a major element in most personality disorders.

➤ The quality of relationships with primary caregivers during the first few years of life teaches people to form strong, trusting attachments or weak, insecure, or ambivalent attachments. These attachments provide models for development of relationships later in life.

➤ Individuals with obsessive-compulsive personality disorder have difficulty showing affection, which may stem from poor development of primary relationships.

SOCIAL FACTORS

Both biological and psychological factors operate in specific social contexts:

➤ Inconsistency in discipline can cause children to become excessively concerned about details in order to avoid punishment from an early age.

➤ Harsh punishment can exaggerate the anxiety of a child with sensitive temperament.

These biological, psychological, and social factors interact to cause problems, as illustrated in the following case:

By the time he reached college, Luis had been diagnosed with obsessive-compulsive personality disorder. His extremely detail-oriented schoolwork resulted in high grades and praise from teachers—when he managed to get his work in on time. But his perfectionism in school was in stark contrast to the neglect of his social life.

The biopsychosocial model explains Luis's problems. Luis was fussy as an infant. Minor changes in routine upset him greatly, and he was hard to settle down when he became fretful. He developed into a highly anxious 3-year-old, who cried easily when scolded. His parents were harsh disciplinarians. From a young age, Luis learned to play with just one toy to avoid his father's yelling at him about "making a mess all over the house." Luis would sometimes rush back into the house on his way to school

to make sure he hadn't left anything lying around. Socially, his parents were rather cold and detached, able to meet Luis's physical needs but less able to meet his needs for love and affection. Luis didn't have many friends, partly because he had never learned the give and take of social relationships from his standoffish parents. As he grew older, Luis became more focused on school, where he met with success, thus reinforcing his behavior and further distancing him from friends.

mations since that time, but the essential features of **obsessive-compulsive personality disorder,** as described in the *DSM-IV,* are not radically different from Freud's description: "preoccupation with orderliness, perfectionism, and mental and interpersonal control, at the expense of flexibility, openness, and efficiency" (American Psychiatric Association, 1994, p. 672).

Individuals with obsessive-compulsive personality disorder are so preoccupied with details, rules, lists, organization, and schedules that they lose sight of the major purposes of their activities. They may spend so many hours getting organized to work, for instance, that the actual work never gets done. Similarly, they are so perfectionistic that they can never complete tasks. A graduate student with this personality disorder took 10 years to finish his doctoral requirements, because with each new publication in his field, he felt that he had to revise his thesis (Salzman, 1985).

The behavioral style of individuals with obsessive-compulsive personality disorder is rigid, stubborn, controlled, and controlling. People with this disorder have inflexible values and are overconscientious about matters of morality and ethics.

Individuals with obsessive-compulsive personality disorder are excessively devoted to their work, excluding leisure activities and friendships. They are classic workaholics, who rarely take vacations and have difficulty relaxing when they do. As parents, they may have the style of a drill sergeant, turning every game into a skill-building lesson and every playful activity into an exercise. Individuals with this disorder are also miserly, often to the point of being hoarders or packrats.

Focus on Critical Thinking

1. Descriptions of people with personality disorders sometimes sound like caricatures or movie characters. Can real people be described so neatly? Why or why not?

2. If you were a clinician, how would you diagnose a patient whose personality is only partly like one of those described in the DSM-IV? (Say, for instance, that your patient is a woman who is excessively emotional, as with histrionic personality disorder, but is not overly attention seeking.)

3. Again, if you were a clinician, how would you diagnose a patient whose personality seems to be a blend of two or more diagnoses? (Say, for instance, that your patient is a man who displays some of the traits of dependent personality disorder; he's submissive, continually seeks advice, and often has others make decisions for him. But he also has an aggressive, demanding style that's more characteristic of narcissistic personality disorder.)

ISSUES AND PROBLEMS IN CATEGORIZING PERSONALITY DISORDERS

Now that you have a basic sense of the characteristics of the various *DSM-IV* personality disorders, let's turn to some important issues that arise when we consider these diagnoses: their epidemiology, reliability, validity, and an alternative system for their diagnosis.

Epidemiology

Prevalence How common are personality disorders? Research into the prevalence of personality disorders has been hampered by the lack of reliable instruments for their assessment. However, a recent review of the world literature on this topic (Weissman, 1993) found remarkably consistent rates of personality disorders cross-nationally, despite broad differences in samples and study methods. Community-based surveys in the United States, Canada, New Zealand, and Scandinavia show that the overall lifetime rate for any personality disorder ranges from about 10 to 13 percent. In other words, 1 out of every 8 or 10 people may be diagnosed with a personality disorder over the course of their lives. (For more information on cross-national concerns in assessing personality disorders, see Thinking about Multicultural Issues.)

obsessive-compulsive personality disorder Characterized by preoccupation with orderliness, perfectionism, and mental and interpersonal control at the cost of flexibility, openness, and efficiency.

In 1979, the World Health Organization (WHO) and the United States Alcohol, Drug Abuse, and Mental Health Administration (ADAMHA) established the Joint Program on the Diagnosis and Classification of Mental Disorders, Alcoholism, and Drug Abuse. The purpose of doing so was to foster a common language for talking about mental disorders and to improve the scientific basis of diagnosis and classification of mental disorders. For instance, the Joint Program has sponsored the development of assessment instruments to compare the types and rates of mental disorders that occur in different cultures (Loranger, Hirschfeld, Sartorius, & Regier, 1991).

In 1984, the Personality Disorder Examination (PDE) (Loranger, 1988)—a semistructured interview being developed for use in the United States—was selected as the basis for the International PDE (IPDE), to be used in the International Pilot Study of Personality Disorders. This interview is divided into six topics: (1) Work, (2) Self, (3) Interpersonal Relationships, (4) Affects, (5) Reality Testing, and (6) Impulse Control. After asking the standard questions, interviewers are free to probe with additional questions before making their own ratings. The behavior (or trait) is rated normal (0), exaggerated (1), or pathological (2).

Although the *DSM* is widely used around the world, the *International Classification of Diseases* (*ICD*) (WHO, 1990) is the official diagnostic manual of the WHO. So the IPDE includes both the *DSM-III-R* criteria for obsessive-compulsive personality disorder and the *ICD-10* (10th edition) criteria. (Both sets of criteria were the most current versions at the time.) Including both sets makes for a long interview of 150 criteria. If the interviewee does not have the trait, it takes about 1 minute per criteria; at this rate, the complete interview requires 2.5 hours. But when an interviewee does have the trait, assessing that criteria can take several minutes. As a result, it can take 3 to 4 hours to administer the entire IPDE. In such cases, the interview is broken up into two sessions in order to keep both the interviewer and interviewee alert and interested throughout.

The IPDE was translated into Dutch, French, German, Hindi, Italian, Japanese, Kannada, Norwegian, Swahili, and Tamil. Great care was taken to make the translations as accurate as possible. A pilot study was then undertaken in Austria, England, Germany, India, Japan, Kenya, Luxembourg, the Netherlands, Norway, Switzerland, and the United States. After extensive training of interviewers, at least 50 patients between the ages of 21 and 55 were interviewed at each site. Altogether, 716 patients were interviewed; 243 were reinterviewed to assess test-retest reliability, and 141 of the interviews were rated by an observer to assess interrater reliability (Loranger, Sartorius, Andreoli, & Berger, 1994). In both evaluations of reliability, results compared favorably with those for other semistructured interviews. That is, it wasn't any more difficult (or any easier) to diagnose personality disorder cross-culturally than within the United States. The two types of personality disorder diagnosed most often worldwide were borderline and avoidant, which are among the most common in the United States, too.

Another important validity issue was what clinicians from other countries thought of the interview. Did the questions make sense in their cultures, or did American ideas about personality disorder seem foreign to them? Surprisingly, a questionnaire that assessed the clinical acceptability of the IPDE found that the only significant reservation clinicians had concerned its length.

Think about the following questions:

1. The diagnostic criteria for personality disorders might seem rather specific to a given culture. For example, "preoccupation with fantasies of unlimited success, power, brilliance, beauty, or ideal love" seems particularly twentieth-century American. How do you explain the surprising results that clinicians from cultures as different as those of Germany, India, Japan, and Kenya had little objection to the IPDE questions?

2. If the IPDE were put into a time capsule and opened in the twenty-third century, would the questions still make sense to clinicians? Explain your answer.

More information is available regarding the prevalence of personality disorders in patient samples. According to a review of eight studies comprising nearly 1,400 patients, rates for specific *DSM-III* disorders ranged from a low of 2 percent for schizoid personality disorder to a high of 21 percent for borderline personality disorder (Widiger & Rogers, 1989). Prevalence among inpatient samples was generally higher than that among outpatient samples—in one study, as high as 64 percent for borderline and schizotypal personality disorders. In the large, single-clinic study mentioned earlier (Fabrega et al., 1991), 13 percent of the individuals who sought psychiatric evaluation over the 7-year period from 1983 to 1989 received a personality disorder diagnosis. Of this group, the most common specific diagnoses were antisocial (20 percent) and borderline (15 percent).

Personality disorders clearly reflect problems in people's long-standing, characteristic behavioral patterns, not just transient or episodic difficulties. Thus, these data indicate that personality disorders represent an important social and clinical problem.

Relation to Axis I Disorders Considerable evidence has also shown that personality disorders overlap with other types of psychological problems. For example, in the Fabrega et al. (1991) study, almost 80 percent of the people with personality disorders also received an Axis I diagnosis. Almost every major class of disorder (Clark, Watson, & Reynolds, 1995) frequently overlaps with personality disorder, including major depression and dysthymia, panic and other anxiety disorders, somatoform disorders, substance abuse disorders, and eating disorders. What's more, the presence of personality disorder is associated with greater social impairment, including poorer social support, greater severity of psychopathology, and slower and worse response to treatment (Pfohl, Black, Noyes, Coryell, & Barrash, 1991). These data support the *DSM* Task Force's decision to draw attention to the personality disorders by placing them on a separate Axis II.

Reliability

As discussed in Chapter 4, to meet scientific standards, a diagnosis must be consistent and replicable. When two clinicians each conduct diagnostic interviews with patients and show good agreement on the diagnoses they assign, **interrater reliability** has been established for that interview. If the diagnostic interviews are then repeated on another occasion, using the same set of patients, and the patients are assigned the same diagnoses, good **test-retest reliability** (also known as **temporal stability**) has been established for both the interview and the diagnoses.

A number of studies of reliability have been carried out for personality disorders. In a review of 15 studies involving 116 tests of interrater reliability, Zimmerman (1994) found that almost 60 percent showed very good reliability and that another 30 percent showed fair to moderate reliability. However, in 9 studies of test-retest reliability, rather different results were obtained (Zimmerman, 1994). In 4 studies in which the retest interval was short (within a week or so), agreement was good about 30 percent of the time and fair to moderate about 40 percent of the time. This means that there was *poor* temporal stability about 30 percent of the time.

This challenges the diagnosis of personality disorder, because (see the *DSM-IV* table, p. 380) a personality disorder should represent "an enduring pattern [that is] stable and of long duration" (American Psychiatric Association, 1994, p. 633). If the diagnosis of personality disorder shows poor temporal stability over the period of a week, how can this represent an enduring pattern?

Five studies of diagnostic test-retest reliability over longer intervals (averaging about 6 months) yielded more disturbing results (Zimmerman, 1994). High test-retest reliability was found only about 10 percent of the time. The temporal stability was fair to moderate about 30 percent of the time, and poor temporal stability was found about 60 percent of the time. Some of this instability may have occurred because the patients were in treatment. But this explanation cannot account for *all* of the unreliability, so these data raise an important question: Do stable patterns representing enduring personality styles really exist?

interrater reliability
Consistency of diagnosis or observational ratings between two or more different interviewers or raters.

test-retest reliability or **temporal stability**
Consistency of diagnosis, test scores, or observational ratings on two or more occasions.

Validity

The validity of the current categorical system of diagnosing personality disorders has been challenged repeatedly since it first appeared in 1980 (Frances, 1980; Widiger, 1993). What is the empirical basis for these challenges? First, type or categorical systems assume that individuals in the same category are highly similar—that is, that they share the essential behavioral features of their common type. However, because of the diagnostic method used in the *DSM-IV*—which stipulates that a person must exhibit at least 5 of 9 criteria—this assumption is often violated.

Let's consider some examples: Suppose that Ann Li engages in the behaviors that are described in criteria 1 through 5 for a certain personality disorder and that Susan engages in the behaviors described in criteria 5 through 9 for that same personality disorder. If that's the case, these two individuals will receive the same diagnosis, even though they have only a single behavioral criterion in common. A related issue is deciding at what point to define the presence versus absence of personality disorder. No study has ever identified any clear distinction.

A second problem with categorizing personality disorder stems from the reasonable assumption that most individuals will clearly fit into a single category. To borrow an example from biology, it's assumed that most animals can be classified as a bird *or* a fish *or* a mammal (and so forth) but not as a bird *and* a fish *and* a mammal or as a half bird/half fish or as a part fish/mostly mammal. This assumption seems reasonable because the features that characterize birds, fish, and mammals are largely nonoverlapping and mutually exclusive. If there were many fish that flew and had fur or many birds that bore live young and could swim, we might question the usefulness of classifying animals in the first place.

Unfortunately, the classification of personality disorders is not so clear cut. According to Widiger and Rogers's (1989) review, most individuals—85 percent—who meet the diagnostic criteria for one personality disorder also meet those for at least one other personality disorder. To complicate matters further, when we look more closely at the 15 percent of individuals that have only one personality disorder, we find that only 1 to 2 percent of them could be considered a **prototype** (Clark et al., 1995). Usually, prototypes are very common category members; in fact, the frequency with which they occur helps define the category. In the case of personality disorders, therefore, the rarity of prototypic cases poses a serious problem.

Another complication in categorizing personality disorders is that the most common diagnosis is actually not one of the ten described in the *DSM-IV*. Instead, the most common diagnosis is the catchall category of **personality disorder–not otherwise specified (PD–NOS).** This is sometimes referred to as *mixed* or *atypical* personality disorder. In the sample of over 18,000 clinic patients mentioned earlier, 30 percent of those with personality disorders were diagnosed as being atypical, which was more than any specific personality disorder (Fabrega et al., 1991). Given this figure, we can readily understand the difficulty of dividing personality disorders into discrete types. It's just not that simple.

Another problem with categorizing personality disorders is that the features of these disorders are hard to define. As a result, there's considerable disagreement in assigning specific diagnoses to individual patients when different methods are used. For example, Skodol, Oldham, Rosnick, Kellman, and Hyler (1991) administered two different standardized interviews for diagnosing personality disorder to 100 inpatients. Although each interview had been shown to have good interrater reliability when used by itself, agreement between the diagnoses assigned based on the two different interviews was no more than fair—only about 50 percent better than would have been obtained by randomly assigning patients to diagnoses. This state of affairs is clearly problematic for both clinical and research purposes. In short, we can have little confidence that a person diagnosed as having a specific personality disorder by one method would be diagnosed as having that same personality disorder using a different method.

Pulling these findings together, then, we can conclude the following about the diagnosis of personality disorder:

1. It's not stable over time.
2. It results in individuals with different characteristics receiving the same diagnosis.

prototype *Particularly good example of a category; one that has almost all the category's features and few features of other categories.*

personality disorder–not otherwise specified (PD–NOS) *Catchall category that includes diagnoses not specific to the ten described in the DSM-IV; sometimes referred to as mixed or atypical personality disorder.*

3. It results in some individuals with similar characteristics not receiving the same diagnosis.
4. It has no clear boundary with normality.
5. It results in most individuals receiving multiple, mixed, or atypical diagnoses.
6. It shows only fair agreement across methods.

Given these observations, we must question the validity of research results on individual personality disorders. More generally, these observations raise the question of whether it wouldn't be better to refer to a single (admittedly broad and varied) domain of personality disorder, rather than specific disorders.

Dimensional Approaches to Describing Personality Disorders

If you wanted to highlight a striking characteristic of someone you know, you might use just one or two words. But to give a full description of an individual's personality, you'd need a much longer set of terms. For example, you might describe a friend as *talkative, outgoing, impish, venturesome, generous, cooperative, helpful, spontaneous, blunt, confident, clever,* and *artistic.*

Many researchers of personality disorder believe that it might be better to use a **dimensional system,** in which an individual's personality is described using traits, rather than diagnostic types. A number of dimensional approaches have been proposed, and they offer several advantages. First is their flexibility in describing the range and complexity of people's personality problems. People who are now diagnosed with several personality disorders (that is, based on a categorical system) would simply be described by a broad range of maladaptive traits. And those persons who now receive mixed or atypical disorders would all have their own individual trait profiles.

A second advantage of dimensional over categorical approaches involves the difficulty in identifying the objective boundary between personality disorder and normality. Dimensional approaches don't solve the problem (which is that no such boundary appears to exist), but at least they explicitly recognize this fact. One intriguing proposal is to separate the assessment of *personality* from the assessment of *distress* and *dysfunction.* The latter would be used to determine the presence or absence of disorder, and the former would be used to describe the person's relevant characteristics (Livesley, Schroeder, Jackson, & Jang, 1994).

A third advantage of dimensional systems is that their use solves the mystery of how personality disorder can be defined as "stable patterns representing enduring personality styles" yet show such poor test-retest reliability. The observed unreliability is not in personality style itself; rather, it's an **artifact** of the use of arbitrary diagnostic thresholds for deciding the presence versus absence of disorder. Loranger, Lenzenweger, and colleagues (1991) tested the stability of personality disorder over a 6-month interval. When they scored their structured interview in the traditional manner, the test-retest reliabilities ranged from poor to moderate. However, when these researchers computed the number of criteria met for each diagnosis, the test-retest reliabilities were considerably higher. Studies that have used self-report questionnaires to assess dimensions of personality disorder also have obtained high test-retest reliabilities (Owen, 1994; Trull, 1993).

At this point in our discussion, it's reasonable to ask: If dimensional approaches are superior, why didn't the *DSM-IV* adopt one? One major problem is that a number of alternative models have been proposed to date, and there is not yet enough evidence to decide which is best. Switching to a dimensional approach actually was considered in developing the *DSM-IV,* but it was finally decided that such a radical change was premature, for both scientific and practical reasons. However, even Allen Frances, Chairperson of the Task Force on *DSM-IV,* has recognized that it's

dimensional system
Method of descriptive classification in which things are described using a specified set of qualities or other continuous variables; in terms of personality disorder, individuals are described according to a designated set of personality traits.

artifact Research finding that reflects a methodological problem, rather than a valid result.

TABLE 12.6 The Five-Factor Approach to Personality and Its Relation to Two Measures of Personality Disorder			
Factor	**Description**	**SNAP**	**DAPP**
Neuroticism	Temperamental *vs.* calm Anxious/depressed Angry	Negative temperament Mistrust Eccentric perceptions Self-harm	Affective lability Suspiciousness Cognitive distortion Self-harming behaviors
Extraversion vs. Introversion	Gregarious *vs.* loner Assertive *vs.* passive Warm *vs.* unfriendly	Detachment *vs.* exhibitionism Positive temperament	Social avoidance Intimacy problems Identity disturbance Restricted expression
(Dis)Agreeableness	Suspicious *vs.* trusting Ruthless *vs.* soft hearted Stingy *vs.* generous	Manipulativeness Entitlement Aggression Mistrust	Callousness Rejection Conduct problems Suspiciousness
Conscientiousness	Hardworking *vs.* lazy (Dis)Organized Oriented to work *vs.* play	Disinhibition Impulsivity *vs.* Workaholism Propriety	Stimulus seeking
Openness to Experience	Imaginative Prone to fantasy Creative	Eccentric perceptions	Cognitive distortion

five-factor approach to personality Currently popular approach to personality that describes five major traits or dimensions: Neuroticism, Extraversion, Agreeableness, Conscientiousness, and Openness to Experience.

Focus on
Critical Thinking

One of the purposes of diagnosis is to guide treatment decisions.

1. If personality diagnoses were replaced with dimensional trait descriptions, how would clinicians know what treatment to apply? Explain your answer.

2. Would insurance companies be willing (and should they be expected) to pay for the treatment of a person described only as extremely high on "Neuroticism" and low on "Conscientiousness"? Why or why not?

just a matter of time before a dimensional system is adopted for diagnosing personality disorder (Frances, 1993).

Recently, researchers of normal-range personality and personality disorder have begun to recognize the commonalities in their work and to collaborate in investigating the entire range of personality (Harkness, 1992; Watson et al., 1994). The approach that's currently most popular—the **five-factor approach to personality**—has been shown to be compatible with many others. For instance, two new multiscale instruments have been developed to assess personality-related pathology: Clark (1993) developed the Schedule for Nonadaptive and Adaptive Personality (SNAP) and Livesley and Jackson (in press) developed the Dimensional Assessment of Personality Problems Questionnaire (DAPP). Table 12.6 provides a brief description of the five-factor approach and illustrates how the more extensive sets of dimensions of the SNAP and DAPP can be aligned with each other and with the five-factor approach (Clark & Livesley, 1994; Clark, Livesley, Schroeder, & Irish, 1995).

*C*AUSES

A biopsychosocial model is quite appropriate when discussing personality disorders. *Personality* itself is often described as the combination of biological temperament and developed character (Akiskal, 1991), and most would agree that both hereditary and environmental factors are important in the development of personality disorder. The difficult part is first to identify the relevant factors in each case and then to describe how their interaction leads to disorder.

Given the tremendous overlap among different personality disorders, it's misleading to discuss the causes of each *DSM-IV* personality disorder individually. Suppose, for example, that research has found that individuals with antisocial personality disorder have histories of parental rejection. Because antisocial personality disorder significantly overlaps with borderline, narcissistic, and histrionic personality disorders, parental rejection will likely be found in the histories of individuals with these disorders, as well.

Moreover, because personality disorders have only recently been recognized formally, the literature on their causes still lacks empirical research and is often highly speculative. Other theories emphasize biological factors that we don't yet know how to measure accurately. Therefore, in discussing the causes of personality disorder, it's more fruitful to consider the various causal models in a broad and general manner, pointing out the various disorders they seem most relevant to and highlighting the data that provide some clues to the origins of these complex disorders.

Biological Factors

Siever and Davis (1991) reviewed the biological and genetic data relevant to personality disorder and outlined a comprehensive psychobiological perspective. They propose four broad dimensions to account for observed links between biological variables and personality disorder diagnoses: (1) cognitive/perceptual organization; (2) impulsivity/aggression; (3) affective instability; and (4) anxiety/inhibition. Each dimension represents a complex of biological and psychological variables. Together, they provide a useful scheme for organizing information about the neuropsychological, physiological, and genetic underpinnings of personality disorder.

1. *Cognitive/perceptual organization*—This dimension underlies the **schizophrenia spectrum**, which includes both schizophrenia and the Cluster A (odd and eccentric) personality disorders (Siever, 1992; Siever & Davis, 1991). Spectrum personality disorders are more common among first-degree relatives (parents, siblings, and children) of individuals with schizophrenia (Nigg & Goldsmith, 1994). Individuals with schizotypal personality disorder also show a particular eye movement impairment seen in schizophrenia (Siever et al., 1990) (see Chapter 13).

Siever and Davis (1991) have also suggested that difficulty in cognitive/perceptual organization could interfere with the development of satisfying relations between infants and their caregivers, which could be the starting point for the social awkwardness seen in certain personality disorders. Moreover, children of schizophrenic parents show attentional abnormalities that are associated with social detachment, another characteristic of the Cluster A personality disorders (Cornblatt & Erlenmeyer-Kimling, 1985).

2. *Impulsivity/aggression*—This dimension reflects individual differences in the degree of responsiveness to stimuli, both internal and external. Zuckerman (1991) has extensively researched a very similar dimension, which he calls *impulsive unsocialized sensation seeking*. According to Siever and Davis (1991), impulsive/aggressive individuals are action oriented and "have difficulty anticipating the effects of their behavior, learning from undesirable consequences of their previous behaviors,

schizophrenia spectrum
Range of disorders, including schizophrenia and the Cluster A (odd) personality disorders (paranoid, schizoid, schizotypal); believed to share an underlying dimension of vulnerability.

and inhibiting or delaying action appropriately" (p. 1650). These are characteristics of certain personality disorders, especially antisocial and borderline. Impulsive behavior has been linked to serious delinquency that is stable over time (White et al., 1994). Also, research has shown that individuals with psychopathic or antisocial personalities have impaired cognitive abilities (Smith, Arnett, & Newman, 1992), fail to learn from negative feedback (Patterson & Newman, 1993), and have difficulty delaying gratification (Sher & Trull, 1994) (see Thinking about Research).

Antisocial behavior in adolescents—a precursor to adult personality disorder— is strongly predicted by neuropsychological deficits (Moffitt, 1993), especially in higher-order (executive) cognitive functions. Neuropsychological dysfunction also has been found in individuals with borderline personality disorder (Judd & Ruff, 1993). Moreover, attention-deficit/hyperactivity disorder (AD/HD) in childhood (see Chapter 14) has been linked to both adolescent conduct disorder (Lilienfeld & Waldman, 1990) and adult antisocial personality disorder (Mannuzza, Klein, Bessler, & Malloy, 1993). A study of 283 male adoptees revealed that having a delinquent or criminal biological parent was associated with increased AD/HD, aggressiveness, and antisocial personality disorder in the adopted sons, suggesting a genetic basis for the observed relations (Cadoret & Stewart, 1991). Finally, both adolescent and adult antisocial (impulsive/aggressive) behaviors have been related to functional abnormalities in the neurotransmitter serotonin (Lahey, Hart, Pliszka, & Applegate, 1993; Siever & Davis, 1991). Taken together, these data describe a pattern of genetically based neurophysiological and neuropsychological abnormalities that are linked with attentional deficits and poor ability to monitor and self-regulate behavior.

Especially intriguing is the question of why more males are diagnosed with antisocial and narcissistic personality disorders whereas more females are diagnosed with borderline and histrionic personality disorders. Perhaps the different socialization experiences of men and women with impulsive/aggressive styles lead to different behavioral expressions of these traits (Lilienfeld, 1992). In any case, it's unlikely that biological factors alone will be able to account for the observed differences, providing further evidence for a biopsychosocial approach.

3. *Affective instability*—Siever and Davis (1991) relate this dimension to the mood disorders on Axis I and the personality disorders in Cluster B (especially borderline and histrionic) on Axis II. As one example of parallel biological findings between these two types of disorders, research documents similar abnormalities in brain functioning during sleep in both mood disorders and affectively unstable personality disorders (for instance, shorter and more variable times between falling asleep and the onset of the rapid eye movements associated with dreaming).

Recall from Chapter 7 on mood disorders that a great deal of research has implicated personality factors in depression. The dimension of affective instability is very similar to dysregulation in the behavioral activation system (BAS). Poor regulation of this system may explain the hyperreactive moodiness of people with Cluster B (dramatic) personality disorders. Recent research has confirmed that individual differences in mood regulation are related to reactivity of the dopaminergic system in the brain, which is involved in regulating the BAS (Depue, Luciana, Arbisi, Collins, & Leon, 1994). Moreover, twin studies have indicated that this broad dimension has a substantial genetic component as well as being influenced by environmental factors (Nigg & Goldsmith, 1994).

Akiskal (1991) proposes that many so-called personality disorders are, in fact, unrecognized manifestations of mood disorders. He describes irritable-cyclothymic and hyperthymic temperaments that closely parallel the *DSM-IV* descriptions of borderline and narcissistic personality disorders, respectively. The following excerpt describes irritable-cyclothymic patients:

> Minor provocation resulted in angry outbursts [and] the emotional storm would not abate for hours or days. . . . Interpersonal crises are further amplified by their

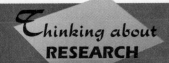
Why do psychopaths or antisocial individuals have difficulty learning from the undesirable consequences of their behaviors? One traditional explanation of psychopaths' failure to learn is that they are less sensitive to negative stimuli. Consequently, they experience little arousal (anxiety) when faced with potential punishment and so are not particularly motivated to learn (Eysenck, 1960). Similarly, Lykken (1957) showed that psychopaths were deficient in *passive-avoidance learning;* that is, they persisted in responding, even when they could avoid punishment by passively doing nothing. More recently, psychopaths have been found to have low physiological reactivity to negative visual images (Patrick, Cuthbert, & Lang, 1994).

However, evidence has shown that psychopaths learn as well as normal individuals under two conditions: (1) if the punishment is something that matters to them, like loss of money (Schmauk, 1970) and (2) if there are no conflicting demands for their attention to the consequences of their behavior (Kosson & Newman, 1986; Newman & Kosson, 1986). When psychopaths had to divide their attention between rewards and punishments or between two tasks, they performed worse than nonpsychopaths; otherwise, they performed just as well.

A second problem with the explanation of underarousal is that some psychopaths do become aroused when stressed. Fowles (1980) found this to be true, observing that psychopaths showed arousal in the form of elevated heartrates, even though they showed little arousal using measures of electrodermal responding (essentially sweating). Fowles hypothesized that these paradoxical findings result from the interaction of two underlying biological systems proposed by Gray (1970, 1987): the behavioral inhibition system (BIS) and the behavioral activation system (BAS) (see Chapter 7).

Electrodermal response is more a function of the BIS, whereas heartrate is more BAS related; thus, Fowles proposed that psychopaths have a deficit in the BIS and a normal or dominant BAS. Because the BAS and BIS are differentially oriented toward positive and negative stimuli, respectively, psychopaths pay more attention to potential rewards than punishments. Setting up the situation to increase psychopaths' attention to the negative consequences of their behavior may increase their learning by activating the BIS more strongly. Fowles's (1980) model thus appears to explain (1) the insensitivity of psychopaths to physical punishment, (2) the greater sensitivity of psychopaths to loss of rewards, (3) the effects of attention on psychopaths' learning, (4) the apparently contradictory findings regarding arousal, and (5) the action-oriented style of psychopaths.

More recently, Fowles (1993b) expanded his model to incorporate the third system Gray (1970, 1987) proposed: the **"fight or flight" system.** Doing so allowed Fowles to account for data indicating that there are two distinct anxiety systems. The first anxiety system is related to the BIS and has been variously termed *anxious apprehension* (Barlow, 1988) or *psychic anxiety* (Schalling, 1978). It may have more in common with the fourth dimension—anxiety/inhibition—proposed by Siever and Davis (1991). The second anxiety system, which is related to Gray's "fight or flight" system, might better be termed a true fear dimension; namely, it represents an unconditioned response to potentially life-threatening situations in which the organism must either fight or flee. Barlow (1988) referred to this response as an *alarm system,* whereas Schalling (1978) used the term *somatic (physical) anxiety.* The connection with psychopathy or antisocial personality disorder is that Schalling found somatic anxiety to be positively correlated with impulsivity.

Upon first impression, it seems paradoxical that psychopaths should have high somatic anxiety, since they score high on self-report measures variously entitled *danger seeking* (Tellegen, 1985), *novelty seeking* (Cloninger, 1987), and *impulsive unsocialized sensation seeking* (Zuckerman, 1991). Perhaps the problem lies in the imprecision and ambiguity of the term *anxiety.* If we discard that term and conceptualize the "fight or flight" system in terms of "readiness to act," then everything seems to fit. That is, psychopaths have a hair-trigger alarm system, are impulsive, and are perpetually ready to act ("fight or flight").

Admittedly, this is all very complicated, and the precise relationships between these systems and the dimensions proposed by Siever and Davis (1991) remain to be clarified. Nonetheless, they do offer seemingly related explanations for the same behavioral data.

Think about the following questions:

1. In psychological research, theories are stated using ordinary language (in contrast to theories in physics, for example, which are stated in mathematical language). In this box, we noted that the use of two ordinary terms—*arousal* and *anxiety*—may have created confusion in research on this topic because they were too imprecise to be used scientifically. Identify other ordinary words used in this box that also may be too imprecise to be appropriate for use in scientific research. How would you solve this problem?

2. This research on psychopaths focuses on its *biological* and *psychological* causes. What *social* influences might contribute further to the development of antisocial personality disorder in someone who is biopsychologically vulnerable to this disorder? On the other hand, what social influences might *inhibit* the development of this disorder in someone with this predisposition? Explain how these different causal factors might interact.

pouting, obtrusive, dysphoric, restless, and impulsive behavior. . . . A tempestuous life-style that creates interpersonal havoc . . . [largely due to] the volatile nature of the moods, and the erratic and high-risk behaviors. (Akiskal, 1991, pp. 47–48)

Akiskal focuses on temperament, which "emphasizes dispositions that are closest to the biological underpinnings of drive, affect, and emotion" (1991, p. 43). Nonetheless, his view is that adult personality represents the individual's adaptation to ongoing environmental experiences, given her biological predispositions. In other words, Akiskal advocates a biopsychosocial model. The case of Luanne, presented at the beginning of this chapter, illustrates how a person's basic temperament may be modified by changing life circumstances:

> At follow-up Luanne was 48 years old, divorced, and living alone in an apartment. She worked full time as a secretary. She was not thrilled with the job but managed to support herself. She was quite active socially, although most of her relationships were rather superficial. She belonged to several theater and singing groups, serving as a "den mother" for members rather than performing. She opened up her home as a "commune" of sorts where young adults who were involved in the groups would stay for short intervals, sometimes up to a month or more. She had two "faithful" women friends whom she could "trust" if she "wanted to," but never risked getting very close with them. She no longer dated, stating that she had "ruled out sex," but did have several men friends. She felt she had good relationships with her sons now that they lived in different localities. She felt much more relaxed since they had left home and were functioning well on their own. Symptomatically, Luanne experienced only slight degrees of anxiety and depression. She drank alcohol occasionally but no longer abusively. (McGlashan, 1993, p. 249)

4. *Anxiety/inhibition*—Siever and Davis (1991) associate this final dimension with the Axis I anxiety disorders and the Axis II, Cluster C personality disorders (anxious, fearful). The data linking social phobia (an anxiety disorder) with avoidant personality disorder are so strong that some argue that they represent points on a continuum, rather than separate diagnoses (Widiger & Shea, 1991).

It's fairly straightforward to match this proposed dimension with the behavioral inhibition system (BIS). As a biological system, the BIS has been linked most clearly with the personality dimension of *negative affectivity* and known as "Neuroticism" in the five-factor approach to personality described in this chapter (Fowles, 1993b). Individuals with marked negative affectivity, which includes anxiety, have an overly strong or active BIS. Because even mild stimuli represent potential threats to these individuals, they are characteristically tense, insecure, and wary. They may also appear timid, shy, cautious, and withdrawn.

The general negative affectivity represented by the anxiety/inhibition dimension appears particularly characteristic of anxiety and related personality disorders. It is not exclusively linked to these diagnoses, however, and has been associated with a wide range of mental disorders (Watson & Clark, 1984, 1994). For example, in a study of 115 patients with either anxiety disorders or recurrent depression, both avoidant and dependent personality disorders occurred with equal frequency, regardless of the Axis I disorder (Mauri et al., 1992).

If individuals with antisocial personality disorder mark one extreme of the BIS dimension and those in Cluster C anchor the other, then there should be low comorbidity between diagnoses of antisocial and Cluster C personalities—in other words, they shouldn't often occur together. Confirmation of this hypothesis was found in Widiger and Rogers's (1989) review, which reported only a 2 percent overlap of avoidant and dependent with antisocial personality disorders.

One of the exciting things about Siever and Davis's model is that it presents an opportunity to map models of personality traits onto a psychobiological

"fight or flight" system
Biological system that responds to unconditioned negative stimuli and directs an organism to action (fleeing or fighting) when threatened.

TABLE 12.7	Convergence of Selected Descriptive Models for Personality and Its Disorders

Psychobiological Models

Investigators	Dimensions			
Siever & Davis (1991)	Anxiety/inhibition	Affective instability	Impulsivity/ aggression	Cognitive/ perceptual organization
Gray (1970, 1987)	Behavioral inhibition system (BIS)	Behavioral activation system (BAS)	"Fight or flight" system	
Cloninger (1987)	Harm avoidance	Reward dependence	Novelty seeking	

Personality Trait Models

Investigators	Dimensions			
Costa & McCrae (1992) Goldberg (1992)	Neuroticism *vs.* emotional stability	Extraversion *or* surgency	Conscientiousness Agreeableness	Openness to experience, intellect, *or* culture
Tellegen (1985)	Negative emotionality	Positive emotionality	Constrait *vs.* disinhibition	

approach. Table 12.7 presents a selection of personality trait models that various researchers have proposed to account for individual differences in both normal-range personality and personality disorders. The table also shows how these models map onto Siever and Davis's psychobiological approach.

In some cases, the researchers themselves have noted parallels between their systems. For example, Tellegen (1985) has compared his dimensions to Gray's (1970, 1987) system, and Cloninger (1987) has compared his system to Tellegen's. In other cases, parallels have been suggested, based on a general understanding of these various models. A great deal of work remains to be done to develop a common system for describing normal and abnormal personality.

Psychosocial Factors

The term *psychosocial* encompasses diverse perspectives, ranging from psychoanalysis to social learning and behavioral models. Psychoanalytic contributions to understanding the development of personality disorders are built on a rich clinical tradition but lack a developed scientific research base. And cognitive-behavioral approaches have tended to rely on studies that provide more information about correlates than causes of these disorders. A psychosocial approach integrates these approaches.

The essence of the psychodynamic view is that personality types—both adaptive and maladaptive—reflect an internal, intrapsychic organization. Personality is built on an inherited constitutional basis and becomes consolidated as a conflict-resolving adaptation to our life experiences (Gunderson, 1991). Personality disorder results when this internal organization develops in a skewed manner and becomes rigidly maladaptive. Such improper development may be the result of excessive exposure to stressful and unhealthy life experiences before the person has developed the psychological resources needed to cope with them.

The *DSM-IV* diagnoses of dependent, obsessive-compulsive, and histrionic personality disorders all have their origins in early psychoanalytic theory, which emphasized conflicts between instinctual (especially sexual) drives and their inhibition through social forces. In addition, narcissistic and borderline personality disorders have been the focus of the recently developed psychoanalytic **object-relations theory,** which emphasizes the influence of early parental relationships in character development (Kernberg, 1993; Kohut, 1990). According to this theory, for example, "dependent personality evolves from parental deprivation; obsessive-compulsive traits are created from control struggles; and hysteric [histrionic] traits derive, in part, from parental seduction and competition" (Gunderson, 1991, p. 9). Moreover, "traumatically unstable parental attachments" lay the foundation for borderline personality disorder, whereas "grossly unempathic parental attachments" are critical in the development of narcissistic personality disorder (p. 9).

Attachment theory (Ainsworth & Bowlby, 1991) has also contributed to modern psychoanalytic thought by emphasizing cognitive factors in development. Current research on attachment looks at how children first form their working models of how close relationships operate. Early concepts of close relationships are then translated into models for later interactions, including those with dating and then marital partners. Children who feel securely attached to their parents handle separation well, whereas those who feel insecurely attached respond with anxiety. In later relationships, children may repeat these attachment patterns (Main & Goldwyn, 1984).

Recently, researchers have begun to investigate attachment theory in relation to personality disorder. In comparison to individuals without personality disorder, those with such disorder report more dysfunctional attachments as adults (West, Keller, Links, & Patrick, 1993) and recall their childhood relationships with their parents as being more dysfunctional (Patrick, Hobson, Castle, & Howard, 1994; Torgersen & Alnaes, 1992). But do these conclusions reflect the reality of the parent/child relationship or distorted recall, based on current psychopathology?

A study looked at relationships between mothers and teen-age daughters who did or did not have borderline personality disorder (Golomb, Ludolph, Westen, & Block, 1994). It found that the mothers of teen-agers with personality disorder tended to view their daughters as need-gratifying objects, rather than as distinct individuals. These mothers also reported more difficult and chaotic family lives than those whose daughters did not have personality disorder.

Kagan (1989b) contributed to the development of attachment theory by emphasizing the role of the child's temperament. Kagan has extensively researched the temperamental extremes of *inhibited* and *uninhibited* children, identifying the precursors of toddlers' shy behavior when they were infants as young as 4 months old (Kagan, Snidman, & Arcus, 1992). These findings further support a biopsychosocial model, because they suggest that both biologically based differences among children as well as parental behavior contribute to the quality of attachments.

Perhaps the best documented psychosocial factor in the development of personality disorder is childhood abuse. Physical, emotional, and especially sexual abuse have all been implicated in causing personality disorder, although the relationship is not at all specific. That is, childhood abuse is a risk factor for a wide range of mental disorders. Most of the research in this area has assessed childhood abuse based on adults' memories of childhood without obtaining corroborative evidence (Frankel, 1993).

Coons (1994), however, obtained objective evidence of abuse that supported the association of severe psychopathology with a history of abuse. Moreover, self-reports of past sexual abuse collected at the beginning of a prospective study predicted self-destructive behaviors (self-cutting and suicide attempts) over the next 4 years in a sample of individuals with personality disorders or bipolar II disorder (Van der Kolk, Perry, & Herman, 1991). Self-destructive behaviors and other personality characteristics of women who have been physically abused in relationships are discussed in Thinking about Social Issues.

object-relations theory
Modern version of psychoanalytic theory that stresses the influence of early parental relationships in personality development.

attachment theory Theory of personality development that emphasizes the quality of the attachment relationship between the child and the primary caregiver.

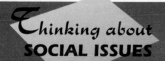

Women in physically abusive relationships are often described as having a dependent and/or self-defeating personality disorder. Many professionals feel that yet another label—the *battered woman syndrome* (Walker, 1993)—is more appropriate because many women who are physically abused don't meet the diagnostic criteria for personality disorder. What's more, use of the word *battered* attributes the disturbance to external forces, not the woman's personality—in other words, it emphasizes that the woman is the victim, not the cause, of the situation. Battered woman syndrome is not listed as a personality disorder in the *DSM-IV*, but the category *physical abuse of adult* may be used to describe a woman who is physically abused by her partner. Such a category allows clinicians to place direct emphasis on the abusive aspect of the *problem*, rather than give the *person* a diagnosis.

Other women who experience domestic violence do show signs and symptoms of depression, anxiety, and dependency. But these commonly observed problems may easily be seen as the consequences of abuse, not necessarily based in a personality disorder. In fact, there is no definitive answer as to which diagnosis, if any, best fits women who are abused. Walker (1993) has argued that the battered woman syndrome is best seen as a subcategory of posttraumatic stress disorder (PTSD), which is characterized by intense distress and intrusive memories of the stressor, accompanied by sleep disturbance and difficulty concentrating. However, only 40 percent of physically abused women have symptoms of PTSD (Cascardi, O'Leary, Lawrence, & Schlee, 1995a).

Most women who are abused lose a great deal of self-esteem, which is a significant part of why they stay in abusive situations. They're also afraid of the greater abuse that will result if they leave their partners. The following case illustrates how such women feel that they're poor wives—in fact, how everything is their fault. In addition, the case depicts how physical abuse by a partner can happen to any woman, regardless of her occupational and social status. Here, a female physician was repeatedly abused, but with a therapist's help, she was able to escape and tell her story to the American Medical Association (Whitehall, 1989, p. 3460):

I'm awake and in a sweat. I don't need to look at the clock; it's about 5 a.m., and I know I won't sleep anymore. I need all the sleep I can get to be alert for this evening. Yet my body demands I wake up and think. So, like on so many previous mornings, I will lie still here for 2 quiet hours.

What to think about? That's easy. No problem. I am unworthy, a poor excuse for a wife, just an anchor on him. But I will change—be more giving, more caring, more something. Something is wrong, and it's my fault, so I must try harder.

But my mind wanders. Get away! Don't come back! I have thought through elaborate escape plans, but I know that when I really need one I can never get away. . . .

To be on guard for tonight I must get more sleep. Silently I turn over, trying to find a more comfortable position. A bolt of pain shoots from my ear to my eyes. It is strange that even for an instant I could forget my raw left ear: For the last 3 days it has ached to use my stethoscope, but the swelling has lessened now; chewing no longer hurts. I don't dare reposition myself again, or he might wake up. I always know the day of the last beating. I always hope it was the last. But it never is. Sometimes 2 or 3 days in a row go by. Or 8 or 10 pass. . . . Then, there it is again. Yet all the beatings and bruises fade and blur with time, as do the reasons. The reason for the last one?

Perhaps I left a towel hanging crooked . . . or did I forget to turn off a light as I left a room? Maybe I wasn't paying enough attention to him while he was talking to me. . . . He says I am selfish. . . . I've been called many things . . . but never selfish! After the bad stuff is over, he tells me I should have known he didn't mean it. . . . Usually just after the beating is all over, he says such nice things. But first he sort of apologizes, something like, "You weren't listening. I had to slap you out of that foggy state. See how you're paying attention now?" Then he tells me he won't ever do it again—unless I do something mean and selfish. And he'll kiss me and say, "You're the gentlest, sweetest, prettiest woman in the world." . . . But I never know how long it will last. And why not forever? I know that's what I want. That's what he wants too, but first I must learn to care more, to love more. Yes, what a poor excuse for a wife I am. . . . Hey, it's working! My ear is just a quiet throb now. . . . Trying not to rustle the blankets, I crawl out of bed, . . . gather up my clothes and slip into the bathroom. I grab my attaché case and sneak a peek at him over my shoulder. So calm and peaceful he looks, still asleep. I will make it to work on time today. . . . I did OK this morning. I will call him at lunchtime to see how his morning has gone.

Janet A. Whitehall, M.D. [A Pseudonym]

Think about the following questions:

1. It seems crazy to remain in a relationship in which you're abused, especially if you have your own means of financial support. What psychosocial factors (other than a psychological disorder) might explain why someone would do so?

2. Some types of abnormal behavior (such as panic attacks) may result simply from being under extreme stress. In such cases, should these behaviors be considered as symptoms of disorders? Explain your answers.

Biopsychosocial Approach

Paris (1993b) proposed that biological factors act both as vulnerabilities and as limiting factors for the type of personality disorder that an individual might acquire. In other words, temperament sets the stage for the range of personality types an individual can develop. Environmental factors then interact with basic temperament to shape behavior. For example, Akiskal (1991) noted that individuals with emotionally reactive temperaments have exaggerated responses to life situations. By overreacting, they often precipitate the next crisis—perhaps an argument with a loved one—to which they again overreact and so forth. It seems likely that similar negative interactive cycles help maintain, if not develop, personality disorder.

Kochanska (1995) has offered a particularly elegant demonstration of the interaction among temperament and interpersonal factors. She demonstrated that the development of conscience in toddlers (2- and 3-year-olds) depends on how each child's temperament interacts with the quality of attachment and the mother's disciplinary style. Anxious children internalized social rules best with gentle maternal discipline, but for nonanxious children, the degree of positive attachment to the mother best predicted internalization.

An inhibited child might develop an obsessive-compulsive style under harsh parental discipline, anxiously trying not to do anything wrong and displease the harsh parent. On the other hand, an uninhibited child with poor parental attachment might fail to internalize social rules and so develop an antisocial behavioral style. The interaction of other psychosocial factors might further modify these pathways so that dependent or narcissistic traits developed, as well.

Paris (1993b) also incorporates social factors into his model. In particular, he notes that social disintegration—family disruption, weak community associations, poverty—has a general relation to psychopathology. Moreover, he speculates that social disintegration might affect certain personality types—for example, the impulsive/aggressive character—more than others. Periods of rapid social change may prove particularly difficult for individuals with a vulnerability on the cognitive/perceptual dimension. Those high on anxiety/inhibition may function poorly in times of ambiguous social rules.

Three key points may be summarized from Paris's (1993b) work. First, personality traits or temperaments have a strong genetic component. Since these traits or temperaments form the basis of personality disorder, it has a genetic component, as well. Second, negative childhood experiences place individuals at risk for various disorders, as shown in the general association of sexual abuse with later psy-

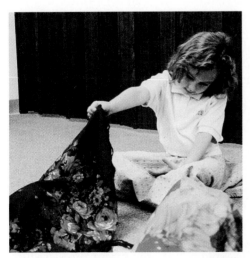 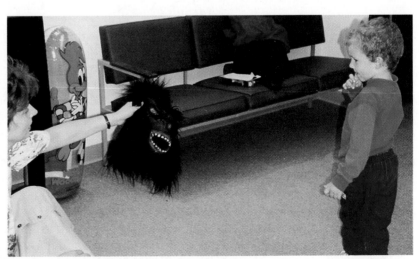

Grazyna Kochanska has studied how temperament, attachment, and maternal discipline interact in the development of conscience. **Left,** *a girl succumbs to the temptation to peek at a hidden toy;* **Right,** *a younger boy expresses some hesitation when Dr. Kochanska shows him a gorilla mask.*

chopathology. Specifically, most people with personality disorder report problems in interactions with their parents. And third, social changes and social disintegration—family disruption, poverty, and weak associations with the community—also place individuals at risk for personality disorder. Particular types of social changes may have different effects on individuals with different vulnerabilities.

For any particular individual, the clinician has to assess the extent to which the biological, psychological, and social factors contribute to the problems that individual reports. Fortunately for individuals with such problems, it's now widely acknowledged that one discipline is usually not enough to understand a particular problem. Therefore, in many psychiatric hospitals, a team approach is used, in which a psychiatrist, a clinical psychologist, and a social worker together address the biological, psychological, and social factors that appear important in each case.

> ### Focus on Critical Thinking
>
> **1.** How could the biopsychosocial approach be used to explain the high degree of overlap among different personality disorders?
>
> **2.** Think of an example from your own experience that illustrates how two people with different personalities adapt differently to the same stressful situation. Now imagine how these two people might turn out differently in the long run if the stressor were chronic. Could one of these people adapt well, while the other developed something like a personality disorder? Or could they both adapt poorly but in different ways? Explain your answers.

TREATMENT

For many years, the most common treatment for personality disorder was psychodynamic psychotherapy. Recently, new types of treatments—both psychosocial and psychopharmacological—have been developed. Although controlled treatment studies are exceedingly rare, several of these new therapies appear promising.

One complication in treating personality disorder is that it occurs with Axis I disorders more often than alone. So in most cases, clinicians are faced with the simultaneous treatment of two or more different types of disorders. Moreover, a recent review (Reich & Vasile, 1993) reported that in study after study, regardless of what the Axis I disorder is—substance abuse, depression, anxiety, eating disorder, and so forth—when the patient has personality disorder, as well, treatment is slower, more difficult, and more likely to result in drop-out. With few exceptions, the clinical and research literature on the treatment of personality disorders has ignored the fact that these disorders are highly overlapping.

Pharmacotherapy

The vast majority of pharmacotherapy (drug treatment) studies for Axis II diagnoses have involved borderline personality disorder. A wide array of drugs have been tested, including neuroleptics (for psychoticlike symptoms), various types of antidepressants, lithium (for manic symptoms), carbamazepine (for behavioral dyscontrol), and benzodiazepines (for anxiety). There may be no drug of choice for treating borderline personality disorder and drugs should be used selectively for the short-term treatment of specific problems, rather than by diagnosis (Soloff, 1993). Affective dysregulation, impulsive aggression, cognitive distortion, and anxiety—the four dimensions discussed by Siever and Davis (1991)—were specifically mentioned as areas in which to target symptoms.

Because generalized social phobia overlaps considerably with avoidant personality disorder, researchers are examining the impact of drug treatments for social phobia on personality features. Monoamine oxidase inhibitors (MAOIs), used in the treatment of depression, have been found effective (Liebowitz, Schneier, Hollander, & Welkowitz, 1991). Traditional antianxiety drugs reduce anxiety symptoms—until the medication is discontinued (Mattick & Newman, 1991). More generally, research suggests that drug maintenance treatment for personality disorder is of limited value (Soloff, 1993).

Because drugs by themselves do not affect the rigid character pathology found in personality disorder, combined pharmacotherapy and psychotherapy is often recommended (Mattick & Newman, 1991; Soloff, Cornelius, & George, 1991; Stein, 1992). When we acknowledge that personality disorders have biopsychosocial origins, it follows that multimodal treatment may be needed to address their diverse problem areas (Stone, 1990).

Psychodynamic Psychotherapy

Freud argued that narcissists could not be helped by psychoanalysis because they were unable to form the necessary close relationship with the therapist. However, modern psychoanalysts, particularly object-relations theorists, have focused primarily on the treatment of narcissistic and borderline personality disorders. Kohut (1990) believed that everyone has narcissistic needs in childhood and that pathological narcissism develops when these needs are not fulfilled. Therapy, therefore, involves getting in touch with and accepting these unfulfilled needs, which have become deeply repressed, "guarded by a wall of shame and vulnerability" (p. 382).

Borderline pathology is viewed as the more serious of the two types, because it involves disintegration of psychic organization, which is the basis for transient psychotic or dissociative episodes and intense swings in mood and interpersonal relations. Kernberg (1993) has summarized several common points of psychoanalytic treatment of this disorder:

1. The rules and boundaries of treatment must be clearly established.
2. Therapists must be active, rather than traditional, passive interpreters.
3. Therapists must tolerate patients' deep sadness and hostility.
4. Therapists must help patients see the connections between actions and feelings.
5. Self-destructive behavior must be discouraged by confrontation.
6. Limits must be set on patients' dangerous, risk-taking behaviors.
7. The emphasis should be on the therapeutic relationship more than the past.
8. Therapists must be alert to their own reactions to patients.

Treatment drop-out is common, and it's increasingly recognized that intermittent, rather than continual, treatment may be the norm for severe personality disorder (Paris, 1993a). Length of continuation in treatment is increased by a positive therapeutic relationship but decreased in more impulsive patients (Yeomans, Gutfreund, Selzer, & Clarkin, 1994). It seems that individuals with borderline personality disorder go in and out of therapy as life's crises—and their ability to handle them—come and go.

Interpersonal Psychotherapy

Interpersonal therapies often trace their origins to Sullivan's (1953) neo-Freudian interpersonal psychiatry. For personality disorders, the most notable application of interpersonal therapy is Benjamin's (1993) structural analysis of social behavior (SASB) approach. In contrast to static trait models, Benjamin's SASB method analyzes the interaction of several intrapsychic and interpersonal dimensions to explain behavioral *processes* involved in personality disorder. The SASB analytical approach is a rich and comprehensive system that has evolved over 20 years of clinical research, but the associated treatment has not yet been subjected to a controlled study of its effectiveness. The treatment stresses:

1. developing a collaborative therapeutic relationship
2. gaining an understanding of one's destructive interaction patterns
3. deciding to give up these destructive patterns and dealing with the negative emotions (sadness, fear) that follow that decision
4. eventual emergence of a new self, defined by more adaptive interpersonal behaviors

Cognitive Therapy

Cognitive therapy has recently been applied to treating people with personality disorder (Beck, Freeman, & Associates, 1990). The core assumption is that particular errors in thinking are responsible for individuals' behavioral and emotional problems. Patient and therapist collaborate in discovering the patient's particular cognitive distortions and replacing them with more adaptive and realistic cognitions. For example, dysfunctional cognitions in an obsessive-compulsive individual might be "I must avoid mistakes to be worthwhile," "Without rules and regulations, I am paralyzed," and "If I'm not positive it's perfect, I'd better do it over."

As cognitive therapy has evolved, it has incorporated behavioral techniques, role-play, imagery, and even reviewing childhood experiences (Beck et al., 1990). Like other therapies for personality disorder, cognitive therapy suffers from the common problem of patient drop-out. Controlled studies evaluating its effectiveness in treating personality disorder remain to be done.

Behavior Therapy

Behavior therapy has been used in more controlled treatment studies of personality disorder than any other treatment. Shea (1993) reports that most of them involved social skills training and/or graduated exposure for individuals with extreme shyness, social avoidance, and other social deficits. Most studies reported improvement among individuals who received treatment. However, changes were sometimes limited to more superficial relationships, and normal levels of functioning and emotional well-being often were not attained.

Treatment outcome may be improved by matching specific patient characteristics with type of treatment (Alden & Capreol, 1993). Specifically, these researchers found that graduated exposure (but not skills training) was helpful for those patients whose interpersonal problems involved mistrust and anger, whereas both procedures helped those who had problems with being controlled by other people. These data again support the idea that trait dimensions, rather than diagnoses per se, provide the most useful information for understanding personality disorder.

Dialectical Behavior Therapy

The most promising new treatment for severely dysfunctional personality pathology is Linehan's (1993) **dialectical behavior therapy (DBT).** DBT is unique in that it blends aspects of psychodynamic, client-centered, strategic, interpersonal, cognitive-behavioral, and crisis intervention approaches into a coherent theoretical orientation (Linehan & Kehrer, 1993). Because it is an explicitly biopsychosocial approach, DBT assumes that personality disorder results from multiple causes. Dysfunction of the emotional regulation system (that is, affective instability) is seen as the core of borderline personality disorder. In order for a personality disorder to develop, though, this constitutional factor must interact with what Linehan has called **invalidating environments**—those that "negate and/or respond erratically and inappropriately to private experience" (Linehan & Kehrer, 1993, p. 402). Parents provide an invalidating environment when they trivialize their children's feelings; continually attribute their children's behavior to laziness, meanness, manipulativeness, or other socially unacceptable characteristics; emphasize the control rather than the appropriate expression of emotions; and oversimplify how easily children should be able to cope with difficult situations. Sexual abuse is the prototypic invalidating experience for individuals with severe personality disorders.

A child who grows up in an invalidating environment has fewer chances to learn how to identify, label, and react appropriately to his own emotional experiences. Thus, a primary emphasis of DBT is *acceptance* of individuals and their

dialectical behavior therapy (DBT) Treatment approach that blends aspects of psychodynamic, client-centered, strategic, interpersonal, cognitive-behavioral, and crisis intervention approaches into a coherent theoretical orientation; assumes that personality disorders result from multiple causes.

invalidating environments Interpersonal environments in which significant others (such as parents) negate and/or respond erratically and inappropriately to an individual's private emotional experiences.

experiences. According to DBT, however, acceptance alone is not sufficient for healing; acceptance must be balanced with a corresponding emphasis on *change*. Use of the word *dialectic* in the title of this therapeutic approach refers particularly to the interplay between acceptance and change.

DBT consists of a pretreatment (commitment) phase and three treatment stages: (1) stability, connection, and safety; (2) exposure and emotional processing of the past; and (3) synthesis. Orienting the individual to therapy is the focus of the pretherapy commitment phase. Recognizing the high drop-out potential of patients with personality disorder, an important goal at this point is to gain the client's commitment.

Stage 1, the first actual therapy stage, has multiple components; completing it successfully can take up to a year or more. Early targets for change include decreasing suicidal behaviors, followed by decreasing behaviors that interfere with therapy (such as not attending sessions) and quality of life (substance abuse, impulsive job switching, participation in abusive relationships) and then increasing a whole range of behavioral/emotional skills: tolerating distress (without feeling the need to make suicidal gestures), dealing with interpersonal conflict, and increasing positive (healthy, enjoyable) behaviors.

Like stage 1, stage 2 is also cognitive-behavioral, but it focuses on remembering and accepting past traumas without intolerably intense rage or self-blame. In particular, stage 2 uses graduated exposure techniques like those for posttraumatic stress disorder (PTSD) and other anxiety disorders. Finally, stage 3, synthesis, most resembles psychodynamic therapy. It focuses on increasing individuals' self-respect and independent goal achievement.

DBT is the only personality disorder treatment study to randomize patients to experimental and control conditions. Long-term follow-up showed DBT to be as or often more effective than "treatment-as-usual in the community" on various outcome measures, such as suicidal attempts and social adjustment (Linehan et al., 1991; Linehan et al., 1994). Moreover, Shearin and Linehan (1992) provided data supporting the theoretical basis of this treatment. Using Benjamin's (1993) SASB technique to assess psychotherapy process, they demonstrated that dialectical techniques balancing acceptance and change were more effective than pure change or pure acceptance techniques in reducing suicidal behavior. This is a very important step in therapy research because it helps us understand *how* therapy works to improve individuals' lives.

Finally, the biopsychosocial orientation of DBT is a model for understanding and treating personality disorder. The integration of concepts and techniques from a wide variety of therapies into a coherent theoretical approach represents a significant advance that deserves broad emulation.

Focus on Critical Thinking

1. Diagnosis is usually very important in deciding on a treatment approach. What role does (and should) diagnosis play in the treatment of personality disorder? Explain your answers.

2. Drop-out is a major problem in treating people with personality disorder. For the purpose of evaluating a treatment, should drop-outs be considered treatment failures? Why or why not?

SUMMARY

Personality and Personality Disorders

■ Personality disorder is diagnosed when an individual's traits are extreme, inflexible, and maladaptive. This type of disorder is hard to treat and may impact every aspect of a person's life—emotional, interpersonal, and occupational.

■ Personality disorder has been studied scientifically since the 1800s.

■ Personality disorders are diagnosed using a categorical system, in which a few prominent characteristics are used to define a limited number of types.

Description

- In the *DSM-IV,* 10 personality disorders are divided into three broad clusters, based on certain descriptive similarities.
- Cluster A (odd and eccentric) includes the paranoid, schizoid, and schizotypal personality disorders.
- Cluster B (dramatic, emotional, and erratic) includes the antisocial, borderline, histrionic, and narcissistic personality disorders.
- Cluster C (anxious and fearful) includes the avoidant, dependent, and obsessive-compulsive personality disorders.

Issues and Problems in Categorizing Personality Disorders

- Personality disorder is fairly common, with a lifetime prevalence of about 10 to 13 percent. Currently, borderline personality disorder is the most commonly diagnosed.
- Personality disorder occurs frequently with nearly every major class of psychopathology. When personality disorder is present, the co-occurring Axis I disorder is usually harder to treat.
- Clinicians tend to agree on personality diagnoses, but only if they use the same diagnostic interview simultaneously. If they use different interviews or interview an individual at different times, diagnostic reliability is only fair.
- There are many problems with the validity of diagnosing personality disorder, especially the findings that few individuals represent clear, prototypic cases and that most individuals with personality disorder either have multiple disorders or are mixed or atypical cases.
- Trait-dimensional approaches to describing personality disorder hold promise, but no one system has yet been agreed on. The five-factor approach to personality is currently the most popular.

Causes

- Siever and Davis (1991) have proposed a comprehensive psychobiological model for personality disorder consisting of four broad dimensions: cognitive/perceptual organization, impulsivity/aggression, affective instability, and anxiety/inhibition.
- Many psychosocial models have been proposed to help explain the origins of personality disorder, but a great deal remains to be learned. Object-relations theory is a modern psychoanalytic model that emphasizes early parental relationships; attachment theory further emphasizes cognitive factors in development.
- Childhood abuse is a powerful negative influence, not only on the development of personality disorder but on many other types of disorder, as well.
- A biopsychosocial approach is especially appropriate for addressing what causes personality disorder; several related models emphasize that temperament and experience interact in the development of both normal and abnormal personality.

Treatment

- Pharmacotherapy is used effectively to treat some symptoms of personality disorder but is not a cure.
- Psychodynamic psychotherapy has long been the treatment of choice for personality disorder and is one of the most developed approaches in theoretical terms. However, in part because it is a long-term treatment, controlled studies of the effectiveness of this approach have not been carried out.
- Interpersonal, cognitive, and behavior therapies all are being used increasingly in treating people with personality disorder. Each approach has generated a small body of research that provides some support for its effectiveness.
- The most promising therapy for severe personality disorder is dialectical behavior therapy (DBT), which has a biopsychosocial theoretical base and research support for its effectiveness.

KEY TERMS

antisocial personality disorder, **p. 383**

artifact, **p. 394**

attachment theory, **p. 401**

avoidant personality disorder, **p. 387**

borderline personality disorder, **p. 384**

categorical system, **p. 381**

dependent personality disorder, **p. 388**

dialectical behavior therapy (DBT), **p. 406**

dimensional system, **p. 394**

"fight or flight" system, **pp. 398–399**

five-factor approach to personality, **p. 395**

histrionic personality disorder, **p. 386**

interrater reliability, **p. 392**

invalidating environments, **p. 406**

narcissistic personality disorder, **p. 386**

object-relations theory, **p. 401**

obsessive-compulsive personality disorder, **p. 390**

paranoid personality disorder, **p. 381**

personality, **p. 380**

personality disorder, **p. 380**

personality disorder–not otherwise specified (PD–NOS), **p. 393**

prototype, **p. 393**

psychopathy, **p. 384**

schizoid personality disorder, **p. 382**

schizophrenia spectrum, **p. 396**

schizotypal personality disorder, **p. 382**

test-retest reliability *or* temporal stability, **p. 392**

CRITICAL THINKING EXERCISE

Consider the following case:

> Jeffrey was a single 21-year-old when admitted to Chestnut Lodge in the mid-1960s. Difficulties became apparent when he was in college, marked by falling grades, anxiety, and difficulty concentrating. Jeffrey was socially isolated, and he alienated peers with his rudeness and arrogant intellectualizing. After being evicted from a dormitory suite, he lived alone. He never dated, nor did he participate in school activities. Jeffrey began outpatient psychotherapy, but after the first of three suicide attempts at age 19, he had to be hospitalized. Eight hospitalizations followed, mostly for manipulative suicidal gestures, in between which he became more and more anxious and nonfunctional. At index admission, Jeffrey was described as unrealistically demanding, rejecting, and unable to tolerate criticism or change. He was often depressed and suicidal and complained of loneliness. Socially, he was initially cold, superficial, and suspicious. Jeffrey was also prone to anxiety attacks and was intensely disturbed by therapy, during which he would regress to abject dependency upon the therapist, whom he would begin calling at all hours of the day and night.
>
> After several months of inpatient treatment, Jeffrey was discharged from Chestnut Lodge while AWOL [absent without leave]. Thereafter, he traveled for 6 months, allegedly to find jobs, but found none. He returned to the Rockville area to visit staff and patients at Chestnut Lodge. After tutoring math at a local university for two years, he returned home and entered college full time. (McGlashan, 1993, p. 242)

Both Jeffrey (described here) and Luanne (from the chapter-opening case) were given the diagnosis of borderline personality disorder by the clinical researchers (McGlashan, 1993) at Chestnut Lodge who treated and studied them throughout their lives.

1. What features of this diagnosis did Jeffrey and Luanne share? How were their personality problems different?

2. Was it useful to diagnose these two people with the same personality disorder? Why or why not?

3. How would each be described using one of the dimensional approaches in Table 12.6?

4. What would be the advantages and disadvantages of a dimensional description in these individuals' cases? Explain your answer.

*C*hapter *13*
SCHIZOPHRENIA

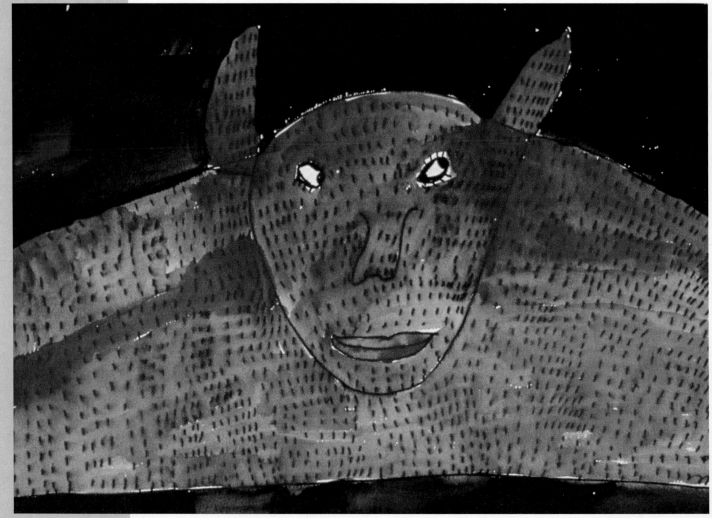

Helen Kossoff, **Untitled,** HAI

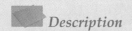

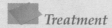
In December 1994, the Nobel Prize in Economics was awarded to John Forbes Nash, Jr. "The award was a miracle. It wasn't just that Nash, one of the mathematical geniuses of the postwar era, was finally getting the recognition he deserved. Or that he was being honored for a slender, twenty-seven-page Ph.D. thesis written almost half a century ago at the tender age of twenty-one.

"The real miracle was that the sixty-six-year-old Nash—tall, gray, with sad eyes and the soft, raspy voice of someone who doesn't talk much—was alive and well enough to receive the prize. For John Nash had been stricken with paranoid schizophrenia more than three decades earlier.

"Nash's terrible illness was an open secret among mathematicians and economists. No sooner had *Fortune* magazine singled him out in July 1958 as America's brilliant young star of the 'new mathematics' than the disease had devastated Nash's personal and professional life. He hadn't published a scientific paper since 1958. He hadn't held an academic post since 1959. Many people had heard, incorrectly, that he had had a lobotomy. Others, mainly those outside Princeton, simply assumed that he was dead.

"He didn't die, but his life, once so full of brightness and promise, became hellish. There were repeated commitments to psychiatric hospitals. Failed treatments. Fearful delusions. A period of wandering around Europe. Stretches in Roanoke, Virginia, where Nash's mother and sister lived. Finally, a return to Princeton, where he had once been the rising star. There he became the Phantom of Fine Hall, home of the mathematics department, a mute figure who scribbled strange equations on blackboards and searched anxiously for secret messages in numbers.

"Then, roughly ten years ago, the terrible fires that fed the delusions and distorted his thinking began to die down. It happened very gradually. But by his mid-fifties, Nash began to come out of his isolation. He started to talk to other mathematicians again. He began to work on mathematical problems that made sense. He made friends with several graduate students. He didn't get a job, or start driving a car, or travel abroad—the things he would have taken for granted if life had taken a different course—but he started to learn new things, like using computers for his research. . . .

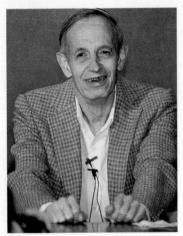

John Nash, a 1994 Nobel Prize winner, who had schizophrenia

"On one level, John Nash's story is the tragedy of any person with schizophrenia. Incurable, incapacitating, and extremely difficult to treat, schizophrenia plays terrible, often terrifying tricks on its victims. Many people with the disease can no longer sort and interpret sensations or reason or feel the full range of emotions. Instead, they suffer from delusions and hear voices.

"But in Nash's case, the tragedy has the added dimensions of his early genius—and of the network of family and friends who valued that genius, wrapping themselves protectively around Nash and providing him with a safe haven while he was ill. There were the former colleagues who tried to get him work. The sister who made heartbreaking choices about his treatment. The loyal wife who stood by him when she no longer was his wife. The economist who argued to the Nobel committee that mental illness shouldn't be a bar to the prize. Princeton itself.

"Together they made sure that Nash did not wind up, as so many victims of schizophrenia do, a patient in a state mental hospital, a homeless nomad, or a suicide" (Nasar, 1994, p. III–1).

As you will soon see, schizophrenia debilitates many people. Like Dr. Nash, they do not function effectively for years. In the 1950s and 1960s, many schizophrenics were hospitalized for decades. However, the prevalent view of a disorder with a continual downward course is changing. Fortunately, like Dr. Nash, many individuals with a schizophrenic disorder eventually function without signs of schizophrenia.

For decades, professionals described schizophrenics as **psychotic**—that is, as not being able to know what is real and what is not real. "They lose touch with reality." For example, often schizophrenics hear "voices," which they experience as real, commanding them to do things. Or they may think people are trying to poison them. According to the fourth edition of the *Diagnostic and Statistical Manual of Mental Disorders (DSM-IV)*, there is no single accepted use of the term *psychotic* (American Psychiatric Association, 1994)—but when one uses the term *psychotic* to describe symptoms of schizophrenia, it refers to delusions (a belief contrary to reality, like "the government is trying to kill me"); hallucinations (perceptions without adequate stimuli, such as hearing voices); disorganized speech; or disorganized behavior.

psychotic Out of touch with reality; showing delusions, hallucinations, and disorganized speech/behavior.

dementia praecox Term coined by Emil Kraepelin, meaning "premature dementia," to describe the psychotic disorder now called schizophrenia.

Description

The story of schizophrenia really begins with Emil Kraepelin (1856–1926), professor of psychiatry in Munich, Germany, who first described schizophrenia. In 1889, Kraepelin grouped several types of mental abnormalities under one heading—**dementia praecox**—the early term for schizophrenia. The term *dementia praecox* literally meant "premature dementia." Kraepelin believed that all dementia praecox involved personality deterioration, and he identified three subtypes: *catatonia*, *hebephrenia* (called *disorganized schizophrenia* in the *DSM-IV*), and *paranoia*. He later adopted a fourth type of dementia praecox from another researcher, Eugen Bleuler, called *simple schizophrenia*. According to Kraepelin (1896; published in 1971), the cause of this disease became evident only during laboratory examination of the brain after the person died (that is, postmortem brain analysis). He believed that changes in the brain were the primary cause of dementia praecox and that psychological factors were of secondary importance in its cause. Kraepelin suggested the disorder started in early adolescence and had a chronic (prolonged) course because of the brain's deterioration.

Modern views about the onset and prognosis of schizophrenia differ from those of Kraepelin. Most hospital admissions for schizophrenia occur in late adolescence and early adulthood, but the first schizophrenic episode can occur at almost any point in life. As you might expect, late-onset schizophrenic patients are more likely to have married, held jobs, and had numerous social interactions (Jeste & Heaton,

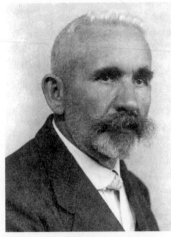

EMIL KRAEPELIN, *a German psychiatrist, coined the term* dementia praecox *and was among the first to classify mental disorders.*

1994). Many individuals with schizophrenia suffer more than one serious episode, although they may also experience long symptom-free periods. Despite inadequacies, Kraepelin's careful descriptions of symptoms and disorders were very influential, as evidenced by the eight editions of his textbook *Clinical Psychiatry* (1915).

Swiss psychiatrist Eugen Bleuler (1857–1939)—who coined the term *schizophrenia* in 1908, disagreed with Kraepelin about some important features of the disorder. Bleuler (1911/1950), who was influenced by Sigmund Freud (1856–1939), argued that schizophrenia does not necessarily have an early onset and that it does not inevitably lead to mental deterioration. In contrast to Kraepelin, Bleuler believed that recovery was possible. Like Kraepelin, however, Bleuler believed an individual's biological makeup plays an important role in causing schizophrenia and that, consequently, the disorder is likely to recur. Bleuler also believed that environmental stress interacts with an individual's biological makeup to produce schizophrenic symptoms. According to this theory, treatment should focus on decreasing the impact of stress on the individual.

Bleuler placed less emphasis on the prognosis of schizophrenia than Kraepelin did, and he attempted to identify an underlying psychological feature of the disorder. Bleuler believed that the common feature in schizophrenia involves a loosening of associations, or connections, between thoughts and feelings. According to Bleuler, the breaking of these hypothetical associations results in the disrupted and unusual behavior observed in schizophrenic patients.

The most common misconception about schizophrenia is that it refers to people with so-called split personalities. The syndrome of split or multiple personalities portrayed in popular movies such as *The Three Faces of Eve* and *Sybil* is extremely rare and differs from schizophrenia. In the *DSM-IV* (American Psychiatric Association, 1994), multiple personality is classified as a *dissociative identity disorder*, in which a person has two or more separate ego states that have little or no contact with each other (see Chapter 6). Each personality exists independently of the others and has a unique set of emotional and behavioral styles. Persons with multiple personalities may complain of being controlled by voices or by other people, as may persons with schizophrenia. However, someone with multiple personalities displays two or more highly developed personalities, as if two or more individuals were coexisting in the same body. In contrast, someone with schizophrenia experiences a splitting of thoughts and feelings.

Prevalence

Approximately 1 percent of the population develops schizophrenia during their lifetime. Although this figure may seem small in comparison to the prevalence of affective disorders (for example, major depressive disorder), schizophrenia has severe negative effects on behavior. People are incapacitated or maintain a low level of functioning because of schizophrenia. People diagnosed with schizophrenia are the major users of psychiatric hospital beds in the United States. To give you a comparison of the prevalence of schizophrenia with that of another very serious psychiatric problem, 1 out of every 200 people (0.5 percent) develops a bipolar mood disorder, but often people with bipolar disorders are not hospitalized.

As noted earlier, schizophrenia most often strikes young people, usually developing between ages 16 and 25. Schizophrenia develops much less frequently after age 35 (Mueser & Gingerich, 1994). The median age of first hospital admission for schizophrenia is in the mid-20s for men and in the late 20s for women (American Psychiatric Association, 1994). (These differences in age of onset between men and women, along with other gender-related topics, are examined more closely in Thinking about Gender Issues.) Recent evidence has indicated that, in contrast to many physical illnesses—in which the symptomatology worsens over time—the symptomatology of schizophrenia tends to decrease with age. That is, persons

Schizophrenia affects approximately equal numbers of males and females. However, the age of first hospital admission in the United States and Europe tends to differ for males and females. Up to age 30, the rates are much higher for males, whereas after age 30, they are much higher for females (Jeste & Heaton, 1994; Zigler & Levine, 1981). In adolescence, the male/female ratio of first admissions is about 2:1, whereas at 55 to 60 years, the male/female ratio is about 1:2 (see Figure 13.1).

Adolescent males are at higher risk for schizophrenia than adolescent females. We don't know why these gender differences in incidence occur in the teen years. Some investigators believe that they result primarily from differential social roles and expectations for young boys and girls in our society. Some experts feel boys are more likely to be hospitalized earlier because parents and teachers may react more strongly to disordered behavior in boys than in girls. Also, adolescent males with schizophrenia are more prone to act aggressively than their female counterparts. Other researchers hypothesize that the later onset for women could be due to biological factors. For example, females may be protected by high levels of estrogen (Jeste & Heaton, 1994). In fact, many women with schizophrenia exhibit a reduction in psychotic symptoms during pregnancy (Chang & Renshaw, 1986).

The course of the disorder also differs for men and women. Women, who tend to have the later onset of schizophrenia, have more mood or depressive symptoms and have a better prognosis. They are more likely to have married and held jobs, and they may have developed better support systems by the time they develop schizophrenia.

Think about the following questions:

1. Which of the five major symptoms of schizophrenia (described earlier) might be better tolerated by females than males? Explain your answer.
2. Which, if any, of the biochemical or hormonal explanations of schizophrenia best explains the different ages of onset for males versus females? Again, explain your answer.

FIGURE 13.1   Male and female admissions

Male and female schizophrenia admissions to psychiatric hospitals differ by age group. At younger ages, males predominate, whereas at older ages, females do.

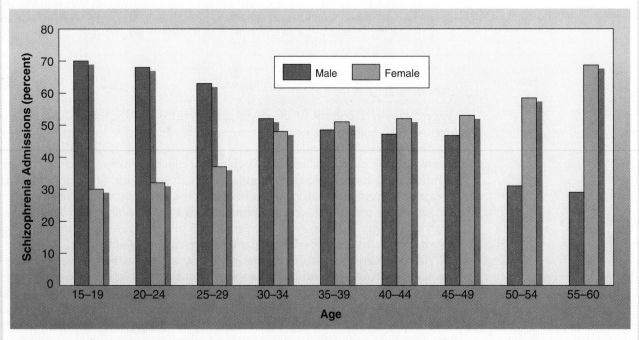

Source: Adapted from D. Rosenthal, "Genetic Research in the Schizophrenic Syndrome," in R. Canero (Ed.), *The Schizophrenic Reactions* (pp. 245–258), 1970, New York: Brunner/Mazel.

414

diagnosed as schizophrenic early in life often exhibit few signs of the disorder by the time they reach their 50s and 60s.

The old view that persons with schizophrenia typically go downhill throughout their lives has been challenged by scientific data collected throughout the world. In a study of the long-term course of schizophrenia in the 1970s, Manfred Bleuler—the son of Eugen Bleuler—found that, on average, individuals diagnosed with schizophrenia showed no further deterioration after five years (Bleuler, 1974). In fact, symptoms tended to improve. In addition, no matter how many years after onset, the proportion of those who improved relative to those who did not improve remained the same as 5 years after onset. But on average, individuals with schizophrenia in the Bleuler study spent about one-third of their lives inside the hospital. Although this may have seemed a grim prospect in the 1970s, it was more promising than previous studies had estimated.

Now consider the follow-up research of social worker Dr. Courtenay Harding and her colleagues (1987) at Yale University and the University of Vermont. Because Vermont is a small state with only one state psychiatric hospital, Harding had excellent access to the records of most Vermont residents who had been hospitalized with schizophrenia in the 1950s. These patients had participated in a specialized vocational rehabilitation program to address their chronic disabilities and resistance to treatment. They were described as "back ward" patients, "middle-aged, poorly-educated, lower class individuals further impoverished by repeated and long hospitalizations" (p. 727). With the introduction of antipsychotic medication, however, most of these patients were eventually discharged from the hospital.

Approximately 25 years later, in the early 1980s, Harding and her colleagues attempted to locate these patients and see how they were doing. Eighty-one of the 118 individuals (70 percent) formerly diagnosed with schizophrenia were interviewed; 28 were deceased, and 4 refused to be interviewed. Those interviewed presented a hopeful picture of the long-term outcome of schizophrenia. When interviewed, most of the individuals had prescriptions for antipsychotic medications, but many were not taking the drugs as prescribed. Only half of the former patients took the antipsychotic medications regularly. Nevertheless, a full 45 percent of the persons interviewed did not exhibit any signs of schizophrenia. Approximately two-thirds of the sample was functioning very well. The majority of the sample were able to meet their daily living needs, met with friends every week or two, and had not been recently hospitalized.

Harding's results seem more hopeful than those of Manfred Bleuler, discussed earlier, because of her depiction of the sample as doing "very well." Further, research from two studies of older individuals who had been diagnosed as schizophrenic has indicated that deterioration usually occurs shortly after the first episode and is often limited to the first 5 to 10 years of the illness (Belitsky & McGlashen, 1993). In sum, schizophrenia is not always a deteriorating illness, and in some cases, there is substantial improvement. Nonetheless, for many individuals, schizophrenia is a severe, chronic disorder.

We've just been discussing how individuals with schizophrenia in the United States often appear to get better with time. Now let's look at some factors that may relate to that recovery in different locales and parts of the world. Long-term outcome is better in persons who develop schizophrenia in non-Western countries (such as Ghana) than in Western ones (Germany, Sweden, United States). A greater proportion of persons with schizophrenia in non-Western countries seem to have complete recovery (Jablensky, 1989). Some argue that the outcome is better in non-Western countries because the responsibility of caring for the individual diagnosed with schizophrenia is often shared by a community. In addition, people in non-Western countries may have greater acceptance of others with unusual behaviors. This acceptance, in turn, may promote recovery.

In the United States, schizophrenia occurs most commonly in the Northeast and Pacific Northwest (Torrey & Bowler, 1990). It's more frequently seen in urban, rather than rural, areas and among people of lower socioeconomic status. Schizophrenia is especially prevalent among the urban poor (Hollingshead & Redlich, 1958; Kohn, 1968; Torrey & Bowler, 1990). Ethnicity does not appear to be a factor in the development of the disorder (Torrey & Bowler, 1990). We'll cover issues of social class and schizophrenia in a separate section, later in this chapter.

Definition and Symptoms

The definition of schizophrenia has been evolving since the early efforts of Kraepelin and Bleuler. The American Psychiatric Association's *DSM-IV* (1994) criteria for a diagnosis of **schizophrenia** include two of the following five classic symptoms, which must be evident for at least 6 months and have a marked effect on social and work relations: (1) delusions, (2) hallucinations, (3) disorganized speech, (4) grossly disorganized or catatonic behavior, and (5) negative symptoms. The complete diagnostic criteria are provided in the *DSM-IV* table. If delusions are bizarre or if hallucinations consist of a running commentary on the person's thoughts or behaviors, only one symptom is required. In addition, if at least two voices converse with one another, this symptom alone is enough to lead to a diagnosis of schizophrenia. Therefore, hallucinations and delusions are quite important in diagnosing schizophrenia, since the presence of either—in particular forms—alone can indicate a schizophrenia diagnosis.

Schizophrenia generally involves impairment in several areas of functioning and multiple symptoms. It's important to note that *there is not one particular psychotic symptom that must be present to make the diagnosis.* Thus, two people may have the disorder and yet have totally different symptoms. In addition, careful diagnosis is especially important because a number of schizophrenia's classic symptoms are also seen in other disorders, such as bipolar illness or substance abuse. Impaired functioning at work or in caring for oneself distinguishes schizophrenia from disorders involving isolated symptoms. For example, a delusional belief may be present in a person who otherwise functions without any impairment at work or in social relations. Interpersonal difficulties are almost always present in schizophrenia, and persons with schizophrenia generally withdraw from others and become emotionally detached. On the other hand, a person with schizophrenia who is overwhelmed with fantasies and illogical thoughts may seek out others for validation of these thoughts. Problems in speci-

schizophrenia Complex mental disorder often characterized by hallucinations (hearing voices) and delusions (holding beliefs not shared by others).

DSM-IV

Diagnostic Criteria for 295 SCHIZOPHRENIA

A. *Characteristic symptoms:* Two or more of the following, each present for a significant period of time during a 1-month period (or less if successfully treated):
(1) delusions
(2) hallucinations
(3) disorganized speech (e.g., frequent derailment or incoherence)
(4) grossly disorganized or catatonic behavior
(5) negative symptoms (i.e., affective flattening, alogia, or avolition)

Note: Only one Criterion A symptom is required if delusions are bizarre or if hallucinations consist of a voice keeping a running commentary on the person's behavior or thoughts, or 2 or more voices are conversing with each other.

B. *Social/occupational dysfunction:* For a significant portion of the time from the onset of the disturbance, the patient is functioning well below their usual level in one or more of the following areas: work, interpersonal relations, and/or self-care.

C. *Duration:* Continuous signs of the disturbance must persist for at least 6 months. This 6-month period must include at least 1 month of symptoms (or less if successfully treated) that meet Criterion A. This 6-month period may also include prodromal or residual periods. During these prodromal or residual periods, only negative symptoms or less severe symptoms in Criterion A may be present.

D. *Schizoaffective and Mood Disorder exclusion:* No Mood Disorders have occurred at the same time as active phase symptoms. If there have been mood episodes, their duration has been briefer than the duration of the active or residual periods.

E. *Substance/medical exclusion:* The disturbance is not due to the direct effects of a drug, medication, or general medical condition.

F. *Relationship to Pervasive Developmental Disorder:* If there is a history of Autistic Disorder or another Pervasive Developmental Disorder, the additional diagnosis of Schizophrenia is made only if prominent delusions or hallucinations are also present for at least a month (or less if successfully treated).

fying and working toward goals are also characteristic of schizophrenia. In brief, persons with schizophrenia often seem unable to initiate activity, and this inability contributes to their impaired functioning in various areas.

We'll now describe the classic symptoms of schizophrenia, as they represent the key elements of this disorder. These symptoms fall into two broad categories: positive and negative. Disorganized speech, delusions, hallucinations, and grossly disorganized behavior are **positive symptoms. Negative symptoms** include little speech, lack of drive, and flat or blunt affect. Positive and negative symptoms do not refer to good and bad symptoms. Rather, positive symptoms refer to symptoms being present, such as hearing voices not heard by others (hallucinations). Negative symptoms refer to the *absence* of behaviors or feelings that most people exhibit—for example, not demonstrating any emotions (blunted affect). We'll discuss the importance of positive and negative symptoms later.

There has been much debate concerning the importance of various symptoms. For example, Bleuler suggested that blunt affect, social withdrawal, indecisiveness, and thought disorder were the hallmark symptoms of schizophrenia, whereas hallucinations, paranoid thinking, delusions of grandeur, and hostility were secondary and therefore less important symptoms. In the 1950s, Schneider stated that the first-rank or most important symptoms of schizophrenia were hallucinations and delusions. According to Schneider, disorganized speech should be considered a second-rank symptom. The *DSM-IV* (American Psychiatric Association, 1994) emphasizes Schneider's first-rank symptoms in its definition of schizophrenia.

Positive Symptoms   Behaviors and feelings in excess of those observed in the general population are positive symptoms. Among those we'll discuss here are delusions, hallucinations, disorganized speech, and disorganized and catatonic behavior.

We all have beliefs that sometimes seem plausible but that we know are probably not true. You may have thought that others were angry with you and are trying to make your life difficult. Or perhaps your boss seemed irritated with you and gave you a series of burdensome tasks that made you think for a few minutes, "He's out to get me." Upon reflection, however, you realized that there was simply a lot of work to get done that week and that large assignments were given to everybody. Fortunately, we discard most of our beliefs that seem unreal. But individuals with schizophrenia hold steadfastly to beliefs that are untrue—even when there's ample evidence to counter the beliefs.

Delusions are false beliefs. Persons with schizophrenia often express unusual beliefs that are not shared by others in their culture. Such expressions tend to lead the average individual to conclude that the person holding the beliefs is crazy. Delusions take various forms. But in general, they include firmly held convictions that most people believe are unusual and false. Delusions are the most colorful and intriguing symptom displayed by persons with schizophrenia. The following are several of the most common types of delusional symptoms:

■ *Delusions of persecution* have a clear central theme: People are out to get me. Approximately 65 percent of persons with schizophrenia have delusions such as these (Sartorius, Shapiro, & Jablensky, 1974):
  —My mom is trying to poison my cereal.
  —The university administration is out to get me; they are trying to drive me out of this university.
  —The FBI has a plan to kill me.

Consider the case of Eileen, whose delusions of persecution developed across the course of her initial year in college:

Eileen was a nearly straight-A high school student with high SAT scores; nevertheless, she found that in her first year of college people were "out to get her."

positive symptoms Presence of behaviors and feelings normally not present, such as hallucinations, delusions, or disorganized speech/behavior.

negative symptoms Absence of behaviors and feelings normally present; for example, little or no speech, social withdrawal, or blunted affect.

delusions False beliefs or unusual misrepresentation of reality, such as delusions of persecution, romance, grandeur, or control.

Moreover, Eileen began to overinterpret minor events. When she could not find her car keys, she believed her dormitory counselor had hidden them. When an instructor said a midterm exam would be difficult and advised students not to rely solely on lecture notes, Eileen believed he was singling her out and that she would be the only one to flunk the exam. And when she walked into a dining hall or a classroom, Eileen felt that people had been talking about her and laughing at her. Because of her fears of others and their opinions of her, Eileen isolated herself almost totally, studying all the time.

Finally, Eileen's paranoid thoughts became focused and so fear provoking that they led to hospitalization. Home from school for the weekend, Eileen became tearful and started to shake and pace on Sunday, the day of her expected return to school. Finally, she confessed that she believed someone was going to take her life if she went back.

"She had been hearing a warning voice, which was an unfamiliar male voice, telling her, 'Don't go back, Don't go back.' She felt that several of the students were playing 'mind games' with her and were controlling her thoughts and actions. For example, even from the distance of fifty miles, she could feel them sending her messages and trying to draw her back like a magnet. She was convinced that when she arrived, she would be physically harmed in some way. Her parents called the dormitory counselor, who indicated that Eileen's fears were obviously unfounded and that Eileen had been behaving in a peculiar and suspicious manner for a number of months, arousing concern in some of the residents that she was having some type of psychiatric problem. Several people, including the counselor, had urged her to see a doctor at Student Health, but she was unwilling to do so. Her parents took her to a local psychiatrist, who recommended hospitalization" (Andreasen, 1984, p. 55).

■ *Delusions of grandeur* include beliefs that you are an especially famous person, such as Jesus Christ, the Queen of England, Elvis Presley, or Michael Jackson. Beliefs that you have special powers—such as the capacity to control the world's destiny—are also considered delusions of grandeur.

■ *Delusions of control* occur when a person believes her thoughts or actions are controlled by external factors, such as forces or people on another planet. Two examples:
—There is a machine in my head that sends me messages every hour.
—My girlfriend controls how I think and she puts thoughts in my head.

■ *Delusions of romance* (erotomania) are false beliefs that someone is in love with or romantically involved with you. John Hinckley—the young man who shot President Reagan in 1981 and was obsessed with actress Jodie Foster—exemplifies how persons with schizophrenia display erotomania. He believed he could win Jodie Foster's love by taking extreme measures to impress her. The romantic delusion may also involve unrealistic expectations about the likelihood of living with a celebrity. Thus, John Hinckley wrote on a postcard to Jodie Foster, "One day you and I will occupy the White House and the peasants will drool with envy" ("Which Is the Real John Hinckley?" 1982, p. 15). Individuals with delusions of erotomania are usually withdrawn and lonely, typically have had few sexual encounters, and tend to focus on people who can give them instant fame by virtue of their superior status or looks (Segal, 1989).

Although striking and colorful, delusions have not been extensively investigated. However, we do know that for those diagnosed with schizophrenia in the United States, men are least likely to have delusions of romance (Segal, 1989); foreign-born Americans are the most prone to have paranoid delusions; and people from higher socioeconomic levels are the most likely to have delusions of grandeur. Delusions vary greatly in terms of the strength of belief, the bizarreness of the conviction, and the extent to which they dominate people's lives. Delusions are not

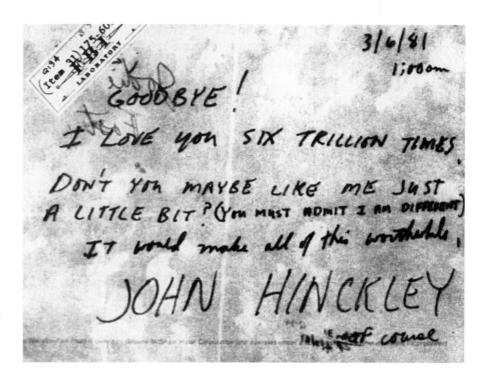

John Hinckley wrote this letter to actress Jodie Foster. He had a romantic delusion called eroto-mania; *he believed that he could win her love. Hinckley was later hospitalized for schizophrenia. How can you tell when a fantasy about a famous person crosses the line and becomes a romantic delusion?*

unique to schizophrenia; for example, people with affective disorders occasionally have delusions of grandeur. The more bizarre the delusions, though, the more characteristic of schizophrenia.

Hallucinations are sensory experiences that occur in the absence of any external environmental stimulation. They are sensations experienced by an individual that are not experienced by others. About 70 percent of persons with schizophrenia have auditory hallucinations, 25 percent have visual hallucinations, and 10 percent have other types of hallucinations (Mueser & Gingerich, 1994). Auditory hallucinations include hearing single or multiple voices (male or female). Even though visual hallucinations are less common, various types occur early in schizophrenia—such as seeing your hands as larger than usual or your penis as smaller. Visual hallucinations of a person's image are unusual, unless associated with alcohol intoxication.

Hallucinations are periodic and are worsened by social isolation (Alpert & Silvers, 1970). In addition, clinical reports of patients during tense or angry periods and continuous monitoring of their autonomic nervous systems indicate heightened emotional arousal associated with hallucinations (Cooklin, Sturgeon, & Leff, 1983). Recent research has also indicated that bloodflow in the speech area of the brain increases during a hallucination and decreases after it (McGuire, Shah, & Murray, 1993). If you ask a nonschizophrenic person to talk to himself (engage in inner speech), activity in this speech area increases. Thus, researchers believe that schizophrenics are unable to tell the difference between inner speech and reality.

Research findings indicate that persons with schizophrenia who are actively engaged in tasks are unlikely to report hallucinations (Margo, Hemsley, & Slade, 1981). Research subjects reported few hallucinations while reading prose or listening to interesting conversations. Self-reports of schizophrenic patients have also suggested that they are less likely to hallucinate when absorbed in activities, as illustrated in the following remark: "Isn't it funny. When I'm shoveling snow, I don't hear voices" (Strauss & Carpenter, 1981). A novel related experiment documents the effect of distraction on hallucinations. When schizophrenic patients were asked to hum while they were distracted (and thus kept their vocal cords occupied), they also reported dramatic reductions in auditory hallucinations (Green & Kinsbourne, 1990).

Another symptom of schizophrenia is speech that's disorganized in a variety of ways. In one type of **disorganized speech**—called *derailment* (slipping off the

hallucinations Sensory experiences in absence of external environmental stimulation; auditory and visual hallucinations are most common.

disorganized speech Symptom of schizophrenia in which the individual's speech is incomprehensible or remotely related to the topic of conversation (such as derailment, tangentiality).

track)—a person moves from one topic to another without any natural transitions. Sometimes, a schizophrenic patient will answer a question in a manner that seems unrelated to the question, a phenomenon called *tangentiality*. An example of derailment and tangentiality is seen in the response of a schizophrenic patient to the question "How are things at home for you?"

> What I'm saying is my mother is too ill. No money. It all comes out of her pocket. My flat's leaking. It's ruined my mattress. It's Lambeth Council. I'd like to know what the caption in the motto under their coat of arms is. It's in Latin. It must mean that you've got semen in you, the spunk to do something. The other thing I'm telling you is my birth certificate. Do you remember when I was in that hospital; I was on my knees. Well I was frightened of those nurses. Well they were stealing. (Cutting, 1985, p. 250)

Illogicality—another symptom often associated with disorganized speech—refers to drawing conclusions that don't follow from what was just said. Consider the following example from a chronic schizophrenic:

> **Doctor:** How long have you been in this hospital?
> **Patient:** 29 years.
> **Doctor:** What's the matter with you?
> **Patient:** Pneumonia.
> **Doctor:** That's a long time to have pneumonia.
> **Patient:** I caught it from a thermometer at Guy's Hospital. The thermometer said that everyone at the age of 20 would get either flu or pneumonia and I got pneumonia.
> **Doctor:** In my view thermometers only measure temperature. They don't actually specify what illness people have.
> **Patient:** Well you better go back and look up your medical books. (Cutting, 1985, p. 250)

Disorganized speech is considered a symptom of schizophrenia only when (1) the disorganization is severe enough to make effective communication nearly impossible and (2) if the disorganized speech occurs in conjunction with another of the five symptoms the *DSM-IV* lists as Criterion A (refer to the *DSM-IV* table).

Finally, two types of specific motor symptoms are also considered positive symptoms of schizophrenia. **Grossly disorganized behavior** is demonstrated in numerous ways, any of which reflect problems in appropriate goal-directed behavior. For example, an individual may not be able to get his dinner prepared. Disorganization also shows up in inappropriate behavior such as masturbating in public or dressing in a highly inappropriate manner (perhaps wearing an overcoat and gloves when it's very hot). It's seen in childlike silliness or highly agitated behavior. A few instances of any of these behaviors does not qualify as grossly disorganized behavior. A clinician looks for a pattern of such behaviors before applying the label.

Catatonic behavior refers to marked motor abnormalities, including motor immobility, excessive motor behaviors, and the maintenance of fixed postures over long periods of time. Some people who are schizophrenic may stand still like tin soldiers. Often, they assume uncomfortable poses, with an arm or leg held out. It appears that people in such poses could be pushed over if touched, yet if you approach them, it becomes apparent that they expend a great deal of energy remaining in this motionless stance. In many ways, individuals displaying this catatonic behavior resemble a military guard standing at attention, refusing to speak, look, or even blink if talked to directly.

Catatonic behavior was once considered rare, and, according to some, it's often inadequately diagnosed today. However, 7 percent of patients admitted to an inpatient psychiatric unit in 1992 had signs of catatonia (Fink, Bush, & Petrides, 1995). Although most diagnostic systems include catatonia as a subtype of schizophrenia, it can also be a feature of other psychiatric disorders, such as brain diseases, drug intoxication, and mood disorders. According to Fink et al., there is almost no con-

grossly disorganized behavior Inability to persist in goal-directed behavior; inappropriate behavior in public.

catatonic behavior Marked motor abnormalities such as bizarre postures, purposeless motor activity, and extreme degree of unawareness.

trolled research on the treatment of catatonia. These researchers found benzodi-azepines quite helpful in bringing 76 percent of patients out of the catatonic state.

Negative Symptoms   Negative symptoms of schizophrenia include three deficits: (1) flat or blunt affect, (2) little speech (*alogia*), and (3) lack of drive (*avolition*). Relatives of individuals with schizophrenia often find the negative symptoms are harder to recognize because they are not as blatant as the positive or excess symptoms (Mueser & Gingerich, 1994). On close examination of an individual, however, the negative symptoms become more apparent. Even though they are characterized by an absence of feelings and behaviors, these symptoms are prominent and quite stable across time.

Flat affect—which refers to lack of emotional expressiveness in gesture, facial expression, and voice tone—is experienced by roughly half or more of persons with schizophrenia (Boeringa & Castellani, 1982; Sartorious, Shapiro, & Jablensky, 1974). But flat affect is also characteristic of patients with mental retardation and organic brain disorders. Therefore, persons with schizophrenia cannot be distinguished from individuals with other problems solely on the basis of blunted affect.

The blunt affect typical of many schizophrenic patients misrepresents their underlying emotional experience (Kring, Kerr, Smith, & Neale, 1993). Although many persons with schizophrenia display blunted emotions, most also experience intense emotions, particularly at their disorder's outset. These emotions commonly arise from the frightening thoughts that affect many persons with schizophrenia. As one schizophrenic explained:

> I think so deep that I am almost out of this world. Then you get frightened that you are going to get in a jam and lose yourself. That's when I get worried and excited. . . . It must look queer to people when I laugh about something that has nothing to do with what I am talking about, but they don't know what is going on inside and how much of it is running round in my head. (Cutting, 1985, p. 236)

Speech disturbances prevalent in schizophrenia were detailed above. Exhibiting little actual speech—a symptom called **alogia,** or poverty of speech—is also characteristic of someone with schizophrenia. The individual talks very little and gives brief, empty replies to questions. Undergraduate visitors and volunteers spending time with schizophrenic patients in psychiatric units often find it difficult to keep conversations going. As noted by Mueser and Gingerich (1994), patients may sometimes not want to talk with visitors or even with relatives, but more often, they simply have little to say.

Another negative symptom, called **avolition,** involves the inability to begin and sustain goal-directed activity. The individual afflicted with schizophrenia often sits for hours, exhibiting little or no interest in activities—even when prompted by family members or ward attendants.

Persons with high levels of negative symptoms tend to have more cognitive deficits, less education, lower intelligence, and greater problems in social functioning than those with predominantly positive symptoms (excess behaviors, such as hallucinations and delusions). High-negative-symptom patients are more impaired at hospital admission and at hospital discharge. In addition, negative symptoms seem to be genetically influenced (Crow, 1985), and it's widely accepted that they are less responsive to antipsychotic medication (Fowles, 1992). In sum, negative symptomatology (such as alogia, avolition, blunt affect) is associated with poorer outcome.

Schizophrenic individuals often display *anhedonia,* or an inability to feel pleasure in activities. But anhedonia is not one of the three negative symptoms of schizophrenia described in the *DSM-IV* (American Psychiatric Association, 1994). Instead, it's listed as a common associated feature. *Physical* anhedonia is a loss of pleasure in eating, drinking, and sexual activities, whereas *social* anhedonia is the loss of pleasure in social contact. Individuals who are schizophrenic display social anhedonia more often than physical anhedonia.

alogia Negative symptom of schizophrenia involving a speech disturbance in which the individual talks very little and gives brief, empty replies to questions.

avolition Negative symptom of schizophrenia that involves the inability to begin and sustain goal-directed activity and the expression of little or no interest in activities.

Phases and Types of Schizophrenia

Do people who develop schizophrenia differ from others in their adolescence? That is, are the signs of schizophrenia evident long before the disorder emerges in its full-blown form? For some, the answer is yes; for others, no.

Many individuals who develop schizophrenia were well adjusted both socially and personally before they became ill (Mueser & Gingerich, 1994). Others had social problems in childhood that were seen by their parents. Two patterns of behavior seem evident in those who had problems in childhood and adolescence: (1) social withdrawal and lack of responsiveness and (2) hyperactivity, conduct problems, and impulsive behavior.

The *DSM-IV* (American Psychiatric Association, 1994) follows the tradition of subtyping persons with schizophrenia into groups of patients displaying different courses of the disorder as well as particular sets of symptoms. After first reviewing the typical phases of schizophrenia, we'll briefly specify the types of the disorder. But because as yet there are few differences in the course, stability, or treatment of the subtypes of schizophrenia, we will only briefly describe these subtypes.

Phases   Schizophrenia is a chronic disorder, as defined by the *DSM-IV* (American Psychiatric Association, 1994), which states that a chronic disturbance must last for at least 6 months. For most people with schizophrenia, symptoms come and go. In general, these individuals have relatively brief periods of high levels of positive psychotic symptoms, such as hallucinations and delusions. Negative symptoms, such as blunt affect and social withdrawal, however, are generally chronic.

Before symptoms of schizophrenia become very apparent, the person's level of functioning deteriorates during the period called the **prodromal phase.** The individual often withdraws socially, neglects his grooming and dress, has difficulty communicating, shows a lack of initiative, and has some bizarre thoughts. During the prodromal phase, parents and friends are apt to notice a personality change in the individual—that he is "no longer the same person." The exact duration of the prodromal phase is often difficult to pinpoint. But if the person gradually withdraws and shows increasingly unusual behavior over many years, the prognosis is poor.

During the **active or acute phase,** the individual exhibits psychotic symptoms, such as delusions, hallucinations, loose associations, and unusual motor behavior. The onset of the active phase may be associated with some life stress such as a move, the birth of a child, the loss of a job, or a promotion. For a formal diagnosis of schizophrenia, signs of disturbance must be present for at least 6 months, including 1 month of active symptoms (which may have been curtailed by treatment prior to the end of the month).

A **residual phase** follows the active phase. Similar to the prodromal phase, this period is also characterized by social withdrawal, inactivity, and bizarre thoughts. Psychotic symptoms such as delusions and hallucinations may persist but are generally unaccompanied by strong affect. During the residual phase, negative symptoms are often predominant, along with impairment in social and vocational functioning.

Types   Now let's look briefly at the five types of schizophrenia: (1) catatonic, (2) disorganized, (3) paranoid, (4) undifferentiated, and (5) residual.

Individuals with the **catatonic type** of schizophrenia have unusual patterns of motor activity. They display rigid postures and refuse to respond to requests or follow instructions. Often, people with catatonic schizophrenia seem to be in a stupor or trancelike state. Occasionally, they alternate between extreme excitement and stupor. Sometimes, they repeat certain words endlessly. On the other hand, mutism (or refusal to speak) is a common feature. Extremes of motor behavior point to the catatonic subtype, and the prominent and unusual symptoms make it easy to diagnose. Onset is usually more sudden than with other types of schizophrenia. Although the catatonic subtype of schizophrenia was seen frequently in the 1950s and 1960s, as noted earlier, professionals now encounter this subtype infrequently.

prodromal phase In schizophrenia, the phase immediately before the active phase of the disorder.

active or acute phase In schizophrenia, phase following the prodromal phase; individual exhibits psychotic symptoms such as delusions, hallucinations, loose associations, and unusual motor behavior.

residual phase In schizophrenia, the phase following the active phase; characterized by social withdrawal, inactivity, and bizarre thoughts; negative symptoms are often predominant, along with impairment in social and vocational functioning.

catatonic type Schizophrenia characterized by unusual patterns of motor activity, such as rigid postures and stupor or trancelike states; speech disturbances such as repetitive chatter or mutism are also common features.

The reasons for this decrease are not known; perhaps the widespread use of antipsychotic medications effectively limits the expression of catatonic symptoms.

The **disorganized type** of schizophrenia is characterized by verbal incoherence, grossly disorganized behavior, marked loosening of associations, and inappropriate affect. Persons with disorganized-type schizophrenia do not display elaborated sets of delusions, as persons with paranoid schizophrenia do. However, they may exhibit delusions or hallucinations whose content is not organized around a consistent theme. Disorganized-type schizophrenics may also display a variety of motor symptoms, such as unusual mannerisms and grimacing, as well as extreme social withdrawal and social impairment. Onset is early in life, and persons with this subtype seldom experience significant remissions or recoveries.

Persons with the **paranoid type** are preoccupied with one or more elaborated sets of delusions. They may also have auditory hallucinations associated with a single theme. Unlike persons with disorganized schizophrenia, those with paranoid schizophrenia don't have grossly inappropriate affect or disorganized behavior, nor do they display the extreme motor symptoms characteristic of the catatonic subtype. Paranoid schizophrenics sometimes show anger and are occasionally violent. If their delusions are intense and they fear physical harm, these individuals may experience severe anxiety and panic. If they don't act on their delusions, they continue to function reasonably well. In fact, according to the *DSM-IV*, the prognosis for persons with paranoid-type schizophrenia may be much better than for those with other types of schizophrenia (American Psychiatric Association, 1994).

The **undifferentiated type** of schizophrenia is characterized by psychotic symptoms, such as delusions, hallucinations, and incoherence. People with undifferentiated-type schizophrenia do not, however, meet the specific criteria for the other subtypes.

Residual-type schizophrenia typically occurs after prominent delusions, hallucinations, or formal thought disorder no longer are being displayed. But the individual with residual-type schizophrenia still speaks very little, shows little affect, has almost no motivation, and experiences some irregular beliefs.

Schizophrenia can vary in many ways, as we've just seen. In addition, schizophrenia can also be mild or severe, acute or chronic. The definitions of schizophrenia have varied across the decades, and different investigators have suggested that different symptoms deserve increased importance. For example, Andreasen and Flaum (1994) have argued for the critical import of negative symptoms. In fact, these researchers have entertained the option of being able to diagnose schizophrenia in individuals having a "pure negative" syndrome. To a student of abnormal psychology, diagnostic changes may seem problematic. However, the specific definitions or subtypes of many disorders do change over time in order to help researchers and clinicians better understand and treat individuals. Indeed, to many researchers, being able to change how a disorder is conceptualized and diagnosed represents one of their greatest challenges.

disorganized type *Schizophrenia characterized by an absence of elaborated sets of delusions and by verbal incoherence, grossly disorganized behavior, marked loosening of associations (disconnected thoughts), and inappropriate affect.*

paranoid type *Schizophrenia characterized by a preoccupation with one or more sets of delusions organized around one or more central themes.*

undifferentiated type *Schizophrenia characterized by psychotic symptoms such as delusions, hallucinations, and incoherence; individuals in this category do not meet the specific criteria for the other subtypes.*

residual type *Schizophrenia that occurs after prominent delusions, hallucinations, or formal thought disorder are no longer displayed but when the individual still speaks very little, shows little affect, has almost no motivation, and experiences some irregular beliefs.*

Focus on Critical Thinking

1. In the United States, schizophrenia is more common in urban areas and among people of lower socioeconomic status. What might explain these differences in prevalence?

2. Based on your answer to the previous question, how would you implement interventions aimed at these different groups?

CAUSES

A variety of biological, psychological, and social factors contribute to an individual's likelihood of developing schizophrenia. Biological factors contributing to schizophrenia include genetic factors, brain dysfunction, and biochemical abnormalities. Psychological factors include communication abnormalities and family dysfunction. Social factors that place people at risk for schizophrenia are low education and income.

Most experts believe that schizophrenia is a disorder with a genetic basis but that environmental factors also appear to contribute to this disorder. Gottesman (1991), a highly respected schizophrenia researcher, summarized the situation as follows: "While the genes are necessary for causing schizophrenia, they are not sufficient or adequate by themselves, and one or more environmental contributors are also necessary for schizophrenia, but they are not specific to it" (p. 164).

Biological Factors

Almost all professionals who assess and treat schizophrenic patients believe that biological factors cause schizophrenia. On the other hand, researchers have not determined the exact nature of these biological causes. We focus here on two major biological causes: genetic predisposition and brain dysfunction. These two types of causes allow an examination of different levels of analyses; they are not contradictory, as a genetic cause is highly likely to exert its influence through a brain dysfunction. We'll also consider briefly a third type of biological factor—biochemical abnormalities.

Genetic Predisposition Compelling evidence suggests a genetic contribution to schizophrenia. As with other disorders, family and twin studies represent the major methods of assessing genetic predisposition to schizophrenia. We will first review the evidence from these family studies and then that from studies of twins and adopted children. Before evaluating the genetic data, we should note that the likelihood of any randomly selected person developing schizophrenia is 1 in 100. This risk for becoming schizophrenic has been known for decades (Book, 1960) and has remained quite constant for more than 30 years in Europe and the United States (Tsuang, Faraone, & Day, 1988; Jones, 1993; Kessler et al., 1994).

The risk of schizophrenia increases with the quantity of genes shared with an already diagnosed individual. Nevertheless, even among first-degree relatives of persons with schizophrenia (parents, siblings, children), the odds are still strong that the family member will not develop the disorder. This suggests the importance of nongenetic factors in the development of the disorder. Some argue that what may be inherited is a vulnerability to the disease—not unlike a predisposition to the development of a physical health problem, such as high blood pressure. This vulnerability may be expressed under specific (stressful) life circumstances.

Family studies have been used longer than any other method to assess genetic predispositions for psychiatric disorders. For centuries, researchers have noted that mental illness runs in families, suggesting that it may be inherited genetically. The family study method compares the risk for a disorder in relatives of someone who has the disorder to the risk in a control sample.

Methodology has become quite sophisticated in family studies of schizophrenia. Many studies have met the following important methodological criteria:

1. They used normal control groups.
2. The assessments used highly defined criteria.
3. The assessors did not know the diagnoses of the individuals.

First-degree relatives of persons with schizophrenia (brothers, sisters, children) have approximately a 5 percent chance of becoming schizophrenic. In contrast, the likelihood of developing schizophrenia in a relative of a normal control was only 0.5 percent (Kendler & Diehl, 1993). Thus, the risk increases approximately 10 times if you have a first-degree relative with schizophrenia. As discussed in earlier chapters, however, shared genes are only one common element among family members. Family members also share experiences, stressors, and behaviors that may be learned from each other and may partly account for the higher risks.

Twin studies are a second major method to assess the role of genetic factors in schizophrenia. Almost no twin studies on schizophrenia have been conducted in the last 10 years or so (Kendler & Diehl, 1993). Thus, we rely on the findings of clas-

family studies Method to assess genetic predispositions for psychiatric disorders in which researchers analyze patterns and prevalence of disorders in families and compare the risk for a disorder in relatives of someone who has the disorder to the risk in a control sample.

twin studies Method to assess genetic predispositions for psychiatric disorders in which researchers compare the prevalence and patterns of disorders in identical and fraternal twins with patterns in nontwin controls.

sic studies, conducted several decades ago. The few recent studies have not produced conclusions substantially different than these earlier studies. Namely, if an identical (monozygotic) twin is schizophrenic, the likelihood (or concordance) that the other twin will also be schizophrenic is roughly 50 percent. If a fraternal (dizygotic) twin is diagnosed as schizophrenic, the likelihood of the other twin developing schizophrenia varies from 15 to 20 percent (Gottesman, 1991; Gottesman & Shields, 1972; Kallmann, 1953; Rosenthal, 1970; Slater, 1953).

Recall that a twin pair is judged as concordant when both individuals meet certain criteria. Estimates of risk are partially determined by how strict or lenient these criteria are. As the criteria for judging concordance become stricter, concordance rates decrease. Conversely, as the criteria become more inclusive, rates increase. Recognizing that varied definitions of concordance will yield different estimates, Gottesman and Shields (1972) devised a three-tier system of concordance criteria. The researchers studied all twin pairs in which at least one twin was hospitalized with a diagnosis of schizophrenia in Maudsley or Betham Hospital in London between 1948 and 1964. The likelihood of identical twin pairs being judged concordant was 79 percent using the very general criterion that the twin of the index case was also "abnormal, but not necessarily hospitalized." The concordance rate dropped to 54 percent if the criterion was "hospitalized, but not necessarily schizophrenic." And the concordance rate fell to 42 percent if the most stringent criteria— "hospitalized and diagnosed schizophrenic"—were used. Concordance rates for both identical and fraternal twin pairs decreased as the criteria for judging concordance became more stringent.

Regardless of the specific method used to judge concordance, however, the rates are much higher for identical than fraternal twins. As will be discussed later, these higher rates of concordance for identical twins are probably due to the greater percentage of genes shared by identical versus fraternal twins. Additionally, concordance rates are higher when the index case presents at least one severe schizophrenic symptom than when the index case presents with only mild symptoms (Gottesman & Shields, 1972).

Adoption studies are a third method of examining the role of genetic factors in the development of schizophrenia. In these studies, subjects are the biological children of persons with schizophrenia but have been raised by nonschizophrenic adoptive parents. Such studies eliminate the confounding of genetic and environmental influences commonly found in traditional family studies, such as modeling of the parent's schizophrenic behaviors, stress associated with the parent's hospitalization and treatment, and inadequate parenting during serious episodes.

While a young resident at the University of Oregon, Heston (1966) conducted an adoption study that has now become classic. He assessed 47 children of schizophrenic mothers; all the children were adopted or placed in foster homes less than 1 month after birth. Of special interest, the Heston study was the first adoption study of schizophrenia. It involved following children separated from their schizophrenic parents in early infancy. The biological mothers gave birth to their children while hospitalized for schizophrenia at the Oregon State Psychiatric Hospital. No attempt was made to assess the fathers' psychiatric status, although none were known to be psychiatric patients. At follow-up, the adopted children were compared to 50 control subjects who had also been reared in foster homes. The average age of individuals in both groups at follow-up assessment was 36 years.

Heston interviewed almost all the index and control cases himself. Two psychiatrists also diagnosed each person and rated him or her on a mental health–sickness scale. Neither psychiatrist knew the nature of the biological mothers' illness or the background of the adult they interviewed. As Table 13.1 shows, the children of schizophrenic mothers were at greater risk than control subjects for developing schizophrenia as well as other mental health problems. None of the control subjects were diagnosed as schizophrenic, whereas 5 of the children of schizophrenic mothers were (see boldfaced numbers in Table 13.1).

adoption studies Method to assess genetic predispositions for psychiatric disorders in which researchers compare the disorders of adopted children with those of their biological and adoptive parents in order to eliminate the confounding of genetic and environmental influences commonly found in traditional family studies.

TABLE 13.1 Risk of Schizophrenia in Adopted Children	Adopted Children of Schizophrenic Mothers	Adopted Children of Nonschizophrenic Mothers
Number of subjects	47	50
Average age at assessment	36 years	36 years
Number diagnosed schizophrenic	**5**	**0**
Number diagnosed sociopathic	9	2
Number diagnosed neurotic	13	7
Number diagnosed mentally defective	4	0
Psychiatric military discharge	8	1

Source: Data from L. L. Heston, "Psychiatric Disorders in Foster Home Reared Children of Schizophrenic Mothers," 1966, *British Journal of Psychiatry, 112,* pp. 819–825. Reprinted by permission.

Several large long-term adoption studies have recently been conducted in Denmark and Finland. A team in Finland under the direction of Tienari (1991) conducted the largest study of individuals who were adopted and lived away from their schizophrenic biological mothers. As you might expect, the research team compared these adoptees to a control group of adopted children contacted for a field study. Based on studying 144 offspring of schizophrenic mothers and 178 offspring of control mothers, the researchers found that 7 of the 144 offspring of schizophrenic mothers (4.9 percent) had schizophrenia, whereas only 2 of the 178 offspring of control mothers (1.1 percent) had schizophrenia. This difference is highly significant. In addition, 8 offspring of schizophrenic mothers had developed some other nonschizophrenic psychosis, whereas none of the children of the control mothers had developed such disorders. Clearly, being the biological child of a schizophrenic mother greatly elevated the risk of developing schizophrenia or some other psychosis.

An adoption study by Kety and colleagues in Copenhagen (Kety et al., 1994) approached this issue differently. They looked at adopted individuals who had been diagnosed with some form of schizophrenia, and they also found a control group of adoptees. They then contacted the adoptive and biological relatives of these adoptees through hospital records and later interviews. As expected, they found schizophrenia to be more common in biological relatives of schizophrenic adoptees than in the biological relatives of the control adoptees. Summarizing all their work in Denmark, Kety and colleagues found schizophrenia in 5 percent of biological relatives of schizophrenic adoptees but in only 0.4 percent of the biological relatives of control subjects.

These recent adoption studies all provide similar evidence. Like Heston's classic work, they show with greater precision that schizophrenia is significantly more common in the biological relatives of schizophrenic individuals. Specific rates of schizophrenia vary from one adoption study to another, but it appears that there is a five- to tenfold increase in risk for biological children of persons with schizophrenia (Kendler & Shields, 1993).

Results from family studies as well as from adoption and twin studies strongly indicate that genetic factors have a key role in the development of schizophrenia. Gottesman (1991) summarized data from 40 European family and twin studies spanning the years 1920 to 1987. As you can see from Figure 13.2, the risk of developing schizophrenia increases as there is greater sharing of genes with the schizophrenic patient. For example, the child of one schizophrenic parent has a 6 percent risk of becoming schizophrenic, whereas the child of two schizophrenic parents has a risk of

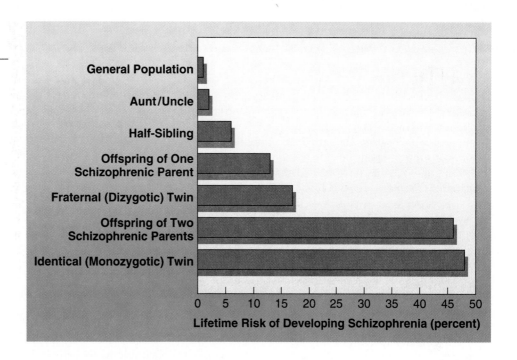

FIGURE 13.2 Lifetime risk for developing schizophrenia

Risks for developing schizophrenia compiled from the family and twin studies conducted in European populations between 1920 and 1987; the degree of risk highly correlates with the degree of genetic relatedness.

SOURCE: *Schizophrenia Genesis* by Gottesman. Copyright © 1991 by Irving I. Gottesman. Used with permission of W. H. Freeman and Company.

48 percent. The exact rates vary somewhat from the studies just reported, as the rates reported by Gottesman summarize studies conducted across a long timespan.

In sum, family studies are generally suggestive of genetic influences in the development of schizophrenia. However, they do not control for environmental influences, which also appear to play a causal role (Gottesman, McGuffin, & Farmer, 1987). Although twin studies strongly suggest that genetic factors are of prime importance in the etiology (causation) of schizophrenia, environmental similarity may be greater for identical than fraternal twins. Adoption studies eliminate the confounding between genetic and environmental factors and show that genetic factors play a very strong role in the development of the disorder.

The disease model of schizophrenia has contributed to the focus on single-gene models of schizophrenia, paying little attention to environmental variables and other genetic models. While the single-gene model of schizophrenia has its proponents (for instance, see review by Pardes, Kaufman, Pincus, & West, 1989), it has been criticized as being distinctly one sided and ignoring environmental influences. For example, a behavioral genetics view clearly supports environmental contributions (Plomin, 1990). Moreover, the data simply do not fit a single-gene model of schizophrenia (Fowles, 1992). Instead, a large number of genes contribute to the overall risk for developing schizophrenia. Family and nonfamily environmental influences also contribute to the genetic risk factors that place the individual at risk for schizophrenia.

This model—in which many genes interact with environmental influences—is called a **multifactorial polygenic model.** It reflects the many factors and many genes that contribute to schizophrenia (Reiss, Plomin, & Hetherington, 1991). The multifactorial polygenic model estimates the overall genetic contribution to be 60 to 70 percent but sees the remaining environmental contribution as very important, too. Fowles (1992), who reviewed a wide range of literature regarding genetic and environmental influences on schizophrenia, has made a point worth remembering when you think of any genetic/environmental interaction: The environmental influence need not be large to contribute importantly to the development of schizophrenia. In fact, the environment exerts its greatest influence on the population of most interest: those genetically at risk for schizophrenia. The majority of people are not at risk or are minimally at risk for schizophrenia; they have so little genetic risk

multifactorial polygenic model Etiological model for psychiatric disorders involving many genes interacting with environmental influences.

Over the last 75 years, various experts have emphasized what they feel is the essential nature of a disorder they call *schizophrenia.* Factors such as positive and negative symptoms, severity, and an acute/chronic dimension have been suggested by some authorities as ways of subtyping this disorder (Andreasen & Carpenter, 1993). Other experts have argued that there is no single disorder of schizophrenia (Garety, 1992).

To provide some closure to the student of abnormal psychology, the *DSM-IV* (American Psychiatric Association, 1994) presents criteria for diagnosis of schizophrenia and for distinguishing among various subtypes and phases of schizophrenia. However, schizophrenia overlaps significantly with other psychotic disorders—especially the affective or mood disorders—and schizophrenia is diagnosed when other psychotic disorders have been ruled out. Naming and defining a disorder does not explain the disorder, and many feel that the *DSM-IV* criteria do not capture the crucial nature of schizophrenia.

Andreasen and Carpenter (1993) described different models to address the variability seen in schizophrenia. These models might be used to conduct research that could help us understand schizophrenia or the symptoms that we have discussed as falling under the diagnosis of schizophrenia:

1. A single disease leads to diverse manifestations or symptoms, as is the case with multiple sclerosis.
2. Varied disorders or diseases lead to schizophrenia by different processes—as is the case with mental retardation, which can be caused by many abnormalities, such as chromosome disorder, oxygen deficiency, or fetal alcohol syndrome.
3. Specific symptom clusters within schizophrenia come together in different ways in different patients. (This method is currently used in the *DSM-IV* diagnostic criteria.)
4. Individuals with schizophrenia could be grouped by physiological or neurological markers (Gooding & Iacono, 1995).

The first model, the single-disease model, is appealing because of its simplicity. And it makes sense if all individuals with a diagnosis of schizophrenia have a central and similar abnormal process operating that produces the symptoms we call *schizophrenia.* However, there are limitations to the single-disease model.

Think about the following questions:

1. What are the limitations of the single-disease model?
2. How might model 2, 3, or 4 be useful in unraveling the mystery of schizophrenia?

that the environment is highly unlikely to bring them to the point of developing schizophrenia. But with a genetic contribution model of 60 to 70 percent, the impact of the environment can be very important.

Polygenic threshold models assume that both genes and environmental factors contribute to the development of schizophrenia. More specifically, many genes contribute to the overall liability or risk for developing schizophrenia; then, for most individuals, whether they become schizophrenic will depend on environmental factors. Fowles (1994) presented a threshold model of schizophrenia that showed that as an individual's genetic liability increased, less environmental stress was necessary for him to develop schizophrenia. Some individuals have little or no genetic risk for developing schizophrenia; however, they may develop the disorder, given extreme amounts of environmental stress. Yet other individuals have a great genetic risk for becoming schizophrenic; these individuals need little or no environmental stress for symptoms to appear.

Andreasen and Carpenter (1993) have also looked at a number of models of schizophrenia to address the variability of symptoms seen in that disorder. Their work is summarized in Thinking about Controversial Issues.

Brain Dysfunction   Some approaches to investigating brain defects in people who are schizophrenic focus directly on brain structure and dysfunction. Another major approach involves assessment of performance on neuropsychological tests; test results can suggest which areas of the brain have some impairment. First, we'll discuss the direct assessment of brain dysfunction; then we'll look at neuropsychological test evaluation of schizophrenic patients.

Investigations that focus directly on brain *structure* assess factors such as reductions in type or amount of brain tissue. Those that look at brain *function* assess brain

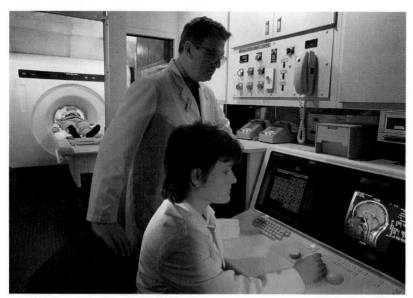

The patient in the background is being moved into the MRI (magnetic resonance imaging) chamber, which allows the physician to take pictures of living tissue. A magnetic field encircling the patient's body enables a computer to produce a three-dimensional picture of body tissue, as seen in the foreground.

activity such as the metabolism of organic compounds. It's likely that, in the end, researchers will find that differences in structure cause differences in functioning.

Magnetic resonance imaging (MRI) provides a view of the brain structure. It takes a picture of living tissue without risk to the patient's health because it uses no radiation. MRI works on the principle that our body cells contain certain elements sensitive to magnetic fields. During the procedure, the patient is placed inside a huge magnet encircling his body. As the magnet passes over the body, a computer creates a three-dimensional picture of body tissue (Kandel & Schwartz, 1985).

MRI research with schizophrenic individuals showed that the ventricles or cavities containing the cerebrospinal fluid were enlarged. In turn, this enlargement correlated with cognitive impairment. In an identical twin study in which one twin was schizophrenic and the other was not, the brain enlargement of the twin with schizophrenia was clearly evident on the brainscan (Suddath, Christison, Torrey, Casanova, & Weinberger, 1990). Some researchers studying postmortem data have suggested that the enlarged ventricles in brains of schizophrenics are caused by abnormal development of the cortex, the thin outer layer of the brain (Weinberger, 1994). Researchers also have directed their attention to specific areas of the brain that might provide keys to this disorder. Decreased brain volume in the temporal region of the brains of schizophrenic patients is related to the severity of hallucinations (especially auditory hallucinations) and disorganized language (Gur & Pearlson, 1993). Decreased brain volume in the frontal area is also significantly associated with blunted affect and lack of motivation (Klausner, Sweeney, Deck, Haas, & Kelly, 1992).

Bloodflow studies permit researchers to study brain function. They provide pictures of cerebral bloodflow, oxygen use, and other brain functions. A major method for such analyses is a **positron emission tomographic (PET) scan.** In a PET scan, radioactive isotopes are bound to compounds of biological interest (such as sugar, water, or neurotransmitters) and injected into the patient's blood vessels. The radioactive isotopes emit particles called *positrons,* revealing how the compound distributes itself in the brain (Kandel & Schwartz, 1985). For example, the PET technique used most frequently involves the injection of glucose (a sugar)

magnetic resonance imaging (MRI) Device providing images of the brain's structure; reveals the chemical composition of the brain.

positron emission tomographic (PET) scan Procedure providing images of the brain's activities by monitoring the activity of radioactive particles injected into the bloodstream.

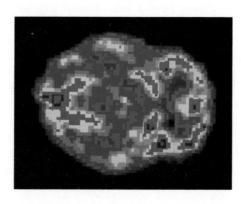
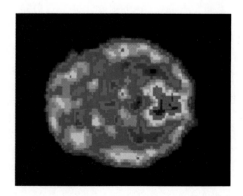

A PET (positron emission tomographic) scan shows how radioactive molecules flow through a patient's blood vessels. **Left** *In the normal subject, many areas of the brain appear active.* **Right** *In the schizophrenic subject, only one area of the brain appears active. Research indicates abnormally low activity in the frontal lobe of the individual who is schizophrenic.*

treated with a positron tracer. Since glucose provides energy in the brain, the positron-emitting glucose allows clinicians and researchers to see which parts of the brain are most active when a person is engaged in a specific activity.

The results of PET scan studies of subjects executing cognitive tasks generally support the view that persons with schizophrenia have abnormally low activity in their frontal lobes, the "executive planning" center of the brain (Berman & Weinberger, 1990; Gur & Pearlson, 1993). For example, when schizophrenic patients in Weinberger's laboratory at the National Institute of Mental Health were performing a task assessing memory and abstract thinking, researchers measured the bloodflow to the patients' frontal lobes. While subjects were performing the task, on average, bloodflow of nonschizophrenic control subjects increased, whereas for the schizophrenic subjects, bloodflow decreased.

Assessing individuals' performance on different neuropsychological tests helps researchers and clinicians determine how particular areas of the brain function. For decades, neuropsychologists have examined the performance of patients with known brain injury from accidents, gunshot wounds, and other traumas. As discussed in Chapter 3, the test performances allowed neuropsychologists to map how different areas of the brain serve particular functions. However, we now know that when certain areas of the brain are damaged, other areas may compensate and begin to serve the function of the damaged area. Thus, we can't simply make a map of a brain and say that this *single* area determines how an individual can function on a test. Nonetheless, as described in Chapter 3, bloodflow in different parts of the brain has allowed neuropsychologists and psychiatrists using PET scan devices to determine that the functioning of many areas of our brain generally governs how we perform on psychological tests.

A research team of psychologists and psychiatrists compared the neuropsychological functioning of individuals with schizophrenia with two groups: (1) the subjects' nonschizophrenic brothers or sisters and (2) a control group of individuals matched for age, race, handedness, and education (Cannon et al., 1994). All the individuals who were assessed took a battery of comprehensive neuropsychological tests. The researchers assessed the schizophrenic people twice to determine the effects of antipsychotic medication on their performance. About half the individuals diagnosed as schizophrenic were not on any medication at the time of the first or second assessment. The other half were not receiving antipsychotic medication at the first assessment, but they were at the second assessment, 2 to 4 weeks later.

As expected, the level of neuropsychological impairment was greatest in the schizophrenic group, intermediate in their brothers and sisters, and lowest in the control group. There were similar patterns of deficits in the test performances of members in each group. Also, the tests indicated that verbal memory, attention, and language were affected most. But schizophrenic subjects did not vary on the tests in the medicated and nonmedicated assessments. These and other results suggest that frontal and temporal lobes (which influence cognitive functions, like memory and language) are part of an inherited substrate of schizophrenia.

We now turn to another dysfunction that leads researchers to believe that some people with schizophrenia have frontal lobe abnormalities. Many schizophrenic individuals have difficulty visually following a continuously moving target, a problem called **smooth-pursuit eye-tracking dysfunction.** This dysfunction is the best biological indicator of genetic liability to develop schizophrenia (Iacono & Clementz, 1992). The dysfunction is stable, and it occurs in long-standing as well as first-episode schizophrenia. Moreover, twin studies also indicate that smooth-pursuit eye-tracking performance is heritable. Several studies have found that frontal lobe dysfunction is associated with poor tracking. However, not all schizophrenic people have eye-tracking deficits; in fact, some appear quite normal in this regard. Thus, Iacono and his colleagues (Gooding & Iacono, 1995) have suggested that one fruitful way to subtype schizophrenics would be on the basis of this abnormality and other brain abnormalities, like those discussed earlier.

smooth-pursuit eye-tracking dysfunction Difficulty visually following a continuously moving target found in many schizophrenic patients; the best biological indicator of genetic liability to develop schizophrenia.

You may recall that Kraepelin thought that schizophrenia was a disorder with a deteriorating course across time. Today, we know that this isn't true. Many patients recover or are less afflicted later in life (Belitsky & McGlashan, 1993), and based on tissue examination in postmortem studies, some schizophrenia experts believe that brain abnormalities of schizophrenia don't increase with time. Nonetheless, until recently, the neuropsychological functions of people with schizophrenia had not been examined for various age groups.

Heaton and colleagues (1994) gave neuropsychological tests to schizophrenic individuals of various ages. Basically, they found that impairment was not related to current age, age of onset of schizophrenia, or the duration of the illness. These results are consistent with the view that schizophrenia is a developmental disorder that may begin sometime between the ages of 3 and 15 years (Gershon & Rieder, 1992). In other words, the individual may gradually experience increasing numbers of symptoms throughout the years until he is fully schizophrenic. Once someone has reached full schizophrenic criteria, he is not likely to deteriorate further but to remain stable or improve. Alternatively, the disorder may have its origins in pregnancy and birth complications; empirical evidence supports the importance of these obstetric or birth complications as well as prenatal exposure to maternal influenza (see review by Gooding and Iacono, 1995). Gooding and Iacono have suggested that an understanding of the concept of sensitive periods is crucial to a developmental perspective in studying schizophrenia.

In summary, based on MRI studies of brain tissue, PET scan studies of brain dysfunction, and neuropsychological testing, researchers conclude that the brains of schizophrenic patients differ from those of normal or nonschizophrenic persons. The ventricles of schizophrenic patients are enlarged, and the frontal and temporal areas of schizophrenic patients are dysfunctional.

Biochemical Abnormalities   As we'll discuss later in this chapter, antipsychotic medication has been used effectively to treat people with schizophrenia since the late 1950s. The medications have a calming effect and diminish the hallucinations and delusions of these individuals. The very notable side effects of the antipsychotic medications, however, alerted physicians to a possible cause of schizophrenic symptoms. The side effects were muscular tremors like those seen in Parkinson patients and, accordingly, became known as Parkinsonian movements. Scientists knew that Parkinson patients had abnormally low levels of the neurotransmitter dopamine and that L-dopa—a chemical related to dopamine—helped reduce tremors in Parkinson patients. It wasn't a big conceptual leap to ask whether schizophrenic patients might suffer from an excessive level of dopamine, because the antipsychotic medication reduced hallucinations and, at the same time, reduced dopamine and led to Parkinsonian tremors.

The ability of the various antipsychotic medications to reduce levels of dopamine in the brain appears to explain much of their clinical potency (Julien, 1995). Certain areas in the brain act as dopamine receptor sites, and the standard antipsychotic medications bind to those same sites, blocking the action of dopamine. The dopamine hypothesis has been the subject of investigations since the 1970s and has stayed relatively strong across the years, despite considerable criticism (Lieberman & Koreen, 1993). This hypothesis stills hold some validity, but comparisons of dopamine levels in schizophrenic patients and nonschizophrenic controls do not reveal differences. According to a National Institute of Mental Health (NIMH) publication, *Special Report: Schizophrenia 1993*, "Clearly no consensus exists about dopamine's role in schizophrenia" (Shore, 1993). This ambiguity exists in part because there are many different dopamine receptors, and different medications have different effects on the various types of receptors. Also, many neurotransmitters appear to be involved in the mechanism of antipsychotic medication, especially some of the new antipsychotic medications that influence serotonin.

Among many other neurotransmitters that may play a role in schizophrenia, two have received considerable attention: serotonin and norepinephrine. It isn't important to describe these neurotransmitters in any detail, because the evidence about them is conflicting and there is no convincing data to support any specific biochemical cause of schizophrenia (Lieberman & Koreen, 1993; Julien, 1995). It appears that progress on the biochemical front may come from subtyping people with schizophrenia, since they differ so markedly in terms of symptoms, severity, and course of the disorder. With such groupings, hopefully, more consistent biochemical data will provide clues to the discovery of new medications for this illness. Research on the roles of serotonin and norepinephrine—in addition to that of dopamine—has already prompted researchers to develop medications that may be more effective for some individuals, as we will see later.

Psychological Factors

Experts in schizophrenia research have held that family stress and communication problems place an individual at risk for developing schizophrenia. This research area began in the mid-1960s, when family researchers became interested in nonbiological aspects of schizophrenia, and it flourished when the focus turned to the high levels of emotion expressed in certain families. This "high-expressed-emotion" (high-EE) research fueled tremendous interest in family variables, both as causes of relapse and as factors that might maintain the length of a schizophrenic episode (Goldstein, 1995). We turn now to this family research, as it evolved across the last three decades.

According to some, the general stress of society leads certain individuals to break down. English psychiatrist Roland D. Laing (1967) argued that people retreat into the refuge of schizophrenia as a way of coping with overwhelming social stress. In the United States, psychiatrist Thomas Szasz took a similar position in his article "The Myth of Mental Illness" (1960). Szasz argued that applying the label "schizophrenia" to certain behavior patterns implies the presence of a disease or illness. In Szasz's view, this label is simply a linguistic practice allowing medical doctors (rather than priests, witch-hunters, or police officers) to control certain behavior deemed unusual or socially unacceptable. Although Szasz's and Laing's ideas did not significantly alter the mainstream view of schizophrenia as a mental disorder, they prompted others to assess the social context of individuals coping with mental illness.

In a review of the literature, Dohrenwend and Egri (1981) stated that recent life events "appear to play a role in both onset and recurrence of schizophrenic episodes, but that we know very little about how the processes differ in the different circumstance of onset and recurrence" (p. 20). Two British researchers, Leff and Vaughn (1989), found that negative life events or a negative family environment appeared to precede the onset of or relapse into schizophrenia. Thirteen weeks before the onset of a schizophrenic episode, the proportion of negative events was 64 percent. In contrast, 3 weeks before an episode, the proportion of undesirable events rose to approximately 77 percent. For some individuals, however, the presence of the negative events alone was not associated with the onset of schizophrenia. "The onset or relapse of schizophrenia is associated either with high EE [high negative emotion in one's family] or with an independent [negative] life event" (p. 387).

Even though family research suggests that family disruption is associated with the onset of schizophrenia, such research does not negate the very strong evidence of a biological risk for developing schizophrenia. Moreover, it's not clear how influential social stress is in predicting the onset of schizophrenia.

Whatever your opinions about Laing and Szasz, deviant family communication was a popular focus of research. We'll examine those communication patterns now.

Communication Abnormalities   In the 1950s, many experts believed that deviant family or parental communication patterns might cause schizophrenia. One concept based on these patterns was the **double-bind hypothesis** (Bateson, Jackson, Haley, & Weakland, 1956). Persons with schizophrenia, the researchers suggested, have experienced intense relationships with parents who sent contradictory messages to them. For example, a mother may complain to her son that he is unaffectionate, yet she may become tense and anxious when he approaches her. Because of the intensity of their feelings, children find it hard to withdraw from such relationships, even though they get contradictory messages from their parents.

Although subsequent researchers did not find empirical support for the double-bind hypothesis, research on communication patterns in schizophrenic families continued. Investigators such as Wynne (1984) and Rodnick, Goldstein, Lewis, and Doane (1984) developed a systems approach to schizophrenia, assigning deviant communication patterns a central role. According to these researchers, a person can be best understood within the social systems in which she lives, such as marriage, the family, and their broader social network. Systems research has shown that communication deviance, a rejecting or indifferent parental style, and a detached family environment are related to schizophrenic behavior. Yet the reasons for the association between family communication problems and schizophrenia are unclear. One possibility for this relationship is that communication problems and family stress result from living with a child who may be preschizophrenic and grossly deviant at a young age.

Deviant communication patterns and family stress could also lead to social withdrawal; in turn, the withdrawal could lead to other problems for an individual with a predisposition for developing schizophrenia. At this point, let's be clear that parents should not be held responsible for the development of schizophrenia in their children, since there is no evidence that parental factors cause schizophrenia.

High-Risk Studies   Studies of childhood records of schizophrenic individuals led researchers to hypothesize that children who are withdrawn, disagreeable, and delinquent are more likely to become schizophrenic than children without these characteristics (Berry, 1967; Watt, 1974). These characteristics, however, are found not only in the childhood records of persons with schizophrenia but also in those of delinquents and criminals. In the search for risk factors of schizophrenia, researchers want to find variables that predict schizophrenia, in particular, rather than mental or social disorders, in general.

High-risk studies for schizophrenia follow children at risk for developing schizophrenia (usually children with a schizophrenic parent) to determine differences between those who become schizophrenic and those who do not. In many of these studies, children with normal parents form the low-risk control group. We include the high-risk studies in this section of the chapter because they can uncover psychological variables that increase a person's likelihood of developing schizophrenia. However, as you will see, these studies can also uncover social and genetic factors that increase the odds of developing schizophrenia.

Many researchers have studied large samples of children at risk for schizophrenia. For example, two researchers, Sarnoff Mednick and Fini Schulsinger (1968), conducted pioneering high-risk studies in Denmark in the early 1960s. They studied 207 high-risk children with adjustment problems whose mothers were schizophrenic. A control group of 104 low-risk subjects whose mothers were not schizophrenic were selected to match the high-risk subjects on variables such as age, sex, race, and socioeconomic status. When the study began, the high-risk subjects averaged 15 years of age (ranging from 9 to 20). By 1972, 17 of the now grown-up high-risk subjects were diagnosed as schizophrenic, whereas none of the low-risk subjects were. Subjects who later became schizophrenic were distinguished from other high-risk subjects by the following characteristics:

1. Their mothers had a more severe course of illness.
2. They were separated from their parents more often and had been placed in children's homes more often.

double-bind hypothesis
Contradictory messages from another person; often the parent, to the child; as when the parent communicates warmth but is cold and withdraws when the child approaches; the child is thus caught in a double bind.

3. They had greater difficulties during the fifth month of pregnancy through the first month of life.
4. Their teachers saw them as more aggressive and easily angered.
5. They had higher autonomic nervous system arousal levels, especially those who eventually suffered from hallucinations and delusions.

As summarized by Watt (1984) in *Children at Risk for Schizophrenia: A Longitudinal Perspective,* some children born to schizophrenic mothers showed more aggressive and disruptive school behavior and had lower intelligence quotients (IQs) than control children. Moreover, their mothers experienced more complications during pregnancy. Recall that Danish researchers had reached similar conclusions approximately 15 years earlier. By the 1980s, however, the high-risk researchers obtained additional information: They learned that different factors predict behavior problems in children of schizophrenic women as compared to children of depressed women. Marital discord, for example, plays an important role in the development of behavior problems in children with depressed mothers but not in children of schizophrenic mothers (Emery, Weintraub, & Neale, 1982). Finally, Mednick and his colleagues have shown that viral infections during pregnancy and other birth traumas appear to trigger schizophrenia in vulnerable people (Barr, Mednick, & Munk-Jorgenson, 1990).

We shouldn't forget that many children of parents with schizophrenia cope extremely effectively. Manfred Bleuler (1984) found that 84 percent of married high-risk subjects in Switzerland had successful marriages. The great majority did not develop the illness and surpassed their parents' social status.

We have discussed family factors as they relate to the development of schizophrenia, and we will return to a discussion of more recent studies on family factors as they influence the relapse rates of schizophrenic patients. Before doing that, however, let's consider larger social issues like education and income, which are also related to schizophrenia.

Social Class Factors

In 1855, a Massachusetts researcher, Edward Jarvis, reported a classic study of the prevalence of psychiatric disorders (1855/1971). Before the term *schizophrenia* had ever been used, Jarvis pointed to the preponderance of cases of what was then called *insanity* in the lowest social classes and the relative absence of insanity in the upper classes. Jarvis was the forerunner of what we now call **epidemiology,** or the study of various disorders in the population and risk factors associated with those

epidemiology Study of disorders or diseases in a population.

TABLE 13.2	Prevalence of Schizophrenia by Social Class (rates per 100,000 in New Haven, Connecticut)	
	Point Prevalence[1]	**Lifetime Prevalence**[2]
Social class I/II (high)	6	111
Social class III	8	168
Social class IV	10	300
Social class V	20	895

[1] Rate per 100,000 individuals who are diagnosed as schizophrenic at a particular assessment point
[2] Rate per 100,000 individuals who ever develop schizophrenia

Source: Data from *Social Class and Mental Illness,* by A. B. Hollingshead and F. C. Redlich, 1958, New York: John Wiley.

Schizophrenia occurs throughout the world (Jablensky, 1989). The odds of developing a first episode of the disorder are approximately equal among people in developed and underdeveloped countries. There are geographical pockets in which schizophrenia is highly prevalent, such as Northern Sweden and Western Ireland (Torrey, 1987). But some investigators see these areas as exceptions to the overall rule of schizophrenia as a culture-free disorder. Schizophrenia appears in all races and among all ethnic groups, although minor symptom variations appear, probably due to cultural factors.

Consider the rates (percentages) per 1,000 in the following countries (Tsuang, Faraone, & Day, 1988):

China	2.1
Denmark	3.3
Finland	15.0
Germany	2.4
Ghana	0.6
India	3.7
Iran	2.1
Ireland	8.3
Japan	2.3

Soviet Union (former)	5.3
Sweden	17.0
United States	7.0

Some investigators who study cultural differences conclude that the differences seen in Sweden may have been due to the particular population studied—that is, people in an isolated area in northern Sweden. The environment was described as austere and perhaps conducive to the isolated style preferred by many schizophrenics (Tsuang, Faraone, & Day, 1988). Generally, these researchers conclude that schizophrenia is not specific to one culture and that it occurs with remarkable consistency across cultures.

Think about the following questions:

1. Even if higher rates of schizophrenia in Sweden and Finland are seen as exceptions, what factors might explain apparent differences in rates between the United States and Ghana or between the United States and China?
2. How would you research the question?
3. How might this influence social policy?

disorders. Let's examine what is now known about the role of social class factors and schizophrenia.

For decades, experts have known that schizophrenia is found most commonly among people from lower socioeconomic groups. In the classic study of social class and mental illness conducted by Hollingshead and Redlich (1958), persons with schizophrenia in New Haven, Connecticut, were three times more likely to be members of the lowest socioeconomic class than of any other class (see Table 13.2). Researchers also found disproportionate numbers of persons with schizophrenia in lower socioeconomic classes in New York City (Srole, Langner, Michael, Opler, & Rennie, 1962) and in Western European countries such as Denmark, England, and Norway (Kohn, 1968). (See Thinking about Multicultural Issues, which looks more closely at the different rates of schizophrenia among countries around the world.) The highest rates of schizophrenia occur in the centers of large cities—areas generally inhabited by members of the lowest socioeconomic classes—except in cities where large urban renewal projects have attracted the upper and middle classes. Thus, despite very different methods of study and different definitions of pathology, the general findings of Jarvis in 1855 still ring true more than 100 years later: People from the lower classes have more severe psychiatric pathology.

Two major hypotheses attempt to explain the fact that schizophrenia is generally much more prevalent in the lower socioeconomic classes. First, the **social causation hypothesis** states that factors associated with being a member of a lower class may contribute to the development of schizophrenia. Such variables might include poor prenatal care; poor nutrition; unequal access to early treatment; and a relative lack of family, social, and medical support. A second hypothesis, the **social selection hypothesis**, is that persons genetically predisposed to schizophrenia drift downward; that is, persons with schizophrenia drift into poor urban neighborhoods. Evidence of downward social mobility is, however, conflicting. Some studies have

social causation hypothesis Hypothesis that factors associated with being a member of a lower socioeconomic class may contribute to the development of schizophrenia.

social selection hypothesis Hypothesis that persons genetically predisposed to schizophrenia drift downward socioeconomically; that is, persons with schizophrenia drift into poor urban neighborhoods.

found such an association (Turner & Wagonfeld, 1967), whereas others have not (Hollingshead & Redlich, 1958).

Examining the occupational status of the parents of persons with schizophrenia is another way to determine the relative merit of the social class and the social selection (downward mobility) hypotheses. For example, if fathers of persons with schizophrenia were from the lowest socioeconomic levels, their children would be born into the same levels; thus, class would precede schizophrenia. If, however, fathers of persons with schizophrenia were from higher socioeconomic classes than their children, schizophrenic offspring could have drifted downward. Research has yielded conflicting findings, depending on the city of the subject population (Faris & Dunham, 1939; Dunham, 1965). A summary (Dohrenwend et al., 1992) of this research concluded that although both theories have presented arguments to support their positions, "no one has demonstrated [previously] that one position is more compelling than the other."

Research in Israel has suggested that social selection—in other words, genetic predisposition—factors contribute more to the development of schizophrenia than socioeconomic class (Dohrenwend et al., 1992). However, it remains to be seen if these results can be replicated. Some factors related to being in a lower class will probably contribute to the development of schizophrenia. And in some cases, individuals predisposed to schizophrenia will withdraw, lose their jobs, and seek the food and housing assistance sometimes available in large cities. Furthermore, because certain parents of schizophrenics may share some similarities with their children, such as withdrawal and lack of social skills, these families may be driven into the lower classes. However, research has suggested that social factors have less value in predicting schizophrenia than genetic predisposition factors.

In accord with this book's biopsychosocial framework, a predisposition to develop schizophrenia may interact with ongoing stressors to increase the risk of schizophrenia. This general interactionist model was developed by Eisenberg (1968), as applied to the concept of schizophrenia, and is now called the **diathesis-stress model** (Zubin & Spring, 1977). The *diathesis* is a person's genetic, biological, and/or psychological vulnerability, whereas the *stress* is current social or interpersonal stress, such as poverty or severe criticism from family members.

Within the biopsychosocial model used throughout this book, we've discussed the interaction of biological, psychological, and social variables in the etiology of many disorders (such as anxiety, depression, alcoholism, and attention-deficit disorders of children). The diathesis-stress model is especially popular in the schizophrenia area, largely as a result of the conceptualization of Eisenberg (1968) and Zubin and Spring (1977). They emphasized the interaction of genetic predisposition and social stressors. For example, Zubin and Spring argued that any individual can be classified according to his vulnerability or predisposition to develop schizophrenia. Some people have almost no likelihood of developing schizophrenia, whereas others may be highly likely. The risk for developing schizophrenia depends, in part, on prenatal and postnatal environmental factors as well as on genetic predisposition. These factors interact with later psychological and social stressors to produce schizophrenia. The diathesis-stress model implies schizophrenia may be preventable or reversible if important stressors are lessened. This theory contrasts with the view that once schizophrenia develops, it will invariably be a lifetime disorder.

The biopsychosocial model of schizophrenia is supported by information presented earlier in this chapter about schizophrenia's episodic nature for some patients—that is, the fact that some people experience symptom-free periods (Bleuler, 1978). Further, as discussed below, schizophrenia is clearly influenced by some social stressors, such as high-expressed emotion among family members. On the other hand, we have also seen that some persons with schizophrenia have structural brain abnormalities that may produce irreversible negative symptoms. Thus,

diathesis-stress model
Model in which preexisting vulnerability interacts with social/environmental stressor in the development of a disorder.

Integrating Perspectives
A Biopsychosocial Model

PERSPECTIVE ON SCHIZOPHRENIA

BIOLOGICAL FACTORS

Biological factors play a key role in the development of schizophrenia:

➤ Genetic factors play a key role in the development of schizophrenia, as reflected in both twin and family studies.

➤ Central nervous system dysfunctions—such as decreased brain volume and low activity in the temporal lobes—are associated with schizophrenia.

➤ Dopamine appears to increase schizophrenic symptoms, and antipsychotic medication that blocks dopamine has definitely been shown to decrease symptoms.

➤ Viral infections and birth trauma may result in at-risk individuals becoming schizophrenic.

PSYCHOLOGICAL FACTORS

Psychological factors interact with biological vulnerabilities in producing or perpetuating symptoms:

➤ Family stressors and communication problems may increase the risk of relapse for individuals recovering from schizophrenia.

➤ High levels of negative affect of family members and guilt-inducing statements toward an individual also increase the risk of relapse.

SOCIAL FACTORS

Both biological and psychological factors operate in certain social contexts:

➤ For over 100 years, individuals with schizophrenia and other psychotic behavior have been disproportionately represented in the lower social classes. Still, the exact role of social context in the development of schizophrenia is uncertain.

➤ Being in a lower social class places infants at risk for birth trauma, which in turn elevates the risk of developing schizophrenia.

These biological, psychological, and social factors interact to cause problems, as illustrated in the following case:

Robert began to show symptoms of social withdrawal and psychotic thoughts as an undergraduate. He avoided all women (including women professors), talked and laughed to himself during the night, and believed that microwave technology was being used to monitor his thoughts. He also heard voices telling him not to go to class, not to trust family and friends, and to cut himself. Soon after his symptoms became severe, Robert's family admitted him to a hospital.

Robert's treatment reflects the biopsychosocial model. Biologically, Robert was treated with Thorazine, an antipsychotic medication known to reduce symptoms of withdrawal and psychotic thoughts. Psychologically, Robert was involved in family therapy, in which he and his family learned about the symptoms of schizophrenia and how family stress could contribute to increases in these symptoms. His family learned how to react supportively and appropriately when Robert displayed decreases in social functioning. In the social area, group therapy was used to help Robert interpret reality and to encourage socialization. By interacting with others, he learned appropriate self-care and teamwork.

the diathesis-stress model's applicability may vary across individuals with this disorder. Psychological and social stressors may play a bigger role in producing the symptoms of some types of schizophrenia than others. For some individuals, it's likely that the vulnerability is a tendency to become overloaded with information and hyperaroused during periods of high stress (Nuechterlein et al., 1992). Under stressful circumstances, the vulnerable person may become overloaded with sensory stimulation, resulting in psychotic symptoms. For other individuals, the vulnerability may be being in a family with very high levels of negative affect and criticism.

Family Variables

As discussed earlier, schizophrenia is a chronic and episodic disorder. Once clinicians rejected Kraepelin's notion that everyone with schizophrenia would have a deteriorating course, they began searching for factors predictive of better and worse outcomes. The two most powerful predictors of good outcomes are medication compliance (taking medication regularly) and family stress levels. Consider the family stress levels reflected in the following comments by two mothers of schizophrenic individuals:

Patient One

Doctor: Does your son have good health habits?

Mother: No, not at all. I have to nag him to death to get him to wash. And he doesn't use deodorant, so he usually stinks. Worse yet, he often sleeps in his clothes!

Patient Two

Doctor: Do you and your daughter generally get along?

Mother: The truth is, she makes me quite angry every day. Just thinking of the mess she makes in the kitchen gets me going! I have to admit, too, that I'm embarrassed by how odd she looks and acts some times—like when she walks downtown.

A pattern of strong negative emotional feelings among family members—like those expressed by these mothers—is a predictor of relapse in hospitalized patients who have been discharged. In England, Brown and his colleagues (Brown, Carstairs, & Topping, 1958; Brown, 1959) noticed that adjustment of schizophrenic patients after release from a hospital seemed to depend on the living group they returned to. Discharged patients living with brothers or sisters did better than those living with parents or spouses. Patients who spent limited amounts of time with family members did better than those who had extensive contact with them.

In a later study, Brown and his colleagues (Brown, Monck, Carstairs, & Wing, 1962) interviewed schizophrenic patients' female relatives upon the patients' first admittance to the hospital. The researchers assessed hostility, dominance, and levels of emotion expressed by the patient and his or her family members. After discharge, patients returning to homes with family members who displayed high levels of expressed emotion (high EE)—that is, who were critical and/or overinvolved with their ill relative—were most likely to relapse and return to the hospital.

In dozens of studies since the early 1970s, high EE has been reliably associated with relapse. In England, the typical relapse rates during the 9-month period following hospital discharge have been approximately 55 percent for high-EE families and 15 percent for low-EE families (Brown, Birley, & Wing, 1972). In the United States, Vaughn and associates (1984) similarly observed that patients discharged to high-EE families had a 56 percent relapse rate after a 9-month follow-up, whereas patients discharged to low-EE families had a 17 percent relapse rate.

We don't know if relatives of persons with schizophrenia have high EE to begin with or whether it develops from their exposure to individuals with schizophrenia. High EE ratings of patients' relatives have, nevertheless, been major predictors of relapse (Hooley, 1985). Hooley (1985) noted that relapse rates of patients discharged to high-EE families appeared to be lessened if they received antipsychotic

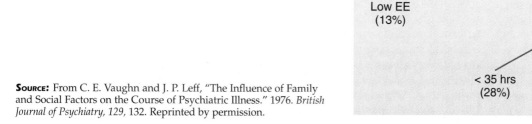

Source: From C. E. Vaughn and J. P. Leff, "The Influence of Family and Social Factors on the Course of Psychiatric Illness." 1976. *British Journal of Psychiatry, 129,* 132. Reprinted by permission.

medication and if they spent fewer than 35 hours per week with family members. The relapse rates of patients spending more or fewer than 35 hours per week with family members are portrayed in Figure 13.3.

High EE has been repeatedly associated with relapse in persons with schizophrenia in the United States, England, France, and other countries. The bulk of the research also strongly suggests that high EE is very important in predicting relapse (Bartlett, Ferrero, Szigethy, Giddey, & Pellizer, 1990; Goldstein, 1995). Other studies in Australia and Germany, however, found no association between relapse rates and high- or low-EE status in the families of discharged persons with schizophrenia (Parker, Johnston, & Hayward, 1988). The reasons for these contradictory findings are unclear.

One possible explanation for the relationship between high EE and relapse is that patients returning to low-EE families may have been less disturbed than those returning to high-EE families. Data on this point are somewhat conflicting. Some studies report that patients from high-EE families have higher levels of symptoms, and others suggest that these differences in symptoms are not factors in explaining outcome (Glynn et al., 1990). It is critical to note, however, that many people view EE as a measure of a family's frustration under the burden of caring for a bizarre, erratic, impaired loved one without adequate community or professional support. In such a model, high EE reflects less about attitudes toward the patient and more about the relatives' own feelings of helplessness and isolation in the face of a devastating, incurable illness. Such an interpretation would be consistent with the lower rates of high-EE families in many non-Western societies, where the notions of community and shared responsibility are often strong and the family is not solely responsible for the care of the ill relative.

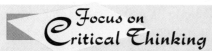

Focus on Critical Thinking

1. As discussed earlier, there are five types of schizophrenia, each characterized by a given set of symptoms. Using the biological, psychological, and social models, what factors explain the development of two types of schizophrenia: catatonic type and paranoid type?

2. Which of the five types of schizophrenia would seem to have the greatest biological/biochemical causes? Explain your answer.

TREATMENT

As we turn our attention to the treatment of schizophrenia, let's recall the chapter-opening case of John Nash. Over the course of 20 years, he was hospitalized a number of times, with little effect:

The months [in hospitalization] did little to arrest the disease. . . . Neuroleptics, the drugs that were used to treat some, but far from all, of the symptoms for the next several decades, were just coming on the scene. And psychoanalysis, which has since been discredited as a means of treating schizophrenia, was still in vogue. . . . As absurd as it now seems, Nash's psychiatrists thought that Mrs. Nash's pregnancy was part of the problem and hoped that he would improve after the baby's birth. (Nasar, 1994, p. III–1)

Like many other serious psychiatric disorders, schizophrenia has been treated with many bizarre interventions. For example, if a man believed he had no head, he might be made to wear a heavy helmet laden with lead until he agreed he had a head. If a woman believed she had snakes in her stomach, she might be given an emetic to cause nausea and vomiting, and a snake might be quickly and secretly placed in the vomit. Early interventions for schizophrenia also included giving opium in high doses and belladonna (a poisonous herb). In the 1800s, Philippe Pinel (1745–1826), a French psychiatrist in charge of several mental hospitals, removed the chains of mental patients and introduced a moral treatment emphasizing dignity, kindness, and sympathy.

In the earlier decades of this century—especially in the 1930s and 1940s—several biological therapies were introduced, including injections of insulin or metrazol (a convulsant), prefrontal leukotomy (the removal of the frontal portion of the brain), and electroconvulsive therapy (ECT). Also during this period, followers of the famous American psychiatrist Harry Stack Sullivan (1892–1949) encouraged the use of psychoanalysis. The first effective treatment for schizophrenia, a neuroleptic medication called chlorpromazine, was developed in the 1950s. (Chlorpromazine is one of a class of medications called *phenothiazines*.)

But during the 1960s—at the time of Vietnam War protests and a rising tide of antiestablishment feelings internationally—a number of clinicians and researchers emphasized social causes of schizophrenia and advocated social as opposed to medical treatments. Issues such as attention problems, language disorders, and family situations, rather than schizophrenia per se, became the focus of treatment for many centers. In the early 1970s, with the rise of community psychology and psychiatry, increased attempts were made to keep persons with schizophrenia at home with their families or in community group homes, as opposed to hospitalizing them. During the 1980s, this movement, called *deinstitutionalization*, began to be reexamined, as many former mental patients became homeless in large metropolitan areas. In part as a response to the obvious need of persons with schizophrenia for more comprehensive care, the 1990s have witnessed the expansion of programs to bring care to the patients (wherever they may be) through assertive community teams. Finally, consumer groups of patients and their relatives assertively strive to better their circumstances and de-stigmatize psychiatric disorders.

Pharmacological, social, and psychological treatments each have some proven efficacy and have been evaluated in many studies throughout the world. Today, drugs are generally regarded as the single most effective treatment for schizophrenic symptoms, but they are now used in combination with psychological and social therapies.

Deinstitutionalization (or release of patients from mental hospitals) has become a hot political issue in many communities. Deinstitutionalization affects the context in which treatments for schizophrenia are now conducted, so we will briefly discuss this topic before discussing pharmacological and psychological treatments. As pressures mounted to release mental patients from hospitals in the 1960s and 1970s, homelessness increased dramatically. Psychiatric facilities seemed to literally dump patients onto the streets. Deinstitutionalization was supposed to be humane, but was it simply a cost-saving measure for states? Follow-up efforts to assess how patients were faring after their transfer from state hospitals to communities were frequently inadequate. In addition, local residents tended to fear or resent patients coming into their communities and often thwarted state planners' efforts to provide patients with homes and hospital aftercare.

deinstitutionalization
Process by which states markedly reduced the population of public psychiatric hospitals by returning patients thought to be able to function outside the hospital to their home communities.

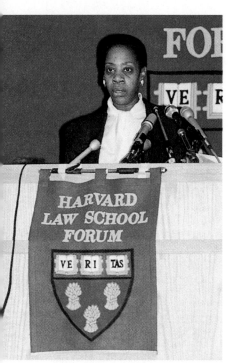

Billy Boggs was a homeless woman in New York City who was institutionalized against her will and diagnosed with schizophrenia. Aided by civil liberties attorneys, she presented her cause in public forums, sued New York City, and won her freedom. What criteria, if any, would you use to remove individuals from the street?

Effective community services for outpatient persons with schizophrenia will require public education about the disorder. Community members will need to understand that persons with schizophrenia don't generally pose a serious threat. The community will also need to accept the unusual behavior, dress, and appearance of some persons who have schizophrenia but are nonetheless able to function outside the hospital. Additionally, successful deinstitutionalization will require staffing of group homes within communities by trained mental health workers who are able to provide support and skills training to people with schizophrenia.

The goal of successful community placement of persons with schizophrenia remains far from realized. In large U.S. cities, homelessness is an acute problem. Only 5 to 10 percent of the housing placements needed for psychiatric patients are available. As a result, people who are psychiatrically impaired are part of an acute problem of homelessness, representing between 25 to 50 percent of the homeless (Mechanic & Aiken, 1987; Julien, 1995).

Pharmacological Treatment

Before the 1950s, mental patients were often as afraid of one another as of the hospital itself. They had good reason to be terrified of the hospital environment. Mental hospitals were often filled with frightening sights and sounds, screams and cries, and unintelligible speech; some patients experienced hallucinations, others were mute and catatonic. Then, as often happens with scientific discoveries, research on a drug for allergies resulted in a very unexpected finding. A French surgeon, Henri Laborit (1951), gave his patients an antihistamine compound in the hope that it would prevent a steep drop in blood pressure during surgery. Although the medication didn't produce the desired effect, Laborit noticed that patients were able to communicate with markedly less anxiety. Laborit's report prompted chemists to experiment with variations of the drug, and these efforts yielded a new medication, chlorpromazine, which had a remarkable calming effect on animals. Laborit then tried chlorpromazine on his patients as a preoperative procedure and found that it kept them calm about the prospects of surgery.

Shortly afterward, two French psychiatrists, Jean Delay and Pierre Deniker (1952), administered chlorpromazine to a variety of psychiatric patients, observing the drug's tranquilizing effect on them. Chlorpromazine not only calmed patients with schizophrenia but also markedly diminished their terrifying hallucinations and delusions, while allowing them to remain alert. Patients who had been ill for years improved significantly on the drug. As a result, many young persons hospitalized with schizophrenia were able to return to their homes, jobs, and families. The news of this development in Paris spread like wildfire: A wonder drug of the mental health field had been discovered. Chlorpromazine became the preferred treatment for schizophrenia, and other antipsychotic drugs began to be developed.

Antipsychotic medications act against the psychotic symptoms. They do not cure or eliminate the disorder, but they reduce and in some cases eliminate many of its symptoms. As the search for new antipsychotic medications progressed, alternatives to drugs like chlorpromazine (brand name Thorazine) were discovered. Other medications developed in the mid-1960s, such as haloperidol (Haldol) became widely used, because they did not have the highly sedating side effects of Thorazine. Because of the use of antipsychotic drugs, within 20 years, approximately one-half of the patients in U.S. mental hospitals were discharged, and even those who remained hospitalized led much improved lives (see Figure 13.4).

In the 1990s, other new antipsychotic medications, such as clozapine (Clozaril) and risperidone (Risperdal), were developed. Clozaril, which affects the serotonin receptors in the brain (Lieberman, 1994), is useful for people who don't respond to other generally available antipsychotic medications; moreover, it doesn't have significant effects on motor functioning. In addition, unlike many other medications,

FIGURE 13.4

Patients in U.S. mental hospitals from 1946 to 1983

Note the dramatic drop of hospitalized patients in 1956 with the introduction of antipsychotic medications.

Source: From *A Primer of Drug Action*, 7th ed., by R. M. Julien. Copyright © 1995 by W. H. Freeman and Company. Used with permission.

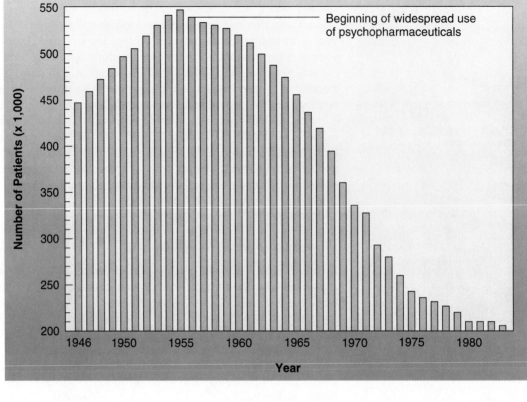

this antipsychotic medication reduces negative symptoms, such as withdrawal and lack of initiation (Meltzer, 1993). However, Clozaril has sedating side effects. In addition, it occasionally causes agranulocytosis, a life-threatening condition in which the white blood cell count is reduced, increasing the likelihood of throat and intestinal tract lesions. For these reasons, physicians need to monitor the level of Clozaril in the blood.

The annual cost of medication with Clozaril is $10,000 (Julien, 1995) because of the requirement that blood be monitored regularly. Any such treatment must be noted in a national registry, and there is mandated education for physicians prescribing it. Although this cost may seem very high, it is less than hospitalization, and, as just noted, Clozaril is clinically useful in many patients who aren't responsive to the other antipsychotic medications. Risperidone (Risperdal) improves both positive and negative symptoms and has a low incidence of motor side effects. It, too, has some side effects, such as insomnia, agitation, and headache; nonetheless, Risperdal is considered as one of the first choices in treating people with schizophrenia (Julien, 1995).

Antipsychotic medications have long-term preventive effects. They deter relapse or reentry into the hospital. A review of more than 35 studies with about 3,500 schizophrenic people showed that only 20 percent of those taking antipsychotic drugs relapsed within 4 to 6 months and had to be rehospitalized, whereas 50 percent of control subjects relapsed within the same period. After a year, 40 percent of persons with schizophrenia taking antipsychotic medications relapsed, whereas 68 percent of controls receiving placebos did (Hogarty, 1984). Despite great strides in brain imaging and neurochemistry, the drugs used to treat schizophrenia have not changed markedly since the early 1960s (Kane & Marder, 1993). The changes in the last decade have been better diagnoses and more effective use of medication to reduce side effects.

Yet like many medications, antipsychotics have undesirable side effects. After treatment with these medications, many schizophrenics develop a severe and largely irreversible side effect called **tardive dyskinesia** (Kane, Woerner, Weinhold,

tardive dyskinesia Largely irreversible side effect of taking antipsychotic medications; characterized by involuntary lip smacking, tongue movements, and chin wagging.

Wegner, & Kinon, 1982). This is an extreme neuromuscular disturbance, usually characterized by involuntary lip smacking, tongue movements, and chin wagging; it can also affect other areas of the body, however. Reviews of antipsychotic drugs' side effects indicate that 3 to 4 percent of patients receiving these medications develop tardive dyskinesia each year and that approximately 20 to 25 percent of any psychiatric population surveyed will experience it (Gilbert, Harris, McAdams, & Jeste, 1995; Jeste & Caliguiri, 1993). Fortunately, doctors are learning to prevent or diminish tardive dyskinesia through low or intermittent doses of medications (Carpenter, Stephens, Rey, Hanlon, & Heinrichs, 1982; Wegner, Catalano, Gilbralter, & Kane, 1985; Jeste & Caliguiri, 1993).

Antipsychotic medications reduce positive symptoms (such as hallucinations) and delusions, and persons with schizophrenia presenting these symptoms are more likely to function effectively after hospitalization. In contrast, despite Clozaril's limited usefulness with negative symptoms, most antipsychotics do not have a major impact on negative symptoms (such as lack of motivation and emotional expressiveness). Structural brain abnormalities are thought to cause these negative symptoms, and some clinical investigators believe they are irreversible (Crow & Johnstone, 1985) and not very susceptible to medication benefits.

The recognition that approximately 30 percent of individuals with schizophrenia who take their medication as prescribed will still relapse, coupled with the limited benefits of medications on negative symptoms and the prominent risk of serious side effects, has spurred work on newer, more effective antipsychotic medications. The two approved most recently by the Food and Drug Administration (FDA) are clozapine (Clozaril) and risperidone (Risperdal). These two new medications seem especially effective on persons who have not benefited from other treatments, thus increasing the hope that even better schizophrenia remission rates will be established in the future (Kane & Marder, 1993).

Psychological Treatments

Psychodynamic Therapy Like Kraepelin, Freud viewed schizophrenia as an organic problem, rather than as primarily a psychological one. In 1938, Freud said, "We must renounce the idea of trying our plan of [psychodynamic] cure upon psychotics" (1935/1964). In contrast, another influential psychoanalyst, Harry Stack Sullivan, had argued in 1924 against the fruitless search for an organic cause of schizophrenia. He felt persons with schizophrenia could respond to a modified version of psychoanalysis.

Sullivan worked with schizophrenic patients at a now famous psychiatric hospital in Maryland called Chestnut Lodge. In his work with young, recent-onset schizophrenic patients during the 1940s and 1950s, Sullivan concluded that their use of language was more a defense than a positive means of communicating. He believed that their speech (or lack of it) served to keep people at a distance, thereby protecting the patients' already low self-esteem. Some patients might maintain their distance by being secretive about their thoughts; others, by talking crazily. Sullivan believed that at least some of this avoidance behavior resulted from a complicated unconscious response to anxiety. In his book *The Psychiatric Interview* (1954), he commented, "People who come to be called schizophrenic are remarkably shy, low in their self-esteem, and rather convinced that they are not appreciated by others. They are faced by the possibility of panic related to their feelings of inferiority, loneliness, and failure in living" (p. 206).

The chief impediment to communicating with a person with schizophrenia, in Sullivan's view, was the patient's anxiety. Therefore, one of the therapist's primary tasks was to avoid provoking unnecessary anxiety in patients during the therapy session. Sullivan believed persons with schizophrenia could benefit if therapists encouraged them to regress or return to early childhood experiences so as to address gradually yet straightforwardly the anxieties experienced at critical points in life. Toward the end of his own life, Sullivan began to emphasize the group or social atmosphere of people with schizophrenia, especially the tension or anxiety experienced in a group. Sullivan was one of the most influential psychiatrists of his time, and the procedures he advocated constituted the standard psychotherapy for schizophrenia in the United States until the 1970s.

Today, few psychodynamic therapists use the specific approaches recommended by Sullivan or by his pupil Freida Fromm-Reichman (1939). Psychodynamic therapies, in general, have become more reality oriented and increasingly focused on current interpersonal relationship patterns (Arieti, 1976). Additionally, since the introduction of clearly effective medication for persons with schizophrenia in the 1950s, most individual psychotherapy approaches have become adjuncts to medication. In a psychodynamic treatment study with over 200 schizophrenic patients, however, May, Tuma, and Dixon (1981) showed that individual psychotherapy was only minimally superior to medication alone in terms of patient adjustment, and that individual psychotherapy did not hasten hospital discharge, either as an adjunct to medication or as the sole treatment. Even though you might expect to find a number of studies evaluating the effects of psychodynamic therapy as compared to those of antipsychotic medication, in fact, a study by May (1968) was the only one that met the standards of a controlled-outcome study in a review of this research. A review of psychodynamic treatment provided no evidence of its effectiveness when offered as the sole treatment. Yet institutions maintain that psychodynamic therapy is a central component of a total treatment program offering various interventions and support services (Mueser & Berenbaum, 1990).

Milieu Therapy   Before the 1960s, the daily care of most persons with schizophrenia centered around routine ward management and custodial care. In earlier years, some experts had intermittently discussed the harmful effects of institutionalization, but in the 1960s, several writers strongly attacked traditional mental hospitals. Sociologist Irving Goffman published a book titled *Asylums* (1961), which depicted the similarities between the life of a mental patient and that of a prisoner. Four years later, psychologists Ullmann and Krasner published *Case Studies in Behavior Modification* (1965), illustrating that the so-called crazy behavior of persons with schizophrenia was sometimes inadvertently reinforced and thus maintained by simple attention from ward attendants. During sessions, too, therapists reinforced "sick talk" by attending to it rather than to "healthy talk." In another influential book, *Institutionalism and Schizophrenia* (1970), British psychiatrists Wing and Brown documented the relationship between a schizophrenic person's environment and mental state. They observed that hospitalized patients were more likely to be withdrawn and apathetic and to speak very little when their living conditions were spartan. The patients' condition was also observed to deteriorate when a new superintendent provided fewer social amenities than the patients previously had.

In sum, these books showed the negative effect on patients of traditional care in mental hospitals. The authors' arguments and findings influenced many professionals to change their attitudes toward the care of persons with schizophrenia. So in the 1960s, clinicians and researchers began to emphasize **milieu treatment** of schizophrenia. Although milieu treatments of persons with schizophrenia vary considerably, they generally emphasize self-care, self-management of ward activities, and group norms for appropriate ward behavior. The new emphasis was on providing as normal a daily routine as possible. People were encouraged to care for themselves, to seek employment if they did not have jobs, and to participate in the variety of social activities the hospitals had begun to provide.

milieu treatment Therapy focusing on the responsibilities of patients to seek employment, care for themselves, and participate in social activities.

Social Learning Approaches   Based on the impetus provided by another book, *The Token Economy: A Motivational System for Therapy and Rehabilitation* by Ayllon and Azrin (1968), behaviorally oriented hospital psychologists began to use reinforcement principles to promote behavior change in persons with schizophrenia. In this kind of social learning approach, for example, attention from ward attendants and opportunities to earn tokens for privileges such as weekend passes were systematically used to motivate persons with schizophrenia to dress appropriately and to participate in group activities.

Paul and Lentz (1977) compared milieu therapy; a social learning approach using reinforcement principles; and a standard hospital regime of occupational therapy, group psychotherapy, and medication as treatments for people with chronic schizophrenia. The social learning approach emphasized prompts, instruction, and reinforcement of desirable behavior on the hospital ward. Individuals matched for age, sex, symptoms, and length of prior hospitalization were assigned to each of the three treatments. Patients in the milieu program and the social learning program showed significantly greater improvement in interpersonal skills, self-care, and ward activities than those receiving routine hospital care. In addition, patients in the social learning program had longer times before they relapsed and had to be readmitted to the hospital than the other two groups.

As Bellack and Mueser (1994) have stated, "Paul and Lentz's study on the effects of a token economy [social learning/reinforcement program] on chronic patients remains a classic to this day." Bellack and Mueser added that the method remains the treatment of choice for many severely ill schizophrenics, even though the results have never been replicated in another setting. Given the results just noted, social learning programs are not as widely used for adult patients as might be expected (Glynn, 1990). Implementation of token reinforcement programs can be very time consuming; they require considerable attention of ward staff and are not suited to the short-term hospitalizations and outpatient care currently predominating in the mental health system (Glynn, 1990; Bellack & Mueser, 1994).

In light of the deinstitutionalization movement, it's not surprising that new treatment approaches were necessary to help patients live independently outside the hospital. In the last decade, social skills training has been one of the most promising treatment developments for schizophrenic patients (Bellack & Mueser, 1994). Programs utilizing behavioral techniques—such as coaching, modeling, role playing, and positive reinforcement—have been designed to change various behaviors—for example, eye contact, smiling, assertiveness, job-interviewing skills, and independent living skills. There are certain problems with the outcome research evaluating social skills training, however, and no study provides unambiguous support for the utility of social skills training (Bellack & Mueser, 1994). Nonetheless, results clearly suggest that persons with schizophrenia can learn new skills. Extra efforts may be required to get schizophrenic individuals to use these skills in the real world where they live. But if they do use the skills, their rates of relapse will decrease and the richness of their lives will be improved (Liberman, Kopelowicz, & Young, 1994).

Family Therapy   As mentioned earlier, periods of hospitalization and other efforts to treat John Nash were largely unsuccessful. "Then came . . . 'a miraculous remission.' It came gradually, almost imperceptibly, starting about . . . when Nash was in his mid-fifties. And as happens in some cases of schizophrenia, the remission was not due to any drug or treatment. [It was] just a question of living a quiet life" (Nasar, 1994, p. III–1).

The "quiet life" Nash lived was made possible by the people around him: his family, friends, and colleagues. They stood by him through 20 years of uncertainty and turmoil, not only making sure he had a place to live but including him as much as possible in regular activities, such as professional projects and seminars.

Family intervention of this type has been one of the most exciting developments of the last two decades in the treatment of schizophrenia. The pioneering work of George Brown and his colleagues (1959, 1972) in England, discussed earlier, led experts to believe that high-EE families may lack the knowledge and skills to assist patients in managing their disorder effectively. In developing interventions to increase knowledge and skills, therapists were careful not to blame the family for the development of a biological disorder. They concentrated on giving families specific techniques that they could use at home, such as how to tell if medication side effects may be too severe, and how to talk with patients so as not to overwhelm them.

The effects of individual social skills training and family therapy were compared by Hogarty and his colleagues (1986, 1991). Schizophrenic subjects were randomly assigned to receive (1) regular outpatient care, (2) social skills training for the individual patient, (3) family intervention for the patient and his or her relatives, or (4) both individual and family treatments. The family intervention and the individual social skills training were conducted for two years. The social skills therapist used the behavioral skills (for instance, coaching, prompting, modeling) discussed in the previous section. The family therapist used advice giving, education, setting of realistic expectations for the individual, and assignment of successive homework activities to help him or her achieve social and vocational independence (Anderson, Reiss, & Hogarty, 1985). Work in the first year was devoted to stress reduction, symptom management, and relapse prevention; the second year was typically focused on enhancing social functioning and autonomy.

The first-year results indicated that both the individual and the family treatment were equally successful at reducing relapse rates. The combined condition was even more effective, with a zero percent relapse rate. In the second year, the benefits of the individual social skills training were reduced; only the family therapy continued to demonstrate significant differences over customary care. Although this study clearly had methodological problems, the results from it and other studies have indicated that family therapy can be a very effective intervention for patients still involved with their relatives (Barrowclough & Tarrier, 1992). In fact, a very large NIMH collaborative treatment study (involving 313 patients) using Falloon's behavioral family therapy along with medication showed significant reductions in relapse rates (Gingerich & Bellack, 1995).

Combined Pharmacological, Psychological, and Social Interventions

Assertive Case Management   From 1955 to 1987, the number of mental patients in public hospitals in the United States fell from 560,000 to approximately 116,000. Following release, these people required many services, including some that were formerly provided by the hospitals. An organized system of community services is still sorely needed. In a review of 14 studies of patients randomly assigned to community treatment or hospitalization, Kiesler and Sibulkin (1987) concluded that community care was more effective than hospitalization on a number of dimensions. As already noted, however, the goal of effective, organized community treatment for the majority of persons with schizophrenia is far from realized.

No single intervention or social service can competently address all the needs of persons with schizophrenia. A critical problem for health specialists is how to organize diverse services in the community (such as medication, family intervention, and social skills training) to benefit these people. To be effective, such services will have to be coordinated with welfare systems, housing authorities, community mental health boards, police departments, and advocacy groups for former mental patients. As Mechanic and Aiken (1987) argued, the solution to the "present crisis and future challenge" of caring for patients who are mentally ill lies in communities' developing coordinated delivery systems for their care.

In the early 1970s, a group of Wisconsin mental health professionals under the guidance of Dr. Leonard Stein began to develop innovative ways to coordinate the delivery of services to patients in their communities and homes. The group organized interdisciplinary teams of public mental health professionals who are jointly responsible for overseeing the total care of specific groups of persons with serious psychiatric illnesses, like schizophrenia. The organizers recognized that individuals coping with serious psychiatric illness such as schizophrenia require continuous,

assertive case management Treatment approach involving multiple systems of intervention, medication, psychological services, and social services; cases are managed through a team of professionals who provide 24-hour services, often in the residence of the patient.

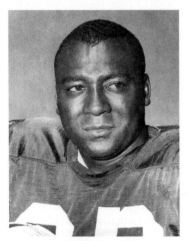

Lionel Aldridge was an All-Pro member of the legendary Green Bay Packer football team. He was also an on-camera commentator for NBC-TV sports, prior to developing schizophrenia at age 33.

reliable, extensive support in order to live successfully in the community. The mental health team either provides the comprehensive array of services the patient requires (such as medication evaluation, 24-hour crisis management, vocational training) or brokers that service from another agency (Social Security benefits, classes at a local technical college). In contrast to other treatment models, services are provided where the individual actually lives or socializes. For instance, a team member may visit the person's home to see where she keeps her medication or may go with her when she has to fix an error made by the bank. This treatment approach, called **assertive case management,** has been found to reduce relapse rates and improve the quality of life of persons with access to these teams (Test, 1992).

In reviewing the research concerning relapse prevention, Barrowclough and Tarrier (1992) found that interventions should focus on the patient and the relatives in the family unit, provide extensive aid on a long-term basis to the family, include mental health professionals in the treatment relationship, and emphasize medication compliance. Efforts are now under way to expand case management approaches nationwide.

The Consumer Movement   Persons with schizophrenia and other psychiatric disorders are beginning to join together to share their techniques to manage symptoms and to work to de-stigmatize mental illness. Rather than labeling themselves as "patients," they consider themselves "consumers" of mental health services and attempt to take a much more active role in managing their circumstances.

Some prominent persons with schizophrenia have taken the lead in sharing how they manage their symptoms and how they try to lead productive lives. Before developing schizophrenia at age 33, Lionel Aldridge was an all-pro member of the legendary Green Bay Packer football team that won Super Bowls I and II. He was also an on-camera commentator for NBC-TV sports. In addition to noting how difficult it is to overcome an illness in which role models are rare, Aldridge has written eloquently about coping with paranoia:

I tell a story about how I learned to handle paranoia. There's a restaurant near my house that has big glass windows in front. And I go there frequently for coffee and to visit with people. But, on some occasions, when I get in front of the windows of that restaurant I start to feel like no one inside wants me in there. If I turn around at that point and go home, I allow the illness to limit my life—to make my world small. So I started to imagine that I love myself, and that took me into the restaurant . . . and sat me down. Not too steady you know. I was a little shaky. But pretty soon the waitress is treating me like she likes me. Somebody else down the counter is talking to me about football. And it becomes apparent to me, real early, that *nobody in the restaurant knew that they didn't want me in there.* So it became real apparent that the whole process was taking place only in my own mind. (Aldridge, 1990, p. 20)

Focus on Critical Thinking

Imagine that you work for a managed care company (HMO) and that your job is to monitor the kind of health care a person with chronic schizophrenia receives, being watchful of the cost as well as the benefit of the treatment. You can choose from drug (pharmacological) therapy, psychotherapy, or assertive case management.

1. Which approach would you decide is most appropriate, and on what would you base your decision?
2. If you only had to consider the successfulness of the intervention, would your choice be the same? Why or why not?

SUMMARY

Description

■ The criteria for a diagnosis of schizophrenia are characterized by a mixture of symptoms that have been present for at least 1 month, including two of the following: delusions, hallucinations, disorganized speech, grossly disorganized or catatonic behavior, and negative symptoms. In order for a diagnosis of schizophrenia to be made, some signs of the disorder must persist for at least 6 months, and the symptoms must be associated with marked social or occupational impairment. Finally, biological factors (such as drug use or a brain tumor) must be ruled out as causes of the symptoms.

■ Positive symptoms of schizophrenia include delusions, hallucinations, disorganized speech, and grossly disorganized or catatonic behavior. Negative symptoms or behavioral deficits are symptoms such as flat affect and alogia.

■ The prodromal phase of schizophrenia, characterized by a deterioration of the individual's functioning, usually precedes the active or acute phase. During the acute phase, the individual exhibits psychotic symptoms. The residual phase follows the acute phase. The residual phase is similar to the prodromal phase in that it is characterized by social withdrawal, inactivity, and bizarre thoughts. Negative symptoms and social and occupational impairments predominate during this phase.

■ Five types of schizophrenia exist: catatonic, disorganized, paranoid, undifferentiated, and residual.

Causes

■ Family and twin studies have repeatedly found that there is a genetic component to schizophrenia. The odds of developing schizophrenia increase with the number of relatives that have this disorder. Research with schizophrenic adopted children has shown that schizophrenia is significantly more common in biological relatives of schizophrenics.

■ Biological research with MRIs and PET scans has shown that people with schizophrenia have structural and functional brain abnormalities, especially in the frontal and temporal areas.

■ Birth trauma and viral infections also appear to be causative factors for some schizophrenic individuals.

■ The role of communication abnormalities in the families of people with schizophrenia is yet to be determined. Research has demonstrated that familial factors may play an influential role in the development of schizophrenia in high-risk individuals.

■ Schizophrenia is more prevalent among people in the lower classes; it appears that schizophrenia causes individuals to drift or move into the lower classes. However, some factors related to being in a lower social class probably contribute to the development of this disorder, as well.

■ Biopsychosocial models of schizophrenia emphasize the interaction of genetic and biochemical factors with the person's environment. Such models imply that schizophrenia may be preventable or reversible, if important stressors are lessened.

■ High expressed emotion (EE) in families has been shown to be a predictor of relapse in discharged schizophrenic patients.

Treatment

■ Antipsychotics (such as chlorpromazine) reduce positive symptoms of schizophrenia and often prevent relapse or reentry into the hospital. The widespread use of antipsychotic medications enabled policy makers to release many patients from hospitals—a change called deinstitutionalization.

■ Despite the advantages of antipsychotics, many individuals who take them develop tardive dyskinesia, an extreme and often irreversible neuromuscular disturbance. Also, standard antipsychotics do not appear to have an impact on negative symptoms. Furthermore, many people who take these medications still relapse. Clozapine and risperidone are new medications that may have fewer side effects.

■ Psychodynamic treatments that focus on interpersonal patterns do not have proven efficacy in studies in different settings.

- Milieu therapy focuses on the responsibilities of individuals to seek employment, to care for themselves, and to participate in social activities. Inpatient social learning programs stress incentive systems for increasing socially appropriate behaviors. Both milieu treatments and social learning programs have been effective on hospital wards, but they are not well suited to the treatment of schizophrenic people in outpatient settings.

- In meeting the challenge of helping schizophrenic individuals who still live with their families in their communities, social skills training and family therapy have proved quite effective.

- In assertive case management, a team of professionals are responsible for overseeing the care of a specific group of persons. Treatment occurs in the schizophrenic person's home and includes an array of services, such as medication evaluation, crisis management, and vocational training. This treatment approach has been shown to improve the quality of life and reduce relapse rates.

KEY TERMS

active or acute phase, **p. 422**
adoption studies, **p. 425**
alogia, **p. 421**
assertive case management, **p. 447**
avolition, **p. 421**
catatonic behavior, **p. 420**
catatonic type, **p. 422**
deinstitutionalization, **p. 440**
delusions, **p. 417**
dementia praecox, **p. 412**
diathesis-stress model, **p. 436**
disorganized speech, **p. 419**
disorganized type, **p. 423**

double-bind hypothesis, **p. 433**
epidemiology, **p. 434**
family studies, **p. 424**
grossly disorganized behavior, **p. 420**
hallucinations, **p. 419**
magnetic resonance imaging (MRI), **p. 429**
milieu treatment, **p. 444**
multifactorial polygenic model, **p. 427**
negative symptoms, **p. 417**
paranoid type, **p. 423**
positive symptoms, **p. 417**
positron emission tomographic (PET) scan, **p. 429**

prodromal phase, **p. 422**
psychotic, **p. 412**
residual phase, **p. 422**
residual type, **p. 423**
schizophrenia, **p. 416**
smooth-pursuit eye-tracking dysfunction, **p. 430**
social causation hypothesis, **p. 435**
social selection hypothesis, **p. 435**
tardive dyskinesia, **p. 442**
twin studies, **p. 424**
undifferentiated type, **p. 423**

CRITICAL THINKING EXERCISE

Suppose you were the director of the National Institute of Mental Health (NIMH). As such, you would have the authority and resources to focus research on the causes of schizophrenia.

1. What would your priorities be? Explain them, based on the information presented in this chapter.

Chapter 14

CHILDHOOD DISORDERS

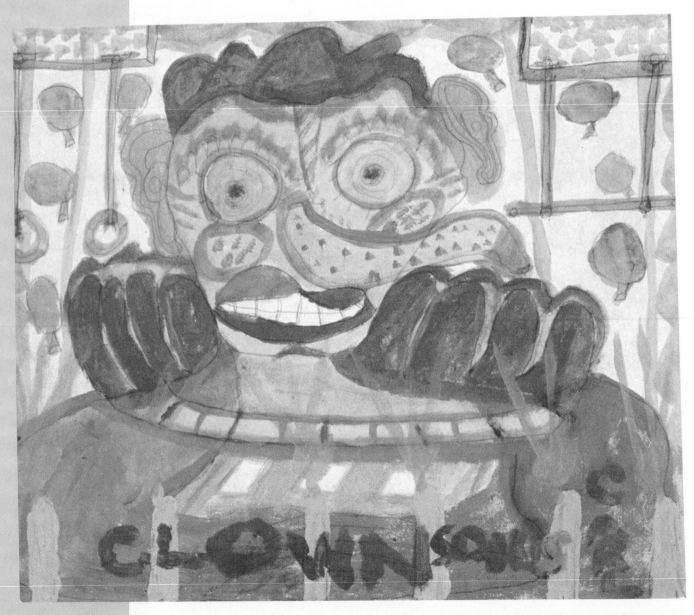

Carl Greenberg, **Clown Songs,** HAI

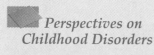

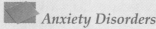

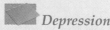

E
ight-year-old Todd fought every day with his 6-year-old brother, Brian. He teased him, threw things at him, and took things from his room. Todd occasionally swore at his mother, but he also was very affectionate to her. Todd's teacher reported that he did adequate work in school. He didn't like school, however, because he found it hard to concentrate. He daydreamed a lot, and he would sometimes get into minor fights.

Todd's mother was often openly angry with his father, who became withdrawn and depressed, fearing that his wife would divorce him. Todd's mother had threatened to leave in Todd's presence. Within 4 months after an initial clinical assessment of Todd, his father left the home at the mother's insistence.

Todd and Brian's visitations with their father were difficult, because he complained that he had little money to take them out. He also made it clear to the boys that their mother had forced him to leave. Using his depression to win the boys' sympathies, he finally convinced the mother to allow him to return home. However, battles quickly started between the parents. During this time, Todd became more and more aggressive. One day, he crawled out a window onto the roof and refused to come inside. The parental conflicts seemed to make his problems worse.

Todd's behavior at home continued to swing from periods of being very good to weeks of hell for his mother. Eventually, the parents divorced, which Todd believed was partly his fault. His mother tried valiantly to provide the love and support that Todd needed. But even with extra help, his schoolwork deteriorated. He and his mother often got into fights over his homework. He began lying to his mother and was even caught stealing from her purse. At times, she threatened to send him to live with his father, though she never followed through with this threat. Todd's angry outbursts were extremely difficult for his mother to handle. She began to fear that her other son would imitate Todd's swearing and fighting.

Todd's case exemplifies several factors common to children with oppositional defiant disorder (ODD). First, they have multiple problems; Todd, for example, had both depressive symptoms and academic difficulty. Second, the pattern of defiance is limited to interactions at home and with children they know well. Third, children with ODD are often from homes with severe marital problems and/or divorce. Finally, parental discipline is lax and often inconsistent.

In this chapter, we'll cover the causes and treatments of some of the major child-hood problems. Using the biopsychosocial orientation, we will review the contributions of biological, psychological, and social factors that place a child at risk for developing various psychological problems. We'll first consider social attitudes toward and prevalence of the major childhood disorders and how these disorders differ for boys and girls. We will then discuss common childhood disorders seen in clinical practice: oppositional defiant disorder and conduct disorder; attention-deficit/hyperactivity disorder; anxiety disorders; enuresis; learning disorders; and childhood depression. (Two other major classes of childhood disorders—mental retardation and pervasive developmental disorders—are addressed in Chapter 15.)

PERSPECTIVES ON CHILDHOOD DISORDERS

Before 1900, society viewed children's psychological and physical abnormalities as downward extensions of adult problems. Children with extreme abnormalities, especially physical disfigurements, went untreated. In general, adults did not enjoy children—normal or abnormal—for their unique childlike qualities. Instead, grown-ups treated the young as little adults (Aries, 1962). Portraiture art from this period mirrors this attitude. For example, the children in *The Maids of Honor*, a painting by Velazquez (1656), wore miniature versions of adult clothing.

A significant change occurred in 1898, when Leightner Witmer, at the University of Pennsylvania, founded the first U.S. psychological clinic for the treatment of children. Witmer believed that the causes of children's problems could be found in their homes, schools, and communities. Then, in 1909, Freud published the story of Little Hans, the first account of the psychoanalytic treatment of a child (Freud, 1909/1955). Another major event was the 1909 establishment of the Healy School (Juvenile Psychopathic Institute) in Chicago, a clinic school for juvenile delinquents. William Healy championed the idea that adolescents' illegal behavior did not have a physical cause. Instead, Healy and his school promoted the notion that children learned such behavior in their subcultures.

By the 1930s, treatment programs had begun for children. State universities established child guidance clinics, and by the 1950s, experts agreed that children's emotional disturbances required consideration separate from adult disturbances.

Children in the 1600s were treated as miniature adults, as evident by their dress and depiction in portraits of this type.

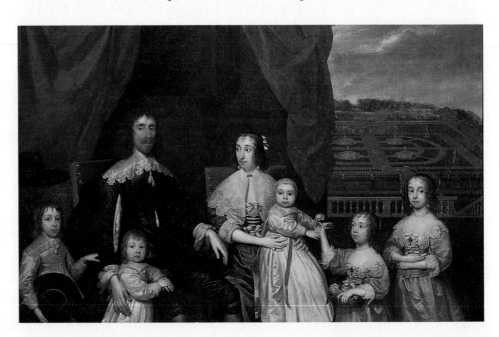

During this time, the field of child psychology expanded, and in the 1970s, many universities started graduate degree programs in developmental psychology. Clinical child psychology became a subspecialty of clinical psychology, and the publication of a prestigious research series, *Advances in Clinical Child Psychology,* began in 1977. Yet mental health professionals specializing in adult disorders still far outnumbered child psychologists and psychiatrists. The history of child psychology journals also reflects the secondary significance attached to the subject. The *Journal of Abnormal Child Psychology* (publishing research on psychological disorders of children) did not emerge until 1973. In contrast, the *Journal of Abnormal Psychology,* focusing primarily on adult disorders, had begun publication in 1906.

The second edition of the *Diagnostic and Statistical Manual of Mental Disorders* (American Psychiatric Association, 1968) had only 6 separate diagnoses. The *DSM-IV* (American Psychiatric Association, 1994) now lists 41 separate diagnoses. Given the number and variety of childhood diagnoses, why then do most abnormal psychology texts devote so little space to them? One reason is that fewer psychologists and psychiatrists specialize in children than in adults. Nonetheless, the number of clinicians and researchers specializing in childhood disorders is growing quickly as evidenced by the recent publication of at least six abnormal psychology texts on childhood disorders. Before 1974 (Ross, 1974), no major publisher had produced an undergraduate text on abnormal child psychology.

Prevalence

Using *DSM-III* (1980) criteria, researchers assessed a representative sample of approximately 800 New Zealand children to ascertain the prevalence of various problems (Anderson, Williams, McGee, & Silva, 1987). The children who were assessed—all nonretarded and between the ages of 11 and 12—were part of an ongoing health and developmental study. Table 14.1 lists the prevalence of various childhood disorders in the New Zealand sample and the male-to-female ratio of each.

About 25 percent of the children received some diagnosis. Almost identical percentages were found in a sample of 15-year-olds (Fergusson, Horwood, & Lynskey, 1993). More than half of those diagnosed had multiple disorders, such as an attention-deficit problem combined with a conduct disorder or oppositional

TABLE 14.1	Prevalence of Childhood Disorders (among approximately 800 New Zealand children)		
Disorder	**N**	**Male/Female Ratio**	**Prevalence**
Attention deficit disorder	53	5.1/1	7%
Oppositional disorder	45	2.2/1	6%
Separation anxiety	28	0.4/1	3%
Conduct disorder/aggressive	27	3.2/1	3%
Overanxious disorder	23	1.7/1	3%
Simple phobia	19	0.6/1	2%
Depressive/dysthymia	17	5.4/1	2%
Social phobia	7	0.2/1	1%
Total	**219**	**1.8/1**	

Source: From Anderson, J. C., Williams, S., McGee, R., & Silva, P. A., "DSM-III disorders in preadolescent children: Prevalence in a large sample from the general population." *Archives of General Psychiatry, 44,* 72. Copyright © 1987 American Medical Association. Reprinted by permission.

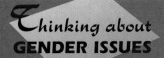

Thinking about GENDER ISSUES — Gender Differences across Disorders

In every major diagnostic category of the children assessed in a New Zealand study, boys far outnumbered girls, with the exception of anxieties and phobias (Anderson et al., 1987). Additionally, for all major disorders except anxious/phobic problems, parents of boys sought help more frequently than parents of girls. Boys' greater vulnerability to most psychological problems, except anxiety, is apparent across cultures in North America, western Europe, Australia, and New Zealand. Moreover, their greater vulnerability to physical problems is evident even before birth and during infancy. For every 100 girls conceived, approximately 140 boys are conceived, but the ratio of boys' births to that of girls is 106/100 (Klug & Cummings, 1986). That is, nearly one-third of boys conceived die before birth. More boys than girls also die from birth defects and diseases in infancy, especially during the first month. By age 3, there are fewer males than females, because of boys' greater susceptibility to physical diseases in utero and in infancy, even though boys outnumber girls by 40 percent at conception.

As they mature, boys are also much more likely to be susceptible to family and marital stress. There are clear associations between parents' marital troubles and their sons' problems. All types of boys' problems assessed were in fact related to tensions or difficulties between parents. Further, U.S. and British studies have repeatedly demonstrated higher associations between marital troubles and boys' problems, especially conduct problems, than between marital troubles and girls' problems (Crockenberg & Covey, 1991; Cummings & Davies, 1994; O'Leary & Emery, 1984).

As children move into adolescence, the distribution of psychological disorders changes. Fifteen-year-old girls begin to have more problems than boys, and anxiety and mood disorders (depression) are among the foremost disorders of teen-age girls (Fergusson, Horwood, & Lynskey, 1993).

Think about the following questions:

1. Why would boys receive more diagnoses for problems in childhood and girls receive more diagnoses in adolescence?
2. Do you think these patterns would change if males and females were treated more similarly at home and in schools? Explain your answer.

---

oppositional defiant disorder (ODD) Characterized by significant defiant and negative child behavior, including frequent anger, temper tantrums, swearing, and defiance of adult rules.

Focus on Critical Thinking

1. Parents of children with conduct disorder or oppositional defiant disorder seek professional help for their children more often than parents of children with other disorders. Why do you think this is so?
2. In your own community, how much professional attention do the psychological problems of children receive compared to those of adults? In your opinion, why?

defiant disorder. Forty-seven percent of the children with an attention-deficit disorder also had a conduct disorder or oppositional disorder. A similar diagnostic overlap occurs among children in the United States (Abikoff & Klein, 1992).

Researchers determine the frequency of various childhood problems in order to obtain data about which problems are most prevalent and the extent to which certain problems overlap. (See the Thinking about Gender Issues box.) The problems that make parents take their children to private practitioners reveal the types of problems parents find most distressing. In the New Zealand study, parents took their children to clinics for the following problems:

1. *Multiple disorders:* 57 percent (primarily conduct [CD]/oppositional [ODD] and anxious/phobic)
2. *Attention-deficit/hyperactivity disorder (AD/HD):* 43 percent
3. *CD/ODD:* 23 percent
4. *Anxious/phobic:* 22 percent
5. *AD/HD and CD/ODD:* 13 percent

Clearly, the majority of the children seen by professionals in the New Zealand study had multiple problems (57 percent). Parents most frequently sought help for their child's conduct problems and hyperactivity.

conduct disorder (CD)
Repetitive and persistent pattern of conduct that violates the basic rights of others and major age-appropriate societal norms or rules.

OPPOSITIONAL DEFIANT AND CONDUCT DISORDERS

Description

All children can be defiant and argumentative. Children diagnosed with **oppositional defiant disorder (ODD),** however, behave defiantly and negatively significantly more frequently than their peers. The diagnostic criteria for ODD specified in the fourth edition of the *Diagnostic and Statistical Manual of Mental Disorders (DSM-IV)* are presented in the first *DSM-IV* table. Children with ODD are often angry, lose their temper, swear, and defy adult rules. Because they usually limit their defiance to situations in the home and with children they know well, they may not show these behaviors during an office visit to a pediatrician or psychologist. Symptoms of oppositional defiant disorder typically appear before the age of 8 and not later than early adolescence (American Psychiatric Association, 1994). In serious cases, they may evolve into conduct disorder, usually diagnosed after age 12.

Children with **conduct disorder (CD)** show a "repetitive and persistent pattern of conduct in which the basic rights of others and major age-appropriate societal norms or rules are violated. The behavior pattern typically is present in a variety of settings such as home, school, or the community" (American Psychiatric Association, 1994). The diagnostic criteria for CD are presented in the *DSM-IV* table on page 456. Children with CD usually display their disorder by verbal and physical aggression but may also destroy others' property or treat animals cruelly. As these children become older, their aggression may take the form of mugging and purse snatching, and in the late teens, sometimes even rape and murder. The following reports of parents exemplify the difficulties of children with conduct problems:

> My boy is always fighting with other kids; he is a bully, and he has a chip on his shoulder. He seems to feel my husband and I don't care for him as much as we do for his brothers and sisters. (O'Leary, 1984, p. 16)

> My ten-year-old boy won't do what I ask him to do unless I threaten him severely; I sometimes wonder whether he has a hearing problem. He refuses to do his homework, yet he is barely passing. I could handle his problems before he went to school, but since first grade he has become unbearable. Now my husband and I argue about how to discipline him, and he is affecting our marriage. (O'Leary, 1984, p. 16)

DSM-IV Diagnostic Criteria for 313.81 OPPOSITIONAL DEFIANT DISORDER

A. A pattern of negativistic, hostile, and defiant behavior lasting at least 6 months, during which four (or more) of the following are present:
   (1) often loses temper
   (2) often argues with adults
   (3) often actively defies or refuses to comply with adults' requests or rules
   (4) often deliberately annoys people
   (5) often blames others for his/her mistakes or behavior
   (6) is often touchy or easily annoyed by others
   (7) is often angry and resentful
   (8) is often spiteful and vindictive

B. The disturbance in behavior causes clinically significant impairment in social, academic, or occupational functioning.

C. The behaviors do not occur exclusively during the course of a Psychotic or Mood Disorder.

D. Criteria are not met for a Conduct Disorder, and if the individual is age 18 years or older, criteria are not met for Antisocial Personality Disorder.

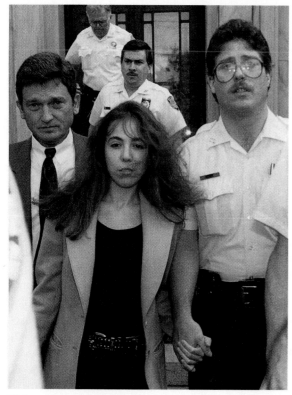

Violence among today's youths is on the rise, and its prevalence is not limited to large cities. Amy Fisher, a teen from a suburb of Long Island, New York, was convicted for attempting to murder the wife of Joey Buttafuoco. Might Amy Fisher, who had sex with Buttafuoco, be diagnosed with any childhood disorder?

DSM-IV   *Diagnostic Criteria for 312.8* **CONDUCT DISORDER**

A. A repetitive and persistent pattern of behavior in which the basic rights of others or major age-appropriate societal norms or rules are violated, as manifested by three (or more) of the following criteria in the past 12 months, with at least one criterion present in the past 6 months:

Aggression to people and animals
(1) often bullies, threatens, or intimidates others
(2) often initiates physical fights
(3) has used a weapon that can cause serious physical harm to others (e.g., a bat, brick, broken bottle, knife, gun)
(4) has been physically cruel to people
(5) has been physically cruel to animals
(6) has stolen while confronting a victim (e.g., mugging, purse snatching, extortion, armed robbery)
(7) has forced someone into sexual activity

Destruction of property
(8) has deliberately engaged in fire setting with the intention of causing serious damage

(9) has deliberately destroyed other people's property (other than by fire setting)

Deceitfulness or theft
(10) has broken into someone else's house, building, or car
(11) often lies to obtain goods or favors or to avoid obligations (i.e., "cons" others)
(12) has stolen items of nontrivial value without confronting a victim (e.g., shoplifting, but without breaking or entering; forgery)

Serious violations of rules
(13) often stays out at night despite parental prohibitions, beginning before age 13 years
(14) has run away from home overnight at least twice while living in parental or guardian home (or once for lengthy time period)
(15) is often truant from school, beginning before age 13 years

B. The disturbance in behavior causes clinically significant impairment in social, academic, or occupational functioning.

C. If age 18 years or older, criteria are not met for Antisocial Personality Disorder.

Violence among young people is often linked to conduct disorder. A person whose conduct disorder pattern persists beyond age 18 often engages in physical fights and reckless behavior, such as driving while intoxicated, speeding or racing cars, promiscuity, and financial irresponsibility. People with conduct disorder lack guilt about their behavior and its negative effects on others. After age 18, such behavior is diagnosed as antisocial personality disorder. We don't know why, but the most blatant forms of antisocial behavior—such as physical fighting and criminal activity—tend to decrease significantly after age 40 in most individuals.

For many persons who develop ODD or CD, a behavior pattern emerges in childhood and becomes serious in the teens and early adulthood. Many children, of course, don't progress from one disorder to another. For example, most juvenile offenders don't move on from minor to more serious crimes. Yet the roots of antisocial personality disorder for males and females can often be traced to conduct disorder in childhood and are clearly evident by puberty or the early teens (see Chapter 12). Also, a disproportionate number of adults diagnosed as drug dependent report symptoms of conduct disorder and attentional problems in childhood (Robins & Price, 1991). Later, we'll discuss some treatments for the various childhood disorders that decrease the possibility of movement from one disorder to another.

Oppositional defiant disorder is more common in boys than in girls. For example, one study found that 5 percent of boys and 3 percent of girls had ODD (Loney, 1987). Overall, the prevalence of conduct disorder in the United States has been estimated at 6 to 16 percent for males and 2 to 9 percent for females younger than 18 years old (American Psychiatric Association, 1994). Although delinquency is not synonymous with having conduct disorder, the two frequently overlap. A **delinquent** is someone under 18 who has committed a legal offense, whereas a young person diagnosed with conduct disorder has a psychological or psychiatric disorder. Most habitual youthful offenders do meet the diagnostic criteria for conduct disorder. Although youthful offenders are usually males, over the last few decades, the percentage of young females committing crimes has increased (Chesney-Lind, 1987; Elliot, 1994).

delinquent Individual under 18 who has committed a legal offense; may not necessarily have a diagnosable psychological or psychiatric disorder.

Causes

Genetic, psychological, and social factors provide some explanations of the causes of oppositional and conduct disorder. Because the common themes in oppositional and conduct problems are anger outbursts, temper problems, and, most significantly, aggression, the etiological question is: What causes extreme anger and aggression in children and adolescents? There are genetic and psychological factors.

Genetic Predisposition   We currently don't have any clear evidence of the specific inheritance of conduct disorders with children. However, twin studies with adults in the United States and Canada provide strong evidence for genetic influences on self-reported aggressive personality styles (Rushton et al., 1986; Telleken et al., 1988).

Researchers have long known that parents of children diagnosed with conduct disorder frequently display an antisocial behavior pattern, such as excessive drinking or criminal activity. Additionally, Robins (1966) found that half the adult males diagnosed as having conduct disorder as children met the criteria for what is now termed antisocial personality disorder. Twin studies have shown that identical (monozygotic) twins have a much higher concordance rate for criminal convictions than fraternal (dizygotic) twins (Cloninger & Gottesman, 1987). Related data have indicated that birth delivery complications predict multiple criminal offenses (Brennan, Mednick, & Kandel, 1991).

Although many children with conduct disorder don't engage in criminal activity in adulthood, it's true that childhood aggressive/impulsive behavior is predictive of antisocial problems in adulthood and that genetic and birth problems as predictors of later aggressive behavior can't be ignored. Indeed, disruptive and antisocial behavior is so stable from childhood to adolescence that there are now research accounts to explain this stability. This research suggests that impulsivity and low levels of anxiety, as rated by kindergarten teachers, seem to best predict later self-reported delinquency scores (Tremblay, Pihl, Vitaro, & Dobkin, 1994).

Psychological Determinants   Learning, cognition, and family factors are clearly related to the development of ODD and CD. We'll now discuss rewards for aggressive behavior, modeling, cognitive misperceptions of hostile intent, harsh punishment, inconsistent and lax discipline, and marital discord and divorce.

Parents and peers often reward aggressive behavior. All children, especially males, are likely to learn of aggression's payoffs. Even 30 years ago, researchers had shown how children were rewarded for aggressive behavior in nursery school (Patterson, Littman, & Bricker, 1967). Specifically, researchers observed nursery school children over a 9-month period and coded consequences of aggression as positive and negative. The positive consequences of aggressive behavior included crying and passivity on the part of the attacked child. (In other words, the aggressive behavior was rewarded and thus encouraged.) Negative consequences included the attacked child's telling the teacher, retaliating, or asking the teacher to intervene. The results of the study showed that the aggressive behaviors of nursery school children were most likely followed by what a child might interpret as positive consequences. (For instance, by having a tantrum, a child might get his way.)

More recent research has confirmed these results with mother-and-child interactions: Stopping a conflict by the mother leads to aggression in the child (Snyder, Edwards, McGraw, Kilmore, & Holton, 1994). In addition, a new wrinkle was discovered: Aggressive boys often match their mothers' punitive behavior with even more negative interactions of their own. In turn, mothers match their sons' negative interactions in almost a tit-for-tat manner. Attempts at deescalation are infrequent.

Children learn to do what they observe others do. Considerable research has been conducted on the effects of observing aggression. Most reviewers of this research have concluded that watching aggression by others in real life and in the media leads some people to act aggressively (Heath, Bresolin, & Rinaldi, 1989;

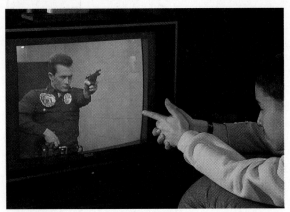

Research has shown that children who observe violence on television are more likely to be aggressive than other children. What restrictions on TV violence would you advocate?

Centerwall, 1992). The impact of television aggression is hotly debated. Given the failure of the TV industry to regulate itself, some 37 percent of TV network executives believe that the portrayal of violence is a serious problem (Guttman, 1994).

In a series of studies, Bandura and his colleagues demonstrated that children readily imitate aggressive filmed models (Bandura, 1977). In a classic study, Lefkowitz, Eron, Walden, and Huesmann (1977) assessed 400 9-year-old boys' viewing habits. Ten years later, when the boys were 19 years old, those who had watched a high level of TV violence at age 9 were more aggressive than those who had not.

Aggressive children misperceive intentions of others as hostile (Crick & Dodge, 1994). Several studies have demonstrated that aggressive children make errors in judging the intent of others when that intent has been manipulated by experimenters. Further, the misperception errors could not be accounted for by verbal intelligence deficits or by general social information deficits.

Parents who tend to resort to strong and frequent punishment tend to have children with conduct problems and delinquent behavior (Bandura & Walters, 1963). Childhood aggression is also associated with the frequency of punishment in the home. When aggressive and nonaggressive children are matched for age and socioeconomic status, parents of aggressive children are found to be more punitive, to disagree with each other more, and to be more cold and rejecting than parents of nonaggressive children (Bandura & Walters, 1959). Children with conduct problems are also more likely to have been physically abused than children referred to clinics who do not have conduct problems (Wolfe, 1987).

Even when parents harshly punish aggressive behavior at home, they often specifically encourage a child's aggression directed at children outside the home (Bandura & Walters, 1959). For example, research has shown that parents who punish their children severely are the same parents who are likely to say to their children, "If anyone makes fun of you at school, don't let them get away with it. Punch them!"

Inconsistent and lax discipline and minimal monitoring or supervision of children's activities are all associated with conduct problems and antisocial behavior. Laxity of discipline and monitoring has been associated with conduct problems (Robins, 1966) and in Patterson and Bank's (1986) complex evaluations of a model of antisocial behavior training, as presented in Figure 14.1. Furthermore, lax and overreactive discipline is also associated with oppositional defiant behaviors of toddlers (Arnold, O'Leary, Wolff, & Acker, 1993).

Inept discipline refers to frequent and severe physical punishment, such as grabbing, hitting, or beating with an object as well as scolding and nagging when trivial problems occur. Most importantly, parents who ineptly discipline their children fail to follow through consistently with their threats. **Inept monitoring** is a failure to provide adequate supervision and attention during child care. Parents considered to be inept monitors often disregard reports by teachers and neighbors of their children's significant misbehavior and have an "out of sight, out of mind" attitude.

Inconsistent discipline often contributes to negative child behavior (Forgatch, 1991). For instance, although children may be punished on occasion for their coercive (demanding) behavior, they also learn that coercive behavior can be rewarding. So they persist in tantrums, arguments, and fighting until they get their way. They manipulate their parents as well as their siblings. In essence, through repeated tantrums and outbursts, they teach their parents to stop making requests.

In Patterson and Bank's (1986) model, inept discipline and inept monitoring lead to antisocial behavior development in children. Inept discipline and coercive child behavior patterns influence each other. Parents who use inept discipline are

inept discipline Frequent and severe physical punishment (such as grabbing, hitting, or beating with an object) as well as scolding and nagging when trivial problems occur, combined with failure to follow through on threats.

inept monitoring Failure to provide adequate supervision and attention during child care.

FIGURE 14.1 Basic training in the home for antisocial behavior

Patterson and Bank's model illustrates the interaction of a number of variables in the home that lead to the development of antisocial behavior in children. The chain starts with inept discipline and often goes on to inept monitoring and coercive (demanding) child interactions. Inept discipline does not always lead to inept monitoring, but parents who are not effective in their use of discipline often do not monitor their children well, either. Both inept monitoring and coercive child interactions lead directly to antisocial behavior.

Source: Reprinted from *Behaviour Research and Therapy, 8,* G. R. Patterson and L. Bank, p. 56. Copyright © 1986 with kind permission from Elsevier Science Ltd. The Boulevard, Langford Lane, Kidlington OX5 1GB UK.

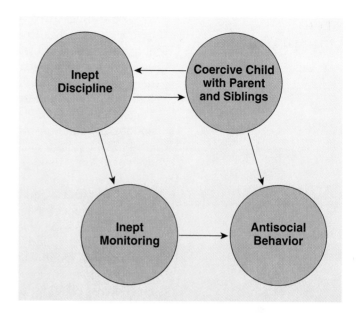

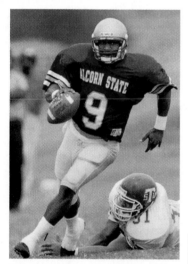

Being raised by a single parent, in itself, certainly does not lead to child behavior problems, in most cases. Steve McNair was raised in extreme poverty by a single parent. He later became a successful football player for Alcorn State and a Heisman Trophy candidate in 1994. What critical factors allow some children in poverty to overcome adversity and succeed in academic and athletic pursuits?

likely to have children who become coercive. And coercive children are likely to produce parental reactions such as severe punishment and failure to follow through on threats. In brief, children and parents cause behaviors in one another.

Marital problems long have been seen as contributing factors to childhood problems, especially conduct disorders. In the 1950s and 1960s, clinicians and researchers noted that teen-agers with divorced parents were more likely to display antisocial behavior and delinquency than those who lived with both parents. Later findings showed that marital discord is a clear risk factor for conduct disorders (Cummings & Davies, 1994; Grych & Fincham, 1990; O'Leary & Emery, 1984; Rutter, 1994). Even so, the correlation between marital discord and antisocial behavior in children is not very large (Fincham, 1994; Jouriles, Bourg, & Farris, 1991; Patterson, Reid, & Dishion, 1992). Subsequent research has also shown that teen-agers from divorced homes have a variety of childhood disorders, not simply conduct problems (Rutter, 1970). Research and theoretical conceptualizations are now directed at trying to determine what aspects of marital conflict are critical risk factors—for example, modeling of hostility and aggression, aggression directed to the child, or poor parent/child relationships (Fincham, Grych, & Osborne, 1994; Rutter, 1994).

In the chapter-opening case, Todd was diagnosed with oppositional defiant disorder, but he also displayed a number of depressive symptoms. He frequently moped around the house, rarely speaking to others. Following visits with his father, he felt so bad that he sometimes cried himself to sleep. The frequent arguments he witnessed between his parents had a negative impact on him. He also suffered from the divorce process. Money problems became obvious to both boys when the family income was split to support two households. At school, Todd's ability to function was impaired by his daydreaming and failure to complete homework. All in all, marital conflict and divorce had an obvious negative impact on Todd.

Still, marital discord and divorce are common in contemporary American society. Many divorced people are able to raise children with little obvious negative impact on them. How can this be?

Parental discord, rather than family structure or divorce, may be the most significant predictor of childhood problems and antisocial behavior (Amato & Keith, 1991; Emery, 1982; Hetherington, Cox, & Cox, 1982; Rutter, 1970). Moreover, children who are subjected to continued or elevated parental fighting after separation or divorce exhibit more behavior problems than those who witness postdivorce reductions in fighting (Long, Slater, Forehand, & Fauber, 1988). Reviews of literature on

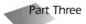

this topic suggest that parental conflict is the central process by which parental divorce negatively affects children (Kitzman & Emery, 1994). Marital discord is probably a marker or correlate of other problems (such as lax discipline, poor supervision, negativity, and scapegoating) that contribute to antisocial behavior. Divorce may also have subtle effects, such as late dating, girls' suspiciousness of men (Wallerstein & Kelly, 1980), and children's taking responsibility for parents' fighting (Cummings, Vogel, Cummings, & El-Sheikh, 1989). Another reaction to marital discord—the "too good" child pattern—is found, more often in girls than in boys (Cummings & Davies, 1994). Even though marital discord and divorce have a negative impact, most children of divorce do not have conduct problems or become delinquents.

Social Factors   Children in lower socioeconomic classes have disproportionate rates of conduct problems and delinquent behavior (Lahey et al., 1995; West, 1982). But social class, like marital discord, seems to be a marker of other factors relating more directly to conduct problems and antisocial behavior, such as large family size, poor parental discipline, and overcrowding. When these variables are controlled for in research, social class has little or no association with antisocial behavior (Robins, 1978). Yet factors such as poor discipline and supervision may be partially caused by the parents' inability to provide or obtain adequate care for their children. Indeed, it appears that low income predicts conduct disorders primarily in young children but not in older children and adolescents (Offord, Boyle, & Racine, 1991; Patterson, Reid, & Dishion, 1992). Research assessing the effects of stress on children's antisocial behavior has indicated that stress plays a much more direct and negative role in families headed by single mothers than in two-parent families (Patterson, Reid, & Dishion, 1992).

Treatment

Patterson and his colleagues at the University of Oregon have repeatedly shown the effectiveness of behavior therapy programs for boys with conduct problems (Kazdin, 1987; Patterson, 1982; Patterson, Dishion, & Chamberlain, 1993). These treatment programs—called *parent training therapy*—teach parents of young children the following:

1. to praise desirable behavior, such as sharing and cooperating
2. to ignore certain annoying undesirable behaviors (for instance, dressing in ways parents disapprove of)
3. to punish other undesired behavior, such as swearing and back talk, through loss of privileges or isolation in the child's room for a fixed period

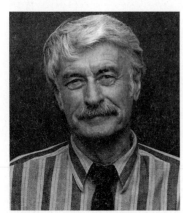

GERALD PATTERSON, *a pioneer in research on the etiology and treatment of conduct disorders, has developed some of the most influential conceptual models of aggression. His treatment research has set the pace in this area for almost three decades.*

Parents of school-age children also receive consultation about methods of helping with homework and learn certain strategies to cope with some of their own problems, such as anger and unreasonable expectations (Miller & Prinz, 1990; Prinz & Miller, 1994). Even though these parent-training programs are effective, Patterson and his colleagues have suggested a shift in emphasis to research on treatment and prevention with younger children, in large part because aggressive behavior of 9- to 12-year-old boys is so difficult to change (Patterson, Dishion, & Chamberlain, 1993). Research shows that the age of the child was the strongest predictor of treatment success—that is, the younger the child, the greater the improvement.

Factors associated with positive treatment outcomes for aggressive children include the absence of parental psychopathology and severe discord, frequent supportive contacts between mothers and their relatives and friends (Dumas & Wahler, 1985), and parental use of social learning concepts (Kazdin, 1987). Outcome studies of similar behavioral treatments for younger children with oppositional and compliance problems have shown that when parents receive brief training in social learning or behavioral principles, their children's behavior improves significantly (Forehand & McMahon, 1981; McCord & Tremblay, 1992).

Another approach to treating aggressive behavior problems in children and adolescents focuses on changing the family system—thus, the name, *behavioral family systems therapy*. Alexander and Parsons (1973) noted that compared to families with normal children, those with problem children are more silent, share talk-time less equally, make fewer positive interruptions, and are less actively engaged in conversation. The researchers argued, therefore, that a treatment goal should be to increase mutual reinforcement, communication, and negotiation.

Thirteen- to 16-year-old delinquents who had been arrested or detained for running away, truancy, and alcohol or drug possession participated in a 12- to 15-week treatment program. In brief, the behavioral family systems therapy approach resulted in a **recidivism** (relapse) rate (26 percent) markedly lower than that of no treatment (50 percent) or alternative treatments. Behavioral family treatment success was associated with more talking, more interruptions (presumably positive) in the family, and more equality of talk-time among members. Additionally, the siblings of adolescents who received the behavioral family treatment had significantly lower rates of referral to juvenile courts than the siblings of children in the no-treatment and alternative treatment groups (Klein, Alexander, & Parsons, 1977).

Related work with adolescent delinquents in a home-style setting with house parents brought about reductions in delinquent behavior and very clear increases in positive social behavior. Unfortunately, a national evaluation of such a home-style treatment program indicated that the gains were lost when the youths returned to their homes (Jones, Weinrott, & Howard, 1981). More recent work indicated that 50 hours of Patterson's parent-training (described earlier) led to reductions in adolescent delinquent behavior—effects that persisted over a 3-year period—and less institutionalization (Bank, Marlowe, Reid, Patterson, & Weinrott, 1991). The message seems clear: Some change in the behavior of adolescents with conduct disorders can be achieved, but it's time consuming and expensive.

A third but related approach uses **problem-solving training** (also called *cognitive skills training*) to treat aggressive children and adolescents. Based on pioneering work by Spivak and Shure (1982), this approach focuses on the individual's cognitive processes, such as expectations, self-statements, taking the perspective of the other, and problem-solving skills (Kendall & Panichelli-Mindel, 1995). Sometimes, the therapist works with the adolescent and her parents (Foster, Prinz, & O'Leary, 1983; Robin & Foster, 1988). If the parents are included, a major focus of the treatment is improving the problem-solving process and the emotional reactions of family members. However, studies that look at outcome measures such as court referrals, classroom observations, and teacher ratings have indicated promising results (Kazdin, 1987; Kendall & Panichelli-Mindel, 1995; Robin & Foster, 1988). The studies have suggested that cognitive style, self-reports of behavior at home, and communication have changed as a result of treatment. Further research is needed to evaluate the effectiveness of this approach.

By now, you should have formed the impression that severe aggression and delinquent behavior are particularly difficult to change (Davidson, Gottschalk, Gensheimer, & Mayer, 1987; Patterson, Reid, & Dishion, 1993). Thus, it's natural to ask which aggressive youths change and which ones do not. Among boys, those who are accepted by their friends despite or perhaps because of their aggression may not be highly motivated to change their aggressive behaviors. Successful bullies may be partly feared and partly liked, sometimes as protectors.

One study of changes resulting from treatment found that aggressive fourth-grade boys who were rejected by their peers were more likely to change following treatment than aggressive boys who were accepted by their peers (Lochman, Lampron, Burch, & Curry, 1985). The treatment was a year-long school-based program that focused on training in social relations. The boys were taught how to solve problems, how to engage positively in play with others, and how to deal with strong negative feelings. As anticipated, the rejected aggressive boys showed greater decreases in parent-rated aggressive behavior than the nonrejected aggressive boys.

recidivism Rate of relapse or repeat offending (that is, return of symptoms or to criminal behavior).

problem-solving training Treatment approach with a focus on cognitive processes, such as expectations, self-statements, taking the perspectives of others, defining problems, and evaluating alternative solutions.

Unfortunately, however, research has not been able to show increases in peer acceptance or decreases in peer ratings of aggressive behavior (Coie, Underwood, & Lochman, 1991; Lochman, Coie, Underwood, & Terry, 1993). Research results repeatedly argue for earlier intervention and/or prevention work with aggressive children.

Medication is used infrequently to treat children with conduct disorder and is highly controversial. Psychostimulants—the medication of choice for children with attention-deficit/hyperactivity disorder—are usually ineffective for children with conduct problems (Campbell, Cohen, Perry, & Small, 1989). Lithium, a medication used to treat bipolar disorder of adults, occasionally has been used in cases of children diagnosed with conduct disorders with severe aggressiveness and explosiveness (Silva, Ernst, & Campbell, 1993).

Focus on Critical Thinking

1. Suppose that you are a child advocate and your goal is to bring children's issues before the state legislature. What issue would be your first priority? Why?

2. Why do you think aggressive behavior in children is so much more difficult to change than anxiety or depression?

ATTENTION-DEFICIT/HYPERACTIVITY DISORDER

Description

Doctors Dorothy Ross and Sheila Ross dedicated their scholarly work *Hyperactivity: Research-Theory-Action* (1976) to "a real stalwart whose warmth, wisdom, and steadfast refusal to accept the school's negative appraisals as final gave a very hyperactive child the support he needed in his troubled years" (p. v). The "stalwart" (a firm, steady individual) was an English nanny; the "hyperactive child" was Winston Churchill, later prime minister of England.

Early in this century, children were not recognized as hyperactive or as having attention-deficit problems. The concept of hyperactivity emerged only as formal schooling became required for all children. Problems categorized today as hyperactivity existed before the invention of this label, but the concept of hyperactivity was not formalized until the 1960s.

Children generally are not diagnosed with **attention-deficit/hyperactivity disorder (AD/HD)** until they reach an age when they are expected to sit still and attend for a significant period of time. The central problems of a child with this disorder are restlessness and difficulty paying attention. These two types of behaviors generally occur together in children (American Psychiatric Association, 1994). In some cases, however, children may have only attentional problems, whereas others may have only activity-level problems (restlessness)—thus, the term *attention-deficit/hyperactivity disorder.*

In classroom settings, when hyperactive children were asked to complete specific assignments at particular times, an observer could easily distinguish the hyperactive from the nonhyperactive children (Jacob, O'Leary, & Rosenblad, 1978).

The diagnostic criteria for AD/HD are shown in the *DSM-IV* table. For a diagnosis, the essential features of AD/HD—inattention, impulsiveness, and hyperactivity—must have existed for at least 6 months. In the *DSM-IV,* clinicians diagnose children who have attention-deficit problems based on three subtypes:

1. AD/HD
2. AD/HD, predominantly inattention type
3. AD/HD, predominantly hyperactive-impulsive type

Although most children have symptoms of both inattention and hyperactivity, this subclassification allows for diagnoses when only one type is predominant.

There is no single test or observation that an expert can make in a short interview to diagnose AD/HD, except perhaps in extreme cases. Because professionals

attention-deficit/hyperactivity disorder (AD/HD)
Childhood disorder in which the central problems are restlessness and difficulty paying attention.

DSM-IV   **Diagnostic Criteria for 314 ATTENTION-DEFICIT/ HYPERACTIVITY DISORDER**

A. Either (1) or (2):

(1) six (or more) of the following symptoms of *inattention* have persisted for at least 6 months to a degree that is maladaptive and inconsistent with developmental level:

Inattention

(a) often fails to give close attention to details or makes careless mistakes in schoolwork, work, or other activities

(b) often has difficulty sustaining attention in tasks or play activities

(c) often does not seem to listen when spoken to directly

(d) often does not follow through on instructions and fails to finish schoolwork, chores, or duties in the workplace (not due to oppositional behavior or failure to understand instructions)

(e) often has difficulty organizing tasks and activities

(f) often avoids, dislikes, or is reluctant to engage in tasks that require sustained mental effort (such as schoolwork or homework)

(g) often loses things necessary for tasks or activities (e.g., toys, school assignments, pencils, books, or tools)

(h) is often easily distracted by extraneous stimuli

(i) is often forgetful in daily activities

(2) six (or more) of the following symptoms of *hyperactivity-impulsivity* have persisted for at least 6 months to a degree that is maladaptive and inconsistent with developmental level:

Hyperactivity

(a) often fidgets with hands or feet or squirms in seat

(b) often leaves seat in classroom or in other situations in which remaining seated is expected

(c) often runs about or climbs excessively in situations in which it is inappropriate (in adolescents or adults, may be linked to subjective feelings of restlessness)

(d) often has difficulty playing or engaging in leisure activities quietly

(e) is often "on the go" or often acts as if "driven by a motor"

(f) often talks excessively

Impulsivity

(g) often blurts out answers before questions have been completed

(h) often has difficulty awaiting turn

(i) often interrupts or intrudes on others (e.g., butts into conversations or games)

B. Some hyperactive-impulsive or inattentive symptoms that caused impairment were present before age 7 years.

C. Some impairment from the symptoms is present in two or more settings (e.g., at school [or work] and at home).

D. There must be clear evidence of clinically significant impairment in social, academic, or occupational functioning.

E. The symptoms do not occur exclusively during the course of a Pervasive Developmental Disorder, Schizophrenia, or other Psychotic Disorder and are not better accounted for by another mental disorder (e.g., Mood Disorder, Anxiety Disorder, Dissociative Disorder, or a Personality Disorder).

often attempt to make such judgments simply on the basis of brief office visits, many of these diagnoses are erroneous. Clinicians also have to differentiate AD/HD from conduct disorder. Approximately half the children with AD/HD also have conduct disorder (Anderson, Williams, McGee, & Silva, 1987). In such cases, clinicians have to decide which is the primary disorder, since the particular diagnosis affects the path of treatment.

Teacher input is essential in determining whether a child has AD/HD. To confirm such a diagnosis, researchers often ask teachers to complete rating forms describing behaviors characteristic of children with AD/HD (Achenbach & Edelbrock, 1986; Conners, 1969, 1990). These rating forms have been standardized with thousands of children and have cutoff points indicating whether a child exhibits more of these behaviors than most children. If a teacher's rating places a child in the upper 5 percent of the population, he would be seriously considered for an AD/HD diagnosis. A child's developmental history is also important in making this diagnosis, since as noted earlier, AD/HD problems are normally apparent before age 7.

A child with AD/HD and symptoms of aggression may later be diagnosed with a conduct disorder or, after 18 years of age, with antisocial personality disorder (Douglas, 1983; Mannuzza, Klein, Bessler, Malloy, & LaPadula, 1993; Weiss & Hechtman, 1986; Wender, 1987). Some children with AD/HD simply have some of

FIGURE 14.2 Long-term follow-up of children with AD/HD

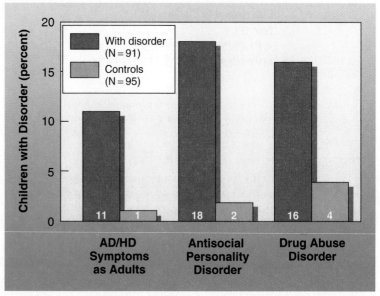

Source: From S. Mannuzza, R. G. Klein, A. Bessler, P. Malloy, & M. LaPadula, 1993, "Adult Outcome of Hyperactive Boys: Educational Achievement, Occupational Rank, and Psychiatric Status," *Archives of General Psychiatry, 50,* 565–576. Copyright 1993 by Archives of General Psychiatry. Reprinted with permission.

the same attentional and hyperactivity problems as adults. Indeed, some professionals see AD/HD as a potentially lifelong problem requiring long-term professional attention and medication (Wender, Reimherr, & Wood, 1980; Wender, 1987). In such circumstances, aggression is a better predictor of how well the individual will function as an adult than are hyperactivity or attention problems (Paternite & Loney, 1980; Weiss & Hechtman, 1986).

Will hyperactive children necessarily be hyperactive or have other significant problems as adults? In one study (Mannuzza et al., 1993), boys who were hyperactive when they were in elementary school were followed approximately 16 years later to find out how many of them had significant problems as adults. Another sample of boys of similar age and race, whose teachers had made no complaints about their school behavior, were also assessed as children and as adults. These two samples were compared. As shown in Figure 14.2, there were major differences between the two in the rates of attention-deficit/hyperactivity disorder symptoms. Of the former hyperactive children, 11 percent had attention-deficit problems as adults, but only 1 percent of the control group had such symptoms. The risk for other problems, however, was even more pronounced. The hyperactive children had a marked risk for developing antisocial personality disorder and drug abuse problems as adults (Mannuzza et al., 1991; Mannuzza et al., 1993; Weiss & Hechtman, 1986).

Causes

Genetic Predisposition Children of active, impulsive, aggressive parents frequently display the same traits. Such parents actually often report that their children inherited their bad characteristics from them. These parental reports led researchers to investigate the role of genetic factors in determining activity levels. Family studies have clearly indicated that both parents and siblings of children with AD/HD have an increased likelihood of having AD/HD (Biederman et al., 1992). Relatives of children with AD/HD had a 16 percent risk for having AD/HD. In addition, studies have also documented that the activity levels of identical (monozygotic) twins are more similar than those of fraternal (dizygotic) twins.

Dietary Influences   In the 1980s, researchers became concerned about the adverse effects of various foods on behavior. One of the first to point to the negative role of dyes and additives in foods, beverages, and medicines was Dr. Benjamin Feingold, whose book *Why Your Child Is Hyperactive* (1975) reached a wide audience. Feingold hypothesized that many of the children he was treating might be hyperactive because of a physiological sensitivity to salicylates (natural aspirinlike compounds in fruits and vegetables), as well as to food additives like red and yellow dye and food preservatives. To test his theory, he placed all his hyperactive child patients on diets free of these substances. According to Feingold, many children had a dramatic positive response to the special diets. Subsequent controlled studies comparing the **Feingold diet** to alternative diets, however, showed no clear evidence that it led to any improvement (Conners, 1980). Nevertheless, comprehensive reviews of the research have indicated that we cannot dismiss the possibility that food coloring has adverse effects on individual children (Prinz, 1985).

Feingold diet Special diet designed for children with AD/HD, whom Dr. Benjamin Feingold believed to be physiologically sensitive to certain substances in food, beverages, and medicines; the diet is free of food additives (like red and yellow dye) and food preservatives.

Lead Poisoning   In old buildings, paint chips containing lead sometimes fall from ceilings and walls. Children who eat these paint chips can suffer lead poisoning, leading to neurological problems and severe hyperactivity. A child may acquire lead poisoning through repeated ingestion of small amounts of lead over several months. In the past, this was a common occurrence in large cities, which had considerable amounts of old and poorly maintained housing. Fortunately, lead-based paints are produced much less frequently today, and when paint contains lead, it is noted on the label.

Children may carry lead in their teeth as well as in their bloodstream. A group of dentists and psychologists found that lead levels in children's baby teeth were related to disruptive behavior and short attention span in school (Needleman et al., 1979). The lead in these children's systems resulted from inhaling fumes that contain lead. The federal government closely monitors industrial pollution from lead- and iron-processing plants. Across the United States, cities and towns are gradually eliminating lead pipes (for domestic water use). Petroleum refiners are also producing lead-free gasolines. These changes were clearly warranted, for the effects of lead poisoning—such as behavioral and neurological problems—persist into young adulthood (Needleman, Schell, Belinger, Leviton, & Allred, 1990).

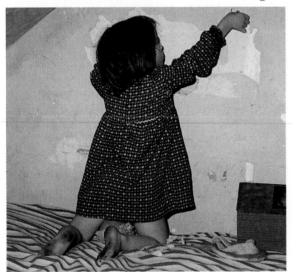

Some children pick paint off the wall and eat the paint chips. If eaten, the lead in old paint causes neurological problems in children.

Brain Dysfunction   In 1902, Dr. George Still observed that children with meningitis (a brain inflammation) and other physical disorders often became overactive. He reasoned correctly that brain damage could cause both hyperactivity and attentional problems. Many professionals, agreeing with Still, began to view brain dysfunction as *the cause* of hyperactivity. After Hans Berger's invention of the electroencephalograph (EEG) in 1929 (Davis, 1992), however, it became apparent that most hyperactive children had no detectable unusual brain-wave patterns. Instead, a significant percentage showed motor coordination problems in writing, in maze tracing, and in the use of small mechanical objects.

The search for what causes motor coordination problems in hyperactive children led medical professionals in the 1960s and 1970s to view hyperactivity as synonymous with **minimal brain dysfunction (MBD).** In other words, although neu-

minimal brain dysfunction (MBD) Term once used synonymously with AD/HD; some medical professionals believed MBD was the cause of children's hyperactivity and motor coordination problems.

rological exams or EEGs revealed no obvious brain dysfunction, researchers hypothesized that some very minor brain dysfunction caused the hyperactivity and motor coordination problems exhibited. Use of the term *MBD* has largely disappeared, but some respected experts believe neurological difficulties are at the root of many children's attentional and activity problems (Conners & Wells, 1986).

Evidence has suggested that neurological dysfunction may indeed cause severe problems of inattention and overactivity. For example, Lou, Henriksen, and Bruhn (1984) monitored bloodflow in hyperactive children's brains and found that it's reduced in the frontal lobes. Other investigators reviewing neuropsychological research in children diagnosed with AD/HD have indicated that there are frontal lobe deficits (Barkley, Grodzinsky, & Dupaul, 1992). In 1990, Zametkin and his colleagues conducted groundbreaking research by studying brain functions of parents of children with AD/HD. The parents were selected for having AD/HD. PET scans of the parents' brains showed abnormalities in the premotor and superior prefrontal cortex, areas thought to control attention and motor activity (Zametkin et al., 1990). Finally, medication used to treat attentional problems results in increased bloodflow to the central frontal areas of the brain, which are thought to regulate attention and impulse control (see review of Lorys-Vernon, Hynd, Lyytinen, & Hern, 1993).

Psychological Causes   Psychological factors may influence the development of attention-deficit/hyperactivity disorders, but such factors are not seen as primary causes. As mentioned, research has suggested that biological factors are likely to be causal factors for most children with serious attentional problems. Recall that there is considerable overlap in the diagnosis of conduct disorder and AD/HD. Thus, some of the same psychological factors that play causal roles in the development of conduct disorders also can influence attention difficulties, hyperactivity, and probably even more importantly, impulsivity.

For two decades, educators believed that praise and other forms of positive teacher attention helped children with hyperactivity and aggression problems. Studies found that children with such problems showed increases in attention and task completion in response to positive feedback (Madsen & Madsen, 1970). Yet evidence gathered in the 1980s and 1990s indicated that praise may not be as effective as earlier thought with children specifically diagnosed with AD/HD. It also seemed that more powerful incentive or reinforcement programs would be required to help many of these children (Kendziora & O'Leary, 1993; Pfiffner & O'Leary, 1993).

Moreover, at least some negative feedback for inappropriate behavior is critical for maintaining appropriate classroom behavior of hyperactive children. One study showed that when teachers of hyperactive children omitted all types of punishment—such as reprimands or loss of recess—the children's attention level dropped markedly over a 5-day period. Yet after the teachers resumed negative feedback for inappropriate behavior, the children's level of attention increased again (Rosen, O'Leary, Joyce, Conway, & Pfiffner, 1984). A series of studies indicated that when teachers of hyperactive children did not use any negative consequences, the hyperactive children engaged in high rates of misbehavior and failed to complete their classwork. These results show that parental and teacher failure to provide negative consequences for hyperactive children's misbehavior contributes to the development or worsening of their problems (Pfiffner & O'Leary, 1993).

Family influences have long been assessed as possible contributors to AD/HD problems. Some researchers have distinguished primary (or *core*) symptoms of AD/HD, such as hyperactivity and inattention, from secondary symptoms, such as aggression and low self-esteem (Paternite, Loney, & Langorne, 1976; Paternite & Loney, 1980). In a sample of over 100 children referred to a clinic for hyperactivity, the primary symptoms of inattention and overactivity were not consistently associated with any family and environmental factors. In contrast, researchers found that the secondary symptoms of aggression and self-esteem problems were related to five family and environmental factors: (1) short temper of father, (2) overly busy parents, (3) poor parent/child relationship, (4) urban residence, and (5) low socioeconomic status.

Of related interest is research about family environment with newborns labeled at risk for having brain dysfunction. These children—so classified because of birth complications such as prematurity and lack of oxygen—were assessed later at age 10 (Werner, 1980). At-risk children whose families were rated as having high emotional support, structure, and organization displayed the lowest rates of behavior problems at age 10. In contrast, at-risk children whose families were characterized by poor parental mental health, poor mother/child relationships, and punitive childrearing practices were more likely to be diagnosed with AD/HD—and to be aggressive in young adulthood (Hechtman, Weiss, Perlman, & Amsel, 1984; Weiss, Minde, Werry, Douglas, & Nemeth, 1971).

Research demonstrates that parental factors and low socioeconomic status predict problems of aggression and hyperactivity in children. In addition, hyperactive children significantly affect their parents' behavior. That is, some of the parental factors previously presumed to be associated with AD/HD may really be due to the AD/HD children's effects on their parents. For example, mothers of hyperactive children behave in more coercive, controlling, and critical ways when their children are unmedicated than when they are medicated.

Yet even when these children become more attentive and compliant, such parents do not increase their rewarding or supportive comments (Barkley & Cunningham, 1979; Mash & Johnston, 1983). Perhaps such children simply elicit fewer positive behaviors from their parents than other children do. One confirmation of this hypothesis is that mothers of children with AD/HD are able to respond well to the appropriate behavior of other children in their family. Precisely how hyperactive children and their parents influence each other is unclear. But obviously, many parents of children with AD/HD have to cope with difficult and often incessant behavior.

psychostimulants

Medication of choice for children with AD/HD; appear to increase certain brain functions that improve attention span and fine motor control.

Ritalin Most common psychostimulant medication prescribed to children for treating AD/HD symptoms.

Treatment

Pharmacological   The most dramatic treatment for children with attention and hyperactivity problems is psychostimulant medication. It generally produces immediate and obvious effects. **Psychostimulants** like **Ritalin** and Cylert appear to increase certain brain functions, which improve attention span and fine motor control (as shown in Figure 14.3). Many well-controlled studies have replicated the original findings of Dr. Charles Bradley (1937), who reported that children with severe behavior problems showed a "great increase in interest in school material" after receiving Ritalin. The children called the medication "arithmetic pills" because they

FIGURE 14.3 Handwriting skills of children on and off medication

Some children who are given psychostimulant medication show dramatic improvements in their motor skills. In this case, handwriting showed great improvement.

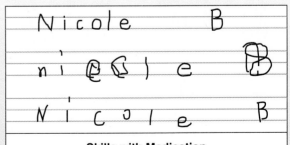

Skills with Medication

These handwriting samples show how medication can help a hyperactive child. The teacher wrote the top line, the child the middle one before taking medication. After taking medication, the child wrote the bottom line—an obvious improvement.

Source: Reprinted by permission of Medical Economics Publishing.

PERSPECTIVE ON ATTENTION-DEFICIT/HYPERACTIVITY DISORDER

BIOLOGICAL FACTORS

Biological factors play a role in the development of AD/HD:

➤ Children who have family members with AD/HD are at elevated risk for developing this disorder.

➤ Children who inhale lead fumes or eat paint chips that are lead based often develop AD/HD and associated neurological problems.

➤ Head injury and spinal meningitis sometimes cause neurological dysfunctions that produce AD/HD.

PSYCHOLOGICAL FACTORS

Psychological factors interact with biological factors in the development of AD/HD:

➤ Failing to provide negative feedback to a child with AD/HD when he engages in highly inattentive and disruptive behavior causes him to quickly become more disruptive.

➤ Children with AD/HD are easiest to distinguish from children without AD/HD in traditional highly structured classrooms. On the other hand, if children can walk around the room and engage in assignments at their own pace, it is often impossible to distinguish them from children without this problem.

➤ Fathers with short tempers and mothers who escalate parent/child conflicts by quickly becoming negative place their children at risk for developing AD/HD.

SOCIAL FACTORS

Both biological and psychological factors operate in specific social contexts:

➤ Children born into families with low levels of income and education are at increased risk for AD/HD.

➤ Inadequate prenatal care places children at risk for developing AD/HD.

➤ Living in an urban environment increases the chance of exposure to lead paint chips and fumes, the ingestion of which has been noted as a cause of AD/HD.

➤ Poor-quality child care can also place children at risk.

These biological, psychological, and social factors interact to cause problems, as illustrated in the following case:

Marcus was diagnosed with AD/HD by a child psychologist after his second-grade teacher suggested an evaluation. Marcus's teacher was sympathetic to his difficulty concentrating, but she maintained a very structured classroom. She wanted Marcus to raise his hand to speak, to sit in an assigned seat, and to complete academic tasks in the same order as all the other children.

The biopsychosocial model helps explain the problem. Marcus's father, a railroad engineer, also had problems sitting still in school and did not read well until junior high. Marcus's mother was very understanding and generally quite positive with him, but his father would blow up at him when he failed to complete his assignments. As a result, his mother had to spend a lot of extra time helping Marcus finish his homework long after he was supposed to be in bed.

felt they could complete their arithmetic assignments more readily when they were taking these pills (Bradley, 1937). Approximately 40 years later, some children still felt that stimulant medication helped them a great deal. Consider this child's feelings:

> **Interviewer:** How can you tell when you forget to take Ritalin?
> **Child:** When I can tell that I'm not concentrating in school. Like she'll [the teacher will] give us a half hour to do a math page, like there's about 20 problems, and I'll get about 6 done in 20 minutes, a half hour. But if I take it, I can get them all done in 10 minutes, 20 minutes, and have 10 minutes free.
> **Interviewer:** This is an "imagination" question. Let's say you stopped taking Ritalin altogether.
> **Child:** Oh wow, I'd stay home from school.
> **Interviewer:** How come?
> **Child:** Because I know what would be happening if I didn't. I wouldn't get my work done at all.
> **Interviewer:** How about your friends?
> **Child:** Nobody would like me then, if I didn't take it. They'd think in their minds, "Gosh, she doesn't even want to play. What a baby!"
> **Interviewer:** Pretend that a friend of yours was about to start taking Ritalin and she asked you what you thought. . . .
> **Child:** They'd ask me, like "What does it do?" I'd just tell them, "Well, it helps you concentrate, get more friends, and you want to join in the games more. And you'd be invited more places." (Whalen & Henker, 1980, pp. 27–28)

After Bradley's initial work, it was hypothesized that children with attentional and hyperactivity problems had deficits (or deviations) in their central nervous system functioning (Clements, 1966; Wender, 1971). Many medical professionals believed that psychostimulant medication stimulated the reticular activating system of the brain, a portion of the central nervous system. They called this the *paradoxical effect* of psychostimulant medication, because it supposedly stimulated or activated a center of the brain yet had a calming effect on the children.

In 1978, this explanation was challenged when children with no attention or overactivity problems were given psychostimulant medication. They showed effects similar to those displayed by children with AD/HD (Rapoport et al., 1978). In other words, attention and fine motor skills improved in children who did not display deficits in these skills before receiving psychostimulant medication.

Psychostimulant medications had their intended clinical effect but not because children with AD/HD have a brain dysfunction that's uniquely treated by psychostimulants. The precise effects of psychostimulant medications are difficult to determine, since these children's neuropsychological problems may vary widely and studies typically measure only one or two problems (Conners & Wells, 1987). In fact, some researchers believe that children with AD/HD may respond to drugs differently according to the nature of their neuropsychological profiles. Brain-imaging studies suggest that individuals with frontal lobe abnormalities show the greatest clinical improvement (Zametkin et al., 1990). Other factors clinicians assessed to predict treatment response include types and severity of the symptoms, developmental and intellectual factors that may interact with diagnoses, the child's medical history, and any family history of psychopathology (Campbell et al., 1989).

Although psychostimulants such as Ritalin remain the drug of choice for treating most AD/HD cases, other medications have been found to be somewhat effective. Many clinicians consider antidepressants as the second-line pharmacological treatment for AD/HD (Elia, Rapoport, & Kirby, 1993). Antidepressants are particularly appropriate for cases in which AD/HD symptoms are seen in combination with those of anxiety and/or depression. Antipsychotics are a third category of medication used in treating AD/HD symptoms. However, both antidepressants and antipsychotics are generally prescribed only as alternatives to psychostimulants, since they are less effective and have some troublesome side effects.

It's important to note that most recent treatment handbooks for AD/HD emphatically proclaim that medication should be offered in combination with some type of behavioral treatment. Such treatment plans that incorporate medication have been found to be more effective than medication by itself (Campbell et al., 1989; Elia, Rapoport, Kirby, 1993; Pelham, 1993).

Behavioral In classrooms—where the difficulties of children with AD/HD are most apparent—behavior therapy interventions have successfully reduced levels of problem behavior and ratings of hyperactivity (O'Leary, 1984; Pfiffner & O'Leary, 1993). In these programs, teachers generally do the following:

1. Praise children's appropriate behavior, such as attending to schoolwork and completing academic problems.
2. Ignore their inappropriate behavior, such as calling out answers.
3. Make the classroom rules explicit and review them daily.
4. Give negative feedback privately to AD/HD children.
5. Set daily goals with AD/HD children each morning.
6. Provide daily feedback to parents on how well their children met the stated goals (daily report system).
7. Request that parents reward children for the daily goals met.

These procedures have been used successfully with AD/HD children who were never medicated, as well as with medicated children whose parents or pediatricians agreed to withdraw medication at the outset of the behavioral intervention (O'Leary & Pelham, 1978; O'Leary, Pelham, Rosenbaum, & Price, 1976).

Combined Pharmacological and Psychological Studies have shown that children with AD/HD who are treated with behavior therapy improve significantly. Studies have also shown that children treated with medication improve significantly. Are the two treatments equally effective, or is one better than the other? A related question is: What would happen if the children received both treatments?

One study examined the effects of psychostimulant medication and behavior therapy on AD/HD children. Those who received medication alone scored better on teacher ratings and independent observations of classroom behavior than children who received behavior therapy alone, even though both groups showed significant improvements. A third group of children, who received a combination of behavior therapy and medication, also did better on teacher ratings of classroom behavior than the group receiving behavior therapy by itself (Gittelman-Klein et al., 1976). In sum, both treatments were helpful for the hyperactive children, but psychostimulant medication had a greater effect on the children's ability to pay attention than did behavior therapy.

One major study conducted a "total push," or *multimodal,* treatment program—that is, a program involving psychostimulant medication and behavior therapy for AD/HD children, along with tutoring, family therapy, and individual therapy for their parents (Satterfield, Cantwell, & Satterfield, 1979; Satterfield, Satterfield, & Cantwell, 1980, 1981). This study showed what can happen in actual clinical practice, since it covered a 2-year period and allowed treatment to be tailored to each family's needs. The researchers reported children achieving academic gains of approximately 1.6 years in mathematics and reading.

Clinicians and researchers have continually debated about the proper treatment for children with AD/HD. The variety of symptoms—which seem to have both biological and environmental causes—appear to indicate that when a child has a full complement of AD/HD problems, including aggression, combinations of behavior therapy and psychostimulant medication are probably most effective (Carlson,

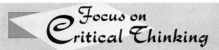

Pelham, Milich & Dixon, 1992; Conners & Wells, 1986; Pelham, 1993; Pelham & Murphy, 1986). Clinical judgment is necessary, however, to aid parents in deciding whether a particular child's treatment should involve behavior therapy, psychostimulant medication, dietary change, tutoring, family therapy, individual therapy for the parents, or some combination of these options. When aggression and conduct problems predominate, clinicians often recommend behavior therapy. When attentional problems and overactivity are most obvious, they will likely suggest psychostimulant medication as the treatment of choice.

ANXIETY DISORDERS

The most commonly discussed childhood anxiety disorders are overanxious disorder and separation anxiety disorder. **Overanxious disorder** involves excessive worry about future situations, and **separation anxiety disorder** is characterized by excessive anxiety concerning separation from home or loved ones. **School phobia** is often seen as a subclass of separation anxiety. We focus here on these three problems..

Description

Fears and worries are common among young children, and girls have more fears and worries than boys (King, 1993; Lapousse & Monk, 1959). In addition, in the United States, children from lower socioeconomic levels have the highest numbers of fears and worries. These children fear guns, switchblades, and whipping, whereas children from higher socioeconomic levels fear car accidents, getting killed, and juvenile delinquents (King, 1993). Similar results have been reported in studies of children in other parts of the world, such as Japan and Europe (Orvaschel & Weissman, 1986). However, anxiety and fears are normally not severe enough to warrant clinical diagnoses. In fact, only 1 to 4 percent of clinical referrals of children in the United States and England occur in response to specific fears (Graziano, DeGiovanni, & Garcia, 1979). Yet children's anxiety problems represent 22 percent of the major problems that make parents seek professional help for their children (Anderson et al., 1987).

Anxieties and fears change during childhood. A classic study by Jersild and Holmes (1935) showed that in the first 2 years of life, fears of noises, strangers, and objects predominate; fears of imaginary creatures and objects, the dark, robbers, and death are much more common between ages 4 and 6. On average, children in both the United States and Australia have shown clear reductions in the number and intensity of fears as they have become older (Ollendick, King, & Frary, 1989).

When some children enter school, however, their worries become more pervasive. Such children are diagnosed as having an overanxious disorder (OD) and are characterized by excessive worry about new and future situations, such as being hurt, doing poorly on a test, or being criticized by others (American Psychiatric Association, 1994). Generally, children with OD feel unable to control their worrying. Children with OD display symptoms such as irritability and difficulty concentrating. These disorders seem to occur in families in which there is high pressure to do well in school; the problem occurs most often in older children (Last, 1989).

overanxious disorder
Childhood anxiety disorder characterized by excessive worrying about new and future situations, such as being hurt, doing poorly on a test, or being criticized by others; a subclass of generalized anxiety disorder.

separation anxiety disorder Characterized by excessive anxiety concerning separation from the home or loved ones.

school phobia Characterized by a child's specific reluctance or refusal to go to school due to fear of separating from parents; a subclass of separation anxiety disorder.

Asking adults with various phobias to report on the fears they experienced as children does not provide consistent evidence of a continuity of anxiety (Klein & Last, 1989; King, 1993). But longitudinal research with children provides very clear evidence of some continuity of childhood anxiety and fearfulness.

As discussed earlier, fears and anxieties usually are more common in girls than in boys in representative samples in diverse cultures (Gittelman, 1986; King, 1993). One reason that boys are taken less frequently than girls to psychological clinics for problems of anxiety may simply be that girls express fears and anxieties more readily than boys. Fearfulness is less acceptable for boys than for girls in U.S. culture.

Perhaps one reason children with fear and anxiety problems are seen less frequently in clinics than those with conduct problems is that the emotions of anxiety are more difficult to recognize than the more overt behavior problems of fighting, temper tantrums, and verbal aggression. Many children don't readily express their worries to their parents. In short, the numbers of children brought to mental health clinics because of anxieties and fears is probably not a reliable indication of the percentage of children suffering significant worries and fears in the population as a whole.

Causes

Genetic Predisposition   Family studies, involving the assessment of relatives of patients with certain disorders, have shown that children of anxious parents express fears more often than children of depressed parents. In addition, parents with specific anxiety disorders (such as a panic disorder with very intense periods of fear and discomfort) are more likely to have children with anxiety symptoms than parents with generalized anxiety problems (Weissman et al., 1984). In a study of parents of children with overanxious and/or separation anxiety disorder seen at a child psychiatric clinic, the vast majority of mothers (83 percent) had lifetime histories of anxiety disorders (Last, Hersen, Kazdin, Francis, & Grubb, 1987).

These family studies don't definitively prove that genetic factors cause children's anxious behaviors, because these behaviors could have resulted from children's modeling their parents' behaviors. But twin studies have provided convincing evidence of genetic factors in the development of fears (Stevenson, Batten, & Cherner, 1992). Further, studies of twins have shown that personality traits like introversion and being anxious have high genetic components (Plomin, 1990). Such research suggests that genetic factors are much more important in personality traits and styles than had been believed a decade or more ago.

Psychological Determinants   For decades, psychological factors have been thought to be influential in the development of anxiety problems of children. Conditioning, modeling, and reinforcement are factors thought to be important.

In 1920, John B. Watson, the famous radical behaviorist, and his graduate student, Rosalie Rayner, published the first experiment on conditioning of emotional behavior (see Chapter 5). In their classic study, "Little Albert," a healthy 9-month-old infant, was repeatedly exposed to the sound of a large hammer striking a steel bar paired with the presence of white furry objects. Since young infants generally display fright in response to loud noises, it was predicted that Albert would react fearfully to the noise of the hammer. It was further predicted that pairing this startling noise with white furry objects (for instance, pieces of cotton, wool, a white rabbit), which Albert was not afraid of, would lead him to fear them, as well.

Albert did show changes in breathing, a startle reflex, and a lip tremble when presented with a series of these objects and the sound of the hammer. One week later, after many pairings of the noise and the white objects, he reacted fearfully to the presence of the objects alone. A month later, when again presented with the white objects alone, Albert showed fearful behavior, though less extreme than pre-

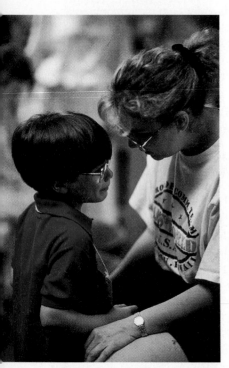

Afraid to leave his mother, this child is comforted by her. To what extent do you think the mother's expression of concern helps the child or maintains his problem?

viously. Thus, Watson and Rayner (1920) believed that fears learned through conditioning could persist and affect an individual's personality throughout life.

In the 1970s, the conditioning view was modified to include the notion that humans are biologically prepared to react fearfully to certain stimuli, such as snakes and spiders, but not to others, such as geometric shapes or wall sockets (Garcia & Koelling, 1966; Seligman, 1971). As discussed in Chapter 5 (Öhman, 1986), some evidence supports the view that humans are genetically *prepared* to react to certain stimuli.

Modeling or observing others displaying fearful behavior increases a child's risk for developing such fears. Clinicians have long known that many children display kinds and numbers of fears similar to those of their mothers (Hagman, 1932). Among a sample of dog-phobic children, 35 percent of their parents also had serious phobias and fears (Bandura & Menlove, 1968). Venn and Short (1973) showed that when children are exposed to filmed models displaying fears of relatively neutral objects, they acquire an avoidance response simply by watching the models.

At times, parents or caregivers may inadvertently reward children for fearful behavior. In turn, the fearful behavior will increase. When a mother praises a child who is afraid of dogs for staying away from them, the child is rewarded for the fear of dogs. Parents of school-phobic children frequently allow them to remain at home and watch TV or engage in other interesting activities (Johnson & Melamed, 1979). This parental behavior fits with psychodynamic interpretations of school phobia, which propose that the supposedly phobic behavior represents a dependency problem reinforced by parental attention.

Treatment

As Mary Cover Jones (1924) demonstrated in a classic study, exposing children to particular feared objects in the presence of peers who are unafraid clearly helps decrease their fear. Since the 1970s, it's been known that observing filmed models of children gradually approaching feared objects helps children overcome fear of surgery or injections (Melamed & Siegel, 1975; Vernon & Bailey, 1974). Therapists have successfully treated fear of the dark by having phobic children recite self-statements—such as "I am brave" or "I can take care of myself when alone"—and then rewarding them for being brave during the night (Graziano & Mooney, 1980). Subsequent research, though, showed that gradual exposure to the dark, not the cognitive component, is the critical treatment ingredient (King, 1993).

Social withdrawal or overanxious disorders are more difficult to treat than specific fears, and the method the clinician chooses will depend on the severity of the problem. One type of treatment that's effective in increasing the social interactions of withdrawn preschool children involves having other children serve as child "therapists" to interact with the withdrawn individuals (Furman, Rahe, & Hartup, 1979). Another treatment involves teaching skill in perspective taking—that is, teaching children how to see another point of view (Gottman, Gonso, & Rasmussen, 1975).

Socially withdrawn children are also not as likely as average children to respond to others' initiations (Hops & Greenwood, 1981). Social skills training programs for withdrawn children teach them skills such as smiling, greeting, joining, inviting, conversing, and complimenting. To master these skills, the children observe model peers, receive coaching, rehearse the behaviors to be used in critical situations, and discuss how they can employ these skills with their classmates. Researchers observed that children who received this treatment initiated more and became less withdrawn compared to children who did not receive this treatment (LaGreca & Santogrossi, 1981). Although children's fearful behavior can clearly be changed, children's popularity or peer acceptance is difficult to change.

Play therapy is a very different approach used by some therapists to treat children with anxiety and withdrawal problems; this approach is evaluated in

$\mathcal{S}$ome therapists use play therapy to engage children and to have the play activities serve as a forum for interpreting the child's behavior. As in all therapies, play therapists differ in their approach and, in particular, in their directiveness. Directive play therapists select toys, state rules, and make interpretations. Play therapy rooms are often equipped with a variety of toys, dolls, playhouses, easels, and chalkboards. If a child acted aggressively toward the father doll, for example, the therapist might interpret that behavior as reflecting the child's angry and hostile feelings toward the father. If a child consistently avoided the mother doll, the therapist would question the child about how the doll felt toward its mother. Presumably, the response might reveal some problem within the mother/child relationship.

As Tuma (1989) stated, "Structured play therapists direct the play activities to focus the sessions on conflict." The play sessions set the stage for releasing unexpressed feelings and inner tensions through specific situations thought to be related to the source of the child's problems. If a child broke a toy and there had been observations of anger toward the mother, the therapist might say, "You are angry at your mom, and you did that to show her how mad you are." As Tuma (1989) emphasized, for many ther-

apists, play therapy is often a technique rather than a general mode of psychotherapy. That is, it's used in conjunction with other therapeutic methods.

In one study, for example, play therapy assessments (Draw Your Family As Animals; Draw Your Family As a Tree), goal setting with the therapist, and family systems procedures were used to treat young children with anxiety and withdrawal problems (Smyrnios & Kirby, 1993). Subjects treated with this combined approach were compared to a control group who had minimal contact with the therapist—primarily assessment and feedback sessions. All groups showed improvement, but there was no evidence that the treated groups improved more than the control group on the main dependent measures.

Think about the following questions:

1. The study described did not demonstrate more improvement for treated children than those whose parents received simply assessment and feedback. However, both groups improved. What do you conclude about the effectiveness of the treatment with a play therapy focus? Explain your answer.

2. For what types of problems, if any, would you suggest play therapy for a child? Why?

Thinking about Research. As noted there, play therapy relies heavily on the therapist's interpretations of the child's behavior.

Researchers are increasingly recognizing the overlap or comorbidity of anxiety disorders and depression, with ranges of overlapping diagnoses often as high as 50 percent (Ollendick & King, 1994). In addition, researchers have realized that the symptoms of anxiety and depression share the mood-based personality factor of negative affectivity in both adults (Watson, Clark, & Carey, 1988) and children (King, Ollendick, & Gullone, 1991). Given this significant overlap, some researchers have suggested that a cognitive-behavioral intervention will best meet the array of the distinctive and overlapping symptoms of anxiety and depression disorders (Kendall, Kortlander, Chansky, & Brady, 1992). Common strategies involved in this treatment include:

1. affective education, in which children learn to understand and differentiate between their feelings
2. behavioral procedures, such as relaxation training and exposure techniques
3. cognitive interventions, to help children improve self-monitoring and self-control
4. social skills training, to help children improve relationships with peers

Parental involvement is also an important component in this treatment.

School phobia is significant because detrimental social and academic consequences often occur if this phobia is not addressed in the early stages. Young children who refuse to go to school after brief illnesses have been successfully treated with variations of a program developed by Kennedy (1965). This treatment involves close collaboration among the therapist, parents, and school personnel. When the child appears to be avoiding school, parents and school personnel promptly begin exerting strong pressure on the child to return to school. The program also includes a physical exam by a school physician and acceptance and support from teachers. This immediate attention to the problem and pressure to return to school has consistently produced positive results (Klein & Last, 1989).

In contrast, adolescents who refuse to go to school, claim they are afraid of it, and come from families characterized by marital discord have not been successfully treated with psychological methods. In one study, the use of tricyclic medication (antidepressants) seemed to be helpful and is based on the notion that children and adolescents with severe anxiety are actually in pain, unhappy, and depressed (Gittelman & Koplewicz, 1986). Although this position is controversial and the outcome results are inconsistent (Barrios & O'Dell, 1989), antidepressant medication appears to allow many school phobics to return to the classroom (Klein & Last, 1989).

At present, there is no one clearly effective treatment for adolescent school phobics that's been used by different investigators in different settings. Clinicians must carefully assess the numerous possible causes of school refusal in adolescents, such as poor academic or social skills, fears of failure or rejection, fear of physical attack, or refusal to leave home because of concerns about parental fighting or sickness. Because school phobias are complex, they require clinicians' utmost skill in the assessment and treatment phases. More specifically, it's sometimes difficult to tell the difference between a child who is really afraid of school and one who simply has gotten his way for years and now doesn't want to go to school.

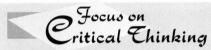

Focus on Critical Thinking

In the 1920s, Watson and Rayner conducted a study with "Little Albert" to demonstrate that fears could be conditioned. But today, their study would not meet the ethical standards of many research committees (see pp. 472–473).

1. Design a study to show how a childhood fear or anxiety could be learned without risking the well-being of the child.

2. List stimuli for which infants may be genetically prepared for developing conditioned responses.

ENURESIS

Description

Enuresis is diagnosed for children of at least 5 years of age when bed-wetting or involuntary urination occurs more than once a week for at least 3 consecutive months. If the frequency is less often, the diagnosis may still be made when the bed-wetting causes significant distress or impairment in the child's functioning (American Psychiatric Association, 1994).

In Western countries, approximately 85 to 90 percent of children learn to be continent (that is, stop wetting their beds) by the age of 5. By the age of 10, approximately 95 percent of youths are continent, and this increases to over 98 percent by adulthood. Like the majority of childhood psychological disorders, enuresis is much more common in boys than in girls. Twice as many boys wet their beds as girls at age 5 (7 percent of boys, 3 percent of girls). Moreover, in adulthood, enuresis is almost nonexistent for females, but approximately 1 to 2 percent of males remain enuretic, as estimated from samples of military recruits (Houts & Liebert, 1984). More children from lower socioeconomic backgrounds than children from higher socioeconomic classes have this disorder. Consistent evidence has also shown that children are more likely to be enuretic if a parent was also enuretic (Doleys, 1989).

Because enuresis generally declines with age, it's reasonable for an enuretic child's parent to wonder how long the bed-wetting will continue. Researchers followed approximately 1,200 bed-wetters between the ages of 5 and 19 over a 15-year period to see how long it took them to become dry without medical or psychological treatment (Forsythe & Redmond, 1974). Their likelihood of a spontaneous cure or simply growing out of the problem was only about 15 percent per year. Parents

enuresis Disorder diagnosed for children of at least 5 years of age when bed-wetting or involuntary discharge of urine occurs more than once a week for at least 3 consecutive months.

of most school-age enuretic children are generally advised to seek treatment for this problem (Houts, Berman, & Abramson, 1994).

Enuresis can be troublesome for children, who can't understand why they wet their beds during sleep. Parents who mistakenly believe that the problem is simply one of laziness often make their children's sense of shame worse. Soiled sheets anger many parents and embarrass many children. Enuretic children tend to avoid visiting friends overnight, going to camp, or staying with relatives. Those who share bedrooms with siblings are often the subject of relentless teasing.

Causes

There are many different causes of enuresis. Parents typically but often mistakenly believe that bed-wetting is caused by emotional problems or by extremely deep sleep that prevents children from detecting bladder pressure (Doleys, 1989). Diseases and infections account for only a small percentage of cases. Most bed-wetters do not have diseases or emotional problems. During sleep or the awaking period, they simply fail to respond to cues from their bladders that it's time to urinate.

Treatment

The most effective and commonly used psychological treatment is the **bell and pad method,** developed in the 1930s (Mowrer & Mowrer, 1938). This alarm device awakens a child immediately upon urination. Parents are encouraged to make certain that the child wakes, goes to the bathroom, and urinates in the toilet. They then instruct the child to return to the bedroom, change the sheets, reset the alarm, and go back to sleep. To monitor the child's progress, the parents keep a daily chart, and for each dry day, they place a gold star on it. Usually, within 3 to 8 weeks of treatment, the child no longer wets the bed. An extensive review of the effectiveness of the bell and pad treatment over the last 30 years has indicated that after treatment, approximately two-thirds of the children had stopped wetting. The researchers also reported that fewer than 1 of every 10 clinic-referred children could be expected to stop bed-wetting if untreated (Houts, Berman, & Abramson, 1994).

A variation on the bell and pad method involves an all-night training program of intensive training in how to become continent (Azrin, Sneed, & Foxx, 1973). This program consists of only one or two extended overnight sessions, with the therapist present. The child drinks large amounts of fluid before going to bed to increase the probability of urinating during the night. Then, throughout the night, the child receives practice and positive reinforcement for getting out of bed to urinate and for urinating in the toilet. The child also receives negative reinforcement for accidents, in the form of reprimands and having to clean and remake the bed. As in the original bell and pad treatment, a chart marks the child's progress.

This all-night training procedure has been used in several studies with 100 percent success, although in some other studies, the success rate has been considerably lower. Another low-cost, one-hour group treatment program for enuretics and their parents—combining the bell and pad and all-night training methods—has been successful in 80 percent of cases (Houts & Liebert, 1984). This program is cost effective and efficient in helping children achieve continence. The relapse rate (23 percent) compares very favorably with other treatment outcomes.

bell and pad method
Alarm device that awakens a bed-wetter immediately upon urination, so the child can rise and continue urination in the bathroom; the most effective and most commonly used psychological treatment for enuresis.

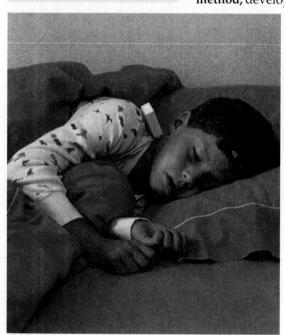

A child using a bed-wetting alarm is equipped with a pouch that attaches to his underwear and contains the urine-sensitive device. In turn, the urine-sensitive device is connected by a small wire to an alarm attached to the child's shoulder with a Velcro strip. When the child urinates, the alarm sounds and he awakens.

Such high success rates, however, do not apply to enuretic children attending mental health clinics because of significant behavioral and emotional problems (O'Leary & Wilson, 1987). Some children with multiple problems who receive enuresis treatment display more behavior problems on days after they wet their beds than on days after they have remained dry (Vivian, Fischel, & Liebert, 1987). Parents and relatives need to be aware that children undergoing enuresis treatment may feel significantly pressured or frustrated when they wet their beds and that successful treatment of those with multiple problems may be a lengthy process.

Regarding the use of medication as a treatment for enuresis: **Imipramine** (brand name Tofranil), an antidepressant, initially seemed effective in treating enuretic children. It's now apparent that even though imipramine does result in decreased frequency of bed-wetting, it's not a cure, in most cases (Houts, Berman, & Abramson, 1994; Houts, Peterson, & Liebert, 1984). Another medication that has received attention in the 1990s is desmopressin acetate (brand name DDVAP). This medication, an antidiuretic hormone that's taken in the form of a nasal spray, has been used for enuretic individuals not responsive to other treatments (Rushton, 1993). But it has not been established as a primary treatment for enuresis that leads to cessation of bed-wetting.

◤ *Focus on* *Critical Thinking*

The bell and pad treatment is clearly one of the most effective treatments for enuresis, but it does have some drawbacks. For instance, if a number of children are sleeping in one room, all of them will hear the alarm. On the other hand, if the child remains a bed-wetter, the smell of nightly urine could lead to other problems, such as complaints from siblings and even physical abuse by parents, in some cases.

1. Suppose that using the bell and pad method helped a child learn to sleep through the night without wetting (which is often the case). What learning mechanisms would account for this treatment success?

2. If you didn't want to use the bell and pad procedure, what alternative intervention would you recommend? Why?

*L*EARNING *D*ISORDERS

Description

Learning disorders (LD) are diagnosed when children show evidence of inadequate development of certain academic, language, speech, and motor skills. However, these disorders are not due to low intelligence or inadequate schooling. For a learning disorder to be diagnosed, a child's skills must be substantially lower than would be expected based on her intellectual capacity (American Psychiatric Association, 1994). Assessment should therefore involve administration of a standardized intelligence test along with a standardized achievement test on the skill area in question.

There are three common learning disorders:

1. *Reading disorder*—This disorder is characterized by impaired word-recognition skills and reading comprehension. The term **dyslexia**, which means "ill words," is often used to describe this disorder. During oral reading, individuals who are dyslexic often omit, add, and distort words. They also tend to read slowly and haltingly.

2. *Mathematics disorder*—Common characteristics of this disorder include difficulty in understanding mathematical terms and operations and/or in recognizing numerical symbols and arithmetic signs. Also common to this disorder is an inability to use mathematical skills such as counting, following sequential steps, and learning multiplication tables.

3. *Disorder of written expression*—The essential feature of this disorder is marked impairment in the development of expressive writing skills. The diagnosis is made only if the impairment interferes significantly with the child's academic achievement or with daily activities that require expres-

imipramine (Tofranil)
Antidepressant medication that is also used to treat enuresis.

learning disorders (LD)
Characterized by academic, language, speech, and motor skills that are substantially lower than would be expected based on a child's intellectual capacity; subcategories include reading disorder, mathematics disorder, and disorder of written expression.

dyslexia Term used for reading disorder; characterized by impaired word-recognition skills and reading comprehension; dyslexics often omit, add, and distort words.

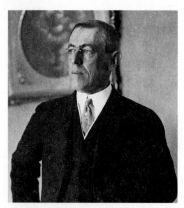

President Woodrow Wilson had a learning disorder, which made it difficult for him to read. These problems plagued him not only in his own schooling but even as a college professor, when he had to read his students' papers.

sive writing skills. When a child with this disorder composes written material, the text is flawed by poor organization and a combination of grammatical, punctuation, and spelling errors. Relatively less is known about this disorder than about other learning disorders. Disorder of written expression is commonly found in combination with reading disorder or mathematics disorder.

Children with learning disorders often have low self-esteem and problems getting along with others. Approximately 40 percent of children with LD drop out of school, and adults with these disorders often have problems at work. Many children with LD also have conduct and oppositional disorders (American Psychiatric Association, 1994). There are also success stories. Many individuals work very hard to overcome their learning disorders and succeed in life despite them. This was the case with President Woodrow Wilson. He didn't learn his letters until he was 12, and he was a very slow reader, both as a child and as an adult (Weinstein, 1981).

Causes

The causes of learning disorders are poorly understood. Some experts believe that children with LD have neuropsychological problems that researchers will eventually detect (Conners & Wells, 1987). Others argue that learning disorders represent the bottom end of the distribution of abilities or are the result of developmental delays (Hynd & Cohen, 1983). Some learning disorders, especially reading disorder, may have a genetic basis (Myers & Hammil, 1990). Recent genetic mapping research has demonstrated that chromosome 6 is partly responsible for the disorder (Cardon et al., 1994).

The *DSM-IV* lists a variety of factors associated with the development of learning disorders: underlying abnormalities in cognitive processing, genetic predisposition, perinatal injury, and several neurological and general medical conditions. However, with the exception of the isolation of chromosome 6 in the development of reading disorders, none of these variables are seen as definitive causes of LD.

Treatment

Treatments for LD vary tremendously and include dietary changes, individual psychotherapy, family therapy, educational tutoring, large muscle training regimens to aid neurological development, and optometric training. According to the most recent federal legislation addressing the needs of exceptional children, schools are required to develop individualized educational programs to meet children's special needs (Gallagher, 1994) (see also Chapter 15). To show improvement, children with LD usually require extensive training in specific skills. A common denominator of treatment for these disorders is educational intervention.

Besides special public school education services, private educational resource centers in many communities provide tutorial or remedial services for children needing this help. Children with reading disorders may also benefit from optometric training to aid them in appropriate visual tracking and focusing.

Focus on Critical Thinking

Schools are now required to provide educational programs for children with LD, and local districts often receive state reimbursement for such programs. Consequently, in some districts, the percentage of children with LD has risen dramatically.

1. How would you determine whether an increase in the prevalence of LD diagnoses is a case of better diagnostic procedures or a means of obtaining state funds at the possible expense of a child who would not have an LD diagnosis?

2. Delayed neurological development possibly prevents some children from learning to read and write at the normal rate. Assuming that's true, special education programs for children with LD may not be worth the time and money allocated. How would you evaluate the long-term usefulness of these programs?

About half the girls in the United States between 15 and 19 years of age are sexually active, and according to various estimates, 40 percent of these teen-age females become pregnant (Marecek, 1987). Among the teen-agers who become pregnant, half—more than 1 million each year—have abortions. Meanwhile, the number of new unmarried mothers, many of them teen-agers, increases each year.

What effect does abortion or childbirth have on a teen-age girl? The American Psychological Association commissioned a panel of experts to address this issue. They concluded that having an abortion in the first 3 months of pregnancy does not cause serious psychological problems for most women. Of course, feelings about having an abortion vary widely. Some women feel regret, sadness, and guilt, but for the majority, severe distress and psychopathology do not follow abortion. In fact, the most common reaction of both adults and minors to abortion is relief. However, if a woman believes that abortion is wrong, if she is not supported in her decision to have the abortion by her male partner and her parents, or if she blames herself for the pregnancy, she will have more difficulty in dealing with her feelings after an abortion (Adler et al., 1990, 1992). For those teen-age girls who decide to have and raise their children, the likelihood of completing school is lessened and future income poten-

tial is diminished. Moreover, if such girls marry, the marriage may be strained by both social and financial pressures (Melton, 1987).

Deciding whether to have an abortion or to give birth is extremely difficult for many teen-agers, and the decision is not based simply on facts. Religious, moral, and family attitudes toward abortion usually weigh heavily in the decision. There is no one right or wrong answer to the question: Should a teen-ager have an abortion? Even with the economic hardships that most teen-age mothers face, many raise their children successfully—usually with the help of understanding and supportive parents. To be sure, when making the decision, the pregnant teen-ager—along with her partner and all their parents, when possible—should consider the impact of religious and moral beliefs and the likely outcomes we have just discussed.

Think about the following questions:

1. If a pregnant teen-ager approached you for advice and support, what positive and negative factors would you encourage her to consider in making her decision? Explain your answer.
2. If you chose to have an abortion, what impact do you think doing so would have on you? Describe both potential short- and long-term effects.

DEPRESSION

Description

Depression has been studied as a childhood disorder only recently because several decades ago, many professionals questioned whether children had the cognitive capacity to become depressed. Depression in children has also been considered controversial because professionals have disagreed about whether it's a unique phenomenon, distinctly different from depression in adults (Cantwell, 1983; Kazdin, 1989). There is increasing recognition that children can be depressed (Kazdin, 1989). Moreover, it's known that rates of **childhood depression** do not differ for boys and girls, although by late adolescence, rates of depression are higher among girls than boys (Fergusson, Horwood, & Lynskey, 1993). In addition, some symptoms are more common in girls than in boys and vice versa. See Thinking about Controversial Issues, which explores one problem associated with depression in teen-age girls—pregnancy and abortion.

The *DSM-IV* does not have a separate diagnostic category for childhood depression. But research on this disorder has increased over the past decade. As with adults, symptoms of childhood depression include depressed mood, low self-esteem, fatigue, somatic complaints, suicidal thoughts, and a sense of hopelessness (Carlson & Cantwell, 1980). However, other factors differentiate depression in adults versus children. For instance, suicide among depressed children is extremely rare. What's more, biological correlates are not identical for children and adults (Kazdin, 1989). And children do not generally show positive responses to treatment

childhood depression

Childhood disorder whose symptoms include depressed mood, low self-esteem, fatigue, somatic complaints, suicidal thoughts, and a sense of hopelessness.

479

TABLE 14.2   **Common Signs of Depression in Children and Adolescents**

While either boys or girls may show these symptoms, they tend to be more common in one sex than the other.

More Common in Girls

■ **Body image distortion.** Feeling "ugly" or otherwise unattractive, when objectively that is not the case.

■ **Loss of appetite and weight.** Losing interest in eating, or eating erratically.

■ **Lack of satisfaction.** Being upset about herself, about life at school and at home and about social life.

More Common in Boys

■ **Irritability.** Being easily angered and hostile; snapping at family, friends and teachers.

■ **Social withdrawal.** Ceasing to spend time with friends; spending most of the time alone.

■ **Drop in school performance.** Loss of interest in and enthusiasm about school, as well as other activities.

SOURCE: From "Common Signs of Depression in Children and Adolescents," *The New York Times,* May 10, 1990. Copyright © 1990 by The New York Times Company. Reprinted by permission.

---

with antidepressant medication. Table 14.2 lists common signs of depression in children and adolescents, noting which are more common in boys versus girls.

The assessment of a child whose parents take him to a mental health clinic for depression generally involves a semistructured interview with the parent or parents present. During this assessment, the clinician asks questions about potential symptoms. The most widely used measure to assess childhood depression is the Children's Depression Inventory (Kovacs & Beck, 1977), a self-report scale that the child completes (Craighead, Curry, & McMillan, 1994; Kazdin, 1989).

Causes

Family Factors   Because close relatives of individuals who are depressed also show increased risk of affective disorders or depression (see Chapter 7), investigators have begun to search for family variables associated with childhood depression. Evidence has suggested that children with depressed parents are more likely to develop problems of depression, substance abuse, poor social functioning, and school functioning than children of control subjects (Weissman et al., 1987).

Researchers found a very low frequency of depression among the young children of depressed parents—namely, less than 1 child in 100. There was, however, a marked increase in the frequency of depression among such children between 15 and 20 years of age, especially for girls. Yet even for adolescents and young adults who had depressed parents, the risk for having a major depressive disorder was relatively low—approximately 1 percent for boys and 4 percent for girls. Family studies of childhood depression, then, do not provide conclusive evidence of the influence of genetic factors on its development. The increased incidence of depression in adolescent relatives of depressed individuals may be simply a function of high stress levels in families of psychiatric patients.

Weintraub and Neale (1984) reported an elevated risk for depression among children of patients with depression or schizophrenia. Comparisons of children of depressed mothers and nondepressed mothers with medical conditions indicate that the children of depressed mothers have more negative thoughts about themselves (Jaenicke et al., 1987). Moreover, the role of criticism by family members is becoming a central focus in much of the research on depression and other psychological disorders, since it appears to be associated with a host of etiological factors in child disorders. To sum up, data suggest that psychosocial stressors and genetic predispositions combine to elevate the risk for childhood depression.

Psychological Factors   Like depressed adults, depressed children often demonstrate a negative self-concept and low sense of self-worth; this, in turn, diminishes their belief that they can accomplish certain goals. Children who are depressed seem to personalize social stressors when exposed to them (for instance, "I'm always in a bad class") and feel unable to cope with such situations successfully. Parental criticism is also highly associated with self-blame and self-critical statements by depressed children (Jaenicke et al., 1987).

Treatment

Psychological and pharmacological therapies have been used with depressed children. Common goals of psychological treatments include changing the negative cognitive style, improving self-esteem, and building social skills. Because children who are depressed exhibit such a variety of associated problems (for example, isolation, anxiety, enuresis), no conclusive evidence has been found of the superiority of any particular form of psychological therapy (Frame, Robinson, & Cuddy, 1992). However, a combination of cognitive-behavioral treatment with a family treatment component appears especially promising. Researchers have noted reductions in depressive symptoms both following treatment and at a 7-month follow-up (Stark, Rouse, & Livingston, 1991).

Rationales for the use of pharmacological treatments for childhood depression are largely based on the findings of drug research with depressed adults. Despite the similarities in the symptoms of depression in children and adults, in general, antidepressant drugs seem to have little or no beneficial effect on children (Craighead, Curry, & McMillan, 1994; Ryan, 1993).

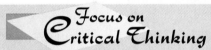

Focus on Critical Thinking

1. Suppose the parents of a 10-year-old girl being treated for depression have come to you for advice. The child's therapist has her participate in play therapy, which the parents think may be doing more harm than good. The parents have voiced their concern, but the therapist rarely talks to them. What do you suggest the parents do?

SUMMARY

Perspectives on Childhood Disorders

■ Psychological disorders of children were not well recognized until the 1950s. Publications such as the *Journal of Abnormal Child Psychology* only began in 1973. However, child clinical psychology is now a recognized subspecialty of clinical psychology.

■ The most prevalent childhood disorders include attention-deficit/hyperactivity disorder, oppositional defiant disorder, conduct disorder, and anxiety disorders (separation anxiety, overanxious disorder, and phobias). More than half of all children with one disorder also have a second. The greatest overlap in childhood disorders is found with attention-deficit disorders and conduct disorders.

■ Boys' problems far outnumber girls' problems in almost every major childhood diagnostic category, except for anxiety and phobias. The reasons for boys' greater vulnerability is unclear, but it's known that boys are more vulnerable than girls to many physical and psychological problems, from conception to adulthood.

Oppositional Defiant and Conduct Disorders

■ Children with oppositional defiant disorder (ODD) are often angry and aggressive, but they limit their defiance to situations in the home and with children they know well. Serious cases of ODD may evolve into conduct disorder (CD). Children with CD are verbally and physically aggressive and violate the rights of others; their behavior is typically present in a variety of settings.

■ As far as we can tell, aggressive behavior is not inherited. Extraversion and fearlessness are, however, and these characteristics may influence the development of aggression.

■ Psychological and social factors such as rewards, modeling, strong punishment, inconsistent discipline, marital discord, and divorce are consistently related to aggressive behavior in children.

■ Effective treatments for ODD and CD include behavior management training for parents, behavioral family systems approaches, emphasis on communication and mutual reinforcement, and problem-solving interventions.

Attention-Deficit/Hyperactivity Disorder

■ In young children, attention-deficit/hyperactivity disorder (AD/HD) is characterized by problems of inattention, distractibility, and overactivity.

■ AD/HD becomes evident when children enter school. For most children, problems of extreme overactivity become less problematic as they reach junior and senior high school, but some youths continue to be restless and have difficulty concentrating even after high school.

■ When aggression and attentional problems coexist, the prognosis is less favorable than if a child has only attentional problems.

■ Both genetic and psychological factors seem significant in the etiology of attentional and aggressive problems. Family and environmental factors are most closely associated with the aggressive symptoms that characterize AD/HD. Neurological problems also appear to play an important role in the development of some children's attentional deficits.

■ Psychological and pharmacological therapies—used individually and in combination—have been quite successful in treating children with problems of attention and overactivity.

Anxiety Disorders

■ Girls are brought to clinics with anxiety problems more frequently than boys. However, it may be that young girls are more likely to express their fears or anxieties than boys.

■ Genetic factors predispose certain children to anxiety disorders, and these disorders are clearly more common in children whose parents had similar problems. Conditioning, modeling, reinforcement, and complex cognitive learning also affect the etiology of anxiety.

■ Psychological therapies involving training anxious children in new cognitive styles and social skills have been effective in reducing anxiety. Both psychological and pharmacological therapies have helped children with severe phobias attend school.

Enuresis

■ A child is more likely to be enuretic if a parent was also enuretic. Although diverse factors (such as small bladder capacities and emotional problems) have been associated with enuresis, the basic problem is one of failing to respond to cues from the bladder to urinate.

■ Programs utilizing a bell and pad device to awaken children when they begin to urinate have successfully trained thousands to become continent.

Learning Disorders

■ Learning disorders (LD) impair the academic functioning of children, and their skill level is substantially lower than would be expected based on their intellectual capacity.

■ We don't know what causes some learning disorders, but chromosome 6 is definitely involved in the development of reading disorders.

■ Treatments for learning disorders include training for visual tracking, neurological programs to develop motor coordination, and psychotherapies. Special training to reduce the specific skill deficits impairing these children's functioning appears essential for promoting improvement.

Depression

■ Professional attention has only recently focused on childhood depression, partly because of uncertainty as to whether it's a syndrome significantly different from adult depression. Despite this problem, childhood depression has become a focus of much research in the last decade.

■ A child has a greater likelihood of developing depression if she has a depressed parent. Significant parental strife and criticism also place children at risk for developing depression, although very few young children actually attempt suicide.

■ Treatment for childhood depression generally involves psychological therapy directed at changing cognitive styles and social skills. Depressed children do not show the same positive response to medication as depressed adults.

KEY TERMS

attention-deficit/hyperactivity disorder (AD/HD), **p. 462**
bell and pad method, **p. 476**
childhood depression, **p. 479**
conduct disorder (CD), **p. 455**
delinquent, **p. 456**
dyslexia, **p. 477**
enuresis, **p. 475**

Feingold diet, **p. 465**
imipramine (Tofranil), **p. 477**
inept discipline, **p. 458**
inept monitoring, **p. 458**
learning disorders (LD), **p. 477**
minimal brain dysfunction (MBD), **p. 465**
oppositional defiant disorder (ODD), **pp. 454–455**

overanxious disorder, **p. 471**
problem-solving training, **p. 461**
psychostimulants, **p. 467**
recidivism, **p. 461**
Ritalin, **p. 467**
school phobia, **p. 471**
separation anxiety disorder, **p. 471**

*C*RITICAL *T*HINKING *E*XERCISE

Early one June morning, Tommy's home burned nearly to the ground after his grandfather fell asleep smoking a cigarette. At the time, Tommy was 7 years old and his sister, Pam, was 10. They lived with their mother and father and maternal grandfather. Tommy's grandfather was rushed to the hospital because of smoke inhalation, but as it turned out, he wasn't hurt.

While the house was being rebuilt, Tommy's parents stayed in a trailer on the premises of the home. But there wasn't enough room for Tommy and his sister, so they stayed with an aunt who lived in the same area. Since Tommy and his sister weren't in school, they went to a community day camp every weekday morning. At camp, Tommy didn't want to play soccer with the other kids his age. Instead, he went to arts and crafts and stayed close to his camp counselor, Marty. Tommy never complained or cried while at camp. But he never smiled or laughed, either.

1. Imagine that you're Marty, Tommy's counselor, and the camp director has asked you to take special notice of Tommy over the next 3 days to see if he's depressed. What would you do? Why?

2. If, based on your observations of Tommy, you concluded that he was depressed, what types of interventions would you recommend? Why?

Chapter 15

MENTAL RETARDATION AND AUTISTIC DISORDER

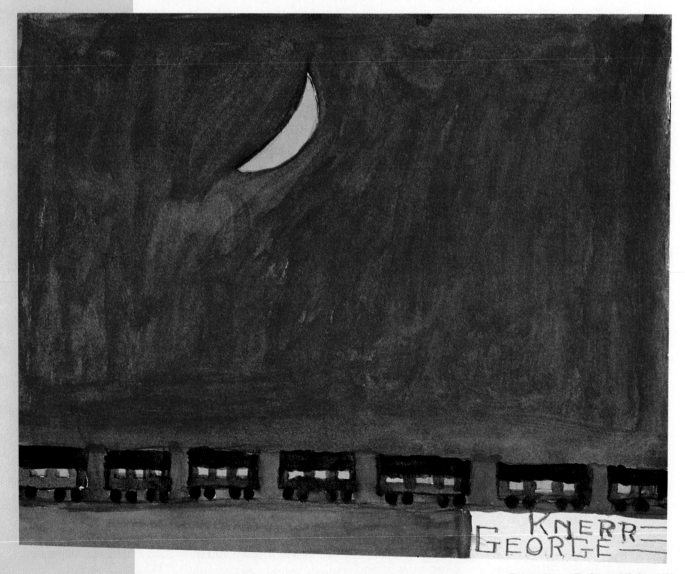

George Knerr, **Train at Night,** HAI

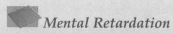
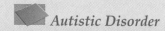
Maria and Mateo Santos waited quite a long time to have their first child. When they married, both were starting graduate school, and although Mateo earned his M.B.A. 2 years later, Maria still had 3 more years to go before earning her doctorate in history. Even when Maria received the Ph.D., she and Mateo decided to wait a while longer, so that she could get a good start on her way up the "academic ladder" at the university where she'd been offered her first teaching job.

As a result, Maria was almost 34 when their first child, David, was born. A smiling, friendly, much loved newborn, David was the realization of Mateo and Maria's most precious dreams. But then, shortly after David's birth, the diagnosis of Down syndrome was confirmed. Mateo reacted to the news by becoming angry and self-pitying; he put emotional distance between himself and David and Maria. For her part, Maria lapsed into depression, blaming herself for having put her career ahead of the family she had always wanted.

As time went on, though, David developed into an affectionate and social child. And when Maria and Mateo stopped mourning what might have been, the Santoses became a family for the first time. It helped that David's grandparents all lived nearby. Not only had they understood and accepted the couple's decision to postpone parenthood, but they became doting grandparents without any apparent effort. Maria and Mateo's solid, loving marriage also helped them get through the postpartum period without blaming and accusing one another. But what helped most was their son, David, who became the beloved focus of their lives, despite the problems they would all have to face.

Mental retardation affects about 1 percent (roughly 2.5 million people) of the U.S. population. Most persons with this diagnosis have intelligence quotients (IQs) of 70 or below, are 18 years or less, and also have other conditions that impair their ability to adapt to social situations and conform to social expectations. Mental retardation can be caused by disease, injury, environmental factors, and chromosomal and genetic conditions that permanently affect brain functioning before, during, or after birth. Although the brain damage responsible for most mental retardation is irreversible, medicine has been increasingly successful in preventing

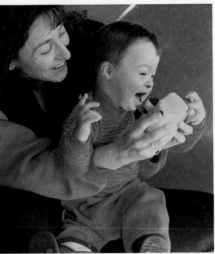

Children born today with mental retardation will likely lead longer, healthier, and more independent lives than similar individuals of even a generation or two ago, due to improvements in health care, special education, and institutional support.

some of the conditions that lead to this disorder. Moreover, advances in institutional and home care in recent years have enabled people who are retarded to live more independently and productively than ever before.

Given the improvements in health care, special education, and institutional support that are now available to individuals who are retarded and their families, Maria and Mateo's son, David, will likely lead a longer, healthier, and more independent life than similar individuals of even a generation or two ago. In this chapter, we'll look at the advances made in diagnosing and preventing mental retardation and in caring for individuals with this disorder. We'll also consider similar topics regarding another much misunderstood condition: autistic disorder.

MENTAL RETARDATION

A Historical Overview

Although such common disorders as schizophrenia, bipolar affective disorder, and alcoholism were recognized by the ancient Greeks and Romans, neither society made much mention of mental retardation. One of the few things we know about the views of the Greeks and Romans on the subject comes from the Father of Medicine, Hippocrates (c. 460–377 B.C.). He made the brief, accurate observation that retardation appeared to result from brain damage taking place before and during birth. And according to some sources, the ancient Spartans and Romans sometimes killed severely mentally retarded infants so as not to be burdened with them throughout life.

Although churchmen, philosophers, and scientists of the Middle Ages were much concerned with psychotics who were possessed by demons, they made little mention of people who were mentally retarded. Still, it seems clear that these individuals were barely tolerated. They were often seen as accidents of nature and sometimes considered in league with the devil. As a result, the mentally retarded were often subjected to the same barbaric treatment that psychotics and alcoholics were during this time.

At the end of the eighteenth century, while Philippe Pinel (1745–1826) was reforming mental hospitals in France, other physicians worked to bring the care and study of people with mental retardation into the realm of medicine. The most famous of these individuals were Frenchmen Jean-Marc-Gaspard Itard (1775–1838) and Édouard Séguin (1812–1880). Their efforts initiated more humane institutional care for people who are mentally retarded, in both Europe and the United States.

By the mid-1800s, the optimism of the late 1700s that had led to efforts to teach the mentally retarded useful skills and to treat them more humanely had turned to pessimism because of the difficulties of doing so. Many of the institutions that had been reformed only a generation earlier again became more custodial than rehabilitative. At about the same time, attempts to manage the problem of mental retardation by eugenic (birth control) means of various kinds began to be considered. Among the options considered was sterilization of people who were severely mentally retarded so they could not reproduce.

The early part of the twentieth century was marked by continued indifference to the problems of the retarded and their families. However, discovery of relationships between inborn errors of metabolism and mental retardation took place shortly thereafter, leading to increased optimism about the prevention and treatment of these forms of mental retardation. In the early 1930s, the discovery of phenylketonuria (a metabolically caused form of mental retardation, which we'll discuss later) raised the possibility that a scientific basis for understanding, preventing, and treating this condition could be established. This initial discovery has

mental retardation Condition characterized by subaverage intelligence beginning before the age of 18, accompanied by impairments in adaptive functioning.

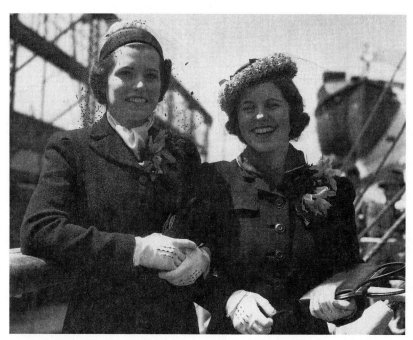

Rosemary Kennedy, President John F. Kennedy's sister, shown on the right in this early photograph with their sister, Eunice. The profound impact of Rosemary's mental retardation was a factor that led President Kennedy to propose legislation early in his term on the education of persons with mental retardation.

been followed by progress in identifying many other metabolic disorders that cause mental retardation, accompanied by rigorous and productive genetics research that reflects the biological basis of most metabolic disorders.

Along with these findings has come a less condemning view of mental retardation. Recall from other chapters that the same change in attitudes toward schizophrenia and manic-depressive disorder occurred during the time of Emil Kraepelin (1856–1926), following recognition that these were real physical disorders. New laws to ensure appropriate care for people who were mentally retarded often coincided with these discoveries. Yet even today, many U.S. institutions for these individuals suffer from legislative and societal neglect.

President John F. Kennedy—whose sister Rosemary was born mentally retarded—sparked a reawakening of Americans' sense of responsibility for retarded people and their families during the early 1960s. That interest and concern is also reflected in the work of the president's sister, Eunice Kennedy Shriver, the founder of the Special Olympics.

Diagnosis of Mental Retardation

The operational criteria for mental retardation provided in the fourth edition of the *Diagnostic and Statistical Manual of Mental Disorders (DSM-IV)* (American Psychiatric Association, 1994) require IQ test information on intellectual functioning and a clinical judgment about level of adaptive functioning (see the *DSM* table).

 Diagnostic Criteria for MENTAL RETARDATION

A. Significantly subaverage intellectual functioning: an IQ of approximately 70 or below on an individually administered IQ test (for infants, a clinical judgment of significantly subaverage intellectual functioning).

B. Concurrent deficits or impairments in present adaptive functioning (i.e., the person's effectiveness in meeting the standards expected for his or her age by his or her cultural group) in at least two of the following areas: communication, self-care, home living, social/interpersonal skills, use of community resources,

self-direction, functional academic skills, work, leisure, health, and safety.

C. The onset is before age 18 years.

Code based on degree of severity reflecting level of intellectual impairment:

Mild Mental Retardation
    IQ level 50–55 to approximately 70

Moderate Mental Retardation
    IQ level 35–40 to 50–55

Severe Mental Retardation
    IQ level 20–25 to 35–40

Profound Mental Retardation
    IQ level below 20 or 25

Mental Retardation, Severity Unspecified: when there is strong presumption of Mental Retardation but the person's intelligence is untestable by standard tests.

As we discussed in Chapter 3, the average IQ score on one of the Wechsler intelligence tests is 100. A score of 70 or below (or 130 or above) is unusual; only 5 percent of the persons taking the test score in these ranges. Yet despite its rarity, an IQ of 70 or below is not sufficient by itself for the diagnosis of mental retardation. Also required are deficits in at least two areas of functioning that interfere with the individual's ability to maintain an independent social, vocational, and personal life. Persons who cannot clearly communicate their needs and desires to others, have been unable to acquire self-care skills, cannot look out for their own health and safety, and don't have the skills to find and hold jobs will have a tough time living independently.

Both of the first two *DSM-IV* diagnostic criteria for mental retardation must have been met before the individual reached the age of 18. When these criteria are only met after that age, the retardation has probably occurred as the result of a serious brain disorder, disease, or injury that caused a variety of serious physical disabilities, as well. In such instances, the person will be diagnosed as having a functional deficit in intelligence and adaptive functioning secondary to the serious physical disorder, disease, or injury.

The *DSM-IV* (American Psychiatric Association, 1994) specifies four degrees of severity of mental retardation:

1. Mild mental retardation (IQ 50–55 to approximately 70): About 85 percent of persons with mental retardation fall into this group. Most develop more or less normal social and communication skills between birth and the time they begin school. They experience few or no obvious impairments in perceptual functions (such as seeing and hearing), and their retardation is often not recognized until they take intelligence tests at school. By their late teens, these individuals might have acquired academic skills comparable to those of a sixth-grade student. As adults, they can usually function independently, although during times of unusual stress, they may require special support. These persons can usually live successfully in the community on their own or in supervised settings.

2. Moderate mental retardation (IQ 35–40 to 50–55): This group includes about 10 percent of the individuals with mental retardation. Most learn to speak as young children. They are often able to benefit from vocational training and, with supervision, can learn to care for themselves. They are able to acquire minimal academic skills, although they generally do not progress beyond the second-grade level. During adolescence, their inability to acquire social and interpersonal skills may interfere with having successful relationships with peers. As adults, these individuals can work at unskilled or semiskilled jobs in sheltered settings in the community.

3. Severe mental retardation (IQ 20–25 to 35–40): This group includes about 3 to 4 percent of persons with mental retardation. They generally acquire little or no speech, even though they can sometimes learn to recite the alphabet, count, and read a few words. They might be able to acquire minimal self-care skills and perform simple tasks in closely supervised environments, but they cannot live independently. Many can, however, live in the community, as long as they are closely supervised.

4. Profound mental retardation (IQ below 20–25): Only 1 to 2 percent of persons with mental retardation fall into this category. Most have an identifiable neurological condition that's responsible for both their mental retardation and associated, often severe, physical deficits. These individuals also have marked perceptual problems that, combined with their extreme intellectual deficits, make it extremely difficult for them to learn. These persons must be cared for throughout their lives in highly structured environments.

Amniocentesis is an important recent advance in our ability to diagnose conditions causing mental retardation. This process involves withdrawing a small amount of **amniotic fluid** (the protective fluid in which the fetus floats within the uterus) toward the end of the fourth month of pregnancy (see Figure 15.1). Fetal cells floating in the amniotic fluid can then be analyzed for signs of various fetal abnormalities, including serious hereditary conditions. Given the test findings, the prospective parents can be informed early enough to consider several options. They may consider a therapeutic abortion if an identified condition poses a threat to the mother's life or would permanently and seriously impair the unborn child's quality of life. Or they may proceed with the pregnancy and use the time to edu-

mild mental retardation Characterized by IQ of between 50–55 and 70; includes 85 percent of persons with mental retardation.

moderate mental retardation Characterized by IQ between 35–40 and 50–55; includes 10 percent of persons with mental retardation.

severe mental retardation Characterized by IQ between 20–25 and 35–40; includes 3–4 percent of persons with mental retardation.

profound mental retardation Characterized by IQ below 20–25; includes 1–2 percent of persons with mental retardation.

amniocentesis Procedure for diagnosing hereditary conditions in fetuses; involves withdrawing a small amount of amniotic fluid to be examined for evidence of chromosomal or genetic disorder in the fetal cells suspended in it.

amniotic fluid Protective fluid the fetus is immersed in.

FIGURE 15.1   Amniocentesis

Amniocentesis involves withdrawing a small amount of amniotic fluid from the uterus—generally toward the end of the fourth month of gestation—so that fetal cells can be examined for indications of abnormalities.

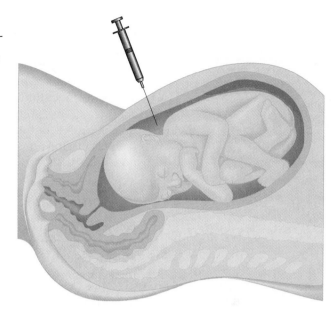

cate and otherwise prepare themselves for the tasks and issues that will be involved with the birth of their child.

The Epidemiology of Mental Retardation

In a 1986 survey of the epidemiology of mental retardation, Munro observed that "mental retardation is the most common lifelong handicap in 'developed' nations and likely consumes more professional and financial resources than any other disabling condition" (1986, p. 593). Although the prevalence of mental retardation in the United States was estimated at 3 percent for many years, more accurate recent epidemiological studies now put the prevalence at 1 percent. This figure is generally accepted as valid throughout most of the world. Thus, with a population of about 250 million, the United States has about 2.5 million citizens with mental retardation. Since all of them—to one extent or another—must receive special care and attention, it's easy to see that the financial and social costs of mental retardation are substantial.

Mental retardation is unevenly distributed across age groups. Fewer than 1 percent of preschool children are recognized as having mental retardation, since only those with one of the most severe forms are diagnosed before schooling begins (Shapiro, Palmer, & Capute, 1987). The greatest prevalence is in school-age children and adolescents between the ages of 10 and 18—the years during which intellectual and academic performance are most intensively evaluated. Prevalence rates then decline steadily through the rest of the life span because many mildly retarded persons disappear into society. Moreover, most of those who are severely or profoundly retarded die before or during middle age. The best estimates are that about 75 percent of people who are retarded are adolescents or younger (Nezu, Nezu, & Gill-Weiss, 1992).

Prevalence studies consistently report higher rates of mental retardation among males than females; the *DSM-IV* (American Psychiatric Association, 1994) puts the ratio at 1.5 males to 1 female. Reasons for this sex difference include males' greater vulnerability to prenatal factors causing retardation, including maternal infections; the significant number of hereditary conditions causing mental retardation that are linked to the male sex chromosome; and the more aggressive social behavior of boys, which brings them to the attention of authorities who might find them to be retarded.

Socioeconomic status and mental retardation are inversely related in the United States: The lower a person's socioeconomic level, the more likely he will be diagnosed with mental retardation. This relationship stems from multiple factors. One is the inferior quality of prenatal care that many poor Americans receive. Similarly, people who are poor are relatively unable to provide their children the same academic stimulation—at home and at school—that middle- and upper-class children receive. Another factor is that school authorities tend to place poor children in classes for the mentally retarded more quickly than other children. For similar reasons, the prevalence of mental retardation in the United States is higher for nonwhites than for whites.

The Nature and Causes of Mental Retardation

Being of limited intelligence does not by itself keep individuals with mental retardation from functioning effectively in the world. Most of these individuals have other problems, in addition to low IQs. Mental retardation caused by prenatal factors, chromosomal abnormalities, and genetic defects typically involves multiple physical problems that affect vision, speech, and locomotion (Koranyi, 1986) as well as intelligence. People who are retarded may also be burdened by a variety of neuropsychological deficits that prevent them from reading, writing, speaking, or perceiving (McCaffrey & Isaac, 1985). Generally, individuals with these deficits fall into the severe and profound categories of mental retardation.

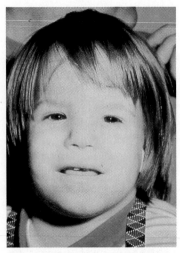

This severely retarded boy's mother drank heavily during her pregnancy. His facial features as well as his retardation are common components of fetal alcohol syndrome.

rubella German measles; major prenatal infectious condition responsible for mental retardation.

Prenatal Factors   Prenatal factors are important causes of mental retardation. A variety of chronic maternal illnesses—including uncontrolled diabetes and high blood pressure—can affect development of the fetus's central nervous system. Chronic alcohol or drug abuse during pregnancy can cause the fetal damage and retardation labeled *fetal alcohol syndrome (FAS)*. Retardation can also be caused by medications taken during pregnancy to induce immunity to disease (for example, antitetanus serum and typhoid vaccine) and by incompatibility between the mother's and child's blood. Likewise, retardation can result from maternal disorders that lead to premature birth and birth injuries, including oxygen deprivation during the birth process.

Infections that occur during pregnancy, especially viral infections, can also seriously damage the developing fetus. The extent of damage depends on the kind of viral infection, its severity, and the age of the developing fetus. (The age of the fetus is significant because it determines which bodily system is developing most rapidly at the time of the infection.) The two maternal infections most likely to lead to mental retardation are rubella (German measles) and syphilis.

Rubella is the major prenatal infection responsible for mental retardation. It also causes serious physical disorders in the developing child, such as heart disease, deafness, and cranial and visual problems. Some 10 to 25 percent of infants born to mothers infected with rubella during the first 3 months of their pregnancies will develop one or more of these serious problems. When the infection occurs during the first month of pregnancy, the risk of serious damage rises to close to 50 percent.

Syphilis is no longer a major cause of mental retardation in the United States because it's now usually detected and treated before it causes fetal damage. However, the bacterium that causes syphilis (Treponema pallidum) has become increasingly resistant to antibiotic treatment. As a result, clinicians have become more concerned that the disease will remain untreated in some pregnant women and cause mental retardation.

Chromosomal Mutations   Chromosomal mutations in the sperm or ova that occur prior to conception produce abnormalities in the genes responsible for the body's form and function. Most often induced by X-rays, these abnormalities are also

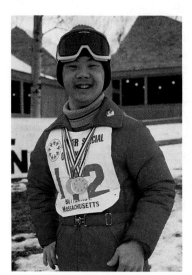

This young skier, with the facial features and stature of Down syndrome, takes understandable pride in the skiing medals he has won.

significantly more common among older mothers and fathers, especially those over 40. Most chromosomal abnormalities that cause mental retardation are located on the autosomal chromosomes, although a few are located on the sex chromosomes.

Down syndrome is due to chromosomal abnormalities. It's one of the most studied forms of mental retardation and was first described almost 125 years ago by English physician J. Langdon Down. Children with this type of retardation have a distinct appearance. They have small, rounded skulls with flattened, moon-shaped faces; the openings for their eyes are narrow and have a downward and inward slope; their noses are short and their tongues are often large and may protrude from their mouths; their cheeks are rosy; and their hair may be coarse, wiry, and sparse. These children are also typically small for their age. This common form of retardation was previously termed *Mongolism* due to the individuals' rather Oriental appearance; that term is no longer used, though, because of its negative racial and ethnic connotations.

The principal causes of Down syndrome are age-related or radiation-induced chromosomal abnormalities. There are probably other causes, as well. Compared to younger mothers, one who's over the age of 32 has at least a seven times greater risk of having a child with Down syndrome (Andreasen & Black, 1995).

Part of the problem of tracing a precise etiology for this disorder derives from the fact that three different chromosomal abnormalities are responsible for it. The most common is **trisomy 21.** Individuals with this abnormality have 3 rather than 2 chromosome number 21s; consequently, they have 47 rather than the usual 46 chromosomes.

The incidence of Down syndrome is estimated at about 1 in every 700 live births. Despite the disorder's severity, only about 10 percent of persons with it live in institutions for people who are mentally retarded (Munro, 1986). Most of the remaining individuals—largely, children and adolescents—remain at home with their parents, as did David Santos, whose story was told at the beginning of this chapter.

Most individuals with Down syndrome fall into the moderate and severe categories of mental retardation; fewer than half have IQs over 50 (American Psychiatric Association, 1994). As children, most are cooperative, friendly, happy, and easy to manage. This explains why they usually live at home with their families and why many are *mainstreamed*, participating with other children in regular public school classrooms. (We'll return to the subjects of education and mainstreaming later in this chapter.)

As children with Down syndrome grow into adolescence, however, emotional and behavioral disorders are more likely to develop (Matson & Sevin, 1994a). The adolescent may perceive more clearly than she did when younger what a profound impact the condition has on her prospects for a normal, independent, happy life. Her increased size and strength—as well as her growing sexual feelings—also contribute to the greater likelihood of antisocial behavior, drug abuse, and sexual promiscuity during this time. Due to these problems, institutionalization becomes an increasingly common option for some individuals by young adulthood.

Maria and Mateo Santos had some of these problems with David. Shortly after his sixteenth birthday, he and his father had a physical confrontation that frightened Maria and Mateo a great deal. The trouble started because David wanted to stay out past his curfew, which was 11 P.M. on weekends. One thing led to another, and eventually David—who was as tall as his father but much heavier—tried to wrestle his father to the ground. Then one Friday night a few weeks later, David came home with alcohol on his breath and proceeded to verbally abuse his mother, saying that she was "so old-fashioned" because she objected to his drinking. The final straw came when David "borrowed" the family car to take his friends to a picnic. Since he hadn't yet learned to drive, the result was predictable: He drove the car into a ditch three blocks from home. No one was hurt, luckily.

Given all this, Maria and Mateo were understandably worried about being able to control David and keep him from harming himself or others. They decided

Down syndrome Common form of mental retardation that's caused by a chromosomal mutation; generally involves moderate and severe categories of retardation.

trisomy 21 Common cause of Down syndrome; individuals have 3 rather than 2 chromosome 21s and thus 47 rather than the usual 46 chromosomes.

to place him in a private school for retarded adolescents in a neighboring state and made arrangements to do so. Fortunately, they could afford the very high fees the school charged. Even though David was initially very angry at being "sent away," within a month, he told his parents that he liked the school very much. He was with young men and women his own age, the schoolwork was made more interesting than it had been in public school, social events were frequently scheduled, and he had the run of the school's grounds, so long as he followed the rules.

Genetic Defects Genetically transmitted conditions account for about 5 percent of all instances of mental retardation (American Psychiatric Association, 1994). **Alkaptonuria**—a disorder of amino acid formation—was the first genetically transmitted source of mental retardation to be identified; it was reported in 1908. Since then, many additional inherited disorders have been described. All are caused by genetically transmitted metabolic errors that result in the accumulation of chemical substances in the brain that prevent its normal functioning.

The most intensively studied inborn error of metabolism is **phenylketonuria (PKU)**, which was discovered in 1934. It's also a disorder of amino acid metabolism. Following its thorough investigation, PKU has become a model for the investigation of other hereditary biochemical disorders.

PKU is transmitted as a simple recessive autosomal trait—in other words, it's only expressed when both parents carry the recessive gene for the disorder. The basic metabolic error deprives the body of the ability to convert phenylalanine (an essential and plentiful amino acid) into another very common substance, tyrosine, because of the inactivity or absence of the liver enzyme responsible for this conversion. As a result, phenylalanine levels rise to between 10 and 25 times their normal amounts in the blood, resulting in a great decrease in levels of the essential brain neurotransmitters serotonin, epinephrine, and norepinephrine. Untreated, PKU emerges between 6 and 12 months after birth, when the child may begin vomiting for unexplained reasons. At about the same time, the infant's urine begins to have an unusual odor, a skin rash or eczema may appear, and unexplained seizures may be experienced (Andreasen & Black, 1995).

PKU ranges in prevalence from between 1 in 10,000 to 1 in 20,000 persons in the United States. Most individuals with this disorder are small in stature, with especially small heads. They tend to be hyperactive and to display temper tantrums and bizarre movements of the body and upper extremities. It's unusual for children with PKU to develop either verbal or nonverbal communication. Most of these individuals ultimately become severely or profoundly retarded. Seizures are a particular hazard (Andreasen & Black, 1995).

An effective screening test designed to detect phenylalanine in the blood is now routinely administered to newborn infants in hospitals in the United States. This has led to early identification of most potential cases of PKU. When placed on a low phenylalanine diet early in life—before blood levels of the substance can rise to abnormal levels—individuals at risk for developing PKU can avoid most or all of the intellectual, behavioral, and physical problems experienced by those whose condition goes untreated. However, since phenylalanine is also an essential amino acid, its total absence from the diet deprives the person of proteins necessary for normal muscle growth and development. That's why a diet containing normal amounts of phenylalanine is reinstituted at around the age of 6, once brain development is complete.

Postnatal Factors Accidents are the leading cause of death and severe disabling injury in the United States; they are also a prime cause of retardation. Head injuries from automobile accidents, falls, and other serious injuries can cause brain damage severe enough to induce seizures and cause mental retardation. Near drowning, accompanied by a prolonged cutoff of the brain's oxygen supply, can

alkaptonuria Disorder of amino acid formation; first genetically transmitted cause of mental retardation to be identified.

phenylketonuria (PKU) Condition that's the result of a disorder of amino acid metabolism; most intensively studied inborn error of metabolism.

Thinking about SOCIAL ISSUES

Does Poverty Lead to Mental Retardation— or the Other Way Around?

Several factors associated with poverty have been implicated in the development of mental retardation. Even though poor people are not alone in suffering from the environmental factors associated with mental retardation, they are clearly at greatest risk because of them. Medical problems that rarely affect middle-class Americans afflict those who are poor, largely because many do not have access to quality medical care.

For instance, pregnant women who are poor are more likely to be malnourished and have little or no prenatal care than women of higher socioeconomic levels. It follows that there's a greater likelihood that these women's unborn children will suffer the consequences of untreated medical problems, including maternal infections, anemia, and birth difficulties—all of which can cause mental retardation. Not surprisingly, mortality and prematurity are highest among infants born to poor women (Borthwick-Duffy, 1994).

Babies born to poor mothers are also less likely to have routine checkups or immunizations. In addition, they are more likely to be treated later, rather than earlier, for serious illnesses. A variety of childhood disorders can cause mental retardation if they are not diagnosed and treated early. Moreover, the infant's nutritional status is probably marginal; severe protein deficiency, caused by dietary deficiencies related to the absence of high-quality food, can cause mental retardation, as well.

As these infants grow, their heightened risk of mental retardation from environmental factors also grows. A common cause of retardation during childhood is lead poisoning. This occurs when children eat paint chips (which taste sweet) from the peeling walls of old tenements that are covered with lead-based paint. Another factor is brain damage from injuries sustained in accidents of various kinds.

Beyond the direct effects that biological and environmental factors have on the central nervous system, poor children in the United States also experience emotional and social problems that affect their ability to learn. Being raised in a family without a father by an undereducated, underemployed, highly stressed mother or by a succession of other caretakers is apt to provide a chaotic learning environment. School attendance is likely to be irregular and parental ability to help in the learning process impaired (Braddock & Fujiura, 1991).

Being poor exposes infants and children to many of the environmental factors that cause mental retardation. Is it any wonder that a substantially higher percentage of the poor in the United States are considered mentally retarded?

Think about the following questions:

1. Much of the material reviewed above links poverty to increased risk for mental retardation. But the relationship might work the other way around in some cases. How might being mentally retarded increase the likelihood of being poor?

2. What do you think would cost society more: comprehensive programs to prevent poor children from developing environmentally caused mental retardation or institutional programs and sheltered environments for children and adults who developed mental retardation from environmental factors? Explain your choice.

---

also lead to the death of enough brain cells to cause retardation, as can lead poisoning, discussed later.

Two serious childhood diseases can also cause brain damage and mental retardation. **Meningitis** is an infection of the membrane covering the brain, and **encephalitis** is an infection of the brain itself. Symptoms of these diseases include a sudden, extreme rise in temperature; vomiting; disorientation; and complaints of a stiff neck. Without early treatment, delirium may develop and acute dementia may follow; permanent effects include mental retardation.

Environmental Factors   Although 1 percent of the U.S. population is mentally retarded, between 10 and 30 percent of this country's poorest citizens meet the criteria for at least mild mental retardation (Braddock & Fujiura, 1991). This finding raises some interesting questions: Are these people poor because they are retarded, or are they retarded because of factors associated with their poverty? These crucial, largely unanswered questions are explored in Thinking about Social Issues.

Mentally retarded children are more likely to be born to mentally retarded parents (Feldman, 1986). **Familial mental retardation** probably accounts for the

meningitis Infection of the membrane covering the brain; untreated, it can cause brain damage and mental retardation.

encephalitis Infection of the brain that, untreated, can cause brain damage and mental retardation.

familial mental retardation Results from having parents who are mentally retarded.

largest single group of mentally retarded people in the United States. These individuals are generally mildly retarded, without demonstrable central nervous system damage. They are simply less able than the rest of us to learn, remember, reason, and function in school and other learning situations. Although they are marginally able to function in the world, they pass on their own borderline intellectual capabilities to their children.

Familial mental retardation is also associated with many other socially unwelcome behaviors: alcohol and drug abuse and dependence, juvenile and adult crime, promiscuity and teenage pregnancy, and early school dropout. Actually, these behaviors are not hard to understand. How would you feel if you were doing badly in school, worried about ever getting a good job, and believed that your peers looked down on you because you were slow? You might well decide to express your frustrations by acting out against society in antisocial ways.

Mental Retardation and Mental Illness

Mental disorder is substantially more prevalent among people with mental retardation (Borthwick-Duffy, 1994). Several reasons explain this co-occurrence. People with mental retardation are more likely to come to the attention of mental health professionals, who might then diagnose mental disorder in addition to mental retardation. Some of the symptoms of mental retardation—especially deficits in adaptive functioning—are also symptoms of mental disorder. And the behavioral and social limitations mental retardation imposes can induce psychopathology (Nezu, Nezu, & Gill-Weiss, 1992).

Yet despite this well-recognized relationship between mental retardation and mental illness, opportunities for outpatient therapy for community-dwelling persons with mental retardation have not been developed in sufficient numbers. Similarly, most therapists have not been trained to understand and treat mental retardation and mental disorder when they co-occur in the same person (Nezu & Nezu, 1994).

Prevention of Mental Retardation and Care for People Who Are Mentally Retarded

No treatments currently available will restore a person with mental retardation to normal intellectual functioning. For that reason, efforts to prevent mental retardation have received a great deal of attention.

Prevention One of the most important first steps in preventing mental retardation is educating people about its nature and causes. For instance, if and when you decide to have children, you should be aware of available genetic counseling services. It's especially important for you to seek genetic counseling before starting a family if your own family has a history of genetically based disease, including disorders associated with mental retardation. And once a child is on the way, what you read here should help you understand why your physician may suggest amniocentesis or other genetic tests. Perhaps reading this chapter will also encourage you to appreciate the importance of good nutrition and good health practices during pregnancy. Finally, what you read here might motivate you to work in your own community—to reduce or eliminate some of the environmental factors causing mental retardation and to increase treatment and support services for persons in the community who have mental retardation.

Concerted efforts to prevent retardation by addressing the factors associated with it are under way in many communities. The most successful approach is early intervention—that is, identifying and modifying or eliminating biological and environmental factors that could cause irreversible brain damage in a child before they actually do so. Discovery of the brain mechanisms responsible for phenylke-

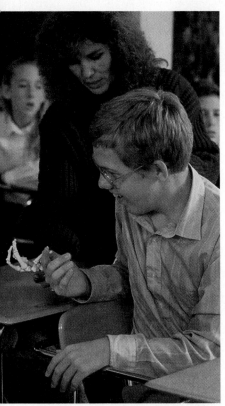

This adolescent with retardation lives at home and goes to his neighborhood junior high school with the friends he grew up with.

tonuria, for example, led to the development of a low phenylalanine diet, discussed earlier. Similarly, recognizing the toxic effects of lead-based paint has led to legislation that requires the elimination of lead from newly manufactured paint. As a result, young children will no longer be at risk of lead poisoning (which causes retardation), should they consume chips of paint.

Care at Home and in Public Schools   Many of us assume that most individuals who are mentally retarded live in institutions and that few live in the community or at home and attend public schools. In fact, though, that's not the case. Approximately 900,000 retarded children attend public school in the United States, compared with only 110,000 children and adults who reside in institutions for people who are mentally retarded (Pfeiffer, 1992). As we've learned in this chapter, the vast majority of people who are retarded are only mildly so, which means that they don't require institutional care. Only persons with severe or profound retardation (and those with marked behavioral problems) cannot live in the community and be integrated into public schools.

Of course, not every child with mental retardation—even mild retardation—can be placed in a regular classroom and be expected to do well, given a little extra attention. For that reason, a variety of means have been developed to keep as many retarded children as possible in society, at home, and in the public schools, including special education teachers, special classes for the educable mentally retarded, programs that make learning easier, associated programs to deal with the emotional problems that frequently accompany retardation, and parent-training programs with much the same purpose (Braddock & Fujiura, 1991).

Most experts agree that the emotional and intellectual development of a child with mental retardation progresses better at home than in an institution. Of course, if the home environment is not appropriate or if the child is physically assaultive or delinquent, residential care may still be the only alternative. In such instances, though, it's the child's antisocial behavior, not his intellectual deficit, that prompts institutionalization. As you may recall, behavioral problems were what ultimately led David Santos's parents to place him in a school for children with retardation.

Psychotherapy is sometimes provided to retarded children to help them deal with the emotional consequences of their condition. Even so, most care and treatment of children with retardation—including those who also suffer from mental illness—is focused and behavioral (Petronko, Harris, & Kormann, 1994; Spreat & Behar, 1994). In line with recent trends in behavior therapy, cognitive-behavioral therapy (CBT) methods have been developed to help individuals with mild and moderate mental retardation who are living in the community achieve the following goals:

- Identify negative self-statements about their intellectual, social, and vocational abilities.
- Adopt more constructive and positive self-statements.
- Incorporate more adaptive interpersonal and cognitive behavior into their behavioral repertoires.

Research into the use of cognitive treatment with these goals has been promising. One study, for example, found that this approach led to improved on-the-job problem solving by two severely retarded adults employed by a janitorial supply company (Hughes & Rusch, 1990). And another study determined that more adequate social and interpersonal behavior developed in three mentally retarded students working in nonsheltered work settings (Park & Gaylord-Ross, 1989).

In recent decades, the U.S. Supreme Court (the principal means by which many of society's most oppressed seek equity) has shown interest in expanding the integration of people who are mentally retarded into society. The 1985 Cleburne decision, for instance, expanded the rights of the mentally retarded. In that case,

PERSPECTIVE ON MENTAL RETARDATION

BIOLOGICAL FACTORS

Biological factors play a key role in many forms of
mental retardation:

➤ In the majority of cases, mental retardation is genetically transmitted.
➤ A variety of structural changes to the brain, responsible for many of the more severe forms of mental retardation, have been identified, including changes caused by
disease, injury, and prenatal factors.

PSYCHOLOGICAL FACTORS

Psychological factors interact with biological
vulnerabilities to influence the development of
accompanying disorders; these factors also
affect response to treatment:

➤ Depression frequently accompanies mental
retardation.
➤ Other psychological and psychiatric conditions
also commonly accompany mental retardation, in
part as the individual's reaction upon realizing
her limitations.

SOCIAL FACTORS

Both biological and psychological factors operate in
certain social contexts:

➤ Environmental factors, many of them associated with
poverty, play important etiologic roles in mental retardation. Limited access to pre- and postnatal health care,
impaired nutrition during pregnancy, exposure to lead
paint, and the increased risks of physical injury and disease during the early years of life are preventable environmental factors that cause mental retardation.
➤ Environmental support from caregivers and supportive communities can facilitate the successful placement
of people who are mentally retarded in group homes
and apartments in the community.

*These biological, psychological, and
social factors interact to cause problems, as illustrated in the following case:*

Shortly after Marcie was born, it
became clear that she had mental retardation. When she started school, Marcie
was placed in a special education class,
along with other children with special
needs. Unlike many of them, Marcie
clearly enjoyed school; she liked being
called on by the teacher and gradually
began to develop relationships with
some of her fellow students. One reason
for her liking school was the quality of
her life at home: Her parents had encouraged Marcie from infancy in much of
what she had done.

Marcie's biologically determined
intellectual deficits set clear limits on her
ultimate achievements. However, her
social skills and psychological strengths
—products of an unusually supportive
family situation—gave her both the
skills and the motivation to extend herself in ways other retarded children
could not.

Justice Thurgood Marshall acknowledged that people who are mentally retarded have historically been subjected to

> a regime of state-mandated segregation and degradation . . . that in its virulence and bigotry rivaled, and indeed paralleled, the worst excesses of Jim Crow. . . . Prejudice, once let loose, is not easily cabined. As of 1979, most States still categorically disqualified "idiots" from voting, without regard to individual capacity and with discretion to exclude left in the hands of low-level election officials. (*City of Cleburne* v. *Cleburne Living Center,* 1985, pp. 462, 464)

Legislation over the past 20 years or so has also addressed the needs of individuals with mental retardation. In 1975, the U.S. Congress passed Public Law (PL) 94-142, the Education for All Handicapped Children Act. It addressed the needs of retarded children as well as those with other disabilities. States that complied with PL 94-142 received increased federal assistance for education. The key provisions of this law granted all children with disabilities between the ages of 3 and 21 rights to the following:

- a free and appropriate educational opportunity
- an individual educational program, reevaluated annually
- education in the least restrictive environment
- due process (if efforts are made to institutionalize them against their wills)

In light of these provisions, PL 94-142 has been called the "mainstreaming law." As you may know, *mainstreaming* is an arrangement in which mildly retarded children participate in regular classrooms with children who are not retarded, bringing educational and social benefits. Happily, most children who are retarded are now mainstreamed in U.S. public schools.

PL 99-457 was enacted in 1986 for the purpose of reauthorizing PL 94-142 and extending its provisions to children younger than school age (that is, 3 to 5 years old). The law provided that services for preschoolers could be offered through private or public agencies, but quality and integration had to be demonstrated. PL 99-457 also emphasized the role of parents and recognized the importance of the family in child development. Finally, this law eliminated the use of labels that categorize people who are retarded, pointing to their stigmatizing effect (Brewer, 1995).

PL 94-142 was updated in 1990 and renamed the Individuals with Disabilities Education Act (IDEA). IDEA expanded what types of children are eligible for special education services, including those with autism (discussed later in this chapter) and traumatic brain injury. The law still requires parental involvement in educational decisions, individualized education programs, and education in the least restrictive environment (Hardman, Drew, Egan, & Wolf, 1993).

In order to help more retarded individuals remain at home and attend public schools, researchers and clinicians have worked hard to develop ways to train those with mild and moderate retardation. One of their most common goals has been to mainstream retarded individuals. Knapczyk (1989) described a project that tested a program designed to help three mildly retarded fourth-graders participate in a regular mathematics class. The three youngsters were shown videotapes of normal children asking questions in the regular mathematics class. They also rehearsed asking questions and received feedback and verbal reinforcement for doing so.

Care in Institutions   Despite their parents' best intentions, most children who are severely or profoundly retarded cannot be cared for at home. Instead, their physical and behavioral disabilities require that they be placed in institutions for the retarded. Most of these institutions are publicly supported. The few private facilities available for people who are retarded are so expensive that, despite the superior care they can provide, they serve only a small number of persons.

In recent years, many public facilities for mentally retarded individuals (like those for mental patients) have made court-ordered improvements in living conditions, staffing, and programs. As a result, these institutions now represent a more adequate alternative to home and community care than was the case even as recently as a decade ago (Spreat & Behar, 1994). Despite these changes, though, many state institutions for the retarded are still overcrowded and underfunded. Too often, the result is a custodial institution that lacks the financial or human resources to make its residents' lives more humane or hopeful.

A notable recent improvement in institutional care for people who are retarded has been a significant decrease in the routine use of major tranquilizers to sedate severely retarded residents (Aman & Singh, 1991). Although the reason usually given for the use of these medications is to protect individuals from harming themselves, they are sometimes used for the convenience of caretakers and, in such cases, can cause residents more harm than good (Aman & Singh, 1991).

Another recent positive change has been the marked increase in availability of transitional and community-based programs for persons with mental retardation. These small, homelike residences house anywhere from 3 or 4 up to 12 mildly and moderately retarded persons who do not need constant supervision and can work in sheltered work settings. Staff in these settings encourage residents to acquire independent living skills, enabling them to enjoy lives that are as independent as possible. Of course, some adults who are mildly retarded live independently in their own homes or apartments, seeing counselors only occasionally.

A recent front-page newspaper story revisited the Southbury Training School in Connecticut. Built more than 50 years ago, Southbury quickly became a model institution for retarded persons who couldn't be cared for at home; today, though, it has become the object of controversy. Thinking about Controversial Issues considers whether Southbury continues to provide a safe residence for individuals who are severely and profoundly retarded or whether smaller, more homelike facilities, located in these individuals' home communities, would serve them better.

Behavioral Treatment of Self-Injury   One of the most serious problems of caring for people who are severely retarded is self-injury. Typical behaviors include repeatedly banging their heads with their hands, slapping their faces, and picking at their skin. Also common are pulling at their ears (sometimes to the point of pulling them off) and poking at their eyes, even blinding themselves. Many individuals run the risk of causing permanent injuries to themselves (Iwata, Zarcone, Vollmer, & Smith, 1994).

Several behavioral treatments have been developed to control self-injurious behavior (Iwata, Zarcone, Vollmer, & Smith, 1994), including:

- withholding social interaction with important persons in the retarded individual's environment as a punishment
- providing the individual with an enriched environment, which distracts him from the temptation to self-injure
- eliminating the sensory feedback for self-injury by making the individual wear heavy clothing, which masks the sensory consequences of self-injury and reduces its reinforcement value
- punishing attempts at self-injury
- communication training

The last approach is based on the assumption that self-injury is communication. This is a cognitive-behavioral treatment that tries to teach the retarded person more effective means to communicate his needs and desires. Although each method for reducing self-injury has its supporters and has proven helpful for some individuals, none has been universally successful in preventing the extremely serious problems associated with self-injury by persons who are severely retarded (Repp & Singh, 1990).

Thinking about CONTROVERSIAL ISSUES   A Safe Haven for the Profoundly Retarded?

The late–twentieth century movement to deinstitutionalize as many people with mental retardation and psychiatric impairment as possible has restored many of these individuals to productive lives outside the institutions they formerly lived in. Today, a new group of persons are threatened with deinstitutionalization, and advocates for them—including their families—are up in arms. They are people who are severely and profoundly retarded, and they have, for the most part, remained in institutions like the Southbury Training School because community-based facilities capable of caring for them have not been available. But now, state financial pressures on the institutions, as well as critics of the care they provide, have led some states to consider alternatives to the institutions:

> More than three decades ago, following the advice of doctors, Edward D. Walen moved to Connecticut so he could place his son in what was regarded as one of the finest institutions for the mentally retarded in the world, the Southbury Training School.
>
> Today, Mr. Walen's son, Jimmy, 43, has the IQ of a 3-year-old, and a physical impairment that precludes him from making noises other than grunts, yelps, and a siren-like squeal. Every morning, he fastidiously sets tables and cleans dishes at the campus cafeteria. At night, he sleeps in a crowded room with eight other men. . . .
>
> "This, in effect, is Jimmy's home," Mr. Walen says of the 1,600-acre campus in western Connecticut. "These advocates are mesmerized by the mystique that all institutions are bad, that the buildings should be razed, the earth bulldozed over and then salt poured on the grounds so it will never rise again."
>
> Increasingly across the country, such parents are finding themselves locked in difficult battle with other advocates for the retarded and civil rights groups. Those advocates are pushing to close Southbury, the state's last large institution for the retarded, and move its 867 residents into group homes. In the last 25 years, as state facility after facility has been closed, the institutionalized population has decreased by 60 percent nationally. (Rabinovitz, 1995, pp. A1, A11)

Those who want to close Southbury and institutions like it claim that many of the patients remaining in these facilities would be able to live more interesting, independent, and productive lives in group homes, where they could also work in sheltered environments. But the parents of Southbury residents have a different view:

> Sarah E. Bondy, president of the Southbury parents' group, the Home and School Association, said: "One of the things that really upsets us is when people talk about our guys going out into the world and holding jobs and going to church and making friends. Then you go into cottage 7A and you'll see people 35 and 40 who are curled up on a mat, and someone is taking a feather, and running it across their cheek just to get the kind of reaction you would want from a 3-month-old child. . . . And they're telling us they can go out? I mean, it's crazy." (Rabinovitz, 1995, p. A11)

Think about the following questions:

1. Based on what you've read in this book, what are the most compelling arguments for and against deinstitutionalization?

2. In your judgment, whose responsibility is it to care for people who are severely retarded: their parents? the state they live in? the federal government? or some combination of these agencies? Explain your answer.

The use of punishment is particularly controversial. Supporters claim that it's sometimes the only way to bring self-injurious behavior under control; opponents, on the other hand, believe it's humiliating, ineffective in the long run, and unnecessary (Matson & Sevin, 1994b).

Behavior Modification in Institutions   Token economies and other behavior modification programs have also been used to manage the behavior of institutionalized persons with severe mental retardation, just as they have been used to manage the behavior of institutionalized psychotic patients. These approaches involve systematic reinforcement of desired patient behaviors—for instance, making their bed or brushing their teeth—through the use of staff attention or tangible reinforcers like candy and food. Unwanted behaviors—such as fighting, poor personal hygiene, or failure to do assigned chores—are either ignored or punished.

A recent application of behavior modification in institutions involved the use of nondisabled peers (essentially, age-mates) who are trained systematically to reinforce appropriate behavior and ignore or punish inappropriate behavior by persons with severe mental retardation. The retarded persons are far more responsive to the nondisabled peers than to ward staff, so their behavior comes under effective control more quickly and tends to stay that way (Pfeiffer, 1992). Although still in an exploratory stage, this approach to behavior modification in institutions for people who are severely retarded clearly holds promise.

Focus on
Critical Thinking

1. Why does the diagnosis of mental retardation require that three diagnostic criteria be met—namely, an IQ of 70 or less, impaired adaptive functioning, and an age of 18 or lower?
2. Consider the four categories of people who are mentally retarded: mild, moderate, severe, and profound (based on IQ level). What role does this categorization play in planning for treatment and making other decisions on behalf of persons with retardation?

Autistic Disorder

The Nature of Autistic Disorder

Autistic disorder, formerly called **infantile autism,** is a profound puzzle, especially to the parents of autistic children and the professionals called on to diagnose and treat them. Consider the following case of Noah, a child with autism:

> While a father pushes his four-year-old son in a cart down the aisle in a supermarket, a friendly woman stops, bends over toward the son, smiles at him and says, "You're beautiful."
>
> "Thank you," says the father. "What's your name?" she asks the boy. He turns his head away making some unintelligible sounds. "What's your name?" she asks again. The boy begins to rock back and forth in the shopping cart. "Don't be shy," the woman continues. "Can't you tell me your name?" "No," says the father, "he can't." . . .
>
> At the age of four [Noah] is neither toilet-trained nor does he feed himself. He seldom speaks expressively, rarely employs his less than dozen word vocabulary. His attention span in a new toy is a matter of split seconds, . . . and he is never interested in other children for very long. His main activities are lint catching, . . . spontaneous giggling, inexplicable crying, . . . jumping, rocking, . . . and incoherent babbling addressed to his finger flexing right hand.
>
> What's the matter with Noah? . . . We'd been told he was mentally retarded, emotionally disturbed, autistic, schizophrenic, possibly brain damaged, or that he was suffering from . . . combinations of these conditions. But we finally discovered that the diagnosis didn't seem to matter. It was all so sadly academic. The medical profession was merely playing . . . games at our expense. For though we live in one of the richest states in the nation, there was no single viable treatment immediately available for Noah, no matter what category he could be assigned to. (Greenfield, 1972, pp. 3–5)

autistic disorder Disorder in the group of pervasive developmental disorders; characterized by marked impairment in social responsiveness, profound communication deficits, and stereotyped or bizarre habits and movements.

infantile autism Term previously used for what is now called autistic disorder.

Noah's parents persisted in their search for treatments and educational teaching methods to help their son. Although they live in New York City, they chose to spend an entire winter at an autism center for behavioral treatment directed by Dr. Ivar Lovaas at the University of California at Los Angeles. At another time, they tried placing Noah on large doses of megavitamins for an extended period of time.

In this section on autistic disorder, we'll cover a number of Noah's behavioral progressions and regressions. Doing so may give you a sense of the overwhelming

Diagnostic Criteria for 299.00 AUTISTIC DISORDER

A. A total of six (or more) items from (1), (2), and (3), with at least two from (1), and one each from (2) and (3).

(1) qualitative impairment in social interaction, as manifested by at least two of the following:

    (a) marked impairment in the use of multiple nonverbal behaviors such as eye-to-eye gaze, facial expression, body postures, and gestures to regulate social interaction

    (b) failure to develop peer relationships appropriate to developmental level

    (c) a lack of spontaneous seeking to share enjoyment, interests, or achievements with other people (e.g., by a lack of showing, bringing, or pointing out objects of interest)

    (d) lack of social or emotional reciprocity

(2) qualitative impairments in communication as manifested by at least one of the following:

    (a) delay in, or total lack of, the development of spoken language (not accompanied by an attempt to compensate through alternative modes of communication such as gesture or mime)

    (b) in individuals with adequate speech, marked impairment in the ability to initiate or sustain a conversation with others

    (c) stereotyped and repetitive use of language or idiosyncratic language

    (d) lack of varied, spontaneous make-believe play or social imitative play appropriate to developmental level

(3) restricted repetitive and stereotyped patterns of behavior, interests, and activities, as manifested by at least one of the following:

    (a) encompassing preoccupation with one or more stereotyped and restricted patterns of interest that is abnormal either in intensity or focus

    (b) apparently inflexible adherence to specific, nonfunctional routines or rituals

    (c) stereotyped and repetitive motor mannerisms (e.g., hand or finger flapping or twisting, or complex whole-body movements)

    (d) persistent preoccupation with parts of objects

B. Delays or abnormal functioning in at least one of the following areas, with onset prior to age 3 years: (1) social interaction, (2) language as used in social communication, or (3) symbolic or imaginative play.

C. The disturbance is not better accounted for by Rett's Disorder or Childhood Disintegrative Disorder.

burdens and frustrations experienced by the parents of autistic children. On the one hand, these parents must constantly scan the environment for potential dangers to their defenseless children; on the other, these parents must be alert to opportunities to teach their children the rudimentary skills they need to survive.

You may also come to understand why dramatic success stories about autistic children are rare. Most parents lack the psychological and financial resources to be able to persist in seeking the expert professional help that Noah's parents finally obtained. At the same time, though, Noah's behavior was quite typical of autistic children, as was his parents' quandary at what to do for him. He could speak only a few words, had to be watched every waking hour, and only rarely acknowledged the presence of his caring parents.

The symptoms of autistic disorder appear before the typical child is 30 months old. One of the most crippling childhood problems, it belongs to a group of rare, serious conditions termed the *pervasive developmental disorders* (American Psychiatric Association, 1994). As the diagnostic criteria for autistic disorder presented in the *DSM* table suggest, children with this condition have severely impaired social and communication skills and stereotyped and repetitive habits and movements.

Understandably, the lack of social responsiveness of autistic children is extremely troubling to their parents. When their parents try to hug them, these children may shrug them off and withdraw. Likewise, when parents try to hold their autistic children, the gesture is rarely returned. Children with autism often seem totally uninterested in people, including their parents and their siblings.

Approximately half of autistic individuals remain mute or speechless all their lives (Smith & Bryson, 1994), making it that much more difficult to relate to them. If they speak at all, they may parrot others' speech. When asked "What's your name?" instead of answering, they may parrot back "What's your name?" This mimicry so resembles in tone and pitch what was originally said to the individual that it's termed *echolalia*. Another distinguishing feature of the speech of individuals with autism is how frequently they use personal pronouns improperly. For example, instead of saying "I rode in the car," the autistic person might say "Him rode in the car." This response further suggests the profound difficulty that the autistic individual has in understanding what it means to be a person.

By the time the autistic child is 3 to 4 years old, it's impossible for her parents to conclude that development has been normal. At this point, the parents will admit that there's a problem yet want to believe that an emotional disturbance has made it difficult for their child to learn to speak and interact socially. They rationalize that if something is wrong emotionally, then it might be possible to enroll the child in some form of intensive therapy that will lead to progress. It's not surprising that parents can cope more easily with the idea that their child has an emotional problem than one that's a genetic defect or a form of mental retardation.

The Course of Autistic Disorder

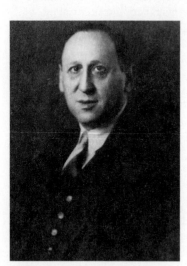

LEO KANNER *was the first to describe what he called* infantile autism *in 1943, explaining that it was caused by emotionally distant parents. Today, we know that autistic disorder results from faulty neurotransmission. How could Kanner have been so wrong in his efforts to explain this condition?*

Leo Kanner, a child psychiatrist at Johns Hopkins University, first described what he called *early infantile autism* in 1943. He distinguished children with this condition on the basis of their inability to relate normally to people, language abnormalities, good cognitive potential based on excellent rote memory (later refuted), repetitive and stereotyped play, and a desire for sameness in the environment (Kanner, 1943).

Autistic disorder occurs in only 2 to 5 children out of 10,000 (American Psychiatric Association, 1994). Because of its rarity and relatively recent discovery, few adults older than 50 were diagnosed with the disorder in infancy. For the same reason, most children diagnosed with this disorder from the 1940s through the 1970s failed to receive the highly specialized educational and psychological programs that are currently available for autistic children. Thus, our knowledge about what happens to autistic children when they age is based on their participation in a variety of unspecialized educational programs—an admittedly inadequate therapeutic setting.

In one sample of autistic individuals, considered by DeMyer and colleagues (1973), 42 percent reported having been institutionalized during childhood or adulthood. A majority were judged to be educationally impaired, 10 to 15 percent were deemed of borderline intelligence, and 1 to 2 percent eventually recovered sufficiently so as to be judged normal. Similar follow-up studies of autistic children have been done more recently in Canada (Wolf & Goldberg, 1986). In one sample, about half the children studied were eventually placed in institutions. Few were ever able to live independently and hold jobs, and most adults diagnosed autistic during childhood functioned in the mentally retarded range of intelligence.

Although general intelligence is a predictor, verbal skill is the best childhood predictor of later functioning for children with autism. Without language skills, many other skills simply cannot be readily acquired. Higher-functioning autistic children—that is, those with more adequate verbal skills—also show fewer of the typical social and behavioral symptoms of autism (Yirmiya & Sigman, 1991). They may even be able to live at home or in a group setting, to complete high school or college, and to maintain some kind of employment (Venter, Lord, & Schopler, 1992).

The original cases of children with autism that Kanner described in 1943 were followed into adulthood by Kanner himself (1971). He reported that those individuals who lived in environments where their condition was well tolerated appeared to fare better than those in less tolerant environments. For example, consider Donald, as described by Kanner:

> In 1942, his parents placed him on a tenant farm about 10 miles from their home. When I visited there in May 1945, I was amazed at the wisdom of the couple who took care of him. They managed to give him goals for his stereotypes. They made him use his preoccupations with measurements by having him dig a well and

report on its depth. When he kept collecting dead birds and bugs, they gave him a spot for a "graveyard" and had him put up markers; on each he wrote a first name, the type of animal as a middle name, and the farmer's last name, e.g., "John Snail Lewis. Born, date unknown. Died (date on which he found the animal)." When he kept counting rows of corn over and over, they had him count the rows while plowing them. On my visit, he plowed six long rows; it was remarkable how well he handled the horse and plow and turned the horse around. It was obvious that Mr. and Mrs. Lewis were very fond of him and just as obvious that they were gently firm. He attended a country school where his peculiarities were accepted and where he made good scholastic progress.

The rest of the story is contained in a letter from [his] mother, dated April 6, 1970: "Don is now 36 years old, a bachelor living at home with us. . . . Since receiving his A.B. degree in 1958, he has worked in the local bank as a teller. He is satisfied to remain a teller, having no real desire for promotion. He meets the public there real well. His chief hobby is golf, playing four or five times a week at the local country club. While he is no pro, he has six trophies won in local competition. . . . Other interests are Kiwanis Club (served as president one term), Jaycees, Investment Club, Secretary of Presbyterian Sunday School. He is dependable, accurate, shows originality in editing the Jaycee program information, is even-tempered but has a mind of his own.

"Don is a fair bridge player but never initiates a game. Lack of initiative seems to be his most serious drawback. He takes very little part in social conversation and shows no interest in the opposite sex." (Kanner, 1971, pp. 121–122)

The few individuals diagnosed with autistic disorder who later assume relatively normal lives offer hope to the parents of autistic children everywhere. The retrospective accounts of such individuals provide insight into their successes and difficulties. One such person is Tony, a 36-year-old man who designs livestock facilities for ranches and meat-packing plants. At the time of the following autobiographical account in 1985, he was enrolled in a doctoral program in animal science at the University of Illinois:

At the age of $1\frac{1}{2}$ to 3 I had many of the standard autistic behaviors such as fixation on spinning objects, refusing to be touched or held, preferring to be alone, destructive behavior, temper tantrums, inability to speak, sensitivity to sudden noises, appearance of deafness, and an intense interest in odors. . . . At the age of 3 to $3\frac{1}{2}$ my behavior greatly improved, but I did not learn to speak until $3\frac{1}{2}$. At the age of 3 to 4 my behavior was more normal until I became tired. When I became tired bouts of impulsive behavior would return. . . .

In college I was on the Dean's honor list, but getting through the foreign language requirement was difficult. I scraped by with Ds and Cs. Learning sequential things such as math was also very hard. My mind is completely visual and spatial work such as drawing is easy. I taught myself drafting in six months. I have designed big steel and concrete cattle facilities, but remembering a phone number or adding up numbers in my head is still difficult. I have to write them down. Every piece of information I have memorized is visual. If I have to remember an abstract concept I "see" the page of the book or my notes in my mind and "read" information from it. Melodies are the only things I can memorize without a visual image. I remember very little that I hear unless it is emotionally arousing or I can form a visual image. In class I take careful notes, because I would forget the auditory material. When I think about abstract concepts such as human relationships between people, they are like a sliding glass door. The door must be opened gently, if it is kicked it may shatter. If I had to learn a foreign language, I would have to do it by reading, and make it visual. (Grandin, 1987, pp. 144–145)

One of the most fascinating and puzzling varieties of people with autism is the **autistic savant.** These rare individuals combine all the usual social, communication, and behavioral deficits of autism with a stunning, often narrowly focused talent or

autistic savant Person who suffers from the full autistic disorder syndrome but also has some singular talent that usually emerges very quickly at an early age.

ability, like drawing, playing a musical instrument, or solving complex mathematical problems. Famed neurologist Oliver Sacks portrays the syndrome as follows: "Such singular talents, usually emerging at a very early age and developing with startling speed, in minds of personalities otherwise deeply defective, appear in about ten per cent of the autistic (and in a smaller number of the retarded, though many savants are both autistic and retarded)" (Sacks, 1995, p. 44).

Causes of Autistic Disorder

Genetic/Biological Factors   Autistic disorder does not have a single cause. Because its symptoms are so unusual and because it does not appear to be caused by environmental factors, it's likely that autism is caused by one or more biochemical defects, perhaps transmitted genetically in some instances.

Evidence in favor of this view comes from a classic study of twins by English psychiatrist Michael Rutter, completed in the 1970s (described in Rutter & Garmezy, 1983). He reported that when an identical twin in his study was diagnosed as being autistic, there was a 32 percent probability that the other twin would receive the same diagnosis—that is, a 32 percent concordance rate. By contrast, if the autistic child was a fraternal twin, the probability that the other twin would have the same diagnosis did not increase; thus, the concordance rate for fraternal twins for autism was zero. When Rutter expanded the diagnostic criteria in his twin study to include severe cognitive problems, he found that concordance for these problems among identical twins increased to 82 percent. In other words, if a child diagnosed with autism has an identical twin, that twin has a concordance rate of 82 percent for severe cognitive impairment; if, however, the twin is fraternal, the likelihood of having a severe cognitive impairment is only 10 percent. Overall, this research provided strong evidence that genetics plays a role in the development of both autistic disorder and other severe cognitive dysfunctions.

The brothers and sisters of children with autism are usually normal, although the occurrence of autism in siblings has been estimated at just under 3 percent—significantly higher than the occurrence in the general population. A history of autism is rare in families with a child who has this disorder (unless, of course, as just noted, the child is a twin). These findings provide additional perspective on the nature of suspected causes of autism (Rutter & Garmezy, 1983). Most instances of autism do not seem to be inherited; instead, they appear to result from a genetic predisposition to develop language and cognitive disorders, of which autism may be one.

Numerous biological variables have been studied as possible keys to understanding autistic disorder. But to date, none has been found to be responsible for the disorder, even in part (Gillberg, 1990). Most authorities believe that the hypothesis with the greatest chance of being confirmed is that several forms of brain dysfunction underlie the syndrome of autistic disorder (Fotheringham, 1991). Because individuals with autism often fail to develop speech or lose what little speech they acquired in early childhood, the left hemisphere of the brain is likely involved, since it houses the brain structures responsible for speech. In fact, only half the autistic population is ever able to speak, which indicates that speech and communication skills are central features of the disorder and possible clues to its cause or causes (Prizant & Wetherby, 1993).

Many children and adults with autism do not imitate the speech of others meaningfully. This helps explain the difficulty children with autism experience learning the skills that normal children acquire with ease during the first 3 years of life. Learning to make certain sounds and to begin to make words depends heavily on the ability to imitate. Moreover, parents of young children are delighted when their children learn to clap their hands in imitation, to play hide and seek behind the high chair (imitating the behavior of the parent), and even to make unusual noises (again, in imitation). These imitated behaviors build the relationship between parent and child on which so much of the child's learning during the early years depends (Prizant & Wetherby, 1993).

Many autistic individuals find learning to speak so difficult that they learn sign language instead, enabling them to ask for food, drink, and necessary help. The fact that sign language can be learned, whereas speech often cannot, further implicates the speech area of the brain as a key to this puzzling disorder.

Endocrinal and chromosomal abnormalities have also been found in some children with autism, but not with enough consistency to suggest that they're involved in causing this condition. Most professionals believe that there are multiple biological causes of autism and that there is no single common pathway by which the disorder develops (Ritvo & Ritvo, 1992). Said another way, "Autistic disorder is a syndrome that represents the final common pathway of a number of different etiologies including biochemical, metabolic, genetic, electrophysiological, and structural abnormalities" (Dawson & Castelloe, 1992, p. 392).

Psychological Factors   Today, few authorities believe that autism is caused by psychological factors. But from the 1950s through the 1970s, psychodynamic and learning theorists argued that autism could, in fact, be caused by psychological variables.

Kanner suggested in 1955 (Kanner & Eisenberg, 1955) that autism was caused by the childrearing practices of detached, emotionally cold parents, whom he termed "emotional refrigerators." Psychoanalyst Bruno Bettelheim (1974) also argued that parents of autistic children were cold and rejecting and that they had unconscious hostility toward their autistic children. To cope with that rejection, Bettelheim advocated placing the children in residential settings, where they could let down their defenses and establish trusting relationships with loving caregivers.

Psychodynamically oriented treatment such as this is rarely employed now for autistic children or their parents. The reason for decline is that few clinicians and educators believe any longer that parents' emotional inadequacies are responsible for their children's autism.

In 1961, behavioral psychologist Charles Ferster suggested that autistic behavior in children was caused by their inability to obtain attention and rewards for appropriate social behavior from their parents. Ferster also believed that the only way in which children with autism differed from normal children was in the amount of attention they received from their parents for such behavior. He was convinced that there were no other differences—biological or genetic. In other words, like Kanner and Bettelheim, Ferster adopted a psychological explanation for autism, rather than a genetic or biological one. This view, like the other psychodynamic views mentioned earlier, has not been supported by scientific evidence.

More recently, experts on child psychopathology—including Dawson and Lewy (1989) and Smith and Bryson (1994)—have hypothesized that autistic children find the demands of complex social and interpersonal interactions incomprehensible due to a basic neurological defect in information processing. These researchers believe that this information-processing defect, which is likely the result of brain dysfunction, is responsible for the autistic person's total social incompetence (Klinger & Dawson, 1992). Burack (1994) has offered experimental data that support this view. He observed that persons with autism found it particularly difficult to pay attention to a stimulus when other distracting stimuli were presented simultaneously. By extension, the distraction of situations involving several people may be too difficult for autistic persons to deal with, thereby explaining their inability to function socially in interpersonal situations.

Treatment of Autistic Disorder

Psychological Methods   Psychological interventions are the primary means of treating children with autism. Behavior therapy programs for such children have proven especially valuable in teaching language, social, and self-help skills, such as dressing and toileting (O'Leary & Wilson, 1987). To be sure, however, teaching even simple skills like these to autistic children can take months and requires extraordinary patience and perseverance. Since children with autism do not initially respond to instructions, first, they have to learn to respond to very simple requests, such as "Come here." To teach the autistic child to comply with such a request, someone must first bring the child to the therapy aid or teacher when the request "Come here" is made. The child is then immediately rewarded with a hug and an edible reward, such as a raisin. Hundreds of such trials must be repeated before the child comes to the teacher entirely on his own (Carr, Robinson, Taylor, & Carlson, 1990).

Similarly, language instruction for the child who is autistic typically begins with efforts to induce him to pay attention to any sounds and then such simple sounds as "ah" or "mmm." After patient hours of work, the child may be prompted to begin to imitate the simple sounds. Only then can additional hours and days be spent in teaching him to model more complex sounds, to combine them, and finally to form words and sentences. Patience, perseverance, and dedication are the keys to success in teaching autistic children who do not speak how to do so (Lord, Bristol, & Schopler, 1993).

Behavior therapist Ivar Lovaas and his colleagues at the University of California at Los Angeles (UCLA) have taught language and self-help skills to hundreds of autistic children for more than two decades. In the Young Autism Project, which is administered by the Department of Psychology at UCLA, Lovaas and his associates (1987, 1993) enlisted the help of scores of undergraduate teaching aids in a large-scale effort that devoted close to 40 hours of teaching a week per autistic child for a period of 2 to 4 years. The encouraging result was that the children could actually learn language and self-help skills. What was discouraging, however, was the regression experienced by most of the children after they no longer received the intensive instruction and frequent rewards for their use of language and social skills.

Lovaas's early intervention program was based on the assumption that if treatment for autistic disorder was begun by the time the child was 2 or 3, greater progress and fewer regressions would result. Most of the children selected for the program had parents or others who were willing to continue the intensive therapeutic program at home after formal treatment ended. This program proved more successful than anticipated. Roughly half the children treated were able to attend regular or special education classes in public schools. As Lovaas noted, 47 percent of the children "made substantial recovery with IQ scores within the normal range of functioning and successful first grade performance in public schools" (Lovaas, 1987, p. 7). Comparisons with a similar group of autistic children treated less intensively (10 hours per week) revealed that only 2 percent of these children had attained the remarkable progress of Lovaas's group.

The message from these treatment results seems clear: Intensive teaching of children with autistic behavior, for 40 hours a week and as long as 4 years, can lead to substantial, positive behavior change. Although teaching efforts of this intensity may seem very costly, remember that the long-term institutionalization of an autistic child can cost as much as $2 million over a lifetime.

Still, it can't be denied that the treatment research of Lovaas and colleagues remains controversial. Some professionals acknowledge that the results are spectacular, but others question the goal of placing autistic children in normal classes if there are other children in the family and extraordinary resources have been used to obtain that goal (Goleman, 1987; Schopler, 1987). Say, for instance, that the autistic child has several siblings. Some individuals would question the parents' decision to spend 8 to 12 hours a day with the autistic child, thereby neglecting the other children. The decision to invest enormous amounts of time and energy in a family's single autistic child is clearly an ethical decision, not a scientific one.

Barry Kaufman (1994) has written about another successful treatment for autism from a unique perspective: as an articulate parent of a child with autism

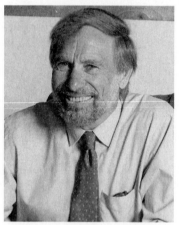

IVAR LOVAAS *developed a time- and person-intensive treatment regimen for children with autistic disorder, which has restored language and self-help skills to literally hundreds of these individuals.*

whose treatment at his parents' hands restored him to a productive, successful life. (We'll look more closely at this case later in this chapter.) Despite major differences between his approach to treatment and that of Lovaas, Kaufman agrees with the growing group of professionals who recognize the value of acquiring fundamental teaching principles before working with children with autism. Kaufman believes that no matter what someone believes about how best to treat an autistic child, to be successful, efforts must be based on the following basic teaching principles:

1. imitating a child's behavior
2. using parents as active teaching resources
3. working one-to-one with the children
4. making aspects of the program home-based
5. embracing a positive attitude as a meaningful component of the healing process

Both Kaufman's and Lovaas's approaches to teaching children with autism reflect the most recent trend toward more humane and dignified treatment and away from the use of punitive measures. The use of punishment in teaching children with autism has been debated for years, as addressed in Thinking about Controversial Issues on page 508.

Pharmacological Methods   Many different medications have been used with children who are autistic, but no medication has been effective with the majority of them (Lyman & Hembree-Kigin, 1994).

Psychostimulant medication has been used to increase the attention span of autistic children. As you may remember from the chapter on childhood disorders (Chapter 14), psychostimulant medication has been used very successfully with children with attention-deficit hyperactivity problems. Even though these medications sometimes increase attention in children with autism, a number of studies have also shown that other symptoms of autism worsen with psychostimulant medication.

For example, haloperidol, an antipsychotic medication, has been used to reduce severe aggressive and self-injurious behavior in children with autism. But it has many negative side effects (such as weight gain) and causes an increased likelihood of seizures; it also does little to address social withdrawal, abnormal interpersonal relationships, and cognitive deficits. Anticonvulsant medication is also often necessary with autistic children, since approximately 25 percent of these children have a seizure disorder. This type of medication is used with autistic children in the same manner that it's used to control seizures in individuals with epilepsy and other disorders involving seizures (Andreasen & Black, 1995).

Several studies have shown that autistic children typically show a 30 to 40 percent elevation of serotonin, a key neurotransmitter, in the bloodstream. Fenfluramine, another antipsychotic medication, has been used to reduce the level of this neurotransmitter. In doing so, it reduces several undesired autistic behaviors (for example, low responsivity to the environment and stereotyped habit patterns) and increases desired behaviors (such as attention and eye contact).

A study conducted at 23 centers for autistic clients (Ritvo et al., 1986) reported a greater than 50 percent drop in serotonin levels on average when fenfluramine was administered. When the drug was no longer given, serotonin levels returned to their previous elevated readings. Approximately one-third of the individuals with autistic behavior who were given the antipsychotic medication showed "strong improvements" in behavior, whereas another half demonstrated "some improvement." Increases in both verbal and performance IQ scores were also observed in treated patients. Unfortunately, other studies have not reported the great degree of behavioral changes following fenfluramine administration to autistic persons as those identified in the Ritvo study, even though equivalent decreases in serotonin levels were reported (Sherman, Factor, Swinson, & Darjes, 1989).

How does the mother or father of an individual with autism cope with repeated, violent temper tantrums at what appear to be the mildest of frustrations? How does a therapist stop life-threatening, self-injurious behavior, like head banging or eye-gouging? What should an institution do if an autistic individual attempts to physically assault a ward attendant every time he appears? What can a parent do when their autistic child insists on smearing feces on every piece of furniture within reach?

Unacceptable, violent, and dangerous behaviors such as these are not unusual among autistic individuals, who often don't speak and can't verbalize their wishes or frustrations. In the past, these types of behaviors brought rather drastic control measures in homes and residential facilities for people who were autistic (Iwata, Zarcone, Vollmer, & Smith, 1994). For instance, major tranquilizers were used to sedate and reduce aggressive behavior. Straight jackets were applied to bind the arms of individuals and prevent assaults on hospital wards. Helmets were put on children to protect them from injuring themselves by hitting their heads on floors, walls, and furniture. And to discipline particularly troublesome, repeated behaviors—and hopefully, to reduce their frequency and intensity—individuals with autism received slaps, mild electric shocks, squirts of ammonia, periods of seclusion, angry shouts, and other punishments.

In recent years, however, psychologists and educators have moved away from highly aversive punishment procedures to try to make autistic individuals' lives more humane and to discourage their maltreatment. The basic thrust of alternative, positive approaches to behavior change involves two parts: (1) to understand why autistic individuals engage in the so-called misbehavior and (2) to try to manipulate the reinforcement of the behavior or the environment it occurs in to make desirable behavior more likely (Dunlap, Robbins, & Kern, 1994). In turn, as desired behaviors increase, undesired behaviors become less likely. Carr, Robinson, Taylor, and Carlson (1990) reviewed over 100 research articles that showed that positive approaches to reducing severe behavior problems, such as aggression and self-injurious behavior, can replace the past maltreatment of autistic individuals.

For example, a careful behavioral assessment of the tantrum behavior of an autistic girl who's being taught to speak may reveal that she has an episode each time the difficulty of the task she's expected to perform is increased. Instead of punishing her for her tantrums, the task difficulty facing her could be decreased and then increased again in very small steps.

Let's consider a few more examples. Observations across a number of days may reveal that when a boy being taught self-help skills is given a small ball of cotton to hold in his hand, he's much less likely to engage in self-injurious behavior involving his hands. Another strategy to avoid the necessity to punish in order to reduce aggressive behavior involves the use of sign language or instruction in pointing to desired things in the environment. This approach is successful because autistic individuals often engage in undesired behaviors when they are trying to communicate something. Teaching such primitive communication skills to nonverbal individuals often reduces aggression.

Think about the following questions:

1. Can you recall how your parents shaped your behavior as you were growing up? As you remember it, did they tend to reward you for desired behavior, punish you for undesired behavior, or use both methods of behavior management? Can you contrast how reward and punishment each made you feel? Was one or the other more effective in getting you to do what your parents wanted?

2. What are some of the reasons that punishment was used in the first place to deal with self-injurious behavior? What are some of the reasons clinicians now appear to have moved away from using it?

Curing Autistic Disorder

All parents of children with autism want to believe that there's a cure for this disorder—or that there will be soon. These desires are identical to those of the parents and other loved ones of people with other serious disorders, like cancer and AIDS.

What would a cure for autism involve? Consider the following criteria for successful treatment of autism:

- All the unusual behaviors are gone.
- The individual speaks.
- The individual initiates social contact.
- The individual interacts with others, like persons of his or her age.

Recall Noah, the 4-year-old child described previously in this chapter. His early years were chronicled by his father, Josh Greenfield, in the book *A Child Called Noah*

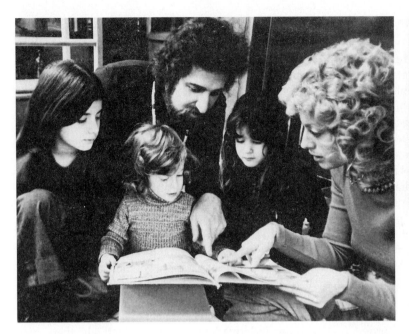

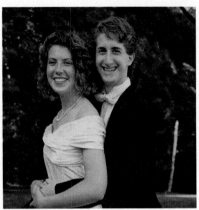

Left *Raun Kaufman, at the age of about 3, with his two sisters, father, and mother. His father Barry's commitment to his intensive treatment was a principal reason Raun was able to rejoin society as he grew older.*
Above *Raun Kaufman as a high school student, with his date for the prom*

(1972), from which the earlier selection was taken. Josh Greenfield also wrote a second book, *A Place for Noah* (1978), about Noah as a 1-year-old. In it, Josh describes his anger and resentment at professionals in the mental health and educational fields who could do so little for Noah. These feelings surfaced in part because Josh had come to believe there was a cure for autism—even though he had never seen a single instance of it with his own eyes. Convinced that the literature leads the parents of autistic children to expect cures, Greenfield felt guilty—and angry—that he had not been able to find a cure for Noah.

In fact, the literature that so angered Josh Greenfield does sometimes describe dramatic successes. Consider the books by Barry Kaufman (1983, 1994), introduced earlier, another author with a child who was diagnosed as autistic. These books were the subject of an award-winning TV special about autism. Kaufman's preschool son, Raun, had an IQ of 30 when it could first be measured. He was almost completely withdrawn, mute, and isolated from his family, even though he lived at home. Barry devoted 12 hours a day to teaching Raun verbal, self-help, and social skills, and when he could not, he hired others to do so.

Raun Kaufman's story represents an inspiring case study of what can happen with those rare autistic children for whom treatment is effective. A clearly autistic child during his early years, Raun ultimately became a highly articulate and social individual with a near-genius IQ. Barry's treatment methods have now been incorporated into a teaching style called the *option process*, which he describes as a "nonjudgmental and accepting therapeutic approach" (Kaufman, 1983, 1994). While this approach has not been subjected to formal evaluation, numerous compelling case studies point to its apparent success.

Focus on Critical Thinking

1. What typical symptoms of autism led to the view that it involves simultaneous deficits in social and communication skills and stereotyped and repetitive habits and movements? Explain your answer.

2. Can you imagine a situation in which punishment would be the most appropriate treatment for an individual showing some of the symptoms of autism? Again, explain your answer.

Is there a cure for autism? The question does not allow a simple yes or no answer. We don't know why Noah made only limited progress and why Raun progressed so spectacularly. Both fathers were successful writers, and both sought out the best experts in the United States. What's more, both sets of parents started teaching their children when they were very young. Why did Raun respond so well and Noah in such a limited way? We don't have the answer.

SUMMARY

Mental Retardation

- Mental retardation affects about 2.5 million people (roughly 1 percent) of the U.S. population.
- Persons diagnosed with mental retardation have IQs of 70 or below, are 18 years of age or less, and have impaired ability to adapt to social situations and conform to social expectations.
- Mental retardation is caused by diseases and injuries that affect brain function as well as by environmental factors and chromosomal and genetic conditions that permanently impair brain functioning before, during, or after birth.
- Although the brain damage responsible for most mental retardation is irreversible, physicians and psychologists have been successful in preventing some of the conditions that lead to mental retardation.
- These prevention activities involve efforts to reduce the incidence of some of the diseases and injuries causing mental retardation, to counsel parents who have the genetic potential to have a child with mental retardation, and to reduce or eliminate some of the environmental causes of mental retardation.
- Advances in institutional and home care in recent years have enabled people who are retarded to live more independently and productively than ever before.

Autistic Disorder

- The symptoms of autistic disorder usually appear before the affected child is 30 months old.
- Autistic disorder occurs in only 2 to 5 children out of every 10,000.
- Children with autistic disorder have severely impaired social and communication skills and stereotyped and repetitive habits and movements.
- Approximately half of all children with autism remain mute or speechless throughout their lives.
- Even when autistic children speak, they may parrot the speech of others; this behavior is termed echolalia.
- Three out of four children diagnosed as autistic are mentally retarded, usually within the moderate range.
- One of the most interesting varieties of autism is the autistic savant, who combines the social, communication, and behavioral deficits of autism with exceptional, often narrowly focused talent or ability.
- Autistic disorder does not have a single cause; it's probably caused by several biochemical defects, one or more of which is likely transmitted genetically.
- Psychological interventions are the primary means of treating autistic children.
- Behavior therapy programs for children with autism have proven especially valuable in teaching language, social, and self-help skills, such as dressing and toileting.
- Teaching even simple skills to autistic children requires extraordinary patience and dedication and can take months and even years.

KEY TERMS

alkaptonuria, **p. 492**

amniocentesis, **p. 488**

amniotic fluid, **p. 488**

autistic disorder, **p. 500**

autistic savant, **p. 503**

Down syndrome, **p. 491**

encephalitis, **p. 493**

familial mental retardation, **p. 493**

infantile autism, **p. 500**

meningitis, **p. 493**

mental retardation, **pp. 485–486**

mild mental retardation, **p. 488**

CRITICAL THINKING EXERCISE

Suppose your older sister and her husband had their second child about 3 months ago. They've been worried because their daughter hasn't been nearly as active or responsive as their first child was at that age, so they've taken her to the pediatrics department at their local university hospital. After half a day of tests, they've just been told that their daughter is probably autistic and might be retarded, as well. Your sister and brother-in-law are distraught. Because you've always been close to your sister and she knows that you have some knowledge about these disorders, she's asked you to answer some questions:

1. Could something that she or her husband did after the baby was born have caused the autistic disorder?
2. Do all children with autism have to be institutionalized before they reach school age?
3. Should she and her husband worry that if they have another child, it will be autistic, too?
4. Is treatment available for children with autism? If so, what is it?

Chapter 16
COGNITIVE DISORDERS

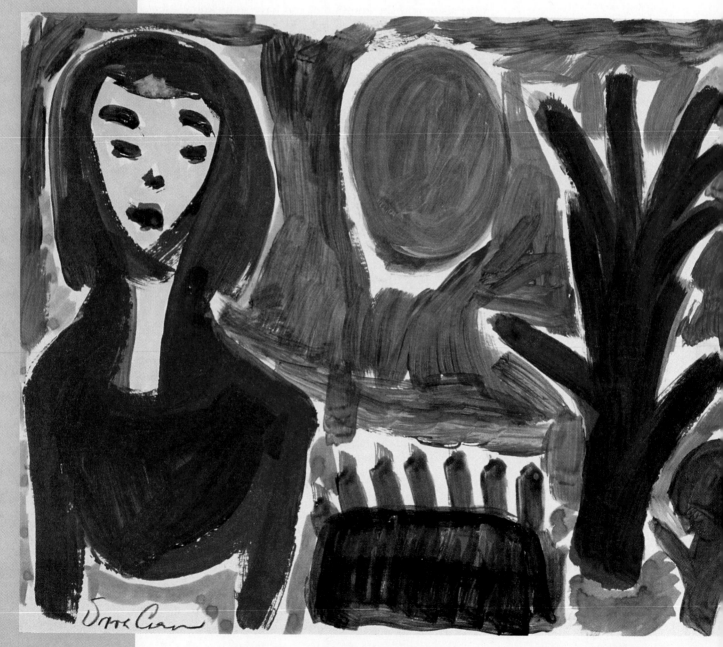

Donna Caesar, **Woman**, HAI

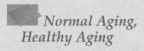
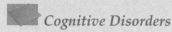
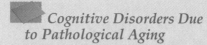
T he material that follows was written by two psychologists—Douglas H. Powell and Dean K. Whitla—who have long-term interests in the changes in cognitive functioning that accompany the normal aging process. Powell and Whitla have also explored differences in how cognition is impacted by normal aging versus **Alzheimer's disease,** a disorder of pathological aging. In the following material (and also in additional material from the same source that follows later), these authors stress the importance of understanding the concerns that older Americans have about their thinking, reasoning, and problem-solving abilities as they age.

Let's look at the following case:

Learning of our research on cognitive aging, a 69-year-old professor came to see us because she wanted to know if she were "losing it." The professor reported that she had difficulty recalling the names of new faculty she had met recently, could not remember the number of her classroom when ordering audiovisual equipment, and just this morning could not think of the name for the thing you turn over eggs with. She went on to say that she had consulted a doctor who, after examining her, told her she was "just fine." She was not reassured. She pressed the physician as to what criteria he was using to assess her mental status and received a vague reply to the effect that she was a great deal sharper than most 69-year-olds he knew, and, besides, she did not exhibit any of the classical signs of Alzheimer's disease.

The professor realized that one of the reasons she was not reassured was that the doctor and the patient had very different frames of reference. The physician had in mind the criteria for Alzheimer's disease and his extensive experience examining other post-65-year-olds when he said she was functioning normally. The professor's frame of reference was herself teaching, but if her symptoms foreshadowed Alzheimer's disease, or something equally ominous, then she would have to begin to make other plans.

The professor's concerns mirror the anxieties of thousands of older individuals at every level of employment and every walk of life who observe in themselves name-number-word finding problems or difficulties with memory, orientation, or calculation skills. They voice the question "Am I normal?" (Powell & Whitla, 1994, pp. 27–28)

This elderly woman's concerns about what's happening to her as she ages are shared by many older Americans. We'll consider those concerns later in this chapter. Most of the discussion will be about the devastating effects on the brain and behavior of pathological changes in central nervous system functioning—many of which are the products of pathological aging. Sad outcomes are common, unfortunately. The effects of brain disease on behavior are great, and treatment efforts overall are not terribly effective. By contrast, we'll also learn in this initial section that not all the news is bad. Today, normal aging is often healthy aging.

$\mathcal{N}$ORMAL AGING, HEALTHY AGING

Almost everyone knows that people today live longer and enjoy better health (Park, 1994). The facts are impressive. In 1900, about 1 American in 25 was over age 65. By the year 2000, only a few years from now, more than 1 in 10 will be older than 65. The population of persons 65 and older is growing much faster than the rest of the U.S. population—at a rate of 21 percent versus 12.5 percent. For those over age 75, the rate of growth is even more rapid—37 percent versus 13 percent. Between 2010 and 2030, the numbers of Americans over age 65 will increase by 73 percent, while the U.S. population under 65 will decrease by 3 percent. As dramatic as these figures are, they will be much more relevant to most of the readers of this book 40 years from now, when they will be reaching late middle age.

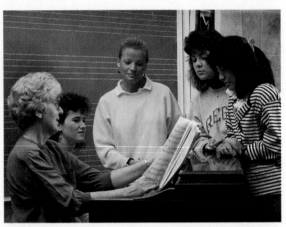

Many older people worry whether changes in cognitive functioning indicate pathological aging disorders, such as Alzheimer's disease.

Why is U.S. society aging so rapidly? Part of the reason is that people are having fewer children. Another is society's growing concern for better nutrition, more exercise, and healthier lifestyles. Advances in medicine are factors, as well. New drugs now available to treat chronic conditions that cause premature deaths, such as cancer and cardiovascular diseases (like hypertension, high cholesterol, and irregular heartrate), have both prolonged our lives and improved their quality.

As we've just observed, Americans today are living longer, healthier lives (Park, 1994). Seventy- and eighty-year-olds live active, productive lives that fifty-year-olds could not have imagined as recently as two generations ago. We're learning that older people who are healthy and vital are fully as interested in learning, producing, and remaining fully involved in society as younger persons. And despite widely held stereotypes, older people don't lose interest in maintaining active sex lives.

To be sure, we have increased the lifespan and substantially extended the productive, healthful years. But we have only begun to recognize the need to develop supportive services to keep pace with the numbers of older people who desire companionship and need specialized housing, transportation, and health care services. The challenge to U.S. society in the future will be to develop cost-effective and humane services for the healthy aged who will increasingly need them.

A number of influential scientific and professional organizations, including the American Psychological Association, have recently joined together to create Vitality for Life: Psychological Research for Productive Aging. This program has been described as a "human capital initiative" that represents "a call to arms on key issues that society will confront as America ages" (Cavanaugh & Park, 1993, p. 8). The initiative seeks intensive research and funding for four key areas of focus:

■ *Health:* We must develop an understanding of how to change behaviors which damage health and how to maintain behaviors which promote health. This will result in productive aging.

Alzheimer's disease Age-related brain disorder characterized by a profound, progressive loss in cognitive ability.

■ *The Very Old:* We can optimize the psychological function of the oldest old (those 75 and older) through both basic research and practical interventions. This will minimize costs of frailty and disability and maintain independent behaviors.

■ *Work:* As our work force ages, we will find that we must use older adults as an important resource to maintain the vitality and productivity of our work force. Understanding how to maximize and maintain productive work behaviors into late adulthood is a necessity.

■ *Psychological Well-Being:* We must develop better techniques for assessing mental health and appropriately treating mental disorders in older adults. This will provide older adults a better chance to achieve vitality throughout their lives. (Cavanaugh & Park, 1993, p. 8)

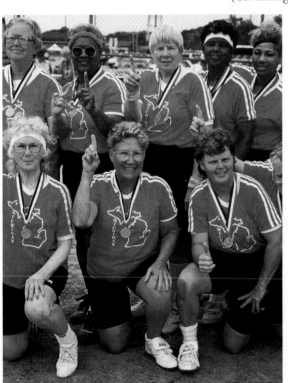

"We're number one!" A number of the key players on this women's softball team are well along in years, proving again that aging is as much a matter of the mind as of the body.

One of the leading private foundations in the United States has undertaken a major research endeavor designed to explore factors contributing to **successful aging.** The MacArthur Foundation Program on Successful Aging reflects the conviction that the nation's focus on the adverse consequences of aging has kept attention from being paid to the millions of individuals over age 70 who lead happy, healthy, productive lives. The principal aim of the initiative is to identify the genetic, physiological, psychological, and social factors associated with successful aging.

An article by two leaders of the MacArthur Foundation Program (Rowe & Kahn, 1987) has acknowledged that age does bring limiting changes in physiology and behavior. But certain people age successfully by dealing effectively with these limitations, whereas others do not. Based on that idea, Rowe and Kahn have asked us to distinguish between *usual* aging and *successful* aging. These authors insist that there is an understudied group of people who age successfully that deserves attention. Rowe and Kahn recommend intensive study of transitions in later life as a uniquely valuable way to understand what factors are involved in successful aging.

In the late 1980s, the U.S. government initially responded to the challenge posed by the aging of America. Through Medicare, substantially increased funding for home health care services was made available, permitting aged persons with chronic but not disabling conditions to remain in their homes; previously, they would have had to enter institutions and give up their independence. Medicare legislation to increase both acute care and long-term coverage was also passed, helping ease the concerns of many elderly individuals that they might outlive their resources.

In 1995, however, the future of Medicare and other programs (perhaps even Social Security) seems to be in jeopardy. Legislators trying to reduce the federal budget and stem the deficit are looking for places to cut, and federal assistance programs such as Medicare seem likely targets. Although President Clinton is opposed to such cuts, he may be forced to consider some reductions in reaching a budget compromise with Congress.

Federal and state governments have also begun confronting **ageism,** which involves prejudicial attitudes, discriminatory practices, and institutional policies directed against certain people solely because of their age. Through new legislation, enhanced enforcement of existing statutes, and social pressure, many communities have begun to address systematic discrimination against people who are aged in areas such as health care, housing, and employment.

Women are especially susceptible to the problems posed by ageism. They live longer than men and, as a result, are more likely to live alone. Moreover, women are more likely than men to fall into poverty in their old age, and they are less likely

successful aging Process in which elderly people deal successfully with the loss of a lifelong partner, a chronic disease, or a change in economic circumstance; concept defined by a MacArthur Foundation group.

ageism Prejudicial attitudes, discriminatory practices, and institutional policies directed against certain people because of their elderly status.

to be aware of available social services and financial aids. Given that women are at particular risk for some of the most difficult problems of old age, social programs to aid aging women have recently been developed in a number of cities.

Powell and Whitla (1994), the researchers mentioned in the chapter-opening, proposed four measures of normal cognitive aging to reassure the 69-year-old professor who feared that she had begun to decline cognitively. *Normal cognitive aging* refers to the normal impact of the aging process on thinking, problem solving, and remembering. Normal cognitive aging is what will happen to each of us—if we are lucky enough to age successfully. Powell and Whitla's measures of normal cognitive aging include:

1. *Age-group normative:* This measure indicates the percentage of the population that is normal cognitively when the percentages of persons with Alzheimer's disease and related disorders are subtracted. The incidence of Alzheimer's disease is about 2.8 percent for men and women aged 65–69 and 11.2 percent for those 75–79. So a 67-year-old scoring in the top 97.2 percent of a test of cognitive ability and a 77-year-old scoring in the upper 88.8 percent of the same measure are both considered normal cognitively. But for people like the professor, this proof of normal cognitive aging would probably not be consoling, since she's always been at the top of her class.

2. *Probably not impaired:* This measure would be more reassuring to the professor. It's based on a test of cognitive skills with proven high levels of sensitivity to and specificity for cognitive impairment. If the professor does well on the test, she will know that she's not in the early stages of Alzheimer's disease; she will not know whether she's still in her intellectual prime, however. For that reassurance, she needs the third and fourth measures.

3. *Reference-group normative:* For this comparison, the professor must take a test of cognitive abilities and then compare her scores to those of a reference group—say, other faculty members aged 45–64. Assuming that almost all the members of the reference group are free from impairment, getting a score that's comparable to younger faculty colleagues (who are presumably in their intellectual prime) ought to be quite reassuring to the professor.

4. *Reference-group plus:* In fact, simply matching the scores of a reference group—however impressive the members of the group might be—won't prove that the professor has retained her unique intellectual strengths. To get that final proof, she will need this fourth measure of normal cognitive aging, in which she will have to meet the standards of the reference group and score no lower than, say, 10 percent below the group mean. Doing so will ensure that her strengths in such key cognitive areas as attention, memory, reasoning, and calculation have all remained more or less intact.

cognitive disorders Clinically significant deficits in cognition or memory that represent significant changes from individuals' previous levels of functioning.

syndrome Distinct, recognizable group of symptoms.

delirium Acute cognitive disorder characterized by a disturbance of consciousness, such that awareness of the environment is reduced; also involves changes in memory, orientation, and perception.

Focus on Critical Thinking

1. Do you have aging parents or grandparents? If so, have they faced serious illnesses or losses that they've successfully recovered from? If so, how were they able to do so? Do they fit Rowe and Kahn's portrayal of successful aging? Explain your answers.

2. Examine your attitudes and those of your friends toward aging and people who are aged. Are you or your friends guilty of ageism in any areas of thinking? Give an example or two of this kind of thinking (whether your own or someone else's).

dementia Chronic cognitive disorder characterized by memory impairment and other cognitive disturbances affecting language, motor abilities, recognition of familiar objects, and planning and organization; causes significant impairment in social or occupational functioning.

COGNITIVE DISORDERS

The preceding section described the impact of normal, healthy aging on cognitive functioning. This discussion affirmed that the changes in thinking that accompany aging don't have to interfere with our quality of life. By contrast, this section—which details the nature, causes, and means of assessment of the cognitive disor-

Diagnostic Criteria for DELIRIUM

A. Disturbance of consciousness (i.e., reduced clarity of awareness of the environment) with reduced ability to focus, sustain, or shift attention.

B. A change in cognition (such as memory deficit, disorientation, language disturbance) or the development of a perceptual disturbance that is not better accounted for by a preexisting, established, or evolving dementia.

C. The disturbance develops over a short period of time (usually hours to days) and tends to fluctuate during the course of the day.

Diagnostic Criteria for DEMENTIA

A. The development of multiple cognitive deficits manifested by both:
  (1) memory impairment (impaired ability to learn new information or to recall previously learned information)
  (2) one (or more) of the following cognitive disturbances:
      (a) aphasia (language disturbance)
      (b) apraxia (impaired ability to carry out motor activities despite intact motor function)
      (c) agnosia (failure to recognize or identify objects despite intact sensory function)
      (d) disturbance in executive functioning (i.e., planning, organizing, sequencing, abstracting)

B. The cognitive deficits in Criteria A1 and A2 each cause significant impairment in social or occupational functioning and represent a significant decline from a previous level of functioning.

amnestic disorder
Cognitive disorder characterized primarily by difficulty in remembering and perceiving.

ders—contains more troubling material. Namely, cognitive disorders *do* impact our quality of life, sometimes very dramatically. Those of you with grandparents who have had strokes or been diagnosed with Alzheimer's disease know full well how marked these changes can be.

The fundamental disturbance in the **cognitive disorders** "is a clinically significant deficit in cognition or memory that represents a significant change from a previous level of functioning" (American Psychiatric Association, 1994, p. 123). This deficit typically involves a *delirium*, a *dementia*, or an *amnestic disorder*; each is a cognitive **syndrome** (that is, a distinct collection of symptoms that often occur together). One or more cognitive syndromes comprise every cognitive disorder.

Delirium and dementia are the most common and most significant cognitive syndromes. When severe, they produce wide-ranging deficits in thinking, reasoning, and problem solving. **Delirium** is caused by brain injury and accompanies metabolic or toxic brain disturbances, including infections that cause high fevers; reduction in oxygen supply to the brain; and alcohol or other drug intoxication. **Dementia** results from strokes (which deprive parts of the brain of oxygen for long enough periods to cause their death); certain serious infections, like syphilis and human immunodeficiency virus (HIV); and brain tumors, brain injury, and chronic, progressive brain diseases.

The diagnostic criteria for these disorders established by the fourth edition of the *Diagnostic and Statistical Manual of Mental Disorders* (American Psychiatric Association, 1994) are presented in individual *DSM-IV* tables. Also review Table 16.1 (page 518), which lists the signs and symptoms that distinguish dementia from delirium.

Persons with delirium often don't know what time it is or where they are. They can pay attention to things for only a few moments and focus on only one thing at a time. They can't relate their present situation to anything that happened to them in the past, and their thinking is disconnected and often preoccupied with imaginary experiences. Individuals with delirium may experience hallucinations of dreamlike scenes that are mainly visual but may also involve the other senses. These individuals are also typically restless and agitated, constantly moving without purpose.

Persons with dementia experience a global deterioration in their intellectual, emotional, and cognitive abilities. They have great difficulty performing tasks that require them to remember, learn, or use facts. Also typical of dementia are changes in personality, emotional balance, and mood. However, memory loss—especially memory for recent events—is usually the initial sign of the syndrome. Attention becomes harder to sustain in dementia, fatigue comes more easily, and a general decline in the normal richness of thought takes place. Paranoid delusions are common as dementia progresses. Despite the paranoia, these individuals seem to have shallow emotions. For instance, during the late stages of dementia, the death of a loved one may prompt surprising indifference.

The primary impairments in **amnestic disorder** are in remembering and perceiving. Individuals who have this disorder typically have problems with both short- and long-term memory. Very remote events (those that happened many years ago) are typically remembered better than those that took place a few days, weeks, or months ago. Sometimes, individuals with this disorder can't learn any new information at all and may be totally unable to remember things that took place only minutes before. The diagnostic criteria for amnestic disorder are presented in the *DSM-IV* table on page 518.

TABLE 16.1	Differential Diagnosis of Delirium and Dementia	
Feature	**Delirium**	**Dementia**
Onset	Rapid, often at night	Usually insidious
Duration	Hours to weeks	Months to years
Course	Fluctuates over 24 hours; worse at night; lucid intervals	Relatively stable
Awareness	Always impaired	Usually normal
Alertness	Reduced or increased; tends to fluctuate	Usually normal
Orientation	Always impaired, at least for time; tendency to mistake unfamiliar for familiar place or person	May be intact; little tendency to confabulate
Memory	Recent impaired; fund of knowledge intact if dementia is absent	Recent and remote impaired; some loss of common knowledge
Thinking	Slow or accelerated; may be dreamlike	Poor in abstraction; impoverished
Perception	Often misperceptions, especially visual	Misperceptions often absent
Sleep-wake cycle	Always disrupted; often drowsiness during the day; insomnia at night	Fragmented sleep
Physical illness or drug toxicity	Usually present	Often absent, especially in primary degenerative dementia

Source: From Z. J. Lipowski, "Cognitive Disorders (Delirium, Acute Confusional States) in the Elderly," *American Journal of Psychiatry, 140,* p. 1432. Copyright 1983, the American Psychiatric Association. Reprinted by permission.

acute cognitive disorders
Cognitive disorders that last only a few minutes or a few hours; recovery from them is almost always complete.

DSM-IV   Operational Criteria for AMNESTIC DISORDER

A. The development of memory impairment as manifested by impairment in the ability to learn new information or the inability to recall previously learned information.

B. The memory disturbance causes significant impairment in social or occupational functioning and represents a significant decline from a previous level of functioning.

C. The memory disturbance does not occur exclusively during the course of a delirium or a dementia.

Amnestic disorder can be caused by head trauma, alcohol abuse, malnutrition, brain surgery, oxygen deprivation, stroke, or brain infection. Research by Butters and Stuss (1989) has localized the brain damage responsible for most amnestic disorders to the medial portions of the diencephalon—specifically, to the dorsomedial nucleus of the thalamus and the mammillary bodies (see Figure 16.1).

Some cognitive disorders are mild, lasting only a few minutes or a few hours. Recovery from them is almost always complete, with only slight or nonexistent permanent effects. Common examples of these reversible conditions—called **acute cognitive disorders**—are the delirium that young children with high fevers sometimes get from infections as well as the disorientation that accompanies substance intoxication and withdrawal. In contrast, other cognitive disorders last much longer. **Chronic cognitive disorders,** like Alzheimer's disease, are typically irreversible and generally have serious behavioral consequences. These disorders may well endure from onset to the end of life.

We'll highlight two kinds of cognitive disorders in this chapter. The first—including dementia of the Alzheimer's type and vascular dementia—is a group of age-related brain disorders characterized by profound, progressive losses in cognitive ability. Aging affects the functioning of many bodily systems. For instance, changes in muscle tone, in the immune system's ability to defend against infection, and in visual and auditory acuity typically accompany the aging process. Aging also causes gradual changes in brain function. Older men and women may find it a bit more difficult to remember new names and faces or to add sums without using paper and pencil. Some individuals may even avoid intellectual challenges, rather than try to confront and overcome these tasks, as they did when they were younger. Occasionally, though, more serious changes in memory, cognitive abil-

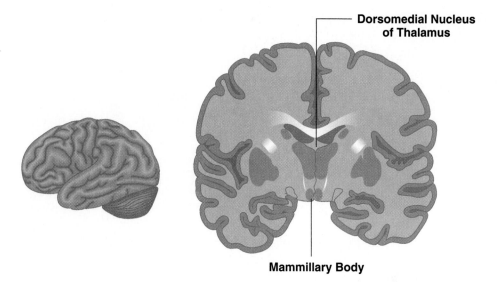

**Dorsomedial Nucleus
of Thalamus**

Mammillary Body

FIGURE 16.1 Brain damage responsible for amnestic disorders

Butters and Stuss (1989) have shown that most amnestic syndromes are caused by damage to the dorsomedial nucleus of the thalamus, the mammillary bodies, or both, shown here.

Source: From "Diencephalic Amnesia," by N. Butters and D. T. Stuss, 1989, in F. Boller and J. Grafman (Eds.), *Handbook of Neuropsychology* (Vol. 3), p. 108. Amsterdam: Elsevier Science Publishers B. V. By permission of the publishers.

ity, personality, and behavior accompany aging. Changes such as these turn a bright, loving, interesting, social person into a dull, unreasonable, insensitive, and isolated one. Such striking changes are commonly associated with Alzheimer's disease and vascular dementia, both of which are common consequences of pathological aging.

The second group of cognitive disorders can be divided into two subgroups. One is substance-induced cognitive disorders. Some of these conditions—like alcohol, heroin, cocaine, and amphetamine intoxication and withdrawal—are short lived, reversible, and of little long-term consequence. Other conditions, however, are permanent, irreversible, and serious enough to compromise quality of life. The chronic effects of drugs of abuse on cognitive functioning include substance intoxication delirium, substance withdrawal delirium, substance-induced persisting dementia, and substance-induced persisting amnestic disorder. Each will be examined separately later in this chapter.

The final group of cognitive disorders are caused by general medical conditions. As mentioned earlier, HIV—the virus that causes acquired immune deficiency syndrome (AIDS)—can also induce pathological changes in brain function with potentially serious behavioral effects. These effects include dementia due to HIV disease, a condition that is occasionally accompanied by delirium due to HIV disease. Other general medical conditions with prominent cognitive consequences include Huntington's disease, Parkinson's disease, and epilepsy. Again, each of these conditions will be discussed briefly later in the chapter.

A Historical Overview

Cognitive disorders that result from pathological aging have been recognized throughout most of history—especially those involving dramatic behavioral changes due to problems with memory and problem solving. Likewise, it's long been recognized that chronic substance abuse and certain physical diseases can impair brain function and cause marked changes in memory, thinking, personality, and consciousness.

Yet for all these types of cognitive disorders, the precise nature of the changes in brain structure and function that cause them has only recently been investigated. After all, it was only slightly more than a century ago that Emil Kraepelin (1856–1926) concluded that the brain was centrally involved in these profound behavioral changes. Since then, tremendous gains have been made through the use of exciting new investigative techniques. In fact, we've acquired more basic knowledge about

chronic cognitive disorders Cognitive disorders that last for a long time, often a lifetime; typically irreversible, they generally have serious behavioral consequences.

FIGURE 16.2   *"Guide to the Principal Zones"*

Spurzheim's 1826 guide shows the precise brain locations of 35 distinct and specific human behaviors. Among the "organs" of the brain are those that control mirthfulness, hope, and combativeness.

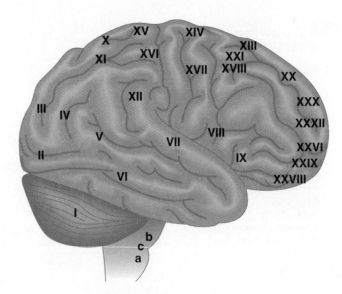

Guide to the Principal Zones

I. Amativeness	XIII. Benevolence	XXV. Weight and Resistance
II. Philoprogenitiveness	XIV. Veneration	XXVI. Colouring
III. Inhabitiveness	XV. Firmness	XXVII. Locality
IV. Adhesiveness	XVI. Conscientiousness	XXVIII. Calculation
V. Combativeness	XVII. Hope	XXIX. Order
VI. Destructiveness	XVIII. Marvellousness	XXX. Eventuality
VII. Secretiveness	XIX. Ideality	XXXI. Time
VIII. Acquisitiveness	XX. Mirthfulness	XXXII. Melody
IX. Constructiveness	XXI. Imitation	XXXIII. Language
X. Self-Esteem	XXII. Individuality	XXXIV. Comparison
XI. Love of Approbation	XXIII. Configuration	XXXV. Causality
XII. Cautiousness	XXIV. Size	

the brain and its workings during the past two decades than in all the centuries preceding. Developments in molecular biology, molecular genetics, and the technology of neuroimaging account for much of this knowledge explosion.

The first focused attempt to understand the brain and its role in behavior is generally traced to the early nineteenth century. Early leaders in this quasi-scientific effort were German **phrenologists** Franz-Joseph Gall (1758–1828) and Johann Gaspar Spurzheim (1776–1832). These researchers mapped protuberances on the head in the belief that these points corresponded to brain centers that controlled such discrete behaviors as love of animals, stubbornness, patriotism, and obedience (see Figure 16.2). Subsequent research, of course, has proven these claims to be false, making Gall and Spurzheim's status as the first scientists of the brain a historical oddity. However foolish their attempts might now seem, though, they did succeed in bringing the brain's central role in behavior to the attention of our skeptical forebears.

Efforts to investigate brain structure and localize brain function advanced significantly in the mid–nineteenth century when French surgeon Paul Broca (1824–1880) took the opportunity to study posthumously the brains of two stroke patients whose ability to speak had been affected. Broca discovered that the posterior third of the inferior frontal convolution in each brain had been severely damaged by the stroke. This led him to conclude that speech is localized in this area of the brain, which has since been called **Broca's area**. Broca's ground-breaking discovery—made more than 100 years ago—is generally considered the first successful effort to localize brain function.

What's more, this discovery continues to stimulate new research. For example, Damasio (1992) has written about a disorder called **Broca's aphasia,** which is a dis-

phrenologist   Quasi-scientists who studied the formation of the skull in the belief that it revealed a person's mental facilities and character.

Broca's area   Posterior third of the inferior frontal convolution in the human brain; controls speech functions.

Broca's aphasia   Disturbance of the comprehension and formulation of language; caused by dysfunction in Broca's area and neighboring brain regions.

turbance in the comprehension and formulation of language caused by a dysfunction in Broca's area and neighboring brain regions. He noted:

> Patients with the disorder have a drastic loss of speech fluency. Their speech is effortful and often slow; pauses between words may outnumber the words themselves. Their manner of speaking is labored and flat, and the melodic modulation that characterizes normal speech is lacking. . . . The hallmark of true Broca's aphasia is agrammatism [that] . . . leads to telegraphic utterances, such as "Go I home tomorrow" [instead of "I will go home tomorrow"]. (Damasio, 1992, pp. 532–533)

A few years after Broca's discovery, German physiologists Georg Fritsch (1838–1927) and Emil Hitzig (1811–1881) conducted research on how the brain controls the body. They reported that when they electrically stimulated specific regions of a dog's cortex, specific voluntary muscles immediately contracted, confirming that specific brain regions control specific body movements. In addition to promoting the electrical stimulation method (a new procedure for studying brain localization in experimental animals), Fritsch and Hitzig's finding motivated clinicians and researchers to widen their study of brain/behavior relationships in animals and humans.

French neurologist Jean Charcot (1825–1893) was another crucial figure in the history of scientific efforts to understand the brain and its disorders. As an influential clinician and teacher, he exerted his greatest influence during the late–nineteenth century, when Sigmund Freud (1856–1939) came to Paris to attend his lectures on neurological diseases. Another Charcot pupil was George Gilles de la Tourette (1857–1904), who, later in his career, discovered a rare and striking neurological syndrome in children (known as *Tourette's syndrome*). Charcot was a keen clinical observer who systematically described the complex interplay of neurological and psychiatric symptoms in delirium, dementia, and other cognitive syndromes. His clinical insights and observations, unparalleled in their day, continue to instruct new generations of neurologists, psychiatrists, and psychologists in training.

The intensive study of relationships between the brain and behavior that was built on these early investigations and continues to the present day has yielded two paradoxical findings. The first is that specific regions of the brain have been found to exert control over various bodily functions. The second is that it's impossible to precisely identify the areas of the brain responsible for many bodily functions. The implications of these two sets of findings are weighed in the Thinking about Controversial Issues box on page 522.

The Nature and Causes of Cognitive Disorders

Every cognitive disorder involves altered brain function; many also involve altered brain structure. Yet as our brief historical overview has suggested, the relationship among kind, severity, and locus of disturbed brain function and the behavioral disturbances associated with them is not completely understood.

Severe disruptions in a person's memory and thinking can result from what appear to be minor changes in the brain—for example, a minor blockage in a key artery can cause profound impairment in memory and reasoning. Correspondingly, striking alterations in the structure and function of the brain—caused by a bullet wound, for instance—can sometimes produce surprisingly small behavioral changes, especially after enough time has elapsed to permit undamaged parts of the brain to take over the functions of damaged ones. Clearly, the form a person's brain disorder takes is based on a number of factors: prior learning history, education, the emotional consequences of the brain injury, chronological and psychological maturity, and the intellectual competence of the person. The nature and extent of the brain damage, however, sets limits within which the other factors are free to operate.

Many cognitive disorders are life threatening. A study of 543 patients hospitalized at a large midwestern university hospital during a 10-year period (Black,

Thinking about CONTROVERSIAL ISSUES — Can Brain Function Be Localized?

Two schools of thought have developed on the paradoxes of brain localization. One group of researchers—the "localizers"—continues to believe (as did Broca, Fritsch, and Hitzig) that brain function can be localized with great specificity, although not to the degree the phrenologists believed possible. Antonio Damasio—a prominent neurologist and authority on aphasia and other disorders of higher brain function—has taken this position, in part because his research focuses on very specific deficits in speech and cognition linked closely to specific lesions of the brain (Damasio, 1992; Damasio & Tranel, 1991). A second group of neurologists have been influenced by German neurologist Kurt Goldstein (1878–1965), who studied the after effects of brain injury in veterans following World War I, and American psychologist Karl Lashley (1890–1958), who examined the ability of rats with experimental brain lesions to solve complex running mazes. These "holists" are impressed by the brain's ability to compensate for even massive injury and reject the idea of specific localization of brain function.

Most researchers today maintain a position somewhere between these two extremes. Psychologist Howard Gardner, author of *The Shattered Mind* (1974)—a graphic depiction of the behavioral consequences resulting from

serious brain injury—describes this middle-of-the-road position as follows:

> Neither the extreme claims of the localizers (in every function its own gyrus, or center) nor those of the holists (all areas of the brain implicated equivalently in all activities) are consonant with the facts. Rather, there is a gradient of neural zones, a cluster of functions, each of which is more likely than not to be associated with a certain brain region; at the same time, there exists considerable variability among individuals and across ages, as well as the strong possibility that a specific kind of impairment may result from a rather wide set of lesions. (Gardner, 1974, p. 26)

Think about the following questions:

1. If the brain "holists" and "localizers" are each correct, to some degree, what adaptive functions does this dual capability of the brain play?
2. Can you separate the brain functions that might be served by brain localization from the distinct and different functions brain plasticity (holism) might play? Explain your answer.

Warrack, & Winokur, 1985) confirmed that patients with cognitive disorders, regardless of their age, were at increased risk of early death. (Death generally comes to patients with Alzheimer's disease, for example, within a decade of the initial appearance of its symptoms.) In this study, patients with cognitive disorders were especially likely to die from natural causes unrelated to their cognitive disorders—for instance, cancer and heart disease among women and influenza and pneumonia among men. During the first two years after the diagnosis of a cognitive disorder, men were also at increased risk of death from accidents and suicide. Unfortunately, the design of this study doesn't permit us to know the direction of causality of these findings. That is, we don't know whether cancer and heart disease among women caused their cognitive disorders (by reducing the brain's oxygen supply, for example) or whether their cognitive disorders influenced the development of cancer and heart disease (perhaps by reducing the frequency of visits to physicians who might have diagnosed these life-threatening diseases earlier).

The increased risk of suicide and accidents among male subjects in this study (Black et al., 1985) parallels the greatly increased risk of depression and other mood disorders experienced by older people with cognitive disorders (Haaland, 1992; Teri, 1992). About 30 percent of patients with Alzheimer's disease meet the *DSM-IV* (American Psychiatric Association, 1994) diagnostic criteria for major depressive disorder, and another large group of Alzheimer's patients exhibit depressive symptoms that do not meet the criteria for a formal diagnosis. (See Chapter 7, pp. 196–198, to review these diagnostic criteria.)

The reasons depression and other emotional disorders so often accompany the cognitive disorders are not hard to understand. Cognitive disorders tend to occur toward the end of life and often seriously impair the quality of those final years. Moreover, some cognitive disorders directly affect the brain areas that control people's experience and expression of mood (Borod, 1992); other disorders bring on such profound changes in personality and behavior that friends and family often become alienated from individuals with these conditions (Prignatano, 1992). Fortunately, many of the psychological consequences of the cognitive disorders diminish when the people who have them receive adequate social support from family and friends.

Assessment of Cognitive Disorders

Neuropsychological Procedures   In the 1930s and 1940s, a growing number of clinical psychologists became interested in assessing the intellectual and emotional consequences of brain damage. The initial development of this subfield of clinical psychology—**clinical neuropsychology**—is generally traced to Ward Halstead (1848–1931). Working at the University of Chicago, he established the first human neuropsychology laboratory. He was strongly influenced by the work of neurologist Kurt Goldstein (1878–1965), who had begun to study the cognitive effects of brain-injured World War I veterans.

As noted in Chapter 3, Halstead developed a neuropsychological test battery— the Halstead-Reitan Neuropsychological Battery—with his student Ralph Reitan (Halstead, 1947; Reitan, 1959; Reitan & Davison, 1974). Despite the development of other neuropsychological test batteries since publication of the Halstead-Reitan Neuropsychological Battery some 50 years ago, it remains the most widely used measure. It assesses the cognitive functions most affected by brain damage, including intelligence, attention, concentration, language, problem solving, abstract thinking, basic reading, spelling, calculating, sensing and perceiving, motor abilities, and vigilance and mental stamina.

Also recall from Chapter 3 the work of Aleksander Luria (1902–1977), the pioneering Soviet neuropsychologist whose major work was done during the early part of the twentieth century. He developed a detailed theory of cortical functioning that has become widely known in the United States during the past 20 years. A standardized set of neuropsychological tests based on concepts and techniques advocated by Luria—the Luria-Nebraska Neuropsychological Battery—was developed in 1980. However, as discussed in Chapter 3, the validity of this instrument and its clinical utility continue to be debated by neuropsychologists (Jones & Butters, 1991).

Neuroimaging Techniques   Much of what we know about how brain injury and disease affect behavior comes from neuropsychological studies of brain damage. They provide information available from no other source on the nature of cognitive deficits brought about by specific forms of brain damage. But we understand much less about how specific changes in brain structure and function cause the behavioral changes that typically accompany them. Our knowledge is lacking in this area for two reasons: (1) Neuropsychological methods are not capable of providing that information, and (2) until very recently, techniques for studying the structure and function of the living brain did not exist.

The X-ray—discovered in the late 1800s by German scientist Wilhelm Roentgen (1845–1923)—was the first technology created to allow us to look inside the living body. The X-ray is much better at imaging dense structures like bones and teeth than softer tissues like the brain. The use of contrast materials like air, however, have extended the X-ray's usefulness for brain scientists. By injecting air into the lumbar space in the spinal cord and positioning the patient so that the air rises to the cerebrum (a technique called the **pneumoencephalogram**), sufficient contrast between

clinical neuropsychology
Subfield of clinical psychology devoted to assessing the intellectual and emotional consequences of brain damage.

pneumoencephalogram
Diagnostic procedure that employs air as an X-ray contrast medium to demonstrate brain contours.

the brain and the skull is induced to reveal differences in brain contours. Because the procedure introduces a foreign substance (air) into the body, however, it runs a modest risk of inducing infection or damage. Moreover, the pneumoencephalogram localizes brain structures with only a modest degree of accuracy and cannot visualize brain function at all.

Computerized axial tomography (CAT, or CAT scan) revolutionized the clinical investigation of many brain diseases because it provides detailed images of the living brain's gross cerebral structure. One of the first achievements of CAT technology was to confirm a long-held suspicion that the lateral and third ventricle spaces and some of the cortical surface markings of the brains of people with Alzheimer's disease were enlarged, whereas the brain tissue surrounding the ventricles was substantially reduced (Brinkman & Largen, 1984). This reduction in brain volume, called *cortical atrophy*, is associated in Alzheimer's disease with the loss of functional brain neurons and their replacement by nonfunctional cells.

Magnetic resonance imaging (MRI)—an even newer neuroimaging method—may ultimately displace CAT as the technique of choice for localizing structural brain abnormalities. MRI provides an extraordinarily clear reconstruction of the brain that, unlike the X-ray and the CAT scan, does not require the use of ionizing radiation. As a result, repeated scans can be made without exposing the body to radiation. MRI has been used to study the brain lesions associated with many cognitive disorders (Damasio & Tranel, 1991).

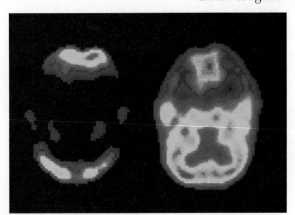

These PET scans of the brains of a person with Alzheimer's disease (left) and a healthy aged adult (right) differ markedly. The excessive dark shading in the left image shows that brain activity has been impaired.

One of the newest noninvasive imaging techniques is positron emission tomography (PET, or PET scan), which provides direct access to information on brain function. When used in conjunction with a CAT or MRI, a PET scan can help localize a structural abnormality in a region of the brain and then test for the functional consequences of the abnormality. These consequences might involve reduced bloodflow or glucose metabolism, signifying reduced cognitive activity levels. Again, as noted in Chapter 3, PET technology brings us closer to realizing the phrenologists' dreams of linking brain regions with behavior by permitting us to study the activity of specific regions of both normal and diseased brains during the execution of specific cognitive tasks.

Focus on Critical Thinking

1. Why are delirium, dementia, and amnestic disorders considered syndromes?
2. Since both dementia and amnestic disorder involve memory loss, what distinguishes one from the other?
3. What differentiates acute from chronic cognitive disorders?

COGNITIVE DISORDERS DUE TO PATHOLOGICAL AGING

There are two principal *DSM-IV* (American Psychiatric Association, 1994) diagnoses describing the pathological effects of aging on the brain: dementia of the Alzheimer's type and vascular dementia. We'll look at each.

Dementia of the Alzheimer's Type

dementia of the Alzheimer's type Age-related cognitive disorder characterized by profound, progressive losses in cognitive ability and marked changes in behavior and personality.

In recent decades, **dementia of the Alzheimer's type** has become a major public health problem in the United States and other developed countries. (It's not as much a problem in less developed countries because their people tend not to live long enough to develop the disease.) Alzheimer's disease will become an even greater problem in the United States in the future, as more and more Americans live long enough to reach the age of greatest risk. Consider these significant facts about this devastating condition:

PERSPECTIVE ON ALZHEIMER'S DISEASE

BIOLOGICAL FACTORS

Biological factors contribute substantially to the development of Alzheimer's disease:

➤ Growing evidence suggests that many individuals with a family history of Alzheimer's carry a genetic predisposition to develop the disease later in life.
➤ Distinctive brain lesions (granulovacuolar bodies, neurofibrillary tangles, and senile plaques) characterize Alzheimer's disease and are responsible for its symptoms.

PSYCHOLOGICAL FACTORS

Psychological factors interact with biological factors in producing symptoms:

➤ The early stages of Alzheimer's disease are often accompanied by anxiety, depression, frustration, and anger, which, along with growing memory loss and personality changes, compound the patient's difficulties in dealing with the symptoms of the disorder. Successful management of these psychological consequences of the disease makes it easier for the patient to manage her own affairs independently.
➤ Denying or underestimating the effects of Alzheimer's disease may help the patient adapt for a time, but doing so might also prevent her from seeking diagnosis and managing her life.

SOCIAL FACTORS

Both social and psychological factors operate in specific social contexts:

➤ Social support from friends and family is crucial in enabling patients with Alzheimer's disease to maintain independence and productivity.

These biological, psychological, and social factors interact to cause problems, as illustrated in the following case:

Thina W. was an 82-year-old retired teacher, as well as a mother, grandmother, and great-grandmother. She had been a widow since her late 40s, which had made her very independent. Although she often visited family and friends, she never stayed long. So it took a year or so for them to notice the problems: memory lapses, personality changes, and moodiness.

The first dramatic sign was an angry outburst from Thina, directed at her daughters. After a visit, they had grown concerned over the dirty condition of Thina's house. When they offered to help clean, Thina became enraged. Soon after, Thina's son got a call from the highway patrol, who had found her driving aimlessly, 50 miles from home. She had become lost when returning from a family gathering. Thina's children persuaded her to have a physical, which brought a diagnosis of Alzheimer's disease.

The biopsychosocial model helps explain Thina's behavior. The role of biological factors is evident in her increasing memory loss, which has left her unable to do routine tasks. Thina's anger and reclusiveness stem from denial over the seriousness and progression of her condition. With social support from family and friends, Thina will be able to live in her own home for several years. A nearby relative will check on her daily, and others will take over her financial and legal affairs.

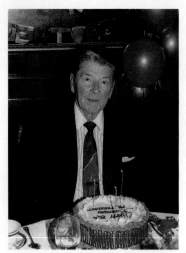

In November 1994, Ronald Reagan, shown here on his 84th birthday, wrote a public letter to the citizens of the United States, announcing that he had been diagnosed with Alzheimer's disease.

■ Alzheimer's disease is the most common cause of cognitive disorder in the elderly; between 2 and 4 percent of the U.S. population over age 65 years is diagnosed with the disease (American Psychiatric Association, 1994).

■ Rates of Alzheimer's disease approximately double every 5 years beyond the age of 65–70. Among elderly people in the United Kingdom, the prevalence rose from 2.3 percent for subjects initially aged 75–79 years, 4.6 percent for those 80–84 years, and 8.5 percent for those 85–89 years (Paykel et al., 1994).

■ The prevalence of Alzheimer's disease in the U.S. population has been estimated at about 10 percent in persons over 65 and 45 percent in persons over 85 (Davies & Wolozin, 1987).

Nature of Dementia of the Alzheimer's Type   As we discussed earlier in this chapter, dementia is an important feature of a number of serious cognitive disorders; prominent among them is Alzheimer's disease. Significantly impaired short- and long-term memory is a conspicuous early symptom of dementia. This memory impairment is commonly accompanied by disturbances in the ability to exercise sound judgment, think abstractly, and plan ahead. Other common features of Alzheimer's disease are:

■ **aphasia**—problems in understanding and using words, even familiar ones
■ **apraxia**—difficulties in moving parts of the body
■ **agnosia**—impairments in the ability to recognize or identify familiar objects

In fact, a recent study (Yesavage, Brooks, Taylor, & Tinklenberg, 1993) reports that Alzheimer's patients who developed aphasia or apraxia deteriorated more rapidly than those without either symptom. This finding suggests the possibility of subtyping the disease by these features and thereby improving the ability to predict how quickly the disease progresses.

Pronounced changes in behavior and personality accompany dementia. Although this condition almost always progresses to the point at which it interferes significantly with work, family, and interpersonal relationships, it generally develops slowly. Even though its course can be stable, it's much more often downward. The duration of dementia is typically lengthy, most often measured in years.

The memory impairment that's usually the first sign of dementia (including dementia of the Alzheimer's type) is sometimes subtle but more often obvious. That was the case with 70-year-old Virginia A., who experienced a typical array of memory problems early in the disorder that was ultimately diagnosed as Alzheimer's disease. But difficulties in remembering were not Mrs. A.'s only problems, as this case illustrates:

Virginia A. was a headstrong, energetic widow with two grown sons, enough money to last a lifetime, a loyal group of friends, and memories of a generally happy life. But in the spring of her seventieth year, she began to complain about her failing memory. Since she was a person who had taken great pride in remembering virtually everything, both good and bad, about almost everyone, Mrs. A. admitted ruefully to her sons that she had begun to forget the names of lifelong friends. She also reported that she sometimes forgot which day of the week it was and the number of the bus she took to go shopping. "I guess age is finally beginning to catch up with me," she complained to her sons, who didn't listen at first.

Virginia's sons took her complaints more seriously when she started calling from public phones downtown to ask what she had gone shopping for and how she should get home. Once, after forgetting which way to walk from the bus stop 3 blocks from the home she had lived in for 45 years, she stopped at a stranger's house and called her older son to come and get her.

Virginia's behavior began to change in other ways, as well. Normally an efficient, upbeat person, she slowly became more and more lethargic, bad tempered, suspicious, and sloppy. Her personal hygiene deteriorated, too, and she didn't

aphasia Disturbance in the comprehension and formulation of language.

apraxia Impairment of movement.

agnosia Impairment in the ability to recognize or identify familiar objects.

seem to notice or care. Even the content of her conversation changed from being far ranging, informed, and thoughtful to focusing more and more on a single topic, which became a preoccupation: her fear that her house would be broken into by men intent on raping her.

Finally convinced that something was seriously wrong, Virginia's sons took her to Dr. K., who specialized in geriatrics. Dr. K. did a variety of tests before she concluded that Virginia was in the early stages of Alzheimer's disease. With live-in help (for which her loving sons arranged), Virginia remained in her own home for another 2 years. After that, however, her disorder became so severe that she was able to do little for herself. That was when, with great reluctance, her sons decided the time had come to close up Virginia's home and place her in a care facility that could do for her what she could no longer do for herself.

As Virginia A.'s case illustrates, changes in other cognitive abilities, judgment, personality, habits, lifelong preferences, and values typically accompany or follow the memory loss that's part of Alzheimer's disease. Because learning and remembering are central to many cognitive tasks, memory deficits create many of the other problems accompanying this disease.

Age-related pathological changes in cognitive functioning range from minimal, barely perceptible differences in reasoning, arithmetic skills, planning, and problem solving—with virtually no discernible effect on functioning—to profound impairment in these processes, resulting in the inability to function independently (George, Landoman, Blazer, & Anthony, 1991). In the early stages of Alzheimer's disease, these cognitive changes are hard to detect. But toward the end of the Alzheimer's process, they are profound and impossible to miss because they affect every aspect of the person's life. And understandably, a person who can't remember where the bathroom in her home is, how to boil soup, or how to call a loved one or the police in an emergency can't live alone.

Deterioration in the quality of judgment frequently accompanies the cognitive deficits of Alzheimer's disease. Virginia A. demonstrated poor judgment when she started going outdoors in the wintertime wearing only a housedress, began eating instant coffee from the jar because she didn't want to go to the trouble of brewing it, and stopped bathing because she decided she wasn't dirty since she never went out. The association between deterioration in judgment and cognitive decline is not surprising, since good judgment requires the ability to choose the best alternative when faced with a range of choices. And making this choice requires the retention of several important cognitive skills, including being able to remember making similar decisions earlier as well as being able to anticipate the consequences of decisions, even unique ones the individual has no experience with.

Many people with Alzheimer's who have impaired judgment behave like Virginia A. Others make absurd accusations or impossible demands in letters to officials, friends, or newspapers, or they spend money on expensive, frivolous, and unnecessary purchases. And still other individuals may stop looking after their health and safety, sometimes with disastrous consequences.

Since problems of forgetfulness affect virtually everyone over the age of 50 or 60, how can we differentiate between normal, age-associated forgetting and the pathological memory impairments associated with Alzheimer's disease? The question is an important one, since many older people who forget things they used to be able to remember worry that they're in the early stages of Alzheimer's disease. (Remember that the elderly professor, discussed at the start of the chapter, had this concern.) Most of the time, these people do not have Alzheimer's—they just have memory lapses.

To help make that determination, an innovative test has been developed to distinguish between normal and pathological aging. See Thinking about Research, which summarizes the findings from a study that developed that test. Any memory problems that concern aging individuals or their family and friends should be brought to

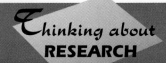
The case at the beginning of this chapter illustrated the importance of differentiating between normal and pathological memory deficits. Recognizing the usefulness of this distinction, Youngjohn, Larrabee, and Crook (1992) tested the capacity of two different kinds of measures—traditional memory tests (such as those described in Chapter 3) and computer-simulated tests of everyday memory. They did so to distinguish between the normal memory decline of age-associated memory impairment (AAMI) and the pathological memory loss of the early stages of Alzheimer's disease (AD). Their subjects were 56 AAMI and 56 AD volunteers.

The computer-simulated tests of everyday memory were created for this study. They included a Misplaced Objects test, which required subjects "to place 20 common objects (for example, a sofa, a bed, and a dining-room table) into a schematic representation of a 12-room house, using the computer touchscreen" (Youngjohn et al., 1992, p. 56). Subjects were then asked to remember where they had placed the objects 40 minutes later. The everyday-memory test battery also included the Name-Face Association measure, in which live, color video recordings of individuals introduced themselves by common first names; subjects were then shown the same recordings in a different order and had to remember the names of the persons shown. The final component of the battery, called Recognition of Faces-Delayed Non-Matching-to-Sample, required subjects to identify the new face added to an array of faces (ultimately numbering 24) shown on the computer screen.

Both test batteries (the traditional memory tests and the computer-simulated everyday-memory tests) discriminated with reasonable accuracy between the two groups. About 7 of 8 subjects in each group were correctly labeled as either "AD" or "AAMI." The most frequent misclassifications by both test batteries were false positives—that is, labeling a subject "AD" when she was "AAMI." AAMI subjects were between 2 and 4 times less likely to show memory deficits on the two test batteries.

The authors of the study explain its clinical relevance as follows:

> The ability to accurately discriminate between AAMI and mild AD with either or both batteries has important clinical implications. Many otherwise healthy older individuals often correctly recognize that they have experienced significant memory decline relative to their younger years (i.e., AAMI). A number of these individuals suffer from fears that they are in the early stages of AD and eventually present in the clinic. Our results demonstrate that their normal cognitive decline can be differentiated from the pathological decline of mild AD with a reasonable degree of accuracy, allowing them to be reassured and their needless anxiety eliminated. (Youngjohn et al., 1992, p. 58)

Think about the following questions:

1. Why is it important to differentiate normal from pathological memory deficits?
2. Why did these investigators utilize both traditional memory tests and computer-simulated tests of everyday memory?
3. What was the point of the Misplaced Objects test?

the attention of a person trained to differentiate among the memory changes associated with normal aging, Alzheimer's disease, dementia from other causes, and serious depression (Conway, 1991). That task is likely to require a mental health professional or physician who specializes in working with people who are aged.

Contrary to widespread belief, Alzheimer's disease is not simply accelerated aging. The effects the disease has on the brain differ markedly from those of normal aging, as does the behavior of the people who get it. Normal age-related forgetfulness and the memory problems associated with Alzheimer's disease can be distinguished. Table 16.2 summarizes some of the ways in which clinicians distinguish between the effects on memory of normal (*benign*) and pathological (*malignant*) aging.

On becoming aware of their lessened ability to reason and remember, many people with Alzheimer's underestimate or deny their deficits for as long as they can. For some reason, women deny their memory deficits more vigorously than men (Sevush & Leve, 1993). Although some persons in the early stages of Alzheimer's disease respond to their growing deficits by underestimating them, many more react with depression, anger, and frustration. Remembering and reasoning are uniquely human qualities that matter greatly to most of us. People for whom reasoning and remembering are of greatest importance over a lifetime—

TABLE 16.2	Differentiating Malignant and Benign Forgetfulness
Malignant	**Benign**
Shortened retention time	Recall failures limited to relatively unimportant facts or parts of an experience (such as name, date, or place)
Inability to recall events of the recent past, including not only unimportant facts but the experience itself	
Distorted recall of some events in the form of confabulations	Details forgotten on one occasion may be recalled at another time
Accompanied by disorientation to place and time and, gradually, to person	"Forgotten" data belong to remote as opposed to recent past
	Subjects are aware of shortcomings and may apologize or compensate

Source: From A. La Rue, "Memory Loss and Aging: Distinguishing Dementia from Benign Senescent Forgetfulness and Depressive Pseudodementia," *Psychiatric Clinics of North America, 5,* 1982, p. 90. Reprinted by permission of W. B. Saunders Company.

teachers, professors, doctors, and lawyers, for example—are most likely to react most negatively to a deterioration in these abilities.

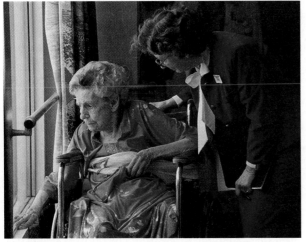

This elderly woman appears to have both dementia and severe depression. Why do the two conditions so often occur simultaneously?

Depression commonly accompanies aging. The increased risk of depression among people who are elderly is understandable, considering the inevitable losses of friends and loved ones as well as the physical infirmities that so often come with the normal aging process (Teri, 1992). However, the risk of depression is substantially higher among Alzheimer's patients. One recent estimate (Teri & Wagner, 1992) put the incidence of clinical depression among people with Alzheimer's disease at 30 percent.

Because many of the symptoms of major depression mimic those of early dementia, differentiating depression from the early stages of dementia in the elderly is sometimes difficult. Diagnosis is also difficult because individuals who are older and severely depressed may demonstrate **depressive pseudodementia.** As the following case summary about Mr. B. suggests, even though the symptoms of this disorder closely resemble those of the cognitive disorders, it's important to differentiate between the two because treating them effectively requires greatly different approaches. If Mr. B.'s depressive pseudodementia had not been diagnosed correctly, he might have been denied the treatment that freed him from his profound depression. Consider the following:

Mr. B. was a 76-year-old man transferred to our mental health center for evaluation of paranoid ideation, social withdrawal, and confusion. His referring physician, an internist, felt that Mr. B. had Alzheimer's disease and commented that "very little reasoning is left in this gentleman." The patient had, in fact, been placed in a nursing home because of his symptoms. His past history was notable for four episodes of depressive illness that had responded to ECT [electroconvulsive shock therapy].

On admission Mr. B. lay curled up in a fetal position. . . . On mental status testing the patient could recall none of three objects after 3 min., was unable to spell "world," was oriented only to person and place, and would not cooperate with further formal testing.

Mr. B. was initially transferred to the medical intensive care unit for treatment of severe dehydration and cardiac arrhythmias. Following resolution of these prob-

depressive pseudodementia Mood disorder in which the symptoms resemble those of dementia, but the condition is not a cognitive disorder.

lems, he showed no improvement in his mental status. B12 and folate levels were normal, as was a [CAT] scan of the brain. Because of his previous psychiatric history, the patient was treated with ECT: he received 10 treatments. He demonstrated a dramatic improvement in mood, appetite, and cognitive abilities and was able to resume a normal life at home without medication. (McAllister & Price, 1982, p. 627)

Causes of Dementia of the Alzheimer's Type   When examined in an autopsy, the brain of an individual with Alzheimer's disease invariably shows two significant features. One is a generalized atrophy of the brain; the brain size of virtually every Alzheimer's patient is decreased. The second feature is the presence of foreign, nonfunctional cells—called *neurofibrillary tangles, senile plaques,* and *granulovacuolar bodies*—that have taken the place of functional brain cells. Although these nonfunctional cells are sometimes found in the brains of other elderly persons, they appear with singular and distinguishing frequency in the brains of those with Alzheimer's.

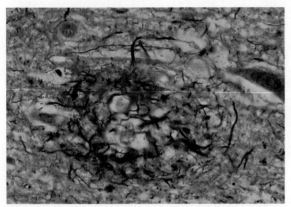

This section from the brain of a 69-year-old man is riddled with the classic lesions of Alzheimer's disease—senile plaques, granulovacuolar bodies, and neurofibrillary tangles.

These pathological cells tend to be concentrated in the base of the forebrain, the brain's uppermost and largest region, as well as throughout the cortical association areas. Cells in this area relay nerve impulses to the cerebral cortex, where most of our cognitive activities are localized, and to the hippocampus, which is vital to the formation of memories. The cells affected in the cerebral cortex and the hippocampus areas rely on the neurotransmitter acetylcholine for communication; this neurotransmitter is found in no other brain area.

Several hypotheses—none fully supported by available data—have been proposed to explain the etiology of Alzheimer's disease. One of the most widely accepted is that this disease is caused by viral infection, perhaps by a **slow virus** (so-called because it takes a very long time following infection for symptoms of disease to develop). This hypothesis is appealing for several reasons. First of all, viral encephalitis is a relatively common acute disease of the brain. In addition, measles virus infection is thought to cause a delayed progressive neurological disease, and postencephalitic Parkinson's disease is considered a late consequence of influenza. The greatest support for this theory, though, comes from the behavioral and pathological resemblance that Alzheimer's disease has to two slow-virus diseases in humans and to one in sheep. Early infection by a slow virus can gradually lead to the development of chronic, dementing disorders similar to Alzheimer's disease.

Other theories about the cause of Alzheimer's disease focus on the presence of certain chemicals in the brain. More than 20 years ago, researchers (Crapper, Kirshnan, & Dalton, 1973) reported elevated levels of aluminum in the brains of Alzheimer's patients. More recently, though, this observation has been found unrelated to factors causing the disease (Schneck, Reisberg, & Ferris, 1982). Other research (Andreasen & Black, 1995) has suggested that the brains of people with Alzheimer's have lower levels of choline, which is an important building block for both cell membranes and the neurotransmitter acetylcholine. While intriguing, these preliminary findings need to be replicated before they can be considered seriously.

Substantial evidence in support of the view that Alzheimer's disease may be a genetic disorder has accumulated during the past decade. There is a growing recognition that the disease runs in families. Additional support derives from the observation that all Down syndrome patients surviving to adulthood eventually develop the brain lesions characteristic of Alzheimer's disease. Down syndrome is caused by a genetic abnormality—most often, an extra chromosome 21. Perhaps information coded on this extra chromosome is also responsible for Alzheimer's disease. Active exploration of genetic explanations for Alzheimer's disease is currently under way (Terry & Katzman, 1992).

slow virus Viral infection so-called because it takes a very long time following infection for symptoms of disease to develop.

Vascular Dementia

Strokes, shocks, and cerebrovascular accidents kill more than 300,000 Americans a year and disable about the same number (Cummings & Mahler, 1991). And among these individuals, the ratio of older to younger people is 6 to 1.

These catastrophic consequences of high blood pressure, arteriosclerosis, and other circulatory diseases are caused either by leakage of blood from an artery into the brain or by blockage of an artery in the brain by a blood clot or arteriosclerotic plaque. In both cases, the part of the brain deprived of oxygen dies. The most common cerebrovascular accident involves a single episode of rupture or blockage—that is, a stroke. About half the people admitted to hospitals with the symptoms of a stroke die within the first 3 weeks. If the individual survives, he is likely to be significantly impaired, although persons with minor, localized strokes may recover almost completely.

A disruption in blood supply to the brain can also cause **vascular dementia.** Instead of having a single rupture or blockage of circulation within the brain, however, patients with this disorder typically have dozens or hundreds of such episodes (strokes) over the course of the illness. In fact, many older persons who never receive the diagnosis still experience one or more interruptions of the blood supply to their brain. Howell (1981) found 506 brain lesions—an average of 10.7 per individual—in 47 elderly patients with histories of cerebrovascular accidents.

It's sometimes difficult to distinguish between the dementia associated with Alzheimer's disease and vascular dementia. This differentiation can sometimes be done on the basis of age (since Alzheimer's disease typically occurs in older persons), but using the basis of behavior or disease course is more reliable. Alzheimer's disease generally begins very gradually, and its course involves a steady, progressive deterioration. By contrast, the deterioration in intellectual functioning, movement, and sensation of vascular dementia follows a characteristic pattern of steps—marked by sudden deterioration in one or more functions—followed by a period of stability and then another abrupt behavioral deterioration. Minor symptoms might surface first, such as temporary concentration problems and balance difficulties; later, mental confusion, emotional instability, and more marked personality changes appear. As time passes, cognitive functions (as well as psychomotor and sensory ones) become progressively more impaired, until the individual reaches a final stage of severe dementia and total disability.

Patients in the early stages of vascular dementia—like those who have experienced single strokes—are usually well aware of its impact on their ability to work, relate to others, and remain independent. The stepwise character of vascular dementia is part of the problem; it gives individuals the time to appreciate both how seriously they have been affected and what future course the disorder will likely take. Depression and suicide are understandable accompaniments of this stage of the disease.

Sultzer and his colleagues (1993) compared psychiatric symptoms of 28 patients with vascular dementia with those of a similarly sized, matched group with Alzheimer's disease. The researchers reported that patients with vascular dementia were more emotionally impaired than patients with Alzheimer's disease with comparable cognitive impairment. Moreover, blunted affect, depressed mood, emotional withdrawal, motor retardation, low motivation, anxiety, unusual thoughts, and somatic concerns occurred in more than one-third of the patients with vascular dementia.

Treatment and Prevention

Because no one has yet found the "fountain of youth," there are still limits on what can be done to treat the effects of both normal and pathological aging. Nonetheless, increased success in preventing and treating the physical diseases associated with aging (which include cancer and heart disease) has helped push the chronological, functional, and psychological thresholds of old age further into the future.

vascular dementia Age-related cognitive disorder caused by a succession of small strokes.

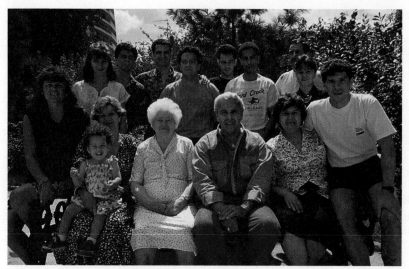

The social support this elderly woman enjoys (she is surrounded by loving children, grandchildren, and great-grandchildren) has helped keep her productive, active, and healthy. Why is social support so important to people who are elderly?

Replacement of worn-out or diseased organs—including the heart, lungs, liver, and kidneys—has become much more common. And prospects are good for the development of mechanical aids that enable people with impaired senses to continue to use them—for instance, far more sensitive hearing aids. In short, as more effective treatments become available to combat age-related diseases and disabilities and as healthier lifestyles push back the onset of old age, more of us will live longer, healthier, and happier lives.

Even despite these advances, until recently, once a dementia associated with pathological aging began, its course could not be altered, although its psychological and psychiatric consequences could sometimes be modified (Teri, 1992; Teri & Wagner, 1992). However, within the last decade, researchers have studied drugs that temporarily reverse the cognitive deficits associated with Alzheimer's disease and vascular dementia. These studies suggest that chemical agents capable of partially restoring the function of damaged or diseased regions of the brain may ultimately be developed, although this will probably be a long and complex process (Moline, 1992). Reports of success using cognitive therapy techniques to remediate memory and cognitive impairments (Larkin, 1992) have also appeared in recent years. These techniques are generally more successful with patients who are younger and have traumatic injuries, in comparison with those who have dementia associated with pathological aging.

Focus on Critical Thinking

1. Biological factors clearly have a very substantial impact on the cognitive disorders due to pathological aging; however, psychological and social factors play important roles in these disorders, as well. From what you have read as well as from personal experience, give examples of the impact of social and psychological factors on these conditions.

2. How do sex, age, and family history affect the likelihood of an individual developing Alzheimer's disease?

Extensive experience has also confirmed the importance of social support for persons who are elderly. Even the symptoms of Alzheimer's disease are lessened when patients' needs for care and concern are satisfied. Families, though, must be thoroughly briefed as early as possible about the disorder so they know what to expect and how to help their loved ones cope with the inevitable loss of function. The task of convincing caregivers not to exhaust themselves is particularly difficult, since the needs of Alzheimer's patients are frequently overwhelming.

OTHER COGNITIVE DISORDERS

Substance-Induced Cognitive Disorders

In this section of the chapter, we'll consider four distinct cognitive disorders, all of them induced by alcohol or drugs:

substance intoxication delirium Substance-induced delirium that occurs during intoxication.

1. Substance intoxication delirium—This diagnosis is made when the cognitive symptoms associated with intoxication (including memory impairment, disorientation, or language disturbance) are greater than usual, a disturbance of consciousness that interferes with the clarity of awareness of the environment is observed, and the symptoms of intoxication are severe enough to call for clinical attention. Substance intoxication delirium arises within minutes to hours after ingesting high doses of drugs like cannabis (marijuana and hashish), cocaine, and the hallucinogens (see Chapter 9). With drugs like alcohol or the barbiturates, several days of intoxication may be required in order for the delirium to develop. The delirium will end with the end of intoxication or a few hours or days after that.

The following describes a substance intoxication delirium that developed when John B.—a college student with little experience with alcohol—consumed a great deal of it in a very short time. Fortunately, the condition subsided after a few hours, and John B. was none the worse for the experience. Here's John's case:

> John B. wasn't much of a drinker. Although he'd experimented with whiskey and beer from time to time as he was growing up, he'd never really developed a taste for alcohol. Many of his high school classmates were regular drinkers, though. Perhaps the fact that John's serious, hard-working parents didn't drink influenced him to generally avoid intoxicating beverages and drugs of all kinds and to devote himself to his schoolwork.
>
> When John got to college, that part of him didn't change much. On weekends, he preferred staying in his room, studying or discussing serious topics with roommates, to going out drinking and partying—that is, until he surprised everyone by agreeing to join most of the occupants of his floor of the residence hall at a friend's apartment. At the party, there was music and dancing and an abundance of alcohol to drink. John sat at a table in the friend's family room with a small group of good friends who, like him, were serious students but much more experienced at drinking. John started off drinking mugs of cold beer; then he progressed to whiskey chasers as the evening wore on. He surprised everyone, especially himself, by keeping up with everyone at the table—beer for beer, chaser for chaser. His friends were even more surprised when John agreed to share some joints of strong marijuana, which someone had started passing around.
>
> After more than 3 hours, it occurred to his tablemates that John had stopped talking and was moving restlessly in his seat, seemingly in an effort to find a comfortable position. At the same time, he constantly looked around the room without seeming to focus on anything for more than a second or two. When his best friend asked him what was going on, John delayed long seconds and then responded, simply, "I don't know." Later, after the conversation at the table had moved beyond him, John broke in abruptly, pleading, "Tell me what I'm doing here . . . and where we are." His gaze shifted repeatedly from the faces at the table to others in the room and then back again, without focus or recognition. He began speaking softly to himself: "I've never felt this way before. I don't know where I am or who these people are. I don't know why I'm here. What's happening to me? I've never . . ."
>
> At that point, John rose from the table and staggered toward the front door of the apartment. His best friend, convinced that John couldn't navigate the city's streets alone, yelled for him to wait. John turned to his friend, closed his eyes, started to say something, and then fell to the floor, unconscious.
>
> John was carried back to the dorm by several friends and put to bed. The next morning, he felt nauseous and remorseful and had a terrific headache. But basically, he was OK. John admitted, though, that he remembered nothing of what had happened the night before.

John B. will never know why a single night of heavy drinking brought on the frightening delirium he experienced. Authorities on the subject can't explain it either. Likewise, they're not sure why heavy drinking results in delirium on one occasion but on many others does not. One thing is certain, however: John B. will think twice about drinking so much next time.

2. **Substance withdrawal delirium**—This condition develops when tissue and fluid concentrations of the substance in the body decrease suddenly after prolonged, heavy substance ingestion. Depending on the substance involved, substance withdrawal delirium can last for only a few hours or as long as several weeks.

substance withdrawal delirium Substance-induced delirium that occurs during withdrawal.

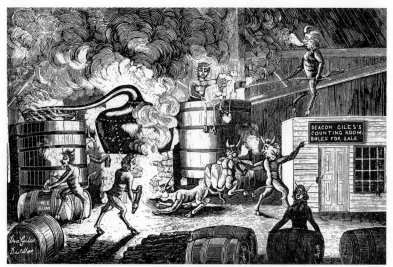

This woodcut from a temperance pamphlet published in Salem, Massachusetts, in the 1830s literally portrays the artist's notion of the demons responsible for the distillation of intoxicating spirits.

Long-term alcohol abusers are at heightened risk for experiencing alcohol withdrawal delirium. More familiarly known as **delirium tremens,** this withdrawal-related phenomenon typically begins a week or so after drinking has stopped. Like the symptoms of other substance withdrawal deliria, those of delirium tremens include difficulty attending to environmental stimuli, constant shifts in attention from one stimulus to another, and disorganized thinking, signaled by rambling or irrelevant speech or incoherence.

People experiencing delirium tremens can develop vivid hallucinations, which may be visual (for instance, seeing pink elephants), auditory (hearing threatening voices of friends or family members), or tactile (feeling insects crawling over the skin). These individuals may also experience paranoid delusions—for example, believing that unknown assailants are planning to harm them.

Untreated, delirium tremens can be life threatening, especially for alcoholics in poor health, who are at greatest risk to develop this condition. Given this dangerous potential, it's important that clinicians recognize as early as possible which alcoholics in withdrawal may be at greatest risk for delirium tremens. These patients can be sedated, thereby preventing development of the syndrome. Fortunately, delirium tremens occurs relatively rarely; most alcoholics, even extremely abusive drinkers, never experience this condition.

3. **Substance-induced persisting dementia**—This cognitive disorder typically follows a sustained period of heavy substance abuse extending over many years. Its symptoms are those of dementia, which include impaired ability to learn new information or recall previously learned information as well as additional cognitive disturbances, such as aphasia, apraxia, agnosia, and deficits in planning or organizing. The cognitive deficits must be substantial enough to cause significant impairment in social or occupational functioning and to represent a decline from previous levels of functioning. The symptoms persist after substance intoxication or withdrawal has ended—often, for a lifetime.

Many people who are homeless have substance-induced persisting dementia, which often co-exists with other serious psychiatric disorders, like schizophrenia or bipolar affective disorder. Because these people go untreated, their psychiatric disorders leave them vulnerable to exploitation and unable to look after their own health and safety. What's more, their suspiciousness and fear of authorities frequently makes them reluctant to seek or accept housing, food, or treatment, even when it's available.

4. **Substance-induced persisting amnestic disorder**—When this serious cognitive disorder follows prolonged, heavy alcohol ingestion and the chronic thiamine deficiency that typically accompanies it, it's termed **Wernicke-Korsakoff syndrome** (or *Wernicke's encephalopathy*). Although thiamine is in ample supply in many foods, alcoholics tend to develop a thiamine deficiency, along with deficiencies in many other vitamins and minerals. This happens because they rely on alcohol, rather than food, for most of their calories (Schuckit, 1995). Unfortunately, alcohol provides so-called empty calories, devoid of vitamins and minerals.

Wernicke-Korsakoff syndrome typically begins with an acute, time-limited episode of confusion, balance and coordination problems, eye movement abnormalities, and other signs of neurological disorder. When these symptoms subside,

delirium tremens Alcohol withdrawal delirium.

substance-induced persisting dementia Chronic cognitive disorder caused by sustained substance abuse.

substance-induced persisting amnestic disorder Chronic, profound, irreversible memory disorder caused by sustained substance abuse.

Wernicke-Korsakoff syndrome Substance-induced persisting amnestic disorder; associated with prolonged, heavy alcohol ingestion, and the chronic thiamine deficiency that typically accompanies it.

the main feature of the chronic phase of the syndrome remains: profound, irreversible memory impairment. This phase of Wernicke-Korsakoff syndrome is marked by four principal cognitive deficits:

a. *anterograde amnesia*—forgetting material learned after onset of the syndrome
b. *retrograde amnesia*—forgetting material learned before onset of the syndrome
c. *visuoperceptual deficits*—difficulties correctly perceiving aspects of the visual environment
d. *problem-solving deficits*—difficulties figuring out how to solve problems, even simple ones, such as putting clothes on in the right order

The severe cognitive deficits experienced by people with Wernicke-Korsakoff syndrome prevent them from living independently. Like individuals who have moderate to severe cases of Alzheimer's disease, they need to be cared for in sheltered environments for the rest of their lives. This was the unfortunate consequence faced by Professor S., whose case follows:

> Professor Ernest S. was a distinguished historian, the author of widely recognized volumes of French history, the recipient of several prestigious awards from the American and French governments, and the holder of an endowed chair in history at a famous U.S. university. But for many years, he'd also been a serious alcoholic.
>
> Because he never drank during the day, Professor S. was able to meet his classes, attend necessary meetings, and pursue his scholarly research. After hours, though, on returning home in the evening, he would consume most or all of a bottle of bourbon. Most of his calories came from the alcohol he consumed, since he ate very little. As a lifelong bachelor, he lived alone, so no one else paid attention to his eating habits. Despite this regimen, which had lasted for more than a decade, Professor S. continued to teach, write, and lecture. Many of his colleagues recognized that he had a drinking problem because of the times they'd seen him overindulge at parties. But few of them thought it affected his thinking.
>
> That all changed when Professor S. developed a brain inflammation, diagnosed as the acute phase of Wernicke-Korsakoff syndrome. One day, he was a distinguished historian, with the detailed minutiae of the French Revolution at his fingertips. Then, just a few weeks later (following resolution of the Wernicke-Korsakoff syndrome), he couldn't remember or learn anything. He couldn't remember how to get from his hospital bed to the bathroom, the name or the face of the doctor he saw every day, which hospital he was in, why he was there, or how long he had been a patient.
>
> Friends and colleagues who came to visit were welcomed with Professor S.'s familiar courtliness. But he had to be reminded how he knew them and what their names were. Oddly, he was ultimately able to remember more about his childhood than he could about what he'd eaten for breakfast or what day of the week it was.
>
> Although Professor S. lived more than a decade after the onset of his disorder, his lost memory never returned to him.

Treatment and Prevention   Much research has been done on medications that increase how quickly individuals with dangerously high levels of intoxication can sober up or detoxify. The shorter the period during which a person maintains a very high blood-alcohol level, the less likely an alcohol intoxication delirium will result. Several substances hasten the removal of ethanol from the blood when they're introduced directly into the bloodstream; the most effective is fructose, a naturally occurring fruit sugar. However, none can be taken by mouth because the oral route to the bloodstream causes chemical alteration of the substances as they pass through the gastrointestinal tract.

Substance withdrawal delirium can be prevented using a combination of tranquilizing drugs (which reduce the intensity of the psychological and psychomotor symptoms experienced during withdrawal) and gradual reduction in the concentration of the abused drug in the blood. If substance withdrawal delirium cannot be prevented, the agitation, anxiety, and hallucinations that accompany it must be treated with substantial doses of tranquilizing drugs. When left untreated, delirium tremens carries a substantial mortality risk.

Roehrich and Goldman (1993) have recently described an innovative program that's designed to teach patients with alcohol-induced persisting amnestic disorder and alcohol-induced persisting dementia how to compensate for their memory impairments. The program might be effective, as well, in treating people with dementias and amnestic disorders from other causes. When allowed to practice on a variety of memory tasks, patients with the memory deficits associated with moderate alcohol-induced persisting dementia significantly improved their performance on the tests. Granted, practice in remembering psychological test items may not always generalize to improvements in memory in the real world, but the possibility that it might do so is intriguing.

Cognitive Disorders Due to General Medical Conditions

Factors other than alcohol, drugs, and pathological aging can disturb the normal functioning of the brain. For instance, infections, tumors, and endocrinal, metabolic, and neurological diseases also affect brain function and behavior. In this section, we review several cognitive disorders that are associated with general medical conditions: delirium and dementia due to HIV disease, dementia due to Huntington's disease, dementia due to Parkinson's disease, and epilepsy, a neurological disorder with prominent psychological and cognitive symptoms.

1. Delirium and dementia due to HIV disease—As you likely know, **acquired immune deficiency syndrome (AIDS)** is transmitted by the **human immunodeficiency virus (HIV),** which is passed from person to person via blood, semen, and other bodily fluids. People at greatest risk for HIV infection habitually exchange bodily fluids with persons already infected by the virus. High-risk individuals include intravenous (IV) drug abusers who share needles contaminated with the blood of previous users and persons who engage in unsafe sexual behaviors with the potential for exposing both partners to shared blood or blood and semen.

From 5 to 35 percent of all persons who become HIV positive ultimately develop **dementia due to HIV disease** (Mapou & Law, 1994). The earliest clinical picture, in such cases, involves depression; this isn't surprising, since to date, HIV infection invariably leads to death (Bornstein et al., 1993). Common cognitive symptoms at this stage of the dementia include forgetfulness and poor concentration. Later, psychomotor retardation, decreased alertness, apathy, withdrawal, diminished interest in work, and loss of interest in sex may develop. Psychosis is an uncommon but serious complication of HIV infection (Sewell et al., 1994). Over the next several months, in cases in which neurological signs and symptoms are most pronounced, confusion, disorientation, seizures, mutism, profound dementia, coma, and death typically ensue. Neurological complications from other AIDS-related causes are also common, including tumors, circulatory problems, and other infections.

The prevalence of **delirium due to HIV disease** is comparable to that of HIV-related dementia. Delirium is characterized by a

acquired immune deficiency syndrome (AIDS) Life-threatening physical disease caused by the human immunodeficiency virus (HIV); sometimes accompanied by cognitive impairment.

human immunodeficiency virus (HIV) Viral infection that causes AIDS as well as delirium and dementia due to HIV.

dementia due to HIV disease Chronic cognitive disorder that can result from infection by the human immunodeficiency virus (HIV).

delirium due to HIV disease Acute cognitive disorder that can result from infection by the human immunodeficiency virus (HIV).

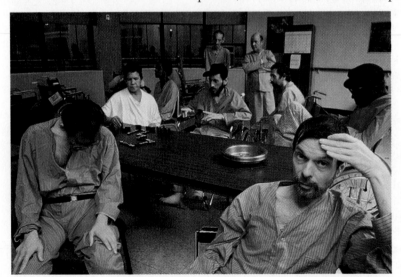

People who become HIV positive sometimes develop a particularly devastating cognitive disorder: HIV-related dementia. Several of these individuals with AIDS have this disorder.

wide variety of symptoms—from feelings of anger, hostility, confusion, and denial to experiencing hallucinations and delusions, some of which involve paranoia.

Not surprisingly, many people who test positive for HIV develop serious psychiatric and psychological complications, including severe depression and anxiety (Bornstein et al., 1993). The fact that the virus is often contracted through socially disapproved behaviors—such as IV drug abuse and unsafe sex—increases the psychological burden of those diagnosed with it. This guilt adds to the difficulty of preventing or treating the psychiatric and psychological consequences of the disease.

At present, no effective treatment has been developed to control the effects of HIV on the central nervous system. As with the other cognitive disorders, however, drugs are available to ease the agitation, depression, and anxiety associated with this life-threatening disease. Support from family and friends is also of inestimable help to people with HIV or AIDS (Hays, Turner, & Coates, 1992). But support and alleviation of symptoms do not constitute a cure. That development remains distant, most likely.

The brain disorders that result from HIV infection are preventable, however. Programs designed to educate one formerly high risk group—homosexuals—on safe-sex practices has led to a marked and sustained reduction in their transmission of HIV (Kelly, Murphy, Sikkema, & Kalichman, 1993). Efforts have not been as successful in inducing IV drug abusers to stop sharing needles, although attempts to bring the message to members of this group continue (Kalichman, Kelly, Hunter, Murphy, & Tyler, 1993). Psychologists are taking the lead in efforts to develop effective prevention programs for IV drug abusers, mainly involving behavioral strategies (Kelly & Murphy, 1992). The Thinking about Multicultural Issues box on page 538 presents research regarding a series of videotapes aimed at reducing rates of HIV and AIDS among yet another high-risk group: African American women living in inner-city Chicago.

2. Dementia due to Huntington's disease—Huntington's disease is a genetic disorder that invariably affects those who inherit the gene—provided they live long enough to develop the disease. Adams and Victor (1981) made a fascinating observation on how the disease came to the United States. They noted that nearly all the people who had this disease in the eastern United States could be traced to about six individuals who had emigrated to this country in 1630 from a tiny village in Suffolk, England.

The defective gene responsible for Huntington's disease ultimately controls the metabolic degeneration of a key group of neurons in the brain. The peak age of onset is 40. The deteriorating course begins with increasingly less subtle changes in personality, intellect, memory, and interpersonal behavior and ultimately leads to **chorea** (involuntary, jerky movements of the face, arms, and legs), depression, dementia, and psychosis. About 90 percent of Huntington's patients ultimately develop dementia during the course of their illness; about 40 percent become clinically depressed. Suicide is common among two groups: those who have the potential to develop the disorder and those who have acquired it.

At present, Huntington's disease is incurable. Treatment is largely supportive; it consists of drugs to control chorea and combat depression. Similarly, no effective treatment exists for Huntington-induced dementia. For these reasons, intensive efforts to prevent Huntington's disease continue. Prevention begins with genetic counseling of persons with family histories of the disorder. Unfortunately, such counseling is often irrelevant, since the disease typically emerges after the peak age of childbearing. Thus, education about the disorder is especially helpful.

3. Dementia due to Parkinson's disease—Parkinson's disease is caused by the destruction of brain cells that produce the neurotransmitter dopamine. The resulting dopamine deficiency results in a degenerative process that involves tremors, muscular rigidity, **bradykinesia** (exaggeratedly slow movement because of muscle rigidity), stooped posture, and a shuffling gait.

Huntington's disease
Autosomal-dominant chronic cognitive disorder with a deteriorating course; characterized by changes in personality, intellect, memory, interpersonal behavior, and movement, typically culminating in dementia; generally begins in midlife.

chorea Involuntary, jerky movements of the face, arms, and legs; a trait of Huntington's disease.

Parkinson's disease Chronic cognitive disorder caused by the destruction of brain cells producing dopamine; results in a degenerative process that includes

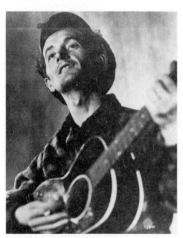

Famed folk singer Woody Guthrie had Huntington's disease, a genetic disorder that almost always results in dementia.

tremor, muscular rigidity, stooped posture, shuffling gait, depression, and dementia.

bradykinesia Exaggeratedly slow movement because of muscle rigidity; a feature of Parkinson's disease.

In the United States, half of all women with AIDS are African American, and most live in urban areas. Yet these very groups of individuals are among the hardest to reach with messages about AIDS education and prevention. The messages designed to reach racial and ethnic minorities must confront greater misinformation about AIDS and a stronger tendency to underestimate the personal risk for HIV infection. How can messages intended to reduce the risk for HIV and AIDS be delivered to members of minority groups in ways that will increase the likelihood they'll be listened to, understood, and acted on?

Kalichman and his colleagues (Kalichman, Kelly, Hunter, Murphy, & Tyler, 1993) recently tested the effectiveness of three different HIV/AIDS risk-reduction videotapes with a group of 106 African American women living in inner-city, low-income housing projects in an area of Chicago with a high incidence of AIDS. The volunteers for this study reported a variety of sexual and drug-using behaviors that put many of them at high risk for HIV infection. Each subject viewed one of three 20-minute videotapes and gave information about risky sexual and drug-using behaviors.

The first videotape, entitled *AIDS: What You Need to Know,* was the *standard public health message condition* presented by the former U.S. Surgeon General C. Everett Koop and two professional broadcasters. This video covered the history, epidemiology, course, risk factors, and common myths and misconceptions about AIDS. The second videotape, *the ethnicity and sex control condition,* presented the same information as the first, in the same format. The only difference between the two was that in the second video, the presenters were African American women.

The third videotape, *the cultural context condition,* was designed to stress culturally relevant values. To develop this video, a focus group of African American women helped provide examples of the three themes that were believed to be culturally and personally relevant to these women: cultural pride, community concern, and family

responsibility. This video provided the same information as the other two, and the information was presented by the same three African American women who presented the material in the second videotape. However, in the third video, the risk-reduction material was systematically linked to the three culturally relevant themes.

All three tapes were viewed in small groups of 6 to 10 women; each woman viewed only one tape. The women who viewed the cultural context (third) tape expressed more fear, anxiety, and concern about AIDS than the women who viewed either of the other two tapes. The women who viewed the third tape also thought that the presenters in it expressed more care and concern than the presenters in the other tapes. On follow-up, in contrast to the women who had viewed the first tape, those who had viewed the second and third tapes (both presented by African American women) were more sensitized to AIDS and more likely to have discussed the disease with friends, to have been tested for HIV infection, and to have asked for condoms.

These findings remind us again of the importance of paying attention to the cultural/environmental context of treatment and prevention programs. Treatment and prevention efforts designed for white Americans may not be nearly as useful for other groups within our multicultural society. We must be alert to the importance of making those efforts relevant for all the groups we wish to reach.

Think about the following questions:

1. How do you explain these findings? Why did the cultural context (third) tape generate more fear and concern about AIDS from the women who viewed it? Why did the tapes with African American presenters lead to more risk-reduction behavior?
2. Put yourself in the place of the women who viewed these videotapes. How do you think you would have reacted to the tapes' different presenters and different cultural contexts? Explain your answer.

The age of onset of Parkinson's disease is between 40 and 60. Although the etiology is often unknown, the disorder can be caused by encephalitis, carbon monoxide poisoning, or head injury. Parkinson's-like symptoms can also be caused by the long-term use of major tranquilizing drugs, such as those used to treat schizophrenia.

Depression and dementia are quite common in Parkinson's disease. Depression affects 50 to 90 percent of these patients, and dementia affects 25 to 50 percent. Some evidence suggests that dementia is more common among individuals who develop Parkinson's disease late in life (Rao, Huber, & Bornstein, 1992).

The drug L-dopa (a precursor of dopamine) is given to Parkinson's patients to increase the level of dopamine in the brain. It helps alleviate the movement disorders associated with the disease. However, L-dopa has significant mental side effects, including confusion and agitation (Boller, 1980), which limit its usefulness.

4. Epilepsy—Epilepsy is a chronic neurological syndrome characterized by repeated and recurrent seizures. A **seizure** is a pathophysiological brain disturbance caused by the spontaneous, excessive discharge of neurons in the cortex. The precise nature and frequency of a seizure depend on where and how the responsible cortical neurons are discharged. A seizure may involve abnormal movement or cessation of movement; an unusual smell, taste, or sight; a behavioral disturbance; or a change in state of consciousness (Dodrill & Matthews, 1992).

Almost any disturbance to the brain can cause epilepsy; as a result, it's considered a cognitive *syndrome,* rather than a cognitive *disorder.* Epileptic seizures may occur at any time; however, they are clearly provoked by stress in certain individuals. Some people with seizure disorders experience several seizures a day, whereas others may have one every few months or less.

One of the most common seizure disorders is **grand mal epilepsy,** involving loss of consciousness and a generalized convulsion of the entire body. Here's a description:

> The patient has a sudden loss of consciousness and falls to the floor or ground. The whole musculature is in spasm; the person may emit a piercing cry and bite the tongue. Breathing stops, the bladder may empty, and the pupils are dilated. This is the tonic phase, which lasts for 10–15 seconds. The clonic stage follows, with rhythmic violent muscular contractions; sweating is pronounced; and the pulse is rapid. After one or two minutes, the jerking stops and breathing resumes. The patient is exhausted, confused, disoriented, and amnesic for the episode. (Parsons & Hart, 1984, p. 896)

Petit mal epilepsy involves a brief disruption in consciousness, generally lasting from 2 to 10 seconds, which may be overlooked by observers. The patient may stare vacantly, with the mouth open and the eyes blinking or turning up.

Jacksonian seizures are signaled by a variety of partial motor symptoms. Initially, these symptoms involve the involuntary movement of a finger or a toe; ultimately, they lead to a period of involuntary jerking of a part of one entire side of the body. Jacksonian seizures typically last from 20 to 30 seconds.

Temporal lobe epilepsy may lead the individual to perform unusual behaviors, which are sometimes quite complicated and may involve episodic violence during the period of the attack. While experiencing a temporal lobe seizure, the individual may drive a car a long distance, get involved in a complex social interaction, or commit a violent crime. And once the seizure ends, she will have no memory of these events.

Personality disturbances are the most common psychiatric complication of epilepsy (Hermann & Whitman, 1992); they most often accompany temporal lobe epilepsy. Symptoms are varied, including changes in sexual behavior (most often involving a dramatic increase or decrease in interest in sex); an increased preoccupation with religion; heightened experience of emotions; and changes in conversation (which becomes ponderous, excessively detailed, and stodgy). Psychosis has also been reported in temporal lobe epileptics between seizures, but this disorder is much less common than the personality disturbance just described.

The advent of effective antiepileptic drugs in recent decades represents a genuine miracle for elderly people with seizure disorders. About 75 percent of individuals with epilepsy experience either complete or substantial remission of seizures when they begin taking one of the antiepileptic drugs. Surgical removal of the diseased portion of the brain responsible for the seizure disorder is another treatment option. However, use of antiepileptic drugs is the treatment of choice (Dodrill & Matthews, 1992).

---

epilepsy Chronic cognitive disorder manifested by repeated, recurrent seizures.

seizure Pathophysiological brain disturbance caused by the spontaneous and excessive discharge of neurons in the cortex.

grand mal epilepsy One of the most common seizure disorders; involves loss of consciousness and a generalized convulsion of the entire body.

petit mal epilepsy Condition involving a brief disruption in consciousness, generally lasting from 2 to 10 seconds; may be overlooked by observers.

Jacksonian seizures Form of epilepsy involving a variety of partial motor symptoms; initially, the involuntary movement of a finger or a toe; ultimately leading to a period of involuntary jerking of a part of an entire side of the body.

temporal lobe epilepsy Form of epilepsy that may lead the individual to perform unusual behaviors during the period of the attack; sometimes quite complicated and sometimes including episodic violence.

Focus on Critical Thinking

1. In most situations, it's obvious that prevention is more cost effective than treatment. Consider this principle with regard to the substance-induced cognitive disorders and the cognitive disorders due to general medical conditions. Give some examples of how preventing these disorders is ultimately less costly than treating them, in both economic and human terms.

2. How do sex, race and ethnicity, and socioeconomic status affect the likelihood of an individual getting substance-induced cognitive disorders and cognitive disorders related to HIV infection?

SUMMARY

Normal Aging, Healthy Aging

■ Because more people throughout the world are living longer, efforts to enable elderly persons to live happier, healthier, and more productive lives are receiving more attention.

■ Research suggests that many supposedly inevitable features of aging may actually be preventable.

Cognitive Disorders

■ Some cognitive disorders are acute and reversible; they often include syndromes involving delirium.

■ Other cognitive disorders, however, are chronic and irreversible. They may involve dementia, which is characterized by serious memory and learning problems, marked changes in personality and behavior, and deterioration in judgment.

■ Cognitive disorders may also involve persisting amnesia, characterized by a profound, irreversible disturbance in memory.

Cognitive Disorders Due to Pathological Aging

■ The most familiar of these conditions are dementia of the Alzheimer's type and vascular dementia, both of which are progressive disorders.

■ Alzheimer's disease—the most common cause of cognitive disorder among the elderly—is initially signaled by impaired short- and long-term memory, accompanied by disturbances in judgment, abstract thinking, and problem solving.

■ Individuals with vascular dementia typically have dozens or hundreds of disruptions in blood supply to the brain, each causing further deterioration in intellectual and cognitive functioning.

■ Although few effective treatments exist for the cognitive disorders of pathological aging, efforts to prevent these conditions from developing in the first place have been substantially more successful.

Other Cognitive Disorders

■ Substance-induced conditions include substance intoxication delirium, substance withdrawal delirium, substance-induced persisting dementia, and substance-induced persisting amnestic disorder.

■ Cognitive disorders due to general medical conditions include delirium due to HIV disease, dementia due to HIV disease, and dementia due to Huntington's disease, Parkinson's disease, and epilepsy.

■ These conditions all represent major problems for society. Even though they cannot be cured, substantial strides have been made in recent years to prevent them.

KEY TERMS AND CONCEPTS

acquired immune deficiency syndrome (AIDS), **p. 536**
acute cognitive disorders, **p. 518**
ageism, **p. 515**
agnosia, **p. 526**
Alzheimer's disease, **pp. 513–514**
amnestic disorder, **p. 517**
aphasia, **p. 526**

apraxia, **p. 526**
bradykinesia, **p. 537**
Broca's aphasia, **p. 520**
Broca's area, **p. 520**
chorea, **p. 537**
chronic cognitive disorders, **pp. 518–519**
clinical neuropsychology, **p. 523**
cognitive disorders, **pp. 516–517**

delirium, **p. 516–517**
delirium due to HIV disease, **p. 536**
delirium tremens, **p. 534**
dementia, **pp. 516–517**
dementia due to HIV disease, **p. 536**
dementia of the Alzheimer's type, **p. 524**
depressive pseudodementia, **p. 529**

$\mathcal{C}$RITICAL THINKING EXERCISE

Suppose you've just come back from visiting your grandmother, who lives 3 blocks from your home. Most of your visit involved listening to her talk about her arthritis, headaches, digestive problems, and susceptibility to colds and the flu. Although you're used to hearing these kinds of complaints from her, this time, she seemed a little different. In addition to her various medical problems, she also talked about her constant fatigue, her growing inability to remember her friends' telephone numbers and addresses (even general locations), and her worries about whether the town's bank is a safe enough place for her money. From what you've heard and read, you wonder whether your 77-year-old grandmother is in the early stages of Alzheimer's disease.

1. What can you tell your parents about the early symptoms of Alzheimer's disease and how they can be distinguished from the effects of normal aging?
2. If your grandmother does have Alzheimer's disease, how can you and your parents make it possible for her to remain independent as long as possible?

Chapter 17

VIOLENCE: PARTNER ABUSE, RAPE, AND CHILD ABUSE

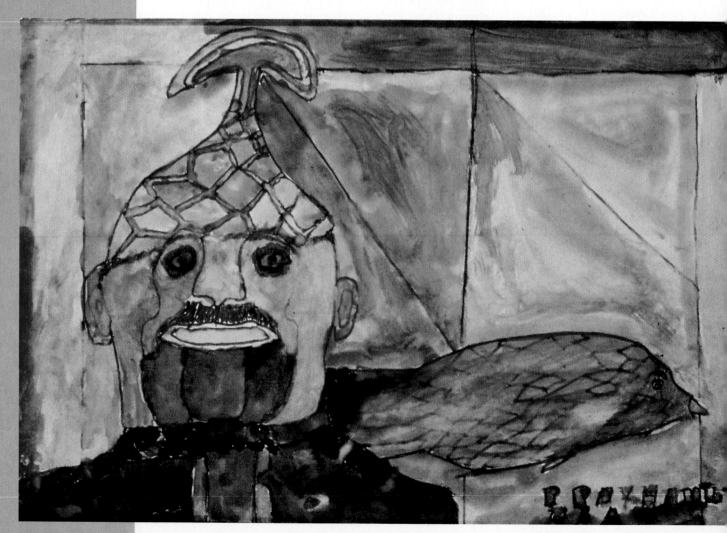

Ray Hamilton, **Man and Fish,** HAI

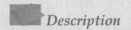

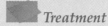
Carolyn Sapp, Miss America 1992, first met Nuu Faaola in 1987 in Kona, Hawaii, when she was Miss Kona Coffee. He was a running back for the New York Jets football team, and they exchanged autographs. She was attracted to the way Nuu interacted with children. Because of their celebrity status and hectic travel schedules, Nuu had to phone Carolyn from everywhere. According to Carolyn, he was romantic and giving. They became lovers, and she decided that she wanted to marry Nuu and have his children.

But matters went rapidly downhill when Nuu was cut from the Jets. One day, while the couple walked in the park, talking about the problem, Nuu reportedly got violently angry. He repeatedly struck Carolyn, kicked her, and threatened to kill her. Nuu had not been drinking and was not using drugs, to Carolyn's knowledge. She blamed herself, thinking she must have provoked him. Carolyn had been known for overcoming odds—she had coped with her parents' divorce and had financed her own education at the University of Hawaii. Nuu's temper was one more challenge to overcome.

After several fights and a separation, Carolyn was tempted to take Nuu back after he was cut from another pro football team. Nuu returned to Hawaii, and he and Carolyn discussed reuniting. But their talk turned into a heated argument. Nuu slammed Carolyn around the room and then took out a knife, pressed it against her face, and threatened to kill her. Fortunately, Nuu's male friend in the next room heard the commotion and came to help Carolyn.

At that point, Carolyn stopped blaming herself and resolved that she would not be beaten by him again. The next day, she went to the police department and filed for an order of protection. Nuu did not hit her again.

Carolyn had dealt with Nuu's physical abuse for several years. Each of the three times Nuu had been cut from a football team, he had become physically abusive to Carolyn—once trying to push her out of a speeding car. Throughout this relationship, Carolyn had the support of her father, a Lutheran minister, and her step-grandparents, who lived in Hawaii. Yet after breaking her engagement and banishing Nuu from her life, she relented and resumed their relationship. She felt

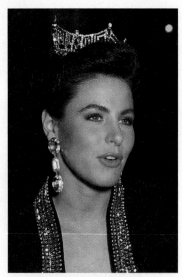

Carolyn Sapp, a former Miss America, was abused for several years by her fiancé, pro-football star Nuu Faaola. Why do you think intelligent, attractive, financially independent women often remain in abusive relationships?

sorry for him. Born in American Samoa, Nuu was one of eight children. His parents separated when he was a toddler, and he was abandoned by his father. Football was his only chance for success. As Carolyn said, "Nuu was my best friend for three years." However, after being beaten again, she realized that she did not deserve this kind of life.

Many people who hear about partner abuse ask the question: Why doesn't she leave? As Carolyn's case illustrates, there is no simple answer. A history of overcoming obstacles; concern for Nuu, who eventually went to work as a cargo handler on the docks; and guilt for pushing Nuu too hard to be what he could not easily be—all kept her from simply walking away.

Description

The violence Carolyn Sapp experienced is a clear example of severe partner abuse. **Abuse**—maltreatment, injury, or neglect—can take many forms. It can be physical, emotional, or sexual in nature. In this chapter, we will focus on physical abuse against a partner or child and rape of a partner or stranger. **Physical abuse** toward a partner or child refers to acts of physical aggression by one individual against the other. Specifically, such acts include slapping, hitting, kicking, biting, and beating. With adult partners, repeated acts of physical aggression and/or isolated acts of physical aggression leading to fear of the aggressor constitute abuse (O'Leary & Jacobson, in press). Physical abuse of children, as will be explained later, is physical aggression or neglect that has injurious effects on a child. Definitions of rape vary somewhat across states, but rape generally refers to unwanted or nonconsensual sexual activity that is forced or coerced against another (Koss, 1993).

Some of you may wonder why violence in the forms of partner abuse, rape, and child abuse is included in an abnormal psychology text. Given the prevalence and mental health impact of such violence, others of you might wonder why these forms of aggression have not been included in abnormal psychology texts before. In fact, violence of these types is not given a separate chapter in most abnormal psychology texts. We include violence in this book because it's becoming recognized as a major health priority by the U.S. Surgeon General (Koop, 1985), the American Medical Association (1992), and the American Psychological Association (Koss et al., 1994; Walker et al., in press). Moreover, in 1994, physical abuse was recognized in the fourth edition of the *Diagnostic and Statistical Manual of Mental Disorders* (*DSM-IV*) (American Psychiatric Association, 1994) as a new diagnostic category, "Problems Related to Abuse or Neglect."

This new category includes diagnoses of four types of severe mistreatment of one individual by another through physical or sexual abuse:

1. physical abuse of a child
2. sexual abuse of a child
3. physical abuse of an adult
4. sexual abuse of an adult

These problems are frequently the focus of clinical attention among individuals in therapy. In using these categories, the clinician should indicate whether the focus is on the perpetrator or victim of these acts. If the victim of these abusive acts is receiving treatment, this must be specified in the diagnosis. A more complete elaboration of the diagnostic criteria is available in the *DSM-IV Sourcebook* (American Psychiatric Association, in press).

New diagnostic classifications regarding abuse were added to the *DSM-IV* because it's become clear that many individuals who engage in these forms of behavior—as well as the people they assault—don't qualify for other diagnostic cat-

abuse Physical or sexual maltreatment or injury, or neglect; see definitions of specific types for more detail.

physical abuse Acts of physical aggression by one individual against another, often leading to fear and/or injury.

egories. For example, many women who are physically abused or raped experience a variety of psychological problems that don't meet the criteria for clinical diagnoses, such as depression or anxiety disorder. Many people who have been raped continue to function; they are able to go to college or work at their jobs. But in many instances, they function much less effectively than they did before the rape. With the official diagnostic recognition of the effects of various forms of abuse, women will be able to receive diagnoses and treatment for the problems associated with abuse. Further, many men who engage in physical abuse against their partners don't have traditional clinical disorders, such as alcoholism or depression. Now, they will be able to receive diagnoses and treatment for their abusive behavior.

Partner Abuse

According to the *DSM-IV* (American Psychiatric Association, 1994), **partner abuse** refers to acts of physical aggression—such as slapping, pushing, shoving, and kicking—that occur more than once per year. It also refers to any act of physical aggression that results in physical injury requiring medical attention. Finally, it can involve physically aggressive acts involving threats and intimidation, such that the victim is almost always fearful of the perpetrator (O'Leary & Jacobson, in press).

According to a national survey of 2,000 women, every year, approximately 12 percent of married or cohabiting women in the United States experience some act of physical aggression against them. These acts of aggression are carried out in anger, and they generally include pushing, slapping, and shoving. Other women experience much more severe aggression. About 4 percent of married or cohabiting women each year experience violence that takes the form of beatings or use of a knife or gun (Straus & Gelles, 1992). Such physical aggression is defined as *physical abuse* in the *DSM-IV* (American Psychiatric Association, 1994).

You may wonder: Why isn't *any* physical aggression against a partner defined as abuse? Certainly, any physically aggressive act against another can be conceptualized as abusive. Basically, the reason is that physical aggression against partners in anger is common, especially slapping among young couples. Therefore, the clinical criteria stipulate more than a single act of aggression against a partner or a single act resulting in injury. For clinical purposes and for purposes of being able to receive treatment for problems of partner abuse, the acts of physical aggression must occur at least twice a year or involve isolated acts of physical aggression that lead to fear of the partner and/or injury.

As you might expect, the lifetime rates of physical aggression against individual partners are much higher than those for any single year. About one-third of all married or cohabiting women in the United States will face some form of physical aggression during their lifetimes. Further, about 10 percent of these women will endure severe and repeated violence at some time in their lives (Straus & Gelles, 1992). Aggression by a husband or boyfriend is one of the most common causes of death for young women. Roughly 2,000 American women are killed each year by their partners or ex-partners (Browne & Williams, 1993). Men and women in their 20s are the people most likely to be in physically abusive relationships; like many other forms of violence, physical aggression in intimate relationships decreases with age.

Are men physically abused by women? Recall that partner abuse includes two acts of physical aggression against a partner and/or isolated acts of physical aggression against a partner that lead her to experience fear and intimidation. A woman whose husband engages in several acts of physical aggression against her in a year usually fears him. In other words, she's afraid that he will use his power and control over her in some fashion. However, even those men who report that their wives unilaterally engage in physical aggression against them (that is, the aggression is one sided) do not generally report that they live in fear of their wives. Thus, the answer to the question of whether men are physically abused by their

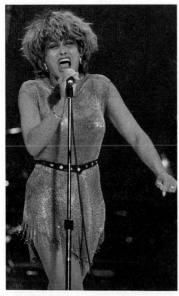

Tina Turner was both physically and sexually abused by her husband/manager. She later made a movie about it, What's Love Got to Do with It?

partner abuse Repeated physical aggression against a partner and/or isolated acts of physical aggression against a partner that lead to fear and/or injury.

Thinking about MULTICULTURAL ISSUES
Prevalence of Wife Abuse in African American and White Couples

Since homicide rates are much higher among African American than among white men, people often ask whether rates of physical aggression within marriage differ according to race. A national survey found that African American men were 1.5 times more likely to engage in physical aggression than white men (Straus, Gelles, & Steinmetz, 1980). More specifically, in the year prior to the survey, 16.9 percent of African American men used physical aggression against their partners, compared to 11.2 percent of white men. But as we'll see later, when the responses were analyzed in terms of respondents' income levels, the differences between African Americans and whites were much less clear (Cazenave & Straus, 1992). Higher rates of physical aggression in African Americans were found only among lower-income respondents.

In another national survey of family violence, Hampton and Gelles (1994) also found that physical aggression was more common in African American men than in white men. Again they found, however, that physical aggression was most common among African Americans in lower-income levels.

In contrast to the results of the above studies, one large survey in Texas found higher rates of being physically beaten in African American than in white women. These findings held even after researchers controlled for age, education, income, and financial stress (Neff, Holaman, & Schluter, 1995). There were two critical differences in the study by Neff and his colleagues. First, the study was conducted with men and women who reported that they were regular drinkers—that is, they drank at least two to three times a month. Second, this study was conducted in only one state, whereas the other studies used nationally representative samples.

Think about the following questions:

1. If rates of wife abuse were reliably higher in African American than in white samples, what factors might account for such differences?
2. In what ways might alcohol use account for differences between the findings of the national surveys and those of the Texas study?

wives is generally not. Nonetheless, even if men don't report being in fear of their partners, men in physically violent relationships report significant negative impact of their wives' aggression (Vivian & Langhinrichsen-Rohling, 1994).

In nationally representative samples, rates of physical aggression by men and women are roughly equal, although women clearly experience more injuries than men in such encounters (Cantos, Neidig, & O'Leary, 1994). You might think that the rates of physical aggression by men and women would be the same, simply because women act in self-defense; however, the most commonly noted reasons college females give for engaging in physical aggression are jealousy, retaliation for emotional injury, and expression of anger (Folingstad, Wright, Lloyd, & Sebastian, 1991; Laner, 1983). In every study of dating aggression in which respondents have had the opportunity to list jealousy as a possible reason for the aggression, it has been the most frequently listed cause (Sugarman & Hotaling, 1989). Further, in the nationally representative community sample of married and cohabiting women, discussed earlier, self-defense was not the primary cause for women's engaging in physical aggression (Straus & Gelles, 1992). In general, in large community samples and even in couples seeking treatment for marital problems, self-defense is often not the reason given by females for engaging in physical aggression.

In couples in which women are severely abused and often injured, however, physical aggression by men is usually much more common than physical aggression by women, and when these women engage in physical aggression, it's generally in self-defense. Finally, many women who eventually murder their husbands have generally made repeated requests for help from the police and state that the murder was in self-defense (Police Foundation, 1976). In short, when men and women engage in lower levels of physical aggression, it often is not in self-defense. But as the frequency and severity of aggression increase, women are more likely to act in self-defense. Moreover, in such cases, women are much more likely than men to be injured (Cantos, Neidig, & O'Leary, 1994).

Do rates of physical aggression within marriage differ according to race or social class? A national survey appeared to indicate that African American men were more likely to engage in physical aggression than white men (Hampton & Gelles, 1994; Straus, Gelles, & Steinmetz, 1980). When the responses were analyzed in terms of the respondents' income levels, however, the differences between African Americans and whites were much less clear (Cazenave & Straus, 1992). Higher rates of physical aggression in African Americans were found only among lower-income respondents. Thinking about Multicultural Issues explores this topic further.

Clearly higher rates of physical aggression are reported among members of lower socioeconomic classes—that is, among people with less education and less income. But the truth is, partner abuse, child abuse, and elder abuse occur in *all* socioeconomic classes. Chief executive officers of large corporations, physicians, and professors may be violent. However, there is an elevated risk of partner abuse, child abuse, and elder abuse among persons who are poor and who hold low-prestige jobs (Gelles, 1993a). One of the explanations offered for higher rates of abuse of all types among people who are poor is the higher levels of stress they face. The more stressful factors an individual has to cope with, the more likely he will be abusive (Straus, 1992). The more stable an individual's living conditions, on the other hand, the less likely he will be to abuse his partner or child (Cazenave & Straus, 1992).

Rape

Definitions of **rape** vary somewhat across states, but generally, rape refers to unwanted or nonconsensual sexual activity that is forced or coerced against another individual (Koss, 1993). Rape victims range from young children to women in their 80s. According to a National Crime Victims Survey ("Unsettling Report," 1992), 1 in every 8 women in the United States is raped at some time in her life. Most of these individuals are young. The national survey revealed that 29 percent were under 11 years old, 32 percent were between ages 11 and 17, and another 22 percent were between ages 18 and 24.

The National Victims Center (NVC) ("Unsettling Report," 1992) surveyed 4,000 women in the United States and found that in almost 80 percent of cases, the woman knew the rapist. The most likely known rapist was an acquaintance; this was true in 29 percent of all cases. The next most likely was a relative (16 percent). Approximately 9 percent of women reported being raped by former or current husbands (see Figure 17.1).

Other findings showing the alarming scope of rape and related sexual aggression have come from a large-scale study of a national sample of 3,187 college students in 32 institutions throughout the United States (Koss, Gidycz, & Wisniewski, 1987). The results showed how widespread sexual aggression is. Approximately 28 percent of college women reported experiencing rape or attempted rape since age 14; approximately 15 percent reported being raped since the age of 14. And 54 percent claimed to have been sexually **victimized** in some way—for example, kissed or petted against their will.

Megan Kanka, an 8-year-old, was one tragic rape victim whose story was highly publicized. Megan lived with her family in the middle-class suburb of Hamilton Township, New Jersey. One Friday afternoon in the summer of 1994, a man who lived across the road from Megan invited her to come and see a new puppy he had bought. Once he had lured her into the house, he attacked her. She screamed and fought back, but she was no match for him. He raped Megan, strangled her to death, and dumped her body in the nearby woods. The man, Jesse Timmendequas, had twice been convicted of sexual assault in the past and had served a 6-year jail term for the second offense. No one in the community knew about his history of sexual violence, however.

rape Unwanted or nonconsensual sexual activity that is forced or coerced against another.

victimized Made the target of another's aggressive behavior.

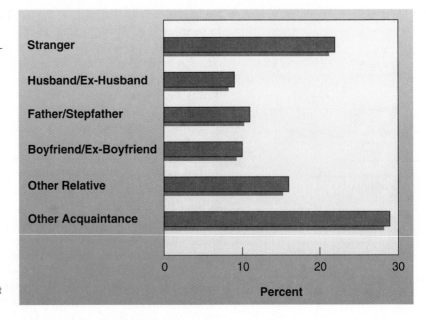

FIGURE 17.1 Relationship of victim and rapist (in percent)

Source: From *Time* Magazine, May 4, 1992. Copyright © 1992 Time, Inc. Reprinted by permission.

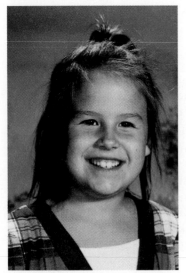

After Megan Kanka's murder, a law was created, mandating that when a child sex offender is released, the community must be forewarned. Although some states enforce such laws, a number have challenged them as being unconstitutional.

Megan's Law A New Jersey law that requires state prisons to notify community officials when convicted rapists and sexual offenders are released from prison and are about to enter the community.

This case enraged the community and led, in part, to **Megan's Law,** a New Jersey law that requires state prisons to notify community officials when convicted rapists and sexual offenders are released from prison and are about to enter the community. This law has been challenged in the courts, but according to New Jersey Assistant Attorney General Jane Grall, variations of it already exist in other states, such as Washington. See Thinking about Social Issues, which looks at societal versus individual rights.

Men are also victims of rape, although data on rapes of nonincarcerated men have been noticeably lacking until recently. Of the men who sought medical services for sexual assault in one study, the vast majority were from prisons; reports of sexual assault on males estimate that 1 to 3 percent of inmates are sexually assaulted (Lipscomb, Murman, Speck, & Mercer, 1992). To put the gender difference in a broader context, of over 1,700 adults seen for medical services at a non-hospital clinic for people who had been sexually assaulted, only 6 percent were males. Rape of men in dating relationships has been studied infrequently, but cases of men being raped by dating partners have been reported (Lane & Gwartney-Gibbs, 1985; Muehlenhard & Cook, 1988).

Throughout history, women in many societies have been considered as property and thus subject to their husbands' control, including sexual control. Even in more egalitarian societies, in which women enjoyed rights and freedoms, they were expected to be available to their husbands sexually, out of a sense of duty or obligation. Given this history, it's been considered virtually impossible for a husband to rape his wife (Whatley, 1993). Indeed, the first prosecution of a man for marital rape didn't occur in the United States until 1978 in Oregon.

A study of marital rape was conducted with a randomly selected sample of 644 women in San Francisco who were surveyed regarding any incident of sexual assault (Russell, 1982, 1990). Of the married women surveyed, 14 percent reported that they had been raped by their husbands. Other studies in the general population have revealed lower rates, ranging from 3 to 9 percent (Finkelhor & Yllo, 1983; Hanneke, Shields, & McCall, 1986; Pan, Neidig, & O'Leary, 1994). The exact percentages vary, in part because of differences in methods and varied definitions of rape. Nonetheless, it's clear that many wives report behaviors that technically meet legal definitions of rape, even though many of these women would not define the behaviors as rape.

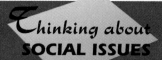

Societal versus Individual Rights:
What to Do with Sex Offenders Released from Prison

After the rape and murder of Megan Kanka, the state of New Jersey passed Megan's Law, which decreed that communities must be notified when sex offenders released from prison have taken up residence in them. Other states are following suit. People in favor of this legislation argue that Megan would still be alive today if her mother had known about the stranger who had moved into the house across the street. She would have ensured that Megan knew never to go into that house.

Opponents, however, denounce the law as an emotional reaction to the crime. They argue that once a rapist has served his time in jail, he should be as free as anyone else. Accordingly, they claim that notifying community residents of the offender's past is a form of discrimination that undermines his civil rights. These opponents point to the case of Melvin Carter, a serial rapist who was released from prison and planned to move to Alturas, California.

When residents found out about this, they threatened to kill Carter. He was barred from living in several communities. In other states, convicted sex offenders have been harassed in their homes. According to a spokesperson for the American Civil Liberties Union, "All these alerts do is cause anxiety among the public and make it impossible for the person to live in the community" (Hall, 1994).

Think about the following questions:

1. Megan's Law has already been challenged in New Jersey, and similar laws have been found unconstitutional in other states. Would you support some form of Megan's Law in your community? Why or why not?
2. What responsibilities, if any, would you place on the offender to notify community officials when there is a change of residence? Explain your answer.

Acquaintance Rape   Most rapes are perpetrated on women by men they know. The most common type of sexual assault by an acquaintance is called **date rape.** Like any other form of rape, date rape is unwanted or nonconsensual sexual activity that is forced or coerced against another (Koss, 1993). Men may use physical force or threaten it, but the most common means of obtaining unwanted sex in a dating relationship is by simply ignoring the woman's refusal, as illustrated in the following account:

> I was 15. I had heard about rape. I knew I was supposed to be careful and not trust strangers, but nobody told me to be afraid of my date. Tom was a senior on the baseball team and was from a nice, White, middle-class family. I didn't recognize it as rape at the time because he didn't hit me or yell at me. He just ignored me. He had sex with me while I was crying and saying no and asking, "Why are you doing this to me?" (Muehlenhard, Julsonnet, Carlson, & Flarity-White, 1989, p. 211)

What if no physical force is involved? What if a man persuades a woman to consent to sex in the heat of passion (perhaps after a few drinks) and then she regrets it the next morning? Is this seduction, or is it rape? *Rape* is defined as sex without consent. But what ensures that consent has been granted? Some critics denounce the idea of so-called politically correct sex. They ridicule the notion that partners should seek informed consent at each stage of a sexual encounter, arguing that this takes the passion and excitement out of lovemaking.

Feminists are divided on this issue. Some argue that prior consent should be obtained for every sexual act, maintaining that the man is totally responsible for sex: "It's the man's penis that is doing the raping, and ultimately he's responsible for where he puts it" (Koss, cited in Gibbs, 1991, p. 53). Other feminists argue that this view demeans women by depicting them as vulnerable and in need of protection against sexual activity (Roiphe, 1993).

date rape *Unwanted or nonconsensual sexual activity that is forced or coerced against a person by her dating partner.*

Table 17.1 lists a number of situations resulting in sex between men and women. Which would you consider rape? Check your opinions against those of the average American man and woman, as polled by *Time* (Gibbs, 1991).

TABLE 17.1	Sexual Situations That May Be Considered Rape			
			Rape	**Not Rape**
A man has sex with a woman who has passed out after drinking too much		FEMALE	88%	9%
		MALE	77%	17%
A married man has sex with his wife even though his wife does not want him to		FEMALE	61%	30%
		MALE	56%	38%
A man argues with a woman who does not want to have sex until she agrees to have sex		FEMALE	42%	53%
		MALE	33%	59%
A man uses emotional pressure, but no physical force, to get a woman to have sex		FEMALE	39%	55%
		MALE	33%	59%
			Yes	**No**
Do you believe that some women like to be talked into having sex?		FEMALE	54%	33%
		MALE	69%	20%

NOTE: Results of a telephone poll of 500 U.S. adults taken for *Time*/CNN on May 8, 1991; sampling error is plus or minus 4.5 percent. ("Not sures" were omitted.)

SOURCE: From *Time* Magazine, June 3, 1991. Copyright © 1991 Time, Inc. Reprinted by permission.

The Impact of Rape   Whether they resist or not, women who are raped are frequently beaten, too (Shields, Resick, & Hanneke, 1990). In some cases, such as that of Megan Kanka, they are even killed. Women who have been raped report more medical problems and visit physicians twice as often as other women (Koss, 1993). Researchers found that one week after a rape, 94 percent of women met criteria for the anxiety disorder called **posttraumatic stress disorder (PTSD);** after 3 months, 47 percent still met full criteria for posttraumatic stress disorder (Resick & Schnicke, 1993; also see Chapter 5). Listen to the psychological pain in the following account, in which a young woman describes her reaction to having been raped repeatedly by her brother's friend:

> When Mark raped me he also raped and manipulated my mind. I no longer trusted anyone, not even myself. I was bitter and angry at the world. I was also very frightened. I didn't feel safe anywhere, unless I was in the woods. I hated my bedroom. It had always been my safest place. It was where I was raped every time. I've been angry at him for taking that from me. For raping me on my own bed. I had to sleep in the bed for two more years. I took nothing with me when I moved out. All of those years of good memories were shattered. I felt nothing was sacred or special. I walked away from childhood, junior high, high school, college, and work friends. . . .
>
> After the rape . . . the world seemed distorted and grotesque. The majority of people are greedy, self-righteous scum. . . . I've turned some of this anger toward myself for letting the rape happen. This inward anger has created a war in my mind. This war took a lot of my self-confidence, esteem, and identity. (Calhoun & Resick, 1993, p. 67)

Child Abuse

Dear Dr. Fontana,

I am presently twenty-nine years old, White, female, married, and the mother of two children: Warren, age seven, and Dawn, age five. . . . To my neighbors I appear to be a well-balanced person, whom they are pleased to have living in their neighborhood.

To my husband, I am an uncommunicative, frigid wife who has no desire to socialize or to be sexually active with him. To my children, I am someone who

posttraumatic stress disorder (PTSD) *Syndrome that may be experienced following exposure to a traumatic stressor, such as rape; symptoms may include intrusive memories, numbing of sensations, and withdrawal.*

barely tolerates their presence; who walks around with the belt in hand, using it every time they step out of line, which is any time they are in my way or not being quiet; who constantly is verbally condemning them for something trivial they may have done; who violently attacks them, using my fists and wire kitchen whisks and kicking them with my feet and then leaving them where they lay, crumpled in pain and misery, to wonder what they could have done to warrant such punishment. Seeing in their eyes the question I asked myself when I was in their position, "How can you do this to me?" I ask myself the same question when I look upon their sleeping faces. "How can I do that to them if I love them?" But how can I love them and hate to be around them at the same time?

I promised God that I would never treat my children the way I was treated. Yet the violent cycle continues. Why can't I stop the wheel of abuse? I do not know. I have tried. (Fontana, 1991, p. 23)

Bedtime sucks when you have a history of being sexually abused. . . . For many kids, like me, the beginning of bedtime starts an inexorable journey down the pathway to hell. The demons wait. They coil behind bedposts, lurk in the doorways, and masquerade as harmless shadows.

At times, fatigue or pure determination will fight them off. You either drift off or raise a defiant shield: "I won't think about the bad stuff tonight. I won't," you proclaim. Sometimes this works. Sometimes.

But sooner or later the demons will clutch your soul and drag you back. Suddenly, you're there, where it all began. The abuse that is.

For me, I'm in my own bed. I can hear my mother's boyfriend, Ronald, swaying up the stairs. Mom's not home—she works the night shift at the post office.

Maybe tonight the drunken bastard will fall and crack his damn neck. But the bedroom door begins to creak open, and the profile of a grizzled, pathetic creature of a man now looms ominously on the bedroom wall. The door stops moving and he begins his approach.

"Gussy, boy—you awake?" (Appelstein, 1994, pp. 61–62)

You have just read about two of the most commonly discussed forms of **child abuse:** physical abuse and sexual abuse. These are the types of abuse that make news when they are discovered. However, the most common form of child abuse rarely makes the headlines, because it does not carry the same drama. The most prevalent form of child abuse is **neglect,** or inadequate supervision and lack of attention to the physical and emotional needs of the child. Another infrequently discussed form is **child emotional abuse,** a term that generally refers to being harsh, critical, and overly demanding of the child.

To be more specific, about half of all child abuse is neglect; approximately 25 percent is physical abuse. Roughly 15 percent of child abuse cases involve **child sexual abuse,** or sexual activity forced or imposed on a child. The remainder of the cases, about 10 percent, involve emotional abuse (Wolfe, 1987). Because physical abuse is the most common type of abusive behavior actively committed against a child and because physical violence is the core subject of this chapter, our major focus here will be on the physical abuse of children.

No specific behaviors define physical abuse of children. In fact, parenting styles vary so considerably across communities that it's necessary to consider the context of the parental behavior being examined. In general, however, physical abuse refers to nonaccidental injuries that result from the behavior of caretakers (Wolfe, 1987).

A very large study surveyed 2,000 parents across the United States about their discipline practices (Straus, 1994). In that survey, approximately 10 percent of parents reported that they engaged in violent behavior toward their children. In 1992, about 1,100 children in the United States died from abuse or neglect (Hansen, Conaway, & Christopher, 1990; Van Biema, 1994). In the same year, the Federal Bureau of Investigation (FBI) indicated that 662 children under 5 years of age were

child abuse Physical abuse, sexual abuse, emotional abuse, and/or neglect directed against a child.

neglect Failure of a parent or caregiver to provide minimal care and support for a child.

child emotional abuse Behavior that is harsh, critical, and overly demanding toward a child.

child sexual abuse Sexual activity imposed or forced on a child.

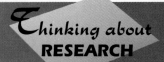

Thinking about RESEARCH — How Do Children Cope with Being Sexually Abused?

As discussed later in the text, being sexually abused clearly places children at risk for mental health problems. The fact is, however, that some sexually abused children show no abnormalities when assessed using common, standardized measures of child psychopathology. Depending on the study, as many as 20 to 50 percent of these children show no problems on such measures (Spaccarelli, 1994). How have these children been able to cope with being abused?

It seems that children who attempt to deal with their abuse directly have fewer problems than those who do not. In a retrospective study of children who had been sexually abused, Leitenberg, Greenwald, and Cado (1992) found that denial and suppression were both highly correlated with having psychological problems. Even though actively disclosing the abuse may be stressful in the short run, it seems beneficial in the long run (Wyatt & Newcomb, 1990). One technique often used in treatment programs is to have those who have been abused express their anger by writing unsent letters to their abusers. No studies have evaluated the usefulness of this therapeutic strategy, however.

Interviews with adults who were sexually abused as children show that they continue to search for meaning about what happened to them for many years; again, though, whether doing so helps them recover remains unclear. Some studies have found that the search for meaning is associated with fewer symptoms in adulthood, but in other studies, individuals who continued to search for meaning had lower levels of self-esteem and greater levels of psychological distress. Generally, women who remain distressed into adulthood require treatment that focuses on their feelings and reactions to the abuse.

Unfortunately, the underreporting of child sexual abuse makes it difficult to draw valid conclusions about how people are affected by this traumatic experience. Keep in mind that the cases of abuse most likely to be reported are those that are most serious, involving injury or repeated incidents. It follows that the children in these cases may be the most severely traumatized, as well. Obviously, from a research standpoint, this may not be a representative population. How to reach those other children poses a challenging problem.

Think about the following questions:

1. How would you design a study to assess the effects of having children who have been sexually abused write unsent letters to their abusers? How would you determine both the positive and negative effects of this technique?

2. How could researchers try to locate children who have been sexually abused but not reported it? Or is the problem of underreporting insurmountable, in terms of identifying a representative sample? Explain your answers.

---

murdered by their parents. In November 1994, Susan Smith confessed to killing her 2 children in Union, South Carolina. Michael Smith was 3 years old; Alex was 14 months. Following a trial that presented Susan's own childhood history of abuse, she was convicted and sentenced to life in prison.

When all types of abuse are considered, biological parents are the individuals most likely to be charged with child maltreatment. However, other caregivers—step-parents, foster parents, relatives—are more likely than parents to abuse children sexually. Women are reported for physical child abuse more than men; approximately 60 percent of reported cases involve abuse by women (Wolfe, 1987). These figures must be interpreted in light of the fact that women have the major child-rearing responsibilities, even in households with two parents. However, as is the case with partner abuse, the likelihood of injury is much higher when child abuse is perpetrated by a man than by a woman. Men are also more likely to sexually abuse children.

intergenerational transmission of violence Passing on of violence within a family from one generation to the next; for example, being the victim of physical abuse as a child increases the likelihood that a person will later engage in violent and/or abusive behaviors.

The Impact of Child Abuse   As noted earlier, children who are physically abused have a greater likelihood of engaging in violent and/or abusive behaviors as adults. It's becoming more evident that children who are exposed to multiple types of violence are most likely to become violent themselves. To put it another way, the probability of **intergenerational transmission of violence** increases with exposure to different types of violence. Individuals who were physically or sexually abused also have higher rates of attempted and completed suicides than others. What's more, the risk of suicide increases with repeated abuse (American Psychological Association, 1994).

Children who experience severe physical or sexual abuse have 3 times the risk of drug and alcohol abuse of the general population. In a study of substance abusers in Maine, 42 percent of the teen-age boys and approximately 80 percent of the teen-age girls reported experiencing sexual and/or physical abuse. Many clinicians have noted that abused children and teen-agers use alcohol and drugs to alleviate their sorrows. Professionals often refer to this pattern as *self-medicating* to cope with feelings of inadequacy and a sense of being different (American Psychological Association, 1994).

Anxiety symptoms in the form of posttraumatic stress disorder are also commonly found in children who have been severely abused. Such symptoms may include memories that intrude into the child's mind, even though they are stressful and unwanted. In addition, a numbing or deadening of sensations often occurs, because allowing sensations to come into consciousness may make the child anxious or depressed. Withdrawal is common, as well. Children who have been sexually abused may show changes in their blood chemistries years after the abuse (Putnam, 1994). For example, in one study, girls who were sexually abused had above-normal levels of cortisol, a hormone that is elevated in people who are depressed.

Children who have been abused typically have more academic problems than those who have not. As early as preschool, differences may be detected in academic performance and intellectual functioning. For example, in one study, abused children had IQ scores that were 20 points lower than those of nonabused children (Wolfe, 1987). As abused children grow older, they often have more school suspensions and more referrals to principals for discipline problems.

Although being abused puts children at greater *risk* for a variety of problems, some children fare better than others in dealing with their trauma. Thinking about Research looks at how children who have been sexually abused are able to cope.

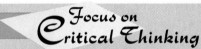

Focus on Critical Thinking

1. How would you design a study to assess whether children who have been physically abused engage in significantly more negative behaviors with their mothers and nonrelatives than nonabused children?

2. In addition, how could you evaluate whether children who are abused appear to push their mothers' emotional limits?

CAUSES

Before we consider some of the causes of partner abuse, note that there will be some overlap in discussing the causes of partner abuse, rape, and child abuse. For example, attitudes that justify physically aggressive behavior are common factors in all three types of violence. Similarly, coming from a violent background and living in poverty are risk factors for all three. On the other hand, a variety of other factors also predict whether a person will engage in one form of violence or another.

Partner Abuse

Let's consider three general perspectives on the causes of partner abuse: feminist accounts, psychological explanations, and biological explanations.

Feminist Accounts   The major tenet of the feminist accounts of partner abuse is that men use their power to gain control over women—and that this practice is supported, both explicitly and implicitly, by the institutions of society. As Bograd (1988) stated, "As feminists we believe that the social institutions of marriage and family are special contexts that may promote, maintain, and even support the men's use of physical force against women" (p. 12). From this perspective, the cause of physical aggression in marriage is the power men derive from their privileged position in society. Indeed, for some, the overarching issue in understanding wife abuse is **patriarchy,** a social system in which males have a dominant position relative to females (Schecter, 1988; Yllo, 1993).

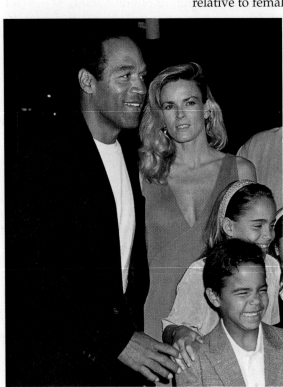

In what's been called the "Trial of the Century," O. J. Simpson was acquitted of murdering his ex-wife, Nicole Brown Simpson, and her friend, Ronald Goldman. In trying to prove its case, the prosecution established a history of partner abuse. To some, the outcome of this case showed society's unwillingness to take wife abuse seriously.

According to Yllo (1993), the general picture that emerges from interviews with women who have been battered is one of domination. This is the picture depicted in the following account of a 31-year-old woman, who described the violence in her home that eventually resulted in her having a miscarriage:

> I didn't even realize he was gaining control and I was too dumb to know any better. . . . He was gaining control bit by bit until he was checking my panty hose when I came home from the supermarket to see if they were inside out. . . . He'd time me. He'd check the mileage on the car. . . . I was living like a prisoner. One day I was at [the store] with him . . . and I was looking at a sweater. He insisted I was looking at a guy. I didn't even know there was a guy in the area, because it got to the point that I had to walk like I had horse blinders on. . . . You don't look anybody in the eye. You don't look up because you're afraid. (Yllo, 1993, p. 56)

After being insulted by one of her husband's friends, she became furious. She remembered the scene as follows:

> I told him, "Who the hell was he?" And I threw a glass of root beer in his face. My husband gave me a back hand, so I just went upstairs to the bedroom and got into a nightgown. And he kept telling me to come downstairs and I said, "No, just leave me alone." . . . He came up and went right through the door. Knocked the whole top panel off the door and got into the room. Ripped the nightgown right off my back, just bounced me off every wall in that bedroom. Then he threw me down the stairs and . . . outside in the snow and just kept kicking me and saying it was too soon for me to be pregnant. . . . His friend was almost rooting him on. (Yllo, 1993, p. 56)

The tendency of men to use **coercion,** or controlling force, appears most evident when the aggression is severe, according to a study of men who requested marital treatment with their partners (Cascardi & Vivian, 1995). However, lesbian violence appears to be as frequent as heterosexual violence, and patriarchy cannot be easily used to explain such aggression (Dutton, 1994). Even Yllo (1993) has noted that a challenge to the feminist position is the question of why so few men batter at all, given the supposed advantages to be gained from battering.

patriarchy A form of social organization in which power is held by and transferred through males.

coercion Threats, force, and other psychological means used to attempt to control another.

Psychological Explanations Psychological explanations of partner abuse have generally been of two varieties: (1) individual accounts about the pathology of the people involved in the physically abusive relationship and (2) relationship accounts of how the interactions of the couple lead to physically abusive acts. These two accounts need not be mutually exclusive. That is, both accounts could help explain why an individual or a couple engages in physically aggressive behavior. In general, however, certain research groups tend to emphasize one account over the other.

Individual Explanations of Women's Behavior   Psychological accounts of partner abuse have changed dramatically across the last few decades. In the 1970s, accounts of wife abuse centered on masochism on the part of the women—that is, women's self-suffering and even self-destructive behavior (Snell, Rosenwald, & Robey, 1964). Specifically, it was believed that battered women had personalities that led them to be with partners who would abuse them. The concept of masochism, or **masochistic personality disorder,** as an explanation for partner abuse has fallen into disrepute for two reasons: The concept was used inappropriately to blame the woman for the abuse she received, and there was no empirical evidence that, in fact, these women were masochistic.

In the 1990s, there was a surge of interest in posttraumatic stress disorder (PTSD). We've already seen that PTSD occurs in veterans of the Vietnam War and in victims of rape. Research on PTSD has also been extended to people who have been physically abused by their mates. About 35 to 45 percent of physically abused women now receive a PTSD diagnosis (Houskamp & Foy, 1991). In women who seek refuge in shelters, the rates of PTSD appear to be even higher. In one study, the types of symptoms most frequently reported by physically abused women with PTSD were irritability or outbursts of anger (94 percent), emotional distress at reminders of the aggressive episode (81 percent), decreased interest in activities (81 percent), detachment from other people (75 percent), and problems concentrating (75 percent). Of physically abused women who were not diagnosed with PTSD, only avoidance of thoughts and feelings associated with abuse (30 percent) and emotional distress at reminders of the abuse occurred with any notable frequency (Cascardi, O'Leary, Schlee, & Lawrence, 1995).

Even though a PTSD diagnosis may be very relevant for certain abused women, it's certainly not relevant for everyone. The other most relevant diagnosis for women who have been physically abused is depression. In one study, approximately 40 percent of physically abused women received a diagnosis of major depressive disorder, a primary depression diagnosis (Cascardi et al., 1995). In addition, evidence is rapidly accumulating that the more severe the abuse, the greater the depression. Finally, evidence has suggested that childhood emotional abuse contributes to current states of depression for women who are in discordant marriages and/or who have been physically abused by their husbands.

Today, diagnosis focuses on the effects the abuse may have had on a woman, such as making her fearful or depressed. Even the use of alcohol and drugs is often thought to be a way for an abused woman to numb herself to her day-to-day negative experiences. Of course, it's also possible that some women may bring their own problems (such as alcohol abuse or depression) to a relationship and that these problems might lead to deterioration of the intimate relationship and eventually to physical abuse. Only longitudinal research will answer that question.

Individual Explanations of Men's Behavior   Several studies in the late 1980s and early 1990s indicated that men who are physically abusive had personality patterns that reflected various types of pathology. As a group, physically abusive men have elevated scores on various measures of personality dysfunction, even though these men cannot be said to exhibit a specific battering profile. Such men score in the pathological range on scales relating to aggressiveness and to a negativistic style of interacting (Hamberger & Hastings, 1991). Further, there is increasing agreement that individuals who engage in minor and isolated acts of physical aggression against their partners are quite different from those who engage in repeated and severe acts of aggression (Holtzworth-Munroe & Stuart, 1994; O'Leary, 1993).

Other analyses have indicated that physically abusive men have very high levels of negative emotion and a great investment in maintaining the marital relationship. In contrast, men who are unhappy in their relationships but are not physically

masochistic personality disorder Former diagnostic label used to characterize self-defeating behavior; individuals with this personality disorder diagnosis (which no longer exists) were thought to be drawn to situations or relationships in which they would suffer.

Integrating Perspectives
A Biopsychosocial Model

PERSPECTIVE ON PARTNER ABUSE

BIOLOGICAL FACTORS

Biological factors contribute to violent behavior but are generally not by themselves sufficient causes of such behavior:

➤ Age is associated with all forms of violent behavior. Younger people engage in violent behavior more frequently than older people.
➤ The rate of head injury is higher than average among men who abuse their partners.
➤ In rare cases, brain tumors can trigger violent behavior.
➤ Alcohol and drug abuse are associated with partner abuse, especially severe cases.

PSYCHOLOGICAL FACTORS

Psychological factors interact with biological factors in producing violent behavior:

➤ Individuals who believe that aggressive actions against others are justified are most likely to engage in various forms of violent behavior.
➤ Men's use of power and control over women is associated with abuse and rape.
➤ Marital discord is highly associated with partner abuse.
➤ Individual psychopathologies—especially personality disorders characterized by aggression—elevate the risk of all forms of violence.

SOCIAL FACTORS

Biological and psychological factors operate in specific social contexts:

➤ Individuals in all socioeconomic classes engage in violent behavior, but poverty and unemployment elevate the risk of abuse.
➤ Patriarchy, a social system in which males have a dominant position relative to females, appears to be a prominent cause of abuse.
➤ The portrayal of violence in the media may encourage or justify a variety of aggressive behaviors but does not cause such behaviors.

These biological, psychological, and social factors interact to cause problems, as illustrated in the following case:

Jack, age 24, had been married only 2 years when he became suspicious of his wife's interest in one of their friends. Jack had lost his job with the closing of an aerospace firm and began to drink heavily several evenings a week. His wife began to work to help pay some of their debts, and occasionally, she'd go out to eat with some of her girlfriends. One night, when she returned at 1:00 A.M., Jack accused her of having an affair. She cursed at him and got "into his face." In turn, he slapped her hard several times. She kicked him and ran out of the house.

Jack's parents divorced when he was 10 years old, and he had seen his parents fight a lot, although only verbally. Nonetheless, his mother told him that one of the reasons for the divorce was fighting and being criticized. Jack vowed not to do that with his wife, but he felt he couldn't stand by and watch his wife have an affair. Though he knew hitting her was wrong, his anger overwhelmed him and he slapped his wife.

The biopsychosocial model helps explain the problem. The role of biological factors is illustrated in Jack's drinking to calm himself yet actually engaging in the aggressive behavior while drinking heavily. Like other aggressive behaviors, physical abuse occurs most often in young men. Psychological factors are most evident in Jack's increasing suspiciousness of an affair and the resulting intense jealousy. In turn, the jealousy often leads to heated arguments with his wife and a marriage marked by serious discord. Finally, unemployment due to the closing of the aerospace firm illustrates the social contribution to Jack's problems.

aggressive toward their wives show moderate levels of negative emotion and much less investment in maintaining their marriages. In brief, it appears that men who are physically abusive resort to coercive control strategies, whereas nonviolent men who are unhappy in their marriages withdraw from such relationships (Murphy, Meyer, & O'Leary, 1994).

The role of alcohol in causing aggression has been debated for years. In fact, the belief that alcohol abuse caused child maltreatment was a factor leading to Prohibition (Gelles, 1993b). Many professionals believe that alcohol is not merely a contributing factor but a cause of abuse of both women and children. The central argument is that alcohol is a disinhibitor, which releases aggressive tendencies. As Gelles (1993b) aptly stated, alcohol is seen as a "superego solvent"—it reduces inhibitions and allows violence to emerge. A large body of data supports the association between alcohol and family violence. For example, if we look at samples of batterers, we'll find that they have rates of alcohol abuse (that is, frequent intoxication and/or negative occupational and family consequences from alcohol use) ranging from approximately 25 to 50 percent. In addition, alcohol consumption and physical aggression against women are associated in large representative community populations.

In a nationally representative sample of approximately 2,500 married and/or cohabiting men and women (Kantor & Straus, 1990), there was a straightforward association between alcohol and man-against-woman aggression. In particular, the men who had "High" (3 or more drinks daily and/or drinks 3 to 4 times per week) or "Binge" (5 or more drinks a day) levels of drinking were definitely at greatest risk for abusing their partners. On the other hand, when investigators assessed whether alcohol was used at the time of a physically aggressive incident, they found that it was used by one or both partners in only 24 percent of the cases.

Cross-cultural data have indicated that in some cultures, men become more aggressive after drinking, whereas in other cultures, they become more passive (MacAndrew & Edgerton, 1969). Thus, alcohol itself is not a necessary or sufficient condition for being physically aggressive against a partner. Many social scientists believe that people behave as they think they are expected to behave when drinking. If the cultural belief is that you should become passive when drinking, you will become passive. If the cultural belief is that alcohol releases violent urges, then people who drink may act violently.

Relationship Explanations   Some researchers have concluded that in physically aggressive relationships, the interactions between the partners are central in the escalation pattern that finally results in physical aggression (Margolin, Sibner, & Gleberman, 1988; Neidig & Friedman, 1984; O'Leary, 1988). Researchers have also noted that marital dissatisfaction is the best predictor of physical aggression in marriage (Pan, Neidig, & O'Leary, 1994). In fact, it's more important than any other social factor (age, class, race) or psychological factor (depression or general stress). Since at least half of all the aggression observed in couples seeking treatment or in community samples is characterized by mutual aggression (that is, both the man and the woman engage in the physical aggression), researchers also believe that the abusive pattern is not likely to stop unless long-term dissatisfaction can be resolved. Numerous studies have indicated that the communication patterns of men and women in physically abusive relationships are different from those of people in nonabusive relationships (Margolin et al., 1988; Vivian & O'Leary, 1987).

Biological Explanations   Mounting evidence suggests that some biological factors may contribute to physical aggression against partners. We'll review five biological variables that are often implicated in the development of partner abuse: (1) brain injury; (2) testosterone; (3) physiological reactivity; (4) evolutionary factors; and (5) genetic factors.

Brain Injury   Family members of men who have brain injuries often report that the injured men have outbursts of rage, irritability, and reduced impulse control. Research has found that men who physically injure their partners are more likely to have had brain injuries than those who have not (Rosenbaum et al., 1994). Specifically, 61 percent of men attending a court-ordered treatment program to decrease battering of their partners had experienced significant head injuries (Rosenbaum & Hoge, 1989). Because this research suggested that brain injury might possibly cause partner abuse, the research team conducted a follow-up study, comparing men who were very unhappy in their relationships and physically abusive toward their partners with men who had very unhappy marriages but were not physically abusive toward their wives (Rosenbaum et al., 1994). The professionals conducting the neurological assessments didn't know which men were abusive and which were not. Fifty-three percent of the batterers, 25 percent of the dissatisfied nonviolent men, and 16 percent of the satisfied nonviolent men had experienced head injuries. Clearly, head injury and partner battering were associated.

Testosterone   Blood analyses have indicated that testosterone levels are 10 times higher in males than in females. The hormone testosterone accounts for a number of male characteristics, such as deepening of the voice and growth of body hair. Castration—that is, removal of the source of testosterone—has been found to reduce aggression in a variety of male animals, and testosterone injections have been found to reinstate aggressive behavior (Huntingford & Turner, 1987). Thus, it was very natural to expect that testosterone would cause or be correlated with aggression in men. However, reviews of the research have indicated that the relationship between testosterone and aggression is weak (Baron & Richardson, 1994).

Physiological Reactivity   Physiological reactivity of physically abusive men has been studied by Jacobson and his colleagues (1994) and by Gottman and his colleagues (1995). They found that, on average, physically abusive men do not differ physiologically from maritally discordant nonabusive men. However, in about 20 percent of the physically abusive men, their heartrates *declined* while they were in heated discussions with their partners about marital problems. These men were also seen as probably being unresponsive to treatment and as being similar to psychopaths in their physiological responding (Goleman, 1994b).

Evolutionary Factors   Another area of research on possible biological causes of partner abuse is in evolutionary analysis of aggressive behavior (Archer, 1994; Daly & Wilson, 1988). The most noted analysis of partner abuse taking this approach was made by Daly and Wilson (1988), who analyzed homicide statistics. The basic premise of their theory is that men and women attempt to maximize their gene potential. That is, they try to maximize the likelihood of having good offspring. In support of this view, the investigators found that men and women kill their step-children more frequently than they kill their own children. The review by Daly and Wilson (1988) also reported data showing that men kill their estranged wives more often than estranged wives kill their husbands. This finding led the investigators to conclude that jealousy is the leading motive in spousal homicide. Data on the murder of wives is consistent with the evolutionary view that males are interested in protecting their own gene pool from being mixed with those of others—that is, "If I can't have her, nobody else can."

The data on homicide are consistent with an evolutionary view; however, other interpretations would also fit these data. First of all, marital dissatisfaction has been found to correlate highly with severe partner abuse. Alcohol and drug abuse have also been found to correlate significantly with severe spouse abuse (Pan, Neidig, & O'Leary, 1994), as has low socioeconomic status (Straus, Gelles, & Steinmetz, 1980). Evolutionary interpretations provide an alternative to the often discussed sociological and psychological views of homicide data. But it remains to be seen whether the evolutionary view can shed light on factors that might help resolve the problem and/or can be linked to variables like jealousy or other psychological variables thought to be crucial to this view.

Genetic Factors   For decades, some researchers have tried to find a genetic explanation for aggressive and violent behavior, whereas others have tried to minimize its role. According to animal behaviorists Huntingford and Turner (1987), some differences in aggressive behavior can be ascribed to genetic influences. However, these researchers have noted that the role of genes in the aggressive behavior of humans is small compared to that of environment. Twin studies in the United States and Canada have provided strong evidence of genetic influences on self-reported aggressive personality traits (Plomin, 1990). Although these studies have not assessed violent behavior directly, most of the data from them regarding self-reported personality styles strongly suggest that violent behavior is influenced by genetic factors. The twin study data on concordance rates for criminal convictions (see Chapter 14) also support this conclusion.

Rape

There are a number of different perspectives regarding what causes rape. In the following sections, we'll consider (1) feminist accounts, (2) deviant sexual arousal, (3) violent pornography, and (4) miscommunication or provocation.

Feminist Accounts   Susan Brownmiller (1975) proposed a feminist view of rape that has influenced much of the thinking in this area. In her view, "Man's discovery that his genitalia could serve as a weapon to generate fear must rank as one of the most important discoveries of prehistoric times, along with the use of fire and the first crude stone axe. From prehistoric times to the present, I believe, rape has played a critical function. It is nothing more or less than a conscious process of

"Take back the night" is the rallying cry of women as they unite to raise awareness about rape.

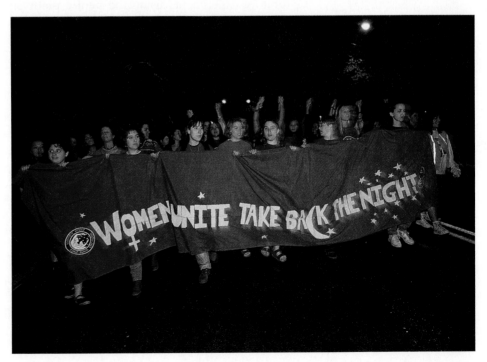

intimidation by which all men keep all women in a state of fear" (p. 5). Brownmiller pointed out that historically, women were punished as often as their attackers and that greater concern existed for women's fathers and husbands than for the women themselves.

Support for this view comes from the recent conflict in Bosnia-Herzogovina. As part of what has been called *ethnic cleansing,* Bosnian Serbs are reported to have systematically raped Muslim women, young and old, by the thousands in order to demoralize and destabilize Bosnian Muslim society. That is, the rapes were intended not just to hurt females but to upset the men and tear apart the family fabric (because women who have been raped may get thrown out of their families).

A major contribution of Brownmiller and other feminist theorists has been to emphasize the violence in rape. The data have supported this *rape-as-violence* view. Rapists are much more likely to have histories of nonsexual criminal and aggressive activity than nonrapists (Hall & Hirschman, 1991). A large proportion of adolescent sex offenders, particularly rapists, have histories of conduct disorder (Becker, 1988).

Malamuth and his colleagues have hypothesized that two main qualities distinguish college men who rape (Malamuth, Sockloskie, Koss, & Tanaka, 1991). The first is what they call *hostile masculinity.* This includes hostility toward women, violent tendencies, a need to dominate women, and arousal to sexually aggressive material. The second quality is early sexual promiscuity, which the researchers have interpreted as reflecting the male's use of frequent sex to prove his masculinity. A study of over 3,000 male college students showed that those rated higher on hostile masculinity and sexual promiscuity had greater rates of sexual aggression (Malamuth et al., 1991).

Rape As Deviant Sexual Arousal?   The rape-as-violence view can be contrasted with the rape-as-deviant-sexual-arousal theory. According to the sexual arousal perspective, the urge to rape is really a **paraphilia,** or arousal or turn-on in response to deviant acts or objects (see Chapter 8). That is, the rapist is aroused by the use of force and humiliation, rather than by attraction or love.

Support for the rape-as-deviant-sexual-arousal hypothesis has come from laboratory experiments using the **penile plethysmograph.** This instrument, which measures features of male erections, has been used to identify specific cues that trigger arousal in rapists (Abel, Barlow, Blanchard, & Guild, 1977). Rapists and nonrapists in one study listened to two different types of audiotapes. One tape gave a detailed description of mutually enjoyable intercourse with an enthusiastic partner. The other described the forcible rape of the same partner, who expressed physical pain and emotional distress. Both the rapists and nonrapists showed sexual arousal to the descriptions of mutually consenting sex. Only the rapists, however, showed significant degrees of **tumescence** (enlargement of penis due to increased bloodflow) in response to the rape cues.

A number of studies have shown that rapists' sexual arousal patterns are different from those of nonrapists (Barbaree, Marshall, & Lanthier, 1979; Quinsey & Chaplin, 1984). For instance, rapists have demonstrated more sexual arousal to rape stories than nonrapists. On the other hand, attempts to replicate these findings have often failed to show differences between rapists and controls in response to cues of sexual violence (Barbaree & Marshall, 1991). One reason for the different results of some studies may be that many sex offenders can voluntarily inhibit their erections to pedophilic (sexual arousal involving children) or rape stimuli (Hall, 1991).

Ellis (1991), however, has cited several findings to support the view that rape is motivated by normal sexual urges. He has argued that men who commit date rape are motivated to have sex and resort to force only as a last resort. Men guilty of date rape are more likely than nonrapists to report histories of using deception

paraphilia Sexual disorder in which the individual is sexually aroused by unconventional acts or odd objects.

penile plethysmograph Device that measures changes in size of the penis during arousal.

tumescence Engorgement of the penis during sexual arousal.

and attempts to get their dates intoxicated so as to have sex (Kanin, 1985). Moreover, many males who coerce women into sex do not report greater hostility toward women or a desire to humiliate them than do males who only engage in mutually consenting sex (Craig, Kalichman, & Follingstad, 1989).

Portrayals of Violent Pornography   Teen-agers commit a disproportionately large number of rapes and other forms of sexual violence (Davis & Leitenberg, 1987). Given this fact, antipornography groups claim that one factor that contributes to rape is the explicit association between sex and violence in movies, rock videos, and music lyrics.

Marshall and his colleagues (cited in Marshall, Seidman, & Barbaree, 1991) studied this possibility in the laboratory. They first exposed male university students to short videotaped scenes of either mutually consenting sex, rape, or nonsexual situations. The researchers then had the students listen to audiotapes of consenting sex and forcible rape while their erectile responses were measured with the penile plethysmograph. The students who had seen the rape videos showed reduced discrimination between the audiotaped rape and the mutually consenting sex stimuli. The researchers have suggested that repeated exposure to violent pornography might reduce the likelihood of a man responding appropriately when the woman indicates that she does not consent to sex.

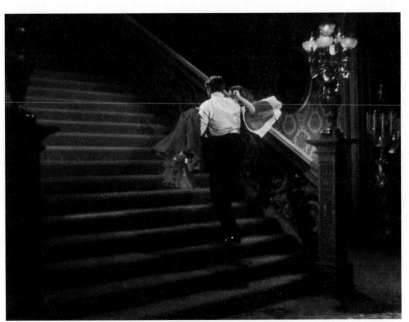

In the movie Gone with the Wind, *the scene in which Rhett Butler (Clark Gable) carries Scarlett O'Hara (Vivian Leigh) up the stairs has been the subject of controversy. How would you interpret this scene: as romantic or as an act of forced sex?*

Miscommunication or Provocation? Is date rape a form of miscommunication between a man and woman? Males are expected to pursue sex; women are expected to offer resistance. The "scenario where a forceful man continues a sexual advance despite a woman's protests, until she melts in compliance" occurs commonly in books and movies. This sexual script, Muehlenhard has contended, may give men the message that although a woman says no, she really means yes (Goleman, 1989).

Decoding these sexual signals may be especially difficult if the couple has been drinking. Some argue that alcohol causes men to be sexually aggressive, whereas women who drink are often believed to be more sexually available (George, Gournic, & McAfee, 1988). However, the explanation given in the previous paragraph does not square with the facts. According to many experts, date rape is sexual violence, not miscommunication.

Child Abuse

The factors that lead to partner abuse and the factors that lead to child abuse have clear similarities. As you might expect, men who abuse their children are more likely to abuse their wives, too (Gelles, 1993a; O'Leary, 1993). On the other hand, many adults engage in abusive behavior toward their children but do not engage in such behavior toward their partners. The following subsections cover several risk factors that have been repeatedly associated with child abuse.

Poverty Child abuse occurs among people of all socioeconomic levels but is most common among people who are poor. Parents who live with the effects of poverty—such as the stress of the phone being removed or the heat being turned off—are much more likely to abuse their children than parents who have sufficient money. Children from families with incomes lower than $15,000 are abused almost 7 times more often than children from higher-income families (Wolfe, 1987).

Neglect, in particular, is strongly associated with poverty. Wolfe (1987) examined physical abuse and neglect reports across the United States and found that 48 percent of the parents charged with neglect were receiving public assistance. In comparison, 34 percent of the parents charged with physical abuse were receiving public assistance. Also, children in the United States are much more likely to live in poverty than children in many other nations comparable on other factors. For example, the U.S. child poverty rate is more than *double* the average of the rates of Canada, England, France, Netherlands, Sweden, and Germany (Children's Defense Fund, 1991). Furthermore, a recent study conducted by researchers in Luxembourg found that children in the United States are worse off economically than children in all 18 Western industrialized nations, except Israel and Ireland (Bradsher, 1995).

The rate of child poverty is disproportionate across racial and ethnic groups in the United States. In 1987, 39 percent of Hispanic children and 45 percent of African American children lived in poverty, compared with just 15 percent of white children (U.S. Department of Commerce, 1987). As you might expect, children in families maintained by a woman with no husband present were most likely to live in poverty. Indeed, more than half of the single-parent families maintained by mothers lived in poverty. Once again, the rates were disproportionate across racial/ethnic groups: 54 percent of African American children lived with single parents compared to 30 percent of Hispanic children and 19 percent of white children. There were similar differences among children living in cities, suburbs, and rural areas. In 1987, 30 percent of the children in cities lived in poverty, compared with 22 percent of those in rural areas and 13 percent of those in suburbs.

Age of Caregiver Young mothers are at greatest risk for abusing their children. In Ontario, Canada, across a 10-year period, 95 percent of mothers reported to a child protection agency for abuse or neglect had become parents before they were 20 years old. This finding and related research have shown that young, single mothers who lack family and social support are at greatest risk for actively abusing their children (Peterson & Brown, 1994). Most parents who are reported for neglect, too, are single parents—most often, mothers.

Caregiver Psychopathology When professionals first wrote about the causes of child abuse, they thought that abusive parents had emotional and psychological problems that led them to hurt their children. But in fact, no particular personality profile describes an abusive parent—just as no specific type of man abuses his wife. On the other hand, research is beginning to show that parents who abuse children and/or their partners may have similar personality styles. Abusive individuals are impulsive and have general problems with anger control (O'Leary, 1993; Wolfe, 1987). In addition, mothers who are very dissatisfied with their marriages or cohabitating relationships and who are depressed are at risk for severely injuring their children. In fact, if mothers are dissatisfied with their relationships or are depressed, their children are 4 times more likely to be abused than children of mothers without these risk factors (Brown & Davidson, 1978).

Alcohol and drug abuse have also been identified as significant risk factors for child abuse. Indeed, research has repeatedly shown that parents who abuse alcohol and drugs are more likely to abuse their children than parents who do not abuse these substances. In a National Clinical Evaluation study, substance abuse was one of the best predictors of child maltreatment (Berkeley Planning Associates, 1983). In another study, approximately 75 percent of women who abuse their children reported having problems with alcohol/ drug abuse (O'Keefe, 1995).

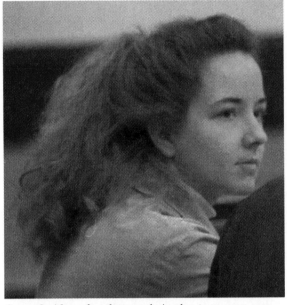

Susan Smith confessed to murdering her two young sons. Her lawyers prepared a defense that emphasized a long history of sexual abuse, depression, and suicidal thoughts. The jury seemed to accept this somewhat and gave her a life sentence, not the death penalty. What would you have done?

Caregiver History of Being Abused As a Child   Parents who abuse their children are more likely to have been abused themselves than parents who do not abuse their children. As mentioned earlier, this phenomenon, which has been found repeatedly, has become known as the *intergenerational transmission of violence*. Basically, the notion is that if a parent abuses a child, the child, in turn, will be more likely to abuse his children. Of course, not every abused child will grow up to be an abuser. Similarly, a boy who observes his father hit his mother will not necessarily abuse his own wife later. The general finding that being abused or observing abuse leads to later abusive behavior is often hotly debated. Many researchers feel that abusers may misinterpret these results as providing an excuse for violent behavior (Gelles & Loseke, 1993).

If you happen to have been abused, it's important to recognize that a risk factor simply *places someone at risk* for developing a problem or engaging in certain behaviors (in this case, abusive behaviors). Having a risk factor for a problem doesn't mean that you necessarily will develop the problem. In fact, some people develop insight about problems they are at risk for and take precautions to minimize the likelihood of developing the problem.

Unrealistic Expectations of Children   Abusive parents tend to overestimate their children's abilities to take care of themselves, to wait patiently, and to behave properly (Azar & Rohrbeck, 1986). These unrealistic expectations lead parents to get angry at their children and become physically abusive when the expectations are not met—for example, if children wet the bed, cry and have temper tantrums, or play with matches. As you might expect, abusive parents are much more likely than nonabusive parents to use harsh verbal and physical punishment when they perceive a child as misbehaving. In addition, insufficient supervision—neglect of parental duties—often leads to injuries of the children.

Child Factors   Parents are most likely to abuse children who are less than 4 years old. Teen-agers are the next most likely age group to be abused and neglected.

Very young children with irregular sleeping patterns and poor eating habits frustrate parents and are at risk for being abused. A child with a conduct disorder who defies authority and has temper outbursts is also at risk for abuse. Children with problems of hyperactivity and distractibility present significant problems for their parents, and they, too, are more likely to be abused. Indeed, impulsivity is one of the most commonly noted characteristics of abused children (Peterson & Brown, 1994).

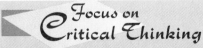

Focus on Critical Thinking

1. Poverty is one of the largest predictors of child abuse, yet lack of money by itself does not cause parents to be abusive. What factors closely associated with poverty might more directly cause child abuse? Explain your answer.

2. Contrast the rape-as-violence view with the rape-as-deviant-sexual-arousal view. Which do you most agree with? Why?

TREATMENT

Partner Abuse

Treatment for problems of partner abuse can be accomplished in several ways. You can treat the woman, the man, or both. In any treatment, safety of the woman is primary; that issue must be addressed first, whether the woman, the man, or the couple is treated.

You may recall that Carolyn Sapp, Miss America of 1992, had great difficulty leaving her physically abusive partner, Nuu Faaola. He struck Carolyn repeatedly and even threatened to kill her. Because, like Carolyn, so many women have difficulty even admitting to being abused, assistance such as that provided by support groups is often needed to recognize the signs of abuse; to develop escape plans, if they are needed; and to begin to look at alternatives to the relationship. Many studies have found that even of those women who seek services in shelters for abused women, at least half return to their partners (Strube, 1988). In some cases, the major problems are financial, but in many, like Carolyn's, the major problem is an emotional tie to the abuser.

A woman may be provided individual and/or group counseling; in some cases, she is provided with a legal advocate, as well. In severe cases, the woman will be provided with a shelter in a secret location so that she may feel free from the harassment of her abuser. Usually, the goals of counseling for the abused woman are to decrease her self-blame for the physical abuse and to help her evaluate her relationship with her partner as it is—as well as alternatives to the relationship. Therapists work to help the woman see that physical aggression against her is never justified, and that even if her partner came from a violent home, he is not excused for any of his violence.

Treatment for a man who has abused his partner has traditionally been conducted in a group of men with similar problems. The goals of such programs are to reduce both the physical and the psychological aggression in the relationship. For the man to take full responsibility for his physical aggression against the woman— no matter what he reports the provocation by the woman to be—is a key first goal of the program. This goal is introduced in the beginning of any program, and because responsibility is so difficult for many men to accept, it's discussed periodically throughout most programs.

Programs also cover anger control techniques, like recognizing small anger cues that occur before the feelings of rage. In addition, they cover the feelings men have while engaging in aggression and the frequent feelings of remorse they have after the aggression. This emphasis on the cycle of feelings is designed to help men recognize the pattern and to help them learn to defuse the anger. Therapists help men understand the thoughts about their partners that make them especially angry ("She was unfaithful to me"; "She is a lazy slob") so that they can decrease the frequency of those thoughts—particularly in the presence of their partners. Aggressive men also learn how to express their feelings without being demanding and aggressive.

Couples treatment for problems of physical aggression is a relatively new phenomenon. It's designed for couples who want to stay together and for couples in which the woman is not afraid to express her opinions in the presence of her partner. It's not for couples in which the woman is terrorized or has been beaten severely and requires medical attention. Rather, couples therapy is for a very large number of couples who engage in low levels of physical aggression and who attend clinics throughout the United States.

In couples treatment, the emphasis is on how *each* partner may be contributing to the escalation of the physical aggression. In turn, each partner must accept responsibility for his or her physical aggression. A significant segment of almost any couples treatment is on increasing communication and enabling each partner to better express his or her feelings. The therapist helps the partners decrease name-calling, cataloging past wrongs, and labeling (for instance, calling the partner crazy, lazy, or evil). The therapist also encourages both the man and the woman to help understand what the real problems are that are contributing to the escalation of violence.

Some evidence supports the effectiveness of both individual treatment for men and women and couples treatment. Members of support groups for women who have experienced physical violence show significant improvements in self-esteem, less traditional attitudes toward marriage, and better relationship functioning (Tutty, Bidgood, & Rothery, 1993). In general, if a man completes a men's program designed to reduce physical aggression, his physical aggression will be lessened (Rosenbaum & Maiuro, 1990). Similarly, if a man completes a couples treatment program, his physical and psychological aggression will be lessened (O'Leary & Neidig, 1993). However, about half of the men who attend several initial treatment sessions never show up for later sessions and thus remain untreated—often even if mandated by the court to receive such therapy. Given the serious difficulty in treating physical aggression in intimate relations, it's important to develop prevention programs for young people when they begin dating.

Rape

Convicted rapists and other sexual offenders usually go to prison, where they are unlikely to receive any treatment. It has been estimated that between 50 and 75 percent of all incarcerated sex offenders get no treatment at all. New Jersey has a correctional institution devoted exclusively to the treatment of adult sex offenders—the Avenel Adult Diagnostic and Treatment Center. But an investigation of this center revealed that one-third of all the inmates refused psychological treatment (Nordheimer, 1994)! Jesse Timmendequas, the man who admitted to raping and killing Megan Kanka, was one of those who refused treatment. After serving his full term, he was released without any supervision or follow up.

What kind of treatment exists for rapists, and how effective is it? The investigation of the Avenel Center in New Jersey revealed that inmates received, on average, 4 hours of group psychotherapy a week (Nordheimer, 1994). Many saw a counselor for 90 minutes a week. Unfortunately, there is no evidence of how effective this minimal treatment is. Indeed, no one has ever evaluated it to see if it works. None of the techniques that have shown some success in treating paraphilias—suppression of deviant sexual arousal, self-control methods, cognitive restructuring, and **relapse prevention training** (see Chapter 10)—are systematically used at Avenel or at most institutions where rapists and other violent sex offenders are held.

Even if the most effective treatment techniques (Abel, Osborn, Anthony, & Gardos, 1992) are used, their long-term results are unclear or significant but small (Hall, 1995). We noted in Chapter 9 that in different studies, relapse rates have varied from 3 to 31 percent, depending on the length of follow-up (Abel et al., 1992). We know that rapists relapse more often than other paraphiliacs, such as child molesters (Pithers, Martin, & Cumming, 1989). And we know that the most violent and dangerous rapists are the least likely to benefit from treatment, although they are the offenders that society should fear the most. Finally, we know that once they are released from prison, violent rapists—who typically have not received any treatment—are very likely to repeat their crimes.

In 1990, the state of Washington did something about this. The state legislature passed the **Sexually Violent Predators (SVP) Law** (Brooks, 1994). It provides for the involuntary civil confinement of dangerous sex offenders after they have completed their prison sentences. During this confinement, the offenders receive treatment. They may eventually be released, if they are judged to be able to control their violent sexual impulses. The SVP Law has proved very controversial and has been

---

relapse prevention training Procedures aimed at reducing the likelihood that an individual will backslide and again begin engaging in an undesired behavior.

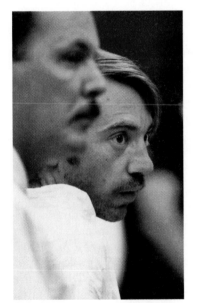

Jesse Timmendequas, the man who raped and murdered 8-year-old Megan Kanka, had already done time for sexual assault. Even though he refused treatment while in prison, he was released without supervision or follow up. Should the community have been forewarned?

Sexually Violent Predators (SVP) Law Involuntary civil confinement of dangerous sex offenders after they have completed their prison sentence.

challenged as unconstitutional. However, the supreme court in the state of Washington has rejected this challenge (Brooks, 1994).

What about rape victims? Their treatment often involves different types of group support and therapy, depending on individuals' needs. One of the most promising approaches involves using elements of exposure and anxiety management. During the exposure phase, the patient writes about the rape and then reads this description to the therapist. Later, the therapist asks the patient for more detail about aspects of the rape that were specified in the original account. The anxiety management involves teaching the patient to track her beliefs about intimacy and self-esteem and then helping her change or restructure beliefs that appear to be detrimental (Foa, Rothbaum, Riggs, & Murdock, 1991; Koss et al., 1994; Resick & Schnicke, 1992).

Child Abuse

Parents Anonymous   Parents Anonymous (PA) is a voluntary program for abusive or potentially abusive parents. PA is modeled after Alcoholics Anonymous (AA), in that the parents don't reveal their full identities; they don't give their last names and can even make up fictitious names. Like AA, PA does not encourage research about its effectiveness. Nevertheless, we note this program here because it exists in many communities throughout the United States. If you know an abusive parent or think you may be or have the potential to be, contact with this program may help you.

One way to deal with the problem of physical abuse and/or neglect of children is to treat people with parenting problems before they actually become abusive. A clear advantage of such an approach is that it's voluntary and does not involve a report about the parents to some child protective agency—unless the parent becomes abusive during the treatment program. You might think that teaching parents new ways of coping with their young children would be an easy task. A review of the literature, however, has indicated otherwise. Young parents who have already encountered serious problems coping with their children do change by decreasing or changing their use of punishment and increasing their use of positive parenting (Kendziora & O'Leary, 1993). However, such changes are often not maintained across time.

A more comprehensive view of dysfunctional parenting places this problem in the context of other factors that must be attended to if parenting programs are to be effective. More specifically, Dumas (1986) found that low income was the biggest factor that predicted poor response to treatment for parenting problems. Similarly, Webster-Stratton (1985) found that a combination of income level and negative events over the past year predicted with 73 percent accuracy whether the parent had met the treatment goal of reducing critical statements and negative behaviors by 50 percent. Discord between partners and depression are also associated with parenting problems. Effective treatment must consider parents in their total environment and the stresses they cope with. Dysfunctional or problem parenting may be only that for some parents—but for the majority of parents it may be one of many problems that require careful clinical assessment and multiple interventions.

In treating the families of children who have been physically abused, the primary focus has been on the parents. If the abuse is not so severe as to require removing the child from the home, treatment can be directed at helping the parents learn better coping and discipline strategies and hopefully preventing any further physical abuse. However, since children who are physically abused are at risk for having social skills deficits as well as problems with anxiety, anger, and aggression, they often need professional attention, as well. Unfortunately, reviews have shown that little systematic research exists on the effectiveness of treatment programs for

Parents Anonymous (PA)
Voluntary program for parents who think they are abusive or have the potential for abusing their child; program is modeled after Alcoholics Anonymous, in that the individuals do not reveal their full identities.

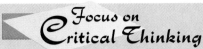

Focus on Critical Thinking

1. How much do you think women who cope successfully with rape think about the incident? Do you think that after a few months, some women simply repress their memories of being raped? Explain your answers.

2. Children who have been physically abused have higher levels of anxiety, depression, and conduct problems. Even so, relatively little research has documented the effectiveness of treatment for such children. Instead, research has focused on the abusive parents with the goal of preventing further abuse. What steps should be taken to ensure that children who are physically abused obtain the services they need?

physically abused children (Hansen, Conaway, & Christopher, 1990).

At the broad policy level, multidisciplinary efforts have been advocated, in which medical, psychological, educational, social, and legal professionals collaborate to help all family members. One such program that has been demonstrated effective was developed by Lutzker and Rice (1984). It provides training for children who are lagging in developmental skills (such as toilet training and bicycle riding), and for parents, it provides self-control training, marital counseling, alcohol treatment referral, social support groups, training in job interview skills, and prevention services for unwed mothers.

SUMMARY

Description

■ About 12 percent of women are abused by their partners each year, and 4 percent are severely battered.

■ Men are also likely to experience physical aggression. Aggression in intimate relationships is often reciprocal; however, women are much more likely to be injured.

■ One in 8 women in the United States is raped in her lifetime. Most are young; more than half are 17 years old or younger.

■ Most women who are raped are attacked by men they know. The most common type of sexual assault by an acquaintance is called *date rape.* Men may use physical force or threaten it to pressure their date, but the most common means of obtaining unwanted sex is by simply ignoring the woman's protests.

■ Although mothers are more likely to physically abuse their children, fathers are more likely to cause injury. Females are more likely to be charged with neglect than males.

Causes

■ Feminists argue that abusive men misuse power and control and that this misuse of control stems from social traditions that condone domination of women.

■ Men who engage in severe violence against their partners are likely to have personality disorders.

■ Two of the factors most highly associated with men's physical abuse of women are alcohol abuse and deep dissatisfaction with the relationship.

■ Communication patterns of men and women in physically abusive relationships are different from those in nonabusive relationships. Both men and women in abusive relationships are verbally aggressive and hostile toward their partners.

■ Biological explanations of aggressive behavior in intimate relationships have begun to receive attention. Brain injury, abnormalities in physiological reactivity, and/or evolutionary or genetic factors may account for some aggression.

■ One major theory holds that rape is a form of male aggression that has served historically to keep women dominated by men. An alternative theory is that rape is a manifestation of deviant sexual arousal—a type of paraphilia in which the man is sexually aroused by the use of force and humiliation.

- Date rape is not a matter of miscommunication between a man and woman. It is sexual violence.
- Risk factors for child abuse include poverty, being young and unmarried, having impulse and control problems, having been abused as a child, and having unrealistic expectations of children.
- Parents physically abuse preschool and teen-age children more than children at other ages.
- Observing violence or being the victim of violence as a child increases the risk of being physically violent toward a partner in adulthood.

Treatment

- Shelters for women who have been battered are the first priority for women in need of protection from their partners.
- Treatment groups for women and separate groups for men are the standard forms of intervention for men and women in abusive relationships.
- Couples treatment also has proved effective for men and women who want to remain together and for women who are not fearful of being in treatment with their partners.
- Convicted rapists and other sexual offenders usually go to prison, where they are unlikely to receive any treatment.
- Even the most effective treatment methods for rapists have questionable results. Rapists show higher relapse rates than other sexual offenders, such as child molesters.
- Treatment for rape victims often involves dealing with their memories of the incident. Exposure therapy—in which the patient writes about and discusses the rape with a therapist—seems to be a critical ingredient of successful treatment. In addition, therapists try to help individuals who have been raped change their beliefs regarding intimacy and self-esteem.
- Treatment programs for abusive parents have proved effective in changing parents' discipline strategies, and sometimes such changes can be maintained. It's difficult to change the behavior of parents who have been repeatedly reported for abuse and who have diverse social and emotional problems.
- Little research exists on the effectiveness of treatment programs for children who have been physically abused. However, these children are known to experience a variety of difficulties, including anxiety, depression, and conduct problems.

KEY TERMS

abuse, **p. 544**
child abuse, **p. 551**
child emotional abuse, **p. 551**
child sexual abuse, **p. 551**
coercion, **p. 554**
date rape, **p. 549**
intergenerational transmission of violence, **p. 552**
masochistic personality disorder, **p. 555**

Megan's Law, **p. 548**
neglect, **p. 551**
paraphilia, **p. 560**
Parents Anonymous (PA), **p. 566**
partner abuse, **p. 545**
patriarchy, **p. 554**
penile plethysmograph, **p. 560**
physical abuse, **p. 544**

posttraumatic stress disorder (PTSD), **p. 550**
rape, **p. 547**
relapse prevention training, **p. 565**
Sexually Violent Predators (SVP) Law, **p. 565**
tumescence, **p. 560**
victimized, **p. 547**

CRITICAL THINKING EXERCISE

Consider the following case and how you believe it should be handled:

Karin is a 26-year-old mother of two children: a 3-year-old and a 5-year-old. Jim, her husband, slaps her when he's frustrated and when they argue about finances. Once, about a year ago, he threw her down on the bed in anger. Karin has not received any injuries from Jim's physical aggression. On several occasions, she slapped him when she thought he was interested in another woman. Occasionally, when her 3-year-old wets his pants, Karin spanks him so hard that she can see print marks on her son for more than an hour. She loves Jim, and at present she has not considered leaving him. Karin and Jim are both high school teachers, but they have no savings. Both came from homes in which they saw physical violence.

1. What traits do you see in this family that are causal factors in both partner abuse and child physical abuse?
2. What types of services do the members of this family need? Consider psychological, medical, legal, and social services. Give reasons for your suggestions.

*C*hapter *18*

INDIVIDUAL PSYCHOLOGICAL THERAPIES

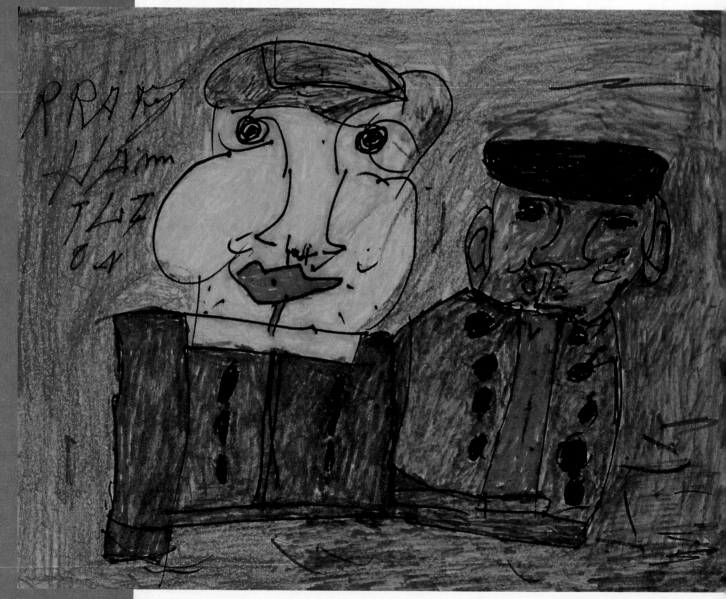

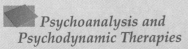

A nita was a 23-year-old schoolteacher who had grown increasingly unhappy over the past few years. She described her problems and what she did about them in the following narrative:

"I had never consulted a psychologist, but when I found myself feeling really miserable and anxious most of the time, a friend urged me to do so. Even though I regard myself as an educated person, I nevertheless felt that only crazy people see psychologists. So instead, I went to my regular doctor, who prescribed tranquilizers. I took them for a few days, but all they did was make me feel more tired. So reluctantly, I decided to see if a psychologist could help. Another friend urged me to call Dr. L., a therapist who had really helped him. So I took the plunge, made the call, and set up an appointment.

"On the day of my visit, I woke up really early with my heart pounding. I knew that I was now doubly anxious because I didn't know what to expect. To make matters worse, I was so uptight that I got lost on my way to the psychologist's office and arrived 10 minutes late. I rang the doorbell, and Dr. L. came to the door. He gave me a pleasant smile, which helped a lot. He invited me in and asked if I would be more comfortable sitting on a sofa or on one of two chairs. I chose a chair. I could feel the sweat on the back of my neck.

"'Let me just take down a few details,' Dr. L. began. He noted my name, address, phone number, age, marital status, and a few other particulars. 'Who referred you to me?' he asked. I told him that he had treated one of my friends, and I mentioned his name. Somehow, I began to settle down and feel more at ease.

"'So how can I be of help to you?' Dr. L. asked. I said I didn't really know but mentioned how anxious and upset I'd been feeling. At the end of the session, I went away feeling a lot calmer and more optimistic. The things Dr. L. had said made sense to me. I liked the fact that he was casual and informal and seemed to have a pleasant disposition. (I've since learned how important it is to have a good relationship with your therapist. If I had not felt comfortable with and confident about Dr. L., it would have made perfect sense for me to have shopped around for another psychologist.)

"We met once a week for about 2 months. I surprised myself by telling Dr. L. really private and personal things that I had never shared with anyone. He had explained to me in our first session that anything we discussed was strictly confidential. But in addition, his nonjudgmental and sincere attitude made it easy for me to trust and open up to him. This doctor was very much like my coach, my trainer. He gave me some books to read, and we chatted about what I got out of them. He also taught me how to use deep muscle relaxation and how to employ positive visualization and imagery when I was feeling uptight. We often role-played difficult discussions I needed to have with people, like my boss, my parents, and my older sister. I really learned a lot about myself and about dealing with the people around me.

"It was approximately 7 months after my first appointment that I went for a session and found that I really had nothing to complain about. I was no longer feeling anxious or depressed. I told Dr. L. how I had handled various thoughts, feelings, and situations, and he congratulated me on each one. I said, 'Maybe I should try going it alone from now on.' He agreed, but added, 'Look, if you ever feel the need to talk to me, the door's always open.' That was about 2 years ago. I haven't needed to go back and am thankful that I overcame my reluctance to consult a psychologist."

The problems that eventually prompted Anita to seek therapy may not seem debilitating, especially compared with some of the disorders we've discussed in this book. In fact, she wasn't even sure what her exact problems were. Yet they affected her life and what she got out of it, so she was wise to get help. Her therapy with Dr. L. taught her how to work through anxiety, how to handle conflicts in relationships, and how to better express her needs and views.

You can probably relate to Anita. Certainly, many of us share some of the same problems. But because we're all individuals—with unique physical and psychological makeup—how we resolve those problems must also be individualized. No single type of treatment is appropriate for the wide variety of psychological disorders that exist nor even necessarily for individuals with the same disorder. Just as we need a broad biopsychosocial model to explain how various disorders develop and are maintained, we also need a range of biological, psychological, and social interventions for preventing or treating them. In this chapter, we'll describe individual psychological therapies.

PSYCHOANALYSIS AND PSYCHODYNAMIC THERAPIES

Psychoanalysis originated with the work of Sigmund Freud (1856–1939) in Vienna, Austria, around the turn of the century. It came to the United States in the 1930s—partly because of the emigration of leading European analysts who were fleeing Nazi persecution—and it was readily accepted. According to Goodwin (1986), "For over 40 years, beginning in the mid-1930s, Freudian psychoanalysis dominated American psychiatry. Almost all the chairmen and professors of psychiatry were psychoanalysts or at least enthusiastic about Freudian theory. Generations of American medical students were taught psychoanalytic theory as received truth" (p. 83). The introduction of psychoanalysis had a similar impact on clinical psychology.

It's important that we distinguish between classical, or pure, psychoanalysis and psychotherapies based on psychoanalytic principles. *Classic psychoanalysis* is an intensive treatment, usually consisting of 4 or more sessions a week for a period of several years. This treatment is conducted by a therapist with formal psychoanalytic training. In today's world, pure psychoanalysis is an infrequent choice of treatment; the length and expense of such long-term therapy place it beyond most people's reach.

Psychotherapies based on psychoanalytic principles vary widely in nature. They differ in content and structure; for instance, some involve only weekly therapy ses-

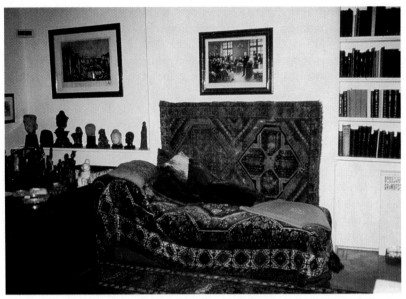

The couch in Freud's office in Vienna. It became customary in psychoanalysis for the patient to recline on a couch while talking to the therapist.

sions and may be relatively brief in duration. But these treatments share some core psychoanalytic concepts:

1. All are concerned with explaining the motives behind why people think, feel, and behave as they do.
2. All assume that early childhood experiences determine personality development. Namely, the bases of subsequent clinical disorders can be found in problems in these early interactions between children and their parents.
3. All recognize that conflict between opposing psychological forces is an inevitable aspect of human development. Among the sources of conflict are those between a person's identity as a biological/instinctual animal versus as a social being as well as those between a person's conscious and unconscious motives.
4. All suggest that the motives behind behavior are mainly unconscious; they remain hidden because our conscious minds find them too threatening or unacceptable. We develop different defense mechanisms to keep these unacceptable motives out of consciousness.
5. All suggest that a critical feature of effective psychotherapy is the establishment and development of a special relationship between the patient and therapist.

Psychoanalytic Concepts and Techniques

Psychoanalytic therapy is characterized by a number of basic theoretical concepts and treatment techniques, which we'll look at in the following sections.

Free Association   With the technique called **free association,** patients talk about whatever feelings and thoughts come to mind—no matter how irrelevant, embarrassing, or personal—without any censoring or editing. This is an indirect means of exploring the unconscious motives that underlie patients' behavior. By remaining passive and letting patients talk, therapists try to minimize any situational influences so that patients' associations are determined mainly by internal or intrapsychic processes. Therapists carefully scrutinize what patients say and how they express themselves for clues to unconscious conflicts and motives.

Resistance   A basic assumption of all psychoanalytic therapy is that patients have an unconscious commitment to maintaining the status quo; that is, they resist personal change. Typical examples of such **resistance** include being unable to free associate, refusing to discuss certain topics, remaining silent, disagreeing with the therapist's interpretations, missing or arriving late for treatment sessions, and failing to pay the therapist.

Resistance occurs despite patients' conscious desires to cooperate with proposed treatment and overcome their problems. The psychoanalytic explanation for resistance is that change is threatening or painful, because in order to change, patients must become aware of previously repressed emotional conflicts. And it's easier to repress or avoid these inner conflicts than to confront them (in the short term, anyway). By directly witnessing patients' characteristic defenses in response to threatening topics, therapists get clues about unconscious conflicts.

free association Technique in psychoanalysis in which patients are encouraged to talk about whatever thoughts or feelings they're experiencing, without any effort to censor.

resistance Unwillingness on the part of a patient to cooperate fully in therapy; for instance, refusing to discuss a certain topic.

Transference The term **transference** describes the developing relationship between the patient and therapist, in which the patient responds to the therapist as he did toward significant individuals in his childhood (usually, his parents). Freud believed that individuals unconsciously reexperience repressed childhood conflicts in the transference relationship, thereby providing the primary means for therapeutic change.

The structure of psychoanalytic therapy actually promotes the development of transference. Patients are dependent on their therapists, who act in an understanding but strictly neutral, nonjudgmental manner. Therapists try to provide a sort of blank slate on which patients can project (that is, *transfer*) their feelings. Patients frequently become frustrated and angry at therapists' apparent unresponsiveness. Such reactions are seen as a necessary and natural part of therapy. The way patients respond to this frustration helps them and their therapists understand how childhood patterns of thinking and feeling influence their behavior. Developing and ultimately working through the transference relationship is the most basic and important element of psychoanalytic therapy (Arlow, 1989).

Interpretation and Denial Once the transference relationship has been established and as treatment develops, the therapist shifts from passively observing to interpreting what the patient has said or done. In making an interpretation, the therapist confronts the individual with information about her behavior that she was previously unaware of. Interpretation makes the individual aware of unconscious conflicts and thereby induces psychological change.

A therapist will usually first interpret the behavior close to the patient's awareness; examples include defense mechanisms and resistance. Only later in treatment will the therapist interpret the content of the unconscious conflicts that give rise to defense mechanisms. These underlying conflicts are less accessible to consciousness and require deeper interpretations.

Dream Interpretation Another important technique in psychoanalytic therapies is **dream interpretation,** in which patients are encouraged to report their dreams. Freud called dreams the "royal road to the unconscious." He assumed the person's ego defense mechanisms were reduced during sleep; this made it more likely that dreams might provide clues about the hidden motives behind clinical disorders and normal behavior. Even so, therapists must still distinguish between the *manifest* content of dreams (what is consciously remembered) and their *latent* content (the hidden expression of unconscious processes).

Insight The goal of all psychoanalytic therapies is to help individuals gain insight into their problems. **Insight** refers to increased awareness of unconscious conflicts and psychological defenses, resulting in more adaptive behavior. Insight is not simply an intellectual awareness. It is an emotional process that occurs only in the context of the unique, emotion-arousing interpersonal interaction that is the transference relationship.

Neo-Freudian Therapies

Freud continued to revise his theory until his death in 1939. Psychoanalytic theory and therapy were also modified and amplified by the *neo-Freudians:* men and women who either had participated in Freud's original Vienna Psychoanalytic Society or had been trained by another member of that distinguished group. Among the most important neo-Freudians were Carl Jung, Alfred Adler, and Harry Stack Sullivan.

Carl Jung (1875–1961) was a psychiatrist who broke ranks with Freud over several basic issues and subsequently developed what has been called *analytic psy-*

transference Special relationship that develops between the patient and therapist in which the patient responds to the therapist as she did toward significant people (usually parents) in her childhood.

dream interpretation Psychoanalytic treatment method in which the unconscious significance of dreams is related to the patient's current problems.

insight In psychodynamic therapy, the awareness patients develop (usually in extended treatment) of their unconscious conflicts and psychological defenses.

chology. Most significantly, Jung rejected Freud's insistence that sexuality is the fundamental source of human motivation. Instead, Jung proposed that sexuality was only one form of a more general psychic energy. In his writings, he focused not only on treating abnormal behavior but also on normal adult development. Consequently, Jung has been regarded as a forerunner of humanistic psychology (discussed later).

Alfred Adler (1870–1937), an original member of the Vienna Psychoanalytic Society, also rejected Freud's view of the primacy of biological/instinctive forces and the overriding importance of sexuality in personality development. Compared with Freud, Adler had a more optimistic conception of human development, in which the self most significantly influenced development. Interestingly, Adler anticipated several developments in the psychological therapies, including the emphasis on the concept of self, a subjective sense of personal worth or adequacy (he coined the phrase *inferiority complex*), and the social context of behavior. Moreover, Adler discussed the influence of patients' beliefs or personal mythology, which he called **basic mistakes.** For example, consider the overgeneralizations we often make, such as "People are hostile" or "Life is dangerous." Another basic mistake is having false or impossible goals, such as "I have to please everybody" (Mosak, 1995, p. 63). Later in this chapter, when we discuss the dysfunctional cognitions of modern-day cognitive behavior therapy, you'll note a similarity between that approach and Adler's notion of basic mistakes.

Harry Stack Sullivan (1892–1949) is credited with emphasizing the interpersonal nature of psychological disorders (Sullivan, 1953). He used the term **parataxic distortions** to describe the effect that troubled interpersonal relationships in childhood have on adults' misperceptions of reality. Although Sullivan emphasized the interpersonal nature of early childhood experiences, the concept of parataxic distortions is consistent with basic Freudian principles: Childhood experiences unconsciously affect later adjustment; the task of therapy is to gain insight into these unconscious influences on present behavior.

Sullivan departed more clearly from orthodox Freudian therapy by introducing the concept of the therapist as a *participant observer.* By this, Sullivan meant that the patient's behavior during therapy sessions was a product not only of her past experience and personality but also of the therapist's subtle influence. His recognition of the therapist's influence as a participant in the treatment process had important therapeutic implications. Whereas Freud insisted that the therapist should remain nondirective and detached, Sullivan felt that the therapist's role should be more directive and focused on events in the here and now.

Ego-Analytic Therapies   A major modification of Freudian psychoanalysis was the development of **ego psychology** and ego-analytic therapies (Erikson, 1959; Hartmann, 1958). The neo-Freudians had moved away from Freud's primary emphasis on intrapsychic conflicts to acknowledge individuals' interactions with their environments. This trend was made even more explicit in the development of ego-analytic therapies. According to Freud's theory, the function of the ego (the conscious part of personality) is to maintain a balance between the opposing forces of the id (primitive, instinctual impulses) and the superego (the conscience). Ego analysts attach greater value than Freud did to current life circumstances and people's ability to adapt to and control their environments. Personal control and adaptive learning are ego functions—hence, the name *ego-analytic therapies.*

Erik Erikson (1902–1994) became one of the best-known ego analysts. He proposed a series of eight psychosocial stages that people pass through over the total lifespan. At each stage, sociocultural reality confronts the maturing person with new challenges. For example, Erikson saw adolescence as the period when a young person is challenged to develop her personal identity or definition of self.

basic mistakes Adler's concept that maladaptive personal beliefs can lead to psychological problems.

parataxic distortions Effects that problematic interpersonal relationships in childhood have on the adult's misperceptions of reality.

ego psychology Psychodynamic approach that stresses the importance of the ego and its defenses in personality development.

Self-Psychology   Another important modification of Freudian psychoanalysis has been Heinz Kohut's development of what's called **self-psychology** (Kohut, 1971). According to this approach, problems between the mother and child early in life leave the child with low self-esteem. So the child grows up trying to compensate for this feeling of vulnerability, which results in an unrealistic and narcissistic striving for expressions of love and approval from others. Therapy founded on self-psychology—which is more directive than classical psychoanalysis—is aimed at restoring the patient's sense of self by providing the acceptance she never had as a child. (See the detailed discussion of the theory and therapy of self-psychology in the description of narcissistic personality disorder in Chapter 11.)

Brief Psychodynamic Therapies

As mentioned earlier, one of the major limitations of orthodox, long-term psycho-dynamic therapy is its length and cost, which few individuals can afford. Thus, the evolution of brief psychodynamic therapies has been an important development. Generally speaking, *brief therapy* in this context means up to 40 hours of treatment.

Only carefully selected patients are considered appropriate for brief psychodynamic psychotherapy. Suitable patients are those with "strong ego resources," namely, "those in whom the behavioral problem is of acute onset; those whose previous adjustment has been good; those with a good ability to relate; those with high initial motivation" (Strupp, 1980, p. 221). Individuals who act out (that is, have problems with impulse control, as in drug or alcohol abuse), are less mature and responsible, are self-destructive, or are poorly motivated are not suitable patients.

Treatment goals in brief therapies tend to be more modest than those in long-term psychoanalysis. Instead of achieving fundamental personality change, the objective of treatment is to resolve the core conflict. Another difference between brief and orthodox psychotherapies is that the therapist in the brief approach is typically more active and directive. In contrast to the more passive and deliberately detached therapist in long-term psychodynamic treatment, in brief treatment, the therapist tries to foster the patient's involvement and collaboration in a working *therapeutic alliance.* In particular, the therapist frequently interprets what the patient says and does. Different brief therapies favor different types of interpretations, but all focus on actively interpreting the focal conflict or central issue behind the patient's problem.

An Evaluation of Psychoanalytic Therapies

Psychodynamic theory and therapy remains influential among mental health professionals in the United States. In addition, its appeal among the broader intellectual community of artists and writers is unrivaled. Several reasons help explain psychoanalytic theory's enormous popularity. One is its breadth, which spans normal behavior and the full range of abnormal behavior. Another strength is that its explanation of the motives behind human behavior is more extensive than that of any other theory. Psychodynamic theory sometimes seems to offer the only comprehensive account of certain disorders. (For example, see Chapter 6 on the somatoform and dissociative disorders.)

Psychodynamic theory and therapy has, nevertheless, been widely criticized on several counts. One such criticism focuses on what some therapists feel are bizarre concepts. In fact, it's easy to be skeptical about some of the more fanciful psychoanalytic notions. Few present-day clinical investigators would agree, for instance, that the reason agoraphobics become anxious upon leaving their homes is because the street represents the place "where it is possible to realize their unconscious wish to be a prostitute" (Arlow, 1989, p. 41). Likewise, few therapists would accept the notion that bulimia nervosa is really a symbolic form of "oral masturbation" (Schwartz, 1988). Yet many therapists are able to reject views such as these and instead point to other contributions of psychodynamic theory, including

self-psychology Modification of psychoanalysis in which the emphasis is on the low self-esteem or vulnerability a child feels because of lack of love; therapy is directed toward restoring the patient's sense of self by providing the acceptance that was missing in childhood.

notions about the importance of early learning and childhood experience, about how much of our functioning is influenced by unconscious processes, and about how personal conflicts can interfere with interpersonal relationships.

Another criticism of psychodynamic theory has to do with its scientific validity. Freud rejected the argument that his treatment had to be tested in controlled empirical research, claiming that each individual patient's success sufficiently proved his theory and its therapeutic value. But this reasoning is unacceptable to clinical researchers. There are problems with drawing conclusions from uncontrolled clinical case studies of the sort Freud reported (see Chapter 4). Judgments of treatment effectiveness must depend on independent investigators' experimental evaluations of treatment outcomes.

Contemporary psychodynamic therapists have been actively researching some of the principles and procedures of psychodynamic treatment. This research falls into two categories: process research and outcome research.

Process Research   Interactions between the therapist and patient during treatment sessions are studied in **process research.** This is the dominant type of research on psychoanalytic therapy. For example, Luborsky (1987) suggested the existence of a consistent, conflict-producing theme in the relationships individuals develop with significant figures in their lives. He called this the *core conflictual relationship theme (CCRT)* and has shown its close resemblance to Freud's concept of transference (Luborsky, Crits-Christoph, & Mellon, 1986). To assess the CCRT, Luborsky records therapy sessions and then examines them for consistencies in patients' narratives (descriptions) of different interpersonal relationships (see Figure 18.1).

process research Research designed to uncover why a particular treatment method has certain effects.

FIGURE 18.1 Schematic summary of a patient's statements about relationships and their core conflictual relationship theme (CCRT)

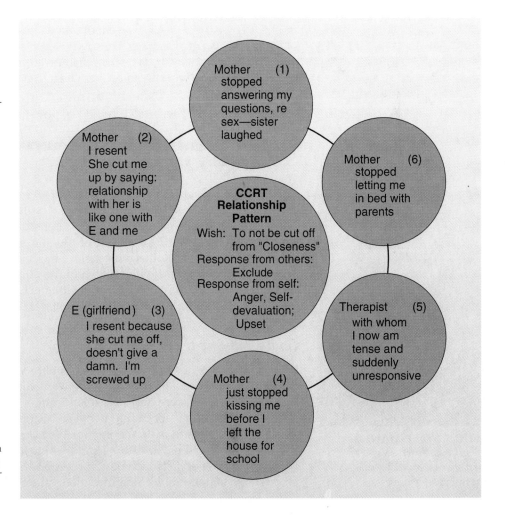

Source: From L. Luborsky, "Research Can Now Affect Clinical Practice—A Happy Turnaround," *Clinical Psychologist,* 1987, *40,* 56–59. Reprinted by permission of Dr. Lester Luborsky.

The numbered circles in Figure 18.1 (page 577) summarize the relationship patterns from a therapy session of an 18-year-old college student who's experiencing anxiety symptoms. Luborsky had clinicians examine these narratives and infer the underlying CCRT. Their interpretation is summarized in the center circle in Figure 18.1. For this type of analysis to be scientifically useful, the clinical judges' interpretations must be reliable—that is, they must agree with each other about the nature of the CCRT.

One of psychoanalytic therapy's basic assumptions is that therapeutic progress depends on therapists accurately interpreting patients' verbal and nonverbal behavior. To study this hypothesis, Luborsky (1987) had one set of clinical judges rate the patient's CCRT and a second set rate the accuracy of the therapist's in-session interpretations of the patient's CCRT. Luborsky was then able to show that the accuracy of the therapist's interpretations correlated significantly with the effects of treatment, thereby providing empirical support for one of the assumptions of psychoanalytic therapy.

outcome research Controlled research designed to evaluate how effective a particular treatment method is.

interpersonal psychotherapy (IPT) Time-limited treatment in which the focus is on understanding and changing interpersonal factors which are thought to maintain the patient's current problems.

Focus on Critical Thinking

Jackson W., age 32, has spent most of the past few therapy sessions talking about his problematic relationships with women. His therapist, Dr. Marcia C., has noted that conflict always seems to occur as soon as Jackson reports becoming emotionally involved with a woman. In the next session, Dr. C. says, "It seems from what you describe that problems arise in a relationship whenever you begin to feel emotionally close to the woman."

1. What psychoanalytic technique is Dr. C. using in this example? Explain your answer.
2. How would psychoanalytic theory explain Jackson W.'s feelings of conflict?

Outcome Research Process research may reveal how treatment works, but this requires evidence of the effectiveness of a particular kind of treatment. **Outcome research** evaluates that effectiveness. To date, little outcome research has been done on psychoanalytic psychotherapy. The exception to this unsatisfactory state of affairs is brief psychodynamic therapy (Crits-Christoph, 1992). A recent task force that evaluated the effectiveness of psychological therapies concluded that brief psychodynamic therapy probably produces the desired effect and urged additional empirical research on this promising form of treatment (Chambless, 1993).

INTERPERSONAL PSYCHOTHERAPY

Interpersonal influences are emphasized by several different forms of current psychotherapy, as well as behavior therapy and multimodal therapy (discussed later). The nature and value of an interpersonal approach is well illustrated by **interpersonal psychotherapy (IPT),** a form of time-limited psychotherapy developed by Klerman, Weissman, Rounsaville, and Chevron (1984). We focus on IPT here because it provides a pure illustration of the interpersonal approach and because controlled empirical research has shown its effectiveness in treating depression (see Chapter 7) and bulimia nervosa (see Chapter 11).

Goals and Strategies

IPT involves three distinct phases: initial, intermediate, and final. In the *initial phase,* the therapist explores the connection between the patient's problem and interpersonal processes. Current and past relationships are examined, together with the patient's expectations about interpersonal relationships and the changes desired.

In the *intermediate phase,* the therapist focuses on different problem areas. The first one is interpersonal disputes. In addressing this problem, the goals are to identify the patient's conflicts with other people and to resolve them by altering expectations or changing faulty communication patterns. The therapist helps the patient

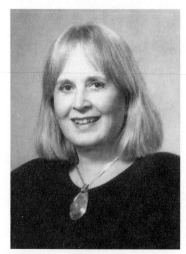

MYRNA WEISSMAN, *one of the individuals who developed interpersonal psychotherapy for the treatment of depression*

to recognize conflicting feelings, to stop avoiding situations that elicit them, and to express himself more directly. Alternative ways of resolving disputes and their likely consequences are analyzed, as well.

A second problem area is role transitions. The therapeutic goals here are to help the patient accept the change or the loss of a previous role and develop self-esteem by acquiring a sense of competence in a new role. These goals are achieved through several means: by exploring the patient's feelings about the role change, by fostering realistic expectations about what's been lost versus what new opportunities now exist, and by encouraging efforts to increase social support for coping with the new role.

A third problem area addressed in the intermediate stage is interpersonal skills. To deal with this problem, goals include identifying the lack of social skills and making the individual aware of how these deficiencies lead to social difficulties. The therapist explores positive and negative aspects of the patient's past relationships and analyzes the current therapist/patient relationship to shed light on other of the patient's relationships.

In the *final phase* of IPT the therapist discusses the termination of therapy and the patient's feelings of loss. The therapist calls attention to evidence of the patient's improvement and to signs of more independent functioning. The goal is to leave the patient with an enhanced sense of self-mastery, enabling her to cope better with life's problems. Future difficulties are anticipated and possible ways of coping are discussed.

An Evaluation of Interpersonal Psychotherapy

Although IPT has much in common with psychodynamic therapy, there are important differences, as well. For instance, in IPT, the therapist recognizes the intrapsychic conflicts that are the focus of psychodynamic therapy but does not interpret the patient's current problems as an expression of these conflicts. Instead, the therapist explores the patient's behavior in connection with her interpersonal relationships. Unlike psychodynamic therapy, which focuses on the transference relationship, IPT does not make the therapeutic relationship the primary focus of treatment.

Psychoanalytically oriented therapists view IPT as a form of supportive therapy—that is, one that fails to address the underlying causes of emotional disorders by focusing primarily on the patient's present problems. Like behavior therapy and other forms of brief therapy, IPT is focused on well-defined problems and time limited. IPT procedures are spelled out in a treatment manual, making evaluation of its effectiveness possible (DeRubeis, Hollon, Evans, & Bemis, 1982). The controlled clinical outcome studies that have been completed have indicated that IPT is an effective form of therapy, particularly in treating people with unipolar depression (Klerman & Weissman, 1993).

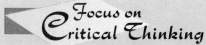

Focus on Critical Thinking

Determine which of the following questions would guide a therapist using IPT (explain your choice):

1. How can I understand the patient's interpersonal fantasies and help her get insight into the origins of the problematic relationships she has with the men she dates? or

2. How can I help the patient clarify her feelings and develop more satisfying relationships with the men she dates?

Humanistic and Existential Psychotherapies

Humanistic and existential psychotherapies have in common with psychoanalytic therapies the core assumption that individuals must develop insight into their underlying needs and conflicts. Yet humanistic therapies differ significantly from Freudian theory and therapy. Person-centered therapy and Gestalt therapy are revealing examples.

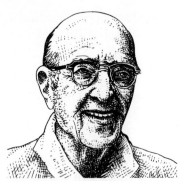

CARL ROGERS, *the founder of person-centered psychotherapy*

Carl Rogers's Person-Centered Therapy

Humanistic therapy is founded on the assumption that people are innately good. Thus, the growth of humanistic psychology and psychotherapy in the 1960s can be seen as a reaction against Freudianism and behaviorism. Carl Rogers (1902–1987)—the best-known personality theorist and psychotherapist within the humanistic tradition—referred to it as the "third force" in psychology. He believed that human behavior is goal directed and purposive; in other words, people are motivated to affect their environments and to achieve personal fulfillment. The tendency toward personal growth is known as **self-actualization.**

Let's look at some contrasts between psychoanalytic and humanistic therapies:

1. Psychoanalytic therapies assume that personality is determined by early childhood experiences. Humanistic therapists believe that people are free to shape their own futures.
2. Psychodynamic therapists act as experts, making interpretations that are designed to give patients insight linking past conflicts to present feelings and actions. Person-centered therapists try to encourage therapeutic relationships in which they listen rather than interpret; what's more, they focus on patients' present experiences without attempting to connect them to childhood traumas.
3. Psychoanalysts foster a transference relationship, whereas person-centered therapists do not. In fact, person-centered therapy rejects techniques that place therapists in control; for example, therapists avoid imposing treatment goals. These techniques are rejected because it's believed they will interfere with patients' experience of self and developing reliance on their own inner resources. This is why Rogers's approach was originally known as *client-centered therapy.*

A radical aspect of Rogers's person-centered therapy is the assumption that the techniques of the various psychological therapies (for instance, psychodynamic interpretations or behavioral methods) are unimportant, for the most part. The only exception is the extent to which different therapies or techniques encourage expression of three personal qualities of therapists:

1. Therapists show **empathy** when they accurately understand each patient's phenomenological world—that is, the way in which the individual perceives and emotionally experiences events. Empathy requires more of therapists than merely understanding patients' words. Specifically, therapists must immerse themselves in their patients' worlds and communicate their understanding to patients at an emotional level.
2. Therapists show **unconditional positive regard** when they warmly accept all aspects of patients' experiences in a completely nonjudgmental fashion, neither probing unnecessarily nor interpreting patients' feelings. Therapists need to simply communicate a sense of trust in patients' own resources for self-understanding.
3. **Genuineness** is hard to separate from empathy and unconditional positive regard. Therapists are genuine (or *congruent*) when they try to experience what patients are experiencing. But genuineness goes beyond intellectual understanding; it's a feel for what others are experiencing emotionally. To be genuine, therapists must first fully trust their own experiences of their relationships with patients. In this way, they allow patients to trust them and to learn from the therapy that they can risk sharing their innermost feelings with another person.

The personal qualities demonstrated by therapists are particularly significant in dealing with people from different ethnic and racial groups. Thinking about Multicultural Issues considers ways of providing culturally sensitive and appro-

self-actualization Term used to describe how people can achieve their unrealized potentials, despite life's inevitable frustrations.

empathy Ability to communicate to another person an understanding of what she's feeling and experiencing.

unconditional positive regard Therapist's nonjudgmental acceptance of the patient's feelings.

genuineness Ability to understand what another person is experiencing emotionally; rooted in the therapist's complete trust of his own experience of his relationships with the patient.

Thinking about MULTICULTURAL ISSUES

Ethnic and Cultural Differences in Psychotherapy

According to the U.S. Bureau of the Census (1990), one-quarter of the U.S. population is defined as being a member of an *ethnic minority*. And predictions are that this percentage will increase rapidly as the demographics of the country continue to change. The prevalence of clinical disorders is as high among people from ethnic minorities as among those from the majority white population. Thus, the growing cultural diversity of the United States has important implications for the practice of psychotherapy (Comas-Diaz, 1992).

One approach to serving the needs of ethnic minorities is to provide ethnic-specific treatment. For example, this might involve treatment designed specifically for African American patients and, most importantly, would be offered by African American therapists. There are several problems with this approach, however. Studies that have assessed the ethnic matching of therapists with patients have yielded mixed results (Sue, Zane, & Young, 1994). Moreover, there are many different ethnic minorities in the United States—including African, Hispanic, and Asian Americans—and considerable heterogeneity within each of these groups.

Another problem with trying to provide ethnic-specific treatment is that stereotypes may unintentionally enter in. Sue et al. (1994) made the point that in contrast to the stereotype of African Americans being poor, roughly half are in the middle and upper classes. We know that socioeconomic status (SES) is a major determinant of health—arguably, more so than ethnicity (see Chapter 10). So it might be more important to design treatment services for people of different SES groups than ethnic groups.

A second, more practical approach would be to train all therapists in cultural sensitivity and other specific

skills for working with culturally diverse groups. In one study, experienced black or white therapists were assigned to either a cultural sensitivity training program or a control condition (Wade & Bernstein, 1991). After that, all therapists treated black patients from the community. In working with these patients, the cultural sensitivity training proved more important than whether the therapist was black or white. Patients rated the therapists who had received training as having greater expertise and empathy. These patients also attended more treatment sessions. Given that the training program involved only 4 hours' time, these positive results encourage the view that all therapists can readily acquire enhanced skills for helping culturally diverse patient groups.

The American Psychological Association accredits training programs in clinical psychology. The criteria for accreditation include an emphasis on cultural diversity. Doctoral programs are required to educate students about the needs of people from ethnic minorities and are strongly encouraged to include members of ethnic minorities among the faculty who train students (American Psychological Association, 1990b).

Think about the following questions:

1. Consider the following statement: "Effective treatment depends more on the therapist's understanding the patient's problem and being a caring and sensitive person than on the therapist's age, sex, sexual orientation, or racial/ethnic identity." Do you agree? Or do you think that, in general, therapists and patients should be matched along personal qualities? Explain your answers.
2. What qualities of psychotherapy require taking special account of a patient's ethnic identity?

priate therapy to individuals from these different groups. This topic clearly has important implications for therapy, given the growing cultural diversity of the United States.

An Evaluation of Person-Centered Therapy   The major contribution of person-centered therapy has been to improve our understanding of how therapists can aid the treatment process. Rogers played an important role in opening up psychotherapy to empirical research in the 1950s. He and his colleagues pioneered the tape recording of entire treatment sessions, which allowed investigators to study the content of sessions and systematically examine interactions between therapists and patients.

As it turned out, however, the collective results of these studies generally failed to support Rogers's theory about the significance of therapist qualities: empathy, unconditional positive regard, and genuineness. It would seem that these qualities would enhance efforts in any helping relationship; indeed, therapists' having these qualities is usually desirable and does help patients improve. But therapists don't necessarily have to demonstrate these qualities to effect change. By themselves, the therapist qualities described by Rogers are simply insufficient to treat major clinical disorders effectively (Rachman & Wilson, 1980). As we've discussed throughout this book, specific psychological and/or pharmacological techniques are needed to treat particular disorders.

Gestalt Therapy

Like person-centered therapists, gestalt therapists believe that human nature is essentially positive and that people can make meaningful choices about their lives and improve themselves. The two approaches differ, however, in terms of what specific therapeutic techniques they use. Gestalt therapists employ a broader range of treatment techniques than their person-centered counterparts.

The founder of gestalt therapy was Frederich (Fritz) Perls (1893–1970), a German who was originally trained in medicine and psychoanalysis. Perls fled Nazi Germany for South Africa and later the United States. In these countries, he was exposed to gestalt psychology and an existential (experiential) perspective, from which he developed gestalt therapy.

Gestalt therapists believe that psychological problems develop when, for whatever reason, an individual's inborn positive potential cannot be freely expressed and developed—in other words, when someone is prevented from being or doing all that she could. To tap that natural potential, gestalt therapy, like other humanistic therapies, focuses on individuals' creative and expressive qualities. *Gestalt* is a German term meaning "whole." Accordingly, gestalt therapy is founded on the principle that individuals need to integrate their experiences of self—their thoughts and feelings—with their environmental circumstances. Any dichotomy between different aspects of functioning (such as conflict between conscious and unconscious parts of the personality) interferes with personal growth and happiness and needs to be healed or integrated.

More than any other approach, gestalt therapy focuses on the here and now. That is, the *process* of experiencing what's happening at any particular moment is more important than the *content* of what's being discussed. The goal of gestalt therapy is increased awareness. Individuals are helped to get in touch with and to be able to integrate and accept both their inner feelings and their external environments. Awareness involves "not only self-knowledge, but a direct knowing of the current situation and how the self is in that situation. . . . Awareness is cognitive, sensory, and affective. . . . The person who is aware knows what he does, how he does it, that he has alternatives, and that he chooses to be as he is" (Yontef & Simkin, 1989, p. 334).

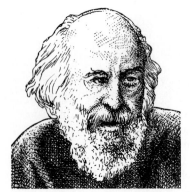

FREDERICK (FRITZ) PERLS,
the founder of Gestalt therapy

Treatment Techniques   Gestalt therapists may use any techniques, provided they are aimed at enhancing awareness and are rooted in the immediate interaction between therapist and patient (Yontef & Simkin, 1989). To keep the patient in the here and now, the therapist often asks basic questions, such as "What are you doing now?" or "How are you feeling now?" When the patient reports a painful or anxiety-provoking thought or feeling, he is encouraged to "stay with it," or experience it more fully, thereby overcoming it. Gestalt therapists instruct patients to communicate directly by talking *to* people, rather than *about* them. To encourage genuineness and personal responsibility for feelings, therapists use "I" statements—for instance, "I think you are hurting right now"—and encourage patients to do the same.

One of the best-known gestalt methods is the *empty chair technique.* Let's suppose a patient is dealing with unresolved emotional conflict about a parent who is dead. Instead of simply talking about her feelings about the parent, the patient is instructed to imagine that the parent is sitting in the empty chair and to talk directly to the parent. The patient might also switch roles, sitting in the empty chair and talking as if she were the parent. The goal of this technique is to take care of unfinished business—to get in touch with a part of the self not yet fully experienced and accepted.

An Evaluation of Gestalt Therapy   Gestalt therapists have traditionally rejected the methodology of quantitative research, claiming that it fails to address change processes within the individual (Yontef & Simkin, 1989). Perls, like Freud before him, argued that the results of therapy don't need empirical confirmation: "We present nothing that you cannot verify for yourself in terms of your own behavior" (Perls, Hefferline, & Goodman, 1951, p. 347).

What research exists on gestalt therapy is process research. Greenberg (1986), for example, has studied the processes involved in the empty chair technique. He found that patients who were rated as achieving greater depth of experiencing during this technique were more successful in resolving conflicts during their sessions. By *experiencing*, gestalt therapists mean *self-exploration*, in which patients are able to verbalize their feelings. Greenberg (1986) also showed that the empty chair technique was more effective in reducing in-session psychological conflict than empathic reflection, the primary technique of Rogerian, person-centered therapists.

Despite its theoretical and empirical weaknesses, gestalt therapy has become a leading therapeutic approach, establishing Perls as one of the best-known psychotherapists. Much of the interest in gestalt therapy focuses on its rich range of treatment techniques. Eclectic therapists use gestalt methods (such as the empty chair technique) within their own conceptual frameworks (Lazarus, 1989). Such practitioners find gestalt methods appealing because of their potential for modifying emotional components of behavior.

Focus on Critical Thinking

The following is a brief excerpt from an interview by Carl Rogers (cited in Raskin & Rogers, 1995):

Patient: I'm having a lot of problems dealing with my daughter. She's 20 years old; she's in college; I'm having a lot of trouble letting her go.

Therapist: A need to hang on so you can kind of make up for the things you feel guilty about—is that part of it?

Patient: Yes. Yes. I also would like to be the kind of mother that could be strong and say, you know, "Go and have a good life," and this is really hard for me to do that.

Therapist: It's very hard to give up something that's been so precious in your life, but also something that I guess has caused you pain. (p. 144)

1. Which of the three therapist qualities of empathy, unconditional positive regard, and genuineness does this interview highlight? Explain your answer.

2. How might a gestalt therapist use the empty chair technique in helping this mother deal with her daughter?

BEHAVIOR THERAPY

The formal beginnings of behavior therapy can be traced to separate but related developments that occurred in three countries during the 1950s. In South Africa, Joseph Wolpe (1958) developed and tested several treatment methods based on experimental research on the principles of learning theory. He shocked the world of psychotherapy by claiming that 90 percent of his patients were either cured or markedly improved. This unprecedented success rate was apparently accomplished not after many years of therapy—as deemed necessary by psychoanalysis—but within a few months or even weeks. At about the same time, in England, Hans J. Eysenck, of the Institute of Psychiatry of London University, defined *behavior therapy* as the application of learning principles and procedures to the treatment of emotional disorders (Eysenck, 1959). According to Eysenck, behavior therapy was an applied science, whose defining feature was that it could be tested and shown to be either valid or false. The third development in behavior therapy occurred in the United States, where principles of operant conditioning were applied to clinical problems (Skinner, 1953).

By the end of the 1960s, behavior therapists had begun to expand their theories and methods. In addition to borrowing from classical and operant conditioning, these clinicians turned to current developments in cognitive, social, and developmental psychology. They were looking for different ways of conceptualizing their activities and for sources of innovative therapeutic strategies. Particularly noteworthy in this regard was Albert Bandura's (1969) social learning theory, which emphasized vicarious learning (modeling), symbolic processes, and self-regulatory mechanisms. (See Chapter 2 for a detailed discussion of social learning theory.)

Today, behavior therapy uses a broad and diverse range of methods, often with different theoretical rationales. Within the broad framework of behavior therapy, it's useful to distinguish among three approaches: (1) applied behavior analysis; (2) a stimulus-response model; and (3) social learning theory. Basically, these three approaches differ in how much they use cognitive concepts and procedures. At one end of the continuum is applied behavior analysis, which focuses exclusively on observable behavior and rejects all cognitive mediating processes. At the other end is social learning theory, which relies heavily on cognitive theories.

Applied Behavior Analysis

Therapists have applied operant conditioning techniques to a wide range of problems in all age groups in clinical and community psychology, education, rehabilitation, and even medicine (Kazdin, 1984). This approach—**applied behavior analysis**—has been found most useful in changing the behavior of chronic mental patients in institutions, young children, and people who are mentally retarded (as described in Chapters 13, 14, and 15, respectively). Nevertheless, most behavior therapists in clinical practice (particularly those working with adult patients) do not describe themselves as applied behavior analysts. Instead, they see themselves as drawing from much broader theoretical and empirical bases (O'Leary & Wilson, 1987).

The Stimulus-Response Approach

The **stimulus-response approach**—drawing on the pioneering contributions of Wolpe and Eysenck—attempts to treat clinical problems by applying the stimulus-response learning theories of Pavlov and other leading learning theorists (such as Clark Hull, Hobart Mowrer, and Neal Miller). Unlike applied behavior analysis and operant conditioning, which focus exclusively on observable behavior, the stimulus-response approach emphasizes unobservable or mediational variables in explaining and modifying human behavior.

A *mediational variable* intervenes between an observable stimulus and response. Anxiety is a mediational variable; it cannot be measured directly but is inferred to explain the effect that an external stimulus has on an observable response. For example, an acrophobic who avoids heights does so because the stimulus (high places) elicits anxiety, which, in turn, mediates the response (behavioral avoidance). The treatment technique of *systematic desensitization,* closely associated with the stimulus-response model, is directed toward extinguishing the underlying anxiety assumed to maintain phobic disorders. The principles and procedures of classical and instrumental conditioning are the backbone of this approach.

Social Learning Theory

The **social learning approach** to behavior therapy depends on the theory that behavior is based on three separate but interacting regulatory systems (Bandura, 1986): (1) external stimulus events; (2) external reinforcement; and, (3) most impor-

applied behavior analysis Application of the principles and procedures of operant conditioning to human problems; the analysis of environmental effects on nature.

stimulus-response approach In behavior therapy, the application of classical conditioning principles to clinical problems.

social learning approach Bandura's theory of complex human learning in which behavior is viewed as a product of both internal cognitive mediating processes (such as self-efficacy and self-regulation) and external stimuli (such as classical and operant conditioning).

tant, cognitive mediational processes. According to the social learning approach, the influence that external, environmental events have on behavior is determined largely by cognitive processes that govern which influences people attend to and how they perceive and interpret them.

Modeling is one of the best-known and most widely used methods derived from social learning theory. In this method, behavior is learned or modified by systematically observing the behavior of someone else—the model. In Chapter 5, for instance, we described how fear is learned by observing the expression of fear in others. The important principle in modeling is that learning occurs even though the observer does not give any response or receive any reinforcement.

Expectations play an important role in social learning theory. Our expectations and hypotheses about what is happening or will happen to us often affect our behavior more than the objective reality of the contingencies associated with the behavior. Clinical problems usually arise when a significant discrepancy develops between our perception of events and objective reality. Social learning theory distinguishes between efficacy and outcome expectations. **Efficacy expectations** refer to our feelings of confidence that we can cope with particular situations. **Outcome expectations** refer to our beliefs that our actions will result in particular outcomes. *Self-efficacy theory* is a critical component of the social learning approach (see Chapter 5).

A social learning approach to behavior therapy also draws heavily on other cognitive concepts. One such concept is *attribution theory,* which accounts for how we typically explain (attribute causes to) our own attitudes and actions as well as those of others (Bandura, 1986). The person is the agent of change. Attribution theory emphasizes the human capacity for self-directed behavior change.

Treatment Methods

In selecting a treatment technique, the behavior therapist relies on empirical evidence about how effective a given technique is when applied to a patient's particular problem. Yet this information is frequently insufficient for guiding therapeutic interventions, because in many cases, the empirical evidence is unclear or largely nonexistent. In these situations, the therapist must rely on accepted clinical practice and the basic logic and philosophy of the approach to human behavior and its modification. In addition, the therapist must often use intuitive skills and clinical savvy in deciding not only what treatment methods are appropriate but also when to use a specific technique. Thus, informed clinical practice draws on both science and art. The most effective therapists are aware of the advantages and limitations of each.

The following sections illustrate the methods likely to be employed by a typical behavior therapist in clinical practice.

Assertiveness and Social Skills Training   Therapists often see patients who seem unable to express their emotions or stand up for their legitimate rights. These individuals are often taken advantage of by others, feel anxiety in social situations, and have low self-esteem. In **assertion training,** therapists model appropriate assertive behavior and then ask patients to rehearse, or role-play, the behavior themselves. Recall the case of Anita from the chapter-opening. Her therapist used role-playing to prepare her for dealing with stressful interactions with her parents, older sister, and boss. In assertion training, attention is focused on developing patients' nonverbal and verbal expressive behavior, such as body posture, voice training, and eye contact. Therapists then encourage patients to carry out these assertive actions in the real world.

In discussing assertion training, it's important that we distinguish among submissive (nonassertive), aggressive, and assertive behavior. *Submissive* people allow others to take advantage of them and then harbor resentment that they don't express openly. *Aggressive* people take advantage of others; they are often selfish

efficacy expectations
People's feelings of confidence that they can cope with particular situations.

outcome expectations
People's beliefs that their actions will result in particular outcomes.

assertion training Behavior therapy technique for helping patients express their feelings in a constructive manner that is neither submissive nor aggressive.

and hurt other individuals. *Assertive* people express their feelings honestly and directly without exploiting others; they have a positive self-image and feel good about themselves. Assertive behavior is more likely to be effective in interpersonal interactions than submissive or aggressive behavior.

In addition to enhancing assertiveness, the instructional, modeling, and feedback components of behavior rehearsal help the patient develop a broader range of communication competencies, including active listening, giving personal feedback, and building trust through self-disclosure. These communication principles, drawn from nonbehavioral approaches to counseling but integrated within a behavioral framework, are a key ingredient of behavioral marital therapy (as described in Chapter 19).

Self-Control Strategies   In behavioral treatment programs, both children and adults are taught that they must be active in determining their treatment goals and implementing their course of therapy. To teach this active participation, behavior therapists use a number of self-control strategies (Bandura, 1986; Kanfer, 1977).

Self-monitoring—a process to make individuals more aware of their specific problems and actions—is fundamental to the successful self-regulation of behavior. In this strategy, the therapist helps the patient set goals or standards to guide her behavior. (You can likely recall examples of self-monitoring that have been discussed in earlier chapters.) To aid in this process, behavioral research has identified certain properties of goals; for example, they should be highly specific, unambiguous, and short term. Setting goals that meet these criteria helps increase the probability that the patient will successfully learn self-control.

After treatment goals have been set, patients self-monitor and evaluate their performance against them. If patients fail to achieve their goals, they get a negative self-evaluation, which motivates them to change their behavior. Success, however, produces self-reinforcement, increasing the likelihood that patients will maintain their self-regulatory behavior.

The idea of self-regulation explains the observation that human behavior is usually maintained and often altered without immediate external reinforcement. People generally make self-rewards or self-punishments conditional on attaining specific standards of performance. The level of self-motivation generated by success or failure in reaching self-imposed goals will vary according to the person's specific performance standards, how he evaluates performance, and the nature of the incentives to perform. An individual's performance standards are a product of his prior learning history.

Cognitive Restructuring   Methods of **cognitive restructuring** are designed to help patients first identify and then modify dysfunctional thinking patterns. We'll describe them more fully in the following section on cognitive therapy. They're mentioned here, as well, because cognitive principles and procedures have been integrated within behavior therapy in an approach called **cognitive-behavioral therapy (CBT)**. Depending on the specific problem of the individual being treated, the cognitive-behavioral therapist will place greater emphasis on either the behavioral or the cognitive component, as appropriate (Hawton, Salkovskis, & Clark, 1989).

An Evaluation of Behavior Therapy

One of the strengths of behavior therapy is that it's founded on the principles and methods of experimental psychology. This means that advances in basic and applied psychological research will continue to inform the clinical practice of behavior therapy. Another asset of this approach is that its treatment methods are carefully specified and thus can be evaluated in experimental research. Numerous well-controlled studies have shown that specific behavioral methods are effective in treating particular clinical disorders, as described throughout this book.

self-monitoring Technique used in behavioral assessment and behavior therapy in which patients are asked to identify and record specific thoughts, feelings, and behaviors.

cognitive restructuring Technique in which patients are helped to identify, challenge, and modify dysfunctional thoughts.

cognitive-behavioral therapy (CBT) Form of psychological therapy that focuses on directly modifying both cognitive processes and behavior; draws heavily on cognitive theory and research as well as more traditional classical and operant conditioning principles.

Behavior therapy has been criticized by some clinicians who feel it's a superficial form of treatment that addresses only the symptoms, not the causes, of people's problems. Furthermore, these critics have alleged that behavioral treatment could lead to **symptom substitution:** the replacement of the treated symptom with another because the underlying problem has not been resolved.

In fact, both behavioral and psychodynamic treatments attempt to deal with the causes of behavior. There is a difference, however, in what these respective approaches see as the causes. Psychodynamic theories focus on historical, unconscious causes of behavior, whereas behavior therapy emphasizes current, ongoing causes. In treating a patient, the psychodynamic therapist asks: Why did he become this kind of person? But the behavior therapist asks: What's causing him to function this way now, and what can be done to change that level of functioning? An adequate behavioral assessment serves as the basis for a multifaceted treatment program that deals with the full range of factors maintaining the problem.

COGNITIVE THERAPY

Cognitive therapies are all based on the assumption that emotional disorders result from maladaptive thought patterns. The task of therapy, therefore, is to restructure these maladaptive cognitions. The two most prominent forms of cognitive treatment are Ellis's rational-emotive therapy (RET) and Beck's (1976) cognitive therapy.

Rational-Emotive Therapy

According to the principles behind **rational-emotive therapy (RET),** emotional disorders are rooted in people's irrational beliefs, which are distortions of objective reality. Ellis (1970) listed 12 irrational core assumptions that could be at the root of most emotional disturbances. Here are a few examples of these irrational ideas:

- It's absolutely necessary to be loved by everyone for everything you do.
- It's easier to avoid life's difficulties and responsibilities than to face them.
- People have virtually no control over their emotions; we can't help feeling certain things.

In everyday situations, individuals don't always consciously or deliberately tell themselves these irrational assumptions. Rather, such assumptions appear to be automatic and pervasive because people repeat them so often that they become overlearned responses. According to RET, then, it's not the experience itself but how the individual perceives that experience that causes neurotic disorders.

This perceptive process is illustrated by Ellis's *A-B-C analysis of depression.* The letter "A" refers to a real-life event—for instance, a broken love affair. "B" symbolizes the person's irrational interpretation of that event, such as believing that nothing has meaning anymore, that there will never be anybody else like him again, and so on. The person greatly exaggerates, or *catastrophizes,* the event's negative meaning. The letter "C" stands for the anxiety and depression the person feels not because of the actual breakup but because of her extremely negative perception of it.

In RET, the therapist helps the patient identify irrational ideas and replace them with more constructive, rational thoughts. In doing so, the therapist must directly challenge the patient's irrational ideas and then model rational reinterpretations of

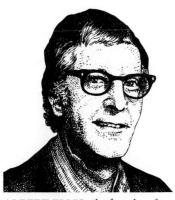

ALBERT ELLIS, *the founder of rational-emotive therapy*

symptom substitution Replacement of one symptom with another following treatment in which the underlying problem is not resolved.

rational-emotive therapy (RET) Therapy aimed at identifying and changing irrational cognitions that are assumed to cause emotional disorders.

disturbing events. The therapist and patient have repeated cognitive rehearsals aimed at substituting rational self-statements for previously irrational interpretations. Additionally, the therapist assigns behavioral tasks that are designed to develop rational reactions to replace the patient's formerly irrational, distress-producing assumptions.

An Evaluation of RET   The effectiveness of RET remains to be proven. Part of the difficulty in doing this lies in specifying the treatment's procedural components. In response to criticism of the conceptual and empirical bases of RET, Ellis has argued that it has been misinterpreted as a treatment approach that's restricted to cognitive restructuring using the techniques of verbal persuasion and logical analysis. He has asserted that RET therapists also use behavior therapy techniques and even methods from other approaches, such as gestalt therapy. In fact, Ellis (1995) has recently renamed his therapy *rational emotive behavior therapy*. The problem, however, with RET becoming so comprehensive—incorporating a wide range of different techniques from other therapies—is that it also becomes difficult to test.

Beck's Cognitive Therapy

The core principle of **Beck's cognitive therapy** (1976) is that holding negative assumptions leads to having negative moods, which, in turn, increases the probability of more negative thinking in what becomes a vicious cycle. Given this, negative assumptions are the target of cognitive therapy. (For further discussion of the foundations of cognitive therapy, see also Chapter 7, the section on the treatment of depression.)

To help patients challenge their dysfunctional assumptions, therapists raise a number of questions. Consider, for example, the case of a patient who felt he was a total failure. Beck, Rush, Shaw, and Emery (1979) listed this series of questions that the therapist would pose:

1. How do you define failure? What are your standards?
2. Have there been degrees of failure: that is, were some failures more total than others?
3. If some experiences were only partial failures, did they also represent partial successes?
4. Were there some areas in your life (friends, family, schoolwork, recreation) in which you did not fail and may, in fact, have reached your goals?
5. Even if you did fail in specific areas, does it follow that you cannot improve and become more successful?
6. Do failures in reaching a goal make you a failure as a person?
7. Should people who have experienced failures be subjected to rejection by other people?
8. Should a person who has suffered defeat subject himself to further pain by rejecting himself? (pp. 195–196)

Cognitive therapists require patients to keep written records of homework assignments that they have both agreed on. For example, patients might be required to identify and challenge the dysfunctional cognitions associated with their problems using **dysfunctional thought records (DTRs).** Figure 18.2 presents an example of a DTR from a patient with bulimia nervosa.

The explicit use of behavioral methods is a fundamental feature of cognitive therapy. Patients do behavioral tasks to help correct dysfunctional cognitions and disprove maladaptive expectations. Instead of arguing with patients about whether their cognitions are valid or helpful, therapists collaborate with them in devising specific behavioral tasks that are framed as experiments to test patients' assumptions. The following excerpt from a treatment session (Clark, 1989) illus-

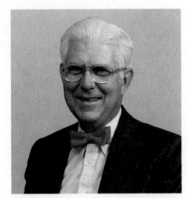

AARON T. BECK, *who developed cognitive therapy for depression*

Beck's cognitive therapy
Form of therapy that helps patients identify and modify dysfunctional thoughts and beliefs.

dysfunctional thought records (DTRs) Records kept by patients between treatment sessions in which they identify dysfunctional thoughts (cognitions) associated with their emotional problems and challenge the validity of those thoughts.

FIGURE 18.2 Example of a dysfunctional thought record (DTR) from a patient with bulimia nervosa

Situation

Describe actual event leading to binge eating (or purging)	My boyfriend and I started discussing what we think is attractive in men and women. I then started feeling fat and as if he couldn't possibly be attracted to me, even though he says he is.

Dysfunctional Thought(s)

Specify the thought(s) that preceded binge eating (or purging)	He'd be much happier and satisfied with another woman who is thinner and more attractive than I am. I need to diet to lose weight.

Challenge Dysfunctional Thought(s)

1. What is the evidence for and against?	Of course he's attracted to me—we've been going out for a long time! I get compliments from other people about my looks.
2. Is there an alternative way of viewing the event?	Just because he says he likes how another woman looks doesn't mean that he thinks I'm unattractive. I admire things in other men—that doesn't mean I don't love him.
3. What is the effect of having this thought?	I know that if I diet, I will probably start binging again. And when that happens, I'll gain more weight.

trates how cognitive therapists prompt patients to examine their assumptions and how behavioral experiments are used to challenge dysfunctional assumptions:

> **Patient [Pt]:** In the middle of a panic attack, I usually think I am going to faint or collapse.
>
> **Therapist [Th]:** How much do you believe that sitting here right now and how much would you believe it if you had the sensations you get in an attack?
>
> **Pt:** 50% now and 90% in an attack.
>
> **Th:** OK, let's look at the evidence you have for this thought. Have you ever fainted in an attack?
>
> **Pt:** No.
>
> **Th:** What is it then that makes you think you might faint?
>
> **Pt:** I feel faint and the feeling can be very strong.
>
> **Th:** So, to summarize, your evidence that you are going to faint is the fact that you feel faint?
>
> **Pt:** Yes.
>
> **Th:** How can you then account for the fact that you have felt faint many hundreds of times and have not yet fainted?
>
> **Pt:** So far, the attacks have always stopped just in time or I have managed to hold onto something to stop myself from collapsing.
>
> **Th:** Right, so one explanation of the fact that you have frequently felt faint, had the thought that you will faint, but have not actually fainted is that you have always done something to save yourself just in time. However, an alternative explanation is that the feeling of faintness that you get in a panic attack will never lead to you collapsing, even if you don't control it.
>
> **Pt:** Yes, I suppose so.
>
> **Th:** In order to decide which of these two possibilities is correct, we need to know what has to happen to your body for you to actually faint. Do you know?

Pt: No.

Th: Your blood pressure needs to drop. Do you know what happens to your blood pressure during a panic attack?

Pt: Well, my pulse is racing. I guess my blood pressure must be up.

Th: That's right. In anxiety, heart rate and blood pressure tend to go together. So, you are actually less likely to faint when you are anxious than when you are not.

Pt: That's very interesting and helpful to know. However, if it's true, why do I feel so faint?

Th: Your feeling of faintness is a sign that your body is reacting in a normal way to the perception of danger. Most of the bodily reactions you are experiencing when anxious were probably designed to deal with the threats experienced by primitive man, such as being approached by a hungry tiger. What would be the best thing to do in that situation?

Pt: Run away as fast as you can.

Th: That's right. And in order to help you run, you need the maximum amount of energy in your muscles. This is achieved by sending more of your blood to your muscles and relatively less to the brain. This means that there is a small drop in oxygen to the brain and that is why you feel faint. However, this feeling is misleading in the sense that it doesn't mean you will actually faint because your overall blood pressure is up, not down.

Pt: That's very clear. So next time I feel faint, I can check out whether I am going to faint by taking my pulse. If it is normal, or quicker than normal, I know I won't faint. (Clark, 1989, pp. 76–77)

An Evaluation of Beck's Cognitive Therapy A major advantage of Beck's cognitive therapy is that it's clearly defined. Because it's adequately implemented and differs procedurally from alternative methods, cognitive therapy has consequently lent itself to research on treatment outcome, which requires such specificity (Hollon & Beck, 1994). We can contrast this explicit identification of treatment procedures and the empirical research that it's permitted with the problems in defining and thus testing RET.

Beck's cognitive therapy has been shown effective in controlled outcome research (Hollon & Beck, 1994). It has been tested extensively in the treatment of depression and consistently produced positive results (see Chapter 7). Evidence has shown that cognitive treatment is also effective in treating anxiety disorders, such as panic disorder (see Chapter 5). However, the reasons for its success in treating these disorders remains to be established.

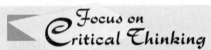

Focus on Critical Thinking

1. Recall from earlier in the chapter Adler's concept of basic mistakes that lead to maladaptive behavior (see p. 575). Consider, as well, that modern cognitive therapies are based on the importance of dysfunctional cognitions. In what ways does Beck's cognitive therapy differ from Adler's approach?

2. Discuss two ways in which Beck's cognitive therapy differs from psychoanalysis.

PSYCHOTHERAPY INTEGRATION

As we've discussed in preceding chapters, a wide range of psychological therapies exist, and they often have conflicting concepts and procedures. But what are the actual practices and attitudes of professionals in the field?

To find out, researchers polled a panel of 75 psychotherapists in 1990 (Norcross, Alford, & DeMichele, 1992). Nearly one-third of the members (31 percent) described their approach as "eclectic," representing an overall trend away from the exclusiveness and narrowness of adhering to a particular system or theory. Another one-third of the panel described their theoretical orientation as either behavioral (18 percent) or psychodynamic (15 percent), and the remaining members categorized themselves as cognitive (10 percent), humanistic (7 percent), or systems (7 percent) therapists.

In contrast with those of the past, today's therapists look for commonalities among different and often conflicting systems. This important development is known as the move toward **psychotherapy integration** (Arkowitz, 1992). The two main directions this quest for integration have taken are *technical eclecticism* and the *common factors approach.* Let's look at each.

Technical Eclecticism

Technical eclecticism allows therapists to draw freely on techniques from all types of psychotherapy without necessarily accepting the theoretical frameworks behind them (Lazarus, Beutler, & Norcross, 1992). This is a practical approach, one that tries to avoid the clash of competing theoretical positions. However, Arnold Lazarus (1989), who founded the technical eclecticism approach, has argued that the field of psychotherapy has not yet reached the stage of development that would permit integrating the different concepts and techniques of varying psychological therapies into a unified whole.

The majority of Lazarus's techniques are standard methods within behavior therapy. This isn't surprising, given that he was one of the clinical pioneers of behavior therapy. But technical eclecticism also uses several nonbehavioral methods. An example is the empty chair technique from gestalt therapy, which Lazarus has adapted as a form of role-playing and role reversal to help individuals modify current maladaptive behavior patterns.

Lazarus (1981) has developed technical eclecticism into what he calls **multimodal therapy.** According to this approach, a patient's problems are assessed across seven different modalities, which are represented by the acronym *BASIC ID:* behavior, affect, sensation, imagery, cognition, interpersonal behavior, and drugs (biology). Comprehensive multimodal therapy requires that interventions be matched to these modalities. Table 18.1 is an example of an assessment profile.

Let's look again at the case of Anita, the 23-year-old teacher described in the chapter-opening. Her therapist, Dr. L., would describe his treatment approach as technical eclecticism. We can identify several different therapeutic strategies that he used in treating Anita.

For example, recall that Anita described how by the end of the first session, Dr. L. had helped her feel more optimistic about life. An important element shared by the different psychotherapies is an initial focus on counteracting the patient's feelings of demoralization or hopelessness. In fact, the first stage of psychotherapy has been called a *remoralization* process. In describing her therapy, Anita also told how she liked the fact that Dr. L. was casual and informal. (Other patients may prefer a more defined, formal style.) She realized the significance that her relationship with Dr. L. had on her benefiting from therapy, which is another core element of all the psychotherapies. Anita felt she could trust Dr. L. and disclose intimate personal details to him because he was nonjudgmental and sincere. These are qualities that a person-centered therapist might describe as *empathy* and *genuineness*. Dr. L. also used specific behavioral techniques in treating Anita, including relaxation training to cope with anxiety and role-playing to become more assertive in interpersonal relationships. In addition, the multimodal nature of Anita's therapy is evident in how Dr. L. focused on her thoughts, imagery, emotions, behaviors, and relationships.

The Common Factors Approach

Goldfried and Castonguay (1992) have advocated the **common factors approach** to integrating psychotherapy. They conceptualize therapy as having different levels of abstraction: the highest consisting of overall theoretical frameworks and the lowest involving specific therapeutic techniques. These clinicians reject both these extremes and instead suggest that the level between theory and practice, which they call *clinical strategies,* offers the possibility of reaching a consensus among different approaches. An example of a clinical strategy that might be common to all

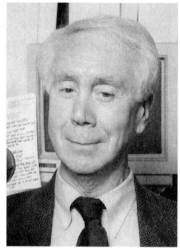

ARNOLD A. LAZARUS, *who has championed the approach of technical eclecticism and multimodal therapy*

psychotherapy integration Process of looking for commonalities among different and often conflicting systems, learning from other perspectives, and integrating divergent methods.

technical eclecticism Form of psychological treatment in which therapists draw on techniques from other systems of psychotherapy without necessarily subscribing to the theories behind the techniques.

multimodal therapy Approach to treatment in which seven modalities of functioning (behavior, affect, sensation, imagery, cognition, interpersonal relations, and biology) are each assessed and then targeted for intervention using an eclectic range of methods; developed by Arnold Lazarus.

common factors approach Approach to psychotherapy integration that emphasizes clinical strategies common to all forms of psychological therapy.

TABLE 18.1	Problem Identification in Multimodal Therapy: A Structured Profile

The following is the structural profile of a 40-year-old man who consulted Arnold Lazarus, complaining of anxiety and panic attacks:

B. Phobic avoidance
Loss of control
Stays in bed when highly anxious (feign illness)

A. Anxious
Panicky
Bouts of depression

S. Abdominal cramps
Headaches
Dizziness
Palpitations
Tension
Numbness
Tremors
Dry mouth
Rapid heart beat

I. Images of helplessness
Pictures himself not coping, losing control, failing
Memories surrounding father's death and funeral
Images of himself dying at age 44 like his father

C. Overvalues Protestant work ethic
Preoccupied with thoughts of death and dying
"My life is controlled by outside forces."
"It is very important to please other people."

I. Overidentified with father
Wife "mothers him for somatic complaints and is critical of his anxieties"

D. Takes tranquilizers
Spastic colon
Smokes about 20 cigarettes a day
Adverse reaction to Tofranil (Psychiatrist had prescribed it to overcome his panic attacks.) (p. 74)

Source: From A. A. Lazarus, *The Practice of Multimodal Therapy.* Copyright © 1981 McGraw-Hill, Inc. Reprinted by permission of McGraw-Hill, Inc.

theoretical orientations is providing the patient with new, corrective emotional experiences. For instance, behavior therapy clearly emphasizes the need for performance-based, corrective learning experiences. Goldfried and Castonguay suggest that other approaches use corrective learning experiences, as well.

Psychodynamic therapists agree about the significance of new learning experiences but differ from behavior therapists as to what experiences are therapeutic. In psychodynamic therapy, the crucial learning experience occurs within the therapeutic relationship: the development and working through of the transference. Even here, though, commonalities have been suggested between psychodynamic and cognitive-behavioral therapy. Psychodynamic therapists believe that transference allows them to uncover patients' childhood conflicts so they can then be resolved. Cognitive therapists, operating from an information-processing framework, might describe transference as the use of that relationship to access and then alter the cognitive-affective processes responsible for patients' problems. Behavior therapists could argue that the patient/therapist relationship brings out anxiety-evoking stimuli that are associated with interpersonal issues, which the patient is then exposed to.

There are two distinct views regarding the status of the common factors approach. One is that there are crucial commonalities that provide a foundation on which we can build a more eclectic and integrated system of psychotherapy (Goldfried & Castonguay, 1992). The second view is that the consensus on the types of strategies identified by Goldfried and others is limited to only the most superficial aspects of treatment. According to this view, the fact that clinicians have fundamentally different perspectives on basic issues means that trying to integrate the diverse forms of psychological therapy is probably futile, at least for the present. An alternative approach would be to concentrate on developing replicable, testable, and effective methods of therapeutic change within each individual system. Once that has been accomplished, it will be easier to determine what elements of different approaches are worthy of integrating into an improved and more comprehensive therapy (Wilson, 1990).

> ### Focus on Critical Thinking
>
> 1. Refer to the most recent discussion of Anita's case on p. 591, where we examined some of the various techniques used by her therapist. Using Lazarus's BASIC ID acronym, determine which modality of functioning each technique addressed.
> 2. Identify and discuss two commonalities between psychoanalytic therapy and behavior therapy.

THE EFFECTIVENESS OF PSYCHOLOGICAL THERAPIES

In 1952, in a landmark paper, Eysenck concluded that there was no acceptable evidence that psychotherapy was more effective than no treatment at all. His challenge ignited a controversy that continues today, as described in Thinking about Controversial Issues (see page 594). Smith, Glass, and Miller (1980) argued the other side of the issue in their widely cited book *The Benefits of Psychotherapy*. They concluded, "Psychotherapy is beneficial, consistently so and in many different ways. Its benefits are on a par with other expensive and ambitious interventions, such as schooling and medicine" (p. 183). Critics, however, have maintained that Eysenck's original assertion cannot be rejected (Prioleau, Murdock, & Brody, 1983).

Even more controversial are claims that some therapeutic approaches are more effective than others. Many clinicians believe that, with few exceptions, no one treatment approach is reliably superior (Beitman, Goldfried, & Norcross, 1989; Lambert & Bergin, 1994). Yet others believe that some therapies are more effective and that specific treatment methods are more effective for particular disorders (Barlow, 1994; Lazarus, 1989). In the preceding chapters, we've described examples of differences in effectiveness among alternative treatments. For example, exposure treatment has repeatedly been found the most effective psychological method for treating phobic disorders. And as we've noted throughout the book, it's now possible to compare the effects of specific psychological methods with those of drug treatments. Depending on the disorder, either a psychological or a drug treatment may be preferable. In some cases, a combined biobehavioral treatment approach is called for.

Another understandably controversial issue is whether therapy can make patients worse. Bergin (1966) used the term *deterioration effect* to describe findings that some patients were, in fact, worse after treatment. Specifically, he examined the results of studies comparing groups of patients receiving psychological treatment with control groups receiving no treatment. The data showed that the variance in treatment outcome was greater for the treatment groups than for the control groups. Bergin interpreted these data to mean that some treated patients improved while others deteriorated. He suggested that either treatment techniques or certain therapists caused patients to become worse. Subsequently, Strupp, Hadley, and Gomes-Schwartz (1977) introduced the term **negative effect** to describe the worsening of patients' problems caused by therapy. To be sure, though, it's hard to establish a causal link between patients' worsening and the therapy they received or the therapists who treated them.

negative effect Outcome of psychotherapy in which the patient's problems have become worse.

The world of psychotherapy was rocked by the recent charge made by highly respected psychologist Robyn Dawes, who said that the "credentials and experience of psychotherapists are unrelated to whether patients benefit from treatment" (1994, p. 38). According to Dawes, any sensitive person can do insight-oriented psychotherapy, provided she can show empathy for patients. Likewise, anyone can do behavior therapy, provided she knows something about behavioral principles.

To become a professional psychologist in the United States, you have to be licensed. Licensure requires earning a doctoral degree, having at least 2 years of supervised postdoctoral experience, and passing written and practical examinations. If correct, Dawes's charge discredits the validity of these licensing requirements. Moreover, Dawes has cast doubt on the value of years of training and practice, which are usually presumed to have a profound effect on the ability to administer competent treatment. Can you imagine the practice of medicine or dentistry being unrelated to years of training?

Believe it or not, the available empirical evidence has generally supported Dawes. Even though the much-cited review of hundreds of studies of psychotherapy outcome by Smith, Glass, and Miller (1980) showed that psychological treatment is effective, it found that therapists' credentials were irrelevant. It made no difference whether the therapist was a psychiatrist (M.D.), a clinical psychologist (Ph.D. or Psy.D.), or a social worker (M.S.W.). Nor did it matter whether the therapist was a recent graduate or an experienced veteran. Several other reviews of the literature have arrived at the same conclusion (Christensen & Jacobson, 1994).

A much earlier, well-known study by Strupp and Hadley (1979) has also illustrated Dawes's point. Patients who experienced primarily anxiety and depression were treated for the same length of time by one of two types of therapists. The first group comprised highly experienced, psychoanalytically oriented psychotherapists, with an average of 23 years' experience. The second group of therapists were liberal arts college professors who were chosen because of their reputations as being warm, understanding, and interested in students; the professors had no training in psychology. At the conclusion of therapy, no differences were found between subjects treated by the two types of therapists.

Critics of Dawes's position recognize that the available evidence has not shown that experienced therapists do better than untrained personnel. But they counter with the following points:

1. The studies on which Dawes's conclusion is based are flawed (Lambert, Shapiro, & Bergin, 1986).
2. Professional psychologists would be more effective with the full range of different patients and disorders than the problems studied to date. Although nonprofessionals might be well suited to treat some problems in some patients, professional therapists are needed to treat other presumably more complicated cases (Berman & Norton, 1985).
3. In some of these studies, the nonprofessionals had been trained and supervised by professional therapists (Weisz, Weiss, Alicke, & Klotz, 1987).

Are these legitimate points? Let's consider each.

First, to try to dismiss the numerous studies that Dawes cites as flawed is not good enough, by itself. Research findings cannot merely be discounted when they don't serve your professional purpose. Similarly, Strupp and Hadley (1979) cannot explain away their own finding by speculating that experience would make a difference with other patients. It might, but we don't have any evidence to prove that.

Regarding the third point, not all the studies involved training nonprofessionals. The college professors in the Strupp and Hadley (1979) study were true novices as far as psychotherapy was concerned. But the concept of training nonprofessionals (or at least professionals with limited credentials) to administer effective treatments is a good one. Research is needed to show how far we can go with such a cost-effective approach.

Think about the following questions:

1. Of all the different psychological therapies described in this chapter, which do you think are most likely to require intensive professional training? Why?
2. Of all the different psychological disorders discussed in this book, which do you think require treatment by a therapist with intensive professional training? Why?

Meta-Analysis

meta-analysis *Quantitative method of integrating the standardized results of a large number of separate studies.*

A new means of evaluating the effects of psychological therapies is a statistical technique known as **meta-analysis,** a quantitative method for integrating the standardized results of different studies (Smith, Glass, & Miller, 1980). The unit of analysis in a meta-analysis is the **effect size (ES),** a statistical index of treatment-produced change. A common way of calculating the ES is to subtract the mean (average) of the control group from that of the treatment group and then divide that difference by the standard deviation of the control group. The larger the ES, the greater the effect of the treatment. ES values from separate studies using different samples and measures can then be combined and analyzed in sophisticated statistical tests of the effects of alternative treatments.

The proponents of meta-analysis have argued that it is superior to traditional qualitative reviews of the research literature because it eliminates or at least minimizes the subjectivity that can bias reviews of research evidence (Smith et al., 1980). Critics have charged, however, that this claim of greater objectivity can be illusory (Erwin, 1986; Paul, 1985). For example, Smith et al. (1980) included all studies in their meta-analysis, regardless of individual quality. They then assigned equal weights in their statistical analyses to studies judged methodologically good versus bad. The problem in doing this is that the relatively small number of well-controlled studies in the literature are swamped by the majority of flawed studies (Wilson, 1985). Smith et al. (1980) nonetheless defended their procedure, claiming that the methodological features of different studies can be systematically related to outcome using statistical techniques. Other experts have asserted that only studies with adequate controls should be included.

Considering these issues, we must ask: Who determines the methodological features of specific studies, and what criteria are used to judge individual studies? Clearly, these are human decisions that inevitably involve subjectivity and often create controversy.

In any meta-analysis, a variety of subjective and arbitrary judgments must be made before the data are entered into the computer, such as what studies to include and what methodological features to emphasize. Nevertheless, the process of examining each study in detail to make these judgments has made more public what was usually a private process in conducting conventional reviews of the therapy outcome literature (Mintz, 1983). This change and the subsequent ability it creates to carry out sophisticated statistical tests are the strengths of meta-analysis.

The meta-analyses done to date have not resolved the controversy about the effectiveness of alternative therapies. Different meta-analyses, even of the same set of studies, have yielded inconsistent findings (Searles, 1985). To a large extent, the difficulty has been in how the method has been used, rather than in the method itself. Despite the controversy, it's widely believed that meta-analysis will fundamentally change how the medical and behavioral sciences process large amounts of data from different studies (Mann, 1990).

◢ ℰ*ocus on* ℰ*ritical Thinking*

Think about the different forms of therapy summarized in this chapter and in the preceding chapters on specific clinical disorders.

1. Do you believe that any single form of psychological therapy is more effective than others? Explain your answer.
2. If you were to seek treatment for a psychological problem, would you prefer any particular form of therapy? Again, explain your answer.

effect size (ES) *Statistical index of the extent of treatment effects; calculated by subtracting the mean of the control group from that of the treatment group and dividing the difference by the standard deviation of the control group.*

ℰ*HE* F*UTURE OF* P*SYCHOTHERAPY*

Health Care Reform

Health care reform was one of the primary issues in the 1992 U.S. presidential election and promises to be again in 1996. Americans have widely different and sometimes antagonistic views about the future of health care in this country. What do psychotherapists think?

This question was asked of the 75-member panel of psychotherapists discussed earlier in this chapter (Norcross et al., 1992). Specifically, when asked to predict what would happen to the practice of psychotherapy in the future, the panel showed impressive consensus, regardless of which therapeutic approaches they personally preferred. The panel predicted that the emphasis would be on present-centered, problem-focused, and time-limited psychological treatments. Although the psychodynamic approach is one of the most commonly used today, the panel predicted that it would be one of the least used in the future. Even the psychodynamic therapists among the group shared this opinion.

The reason this shift in therapeutic emphasis will likely occur is one of the central issues in health care reform. Most people anticipate that in the future, government or private insurance programs will reimburse patients only for time-limited treatments. Moreover, it's likely that certain kinds of therapy will not be covered and that patients will not have as much freedom in selecting therapists. Similar limits are already in place in many insurance programs for health care of all kinds. This development is often blamed on the so-called **managed care movement**—represented by health maintenance organizations (HMOs)—in which all medical costs and procedures are tightly controlled (Hoyt & Austad, 1992).

Women's issues will also likely be addressed in health care reform. As noted in Thinking about Gender Issues, more and more women are going into psychology, especially clinical psychology. The greater presence of women in the field will undoubtedly direct attention to women's issues, which often means children's issues, as well.

Psychotherapy and High Technology

Technological advances, especially in electronics, continually change the world we live in. Is it too farfetched to imagine something called **electronic therapy?**

It all started with the telephone. For many years, suicide hotlines have provided a useful source of crisis intervention for callers who reach out for help. Similar call-in services exist for people who have experienced various types of abuse, including women and children who have been physically or sexually abused. Many therapists also take emergency calls from patients in extreme situations. In addition, many therapists maintain regular telephone contact with their patients, such as brief check-ins between therapy sessions.

But within the past few years, we've seen the telephone used in a new way: National networks of "telephone therapists" have been created to treat people for $3 to $4 per minute (Newman, 1994). Most professional therapists are understandably apprehensive about this development, which has raised a number of questions: What problems can be handled appropriately through telephone therapists? How can people with problems that are appropriate for telephone therapy be differentiated from those whose problems are not—say, someone in a psychotic state? What sort of training is necessary to qualify an effective telephone therapist?

Today, we see the telephone combined with the computer to create "e-mail therapy." As Newman (1994) describes, "For a monthly subscription fee (plus the cost of computer time), computer aficionados [can] have access to keyboard-equipped therapists poised for empathic responding virtually anywhere in the world" (p. 25). Newman, who is a professional psychotherapist, has negative views about these developments. He points out that the potential for misuse is staggering. Yet given that this technology exists, the profession of clinical psychology must face how to avoid misusing it as well as how to utilize whatever advantages electronic therapy offers.

Another quite remarkable use of computer technology with possible therapeutic uses is *virtual reality*, which refers to a means of manipulating the environment you experience. In most applications, the individual wears a helmet that covers his eyes and blocks out his peripheral vision. The helmet also contains a small computer screen that displays a computer graphics environment. This is the environment the individual experiences; it seems real, in all respects. By controlling what appears on the screen, the individual can control this perceived environment.

managed care movement
System of health care in which all costs, options, and procedures are tightly controlled by health maintenance organizations (HMOs).

electronic therapy Treatment delivered via the telephone or computers, such as hotlines, telephone networks, and electronic mail (e-mail).

Thinking about GENDER ISSUES   The Feminization of Psychotherapy

For the past decade, more than half of all doctoral degrees in psychology awarded in the United States have gone to women (Goodheart & Markham, 1992). This trend toward the feminization of psychology is especially strong in clinical psychology training programs. In many of these, three-quarters or more of the students are women.

Psychology and psychotherapy have been dominated by men over the past 100 years. Considering this history, some observers see the rapidly growing number of women in the profession as a social success story. The profession has opened up to women. But not everyone sees it this way. Both male and female psychotherapists have expressed concern that the feminization of the field will devalue its status and importance. Goodheart and Markham (1992) have predicted that as women disproportionately dominate clinical psychology, the entire profession will be devalued. As a result, clinical psychologists will earn less and be less respected.

The more positive side to the increasing number of women professionals within clinical psychology is that the field will be diversified to the benefit of both women and men. The greater presence of women will also ensure that attention is given to women's issues, which many feel might have been deemphasized in the past.

Think about the following question:

1. In response to the trend toward feminization, some clinical training programs have discussed preferentially selecting male graduate students to admit equal num-

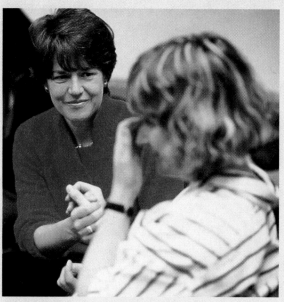

The majority of graduate students in clinical psychology today are women. More and more women are becoming psychotherapists.

bers of each sex. This amounts to affirmative action for men. Is this policy sensible or fair? Should a more qualified woman be denied admission in favor of a less qualified man simply to meet sexual quotas? Explain your answers.

---

virtual reality therapy
Computer-based means of manipulating the environment an individual experiences.

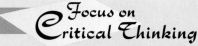 *Focus on* Critical Thinking

1. A common denominator of all psychological therapies is the relationship between therapist and patient. As described in this chapter, that relationship is the most important feature of psychotherapy. Can a patient develop a therapeutic relationship with a telephone (electronic) therapist whom she never actually sees? If so, how would it differ from the traditional therapeutic relationship? Explain your answer(s).

2. What problems other than phobias might virtual reality therapy be suitable for? Might this treatment make some problems worse? Again, explain your answers.

Virtual reality therapy has been used to treat patients with phobic disorders. For example, someone who is afraid of heights can create an environment in which she is exposed to specific situations that elicit anxiety, such as climbing a fire escape or walking across the Golden Gate Bridge. From what we know about the effectiveness of exposure treatment in treating people with phobias (see Chapter 5), virtual reality therapy makes sense. Also consider that therapists often have to use imaginal exposure. Some patients aren't good at generating vivid imagery, and real-life exposure is often inconvenient, dangerous, or even impossible. Virtual reality provides a more powerful and convenient means of achieving exposure.

The initial clinical reports about the use of virtual reality therapy are promising (Steven, 1995). Controlled studies are still needed, however, to verify if this treatment is really more efficient and effective than current methods.

Psychoanalysis and Psychodynamic Therapies

■ Psychoanalytic therapies remain a prevalent treatment approach for people with abnormal behavior. Core psychoanalytic concepts emphasize the unconscious motives behind behavior, early childhood experiences, and intrapsychic conflicts.

■ Traditional Freudian psychoanalysis is relatively rare today. The more commonly used methods are ego-analytic and brief psychodynamic offshoots of Freud's approach. Despite their popularity, however, psychoanalytic therapies enjoy only limited empirical support.

Interpersonal Psychotherapy

■ Interpersonal psychotherapy (IPT) focuses primarily on interpersonal relationships.

■ The goals of IPT are to identify patients' conflicts with others and to help them resolve these conflicts, to help patients move into new roles, and to remedy deficits in interpersonal skills.

Humanistic and Existential Psychotherapies

■ Humanistic and existential therapies assume that people are innately motivated to affect their environments and achieve personal fulfillment.

■ Rogers's person-centered therapy assumes that if therapists are empathic and genuine and express unconditional positive regard for their patients, personal growth will occur. Therapists who do not express these relationship qualities may make patients' problems worse.

■ Gestalt therapy is a humanistic/existential approach focusing on the here and now. The goal of therapy is for individuals to gain increased awareness of their inner feelings and environmental influences and to take personal responsibility for their feelings and actions. Gestalt therapists are more directive than Rogerians and use a range of different techniques to promote awareness.

Behavior Therapy

■ Behavior therapy is the application of the principles and procedures of experimental psychology to clinical problems. It focuses primarily on the current determinants of behavior, rather than the historical origins of problems.

■ Behavior therapy encompasses a wide range of techniques, variously based on the principles of classical and operant conditioning, on the one hand, and cognitive psychology, on the other. The increasing emphasis on cognitive principles and procedures has led to use of the term *cognitive-behavioral therapy (CBT)* to describe the approach.

■ Behavior therapy techniques have been extensively evaluated and are broadly applicable to a wide range of problems in diverse patient populations.

Cognitive Therapy

■ Cognitive therapy is based on the assumption that emotional disorders result from dysfunctional thinking. The treatment goal is to identify and then alter the maladaptive thoughts.

■ Both Ellis's rational-emotive therapy (RET) and Beck's cognitive therapy prompt patients to challenge their dysfunctional thoughts. Beck's approach, however, relies more heavily on behavioral methods to correct those thoughts. Therapists collaborate with patients in devising specific behavioral tasks to test patients' assumptions.

■ Beck's cognitive therapy has been found effective in the treatment of anxiety disorders and depression, whereas RET has received little direct empirical support.

Psychotherapy Integration

■ Therapists today try to find commonalities among different and often conflicting systems, to learn from other perspectives, and to integrate divergent methods.

■ In technical eclecticism, Lazarus combines techniques from other systems with cognitive-behavioral therapy to address seven different modalities of functioning: behavior, affect, sensation, imagery, cognition, interpersonal behavior, and drugs (biology). In order, these modalities form the acronym *BASIC ID.*

The Effectiveness of Psychological Therapies

■ Evaluation of the effectiveness of psychological treatments remains controversial. One group of investigators believes that psychological therapy has been shown to be effective and that no differences exist among different psychotherapeutic approaches. Another group argues that some therapies are more effective than others and that specific treatment methods are more effective for particular disorders than others.

The Future of Psychotherapy

■ The majority of psychologists believe that future pressures to reduce costs will result in their providing psychological treatment that is present centered, problem focused, and time limited.

■ Advances in electronics, involving primarily telephone and computer technologies, have already led to the development of new and sometimes controversial therapeutic methods—a trend that will likely continue.

KEY TERMS

applied behavior analysis, **p. 584**
assertion training, **p. 585**
basic mistakes, **p. 575**
Beck's cognitive therapy, **p. 588**
cognitive-behavioral therapy (CBT), **p. 586**
cognitive restructuring, **p. 586**
common factors approach, **p. 591**
dream interpretation, **p. 574**
dysfunctional thought records (DTRs), **p. 588**
effect size (ES), **pp. 594–595**
efficacy expectations, **p. 585**
ego psychology, **p. 575**
electronic therapy, **p. 596**

empathy, **p. 580**
free association, **p. 573**
genuineness, **p. 580**
insight, **p. 574**
interpersonal psychotherapy (IPT), **p. 578**
managed care movement, **p. 596**
meta-analysis, **p. 594**
multimodal therapy, **p. 591**
negative effect, **p. 593**
outcome expectations, **p. 585**
outcome research, **p. 578**
parataxic distortions, **p. 575**
process research, **p. 577**
psychotherapy integration, **p. 591**

rational-emotive therapy (RET), **p. 587**
resistance, **p. 573**
self-actualization, **p. 580**
self-monitoring, **p. 586**
self-psychology, **p. 576**
social learning approach, **p. 584**
stimulus-response approach, **p. 584**
symptom substitution, **p. 587**
technical eclecticism, **p. 591**
transference, **p. 574**
unconditional positive regard, **p. 580**
virtual reality therapy, **p. 597**

CRITICAL THINKING EXERCISE

Return to the case of Anita, from the opening of this chapter. In it, she describes briefly how she was treated by Dr. L., who practices multimodal therapy. Now put yourself in the place of a psychodynamic therapist.

1. What would your approach be in treating Anita?

2. Describe the most important ways in which a psychodynamic treatment approach would differ from the multimodal approach used by Dr. L.

Chapter 19

MARITAL, FAMILY, GROUP, AND COMMUNITY THERAPIES

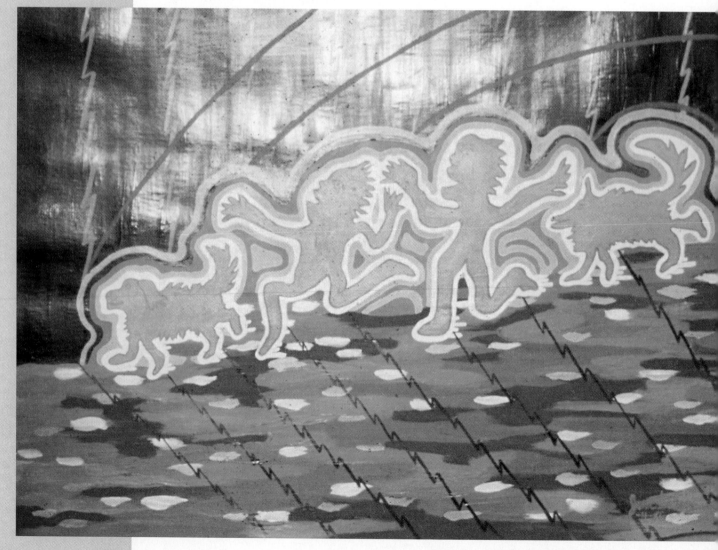

Jane Gerus, **Friends,** 1986, Very Special Arts Gallery

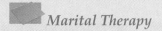
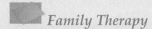
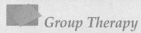
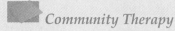
Kim and Lenny were married 25 years ago. Lenny had a good job with a local contracting firm and had worked there for 20 years. While their two children were growing up, Kim didn't work outside the home. When the children began high school, however, Kim began working for a real estate firm. Lenny complained that Kim "retired" from her household responsibilities after she took the job. And indeed, Kim refused to continue doing everything that she had done before she started working outside the home. She now worked almost the same number of hours as Lenny, and she thought he should share equally in the household chores. Lenny was angry that Kim spent considerable time making herself look good to go to work and that she gave her full energy to her job. Although she and Lenny argued a lot, Kim could forget about their disagreements, usually by later in the same day. In contrast, she felt that Lenny was spiteful and could not "forgive and forget." Lenny's resentment was clearly building. Jealousy was not discussed openly, but it was obviously present. Last year, Lenny slapped Kim twice when she came home from the movies with her girlfriends one night at 1:00 A.M.

After the slapping incident, Kim sometimes called Lenny lazy and selfish. In turn, Lenny would refuse to talk at all with Kim for several days. He withdrew from social interactions with her, and they spent very little time talking, although they were both at home most evenings. He was generally unhappy. He slept 10 to 12 hours per day on weekends. Like Lenny, Kim had symptoms of depression. She said she generally felt "down" at home. She had little energy to do things around the house, and she was rarely interested in sex. According to Kim, Lenny hugged and kissed her only when he wanted sex. According to Lenny, intercourse was great when it occurred—about once every 8 weeks. (Kim said he had a poor memory about sex, since her recollection was that they had sex once every 3 to 4 weeks.)

Kim said that Lenny was thoughtful and a great dad. She enjoyed walking on the beach with him, and she liked to talk about what they read. She definitely wanted to stay in the marriage. As she said, "At 52, where am I going to find a man?" Occasionally, Lenny wasn't sure whether he wanted to remain married. He threatened Kim with divorce and left home twice. (Kim said that they never really had a separation, because he just went to his mother's house and stayed there only a week each time.) When asked whether he loved Kim, Lenny said, "Yes, but we can't go on like this. Things have to change, or I am going to leave for good."

What's typical about Kim and Lenny's marital troubles? Couples say communication is their most important problem, and they rank lack of love as second. Kim and Lenny have both these problems, and their interactions are like those of many distressed couples. Often, for example, when women bring up issues they feel must be addressed, such as sharing household responsibilities, men withdraw—even refuse to talk at all. Changes in the roles of men and women in recent decades have contributed to marital problems; many men have difficulty with the idea of their wives working outside the home, just as Lenny did. Frequently, too, the husband, the wife, or both have individual problems such as depression that influence the marriage. Lenny often felt depressed, and Kim did, as well.

Can a marriage like this be helped? As we'll see in this chapter, unhappy marriages can generally be improved, at least to some degree. One of the most successful ways of making this change is through marital therapy, in which a couple works through their problems together. As you may recall, in the last chapter, we discussed individual approaches to treating psychological disorders. Critics of individual forms of treatment suggest that they are far too expensive to adequately address the vast number of psychological problems that affect people in U.S. society. However, the argument for moving beyond individual therapy isn't simply a matter of cost. Many contend that the individual is often the wrong focus of treatment. In this chapter, we'll address four types of therapy that focus on more than one individual: marital, family, group, and community therapies.

MARITAL THERAPY

Each day, thousands of Americans go to therapists for help with marital problems per se, not because of marital trouble brought about by some other issue, such as depression or alcoholism. People go to marital therapists for help in maintaining their marriages and families. Thus, we'll briefly discuss the prevalence and impact of marital problems themselves in order to clarify the importance of marital therapy.

Prevalence and Impact of Marital Problems

Of all the difficulties people face, divorce and marital separation rank second and third, respectively, as the most significant life stressors, exceeded only by the death of a spouse (Holmes & Rahe, 1967). At least half of the depressed women who seek treatment (see Chapter 7) have clinically significant marital difficulties. Further, most couples with sexual problems (such as low sexual desire, situational impotency, and orgasmic dysfunction) have marital trouble. In addition, if one spouse has alcohol or drug-dependency problems, significant marital disruptions are usually present. In some cases, marital difficulties may result from other problems, such as substance abuse or schizophrenia; in others, they may lead to the individual psychological problems mentioned earlier, such as depression. In light of the growing awareness that marital distress can cause or magnify individual problems (Gotlib & McCabe, 1990), many researchers have concentrated on developing marital therapy either as a primary treatment or as a supplement to other therapies.

Divorce and separation have widespread consequences for many other social and mental health problems. For instance, depression and suicide among adolescents and young adults are higher today than they have ever been. Experts in depression research believe that one reason for these increases is the rise in divorce and the dissolution of family support (Klerman & Weissman, 1990). According to the U.S. Census Bureau (Norton & Miller, 1992), in 1990, the United States had the

Thinking about GENDER ISSUES   **Why Get Married?**

$\mathcal{Y}$ears ago, sociologist Jesse Bernard (1972) argued that marriage was good for men but bad for women. Many people still wonder whether she was correct.

Married women who stay home to take care of their children sometimes feel trapped. Some suggest that marriage is a convenient way for men to have their meals cooked, their laundry done, and their children raised. Even in the 1990s, we are not on the fast track to gender equality when it comes to work done at home. Women still do at least twice as much of the household work and chores as men (Schor, 1991). In the United States today, twice as many men as women report having affairs (Lauman, Gagnon, Michael, & Michaels, 1994). As might be expected, in numerous studies, wives report being less satisfied with their marriages than their husbands do (Margolin, Talovic, & Weinstein, 1983). And although marriage does protect people against dying young, it protects men more than women (Lillard & Waite, 1995).

If more than 40 percent of young couples divorce, many might question the idea of marriage. Young people are clearly delaying the age at which they get married.

However, at least 90 percent of high school students say they want to marry. And, in fact, about 90 to 95 percent of all men and women do marry (Norton & Miller, 1992). Even of those who divorce, most want to remarry. Approximately 70 to 75 percent of those whose first marriages end in divorce do remarry.

Despite the disadvantages of marriage, for many people, it provides a lifelong companion. For others, marriage and family are among the most satisfying aspects of life. Research has shown that married men and women are happier (O'Leary & Wilson, 1987) and live longer than unmarried people. Finally, when a marriage is good, it provides a buffer against many of the psychological abnormalities described in this text.

Think about the following questions:

1. In American society, increasing numbers of women are employed outside the home. How might this development affect the psychological and physical benefits of marriage for women?
2. What types of benefits do men *and* women receive from marriage? Explain your answers.

largest percentage of children living in single-parent families among major industrialized countries—Australia, Canada, Germany, France, Italy, and Japan. Specifically, in that year, 25 percent of all U.S. children lived in families headed by single parents, and 55 percent of all black children lived in such families (Norton & Miller, 1992).

Marital problems are also associated with decreases in biological functioning, according to a number of studies. More specifically, both divorce and marital disruption appear to lead to decreases in immune function (Kiecolt-Glaser & Glaser, 1992). It isn't clear that the reductions in immune function associated with marital distress influence individuals' likelihood of developing infections or other diseases. However, many clinicians presume that the likelihood of infections and diseases does increase if the stressors are intense and occur over a long period. Perhaps even more striking are the data showing that married men and women live longer than those who are not married. As found recently in a sample of 11,112 individuals, "Marriage appears to protect its incumbents against many of life's blows. The married, especially men, show lower levels of alcohol and cigarette consumption, higher earnings, and perhaps as a consequence, lower levels of [premature] mortality than the unmarried" (Lillard & Waite, 1995, p. 1131). Related research following up 1,500 gifted individuals showed that marital instability was predictive of premature death (Friedman et al., 1995).

Some researchers have suggested that marriage benefits men more than women (a notion that's shared by some people in the general public, as well). Thinking about Gender Issues considers what men and women get out of marriage in answering the question: Why get married?

Treatment of Marital/Relationship Problems

Marital therapy aims to help couples improve their communication; develop insight into their problems; explore the feelings they experience in their typical negative interactions; and, hopefully, rekindle some of the sparks that existed in the relationship at an earlier time. Marital or relationship therapies are used not only with young married couples but with unmarried couples, gay or lesbian couples, and now often with elderly couples. Marital therapists also treat couples who wish to separate and divorce on amicable terms so as to minimize the negative impact of the parental split on the children.

Before the start of marital therapy, therapists usually meet with each partner separately. These individual sessions allow the therapist to obtain a sense of the different perspectives that the partners have about the relationship. In addition, the individual assessment sessions are necessary to establish whether there are alcohol, drug, spouse abuse, and/or infidelity issues that might interfere significantly with marital therapy. If any of these issues pose problems, the therapist will often suggest individual therapy prior to or in conjunction with marital therapy. (See Chapter 18 for a discussion of individual therapy.)

Following the individual assessment sessions, the therapist begins sessions with both partners together, called **conjoint sessions.** Sometimes, the therapist uses the first conjoint session to get some sense of the interaction between the partners—that is, to see how they communicate with each other. Unfortunately, both partners are not always willing to attend marital therapy sessions. The unwillingness of a partner to participate in marital therapy often reflects a lack of commitment to the relationship. And understandably, treating only one partner is less effective than treating both (Gurman & Kniskern, 1986).

The couples who profit most from marital therapy are those who have some commitment to remaining together and some love or caring for each other. Often, as illustrated in the case of Kim and Lenny at the beginning of this chapter, either the husband or the wife may be questioning whether to remain in the marriage.

marital therapy Intervention designed to help couples improve their communication, develop insight into their problems, and explore their feelings.

conjoint sessions Marital therapy sessions in which both partners are present.

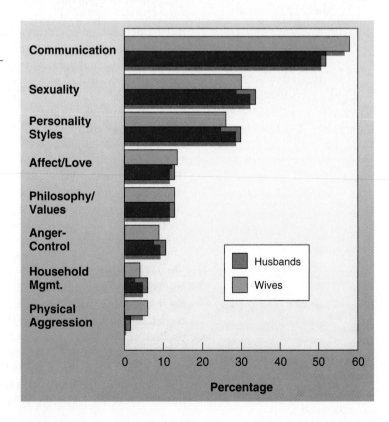

FIGURE 19.1 Men and women reporting problems at the initial marital assessment (in percent)

Source: Reprinted from *Behaviour Research and Therapy, 14,* O'Leary et al., "Assessment of Physical Aggression in Marriage: The Need for Multimodal Assessment." Copyright © 1992 with kind permission from Elsevier Science, Ltd., The Boulevard, Langford Lane, Kiddlington OX5 1GB, UK.

However, if the couple share some desire to remain together, marital therapy can help clarify their options. In assessment sessions, more than 50 percent of men and women say that their main problem is communication (see Figure 19.1). About one-third of men and women report decreased interest in sexual interactions and conflicting personality styles. Lack of affection and love is reported as the main problem in about 10 percent of relationships (O'Leary, Vivian, & Malone, 1992).

The marital therapies we'll describe in this chapter have been used to treat a wide variety of relationship problems, including infrequent sexual interactions, infidelity, and differences over finances, childrearing, and gender roles. Marital therapies have also been used when one partner has a specific mental disorder, such as substance abuse, depression, and hypochondria. In these cases, marital therapy is adapted to the particular needs of the partner with the disorder. In brief, marital therapy has proved quite useful with diverse groups in the United States and Europe, either as a treatment itself or in combination with individual therapy for specific disorders (Beach, Whisman, & O'Leary, 1994; Hahlweg, 1988).

Changing Patterns of Communication   Regardless of theoretical orientation, most marital therapies attempt to analyze and change couples' communication patterns. The key to mending the communication process is getting each partner to listen to the other with concern and understanding. Generally, such understanding occurs after the husband and wife ask for clarification of certain statements. In the beginning, the therapist often works to clarify meanings, feelings, and messages sent, but as therapy progresses, clarification and restatement of problems come directly from the partners. To develop mutual understanding, the therapist helps each partner express empathy for the other's feelings and needs. Partners learn that agreeing with each other isn't always necessary. Once they understand and empathize with each other, the couple can begin to resolve differences and find ways to satisfy each other's needs.

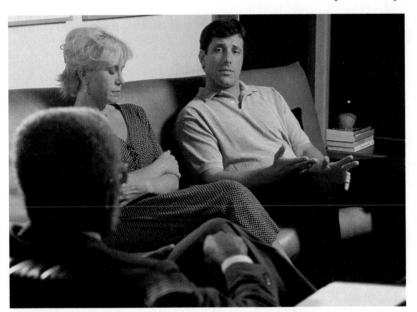

Therapists at SUNY Stony Brook conduct marital therapy and have demonstrated that communication problems are central to marital difficulties. What stressors are most likely to affect marriages of young men and women?

Some couples tend to avoid discussing problems altogether. Others are apt to become angry and critical; although they may finally disclose negative feelings, they often make no progress toward solving problems. Therapists encourage all couples to communicate their feelings and needs directly. Partners are taught to avoid general, sweeping criticisms ("You're a lazy bum") and to replace them with specific requests and suggestions ("I'd really appreciate your help with the dishes"). They learn to substitute direct expression of their own feelings and desires ("I would love to go dancing this weekend") for negative or coercive attempts to get their way ("Are you going to sit in front of that stupid TV all weekend again?").

Once the partners begin to communicate feelings and desires more effectively and learn to empathize with each other, therapy often turns to problem-solving skills. The partners are encouraged to define a problem and then brainstorm possible solutions. Next, they evaluate the possible solutions and decide which to implement. Often, partners need to negotiate compromises—for instance, "I'll stay home with the kids while you do aerobics on Wednesday if I can go bowling on

Thursday." Sometimes, they have to choose a solution that is only partly satisfactory for each person, in order to avoid solutions that are completely satisfactory for one partner but unsatisfactory for the other.

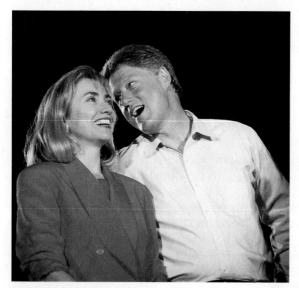

In a television address before the 1992 presidential campaign, Bill Clinton publicly addressed the marital problems he and his wife had.

Changing Attitudes   Many dissatisfied husbands and wives have irrational attitudes and/or unrealistic expectations of their partners and of marriage. One common unrealistic expectation is: My spouse should always agree with me; otherwise, he doesn't love me. Another is: My partner should know what I'm thinking or feeling without me having to tell her (Baucom & Epstein, 1990; Eidelson & Epstein, 1982).

People in distressed marriages often believe that marriage should satisfy all their needs. They may even perceive friendships or interests outside the marital relationship as threatening or upsetting. Unhappy husbands and wives also frequently attribute their partner's negative behaviors to stable traits ("He is basically a mean person"). This attitude can lead spouses to ignore the changes the partner makes in therapy. The therapist prompts each partner to discover and change unreasonable beliefs or thoughts that produce distressing feelings. According to Epstein, Schlesinger, and Dryden (1988), the therapist should try to get the partners involved in a discovery process by having them adopt certain attitudes for specified periods. The idea is to let couples see how changing their attitudes affects their feelings and behavior.

Changing Behavior   Many therapists also directly attempt to change the daily interactions of the couple—especially to reduce criticism and increase positive, supportive comments and actions. To increase positive behaviors, the therapist might have each partner focus on the other for a day at a time, showing love through daily actions. The concept of **love days** was developed by Weiss, Hops, and Patterson (1973) and extended by Stuart (1980) as **caring days;** it is still implemented by many therapists (Baucom & Epstein, 1990). As each partner shows the other caring by everyday actions, the husband and wife begin to feel better about each other.

The first step in the caring days procedure is for each spouse to list things that the other partner could do to demonstrate caring. This list is usually made for a week. Once the caring days list has been agreed on, the therapist emphasizes that each person is responsible for carrying out some of his or her partner's requests on certain days, regardless of the partner's behavior. This is not a tit-for-tat agreement. The husband, for example, agrees to do nice things for his wife on particular days, even if she fails to do the things he requested. An individual may have trouble doing some of the nice things on the caring days list for many reasons, and these are discussed with the therapist at the weekly session. When a husband or wife resists doing things on the list, the therapist uses this resistance to clarify underlying issues, such as jealousy, unresolved anger about past events, or bitterness toward a child or stepchild. These problems are discussed while the couple learns to communicate more effectively.

love days or caring days
Technique used in couples therapy to increase daily positive interactions between partners; each person agrees to engage in specific behaviors that please his or her partner.

Effectiveness of Marital Therapy

If increasing marital satisfaction is the goal of therapy, then insight-oriented therapies focusing on *unconscious* factors that influence choice of mate and later marital conflicts are not effective (Beach & O'Leary, 1985; Boelens, Emmelkamp, MacGillavry, & Markvoort, 1980). On the other hand, if the insight concerns the kinds of *behaviors* that should be changed to make the marriage better, then marital therapy is successful in increasing marital satisfaction. Insight alone, therefore, may be beneficial to couples if it involves current interaction patterns and individual personality styles (Boelens et al., 1980; Snyder & Wills, 1989). In fact, a comparison of the results of insight-oriented marital therapy with those of behavioral marital therapy indicated that couples who engaged in insight-oriented therapy fared much better at follow-up (Snyder, Wills, & Grady-Fletcher, 1991).

In most studies, couples begin therapy feeling quite dissatisfied with their marriages. They say therapy significantly improves their marriages, but they still rate the relationships as slightly dissatisfying. Is this amount of change enough to keep husbands and wives together? Apparently, it is. In summarizing over two dozen treatment studies, Jacobson and Addis (1993) reported that therapy consistently increases marital satisfaction. Usually, after 4 to 5 months of weekly meetings with a therapist, clients are more satisfied with their relationships. Couples given marital therapy consistently experience greater improvement in marital satisfaction than no-treatment couples (Shadish et al., 1993). Even trained undergraduates hear improvement when they listen to audiotapes of couples in therapy attempting to solve problems. Moreover, husbands and wives who receive marital therapy typically feel more love and caring for their partners (O'Leary & Arias, 1983).

On the other hand, after treatment, a substantial number of couples feel their relationship is unchanged, and only 50 percent say that they are happily married. Depending on the study, between 60 and 95 percent of the couples who receive marital therapy stay married several years after treatment (Jacobson & Addis, 1993).

Keeping couples married is not necessarily the primary goal of marital therapy, however. For some couples, separation or divorce may be a more desirable outcome than remaining together in a stable but highly unsatisfactory marriage. For instance, if a woman is repeatedly physically abused or if a man is criticized and humiliated daily—and the partners are unwilling to change—marriage may not be psychologically healthy for either spouse. However, as noted earlier, when partners sincerely desire to remain together, both partners can change. And in doing so, they may also feel better about themselves and the relationship. Moreover, strong evidence exists that increased marital satisfaction results in less depression and anxiety (Beach et al., 1994; Snyder & Wills, 1989).

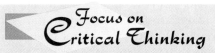

Focus on Critical Thinking

A recent focus in some marital and other therapies is to help men and women accept certain aspects of their partners and family members that simply may not change (Christensen, Jacobson, & Babcock, 1995; Goldfried & Davison, 1994; Seligman, 1994).

1. Under what conditions is this therapeutic strategy of encouraging acceptance realistic and advisable, and under what conditions does it seem like a cop-out?

2. How might a therapist turn a conflict about a marital or other long-standing intimate relationship into an opportunity for better communication and intimacy?

Family Therapy

The central theme for all family therapy is treatment of the family as a whole unit. Like marital therapy, family therapy can be used by therapists of different theoretical orientations, on the general premise that family issues affect us all at points in our lives. Two prominent approaches to family intervention are family systems therapy and problem-solving therapy. We'll cover both in this section.

Family Systems Therapy

family systems therapy
Therapy treating the family as a dynamic system in which each member's role affects each other member and the system as a whole; relationships among family members are emphasized more than the specific difficulties of individual family members.

In **family systems therapy**—the most common approach to treating families—therapists see the family as a dynamic system in which each member has a major role. Thus, if one family member's behavior changes, the whole system of family relationships can change. Given this premise, the family system as a whole becomes the focus of understanding the family and its members. Therapists try to see all members of the family for assessment and treatment.

The relationships among family members are emphasized more than individual family members' specific difficulties. For example, rather than viewing an aggressive child as the problem and treating him alone, a family systems therapist expects every family member to attend treatment sessions, because the child may be reflecting pathology within the family unit or system. According to this approach, problems do not simply flow from one person to another—for instance, from parent to child. All family members, even children, influence one another in complex ways.

The particular roles that family members determine for each other affect their mental health. Let's consider an example: A mother who has defined herself solely as her children's caretaker may begin to feel unimportant or unwanted when the children "leave the nest." In this situation, she may attempt to find new roles within or outside the family; for example, she might take a job outside the home. This, in turn, may cause stresses among family members. A family therapist would avoid blaming any particular individual for the mother's feelings. The therapist would emphasize instead that everyone in the family has shaped the mother's role across many years. This example illustrates why the therapist may ask all the family members to join the therapy sessions, should the mother's changing role disrupt family interactions.

Certain boundaries normally separate parents and children. But such boundaries often become blurred when two family members from different generations form a tight bond and exclude another member. For example, both a mother and a son may harbor resentment against the husband/father for his temper outbursts and physical abuse of the son. The mother and son may then form an alliance, excluding the husband/father in a coalition against a common enemy. In turn, the father will feel more alienated, defensive, and unsupported and become even more easily angered. The system becomes stable, taking on a life of its own.

Another frequently described problem related to boundaries within the family occurs when parents are locked in intense conflict. In an effort to take the pressure off themselves, they may draw a third member—usually, a child—into their system by making her a target of criticism. That is, the child becomes a scapegoat. Instead of addressing the problems between themselves, the parents may yell at their daughter for minor things (not picking up toys, teasing friends) and may provide inconsistent discipline. The parents may even blame the daughter for their own frustration and fights and thus avoid addressing difficult conflicts between themselves.

In all these kinds of difficulties, a family therapist will try to make the family the unit of change, even though one family member may be seen by the others as the problem. To accomplish change, family systems therapists employ a wide variety of strategies. The particular strategies emphasized in a family therapy session will vary, depending on the type of training the therapist has had. Salvadore Minuchin and Virginia Satir pioneered developments in family therapy in the 1960s and 1970s; here, we provide some examples of strategies used by these pioneers and many who followed them.

Reframing   **Reframing** means conceptualizing of a problem in a new way. If you sought help from a family therapist, he would ask you and each family member to get a new picture—a new "framing"—of the problems existing within your family. The therapist would reframe each individual problem as a family problem, removing blame from the person seen as causing or having the problem. Even though one family member may be hurting the most psychologically, that individual will not be the focus of the family therapy.

The general purpose of reframing is to lessen the negative views or attributions that individuals have about the person usually identified as "the problem" or the

reframing Conceptualizing a problem in a new way.

one in need of psychological help. For example, a therapist may reframe an adolescent's anger and acting out as expressions of insecurity, not hostility. Similarly, a therapist might help a family who's upset over Mom's return to work, showing them that this change reflects her need for self-development, not her desire to become distant from the family.

Validation   Validation means expressing an understanding of individual family members' feelings and desires (Satir, 1967). For example, consider an adolescent who says to his father, "You're always mean to me. You criticize me for coming home late from the restaurant [where he works], and I don't have a thing to do with the work schedule. And to rub it in, you won't give me a cent for spending money." To validate this boy's feelings, the therapist may try to convey understanding by saying, "It seems that you resent not getting lunch money from your father simply because you now have a job. It also angers you when he criticizes you if you are late, because you don't determine the hour when you are able to finish." By validating the feelings of the teen-ager, the therapist serves as a model—teaching family members to validate each other's feelings. This kind of understanding is necessary before changes in family dynamics can take place. Unfortunately, parents often enforce rules and restrictions before they even hear, much less validate, why their children may not have done what was expected of them.

Communication   In family therapy, the therapist provides guidelines for communicating with "I feel" statements. Many problems arise when family members assume they know each other's feelings and desires. This kind of assumption, called *mind reading*, is expressed by comments starting with "You feel . . ." or "You make me . . ." For example, suppose that a college sophomore who's been fighting with his parents makes this statement: "Both of you think I am a lazy bum, sponging off you, drinking, and sleeping until noon." Instead of expressing his own anger or resentment directly, he assumes he knows what his parents feel and blames them for their feelings. But with a therapist's help, he can rephrase his remarks: "I have been angry because I have the feeling that you think I blow off my studies and stay out drinking. You should know that I work until 3:00 or 4:00 A.M. in the local pizza joint." As you can see, the rephrased statement avoids mind reading. Instead of forcing his parents to respond defensively, the rephrasing makes their response more likely to be empathic.

A second communication guideline involves so-called fair-fighting exercises. These exercises specify times when members can vent or release their feelings. During these periods, one person may be a "yeller," while the other family members remain "listeners."

The therapist also teaches individual family members to analyze why they hear certain messages sent by other members in ways that may have been unintended. The therapist asks individuals to distinguish between the *intent* of these messages and the *impact* they have. For example, the meaning of a parent's remark to a teen-ager—such as "Why are you so late?"—could have a very different impact than the parent intended. Parental voice inflection and intensity, as well as the teen-ager's perception of the intent, can dramatically influence the gap between the intent of the parent and the impact on the teen-ager.

Paradoxical Directives   A therapist using a **paradoxical directive** prescribes the symptom. Salvadore Minuchin, a noted family therapist, used this strategy in planning a therapy session with the family of a 13-year-old girl with anorexia nervosa. The girl and her parents, brothers, and sisters attended the session. Minuchin suggested that the family have lunch so that he could observe their relationships to each other.

validation Expressing an understanding of other family members' feelings and desires.

paradoxical directive Technique in which the therapist encourages the client to do something that seems contradictory, such as prescribing the actual symptom the client wishes to eliminate.

Dr. Minuchin: I don't think that we have any problem with Laura's eating—she will eat. At the point at which you are 14, Laura, you will eat without any problems. . . . But I think that it is good that you are not eating now, because I think that what is happening is that this is the only area in your family, Laura, in which you have a say-so. And at 14 you'll need to have a say-so in another way. . . . What about—there are some other things, Laura, about which you have a say-so? . . . Around food, at least you can fight. You can say, "That's my body, and that's what I want to eat." Isn't that what you are saying?

Laura: Um hmm. (Aponte & Hoffman, 1973, p. 525)

Instead of forcing the teen-age girl to eat, Minuchin tried to help her feel in control of some part of her life, other than eating. He organized the entire family in Laura's presence, giving her permission and even suggesting that she should not eat. In this directive, there is also an implicit directive for Laura's family to get off her back for not eating. (Of course, the paradoxical directive approach can be dangerous in certain cases. In the case presented earlier, however, the therapist had assessed Laura's health and recognized that she was not in danger. Therefore, he felt that this approach was worth the risk—and indeed, it worked well.) To many clients' surprise, the effect of these paradoxical directives—when they are chosen carefully—is to remove the patient's need to have the problem (such as not eating or fighting). Paradoxical directives have been especially effective with resistant teen-agers and young adults, particularly those who have problems with procrastination, insomnia, and nail biting (Lopez & Wambach, 1982).

Family therapy approaches have not yet been evaluated as rigorously as have other treatments, such as marital and individual therapies. They have, however, been proven effective when a family member has a drug abuse problem. For example, Stanton and Todd (1982) evaluated **structural family therapy,** a type of family systems therapy, as a supplement to the standard drug treatment program in a Veterans Administration hospital. The standard drug treatment program consisted of detoxification, methadone maintenance, drug counseling, and occupational therapy. Six months after treatment, the group of patients who received the standard program plus structural family therapy were more likely to be employed and less likely to be using drugs than the standard treatment group. In addition to the promising results obtained in treating drug abuse, structural family therapy approaches have proved useful in treating individuals with anorexia, bulimia, and certain types of diabetes (Nichols & Schwartz, 1991).

Initial reviews of the effectiveness of family therapy suggested that 65 to 76 percent of all clients show improvements (Gurman & Kniskern, 1986; Wells & Dezen, 1978). These reviews, however, often used case studies, and those subjects who received therapy were not compared with subjects from control groups. Therefore, these studies provided only suggestive evidence (Ganahl, Ferguson, & L'Abate, 1985). On the other hand, an experimental study by Markus, Lange, and Pettigrew (1990) provided statistical evidence that family therapy was more effective than an alternative treatment (often individual psychotherapy), a minimal treatment, or no treatment. Further, these researchers' data suggested that family therapy had better results 10 months after treatment than the alternative treatments, even though the effects were quite variable across studies.

Recently, a research team (Szapocznik et al., 1991) developed the Structural Family Rating Scale to evaluate the functioning of the whole family unit. This assessment measure involves the whole family in three tasks: planning a meal, discussing what other family members do that pleases and displeases each person, and recalling and evaluating a recent family argument. Different raters can reach agreement using the Structured Family Rating Scale, and in therapy with Hispanic American boys (ages 6 to 12) with behavioral and emotional problems, the scale has proved sensitive to changes. More specifically, the assessment measure showed

structural family therapy
Treatment approach in which the family is viewed as the unit to change; the therapist's main goal is to alter the entire family system by assessing and restructuring the roles of and relationships between family members.

that the boys who received structural family therapy underwent more promising changes than did boys in individual child psychotherapy or a control group who simply participated in structured recreational activities (Szapocznik et al., 1991).

Problem-Solving Therapy

The second major treatment approach directed at changing families is **problem-solving therapy.** Problem-solving approaches have somewhat more focused goals than family systems therapy. Although both approaches treat the family as the unit to change, changes in communication or behavior for a dyad (such as mother/daughter) or an individual (for instance, a child or teen-ager) are acceptable goals for problem-solving therapy. Robin and Foster (1988) reviewed problem-solving treatments for families with parent/adolescent conflict and found them useful in changing communication patterns, parental reports of problem behaviors by the adolescent, and adolescent reports of parental hostility and criticism. Problem-solving approaches are built on the base of family system therapy but particularly emphasize problem solving and communication.

Problem-solving approaches consist of guidance for the family in four basic phases:

1. defining the problem
2. generating alternative solutions to the defined problem before family members criticize solutions (sometimes called *brainstorming*)
3. evaluating the alternative solutions
4. implementing the best available solutions

problem-solving therapy
Approach in which the therapist focuses on improving the family's process of solving problems by teaching family members to define each problem, generate alternative solutions, evaluate those alternatives, and implement the best alternative.

In this approach, the therapist uses her clinical skill to help the family reduce intense emotional conflicts through problem solving. For example, suppose a couple tells their therapist that their problem is their teen-age daughter's being led astray by her boyfriend. The father adds, in a hostile tone of voice, "I think the guy is a waste." The daughter then retorts, "He's no more a waste than you, when you came home drunk from your pool party and swore at Mom!"

At this point, the therapist quickly intervenes to stop the escalating argument and help the family understand their dysfunctional communication patterns. In this case, for example, the therapist may point out the father's and daughter's tendencies to trade criticisms without defining problems or looking for solutions. Then the therapist may help the parents articulate what really concerns them about their daughter—her coming home late or failing to do homework, perhaps, or their fear that she is having sex. The therapist may also try to define the problem from the daughter's vantage point: "Mom and Dad don't treat my boyfriend with respect; they don't even say hello to him when he comes to pick me up; they are critical of his home."

After defining the problem, the next step is to come up with alternative solutions. The therapist will encourage the parents and daughter to brainstorm possibilities. Perhaps the daughter will agree to do her homework and keep her curfew, and the parents will say hello to her boyfriend and invite him over for dinner with the family once a month. After an agreed on trial period (say, 3 months), the parents and daughter will move to the next step: evaluating the alternative solutions. Finally, based on this evaluation, the best available solutions will be implemented.

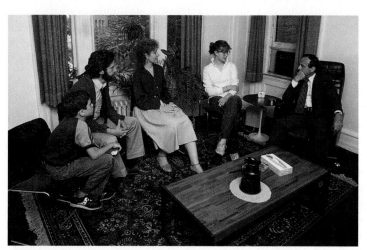

Problem-solving therapy is a type of family intervention that focuses on helping family members understand illnesses like schizophrenia. Family members also learn to decrease criticism of the patient, a factor that places the patient at risk for readmission.

Problem-solving therapies with families have helped to improve the functioning and social skills of people who are depressed and schizophrenic. In one family therapy intervention, Falloon and associates (1985) treated schizophrenic patients as members of family units. They emphasized that the schizophrenic patient should not necessarily be seen as the most disabled, and they treated the patient's needs within the context of the whole family system. Families of individuals with schizophrenia were trained to solve problems in a structured manner: outlining possible solutions, choosing workable solutions, and making detailed plans to implement them.

Many successful programs that aid the families of people with schizophrenia share these key elements: (1) giving the families information about the nature of the disorder; (2) helping them cope with the schizophrenic member's problems; and (3) decreasing the intensity of conflict within the family (Goldstein, 1995). In several studies combining family therapy with medication, only about 10 percent of schizophrenic patients treated were readmitted to the hospital within 9 months after treatment. In contrast, individuals in control groups who received individual supportive therapy and medication had rehospitalization rates of approximately 50 percent (Goldstein, 1984).

Integration of Family and Behavior Therapy

Sometimes, behavior therapy strategies are more effective when combined with family therapies. As early as 1973, Alexander and Parsons developed a *systems-behavioral approach* to dealing with delinquent children and their families. This model evolved from a behavioral perspective with an emphasis on parental disciplinary strategies, and it has become a dominant force in integrating various therapeutic approaches (Alexander, Mas, & Waldron, 1988). The systems perspective added the view that the delinquent and his parents were actively trying to change or influence each other. Within this perspective, the therapist tries to help families identify the function or value of the problematic and adaptive behaviors within the family context.

For some problems, each approach appears to affect different behavior or attitude domains. Consider a study comparing three different family treatments for child abuse and neglect: (1) behaviorally based parent-training programs; (2) family systems approaches; and (3) an integration of the behavioral parent-training and family systems approaches. The study showed parent training to be more effective in reducing children's specific social problems. Systems therapy was more effective in restructuring parent/child relations. However, families receiving both therapies showed these benefits as well as reduced overall stress and fewer psychological problems among parents (Brunk, Henggler, & Whelan, 1987).

Family therapy has also proved effective with populations that have been difficult to reach and treat successfully. For example, to the surprise of many, in one study (Henggler, Melton, & Smith, 1992), a family therapy approach was an effective treatment for serious juvenile offenders in inner-city Charleston, South Carolina. The youths had an average of 3.5 previous arrests; 54 percent of the offenders had at least 1 arrest for a violent crime. Compared to the usual intervention—namely, meeting with a probation officer once a month—family therapy led to fewer arrests, fewer self-reported offenses, and less incarceration. The family therapy sessions were usually conducted in the clients' homes. The treatment lasted approximately 4 months, and the therapists spent an average of 33 hours per case. The therapists had frequent contact with the clients by phone, if necessary, and the cost of the family therapy was about $2,800 per client. In contrast, at the time the study was conducted (1992), it cost $16,300 for the average institutional placement in South Carolina.

Another special challenge is designing family therapy that takes into account the cultural values and traditions of specific subgroups in the American population. Thinking about Multicultural Issues addresses one such issue.

Thinking about MULTICULTURAL ISSUES — Designing Mental Health Services That Address Hispanic Family Values

The values and lifestyles of Hispanic families in the United States differ greatly, depending on the particular countries from which the couple or their parents came. Even within this diversity, however, some characteristics are evident among Hispanic families, regardless of their countries of origin.

Familism—or maintaining close ties with the extended family and respecting authorities within the family structure—is a characteristic found both in Mexican American families and in families with origins in Puerto Rico (Vega, 1990). Familism can function to maintain traditional values and to influence the conduct of family members. Having large family networks can also buffer the effects of stress associated with the loss of a job or coping with illness (Zayas & Palleja, 1988). In short, Hispanic family values provide structure, support, and a sense of community.

Familism also influences gender roles within the family. In traditional Hispanic families, men were dominant and women were submissive to their husbands. These gender roles were heavily influenced by religious and spiritual (Catholic) beliefs (Ramirez, 1991). The concept of *machismo* embodies the traditional belief of the man as dominant. On the other hand, *marianismo* is a role thought to be played by a traditional Hispanic woman; women who follow this model are described as being subservient to their husbands and as putting family concerns before their own (like the Virgin Mary; thus, the term *marianismo*). Such role models and family dynamics also seem to operate, and indeed may also be influential, in American non-Hispanic families. In fact, when researchers looked at decision making within families, there were no differences among Hispanic, white, and black families. However, other researchers found differences between generations of Hispanic families. That is, the longer a Hispanic family had been exposed to U.S. culture, the more egalitarian the family members' decision-making processes (Cooney, Rogler, Hurrell, & Ortiz, 1982).

Think about the following questions:

1. If you were designing a mental health agency in a Hispanic neighborhood, how would you use the concepts of *familism*, *machismo*, and *marianismo* in planning types of marital, family, and group treatments?
2. Which types of therapy would seem most appropriate for Hispanic Americans? Why?
3. What types of support groups could be offered by community volunteers, given the roles of the family and the church in Hispanic culture? Why?

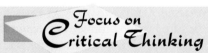

Focus on Critical Thinking

1. Under what conditions would you not want family members present when dealing with a childhood problem? Why?
2. Under what conditions would you not want family members present when dealing with a teen-ager's problem? Why?

Dr. Gerald Patterson, a behavior therapist who has also incorporated family therapy or family systems views into his conceptualization, has argued that children who display deviant behavior are the victims as well as the architects of their situations (Patterson, Dishion, & Chamberlain, 1993). Interventions combining family systems and behavioral approaches effectively change aggressive and delinquent children's behavior (Alexander et al., 1988; Patterson et al., 1993) and are likely to become increasingly useful.

GROUP THERAPY

group therapy Treatment approach in which a small group of individuals meets to obtain mutual support and guidance in coping with psychological problems.

Group therapy consists of meetings of a small group of individuals to obtain and provide mutual support and guidance in coping with psychological problems. In contrast to family therapy, group therapy is usually conducted with individuals who are not related to one another. Some groups are led by mental health professionals or members of the clergy, whereas others are strictly self-help (that is, organized and facilitated by group members). Small-group approaches that you probably have heard

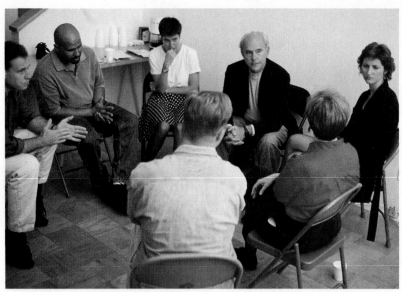

Group programs—such as Weight Watchers, Alcoholics Anonymous, and patient support groups for cancer patients—help individuals cope with a wide variety of psychological and health problems. What factors may deter people from participating in support groups?

about include Alcoholics Anonymous (AA) and Gamblers Anonymous. In addition, many residential programs for drug addiction emphasize small-group treatments.

Although the programs just mentioned all treat addictive problems, group approaches are employed for almost every type of psychological problem (Yalom, 1985). For example, groups exist for assertiveness training, parent training, and couple communication. Support groups have also emerged in recent decades for many of the major physical diseases, such as cancer, heart disease, acquired immune deficiency syndrome (AIDS), and kidney failure.

According to one survey, more Americans engage in some form of group therapy than in any other type of therapy. Approximately 5 percent of Americans have participated in self-help/support groups such as AA, 6 percent in group therapy sessions conducted by mental health professionals, and 5 percent in group therapy conducted by members of the clergy ("Group Therapy," 1989).

Group therapies are popular partly because they are less costly than individual treatment. Participation in groups like AA, Parents Anonymous, and Gamblers Anonymous is free. Participating in group therapy conducted by a professional usually costs only one-third as much as individual therapy. Also, group approaches help individuals with problems that are very difficult to treat individually, such as alcoholism and partner abuse. In general, an individual therapist cannot generate as much pressure to change behavior as a group can. Sometimes, too, being with others dealing with the same problems offers comfort an individual therapist cannot provide.

Gestalt Therapy

One type of group therapy is **gestalt therapy.** *Gestalt* is a German word meaning "whole," and it's natural to see wholeness or closure in many things. For example, we naturally perceive a set of dots as a line. In human relations, the closure is not usually so simple, but gestalt therapists argue that "what we really want and what we are looking for in our lives are complete experiences" (Korb, Gorrell, & Van De Reit, 1989, p. 9).

Gestalt therapy encourages participants to complete "unfinished business." In other words, it encourages them to examine the past for unresolved conflicts and to explore their feelings about those conflicts. Because gestalt therapists encourage examining feelings about past relationships, gestalt groups differ from encounter groups, which focus on the here and now.

gestalt therapy Humanistically oriented therapy in which participants are encouraged to complete "unfinished business" by examining the past for unresolved conflicts yet deal with current life issues and make the most of each day.

Gestalt therapy, like many other therapies, takes place in groups and in one-to-one therapist/client settings. We focus here on the group format of gestalt therapy, which was made very popular by Fritz Perls. Gestalt therapy is a form of humanistically oriented therapy; in accord with that approach, the emphasis is decidedly positive. Clients are encouraged to grow as they interact with other group members and as they express a wide range of emotions with those individuals, who accept and express whatever they feel. All group members are encouraged to respond similarly. In short, gestalt therapists encourage awareness, expression, and acceptance.

In contrast to other types of therapy, gestalt therapy places extremely strong emphasis on the intuition, or the feelings and hunches, of the therapist. As Naranjo (1993) noted, "Gestalt therapy is unique among the major schools of psychotherapy because of the extent to which this is a system built upon intuitive understanding rather than theory" (p. 5). Perls said that being a therapist meant being yourself (Perls, Hefferline, & Goodman, 1951).

Gestalt therapy is as much an attitude about life as a set of highly developed principles. Even though gestalt therapists encourage clients to examine the past and to complete their unfinished business (unresolved conflicts), they also stress the need to deal with current life issues and to make the most of each day. This latter attitude of gestalt therapy is conveyed in the following statements (adapted from Naranjo, 1993):

1. Live now; be concerned with the present, rather than the past or future.
2. Live here; deal with the present rather than what is absent.
3. Stop imagining; experience the real.
4. Accept no "should" or "ought" other than your own.
5. Surrender to being who you are.

Many books on gestalt therapy provide little or no empirical data about the effectiveness of this form of therapy (Korb et al., 1989; Naranjo, 1993). This may not surprise you, after reading about gestalt therapy approaches. Indeed, gestalt therapists are not highly concerned about evaluation of change. What's more, they do not accept the overt goal of changing particular problems. Perls even argued that it's not necessary to validate gestalt therapy empirically (Perls et al., 1951; see also Chapter 18). Instead, gestalt therapists show great concern about how an individual feels about life and relationships.

Although little research has evaluated gestalt therapy, thousands of people have testified to its value. Moreover, gestalt therapy (or variations of it) has been shown to be effective in specific areas—for instance, marital therapy or marital enrichment (Greenberg & Johnson, 1988). Gestalt therapy has also had promising initial results in some areas, such as decision making and depression (Greenberg, Rice, & Elliot, 1993).

Alcoholics Anonymous

Alcoholics Anonymous (AA) has been helping alcoholics throughout the world for decades. In the United States, AA programs are available within 30 miles of almost anyone. AA is a form of group therapy that relies on a "buddy," or sponsor, system (see Chapter 9). The sponsor, a member of AA who has been able to remain sober for some time, provides support and encouragement to a new AA member who's trying to stop drinking. As the name of the organization implies, the *anonymity* of the individuals attending meetings is preserved. Thus, only first names are used at AA meetings.

Two men from Akron, Ohio—Dr. Bob and Bill W.—founded AA in 1935. A sense of spiritual change helped Bill recover from alcoholism, and he then helped Dr. Bob recover. In turn, they both sought to help other alcoholics by starting an organization that has grown to millions of members. AA's basic aim is lifelong abstinence—that is, not having a single drink, ever again. At AA meetings, members "tell their stories"; they tell what their lives were like while they were dependent on alcohol and what their lives are like without it. Much of the meeting time is spent on problem-focused discussions about how to resist drinking. AA members are encouraged to accept most, if not all, of a 12-step program. Most important, AA members encourage new recruits to admit that they cannot control themselves if they use alcohol and to say, "I am an alcoholic" (see also Chapter 9).

Alcoholics Anonymous (AA) Volunteer self-help organization designed to help individuals maintain sobriety; basic principles include anonymity, "buddy" system, and 12-step program.

AA provides four critical treatment ingredients (Vaillant, 1988):

1. It offers a substitute for drinking at bars, because AA meetings are held at hours that compete with those of bars.
2. AA makes it clear that the alcoholic cannot drink without becoming dependent.
3. It teaches the individual how to cope with feelings of loneliness.
4. It offers role models, in the form of sober people who have successfully coped with their desire to have alcohol.

AA's effects are difficult to ascertain (McCrady & Miller, 1993). Even though AA has been a major force in treating alcoholism for more than 50 years, there are few controlled evaluations of this treatment approach. The small amount of research that has been completed leads to the conclusion that between 25 to 50 percent of individuals who stay in the program remain sober after 1 year (NIAAA, 1993). A survey of AA members reported that, on average, members who regularly attended meetings (about 4 meetings per week) remained sober for 50 months (Alcoholics Anonymous, 1993). About half of the members do not attend meetings with this regularity, however.

Whatever the overall effectiveness of AA, millions of people throughout the world find it helpful. It gives members daily social support for resisting that first drink, and, for many, it provides an alternative social network to the bar scene, formerly used as a base for their social life.

> ## Focus on Critical Thinking
>
> 1. Under what conditions is obtaining individual treatment from a mental health professional defensible if support groups are able to provide the same types of benefits?
> 2. Some people are reluctant to join groups of any kind. But suppose that insurance companies required every therapist to have a certain percentage of his clients in groups. Do you think that this would be a reasonable requirement? Explain your answer.

COMMUNITY THERAPY

In discussing community therapy, we'll look at two very different kinds of approaches. The first is the therapeutic community, which is a homelike program for psychiatric patients. In addition, we'll look at preventive programs aimed at forestalling psychological problems in the larger community.

Therapeutic Communities

In the 1950s and 1960s, tremendous dissatisfaction arose concerning the apathy and listlessness of patients in most mental hospital wards. Goffman (1961) showed that patients learned to become dependent and docile, taking on what he called "sick roles." Some critics even asserted that hospitals taught patients to become mentally incompetent so they would remain in them. These criticisms became so powerful that a new approach emerged: the **therapeutic community.**

A therapeutic community generally revolves around regular meetings in a homelike atmosphere. Everyone shares in the work of running the community. Patients, or *clients,* are on an equal footing with staff members in their ability to influence the behavior of other community members. Part of the therapeutic community's effectiveness lies in its ongoing influence. A great deal of therapy occurs during unofficial meetings and leisure activities. Therapeutic communities differ in their therapeutic emphasis, however: Some favor active confrontation, whereas others simply focus on patients' responsibility for their behavior.

The therapeutic community approach became a model for many halfway houses. A **halfway house** is a facility for individuals who have been released from

therapeutic community Treatment approach in which patients in an institutional setting are treated as normally as possible; they live in a family-style environment and are encouraged to develop routines and participate in chores.

halfway house Facility for individuals released from a hospital or other treatment program who need more supervision and monitoring than their families can provide before they can live on their own.

a hospital or other treatment program and who need more supervision and monitoring than their homes and families can provide. Thus, as the term implies, the individual is halfway between the hospital and home. Halfway houses are usually located in large, private residences within communities. Clients sleep and eat in the halfway house and are supervised by one or two people—often, a husband and wife—living at the residence. Well-run halfway houses provide skills training in a number of areas. For instance, the staff help clients develop and maintain daily routines such as cleaning, meal preparation, and laundry and also assist with school and/or job problems. Finally, even after a client returns to his family, follow-up by the halfway house staff is often necessary.

If there is adequate community follow-up, halfway houses or group homes are effective in facilitating patients' return to the community. Compared to standard hospital aftercare, halfway houses for mental patients result in less frequent readmittance to mental hospitals and more employment. Yet despite this demonstrated effectiveness, establishing a halfway house is no easy task. Groundwork with local leaders is critical, because there is often intense opposition from neighbors or community members. The common sentiment is "Not in my backyard."

Community Psychology

Therapeutic communities and group approaches such as AA focus primarily on changing problematic behaviors or conditions. In contrast, **community psychology** attempts to prevent problems and to teach new skills (Heller & Monahan, 1977). Community psychology developed in the 1960s and 1970s simultaneously with an increased awareness of the roles of racial discrimination and poverty in the development of psychological problems. Community programs have involved television programs and commercials to foster health-promoting behaviors, such as eating properly, exercising, reducing high-risk sexual behaviors, and quitting smoking. Similarly, police arrests for partner abuse are a relatively recent strategy designed to prevent and reduce family violence at the community and city level; these arrest programs serve as a warning or deterrent (Berk, 1993). Community interventions promote competencies, rather than remedy long-standing deficits or problems. These interventions may be small or large and range from small groups, such as groups of parents, to police departments, Head Start programs, or entire communities.

As mentioned earlier, prevention has always been a major focus of community psychology. There are three basic types of prevention programs:

1. Primary prevention programs attempt to prevent the development of new problems in a population. Basically, primary prevention focuses on education. For example, some primary prevention programs attempt to prevent adolescent parenthood. Adolescent parenthood is not a psychological disorder, but it is a tremendous social problem that has widespread psychological consequences. Unwed teen-age mothers are often depressed, often do not complete high school, have lower school achievement, and are more likely to be on welfare than mothers who have their first child at a later age. Teen-age mothers are also more likely to use cigarettes, marijuana, and alcohol during their first pregnancies (Abma & Mott, 1991).

One program was designed to help adolescent girls say no to sex without hurting boys' feelings (Howard & McCabe, 1990). The four-session program incorporated peer counseling and role-playing—all designed to delay sexual involvement. It also included a 3-month follow-up to encourage and support girls who were delaying sexual activity. Approximately 400 girls received the program in eighth grade; a control group of girls did not receive the program. The experimental group reported less sexual activity than the control group, but the effect seemed greatest with those girls who had not begun having intercourse before participating in the program. About 19 percent of those girls exposed to the program had intercourse by the ninth grade, as compared to 27 percent of girls who did not have the program.

community psychology
Programs designed to prevent problems and to teach new skills; examples include television messages, preventive policing, and community meetings to foster health-promoting behaviors.

primary prevention Efforts to reduce the occurrence of new problems in a population.

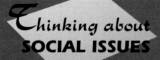

A Call for Primary Prevention of Dating Violence

*L*et's consider the need for community-level interventions and primary prevention by looking at partner abuse. Physical violence toward a partner occurs in at least 25 percent of all college dating couples and in almost half of engaged couples (O'Leary et al., 1989; Pirog-Good & Stets, 1989). Physical aggression in extreme forms—called *partner abuse*—occurs in about 10 percent of all couples in the United States (Straus & Gelles, 1992).

Partner abuse can be treated with a combination of individual and marital/relationship therapy. But with a problem so pervasive, attitudes of men toward hitting women (and vice versa) need to be changed before the violence begins, at an age when dating starts regularly—that is, in high school and college. Men's perceived need for power is of considerable importance. Many men become aggressive when their power or control seems threatened. In addition, it is now well known that a cycle of violence exists across generations. Individuals who observe their parents hit each other or who were themselves abused as children are more likely to engage in physical aggression with their own partners as adults

(Straus & Gelles, 1992). Unfortunately, therapists often have to treat couples with long histories of abuse. In many of those cases, the therapy comes too late.

Thus, we need primary prevention efforts directed at teen-agers and young adults to help them establish relationships that are violence free. At this point, it's clear that attitudes justifying violence toward a partner can be reduced (Avery-Leaf, Cano, Cascardi, & O'Leary, 1995). But there is no evidence that physically aggressive behaviors toward dating partners can be prevented or reduced.

Think about the following questions:

1. What factors would you target to change the physically aggressive behaviors of teen-age dating males? females? Explain your answers.
2. Is adolescence too late to initiate programs for preventing physical aggression against partners? Would it be better to start sooner, with younger children? If so, how young? What can parents do to teach their children nonviolent ways of solving problems and disagreements?

Another important area for primary prevention is the widespread problem of partner abuse (see Chapter 17). Thinking about Social Issues discusses this subject.

2. Secondary prevention programs attempt to detect problems early on in order to reduce their intensity and prevent further escalation. One example is the *diversion program* approach for juvenile offenders. Because rehabilitation within the juvenile justice system has not proved successful, the diversion approach attempts to steer adolescents away from jail or juvenile detention facilities. Diversion programs help adolescents with conduct problems avoid the harmful effect of being labeled "juvenile delinquents."

In one study of diversion programs (Davidson, Redner, Blakely, Mitchell, & Emshoff, 1987), subjects were primarily teen-age male offenders arrested for stealing and breaking and entering. College students worked one on one with each juvenile offender for 6 to 8 hours per week over the course of several months, helping the boy learn communication skills and use community resources such as job placement and recreational services. The results were impressive: The youths diverted from the juvenile courts were significantly less likely to engage in delinquent acts than those who were part of the normal court-processing system. Typically, courts would place these teen-agers in juvenile detention facilities or simply put them on probation for fixed periods, often without any systematic help for the juvenile or his family.

3. Tertiary prevention aims to reduce the long-term damage caused by a problem. This type of prevention is exemplified by programs that help mental patients when they are released from a hospital. For example, *Training in Community Living* involves intensive management of cases to improve former patients' quality of life and to reduce rehospitalization. The program was devel-

secondary prevention
Efforts to detect problems early in their onset and to reduce their intensity.

tertiary prevention Efforts to reduce long-term damage caused by a problem.

oped in Madison, Wisconsin, in the 1970s, and by the early 1990s, it had been used in many states (Surles, Blanch, Shern, & Donahue, 1992). The ratio of staff to clients is small (1:10), and contact with each client is made directly at her residence. The staff of Training in Community Living programs make themselves available during evenings and weekends. Emphasis is on teaching the client social skills so she can operate in the new residence and community, not on reducing psychological symptoms. This type of program is labor intensive and relatively expensive, but it has been recognized as a particularly good alternative to hospitalization for young people and for individuals who are homeless and mentally ill. The program leads to a reduction in hospital usage and has been used successfully in many different communities (Levine, Toro, & Perkins, 1993).

Another tertiary program, *Man to Man,* allows men to talk about their problems in dealing with prostate cancer and the effects of treatment for this disease. (Temporary or permanent impotence and incontinence are among the most negative consequences of surgery for prostate cancer.) Hundreds of Man to Man groups now operate with the help of the American Cancer Society (Brody, 1994). The groups sponsor talks by professionals and small-group sessions in which men talk about issues like the need for adult diapers, the inability to have an erection, and the question of whether to have a penile implant (which would be needed to have an erection). Wives can participate in a parallel group called *Side by Side,* and every 3 months, the groups for men and their partners meet together.

Like other groups for particular problems, Man to Man provides men with the sense that they are not alone. James Mullen, who founded Man to Man in Sarasota, Florida, put it this way: "When a person faces cancer, he tends to think of it as a death sentence. He needs someone to talk to who's been through it. Just like in combat, you always want to be with a veteran. In a support group, he'll see other men who came through it, survived and are coping with the side effects and leading full, meaningful lives" (Brody, 1994, p. C12).

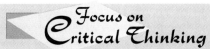

Focus on Critical Thinking

1. How can the "not in my backyard" attitude against halfway houses be overcome?
2. Describe one problem in your community that you feel calls for a prevention approach.

SUMMARY

Marital Therapy

■ Of all the difficulties people face, divorce and marital separation rank second and third, respectively, as the most significant life stressors, exceeded only by the death of a spouse. At least half of depressed women seeking treatment have clinically significant marital problems.

■ Marital therapy helps couples improve their communication, gain insight, and explore feelings.

■ Marital or relationship therapies are used with unmarried couples, gay or lesbian couples, and often with elderly couples. In addition, the goal of therapy may be to make a separation or divorce more amicable, particularly if children are involved.

■ Marital therapies include both insight-oriented and behavioral approaches. In clinical practice, the goals of therapy include changing attitudes and behaviors as well as gaining insight and improving communication.

Family Therapy

■ Family systems therapy is the most common approach to treating families. Rather than viewing the individual as "the problem," the therapist sees the family or the system as playing a role in maintaining the problem behavior. The therapist teaches the family techniques such as reframing, validation, and paradoxical directives and gives guidelines for communication. Structural family therapy—one form of family systems treatment—has proved useful in treating drug abuse, anorexia, bulimia, and certain types of diabetes.

■ Problem-solving therapy, another type of treatment for families, helps family members learn four basic skills: defining the problem, generating alternative solutions (brainstorming), evaluating the alternative solutions, and implementing the best available solutions.

■ In many situations, interventions combining family systems and behavioral approaches are becoming very useful. Each approach appears to change different behavior or attitude domains.

Group Therapy

■ Group therapy is a treatment approach in which a small group of individuals meets to obtain mutual support and guidance in coping with psychological problems. The group may be self-directed or led by a mental health professional or clergy member.

■ Gestalt therapy is a humanistically oriented therapy. It encourages participants to complete "unfinished business" and resolve feelings about past relationships while also emphasizing the need to make the most of each day. Participants in gestalt therapy are encouraged to become more aware of their emotions and to accept and express whatever they feel. This type of therapy (or variations thereof) has proved effective in treating marital problems and offers promise in treating depression.

■ Alcoholics Anonymous (AA) is a form of group therapy for people with drinking problems. Each member has a sponsor, a member of AA who has been able to remain sober and can be supportive and encouraging. Anonymity is maintained. The basic aim of AA is abstinence. The effectiveness of AA is very difficult to determine, as little research has been done on this population; but hundreds of thousands of individuals have been helped by AA.

Community Therapy

■ Therapeutic communities grew out of dissatisfaction with the limitations of traditional mental hospital treatments. In a therapeutic community, patients are treated with dignity and respect and are encouraged to develop routines and participate in chores. Halfway houses and other nonhospital treatments rely on many of the principles used in the therapeutic community approach.

■ Community psychology attempts to prevent problems and to teach new skills. Community interventions foster health-promoting behaviors and promote competencies rather than remedy long-standing deficits or problems.

KEY TERMS

Alcoholics Anonymous
   (AA), **p. 615**
community psychology,
   p. 617
conjoint sessions, **p. 604**
family systems therapy,
   p. 607
gestalt therapy, **p. 614**
group therapy, **p. 613**

halfway house, **p. 616**
love days *or* caring days,
   p. 606
marital therapy, **p. 604**
paradoxical directive, **p. 609**
primary prevention, **p. 617**
problem-solving therapy,
   p. 611
reframing, **p. 608**

secondary prevention,
   p. 618
structural family therapy,
   p. 610
tertiary prevention, **p. 618**
therapeutic community,
   p. 616
validation, **p. 609**

CRITICAL THINKING EXERCISE

Kim and Lenny—the couple in the chapter-opening case—had significant marital problems. To help work through these problems, they decided to see an individual therapist. But they had also considered group marital therapy, as there is some evidence that this approach helps improve relationships, as well. In fact, as noted in this chapter, some professionals believe that group approaches are the most helpful in treating certain problems.

1. What types of marital problems, if any, might not be appropriate for group therapy? Why?

2. What types of nonmarital problems would be best addressed by group therapy or support groups? Why?

*C*hapter **20**

BIOLOGICAL THERAPIES

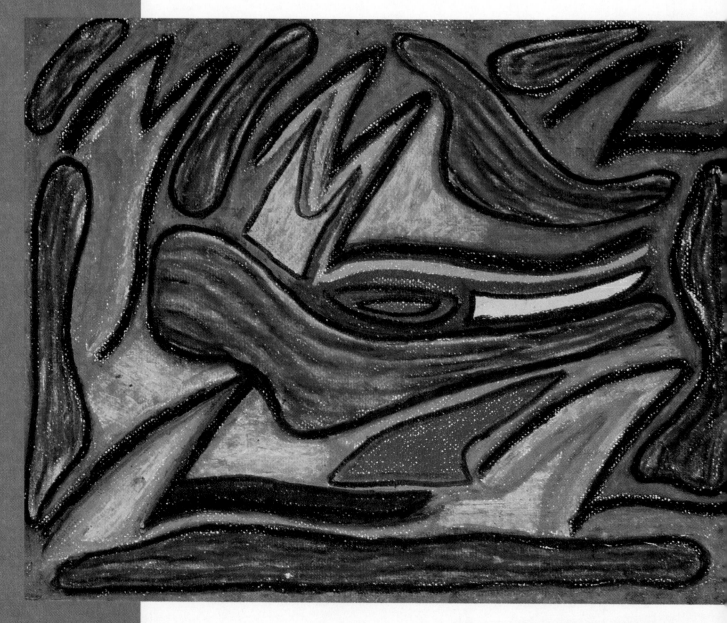

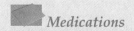 **Medications**

Antidepressants

***Thinking about
Multicultural Issues***

Lithium

Antianxiety Medications

Thinking about Gender Issues

Antipsychotic Medications

Psychostimulants

Thinking about Social Issues

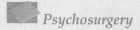 *Electroconvulsive
Therapy*

Discovery

Current Use

Psychosurgery

S am, an architect, had daily feelings of intense sadness. He went to work, but he doubted his ability to be productive. He drew sketch after sketch of various buildings, usually throwing them all away. These doubts were not fleeting fears of incompetence but pervasive and nagging intrusions on every aspect of his life. About the time Sam turned 40, his father died. Not long afterward, his mother died, and his business went sour. Before his parents died, he had often fought with them, but he had had hopes of renovating the family farm and getting on good terms with his mom and dad.

Many months later, Sam began psychotherapy with Dr. Kramer to try to understand the factors that appeared to lead to his depression. The depression persisted, however. Sam tried taking an antidepressant medication (which Dr. Kramer prescribed), but this treatment was only partially successful.

In therapy sessions Sam described his obsessional personality style as a child. He used to worry about death, and he arranged and rearranged his various collections—stamps, coins, bottle caps, and coasters. Even though this style had faded as Sam became an adult, Dr. Kramer thought about the use of Prozac, which had been thought by some to reduce obsessional thoughts as well as depressed moods. Dr. Kramer discussed Prozac with Sam, and they agreed to give it a try. Dr. Kramer described the effects of this treatment as follows:

> The change, when it came, was remarkable: Sam not only recovered from his depression, he declared himself "better than well." He felt unencumbered, more vitally alive, less pessimistic. Now he could complete projects in one draft, whereas before he had sketched again and again. His memory was more reliable, his concentration keener. Every aspect of his work went more smoothly. He appeared more poised, more thoughtful, less distracted. He was able to speak at professional meetings without notes. (Kramer, 1993, p. x)

Sam had had a blustering, sometimes rough-edged manner, but that quality now seemed to disappear; he began to believe that what he described as "independence of spirit" was a biological abnormality. His mood lifted remarkably; his interest increased in a broad range of activities; he felt less obsessional; and he regained his feeling of competence as an architect.

Dr. Kramer (1993) stated his view quite clearly: "Spending time with patients who had responded to Prozac had transformed my views about what makes people the way they are. I had come to see inborn, biologically determined temperament where before I had seen slowly acquired, history laden character" (p. xv).

623

Prozac changed both Sam and Dr. Kramer. Sam became a different person on Prozac. He felt better than he ever had in his life. In turn, Dr. Kramer saw changes in Sam that he had thought would be almost impossible to achieve. He had believed that Sam's personality patterns were at least partly due to well-established character traits. But after giving Prozac to Sam and many other patients, Dr. Kramer strongly believed that many people who are depressed have a biological abnormality (Kramer, 1993).

Sam received a biological treatment designed to alter his biochemical state. In turn, the changed biochemical state was believed to alter Sam's mood. Individuals who are seeking relief from various problems will often try to find some way to alter their biochemical state. Some people may try ingesting different foods, drinks, and other substances; engaging in exercise regimens; or taking various vitamins. Others seek the aid of physicians to prescribe medication. A much smaller group with very severe psychiatric symptoms will receive electroconvulsive therapy or brain surgery. The alternative methods people use to change their biological and/or biochemical state are the focus of this chapter.

$\mathcal{M}$EDICATIONS

In the chapters on specific disorders, we briefly discussed various biological therapies, such as the use of antianxiety and antidepressant medications. We will now focus in more detail on these attempts to alter behavior by changing the patient's biochemical makeup. We'll look at the general effects of various medications, because single drugs are often used to treat a number of different disorders, not just specific problems. For example, antidepressant medication is used not only to treat depression but also anxiety and obsessive-compulsive disorders.

In this chapter, we will cover three major classes of biological treatments: medication (antidepressants, lithium, antianxiety medications, antipsychotic medications, and psychostimulants); electroconvulsive therapy (ECT); and psychosurgery. Medications are by far the most commonly used biological treatments today for psychiatric problems, and they will receive the greatest attention in this chapter.

Throughout this section, we'll provide tables of the commonly used **psychotropic medications**—that is, medications used to change feelings, thoughts, and behavior. The tables list the classes and generic names of the medications, along with their brand names. This information will help you recognize the medications by one name or another, so that if you read or hear about one of these commonly used psychotropic medications, you will be able to determine its treatment effects and side effects.

Antidepressants

As has happened with many medications, physicians discovered antidepressants while treating a problem other than depression. In the 1950s, a medication first used to treat tuberculosis had broad-based effects. The medication, a monoamine oxidase inhibitor (MAOI), caused a reduction in the bacteria that caused tuberculosis, but importantly, it also had an energizing effect on patients (Kramer, 1993). In brief, the tuberculosis medication was found to be a "psychic energizer."

The antitubercular medication was quickly adopted as an antidepressant in 1957, after its success in treating depression was reported in *The New York Times*. However, it was soon found that some depressed patients taking the antituberculosis medication to cope with their depression developed a liver disorder. The producer quickly stopped making the medication. Despite the brief use of this antituberculosis medication for depression, the discovery prompted the search for a true antidepressant medication. The search was intense, because in the late 1950s, there was no pharma-

psychotropic medications
Drugs used to alter feelings, thoughts, and behavior.

TABLE 20.1   Antidepressants

Brand Name (generic name)

Selective Serotonin Reuptake Inhibitors (SSRIs)
Effexor* (venlafaxine)
Paxil (paroxetine hydrochloride)
Prozac (fluoxetine)
Zoloft (sertraline hydrochloride)

Tricyclic Antidepressants (TCAs)
Anafranil (clomipramine)
Asendin (amoxapine)
Elavil (amitriptyline)
Norpramin (desipramine)
Pamelor (nortriptyline)
Sinequan (doxepin)
Surmontil (trimipramine)
Tofranil (imipramine)

Monoamine Oxidase Inhibitors (MAOIs)
Marplan (isocarboxazid)
Nardil (phenelzine)
Parnate (tranylcypromine)

Others
Desyrel (trazodone)
Serzone (nefazodone hydrochloride)
Wellbutrin (bupropion)

*A structurally novel antidepressant that is chemically unrelated to other antidepressants. Suggested mechanisms of action include inhibiting the uptake of both serotonin and norepinephrine (Wyeth-Ayerst Laboratories, 1994).

selective serotonin reuptake inhibitors (SSRIs)

Class of drugs that selectively prevent the reuptake of serotonin without affecting the uptake of other neurotransmitters.

cological treatment for depression. This void was significant, considering that between 10 and 25 percent of women and 5 to 10 percent of men develop a major depressive disorder at some point in their life (American Psychiatric Association, 1994).

Since that time, several types of medications have been developed for use in treating depression. They can be grouped in various ways (Gitlin, 1990; Julien, 1995; Salzman, 1991; Yudofsky, Hales, & Ferguson, 1991), but we present them under three classes:

1. selective serotonin reuptake inhibitors (SSRIs)
2. tricyclic antidepressants (TCAs)
3. MAO inhibitors (MAOIs)

Table 20.1 lists these classes with the brand and generic names (respectively) of some commonly used antidepressant medications.

Selective Serotonin Reuptake Inhibitors   Prozac is the most commonly used drug of the category **selective serotonin reuptake inhibitors (SSRIs)** (Yudofsky et al., 1991). The SSRIs are called *selective* serotonin reuptake inhibitors because they are said to impact serotonin while having very little effect on other neurotransmitters (Breggin, 1994; Kaplan & Sadock, 1993). Two new SSRI medications, Zoloft and Paxil, are also grouped with Prozac. Even though Prozac is quite controversial, many professionals feel that it's the "wonder drug" of mental health; it's very effective in treating depression and has few side effects. Even more important, many patients—like Sam, discussed in the introduction to this chapter—report that when they take Prozac, they feel better than they have ever felt in their lives.

The exact biochemical causes of depression are not clearly known (Kramer, 1993). It's believed, however, that the levels of serotonin and norepinephrine are depleted in depressed individuals. In fact, there is debate about how Prozac and the other SSRIs actually work. Some experts believe that Prozac makes more serotonin available by blocking the reuptake or reabsorption of serotonin at the nerve cell (Julien, 1995; Kramer, 1993). Other researchers have argued that these drugs are not at all as *selective* in their effects as the advertisements for them indicate (Breggin, 1994; Gilman, Goodman, Rall, Nies, & Taylor, 1991). Regardless of the exact biochemical mechanism of Prozac and the SSRIs, they are quite effective in treating individuals who are depressed.

Not long after Prozac was first marketed, Teicher, Glod, and Cole (1990) reported in a major psychiatry journal the cases of six patients who had intense suicidal thoughts while taking the medication. As you might expect, there was a flurry of research on the topic. Numerous reviews showed that Prozac was safe for treating depression. Patients have as few suicidal thoughts while on Prozac as on any antidepressant medication. In fact, the risk appears less for patients receiving Prozac than for patients receiving many standard antidepressant medications (Kapur, Mieczkowski, & Mann, 1992). Moreover, taking antidepressant medication often leads to *decreases* in suicidal thoughts.

Another concern about taking Prozac has been the loss of sexual desire and inhibited orgasm reported by some individuals. The *Physicians' Desk Reference* (1994) listed these adverse reactions as occurring in 1.9 percent of the people taking this medication. The exact frequency of these problems is actually unclear, because sexual problems often are not discussed with physicians. However, many clinicians who treat depression have heard such reports. If patients have sexual problems after taking Prozac, switching to a non-SSRI antidepressant, Wellbutrin, appears to lead to increased sexual satisfaction in both men and women without increases in depression (Walker et al., 1993).

FIGURE 20.1 The three-ring structure of tricyclics

As shown here, certain antidepressant medications are called tricyclic compounds because of their structure: two benzene rings (6-sided rings) joined by a central compound ring.

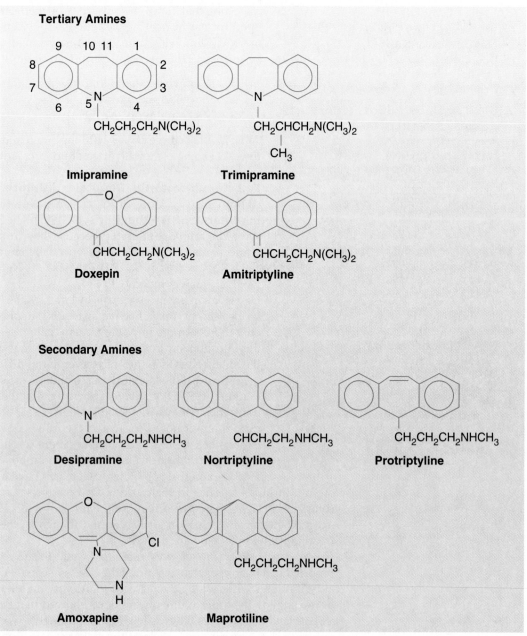

SOURCE: Reprinted by permission of the publishers from *The New Harvard Guide to Psychiatry,* edited by Armand Nicholi, Cambridge, Mass: The Belknap Press of Harvard University Press, Copyright © 1988 by the President and Fellows of Harvard College.

Some clinicians believe that among the SSRIs, Prozac "has the fewest side effects of any antidepressant currently available"; it is also appealing because it can be given at the same dosage over the entire course of treatment (Julien, 1995, p. 157). Even so, Prozac produces insomnia, nervousness, restlessness, and anxiety in 21 percent of individuals who take it (Kaplan & Sadock, 1993, p. 161). A few clinicians even question whether Prozac has fewer side effects than other antidepressants, because in con-

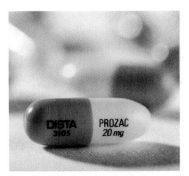

Prozac, the most commonly used antidepressant medication, has also been found effective in treating PMS (premenstrual syndrome). If Prozac serves the PMS market, to what extent will women be likely to take it as an all-purpose medication for well-being?

trolled trials, patients reportedly can tell whether they are receiving Prozac (or many other medications) or a placebo because of the side effects (Greenberg, Bornstein, Greenberg, & Fisher, 1994).

Regardless of the outcome of the debate about Prozac, drug manufacturers will continue to try to develop new antidepressant medications with as few side effects as possible. In fact, in 1994, yet another SSRI antidepressant medication, Effexor, was introduced. It appears to compare favorably with the other SSRIs, producing relatively immediate clinical effects. And based on initial data, it too has few side effects (Julien, 1995).

Tricyclic Antidepressants   The effects of the **tricyclic antidepressants (TCAs)** were discovered almost accidentally. The TCAs have a three-ring molecular structure similar to that of certain drugs used to treat patients with schizophrenia (see Figure 20.1). Indeed, doctors originally gave tricyclics to schizophrenics. Although these drugs did not reduce psychotic thinking, the patients taking them showed some mood improvement. Consequently, researchers began to use TCAs to treat depression. And in 1957, they found that the tricyclic medication imipramine (Tofranil) had antidepressant effects in people with depression (Kuhn, 1958). This was almost the same time that researchers found that the antitubercular medication had antidepressant qualities. Thus, while trying to treat schizophrenia and tuberculosis, physicians noted the antidepressant qualities of medications, pushing the search for a true antidepressant.

Researchers believe that the TCAs interfere with or block the reuptake of norepinephrine and serotonin at the nerve cell after it has fired. As mentioned earlier, deficiencies in brain levels of norepinephrine and serotonin are believed to cause depression (see Chapter 7). This theory is what is guiding researchers today, but it certainly isn't the whole story. There is general agreement that a neurochemical balance is involved, and depression often seems to be genetically determined. Nonetheless, researchers don't know exactly *why* the antidepressants work (Julien, 1995, p. 186).

Whatever their exact mechanism is determined to be, tricyclic antidepressants clearly have a positive mood-elevating effect on many depressed individuals. The initial effects on sleep and appetite usually occur after 1 or 2 weeks of treatment. However, the antidepressant effects may not be achieved until the third or fourth week, and a complete evaluation should last 6 weeks (Kaplan & Sadock, 1993). The most common side effects of taking TCAs are dry mouth, fatigue, constipation, difficulty in urination, memory difficulty, dizziness, and weight gain. The optimal duration of treatment is 4 to 6 months for an acute episode of depression; gradual withdrawal of medication is advised 3 to 5 months after the initial antidepressant effects of the medication have been observed (Kaplan & Sadock, 1993).

Combined Effects of Antidepressant Medication and Psychotherapy

Some individuals who are depressed respond well to antidepressant medication alone, and some respond well to psychotherapy alone, especially cognitive-behavioral therapy. Fortunately, both the pharmacological and psychological treatments of unipolar depression work well (Murphy, Simons, Wetzel, & Lustman, 1984). There is continuing debate about which treatment is better for severe depression. Even though one study showed that severely depressed patients respond best to medication (Elkin et al., 1989), other studies have shown no differences in the effectiveness of medication and psychological treatments (Hollon, DeRubeis, & Seligman, 1992; McLean & Taylor, 1992).

The official guidelines of the American Psychiatric Association (1993) and of the Agency for Health Care Policy and Research (Depression Guideline Panel, 1993b) (which provides federal documents to primary care physicians) both argue for the use of antidepressant medication as a treatment of choice for depression. On the other hand, some psychologists argue that the evidence does not support this

tricyclic antidepressants
Class of drugs with a 3-ring molecular structure that block or interfere with the reuptake of norepinephrine and serotonin.

position (Muñoz, Hollon, McGrath, Rehm, & Vandenbos, 1994; Persons, Thase, & Crits-Christoph, in press). Choice of treatment is often influenced by the professional training of the clinician and the personal preferences of the patient. Whether a pharmacological or psychological treatment is used or a combination of both, it's best to remember that the two types of therapies generally affect different targets. *Medication* is designed to elevate mood and increase energy directly; *psychotherapy* is intended to elevate mood through enhancing interpersonal skills or changing thought patterns.

Combinations of medication and psychotherapy are often seen as the most effective way to treat depression (Julien, 1995; Kaplan & Sadock, 1993; NIMH, 1989). Indeed, Schulberg and Rush (1994) have argued that persons with severe or chronic depression who are partial responders to either treatment alone (psychotherapy or medication) may benefit from combining psychological and pharmacological treatments. In fact, combining the two approaches appears to reduce relapse of depression by as much as 50 percent during the year following treatment termination (Miller, Norman, & Keitner, 1989). However, evidence has not been consistent about the value of combining medication and psychotherapy, and where combined effects are superior, patients are severely depressed (Persons et al., in press).

MAO Inhibitors   The **monoamine oxidase inhibitors (MAOIs),** which appear to block the action of monoamine oxidase (MAO), are the third major type of medication used to treat depression. Because of the potential negative side effects of MAOIs, they are used primarily with individuals who do not respond to other antidepressant medications (Gitlin, 1990). The MAOIs prevent the breakdown of the neurotransmitters norepinephrine and serotonin, thereby keeping more of these substances available for uptake. Their availability, in turn, reduces depression. As with the tricyclic medications, the antidepressant effects of MAOIs were discovered accidentally, when these drugs were found to elevate the mood of tuberculosis patients.

When MAO inhibitors are taken with certain common foods that are high in tyramine (such as yeast, chocolate, beer, and various wines), serious physical reactions can occur, including severe headaches, heart palpitations, stroke, or even death. These side effects occur because tyramine is absorbed rapidly in combination with the MAOIs, leading to a life-threatening increase in blood pressure (Julien, 1995; Yudofsky et al., 1991). Therefore, people taking MAOIs cannot eat even small amounts of certain foods. In addition, many people taking MAO inhibitors become dizzy when they get up from a sitting position (Gitlin, 1990). Because of the potentially lethal side effects of the MAOIs, doctors generally use them only for individuals who don't respond to other available medications. Even then, however, their use must be carefully monitored, and the patient must be informed of the toxic interaction of the medication with various foods, as well as other side effects.

Other Antidepressants   Before we leave the discussion of the various types of antidepressant medications, we should discuss two additional medications: Wellbutrin and Desyrel. Neither is included among the three classes of medications discussed so far. These two drugs are listed in Table 20.1 under the class "Others."

Wellbutrin does not affect the neurotransmitter serotonin. It is chemically unrelated to the other antidepressant drugs (Yudofsky et al., 1991). Some clinicians believe that it increases the amount of norepinephrine in the brain (Salzman, 1991), whereas others argue that it selectively inhibits the neurotransmitter dopamine (Julien, 1995). Unfortunately, Wellbutrin sometimes produces seizures—particularly at the higher doses—so it must be used with extreme caution. As noted earlier, though, Wellbutrin is sometimes used as an alternative to Prozac for patients who experience sexual problems.

monoamine oxidase inhibitors (MAOIs) Class of drugs used to treat depression that act by increasing the amount of available norepinephrine and serotonin; prescribed less often than other antidepressant medications because of their potentially lethal interactions with certain foods.

Desyrel, another effective antidepressant, does not block serotonin reuptake. Its mechanism of antidepressant action is unclear (Julien, 1995), but clinically, it produces drowsiness in about 20 percent of patients (Kaplan & Sadock, 1993; Salzman, 1991). This sedative quality makes it effective in helping patients sleep at night, so Desyrel is sometimes used in combination with Prozac to counter the insomnia that Prozac may produce (Gitlin, 1990). However, clinicians have repeatedly noted that Desyrel seems less effective than other antidepressants in treating severe depression. And it can have a very painful, though rare, side effect: a constant erection (Gitlin, 1990).

One of the newest antidepressant medications—Serzone (nefazodone hydrochloride)—is structurally different from the other major classes of antidepressants (the SSRIs, TCAs, and MAOIs). Serzone was introduced in 1995 as an antidepressant that led to improvement of depressive symptoms as well as anxiety symptoms associated with depression. In one study of patients taking this drug, it appeared that sexual dysfunction was not a significant side effect. Namely, sexual dysfunction didn't occur any more frequently among patients taking the drug than among those taking placebos (Bristol-Myers Squibb, 1995).

Secondary Clinical Uses of Antidepressant Medication   Antidepressant medications are also used to treat other conditions: panic disorder with agoraphobia, obsessive-compulsive disorders, bulimia nervosa, and aggressive-impulsive behavior.

Antidepressants may do more than treat the symptoms of depression often found to coexist with these disorders. MAO inhibitors help some agoraphobics (Sheehan, Ballenger, & Jacobson, 1980). The tricyclic antidepressant Anafranil has reduced the symptoms of obsessive-compulsive children and adults (Leonard et al., 1989). In many studies, treatment with Prozac has led to significant reductions in obsessions and compulsions (Tollefson et al., 1994). Indeed, many physicians believe that antidepressants are the first choice of treatment for individuals with obsessive-compulsive disorder and panic disorder with agoraphobia (Salzman, 1991; Yudofsky et al., 1991).

Antidepressants are also used to treat eating disorders such as bulimia nervosa. They work better than placebos and, as noted in Chapter 11, reduce the depression commonly associated with bulimia nervosa. However, cognitive-behavioral therapy is more effective than pharmacotherapy in the treatment of bulimia, although research has shown that a combination may be more effective than cognitive-behavioral therapy alone in some patients (Mitchell & de Zwaan, 1993).

The use of antidepressant medication to treat individuals with primary disorders other than depression can help us learn more about these disorders. For example, the use of Anafranil has sparked interest in the idea that people who are obsessive-compulsive have a serotonin deficiency. Therefore, researchers are evaluating antidepressant medications and other chemical compounds directly affecting the body's use of serotonin in people with obsessive-compulsive disorder to try to understand that disorder's mystery (Charney et al., 1988; Zohar, Insel, Zohar-Kadouch, Hill, & Murphy, 1988). In fact, depression and/or a serotonin deficiency may underlie not only some compulsions but some aggressive disorders, as well. Indeed, giving medications that increase serotonin functioning significantly reduces aggressive behavior (Coccaro, 1993). Some professionals believe that it may be helpful to view a variety of problems, like depression and obsessions, as disorders that are caused at least in part by depressed mood (Hudson & Pope, 1990) and/or reduced serotonin system function.

Another interesting topic in research on the use of medications to treat psychological disorders concerns multicultural differences. Thinking about Multicultural Issues examines evidence that certain medications affect Asians differently than people from other racial and ethnic groups.

iven the increasing interest in ethnic issues in mental health, we might ask if certain chemical compounds or medications affect racial/ethnic groups differently. Alcohol is an example of a common chemical compound that's metabolized differently by people of some racial/ethnic groups. For example, Native Americans and Asians seem to have lower tolerances for alcohol than other groups. Similarly, milk sugar has very different effects on African Americans and Asian Americans than on Americans of northern European descent. People lacking the enzyme lactase, which allows us to digest milk sugar (lactose), experience difficulty digesting milk products. Indeed, the differences in lactose intolerance are very dramatic. Lactose intolerance has been reported in 94 percent of Asians and 75 percent of African Americans, but it's reported by only 15 percent of white Americans (Chien, 1993).

What about medications? Some evidence has suggested that Asians respond differently to medications than other groups. Dr. Keh-Ming Lin, a research scientist and psychiatrist from Taiwan, came to the United States in 1974 and was struck by the fact that Americans were receiving doses of antipsychotic medications that were considerably higher than those prescribed to patients in Taiwan. Subsequent research by Lin and Finder (1983) indicated that East Asian patients who were being treated for schizophrenia with the antipsychotic medication haloperidol (Haldol) not only received lower doses than most Americans but also displayed optimal response to lower doses. Moreover, the different dosages did not seem to be the result of environmental or lifestyle differences; lower doses of medications were given to both American and foreign-born East Asians. On the other hand, a recent summary of antipsychotic medication use with Asian populations has indicated that doses now given are much higher than they were many years ago (Chien, 1993). Even though there is some evidence of different metabolism of medications by Asian and non-Asian groups, there also appear to be changes in prescription practices by Asian psychiatrists.

Pharmacological treatment of certain anxiety and mood disorders in Asian populations also appears to differ from the treatment of other groups. In a survey of Asians in 10 countries, daily doses of antidepressant medication were about half of what white Americans received. These lower dosages taken by Asians produced effects similar to those seen in white populations. Although the number of studies is limited, research has also suggested that Asians require lower doses of antianxiety medications (benzodiazepines) then their white American counterparts (Chien, 1993).

Think about the following questions:

1. Should drug companies be required to conduct clinical trials with people from different racial and ethnic groups before allowing medications to be used on populations other than those that were part of the drug testing (often white males)? Why or why not?

2. If not, should warnings be placed on medications to alert people from different major ethnic and racial groups that the medications were not tested in clinical trials with such groups? Again, why or why not?

Lithium

Lithium (lithium chloride) is a naturally occurring salt, similar to table salt. Because of its availability in natural forms, lithium has been used by native spiritual healers and snake-oil peddlers as well as by modern pharmacologists. In the 1800s, Lithia Water was sold in the United States to treat a variety of nervous and mental problems and for gout, a disease of the joints (Bernstein, 1988). The popularity of Lithia Water declined shortly after the turn of the century, when it was observed that preparations of it led to nausea, giddiness, and even poisoning.

In the 1940s, Australian psychiatrist John Cade noted that when lithium was given to guinea pigs, they became quite calm. After observing this, Cade gave lithium to agitated psychotic patients and saw the same quieting effect. Today, physicians frequently prescribe lithium to treat individuals who have manic episodes of bipolar disorder, because the drug normalizes their moods. Without medical treatment, manic episodes are unpredictable and uncontrollable. Lithium prevents the characteristic swings from extreme highs to extreme lows (Baldessarini & Cole, 1988; Kaplan & Sadock, 1993).

lithium Naturally occurring salt that is the drug of choice for treating bipolar disorder; normalizes mood, especially manic highs.

TABLE 20.2	Adverse Side Effects of Lithium

Effects of Therapeutic Dosage
  Nausea
  Dizziness
  Weight gain
  Mild diarrhea

Effects of Near Toxic Dosage
  Nausea and vomiting
  Hand tremors
  Sleepiness
  Vertigo

Effects of Toxic Dosage
  Heart problems
  Convulsions
  Coma

Lithium is clearly the treatment of choice for patients with manic-depressive disorder. It's effective in approximately 60 to 70 percent of cases (Julien, 1995). Because many individuals with bipolar disorder are frequently quite agitated and even psychotic, doctors often prescribe antipsychotic medication in addition to lithium. If, on the other hand, an individual is in the depressive phase of a bipolar disorder, antidepressant medication is given together with lithium (Julien, 1995). By itself, lithium is generally not useful in treating major depression; antidepressants are the treatment of choice for that disorder. In fact, a significant percentage of bipolar patients become manic if given antidepressant medication alone.

Like most chemical treatments for psychiatric disorders, lithium has some adverse side effects (see Table 20.2). It has even led to the deaths of cardiac patients who used large amounts as a salt substitute. Lithium has a very small "therapeutic window," or dose level that is therapeutic rather than toxic. Consequently, lithium should be prescribed with a careful plan for monitoring the amount of the drug in the blood. Monitored appropriately, however, lithium often provides therapeutic effects directly related to its level in the blood (Julien, 1995).

In addition to concerns about side effects, some manic-depressive individuals may not want to take lithium because they find their "highs" (or manic phases) pleasant and exciting. Evidence has indicated that artists and authors such as Robert Schumann and William James suffered from bipolar illness (Jamison, 1993). Based on the belief that mania can trigger creativity, some people may simply refuse to take medication that might prevent their manic episodes.

Exactly how lithium works is a matter of speculation. At least six possible mechanisms have been hypothesized (Julien, 1995); among these, theories that suggest alterations in brain levels of serotonin and norepinephrine are most prominent (see Chapter 7). Despite theoretical differences about how lithium works, there is general agreement that a biochemical abnormality produces bipolar disorder. Since 30 to 40 percent of bipolar patients do not respond to lithium, other medications are currently being assessed for their possible therapeutic benefits. One group of medications that have proved useful in treating bipolar disorder are the anticonvulsant drugs Tegretol (carbamazepine) and Depakote (valproic acid). Indeed, both these medications are alternatives to lithium for patients with rapid-cycling bipolar disorder (Julien, 1995).

Antianxiety Medications

For more than 100 years, investigators have tried to find a chemical that would calm people but not cause addiction. In 1869, just after the Civil War, scientists discovered a sedative/hypnotic, chloral hydrate (Noctec); this medication is still used occasionally for treating insomnia (Kaplan & Sadock, 1993). In

Chloral hydrate, a sedative/hypnotic, was discovered in 1869, just after the Civil War. Before that, surgeries and amputations were performed without pain-killing drugs in hospital tents like that pictured here.

Thinking about GENDER ISSUES   Gender Differences in Drug Prescriptions

*W*omen far exceed men in their consumption of prescribed psychoactive drugs. Although women make slightly over half of all visits to physicians' offices, they receive 73 percent of all prescriptions written for psychiatric drugs (Laurence & Weinhouse, 1994; Rossiter, 1983). Also, male psychiatrists prescribe drugs twice as often as female psychiatrists (Cypress, 1980).

In a study of outpatient services, female patients were 37 percent more likely than males to receive minor tranquilizers (benzodiazepines) and 62 percent more likely to receive antidepressants. (Men and women were equally likely to receive antipsychotic medication: 0.08 percent of all male patients versus 0.10 percent of all female patients [Hohmann, Larson, Thompson, & Beardsley, 1988].) Are these discrepancies a result of sexist attitudes? To try to answer this, let's first consider what happens when men and women present with similar symptoms, such as depression. Women make up 66 percent of the total number of patients who are depressed—but women receive up to 83 percent of the prescriptions for antidepressant medication (Laurence & Weinhouse, 1994).

Why does this happen? Instead of suggesting other therapies that may work as well, physicians (especially males) may offer female patients a quick fix rather than attempting to deal with the psychosocial issues underlying the depression and anxiety. The contemporary psychosocial stressors of differential pay in the workforce, partner abuse, marital discord, and single parenthood can cause some women to become anxious and depressed. These problems, however, require much more than a temporary solution. Yet some psychiatrists argue that a number of anxiety patients are undertreated and are made to suffer unnecessarily because of fears of dependence on medication.

To sum up, women receive more antianxiety and antidepressant medications than men, given the rates of anxiety and depression in the populations. However, perhaps women ask their physicians for medications to help them become less anxious or depressed.

Think about the following questions:

1. Is it a physician's job to discourage women from taking medications that may be effective in alleviating some of their symptoms? Why or why not?

2. Why do you think male psychiatrists are more likely to give medications for problems of anxiety and depression than female psychiatrists?

1912, drug companies introduced the barbiturate sedative phenobarbital. Sedatives like meprobamate (Miltown) arrived on the market in the 1950s, and by 1963, minor tranquilizers like diazepam (Valium) were available for public use.

With each new drug, the goal was to develop a perfect tranquilizer. Although each came closer to the ideal, none ever reached the goal. Chloral hydrate was used as a sleeping agent in the late 1800s, but many people became addicted to it. Barbiturates dominated the treatment of anxiety in the first half of this century, but they are also highly addictive; what's more, they are sedating and impair coordination. Miltown and Valium were used to treat anxiety and insomnia in the 1960s but, like their predecessors, were addictive—though less so than the barbiturates. In 1979, the quest led to the discovery of Buspirone (BuSpar), a medication with less addictive properties than its predecessors and thus one that may become the treatment of choice for anxiety (Yudofsky et al., 1991).

The most commonly used class of antianxiety medications are the benzodiazepines, often called minor tranquilizers (Yudofsky et al., 1991). This group of popular medications includes 6 of 25 best-selling prescription drugs in the United States. However, because of publicity about the addictive properties of these tranquilizers, their use in this country has been declining modestly since the mid-1970s (Julien, 1995). Interestingly, women are more likely than men to be given prescriptions for tranquilizers and some other psychotropic drugs. This and other gender differences in drug prescriptions are considered in Thinking about Gender Issues.

In any case, the market for antianxiety medications is huge. And although their use in the United States has declined, in some other countries, such as France, their use has escalated (Breggin, 1991). Some clinicians would argue that the increasing use of antianxiety medications is understandable, as many individuals with anxiety disorders never receive any treatment. For example, only 3 out of 4 individuals with panic disorder receive any treatment at all (NIMH, 1991), and many probably receive ineffective treatments.

TABLE 20.3	Eight Most Frequently Prescribed (Ranked) Benzodiazepines

Brand Name (generic name)
  Xanax (alprazolam)
  Valium (diazepam)
  Tranxene (chlorazepate)
  Ativan (lorazepam)
  Serax (oxazepam)
  Centrax (prazepam)
  Librium (chlordiazepoxide)
  Paxipam (halazepam)

Source: From Yudofsky, S., Hales, R. E., and Ferguson, T., *What You Need to Know about Psychiatric Drugs*, p. 86. Copyright 1991 Grove/Atlantic, Inc. Reprinted by permission.

Benzodiazepines   The **benzodiazepines** are a class of antianxiety medications that includes Valium, Xanax, and Halcion. All the medications in this class are equally effective in treating anxiety (Gitlin, 1990). The eight most frequently prescribed benzodiazepines are listed in Table 20.3.

Because different terms are sometimes used for the benzodiazepines, let us note several alternative labels for these medications. For a long time, they were called the *minor tranquilizers.* For example, until 1990, the *Physicians' Desk Reference* (1994) used the term **tranquilizers** as the heading for medications that include the antianxiety agents. The *Essential Guide to Prescription Drugs* (Long & Rybacki, 1994) uses the term *mild tranquilizers* to describe the class of many of the antianxiety medications, such as Valium and Xanax. Finally, many researchers call the benzodiazepines by a more technical name, *anxiolytics*, literally meaning "anxiety looseners."

benzodiazepines Most commonly used class of antianxiety medication.

tranquilizers Class of drugs that includes the antianxiety medications, benzodiazepines; have a calming effect on mood.

Positive Effects   Taken in appropriate doses, the benzodiazepines have calming effects. If you take these drugs, you will feel calmer and less nervous and worried. Life will seem better. If you have a sleeping problem, you may fall asleep more quickly.

Approximately 65 to 70 percent of individuals who take benzodiazepines report these desired effects. Unfortunately, there's no way to predict which individuals will benefit and which ones will not. However, those who *do* experience the desired effects of taking this medication will usually do so within the first week. Overall, the benzodiazepines have been used successfully in treating people with situational anxiety, generalized anxiety, and panic attacks (Gitlin, 1990).

Negative Effects   The benzodiazepines frequently cause drowsiness and lack of coordination early in treatment, and they affect walking or driving. In fact, a study of automobile accidents in older drivers, aged 65 to 84, found that a significant number of accidents were due to the drivers' taking benzodiazepines (Ray, Fought, & Decker, 1992). Because benzodiazepines (such as Xanax) and alcohol together decrease alertness and central nervous system activity, their combined use is very dangerous and can be fatal. Many medical professionals are also concerned about the risk of dependency, abuse, and addiction with the benzodiazepines (Baldessarini & Cole, 1988; Hayward, Wardle, & Higgitt, 1989). Tolerance and withdrawal symptoms that appear on abrupt termination of use are additional problems with these medications (Rickels, Case, Downing, & Winoker, 1983).

Benzodiazepines like Valium generally inhibit the central nervous system. They act on specific receptor sites that affect neurotransmitters in the brain, leading to reduced nerve cell firing (Hayward et al., 1989). Relief from anxiety is almost directly proportional to the dosage taken. As the body develops increasing tolerance, the dosage must be increased to obtain the same level of anxiety reduction. Physiological and psychological depen-

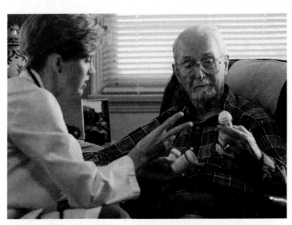

Elderly individuals often misuse antianxiety medications. What sources or reference books would you consult to find out if a relative or friend was taking medication properly?

dency on the benzodiazepines may develop from this increased tolerance. Whether this happens will vary with the specific drug, the dosage level, and the length of time a person is on the drug, but physical dependence can occur within 2 to 4 weeks.

Regardless, individuals taking these medications should withdraw from them gradually (Yudofsky et al., 1991). The most common withdrawal effects from the benzodiazepines (after having taken them for over a month) are anxiety, irritability, sleep disturbance, and impaired memory. A small percentage of patients experience panic, but these feelings generally subside in 2 to 4 weeks. Sometimes, these symptoms are present before using the antianxiety medications, so it's not clear whether their presence represents a recurrence or a response to the medication. Because the benzodiazepines are potentially addictive, psychological therapies should always be considered as alternatives or adjuncts to any long-term use.

The benzodiazepines are also used in clinical settings by nonpsychiatrists. In 1988, general practitioners and family physicians accounted for 52 percent of prescriptions given for tranquilizers or benzodiazepines in the United States, whereas psychiatrists accounted for only 28 percent (Beardsley, Gardocki, Larson, & Hidalgo, 1988). One reason for this difference is that nonpsychiatrists co-prescribe tranquilizers (that is, they prescribe them together with other medications) when symptoms of anxiety are thought to aggravate gastrointestinal or respiratory disorders and to treat insomnia and stress associated with a variety of illnesses.

Heated debate continues about whether the symptom relief produced by the benzodiazepines may actually hamper our understanding of the factors that cause anxiety. Critics of their use argue that these drugs are merely a crutch. Supporters, on the other hand, contend they are useful crutches that help people regain control at times of severe stress.

Buspirone   Buspirone (BuSpar), introduced in 1979, is an antianxiety medication that is chemically unrelated to the benzodiazepines; its mechanisms of action are unknown. Most importantly, physicians are interested in this drug because it does not have the potential for addiction that the benzodiazepines have. Proponents of BuSpar see it as an effective antianxiety medication that does not have significant sedating effects or a risk of dependence. It does not impair coordination and people taking it can drive without risk of accidents. Further, it does not interact dangerously with alcohol (Yudofsky et al., 1991). Because of its nonaddictive properties, BuSpar is advertised as being useful in treating alcoholics and other addiction-prone people. Since it is less sedating than the benzodiazepines, it is also often used with people who are elderly (Long & Rybacki, 1994).

BuSpar has some negative side effects, however, including dizziness, faintness, and mild drowsiness (Long & Rybacki, 1994). In addition, there is a lag of 1 to 3 weeks between when BuSpar is first taken and when it begins to have a clinical effect; thus, it cannot be used to produce immediate benefits. Finally, this drug is generally not useful for individuals who have not responded to the benzodiazepines.

Antipsychotic Medications

The word *psychotic* has many meanings, but in the mental health professions, it's used to describe someone who's unable to tell the difference between what is and is not real. The ability of **antipsychotic medications** to reduce symptoms of psychosis, like hallucinations and delusions, is the key criterion for their effectiveness, since changing these symptoms is a primary goal of mental health professionals working with psychotic patients.

Antipsychotic medications are sometimes called *major tranquilizers,* because one of their most common side effects is sedation. Antipsychotics are also sometimes called *neuroleptics,* because they have side effects that influence the neurological system. Neither label—major tranquilizers or neuroleptics—is correct, how-

antipsychotic medications Medications used to reduce symptoms of psychosis, like hallucinations and delusions; sometimes called major tranquilizers because of their sedating effect.

ever. Medications are classified according to their primary targets, and in the case of antipsychotic medications, the primary target is psychotic thought.

Psychotic symptoms can occur in several different disorders, among them alcoholism, depression, and schizophrenia. Here, however, we'll focus on the treatment of psychotic symptoms in schizophrenia. Psychotic thought is a defining feature of this disorder, whereas it is not a key feature of alcoholism or depression (American Psychiatric Association, 1994). We'll discuss the discovery of antipsychotic medications, positive and negative effects of these medications, the search for antipsychotic medications with few negative side effects, and the need for family therapy with schizophrenic patients taking antipsychotic drugs.

Discovery of Antipsychotic Drugs   As was the case with the antidepressant medications, use of antipsychotic medications arose from work on a problem other than psychosis. French surgeon Henri Laborit used a medication to try to reduce blood pressure in patients before surgery. But instead of seeing a drop in blood pressure, he observed that the patients were markedly less anxious. In 1952, French psychiatrists Jean Delay and Pierre Deniker gave Thorazine (chlorpromazine), a variation of the medication used by Laborit, to a group of psychiatric patients. Many of the patients showed reductions in anxiety. And of special importance, the schizophrenic individuals in this psychiatric sample reported a marked decrease of hallucinations and delusions. Delay and Deniker's observation led to the commercial use of Thorazine. Professionals saw this medication as a wonder drug, as it was the first medication known to decrease psychotic symptoms. Although other antipsychotic medications have been developed since 1952, no new medication has been found more effective than Thorazine in reducing psychotic thought (Gitlin, 1990).

Thorazine was the first antipsychotic produced commercially and therefore is often used as a *reference drug;* that is, all other antipsychotics are compared to it. Some of those medications are listed in Table 20.4. In this section, we will discuss the use of Thorazine as the primary example of antipsychotic medication because it was the first medication to reduce symptoms of schizophrenia. Even though Thorazine was used extensively, it does have negative side effects, so other medications (such as Haldol) are now often used instead.

TABLE 20.4   Antipsychotic Medications
Brand Name (generic name)
Clozaril (clozapine)
Haldol (haloperidol)
Mellaril (thioridazine)
Navane (thiothixene)
Risperdal (risperidone)
Stelazine (trifluoperazine)
Thorazine (chlorpromazine)

Positive Effects   After Thorazine became available, many schizophrenic people who had been hospitalized for years were able to return to their jobs and families (see Chapter 13). In fact, many of these people returned to their families and communities as part of the **deinstitutionalization** trend that began in the 1960s. Part of the reason these people were released from mental hospitals was that antipsychotic medications had been shown to reduce or eliminate psychotic thoughts. If you walk the streets of some large U.S. cities today and see homeless people who appear psychotic, you may question whether the release of schizophrenic patients from hospitals was a positive development. In certain instances, deinstitutionalization has clearly brought new problems. We must remember, however, that thanks to antipsychotic drugs, many schizophrenic individuals can now live with their families or in small-group homes in the community.

The positive effects of antipsychotic medications like Thorazine occur in about 80 to 90 percent of people who are schizophrenic. In addition, the antipsychotic medications also reduce the need for readmission to psychiatric hospitals (Hogarty, 1984; Mueser & Glynn, 1995). Of those patients who initially respond to the drugs, 20 to 30 percent relapse during the first year or two on medication after their release from the hospital (Kane et al., 1988). It's not clear why patients relapse while taking medication. In some cases, they may simply no longer be responsive to the medication. In other instances, they may encounter new stressors that they cannot handle, such as job problems or family difficulties. Finally, some may not take the medication as prescribed.

deinstitutionalization
Trend started in the 1960s, in which hospitals markedly reduced the populations of psychiatric wards by returning to the community patients judged capable of functioning outside the hospital.

Negative Effects Antipsychotic medications like Thorazine produce negative side effects, such as muscle rigidity, stooped posture, an unusual shuffling gait, and even occasional drooling. These negative side effects are similar to the symptoms of Parkinson's disease and thus are called **Parkinsonian effects.** If these problems are to emerge in a patient, they usually appear in the first few weeks of treatment. Anti-Parkinsonian medications can reduce these side effects, but their use is controversial because of their own side effects. Anti-Parkinsonian medications must be monitored carefully; they can lead to drug-induced states of confusion that are difficult to recognize in schizophrenic patients.

A related side effect of antipsychotic medications is **tardive dyskinesia,** which is characterized by slowed movements of the face, tongue, and neck muscles. These symptoms often start as small eye twitches or unusual finger movements. Occasionally, they are accompanied by strange tongue-thrusting movements. Such movements not only occur while patients are taking antipsychotic drugs but are often observed after patients withdraw from medication. And for many patients, these motor abnormalities are irreversible. When patients stop taking antipsychotic drugs, there may be about a 50 percent reduction in symptoms of tardive dyskinesia (Yudofsky et al., 1991). But some patients show little or no change.

There is currently significant debate about the exact percentage of schizophrenic individuals who develop tardive dyskinesia as a result of taking antipsychotic medication and about the exact number for whom symptoms are reversible. It has generally been estimated that 15 to 20 percent of those persons who receive antipsychotic medications for 6 months to 2 years develop tardive dyskinesia (Breggin, 1991; Gitlin, 1990). In one study, approximately 60 percent of older patients who were on the medication for many years developed tardive dyskinesia (Yassa, Nastase, Dupont, & Thibeau, 1992). Finally, *Clinical Psychiatry News* (cited in Breggin, 1991) reported information that raised even greater concern: that prolonged use of Thorazine almost certainly leads to developing tardive dyskinesia.

Researchers recently found that some types of movement disorders like tardive dyskinesia occur in approximately 25 percent of schizophrenic individuals who never took antipsychotic medications (Fenton, Wyatt, & McGlashan, 1994). Therefore, some patients taking these medications who had tardive dyskinesia may not have developed the dyskinesia because of the medication. Even with this finding, however, researchers noted that any patient taking antipsychotics should be warned about the risks of developing tardive dyskinesia.

Because schizophrenia is a chronic illness for which there is no cure, many people with this disorder may have to take antipsychotic medications throughout much of their lives (Meuser & Glynn, 1995). And because there is no known effective treatment for tardive dyskinesia, physicians must carefully observe patients on antipsychotic drugs so as to catch the problem when it first begins. Physicians can minimize the effects by finding the lowest efficient dosage to reduce patients' psychotic thoughts.

Parkinsonian effects Side effects of antipsychotic medications; typically include muscle rigidity, stooped posture, an unusual shuffling gait, and drooling.

tardive dyskinesia Sometimes irreversible side effect of antipsychotic medication; characterized by slow movements of the tongue, face, and neck muscles.

Search for Antipsychotics with Few Negative Effects The serious side effects of many antipsychotic medications and the fact that some patients do not respond to antipsychotic medications have led researchers to search for alternatives. Clozaril (clozapine) appears useful for some of the 10 to 20 percent of schizophrenic persons who are unresponsive to generally available antipsychotic medications. Clozaril does not have significant negative effects on motor functioning (Brier, Buchanan, Irish, & Carpenter, 1993; Kane et al., 1988). However, it causes diminished white blood cell (WBC) count in about 2 percent of patients (Julien, 1995; Marder & Van Putten, 1988). Partly because of the risks associated with lowered WBC counts, Clozaril is recommended only for treatment-resistant patients. Further, its use is restricted to certain medical centers. All patients must have their blood count taken weekly, physicians can receive only limited supplies of the medication for a patient, and the producer of Clozaril monitors its use. In 1991, a year's supply of this medication and its monitoring cost $10,000 (Julien, 1995). This cost may seem extremely high, but as noted in Chapter 13, the cost of this medication is far less than the cost of psychiatric hospitalization (Meltzer, 1993).

An additional antipsychotic medication, Risperdal (risperidone), was introduced in the United States in 1994. It inhibits both dopamine and serotonin, and it reduces both positive and negative symptoms of schizophrenia (see Chapter 13). Because it has a low incidence of motor side effects (tardive dyskinesia), Risperdal is increasingly becoming one of the medications of choice in treating people who are schizophrenic (Julien, 1995).

Combined Use of Antipsychotic Medication and Family Therapy   Antipsychotic medications have led to dramatic changes in the lives of schizophrenic individuals, but their positive effects should not mask the psychological needs of these people and their families. Psychological counseling can be very effective with families of schizophrenic patients who have been released from hospitals while these patients continue to take some antipsychotic medication. A family psychoeducational approach often leads to a reduction of criticism. This in turn brings about a highly significant reduction in the rehospitalization of patients (Hogarty et al., 1991; Meuser & Glynn, 1995). (See Chapter 13 regarding the impact of emotional and family variables on the functioning of people with schizophrenia.)

Psychostimulants

Psychostimulants have been used for decades to treat a variety of clinical problems (Klein, 1995). Most important, they have been used to increase the attention span in children with attention-deficit disorders. Approximately 5 percent of children are diagnosed with attention-deficit/hyperactivity disorder, and adults can be diagnosed with the problem, as well. As more and more people are diagnosed, the use of psychostimulant medication soars. In fact, from 1990 to 1994, prescriptions for the most commonly used psychostimulant medication, Ritalin, jumped 390 percent (Wallis, 1994). In addition, physicians prescribe psychostimulants for a sleeping disorder, narcolepsy. (We'll discuss this later in the chapter.)

In this section, we'll discuss the discovery of psychostimulants' capacity to increase attention, their positive and negative effects, and varied psychostimulant treatments for problems other than attentional problems and hyperactivity of children.

Psychostimulants' Capacity to Increase Attention   In 1937, Dr. Charles Bradley gave children in a psychiatric hospital a psychostimulant in an effort to decrease their headaches. But instead of curing headaches, he made an observation that led to a new treatment for children. Namely, he found that children who were aggressive and hyperactive responded favorably to a psychostimulant, Benzedrine. (Note that children previously diagnosed with *hyperactivity* are classified as having *attention-deficit/hyperactivity disorder* in the *DSM-IV* [see Chapter 14]. We will use both terms interchangeably in this chapter.) The children called the medication "arithmetic pills," because they felt they could complete arithmetic assignments more readily when taking their medication. Thus, Bradley joined the long list of clinicians and researchers who have made important medical discoveries accidentally.

In the 1940s, researchers noted that psychostimulant medications—especially amphetamines—increased alertness, motor skills, and general arousal in laboratory situations with adults. Based on these results, pilots, scouts, and foot soldiers fighting in World War II were equipped with survival kits containing stimulants. The soldiers took the medication if they were in foxholes and had to remain awake or if they had to flee from their enemies.

psychostimulants
Medications used primarily to increase attention span and decrease restlessness in children.

Neither the discovery by Bradley nor the military use of psychostimulants led to any major use of these medications until the late 1960s. Then, research by psychologist Keith Conners showed that children with hyperactivity and attentional problems showed a positive response to psychostimulant medication (Conners, 1969). As a result of that research and many other studies showing the same positive effects, psychostimulants became the most frequently prescribed medication for treating children with psychological problems. The three most commonly used psychostimulant medications are listed in Table 20.5. Although they are all generally equally effective, Ritalin is used most commonly with children.

TABLE 20.5   **Common Psychostimulant Medications**
Brand Name (generic name)
Ritalin (methylphenidate)
Dexedrine (dextroamphetamine)
Cylert (magnesium pemoline)

Positive Effects   Children's attention and activity problems become most apparent in structured situations like the classroom. Taking psychostimulants has been shown to decrease children's restlessness and increase their attention span. In more than two dozen studies, teachers and classroom observers have consistently noted increased focus and attention in hyperactive children on psychostimulants. Social behavior in the classroom also shows significant improvement. Decreases in fidgeting and walking around the classroom have been repeatedly observed (Conners & Wells, 1986). Psychostimulants' effect on motor skills is also often positive. Researchers found that 50 percent of hyperactive children receiving psychostimulants improved in their handwriting, whereas only 5 percent who received a placebo showed handwriting improvement (Lerer, Lerer, & Artner, 1977).

Negative Effects   In the late 1960s and early 1970s, a number of studies demonstrated physiological side effects of psychostimulants in children and adults. For instance, these drugs increased heartrate, blood pressure, and central nervous system responsivity. And in adults specifically, psychostimulants also produced marked feelings of euphoria and increased energy levels and attention span. This increased energy resulted in giving the nickname "speed" to various psychostimulants. Thinking about Social Issues looks more closely at the use of these drugs to enhance performance on physical and intellectual tasks.

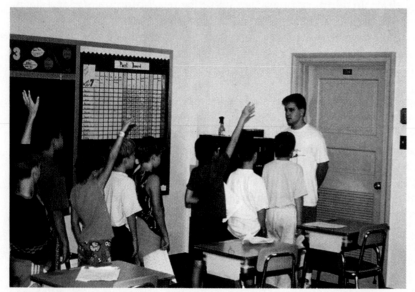

The Pittsburgh Summer Treatment program, directed by Dr. William Pelham, specializes in the treatment of children with AD/HD. In this program, psychostimulant medication (Ritalin) is used alone and in combination with token reinforcement programs to help children with AD/HD increase attention span and academic productivity.

Unfortunately, psychostimulants were misused by many young adults, especially in the 1960s and 1970s. Gradually, it became clear that the drugs were addictive and dangerous for adults. Thus, psychostimulants are now classified by the federal government as Schedule II Drugs, which have the highest abuse potential (Long & Rybacki, 1994). Because of this abuse potential, the federal government scrutinizes prescriptions for psychostimulants. In other countries, such as Sweden, use of these medications is restricted, and in Italy, Spain, and China, the use of psychostimulants with children is highly unusual (O'Leary, 1984; O'Leary, Vivian, & Nisi, 1985). Even advocates of giving psychostimulant medication to adults with AD/HD admit that it's unclear whether an adult taking therapeutic doses of psychostimulants may experience the highs and the addictive effects felt by others who abuse the drugs (Wender, 1987).

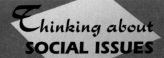

Should We All Get Psychostimulants?

Basic research has repeatedly proved that various psychostimulants enhance the attention and motor skills of normal adults. As early as 1966, Laties and Weiss stated, "There is little doubt that amphetamines can improve performance on a wide variety of tasks, especially on those involving an element of fatigue or boredom" (p. 806). These researchers reviewed evidence indicating that swimmers and runners could enhance their speed and endurance by using psychostimulants. Laties and Weiss also indicated that performance on simple intellectual tasks, such as completing rote arithmetic problems, could be improved with psychostimulants. Nevertheless, they concluded that many other ways besides drugs exist to improve performance.

In the past, many experts believed that hyperactive children with attentional problems had a brain dysfunction. In fact, the terms *minimal brain dysfunction* and *hyperactivity* were used interchangeably in the 1970s and early 1980s. Even though some research with PET scans and new magnetic imaging procedures has suggested that there may be subtle differences in the brains of children with AD/HD, even the researchers who conducted these studies admit that it's not clear what these differences mean (Wallis, 1994). It's possible that brain-imaging procedures cannot capture small or subtle differences—sometimes called *soft neurological signs*—that might exist in the brains of children with attention-deficit/hyperactivity disorder.

However, some hyperactive children may not have any brain disorder. In addition, it's now clear that children with normal activity levels and attention spans display the same type of response to psychostimulants as hyperactive children (Rapoport et al., 1978). All children—hyperactive and normal children—show increased attention spans and somewhat greater fine motor control if they take psychostimulant medication.

So, if psychostimulants improve adult performance on a variety of tasks and if hyperactive children have no well-documented brain dysfunction addressed by stimulant medication and respond no differently to stimulants than other children, should we all take psychostimulants? Consider that, as you read this text, you might be able to stay up later, sit stiller, and concentrate longer if you were taking psychostimulants.

Think about the following questions:

1. Suppose that Marcus, who's 11 years old, has taken a psychostimulant medication for 5 years to treat his hyperactivity. Beyond the desired calming effect of the drug, what effect would taking it have on his thoughts about his ability to concentrate and work efficiently without medication? Explain your answer.

2. If psychostimulant medications were not addictive and could be taken in small doses to keep us more attentive as we work or drive our vehicles, should the public have access to such medication?

When administered appropriately, however, psychostimulants are not addictive to children.

Combined Use of Psychostimulants and Other Therapy   Although psychostimulants help children with attentional problems, to the surprise of many professionals, the use of these drugs has not been associated with increases in academic performance as reflected on standard achievement tests (Barkley & Cunningham, 1978). One study also found that hyperactive children who received psychostimulant medication for several years did not fare better academically than unmedicated hyperactive children (Weiss, Hechtman, Perlman, Hopkins, & Wener, 1979). These findings led professionals to believe that the critical problems of hyperactive children in learning new academic and social skills cannot be addressed simply with medication. Other professionals questioned the widespread use of psychostimulant medication, given the positive effects of behavior therapy on social and academic behaviors (O'Leary, 1980).

A combined approach using medication and behavior therapy or family therapy, then, may be the treatment of choice for some children with AD/HD. Support is increasing for the combination of a low dose of psychostimulant medication and psychological therapies, especially if a child does not respond to psychological and educational interventions alone (Pelham, 1993; Pelham et al., 1991; Satterfield, Satterfield, & Cantwell, 1980). For example, in reviewing the effects of psychostimulant medication for children, Pelham (1993) suggested that parent training, psychological consultation with the teachers of the AD/HD child, and tutoring should be considered before using medication. If these interventions are insufficient, Pelham has advocated adding psychostimulant medication to the treatment. In 1994, the National Institute of Mental Health launched a 6-site study comparing psychostimulants alone with behavior therapy; by 1998 to 2002, we'll know much more about how these two approaches work in practice.

Secondary Clinical Uses   Psychostimulants have been used for decades to treat *narcolepsy,* a rare sleep disorder that occurs in approximately 1 out of 1,000 people. Individuals with this problem fall asleep suddenly at inappropriate times and places. Narcolepsy usually begins when a person is between 15 and 25 years of age and lasts for the remainder of the person's life. Because psychostimulants increase central nervous system activity, these drugs may energize the reticular activating system of the brain and help maintain alertness. Psychostimulants often decrease the frequency of narcoleptic sleep attacks and drowsiness. Approximately 70 to 80 percent of narcoleptics improve with medication and can resume active normal lives (Roth, 1980).

Psychostimulants are sometimes used to help people who are depressed and do not respond to antidepressants and who have adverse reactions to antidepressants; these drugs are sometimes used for elderly patients, as well (Gitlin, 1990; Satel & Nelson, 1989). Psychostimulant treatment for depression is problematic, however, because the physician must find a dosage level to reduce the depressed mood without producing the emotional high associated with psychological and physical addiction (Gitlin, 1990).

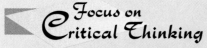

Focus on Critical Thinking

1. What factors would be important in your decision to recommend that a relative or friend with schizophrenia undergo a trial of Clozaril? Explain your answer.

2. What risk factors are involved with taking Clozaril?

ELECTROCONVULSIVE THERAPY

Electroshock treatment, or electroconvulsive therapy (ECT), is the application of an electrical current through the brain to produce a brief convulsion. The mere use of the words *shock therapy* and *electroshock therapy* usually draws very negative reactions. The phrases remind us of ancient practices and torture. Nonetheless, today ECT is seen by many psychiatrists as "among the safest and most effective forms of treatment" (Yudofsky et al., 1993, p. 331).

Discovery

electroshock treatment
Passage of electrical current through the brain to produce a convulsion; used to alleviate severe depression; also known as electroconvulsive therapy (ECT).

As early as the 1700s, doctors knew that severe bodily stresses alleviated mental illness. These observations eventually led to medical interventions such as inducing fever and convulsions for mental patients. In 1938, two Italian physicians, Cerlutti and Bini, began to induce convulsions electrically, initiating the treatment known today as electroconvulsive therapy (ECT). From the 1940s through the mid-1960s, ECT became accepted in treating schizophrenia. Then, as psychiatrists became optimistic about its use, they started using it to treat many mental disorders, especially

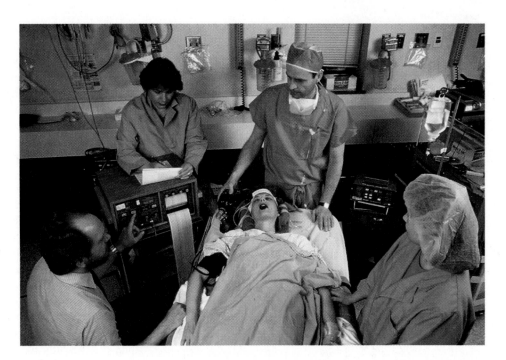

Although the administration of ECT may look scary, recently modified techniques have helped many individuals overcome severe depression. Which of the ECT safeguards mentioned in this chapter appear to be utilized in treating this patient?

severe depression. In the 1950s, however, concern mounted as doctors began to observe bone fractures, memory loss, and heart complications in patients receiving ECT. Anesthesia helped prevent the bone fractures associated with convulsions, but this didn't stop the criticism. Reviews of hospital records revealed that ECT had been used on some individuals hundreds of times. Critics argued that each shock treatment killed brain cells. In addition, many contended that ECT was misused to control violent and aggressive patients on hospital wards (Breggin, 1991).

In some parts of the United States, concern about electroshock treatment resulted in hearings and court battles, in which opponents attempted unsuccessfully to ban it. Further, public outcry led to federal panels adopting specific guidelines concerning its use. At the same time, the advent of antidepressant medication and the use of lithium in treating manic depression led to decreased interest in ECT. By the mid-1960s, many hospital ECT facilities were closed.

Research in the 1960s and 1970s led to safer and more effective ECT treatment. Brief electrical impulses were used, at lower dosages than in earlier decades. In addition, placing electrodes on only one side of the head resulted in fewer side effects (such as memory loss) than when electrodes were used on both sides ("Effective Treatment," 1994). Any memory loss is usually temporary. It's unknown whether occasional long-term memory losses with unilateral placements are due to ECT or other factors (NIMH Consensus Statement, 1985). With careful monitoring, ECT is generally safe, rapid, and effective in alleviating depression (Yudofsky et al., 1993).

Current Use

Patients undergoing ECT today receive a light, general anesthesia to make them sleep before treatment (see Chapter 7) and are injected with a muscle relaxant to prevent violent muscle contractions. Blood pressure and heartrate are monitored, and oxygen is administered ("Johns Hopkins Medical Letter," 1994). The doctor then induces a seizure by passing 150 volts of electricity through electrodes placed just above the patient's temples. The seizure is detectable by use of an electroencephalograph (EEG), which monitors brain-wave activity. After 1 minute, the seizure is over, and within 5 to 10 minutes, the patient awakens. Most patients receive six to eight ECT treatments over a 3-week period.

Today, ECT is most commonly used in treating patients with severe, long-lasting depression who have not responded to or cannot tolerate the side effects of various antidepressant medications; often these are elderly patients. Electroshock therapy can be especially useful in treating cases of severe depression in which there is a risk of suicide (Fink, 1994).

Consider the case of Roland Kolhoff, principal timpanist with the New York Philharmonic Orchestra. He had such severe depression that he had to stop performing. Kolhoff stated, "I could feel it coming on. My chemistry was going out and I was totally helpless. You don't want to get out of bed. It's very hard to do anything. What I think [ECT] did was to act like a Roto-Rooter on the depression. It just reamed me clear and the depression was gone" (Foderaro, 1993, p. 7).

A review of 16 studies showed no credible evidence that ECT causes structural brain damage (Devanand, Dwork, Hutchinson, Blowig, & Sackheim, 1994). Even though many people report being somewhat fearful of ECT, a survey of ECT patients indicated that nearly 80 percent felt that they had been helped by ECT and would not be reluctant to have the treatment again, if needed (Andreasen & Black, 1991).

Despite decades of research, however, we do not actually know how ECT works. Evidence has suggested that the hormone cortisol—which may lead to depression—is suppressed in patients who receive ECT (Grunhaus et al., 1987).

> ### Focus on Critical Thinking
>
> **1.** Do you think that the minimal memory loss associated with ECT is preferable to some of the side effects of drug therapies—such as insomnia, weight gain, food restrictions, and decreased sexual interest? Why or why not?
>
> **2.** For what types of depression and for which groups of people do you think ECT is most appropriate? Why?

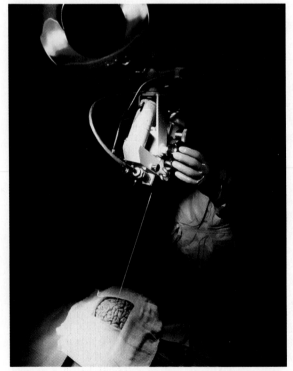

Laser surgery can be directed at extremely small areas of the brain. To what extent can laser surgery replace the removal of brain tissue with operations such as prefrontal lobotomy?

PSYCHOSURGERY

Of all the treatments for psychiatric disorders, the most controversial is **psychosurgery,** which involves the selective surgical removal of part of the brain or the destruction of nerve pathways to influence behavior. These procedures were developed before the discovery of effective antipsychotic medications, at a time when no effective treatments existed for many psychiatric disorders.

The earliest psychosurgeries removed the frontal lobes from patients with schizophrenia. In an operation known as **prefrontal lobotomy,** Dr. Moniz and a colleague, Dr. Lima, removed frontal lobe tissue from each side of the brains of schizophrenic patients. The two surgeons performed these operations on hundreds of patients for whom other treatments should have been sought. As a result, many patients became apathetic and inactive; over half became mute. It's now estimated that over the years, thousands of patients were permanently brain injured by this procedure. Nonetheless, in 1949, Moniz received the Nobel Prize in Medicine for developing the prefrontal lobotomy.

Early reports by neurosurgeons indicated that most patients improved. Further, a study citing more than 60 clinical investigators—recognized experts in the field—found no evidence of an association between the early psychosurgery and any permanent memory loss or ability impairment (Freeman & Watts, 1942). But this early clinical evaluation had no control group, and the evaluation's emphasis was on eliminating the undesirable behavior, not on the lobotomized person's quality of life. This attitude is illustrated by Freeman and Watts's comment on one of their cases: "She is not noisy and is now easy to manage" (p. 241).

Today, doctors perform very limited forms of psychosurgery on people with specific severe and intractable disorders. Some psychosurgery involves selective cutting of an extremely small area of the brain that provides stimulation to the limbic system. Researchers believe this operation slows the neural firing of the limbic system, which is believed to cause the emotional stimulation that causes some obsessions (Andreasen, 1984). This type of surgery is largely confined to the treatment of severely obsessive-compulsive individuals or of patients with incapacitating depression associated with severe anxiety. Even current surgical procedures, however, are controversial as treatments for obsessive-compulsive behavior. Nonetheless, the operation holds hope for some people whose lives have been severely restricted by obsessions and compulsions. More specifically, this surgery appears to help about 50 to 60 percent of obsessive-compulsive individuals who have not responded to any other treatment (Andreasen, 1984; Jenike et al., 1991).

A new form of psychosurgery, *videolaserscopy*, allows surgeons to use a video camera to guide laser surgery in repairing blood vessels in the brain and making cuts smaller than 1 millimeter. Such surgery may completely replace the scalpel as a neurosurgical technique (Cowley, 1990). Whatever the method of destroying brain tissue—even if the destruction is minuscule—such procedures are last-resort treatments for psychological disorders.

psychosurgery Selective surgical removal of part of the brain or destruction of nerve pathways to influence behavior.

prefrontal lobotomy Surgical operation involving cutting fibers of the anterior portion of the frontal lobe of the brain.

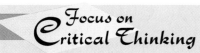
Focus on Critical Thinking

1. Psychosurgery is currently used as a last-resort treatment for patients with severe obsessions; recently, it's also been used to repair extremely small blood vessels. If a child or an adult were very aggressive toward others, under what conditions, if any, would psychosurgery be justified? Why?
2. When is it justified to cut portions of the human brain? Why?

SUMMARY

Medications
- Antidepressants can be grouped in three classes: selective serotonin reuptake inhibitors (SSRIs), tricyclic antidepressants (TCAs), and monoamine oxidase inhibitors (MAOIs).
- One of the SSRIs, Prozac, is very effective in alleviating depression and seems to have relatively few side effects. Tricyclic antidepressants such as Tofranil, like other antidepressants, appear to elevate mood by blocking the reuptake of serotonin and norepinephrine. MAO inhibitors can have serious side effects when they are taken with certain foods.
- Lithium is the drug of choice for treating bipolar disorder. It's effective in preventing the characteristic mood swings in approximately 60 to 70 percent of patients. Tegretol (carbamazepine) and Depakote (valproic acid) are anticonvulsant drugs that can be used as alternative treatments for bipolar disorder.
- The benzodiazepines are the most commonly used class of antianxiety drugs, or tranquilizers. These drugs have calming effects, reducing anxiety and nervousness. Side effects include drowsiness, dizziness, and decreased alertness. Tolerance and physical dependence (addiction) may occur within 2 to 4 weeks.
- Buspirone (BuSpar) is an antianxiety medication chemically unrelated to the benzodiazepines. BuSpar is nonaddictive; as a result, it can be useful in treat-

ing addiction-prone patients such as alcoholics. It also is often used with people who are elderly, because it is less sedating than the benzodiazepines.

■ Antipsychotic medications such as Thorazine are used to reduce hallucinations and delusions and are effective in 80 to 90 percent of patients. There are common side effects, however. Parkinsonian effects include muscle rigidity, stooped posture, unusual shuffling gait, and drooling. Tardive dyskinesia is a sometimes irreversible side effect that is characterized by involuntary movements of the tongue and face.

■ Clozaril, a new antipsychotic medication, appears to be effective with 10 to 20 percent of people who do not respond to standard antipsychotic drugs. Clozaril has fewer negative effects on motor functioning than conventional antipsychotic drugs.

■ Psychostimulants enable children with attention-deficit/hyperactivity disorder to attend to tasks and become less restless. These drugs are also prescribed to some adults with attentional problems, although this use is controversial. Psychostimulants also enable individuals with narcolepsy to avoid falling asleep unpredictably.

Electroconvulsive Therapy

■ Electroconvulsive or electroshock therapy involves the passage of an electrical current through the brain to induce convulsions. It is a highly effective treatment for people with severe depression and for those who don't respond to drug therapy or who are at risk for suicide. Side effects may include temporary memory loss.

Psychosurgery

■ Psychosurgery is rarely used today. This type of surgery involves cutting out part of the brain or severing nerve fibers in order to influence behavior. It's currently used to treat individuals with severe obsessive-compulsive disorder who have not responded to medication or psychotherapy.

KEY TERMS

antipsychotic medications, **p. 634**
benzodiazepines, **p. 633**
deinstitutionalization, **p. 635**
electroshock treatment, **p. 640**
lithium, **p. 630**

monoamine oxidase inhibitors (MAOIs), **p. 628**
Parkinsonian effects, **p. 636**
prefrontal lobotomy, **pp. 642–643**
psychostimulants, **p. 637**
psychosurgery, **pp. 642–643**

psychotropic medications, **p. 624**
selective serotonin reuptake inhibitors (SSRIs), **p. 625**
tardive dyskinesia, **p. 636**
tranquilizers, **p. 633**
tricyclic antidepressants (TCAs), **p. 627**

CRITICAL THINKING EXERCISE

As we've discussed elsewhere in this book, placebos (pills that are basically sugar pills) are used as a means of testing whether a medication can produce meaningful clinical changes. In many studies with antianxiety medications, antidepressant medications, and psychostimulants, placebos have been used as alternatives to the real medication. And generally, the results have favored the real medication.

However, if there are often side effects with certain medications, the individuals receiving the real medication may know they are not getting the placebo. For example, if a man developed insomnia or erectile problems after taking a medication but had never had such problems before, it would be difficult to conceal the fact that the individual was given the real medication.

1. Why have researchers felt that placebo groups are necessary?
2. If side effects of certain medications are quite well known and occur in at least 30 to 40 percent of individuals receiving the medication, how would you design a placebo study to test the effectiveness of the real medication?

Chapter 21
LEGAL AND ETHICAL ISSUES

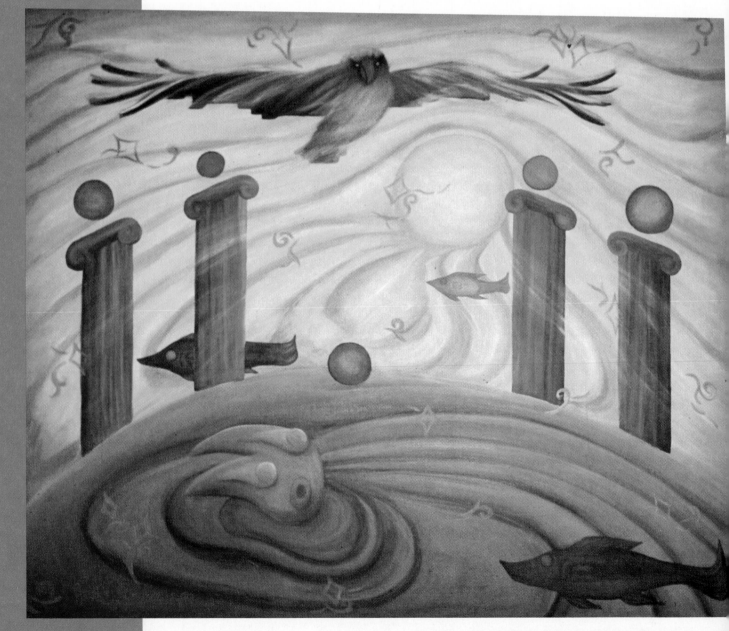

Jane Gerus, **The Arrival,** 1989, Very Special Arts Gallery

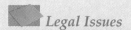

Legal Issues

Mental Health Professionals
and the Law

Dangerousness and the
Duty to Warn

Civil Commitment

Thinking about Social Issues

Patients' Rights

Competency and Responsibility

*Thinking about
Multicultural Issues*

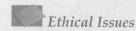

Ethical Issues

Professional Ethics

*Thinking about
Controversial Issues*

Ethical Issues in Research

Ethical Standards and the Law

Sometime in 1969, Prosenjit Poddar, a graduate student at the University of California, Berkeley, became preoccupied with fellow student Tatiana Tarasoff after meeting her at a student mixer. His growing obsession for Tarasoff led Poddar to tape-record his conversations with her and then spend many hours listening to the tapes, trying to determine whether she'd begun to return his strong feelings of attraction. A friend, worried about the obsession, urged Poddar to seek treatment at the student health service of the university. After an initial evaluation by Dr. Gold, a psychiatrist, Poddar was assigned to Dr. Moore, a psychologist. Poddar participated in weekly psychotherapy sessions and was given a tranquilizing medication. Neither Dr. Gold nor Dr. Moore thought that Poddar needed hospitalization.

Once in therapy, Poddar revealed that he had thoughts of harming—even killing—Tarasoff because she didn't return his affections. Dr. Moore also learned from one of Poddar's friends that he was considering buying a gun. Shortly thereafter, Poddar dropped out of therapy. At this point, Drs. Moore and Gold agreed that Poddar should be hospitalized. They asked the campus police to bring him to the student health service for evaluation. The campus police went to Poddar's apartment and asked him about his plans; when he denied any intention to hurt Tarasoff, they left.

Two months later, Poddar stabbed Tarasoff to death. He was indicted for first-degree murder and ultimately convicted of second-degree murder. When that conviction was overturned on technical grounds (the judge had given improper instructions to the jury), Poddar returned home to India. Subsequently, Tarasoff's family brought suit for negligence against the university, including Drs. Gold and Moore as well as the university police in their suit.

In 1974, the California Supreme Court decided that if the facts in the case were as alleged, Drs. Gold and Moore had had a duty to warn Tarasoff. However, the court did not find either doctor or the university police liable for failing to hospitalize Poddar. This judicial decision established for the first time the legal responsibility of psychotherapists to warn persons threatened during the course of psychotherapy— a responsibility that's now called the *Tarasoff standard* (adapted from Mills, Sullivan, & Eth, 1987, pp. 69–70) (We'll return to this decision later in the chapter.)

Despite the significance of this standard, legal questions still remain about the rights and responsibilities involved in the diagnosis and treatment of persons with emotional disorders. Think about the issues raised in each of the following cases:

Your grandfather has begun to forget more than he remembers. He loses his way between the grocery store and the house he and your grandmother have lived in for more than 40 years. He's also become extremely quick to lose his temper; on

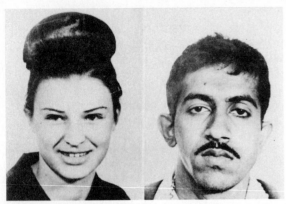

Tatiana Tarasoff and Prosenjit Poddar, whose lethal interaction tragically led to enactment of the Tarasoff *standard, which involves "the duty to warn and to protect"*

several occasions, he's reduced salespeople to tears at the grocery store. Although he denies that he has a problem, your grandmother strongly disagrees. She's not sure she can continue to care for him and wonders whether he can be placed in a nursing home against his will. Can she have him committed?

After 22 years of marriage, your best friend's parents have decided to divorce. Your friend is away at college, but her younger siblings—ages 14, 12, and 8—have become the subjects of a custody dispute between their mother and father. Each parent claims to be able to provide the best home. How will custody be decided? What rights and responsibilities does your friend have in protecting her own interests, as well as those of her brothers and sisters?

Infuriated by an article in the local paper, questioning the integrity of his best friend, your uncle—the mayor—goes to the newspaper office and physically assaults the paper's editor. Prone to epileptic seizures all his life, your uncle later claims he was in the midst of a psychomotor seizure when he attacked the editor. For this reason, he has decided to plead not guilty by reason of temporary insanity to the assault charge. His lawyer has hired a consulting psychologist who will testify that violent behavior is typical during an epileptic seizure. Is this a legitimate defense? Is it ethical for psychologists to serve as paid consultants in this way?

This chapter is about how questions like these and countless others like them are asked—and answered—every day in courts throughout the United States. Human beings have energetically debated these matters throughout history. Not only does every generation reach its own conclusions on how to settle such vexing questions; each inevitably argues and resolves them anew. Sometimes, new conclusions are reached and those of the previous generation are tossed out; sometimes, they are not.

Today, we seem to be confronting a wider array of questions than has been asked in past years. And in addressing them, we seem to be trying to entirely rethink them, perhaps because of the complex society in which we live. We'll consider this variety of questions in looking at two general topics: legal issues and ethical issues.

ℒEGAL ISSUES

Legal issues concern the rights and freedoms that all persons—including those who are mentally or medically impaired—can expect from U.S. society and what society, in turn, can expect from them. Some of these issues are as old as recorded history. For example, the question of what society can do to protect itself from dangerous persons (including those with mental disorders) goes back to antiquity. So does the issue of individual competency to stand trial. More than 600 years ago, Western society vigorously debated whether it was appropriate to try a person for a crime committed during a psychotic episode.

Some of the other issues considered in this chapter, however, are more specific to the age and place we live in today. They reflect the strong commitment of the United States to civil liberties and civil rights—a pledge that's uncommon even among modern Western democracies. A good example of this commitment is the issue of patients' rights, which has only been pursued during the past two decades in the United States. Do psychiatric patients who are committed to hospitals against their will have a right to expect treatment, to be treated in the least restrictive environment, and to be free to refuse possibly harmful treatments? These questions reflect the growing conviction in the United States that even persons who are seriously disturbed have civil rights that cannot be ignored. Our country seems intent on continuing its legal efforts to humanize the care of psychiatric patients, to protect them against unfair or biased efforts to confine them against their will, and to assess their competency to stand trial and their responsibility for their actions in an enlightened and humane manner.

Mental Health Professionals and the Law

Mental health professionals—mostly psychiatrists and psychologists—are routinely called as expert witnesses during court proceedings. They help answer such difficult questions as whether a defendant is competent to stand trial, is dangerous and should be involuntarily committed for psychiatric treatment, or was psychologically incapacitated when the crime he is accused of was committed. Mental health professionals also testify in family court matters—for instance, recommending which parent should be awarded custody of children in a disputed custody suit. Finally, these professionals may be called on for advice regarding whether a mental patient is receiving appropriate treatment in an institution or by an individual practitioner (Hiday & Scheid-Cook, 1991; Turkheimer & Parry, 1992).

Although it's the ultimate responsibility of the judge—and in cases involving one, the jury—to decide on these matters, psychologists and psychiatrists are often asked their opinions as experts on behavior before decisions are made. In fact, the involvement of mental health professionals is legally mandated for certain cases in all states (DeAngelis, 1994). But just how useful are mental health professionals in helping the courts decide such complex issues? Nearly everyone agrees that they have important roles to play; however, the quality of their judgments has been disappointing, for several reasons:

1. Psychologists and psychiatrists who serve as expert witnesses are typically asked to answer some of the hardest human questions imaginable (DeAngelis, 1994). For instance, they're often asked to predict the likelihood that a person will be dangerous to society or to herself in the future on the basis of clues from past and present behavior (McNiel & Binder, 1991; Rosenthal, 1993). Likewise, psychologists and psychiatrists are often called on to decide which of two loving parents will provide the best care for a child or children over a 10- to 15-year period (Melton & Limber, 1991) or to judge whether someone's current mental state prevents her from understanding the criminal charges against her, from defending herself against those charges, or both (Margolick, 1994).

2. The adversarial nature of the U.S. legal system requires each side in a civil or criminal matter to try to convince a judge (and often a jury) that their viewpoint is correct. In those cases in which a judgment call, rather than definitive evidence, must be relied on, each side can usually find a mental health professional who is willing to support its contention—whatever that may be. It's so easy to find psychologists and psychiatrists willing to testify in disputes over custody, competency, and dangerousness that some people (Shah & McGarry, 1986) are convinced that so-called expert testimony is of little use. But others feel just as strongly that psychologists and psychiatrists have important insights to share with judges and juries—insights that are available from no other source (Boyer, 1990; Clark, 1990).

3. The extensive training and experience required to produce a competent expert witness is another issue (Garb, 1992; Grisso, 1987). Garb (1992), a psychologist and authority on such training, believes that psychologists and psychiatrists

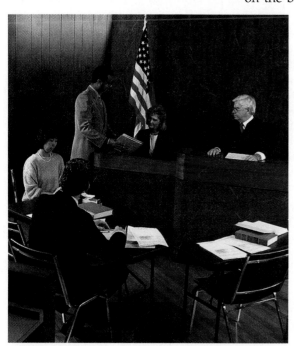

The adversarial nature of the U.S. legal system requires both sides in a civil or criminal matter to try to convince a judge and sometimes a jury of the correctness of their opposing viewpoints.

are "able to make reliable and valid judgments for many tasks" and that "their judgments are frequently more valid than judgments made by laypersons" (p. 462). An extensive review of the voluminous literature on this subject convinced Garb that psychologists are best at three things: (a) detecting **malingering** (faking an illness or disorder); (b) predicting violent behavior, especially on a short-term basis; and (c) evaluating competency to stand trial. However, Garb noted that successful expert witnesses must have the appropriate background, experience, and training to do the job and must also be aware of the limitations of their expertise.

Dangerousness and the Duty to Warn

Predicting Dangerousness Judgments about **dangerousness** are among the most frequently sought, important, and difficult of those mental health professionals are asked to make. These judgments are difficult because mental health professionals often don't receive all the information necessary to make a sure call. What's more, they're often asked to make decisions quickly, without the luxury of time for reflection. Consider the moral and professional dilemmas faced by a therapist, Dr. Fowler, in the following case:

> Dr. Fowler has been treating Professor Harris, a 45-year-old nuclear physicist specializing in nuclear weapons development, with individual psychotherapy during the past 3 months. Professor Harris developed a reactive depression after the breakup of a love affair. . . . [His] initial depression abated when he was asked to take an important research position with a prestigious institution engaged in the development of nuclear weapons. Although uncertain about whether to work in weapons development, he eventually decided to take the position. Professor Harris created a breakthrough with his discovery and development of low-yield tactical nuclear weapons. These weapons were found to be extremely valuable for use in military war games and against selected targets where highly circumscribed lethality was required. . . .
>
> While working on this project, [Professor Harris] became enamored of his secretary. Twenty years younger than him, she had worked for [Harris] about a year before their personal relationship developed. . . . Six months after the relationship began, it dissolved when she resigned her position as his secretary and refused to see Professor Harris. She was frightened by his jealous rages and his desire for bondage and other sadistic practices in their sexual relationship. Professor Harris was devastated and slipped back into depression. . . . [He] developed the delusion that death by cancer is imminent.
>
> Dr. Fowler is alarmed by Professor Harris's ideas that his former girlfriend, her parents, and his former department head at the university are gloating over his imminent demise. He has never been able to settle his guilt over developing nuclear weapons. Professor Harris now feels that his imminent death is a just punishment. . . . He tells Dr. Fowler that perhaps he should die by the very weapons he has engineered and "take some of these other worthless people with me." Also, during the past week, he [has made] threatening calls to his former girlfriend, her parents, and his former departmental chairman, fully identifying himself. . . .
>
> Dr. Fowler proposes that her patient return to three-times-a-week psychotherapy and begin taking antidepressant medication. He refuses both suggestions, stating, "I am going to die soon anyway." Professor Harris does not want medication to confuse his thinking or interfere with making his "final plans." Dr. Fowler's recommendation of psychiatric hospitalization is viewed by Professor Harris as a plot by his enemies to "foil me." Dr. Fowler knows that Professor Harris has access to low-yield tactical nuclear weapons with a force of approximately 1,000 pounds of TNT that could kill anyone within 500 feet of ground zero. . . . Also, for the first time, Professor Harris is considering carrying a .38 caliber Beretta pistol. He is no longer eating, having lost 10 pounds in the past week. He spends much of each night "pacing and plotting." . . .

malingering Falsely claiming an illness or disorder in order to obtain some reward or to avoid an unpleasant situation.

dangerousness Legal concept that refers to the likelihood a person is or will be a danger to herself or others.

Dr. Fowler assesses her patient's risk of violence as high. This assessment is based upon the severity of Professor Harris' psychotic depression, threats of violence toward identifiable victims, access to weapons of mass destruction, a clear motive of revenge, and a deteriorating therapeutic alliance. . . . Dr. Fowler considers her options. She reasons that because no duty to warn exists in her state and because the three individuals threatened are fully aware of the threats made against them by Professor Harris, no duty to warn these three individuals exists. However, she decides that the danger to the public is so great that ethically, morally, and professionally she must inform the police. . . . Dr. Fowler immediately signs medical certification papers for the involuntary hospitalization of Professor Harris, which permits the police to apprehend and take him to a designated psychiatric hospital. (Simon, 1992, pp. 297–299)

As we've already noted, the data on the ability of mental health professionals to predict long-term dangerousness have tended to be discouraging. The primary reason for this lack of predictive ability is that the likelihood of violent acts seems to depend more on the immediate circumstances preceding the violence than on the attacker's personality. However, Appelbaum and Rosenbaum (1989) have reported that the more extensive the behavioral data on individuals who might be dangerous, the greater the accuracy of the dangerousness predictions. John Monahan—a professor of both law and psychology and director of a large-scale study of violence in the mentally ill—has agreed (Rosenthal, 1993). He and his group have begun to explore four kinds of risk factors for violence:

1. *factors in the patient's current behavior*—anger control capacity and ability to meet threats without violence
2. *factors in the patient's past*—arrest and conviction history and history of diligence in keeping psychiatric treatment appointments
3. *factors in the patient's environment*—living arrangements and family situation
4. *factors in the patient's illness*—delusions, hallucinations, and fantasies of violence

More and more often these days, urban general hospitals are having to confront the problem posed by violent patients. Columbia-Presbyterian Medical Center, which serves a large, urban, impoverished area of New York City, deals with this problem after every weekend. A recent front-page story in the *New York Times* (Rosenthal, 1993) described the situation:

Early on a Monday morning in the Columbia-Presbyterian Medical Center emergency room, nine psychiatric patients with recent histories of violent behavior lounged on stretchers and armchairs, awaiting a doctor's decision about who would be committed and who discharged. One man had threatened to murder his girlfriend and another, hearing voices urging him to kill a prostitute, had grazed a woman's neck with a knife. A 51-year-old woman, while high on crack, had tried to place her young niece in the oven for being disobedient.

"The normal complement after a weekend," said Dr. Ellen M. Stevenson, the psychiatrist in charge of the hospital's emergency services. "The knife and gun club. The crack. The threats. The temper tantrums gone bad." (p. B6)

What strategy have Dr. Stevenson and her colleagues (Rosenthal, 1993) adopted to decide which of these patients will be committed to the hospital—for their own safety or that of others—and which can be safely released back to the streets?

The strategy includes extensive dredging of the person's past for patterns of violence, instead of relying primarily on interviews with the patient. The new method has allowed emergency room staff to make far better determinations about violent potential. . . . There is tremendous pressure to improve since, rightly or wrongly, the courts and public have frequently held therapists accountable for a patient's violent acts. (p. B6)

Looking 5 or 10 years into the future, it's very hard to know whether intensive treatment for an anger-control problem will help a person with a past history of violence. Who knows what life has in store for him? Will he be able to withstand serious marital discord or continuing stress on the job without resorting to violence? The further into the future a professional is called on to predict behavior, the less likely she will be able to account for the factors most likely to influence that behavior. Thus, experts agree that predicting immediate dangerousness is much easier than predicting dangerousness well into the future (McNiel & Binder, 1987, 1991).

Even the U.S. Supreme Court has recognized the difficulty of predicting dangerousness by estimating, at best, one correct prediction of dangerousness out of three. In *Barefoot v. Estelle* (1983), the Court ruled on a case involving a convicted murderer found to be dangerous by a psychiatrist. That finding had influenced a jury's deliberations over assigning the death penalty. The Court concluded that "neither petitioner (Barefoot) nor the [American Psychiatric] Association suggests that psychiatrists are always wrong with respect to future dangerousness, only most of the time" (*Barefoot v. Estelle*, 1983). In this decision, the highest court in the United States went on record to express its skepticism about the ability of psychiatrists to make the all-important prediction of dangerousness.

Tarasoff and the Duty to Warn and Protect   Despite the hazards of predicting dangerousness over the long term, psychologists and psychiatrists are called on to make this prediction at times. The importance of this judgment to mental health professionals has become substantially greater since 1974, when the California Supreme Court handed down the decision on *Tarasoff v. Regents of the University of California* (1976). As mentioned in the chapter-opening case, this judicial decision established for the first time the legal responsibility of psychotherapists to warn persons threatened during the course of psychotherapy (Mills, Sullivan, & Eth, 1987, pp. 69–70). That decision—the ***Tarasoff* standard**—states:

> When a therapist determines, or pursuant to the standards of his profession should determine, that his patient presents a serious danger of violence to another, he incurs an obligation to use reasonable care to protect the intended victim against such danger. The discharge of this duty may require the therapist to take one or more of the various steps . . . [such as] to warn the intended victim or others likely to apprise the victim of the danger, to notify the police, or take whatever other steps are reasonably necessary under the circumstances. (*Tarasoff v. Regents of University of California*, 1976)

In its decision on *Tarasoff*, the court specified that only therapists have the clear duty to warn, presumably on the assumption that they know their patients better and can thus make the difficult judgment of dangerousness more accurately than anyone else. Fearful of *Tarasoff* liability suits in those states that have adopted the standard, some therapists have begun hospitalizing patients to prevent violence, even though they don't really require inpatient treatment. According to Appelbaum (1988b), these actions amount to "preventive detention" that uses scarce mental health resources to deal with what is actually the responsibility of the criminal justice system. Some states have responded to protests from therapists by limiting therapists' liability, so long as they take prescribed steps to warn or protect. Other states have backed away altogether from the *Tarasoff* decision and do not hold therapists responsible to warn or protect (Stromberg, Schneider, & Joondeph, 1993). For their part, professional organizations have begun to develop standards that help therapists limit their *Tarasoff* liability by reducing their risks when they have or expect to have potentially dangerous patients in treatment (Monahan, 1993).

Predicting Suicide   Clinicians are more confident that they can accurately predict the seriousness of a suicide threat or attempt, but as with dangerousness, data supporting that conviction are not completely convincing. Nevertheless, psycholo-

Tarasoff standard Established the duty of therapists to warn and protect persons threatened by their patients.

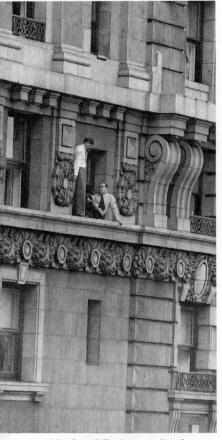

It's often difficult to predict the seriousness of a suicide threat or attempt; however, the person shown in this photo standing on the ledge of a building seems quite serious about wanting to end his life.

TABLE 21.1   Predictors of Completed Suicide

1. The absence of a close and effective relationship with the therapist
2. Ending formerly meaningful relationships and failing to substitute new ones
3. The existence of severe depression
4. The presence of psychosis, particularly if auditory hallucinations that command particular actions are present
5. Prior suicide attempts, particularly a recent attempt
6. Improvement from a psychotic episode but continuance of secondary depression
7. Advancing age, personal loss, or physical illness, particularly if the latter is chronic
8. Single or divorced
9. High lethality potential (dangerousness) of the method used to attempt suicide (Jumping from a high bridge is more dangerous than consuming four aspirin tablets.)
10. Behavior possibly indicative of a finalized decision to die (for example, writing a farewell note to children, spouse, or friends)
11. Presence of a specific plan
12. Availability of a lethal (deadly) means
13. A family history of suicide
14. Chronic alcoholism
15. Drug addiction
16. In the age group of 15–24
17. Mental incompetence prevents development of an effective therapeutic relationship

Source: From T. R. Simon, *Clinical Psychiatry and the Law,* 2nd ed., p. 259. Copyright © 1992 American Psychiatric Press. Reprinted with permission of the American Psychiatric Association.

gists and psychiatrists have developed criteria for making this judgment, which many professionals depend on. Table 21.1 summarizes a comprehensive list of predictors of completed (or successful) suicides; the list highlights factors found to be associated with such suicides. If you have a friend or family member who is seriously depressed, you should read this list carefully.

Civil Commitment

What Is Civil Commitment? Despite the turmoil and confusion they may be experiencing, individuals whose behavior represents a danger to themselves or others are often willing to consent to hospitalization. But what about cases in which someone cannot or will not agree to voluntary hospitalization? When hospitalization is clearly indicated but the patient refuses to comply, **civil commitment** (or involuntary hospitalization) may be necessary.

Civil commitment presents several dilemmas that most psychologists and psychiatrists would prefer to avoid. First, the formal process of civil commitment is time consuming and expensive. In addition, it often pits patients against their families, mental health professionals, or both. Finally, a state's legal guidelines for commitment may be unclear and confusing, so professionals might be uncertain about what the circumstances require. There are certain times and instances, however, when most mental health professionals would agree that civil commitment is the

civil commitment Involuntary, enforced inpatient or outpatient treatment; necessary when clearly indicated for a psychiatric condition a patient refuses treatment for.

only alternative to allowing persons who are frightened, psychotic, or potentially dangerous to resolve their own problems.

The following case illustrates some of the complexities—legal, professional, and human—of civil commitment:

> Mr. C., a 34-year-old single computer operator, was evaluated in a general hospital emergency room for feelings of depression and, at times, anger and rage at his ex-wife. Dr. V., the examining psychiatrist, determined that the symptoms first appeared when Mr. C. learned that his ex-wife—from whom he had been divorced for three years—had begun to date. Dr. V. also found out that Mr. C. had consulted a psychologist and a psychiatrist for depression, uncontrollable anger, and alcohol and drug abuse on several previous occasions (including during the last 6 months) and that he had a lengthy police record extending back to his early adolescence for assault, petty theft, and minor drug offenses. Mr. C. was currently on probation for possession of a controlled substance.
>
> Dr. V. had determined that Mr. C. was not psychotic; he did not demonstrate hallucinations, delusions, disordered thinking, or bizarre behavior. He was moderately depressed but not suicidal. On checking past hospital records, Dr. V. learned that Mr. C. had been diagnosed with an antisocial personality disorder. This diagnosis confirmed Dr. V.'s clinical impression.
>
> Mr. C. was genuinely concerned for the consequences of his uncontrollable anger, his fear that he might hurt someone, and his lingering depression. In addition, his ex-wife had spoken to him several times and believed he might harm her. Given all this, Mr. C. agreed to voluntary admission to the psychiatric ward that Dr. V. oversaw. However, after less than 24 hours, Mr. C. requested discharge. He felt "cooped up" in the hospital, believed that he had achieved a better understanding of his anger, and reported that he was no longer depressed.
>
> However, staff on the ward discovered a discarded suicide note, written by Mr. C., which suggested that he was planning to kill his ex-wife before taking his own life. Dr. V. decided to seek an emergency involuntary commitment of Mr. C.; his primary reason for doing so was fear for the ex-wife's safety. The state commitment regulations specify, however, that an emergency civil commitment will only be granted if a recent act of violence had taken place that has proven the patient's dangerousness. (*Recent* is defined as within 60 days of the request for commitment.) Although Mr. C. had threatened violence against his ex-wife on numerous recent occasions, his only violent acts against her took place during their marriage and the first several months after they were separated. During the hearing on Dr. V.'s commitment request, the judge concluded that the psychiatrist had not met the regulations for commitment and refused to sign the commitment papers. Mr. C. was freed.
>
> Four days later, Mr. C. was found dead in an automobile outside his ex-wife's home, with a .38 caliber bullet hole in his skull. Next to him was his ex-wife, who had been killed the same way. No suicide note was found.

Civil Commitment Criteria Few legal or ethical issues of concern to mental health professionals have been debated for as long or with such passion as civil commitment. Similarly, few issues have generated such a volume of rhetoric, and partly because of this continuing debate, few have caused such radical changes in public and professional attitudes over the past two decades (Turkheimer & Parry, 1992).

In the past, before someone could be committed to a psychiatric hospital, she had to be judged mentally ill, dangerous to herself or to others, or gravely disabled. She also had to be unwilling to enter a hospital voluntarily and capable of benefiting from treatment or sufficiently disturbed that hospitalization represented the *least restrictive alternative* (which we'll discuss later in this section). Additionally, some states required that the person lack the capacity to make a reasoned decision about her need for treatment. But today, civil commitment statutes are based solely on a combination of criteria regarding dangerousness and *grave disability* (again, see later in this section), using the latter most frequently (Turkheimer & Parry, 1992).

Prior to the 1960s, proof of mental illness alone was sufficient to justify most involuntary commitments. As a result, many persons who could have managed on their own or in sheltered environments outside hospitals were forced to spend some, much, or all their lives in psychiatric hospitals—simply because someone concluded they were mentally ill and in need of treatment. Following a California Supreme Court decision in 1969, however, one state court after another agreed that mental illness alone was insufficient to justify involuntary hospitalization. As was decided in California, proof was required that the person was either dangerous to herself or to others or gravely disabled.

Mental health professionals and judges alike must ask themselves a series of questions to evaluate dangerousness:

- How serious is the danger? For example, is a person who occasionally exposes his genitals in public dangerous enough to society to justify his civil commitment? Is a person who steals but has never committed a violent crime against another person dangerous enough to be committed?
- How imminent is the danger? If a person threatens to harm someone years after making the threat, is that threat imminent enough to justify commitment?
- How real is the threat? How probable is it that a threat against someone else will be carried out?
- How can mental health professionals be trained to agree on commitment criteria, including dangerousness?

This final question has been studied. Relatively recent research has encouraged the view that mental health professionals working in hospital emergency rooms can be trained to agree on assessments of dangerousness (Phillips, Wolf, & Coons, 1988). Another study has reported on the development of a questionnaire—the Index of Dangerousness Indicators (TRIAD)—designed to enable clinicians to evaluate dangerousness (to self and others) and grave disability more reliably and validly than through clinical interviews alone (Segal, Watson, Goldfinger, & Averbuck, 1988a, 1988b). Research with the TRIAD reveals that clinicians' ratings of dangerousness and of severity of mental illness are highly correlated (Segal, Watson, Goldfinger, & Averbuck, 1988c). This finding disputes those who claim that an overemphasis on dangerousness as a prime criterion for commitment neglects persons who are severely mentally ill in favor of those less ill but dangerous.

Individuals who do not meet the dangerousness criterion but clearly do require and would benefit from treatment can be committed if they cannot exercise the good judgment required to know they are sick, incapacitated, and in need of treatment—in other words, because they are gravely disabled. Examples of persons who are gravely disabled include those who are clearly suicidal (and thus dangers to themselves), those who are suffering from paranoid delusions that might cause them to harm other people (making them dangers to others), and those who are so confused, psychotic, or demented that they cannot provide for their own basic physical needs for food and shelter or look after their own safety. **Grave disability** has become the most frequent basis for civil commitment. A review of seven studies by Turkheimer and Parry (1992) found that 78 percent of those participating in commitment hearings were committed on the basis of grave disability. Some of these persons were also judged dangerous; others were not.

As we've discussed, it's proven difficult to get reliable assessments of dangerousness and diagnoses of mental illness. Yet getting clinicians to agree that someone is gravely disabled and cannot provide for his own needs has proven even more difficult. Lidz and his colleagues (Lidz, Mulvey, Appelbaum, & Cleveland, 1989) have reported that judgments on ability to care for oneself (which is a measure of the extent of grave disability) are only moderately reliable (0.44)—substantially less so than those on dangerousness or suicidality (0.67 and 0.66, respectively). At the same time, two other studies have shown that patients' ability to care

grave disability Principal criterion for civil commitment that depends above all on the patient's ability to care for herself.

for themselves had a greater impact on clinicians' commitment recommendations than either dangerousness or mental illness (Appelbaum & Hamm, 1982).

The courts in most states must approve a plan for civil commitment that involves the **least restrictive alternative**—that is, the arrangement that will be least restrictive of a patient's freedom and civil rights. For instance, a brief period of hospitalization for the purpose of establishing a patient on effective antipsychotic medication may actually prove least restrictive over the long run. On the other hand, a short period of inpatient treatment might be less restrictive than no hospitalization and no treatment over the long term, if the hospitalization and medication permit the patient to resume a productive and meaningful place in society rather than begin a cycle of repeated hospitalizations for chronic psychosis.

In the few communities that have them, other less restrictive alternatives include community residential treatment facilities. These supervised group units provide less restrictive and regimented living environments than large psychiatric hospitals. Although most local political leaders favor such alternatives to hospitalization, as our discussion in Chapter 2 and later in this chapter suggests, many have been unable to assemble the necessary public funds and locate suitable places in the community. The result has been a dramatic increase in rates of homelessness.

Most states now permit commitment to outpatient treatment (McCafferty & Dooley, 1990). One of the advantages of this arrangement is that it gives the courts a greater choice of least restrictive alternatives. Another advantage is that the flow of patients back to the state hospitals is restricted. So why are commitments to outpatient treatment so rare?

One reason is that many acute psychotic conditions require a period of hospitalization in order for patients to receive antipsychotic medication and to be monitored for dangerous side effects. Another issue is significant concern over the efficacy of forced treatment, especially forced outpatient treatment (Lamb, Weinberger, & Gross, 1988). Whereas the effectiveness of antipsychotic medication is independent of whether a patient is in a hospital voluntarily or due to commitment, the effectiveness of the psychotherapy that often accompanies the medication given to outpatients does vary with motivation for treatment. And that motivation depends a great deal on whether individuals have freely chosen to participate in treatment.

History of the Concept of Civil Commitment   The laws governing civil commitment have changed a great deal over the past 25 years. Prior to 1969, involuntary hospitalization of mental patients in most states simply required that patients be judged "in need of treatment" (Appelbaum, 1985; Simon, 1992). It was assumed that being committed to a hospital for treatment was a benevolent act, in the best interests of everyone concerned. Based on that assumption, most courts agreed that basic legal protections were unnecessary, including **due process,** which includes being able to confront the person responsible for the commitment request, to have a hearing before a judge, and to be represented at the hearing by an attorney. Police, families, and society agreed that the best place for many psychotic persons was the state hospital. Even if treatment wasn't provided, at least the person would be taken care of and out of sight (Brakel, 1986; Turkheimer & Parry, 1992).

During the early 1960s, however, more and more people—especially young people—began to question many U.S. social institutions, including long-held views about the rights of people with mental disorders. Americans were inspired by articles like Thomas Szasz's "Myth of Mental Illness" (1960; see also Chapter 1), movies like *One Flew Over the Cuckoo's Nest,* and general dissatisfaction with the status quo brought on by the Vietnam War and the civil rights movement. In short, people began to question both the goals of civil commitment and the relative ease with which it could be accomplished (Meisel, 1982).

In 1969, California adopted a radically different commitment standard. To be committed, an individual had to be judged dangerous to himself or others or

least restrictive alternative Arrangement in a plan for civil commitment that will be least restrictive of a patient's freedom and civil rights.

due process During commitment proceedings, mental patients must be accorded specific rights: the right to confront the person responsible for the commitment request, to have a hearing before a judge, and to be represented by an attorney at the hearing.

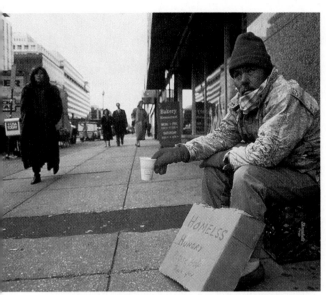

One of the most distressing consequences of deinstitutionalization has been a dramatic increase in the number of mentally ill people who are homeless. In the past, many of these individuals would have been sheltered, fed, and cared for in public institutions.

deinstitutionalization

Process begun in the late 1960s in which many thousands of chronic mental patients have been released from state hospitals across the United States.

gravely disabled. It was no longer possible to commit someone to involuntary hospitalization simply because treatment was indicated or mental illness had been detected. Since then, virtually every state has followed California's lead and adopted the so-called dangerousness criterion (Hoge, Appelbaum, & Greer, 1989). Consequently, the authority of psychiatrists and psychologists, police, and judges to commit individuals has been severely narrowed (Hoge, Sachs, Appelbaum, Greer, & Gordon, 1988). Legal protections have also been enacted for individuals under threat of commitment, comparable to those protections long available to persons accused of crimes. We'll look at these in the next section on patients' rights.

Following years of concern by psychiatric reformers, the living conditions in many state hospitals in the United States became another major legal battleground in the 1960s. One of the most important results of these concerns was the decision to emphasize the benefits of **deinstitutionalization,** the movement to empty the state psychiatric hospitals of as many psychiatric patients as possible (Peters, Miller, Schmidt, & Meeter, 1987). Today, more than 30 years later, we can see the effects of massive deinstitutionalization: More than four-fifths of the involuntary (committed) psychiatric patients who lived in public psychiatric hospitals at the beginning of the 1960s have been released into the community.

As a result, many public psychiatric hospitals have closed, and the total population of patients living in the remaining facilities represents a small fraction of the number living there four decades ago (see Figure 21.1). On an average day in 1955, 560,000 Americans were involuntarily confined in state and county mental hospitals. By 1972, because of deinstitutionalization and much tougher laws governing involuntary commitment (Appelbaum & Gutheil, 1991), that number had declined

FIGURE 21.1 The number of patients in U.S. mental hospitals

This number peaked at just over 500,000 in the early 1950s. Since then, the discovery of antipsychotic medications and changes in civil commitment policies have led to a significant decline in patients—a trend that continues to this day.

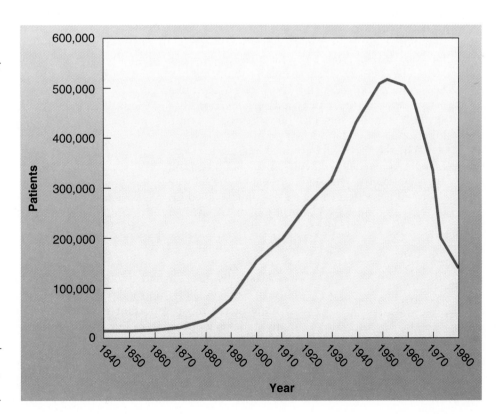

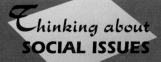

Thinking about SOCIAL ISSUES

People Who Are Homeless and Mentally Ill

*I*f you've spent much time in a large U.S. city, you've probably seen people who are homeless sleeping in doorways, begging for money, walking the streets, and occasionally committing crimes. Many of the urban homeless—though by no means all of them—have problems with mental illness, substance abuse, or both. As we've discussed in this chapter, many of these individuals would be living in state hospitals or other institutional settings had the great wave of deinstitutionalization not begun in the 1960s.

Who are the homeless? How did they get that way? A recent article in *New York Times Magazine* (Dawidoff, 1994) looked at New York City subway beggars, almost all of whom are homeless. This article painted a vivid picture of some of these people:

> An alcoholic panhandler named Roy Jackson (he drinks 12 40-ounce beers a day) spends his weekend at his mother's home, where he washes his clothes, and then returns to a steam grate on a Vanderbilt Avenue sidewalk near 45th Street, where he sleeps all week in a cardboard box. He does this, he says, because he "doesn't want to be a burden."
>
> [Rico] is a garrulous man who seems incapable of embarrassment, two helpful traits in the begging game. One afternoon I rode the train with him, watching him work. Rico sometimes urges people who don't give to him to "have a rotten day," but he didn't do this in front of me. He did, however, talk a lot. Rico makes about $30 a day. He could make more, but he is lazy, which he doesn't admit. Instead, he is convinced that Satan is conspiring against him by whispering to subway passengers that Rico spends the money they give him on drugs, prompting them to refuse him.
>
> When I tried to introduce myself to Dean Mandel, a panhandler with blood-shot eyes and angry red boils on his skull, he spat on the subway floor and began screaming. "Dean almost killed his father," an undercover transit policeman named

Armando D'Andrea later told me. "He took angel dust and started hallucinating. Dean has this thing against women. He's taking out his rage. If a woman only gives him a nickel, he'll throw it right back and spit on her."

> Tom has been living in the New York subways for four years, sleeping in the cars or in subway stations. It wasn't always this way. He says he graduated from Bergen Community College and once was a computer technician in Teaneck, N.J. "I had depression, and then I got sick (with the AIDS virus) within the past year," he says. Tom says he believes he became infected while sharing syringes of heroin with other addicts. (pp. 37, 38)

What happens to men who are homeless and mentally ill? As these brief stories suggest, they become or remain substance abusers, get sick with AIDS or other physical diseases, and are victimized by others who are stronger or smarter than they are. What tends *not* to happen to them, apparently, is that they stop being homeless. That was precisely the point made by a recent study of 42 homeless, mentally ill, substance-abusing men (Caton, Wyatt, Felix, Grunberg, & Dominguez, 1993), who participated in a treatment program for homeless mentally ill men living in shelters. Eighteen months after treatment, almost half the men were again homeless and more had gotten involved in criminal activities than before treatment. These people don't find homes, and for the most part, they don't get better.

Think about the following questions:

1. Why are so many homeless people on U.S. streets mentally ill?
2. Why does the United States have a greater homelessness problem than other industrialized countries?
3. Why doesn't the widespread availability of antipsychotic medication help control homelessness among people who are mentally ill?

to 276,000. By 1981, it had dwindled to 138,000 (U.S. Department of Health & Human Services, 1981), and today, it probably totals less than 100,000.

One of the most important goals of deinstitutionalization was to enable as many patients as possible to live closer to family and friends in apartments and group homes in their own communities, rather than in large, impersonal public hospitals (Shadish, 1984). Idealistically and theoretically, this would seem to represent a great step forward; yet deinstitutionalization has been only modestly successful in practice. One of the most important reasons for this limited success has been the failure of most states to plan and pay for alternative programs for psychiatric patients released from hospitals to their home communities (Miller, 1987).

Today, there are too few community residences, too few community mental health centers with staff workers willing and able to care for chronic mental patients, and too few sheltered work environments. Having nowhere else to go, many individuals with mental disorders have literally ended up on the streets. With the decline of hospitalized mental patients has come an explosion in the number of people who are homeless, encumbering virtually every U.S. city. Precise numbers are hard to come by, since the homeless, by definition, don't have addresses and phone numbers.

A study of 529 homeless adults in Los Angeles (Gelberg, Linn, & Leake, 1988), completed in the late 1980s, revealed some of the consequences of the failure of U.S. society to care for people who are mentally ill and homeless. Within the total sample, there were 232 persons with histories of previous psychiatric hospitalization. These individuals:

■ were least likely to use emergency shelters
■ had been homeless almost twice as long as subjects without that history
■ had the worst mental health status
■ abused alcohol and drugs the most
■ were most involved in criminal activities

Another study of people who are homeless (Bachrach, 1984) focused on the special problems of mentally ill women, who may face even more problems than comparable men. The research confirmed that women who are homeless and mentally ill are especially likely to be sexually exploited, targeted as objects of violence, involved in crime, and stigmatized for their mental disorders. Some of the specific problems facing homeless men are examined in Thinking about Social Issues.

Patients' Rights

In addition to deinstitutionalization, another consequence of U.S. society's dissatisfaction with the treatment of people who are mentally ill was the patients' rights movement. Activists in the 1960s believed that it was bad enough that institutionalized patients still lived in filth and squalor, as they had for centuries before. But did they also have to be denied most of the civil and legal rights and privileges enjoyed by others in society, simply because they had psychiatric disorders? At about the same time, researchers began to report data that indicated more and more strongly that some of the most serious psychiatric disorders might have genetic and biochemical bases. The essential unfairness of denying basic human rights to persons with disorders due to physical causes—over which they had no control—made these reform efforts even more compelling (Appelbaum & Gutheil, 1991; Simon, 1992).

Accordingly, when asked to consider the rights of patients committed to public psychiatric hospitals, state courts in the 1960s and 1970s increasingly concluded that patients had a right to treatment. This right stemmed from the state's obligation as part of the hospitalization contract. The courts also ruled that patients committed to public institutions deserved humane living conditions and, when possible, privacy. Many judges decided, as well, that even committed psychiatric patients had a right to many of the same legal safeguards the Constitution guaranteed defendants in criminal cases. As indicated earlier in this chapter, among these were due process rights—namely, to confront witnesses whose testimony threatens one's freedom, to be represented by an attorney, and to have a hearing before a judge.

Civil Rights of Patients in Mental Hospitals Today, being either a voluntary or an involuntary patient in a mental hospital does not by itself deprive you of your civil rights or prove you incapable of exercising them. Although these protections have not always been extended to patients in mental hospitals, most courts today firmly uphold them (Appelbaum & Gutheil, 1991). These rights, however, do not guarantee that you may not be judged incapable of doing such things as driving a car, making certain business or legal decisions, or exercising parental rights and responsibilities.

In sum, patients in mental hospitals have four basic rights:

1. Right to treatment—Common sense may tell us that mental patients have the right to treatment. However, a court first recognized this only in 1971, in the well-known *Wyatt v. Stickney* decision of an Alabama federal district court. Before *Wyatt*, many patients who had been involuntarily committed to underfunded public institutions did not receive treatment. Instead, they languished in institutions for months or years, receiving no treatment yet remaining hospitalized because no one else would assume responsibility for them. In part, the *Wyatt* decision said that "to deprive any person of his or her liberty upon the altruistic theory that the confinement is for humane therapeutic reasons and then fail to provide adequate treatment violates the very fundamentals of due process" (*Wyatt v. Stickney*, 1971).

Before this case, living conditions for patients in Alabama state hospitals had been particularly deplorable. A long history of inadequate state funding for the care of Alabama's state hospital patients had resulted in deteriorating buildings and leaking roofs; poorly paid, poorly trained, and poorly motivated hospital workers; few fully trained mental health professionals; frequently inedible food; and filthy bedclothes. Worst of all, state funding inadequacies had condemned most patients to long days with nothing to do—and no treatment for the disorders that had brought them to hospitals in the first place. No occupational or recreational therapy and little or no individual or group therapy were offered because the persons trained to provide them could not be hired. Instead, patients were usually heavily dosed with sedating drugs so they could be managed by the few employees in each ward.

Wyatt v. Stickney represented an effort to force the state of Alabama to meet its responsibilities to these committed patients. The most important issue in the case was deemed to be the right to treatment, but *Wyatt* also emphasized the right to *adequate* treatment. This right was designed to ensure that the administration of antipsychotic medications to psychotic patients would conform to sound medical practice. It's unacceptable to give massive doses of sedating drugs to aggressive psychotic patients when the purpose of doing so is only to protect staff, not to benefit patients. *Wyatt* also mandated the right of patients to wear clothing of their choice, to interact with the opposite sex (under controlled conditions), and to be free from physical restraints, except in psychiatric emergencies.

Despite *Wyatt* and subsequent decisions requiring improvements in the quality of life in public mental hospitals, the courts' ability to enforce these improvements in grossly underfunded public institutions remains limited. (A visit to a public mental hospital in your state will doubtless demonstrate this reality.) In most instances, the courts cannot force legislatures to provide funds, even for mandated improvements in hospital care. Too often, a standoff has resulted between a federal or state court and a state legislature that claims to be unable to bear the additional burden of the funds needed to improve services for patients in state mental hospitals (O'Reilly & Sales, 1987).

2. Right to least restrictive alternative—The concerns about humane care for mental patients mobilized by *Wyatt* were also

right to treatment People who are mentally ill have a right to receive treatment.

right to least restrictive alternative People who are mentally ill cannot be confined to psychiatric hospitals for indefinite custodial periods simply because no one can or will assume responsibility for them outside the hospital; also applies to the regimens of locked wards, seclusion, and restraint by which committed patients are managed.

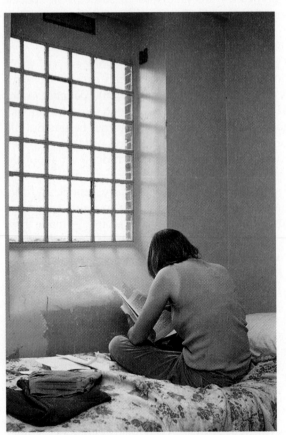

Squalor, degradation, and boredom still characterize most public psychiatric hospitals in the United States, making them a source of national concern and embarrassment.

responsible for *Donaldson v. O'Connor* (1975). This court decision established that people who are mentally ill cannot be confined to psychiatric hospitals for indefinite custodial periods simply because no one else can or will assume responsibility for them.

At least three-quarters of the states have now adopted laws based on a related suit, *Youngberg v. Romeo* (1982), which affirmed that the right to the least restrictive alternative also applies to the locked wards in which committed patients were previously kept. A number of questions were raised: Do hostile, threatening patients confined to locked wards need to be in restraints or in "quiet rooms," or is there another, less restrictive alternative? How long must these individuals remain on locked wards after medication and secure environments have helped them calm down? And when can they return to the community, where they can come and go as their caretakers and they agree is appropriate?

Court decisions on least restrictive alternative have answered some of these questions. For example, the question of behavior within a *specific social context* has been addressed. This phrase refers to the fact that a patient might be considered dangerous if allowed to live alone but not dangerous if she lives in a supervised group home and takes daily antipsychotic medication. Unfortunately, least restrictive alternative also depends on the state's limited capacity to fund housing and other community services for deinstitutionalized patients. If that housing is unavailable, patients must either remain institutionalized or, on being released from the hospital, join the ranks of the homeless.

As mentioned earlier, almost every state now permits involuntary commitment to outpatient treatment as a new type of least restrictive alternative (McCafferty & Dooley, 1990; Miller, 1991). Despite its appeal from cost savings and patient rights perspectives, most states employ this alternative relatively rarely because of the difficulty in supervising and guaranteeing it. One study conducted a 5-year follow-up of 79 defendants found "not guilty by reason of insanity" and referred to court-mandated outpatient treatment in Los Angeles (Lamb et al., 1988). It found that 25 of the subjects (32 percent) had been rearrested during the follow-up period—18 of them (72 percent) for committing violent crimes. In addition, 37 of the 79 had been rehospitalized, and 38 had had their conditional release from jail revoked. By any standard, these outcome figures are discouraging.

3. Right to refuse treatment—Considering the lengthy history of efforts to ensure mental patients' right to treatment, you may find it surprising that these individuals also have the right to *refuse* treatment. In fact, though, the theory that committed patients have the right to refuse specific treatments makes complete sense.

The history of this right dates back to 1914, when Supreme Court Justice Benjamin Cardozo stated, "Every human being of adult years and sound mind has a right to determine what shall be done with his own body, and a surgeon who performs an operation without his patient's consent commits an assault, for which he is liable for damages." Although this statement originally referred to general treatment of physical disorders, it's also been applied to mental disorders. For years, agitated and troublesome psychotic patients were forced to take massive doses of powerful antipsychotic drugs or to submit to psychosurgery or electric shock therapy to make them more manageable. (Obviously, these individuals were also forced to endure the sometimes serious side effects of these treatments.) The courts consequently gave involuntary patients the right to resist inappropriate or dangerous treatments, under certain circumstances (Appelbaum, 1988a; Deland & Borenstein, 1990).

In *Rennie v. Klein*, decided by the New Jersey Supreme Court in 1978, a depressed schizophrenic patient was given the qualified right to refuse antipsychotic medication that he feared would cause him permanent harm. The judge imposed qualifications, however, that required determining (a) whether the patient would be more likely to injure himself or others if he were not medicated,

right to refuse treatment

People who are mentally ill have the legal right to refuse treatment (usually medication or another somatic treatment) under certain specified circumstances.

(b) whether other effective treatments were available, and (c) whether the patient's belief that the medications prescribed for him were potentially dangerous was valid. The judge also established a process by which both the patient and hospital could appeal a treatment or its refusal, if they wished.

A subsequent U.S. Supreme Court decision, *Rogers v. Okin* (1979), questioned the *Rennie* precedent, in view of the proven efficacy of the medications now given to committed psychotic patients. This decision moved the issue back to the state courts, which subsequently took a number of diverse and, at times, conflicting positions on the right to refuse treatment. Many mental health professionals believe the right to refuse treatment is of questionable logic, under certain circumstances. One such circumstance, for instance, occurs when people who are seriously disturbed and have impaired judgment can refuse treatment that would actually restore their health (Binder & McNiel, 1991).

4. Right to privacy—Privacy, the broadest of the legal concepts discussed here, refers to the right each of us has to enjoy our own homes and personal lives (Stromberg, 1993). Most of us value this right for ourselves and respect it for others. Thus, we wouldn't ask strangers or casual acquaintances intimate details about their lives, nor would we expect them to ask us about ours. Despite the widely held belief that the right to privacy is enshrined in the Constitution, it's not explicitly mentioned. Instead, it's been inferred to be within the scope of certain other explicit constitutional rights.

Psychiatric patients have the right to expect the professionals who care for them to respect their privacy by entering only those areas of their lives directly relevant to the clinical situation (Stromberg, 1993). Because it's not always possible to distinguish what is relevant in the personal history of a patient from what is not, patients and psychologists may disagree about where to draw that line. Consider the following situation:

> Mr. Grant, a 55-year-old businessman, dies suddenly under suspicious circumstances. At the time of his death, he was being treated with twice-a-week psychotherapy by Dr. Bellows, a psychiatrist. Mr. Grant suffered a depression secondary to recent business reversals. The depression was interfering with the patient's ability to concentrate, causing difficulties with his business partners, who noticed that Mr. Grant had become indecisive. While previously Mr. Grant was a very successful businessman, his productivity recently had markedly diminished. . . .
>
> The therapy sessions were utilized by Mr. Grant to talk about his depression and rage at his business partners. He accused a senior partner of embezzlement. Mr. Grant felt that certain irregularities in the company's finances had surfaced at the same time that this partner bought a very expensive foreign car. In addition, he was certain that another partner profited from fraudulently misrepresenting to wealthy investors a limited partnership that eventually went bankrupt. Dr. Bellows, who keeps meticulous records, noted in detail the comments made by his patient. . . .
>
> Six months after starting therapy, Mr. Grant is found at home dead in bed. There are no antidepressants left in his medication bottle. Liquor bottles are found strewn about his apartment. The partners of his business firm hold key life insurance policies on each other in case of untimely death. Because the circumstances of Mr. Grant's death are unclear, the insurance carrier is unwilling to make payment on the life insurance policy until a final decision is reached as to the cause of Mr. Grant's death. Attorneys for the partners request and, under threat of a subpoena, receive Mr. Grant's psychiatric records from Dr. Bellows. Because of the trauma surrounding the death of his patient, Dr. Bellows is eager to avoid any more personal turmoil and readily provides the records. He is worried and intimidated by the subpoena. The state confidentiality statute prohibits such a disclosure. Mr. Grant's former business partners are outraged when they discover accusations of

right to privacy People who are mentally ill have the right to decide the time, place, manner, and extent of sharing themselves with others.

embezzlement and fraud written about them in the medical records. They threaten Dr. Bellows with a suit for defamation of character. (Simon, 1992, pp. 79–80)

Certain kinds of behaviors by mental health professionals that infringe on patients' privacy are always out of bounds. These include unnecessarily calling patients at home or inquiring about intimate details of patients' sexual histories when they have sought treatment for entirely different problems. Research subjects also have the right to privacy (Adair, Dushenko, & Lindsay, 1985; Stanley, Sieber, & Melton, 1987). Above all, they have the right to expect that their responses to questionnaires, performance on personality tests, and answers to interview questions will not be disclosed to others or published in such a way as to reveal their identity.

Mental health professionals also have both socially agreed on and legal rights to privacy. For instance, patients are not supposed to try to involve themselves in their therapists' personal lives—even though they are often extremely curious and eager to do so.

Social convention usually assures that patients and mental health professionals respect each other's rights to privacy. Sometimes, though, the ordinary, unspoken rules of society are not enough. In these cases, legal sanctions can be invoked to protect whomever is threatened by the invasion of privacy.

The ethical standards of the four core mental health professions specifically uphold the right to privacy. For example, the American Psychological Association's "Ethical Principles of Psychologists" (1992) state:

> Psychologists discuss confidential information obtained in clinical or consulting relationships, or evaluative data concerning patients, individual or organizational clients, students, research participants, supervisees, and employees, only for appropriate scientific or professional purposes and only with persons clearly concerned with such matters. (Standard 5.03[b])

Confidentiality   When applied to relationships between patients and therapists, the term **confidentiality** has a very specific meaning. Like those between attorneys and their clients, these are **privileged relationships.** Only under very special, restricted circumstances can therapists reveal the contents of conversations or other information about patients gathered during therapy. Without this protection, it's likely that many patients would be unwilling to reveal the information about themselves necessary for thorough diagnosis and effective treatment. Based on this assumption, the "Ethical Principles of Psychologists" (American Psychological Association, 1992) specifically instructs psychologists to inform patients as early in therapy as possible about the limits to the confidentiality of their communications— that is, the few circumstances under which therapists are required or can be forced to break this confidentiality.

confidentiality Legal term that refers to the very special, restricted circumstances in which a therapist can reveal the content of conversations or other information about a patient gathered during assessment or therapy.

privileged relationships Therapist/patient relationships are privileged because the confidentiality of communication in them is protected by legal statute.

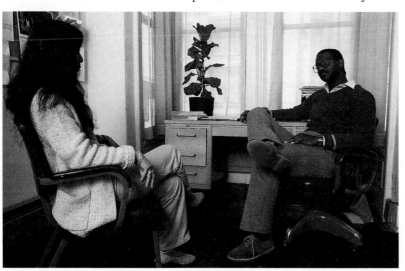

Only under very special and unusual circumstances can the confidentiality that protects communication between a patient and her therapist be breached. Why is confidentiality so essential to the therapeutic relationship?

Confidentiality extends to virtually all the materials about patients that mental health professionals gather to perform their jobs. This includes information about a schoolchild, gathered by a school psychologist while assessing the child's ability to benefit from special classroom placement. Likewise, material about a corporation's employees, solicited by an industrial psychologist evaluating management potential, is considered confidential. And so are intimate details about a student seen in therapy at a college counseling center and data from a consultant psychiatrist's evaluation of the fitness of a group of candidates for a city's police force.

However, in some situations, mental health professionals may have to breach confidentiality:

■ If the patient agrees that information can be released, the therapist will release it. For example, if a prospective employer requests information about a patient's previous hospitalization or if the patient's insurance company wants to know the length and focus of treatment, this information may be released—but only with the patient's permission.

■ When the law requires disclosure of information acquired by a mental health professional, it must be provided. Most states now require the reporting of any suspicion of physical or sexual abuse or neglect of a child within 36 hours. Accordingly, if an adult client reports having abused a child or having seen or been aware of abuse or if a child client reports having been abused, this information must immediately be reported to local authorities. The critical issue is whether, in the psychologist's professional judgment, he has reason to believe abuse has taken place or will take place. Failure on the psychologist's part to report suspected abuse can result in criminal penalties.

■ Disclosure of confidential material is also permitted when the clinician is bound by the duty to warn. In states that have adopted the *Tarasoff* standard, as discussed earlier, professionals who learn of a serious threat to another person in a confidential relationship (such as during treatment) are legally required to warn the threatened person and, if appropriate, to alert the police.

■ When disclosure of confidential information is required for legal reasons, it must be disclosed. For example, federal and state laws governing Medicare and Medicaid programs, which pay mental health professionals for providing services to patients in particular groups, require information on the names and addresses of patients, their Medicare or Medicaid numbers, the dates of services, and the nature of services. Sometimes a diagnosis is also requested. Therapists must supply this information to be paid for their services.

■ Confidentiality is not absolute when a patient brings a lawsuit. The female patient who sues an employer for sexual harassment should know that her therapist can be asked to testify about its emotional consequences on her. Similarly, the passenger who has experienced irreversible brain damage in an automobile accident should expect the examining neuropsychologist to report on her findings in a suit for damages.

■ Confidential information can also be released in an emergency. For example, if a patient receiving drug therapy for a serious psychiatric disorder is injured in an automobile accident, her attending physicians must know the drug and its dosage before they can treat her injuries.

■ A 1991 California appellate court decision (*Rittenhouse v. Superior Court*, 1991) confirmed that confidentiality survives the death of a patient. The ruling established that the death of a patient does not invalidate the sanctity of the confidentiality accorded the patient/therapist relationship. The ruling is important because in its absence, patients might withhold important information from therapists out of fear it will not be treated confidentially following their death.

Issues regarding acquired immune deficiency syndrome (AIDS) present a whole new set of questions: Does the duty to warn extend to the spouse or lover of a patient infected with the AIDS virus (Knapp & VandeCreek, 1990)? Does a therapist who learns that a patient has AIDS have the duty to inform the patient's lover or spouse that he is in clear danger (Totten, Lamb, & Reeder, 1990)? Are research data gathered on people with AIDS protected by confidentiality statutes?

Because the AIDS epidemic is so recent, most states have not taken positions on these matters (Gray & Melton, 1985; Melton & Gray, 1988). However, the 1989 action of a California court may have set a new legal precedent. It found the estate of Rock Hudson and his long-time business manager liable for damages totaling more than $24 million for failing to inform Hudson's lover of his disease and the risk it presented him.

Competency and Responsibility

Much of our discussion to this point has concerned the rights of mental patients, including the behavior they are entitled to expect from mental health professionals. Now, we will consider a different set of responsibilities—those of the criminal and civil justice system—as well as a different set of rights—those of persons accused of civil or criminal violations.

The accused have well-established rights enshrined in the Constitution, including the right to know the charges against them, to understand and participate in the court proceedings considering those charges, and to engage an attorney to defend them. Accused persons with mental disorders, however, are dealt with a bit differently by the criminal and civil justice systems. In particular, their competency to stand trial and their responsibility for their actions must also be taken into account by judge and jury. These are the central issues considered in weighing the merits of an insanity defense.

Competency to Stand Trial   The accused's mental condition at the time he's tried is referred to as **competency to stand trial.** Presumably, accused persons cannot take advantage of their constitutional rights unless they are competent to stand trial. If they are not, they will not be able to assist in their own defense, as the Constitution says they must. The usual standard employed to assess competency was first stated in 1960, in *Dusky v. United States* (1960): "The test must be whether he [the defendant] has sufficient present ability to consult with his lawyer with a reasonable degree of rational understanding and whether he has a rational as well as factual understanding of the proceedings against him."

Despite the widespread acceptance of this standard, assessment of competency to stand trial remains problematic, time consuming, and controversial. Some mental health professionals prefer to leave this determination to the courts because they believe the judgment is a legal one, not a psychological or psychiatric one. Other psychologists and psychiatrists refuse to participate in competency assessments because they view them as too often arbitrary and unpredictable and thus at variance with their professional standards. Still others consider competency assessments an unpleasant but necessary part of their jobs as mental health professionals and, when asked, will perform them.

The Insanity Defense   Of the legal issues considered in this chapter, the **insanity defense** is one of the best known and most controversial. You've no doubt read about famous insanity defenses in books and newspapers or seen them portrayed on television and in the movies. The deliberations of a jury on whether a defendant ought to be judged not guilty by reason of insanity are among the most dramatic events in criminal trials.

Because of the drama and notoriety of the insanity defense, we assume it's a common event. In fact, though, that doesn't appear to be true. On reviewing police records, court reports, and clinical files for 2,735 psychiatric referrals from Alaska's criminal justice system from 1977 through 1981, Phillips, Wolf, and Coons (1988) reported that a successful insanity defense was used in 0.1 percent (1 in 1,000) or less of all criminal cases. In another study in Wyoming (cited in Stromberg et al., 1988), people were asked to estimate how many criminal cases involved an insanity

competency to stand trial Legal concept that asks whether the accused is able to understand the charges against him and participate fully in his own defense.

insanity defense Legal defense that asserts the defendant is not guilty of a crime by reason of insanity.

Thinking about MULTICULTURAL ISSUES

Who Says Justice Is Blind?

Two recent criminal trials that took place in the same courtroom, both involving defendants who sought to explain violent behavior as a product of temporary insanity, recently caught law reporter David Margolick's attention (1994). They did so because the temporary insanity defense worked very well for one defendant—a well-educated, middle-class white woman named Lorena Bobbitt—but not at all for the other—a poorly educated, lower-class black man named Lonnie Weeks. Margolick asked himself why the outcomes of the two trials differed so much when the defenses were so similar. His conclusion: Differences in race, education, and the resources required to hire a competent attorney explained the difference in outcome. We might ask: Is justice blind? Based on evidence from these two cases, Margolick would say that it's not.

You probably know of the sensational case of Lorena Bobbitt, who was on trial for cutting off her estranged husband's penis while he was sleeping; she claimed that he had just raped her. During her trial, Ms. Bobbitt told how her husband had abused, degraded, and threatened her physically and emotionally throughout their marriage. Explaining her unorthodox act of retribution, Ms. Bobbitt "said her mind went blank when she committed the act for which she had been charged. She said she had been forced to figure out what happened from the evidence she found herself holding afterwards—the kitchen knife and her husband's severed penis" (Margolick, 1994, p. B11). As it turned out, the jury cleared Ms. Bobbitt of all criminal charges, concluding that she had been temporarily insane when she assaulted her husband.

Lonnie Weeks was on trial in the same courtroom in Manassas, Virginia, for killing a state trooper when his sentencing hearing was interrupted by the Bobbitt trial. As Margolick described it, "Mr. Weeks . . . did not actually plead insanity but suggested that it accounted for his conduct last Feb. 23, when Officer Jose Cavazos pulled him over for speeding. 'I just remember afterwards, not at the time, that I started firing the gun,' he told the jury. When the shooting stopped, he testified, 'I was standing there

looking at the trooper, and I was just in a daze—couldn't believe what just happened'" (p. B11). The jury hearing the case convicted Weeks and recommended the death penalty; the judge confirmed it.

Of course, other differences in addition to race, education, and defendants' resources distinguish the Weeks and Bobbitt cases: Weeks killed a man whereas Bobbitt only maimed one; Bobbitt's

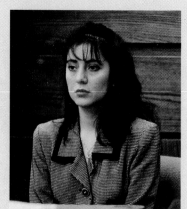

Lorena Bobbitt, who claimed at her trial that she mutilated her estranged husband while he was sleeping because she was "temporarily insane"

victim was an unsympathetic bully, but Weeks's was a state trooper. Margolick discounts the impact of these differences, however. Referring to what he calls "the strikingly similar excuses and starkly different fates of Mr. Weeks and Ms. Bobbitt," Margolick observed instead, "While it helps to have an unsympathetic victim who was harmed in an unorthodox but nonfatal fashion, . . . it helps, too, to have money to pay for lawyers, expert witnesses and investigators" (p. B11).

And so we ask again: Is justice blind? Lonnie Weeks, sitting in his cell on death row in Petersburg, Virginia, would strongly disagree.

Think about the following questions:

1. Why did use of the insanity plea in these two cases have such different outcomes? Give a few reasons.
2. Why is the insanity plea so difficult to support?
3. Why has use of the insanity plea become confined largely to poor, often minority defendants in criminal cases?

defense. Average citizens estimated 43 percent, students guessed 37 percent, and state legislators said 21 percent. The actual figure was less than 0.5 percent. And after an exhaustive survey of all offenders with mental disorders in federal, state, and local correctional facilities, Steadman and his colleagues (1982) found that only 8.1 percent had mounted a successful insanity defense.

Despite its infrequent use, the insanity defense continues to generate heated debate. Widespread opinion holds that it's a clever strategy used by highly paid lawyers to defend rich clients charged with serious offenses. Actually, today the insanity defense is used mainly by poor persons defended by public defenders and accused of nonviolent or marginally violent crimes (Phillips et al., 1988). Some of these topics are raised in Thinking about Multicultural Issues, which compares uses of the insanity defense in the criminal trials of Lorena Bobbitt and Lonnie Weeks. As demonstrated by Weeks's case, this strategy is not always successful. And even when it is successful, the usual outcome is commitment to a state hospital's forensic unit for an indeterminate time, which usually turns out to be as long or longer than the prison sentence the accused would otherwise have served.

There's a long history on Western society's views of the fairness of trying someone who's insane for actions she has no rational control over (Finkel, 1988). Insanity as a defense against criminal charges dates back at least to the thirteenth century. Since that time, the belief has evolved that it's unfair to accuse someone of something she cannot comprehend or to convict her of a crime she may not have intended to commit. This notion of **responsibility for one's actions** has evolved into an important humane value (despite the relatively small numbers of persons who have been relieved of criminal responsibility by employing it).

For a time, this long-term trend was countered by fallout from the verdict of not guilty by reason of insanity in the trial of John Hinckley, Jr. As you may recall, he was the young man who attempted to assassinate President Ronald Reagan in 1981 in order to draw attention to himself. Right after the verdict, several legislators and professionals argued for restrictions on the insanity defense, for several reasons. Namely, they felt the Hinckley jury had failed to serve justice, and they feared the verdict would promote an outpouring of similar efforts to gain attention at the expense of public figures. But the Hinckley jury may have acted quite rationally. They might well have had a reasonable doubt about the defendant's sanity, based on testimony during the trial from five different psychiatrists, who described 13 diagnoses of mental disorders that they thought could apply to Hinckley.

Over the last 150 years, four standards have guided U.S. courts and judges in deciding criminal cases involving the insanity defense:

1. *M'Naughten* standard—In 1843, Daniel M'Naughten mistakenly shot at the secretary to the prime minister of England, Robert Peel. (He had intended to shoot the prime minister.) When M'Naughten was subsequently found not guilty

responsibility for one's actions Legal concept that asks whether the accused was responsible for the actions taking place at the time she committed the crime she is accused of.

M'Naughten standard Establishes that the accused cannot be held criminally responsible if, at the time the crime was committed, he was laboring under such a defect of reason from mental disorder as not to know the nature and quality of what he was doing.

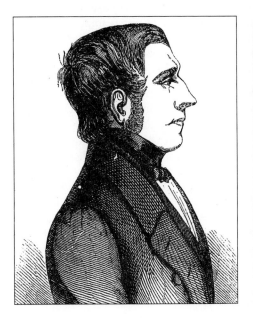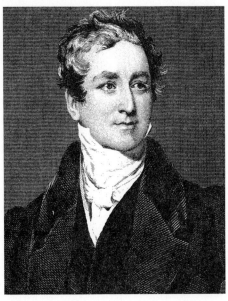

Daniel M'Naughten's (left) *unsuccessful attempt in 1843 to kill Sir Robert Peel* (right), *the British prime minister, led to development of the* M'Naughten *standard, after M'Naughten was found not guilty by reason of insanity.*

by reason of insanity, the public was outraged and a great debate ensued. The House of Lords asked a group of distinguished judges to suggest a more acceptable basis for making such determinations in the future. Their recommendations included the following:

> Every man is to be presumed sane, and . . . to establish a defense on the ground of insanity, it must be clearly proved that, at the time of committing of the act, the party accused was laboring under such a defect of reason, from disease of the mind, as not to know the nature and quality of the act he was doing; or if he did know it, that he did not know he was doing what was wrong. (M'Naughten, 1843)

The *M'Naughten* standard was soon taken up as the guiding principle of the insanity defense by courts throughout the United States. And 150 years later, it remains the exclusive standard for the insanity defense in about one-third of the states.

2. Irresistible impulse standard—Over the past several decades, several inadequacies in the *M'Naughten* standard have become more widely recognized—especially its emphasis on cognitive factors (knowing) and corresponding deemphasis on feeling, wanting, or being able to control impulses. As a result, many states have adopted what's called the *irresistible impulse standard* as an alternative. It asks:

> Did he know right from wrong, as applied to the particular act in question? . . . If he did have such knowledge, he may nevertheless not be legally responsible if the two following conditions concur: (1) If, by reason of the duress of such mental disease, he had so far lost the power to choose between right and wrong, and to avoid doing the act in question, that his free agency was at the time destroyed; (2) and if, at the same time, the alleged crime was so connected with such mental disease, in the relation of cause and effect, as to have been the product of it. (*Parsons v. State*, 1886)

This standard became attractive to the courts because judges and juries could easily apply it to the facts they were called on to judge in insanity defense cases.

3. *Durham* standard—A 1954 case, *Durham v. United States*, led Presiding Justice David Bazelon, of the United States Court of Appeals, to propose the following even broader standard of insanity defense:

> An accused is not criminally responsible if his unlawful act was the product of mental disease or defect. We use "disease" in the sense of a condition which is not considered capable of either improving or deteriorating. We use "defect" in the sense of a condition which is not considered capable of either improving or deteriorating, and which may be either congenital, or the result of injury, or the residual effect of a physical or mental disease. (*Durham v. United States*, 1954)

The effect of the *Durham* standard was to shift the focus of the criminal defense from whether the defendant knew the difference between right and wrong (as with the *M'Naughten* standard) or had lost the power to choose between right and wrong (as with the irresistible impulses standard) to a single clinical judgment: Was the crime a product of mental disorder?

4. American Law Institute (ALI) standard—*M'Naughten* continues to be an influential standard, despite its antiquity and the problems associated with it. However, the ALI standard—first proposed in 1962 and considered an improvement in clarity and ease of use over its predecessors—has become the insanity defense standard of choice in many states (even though successful use of the ALI standard by attorneys for John Hinckley caused it to be replaced in some states by the *M'Naughten* standard). The ALI standard provides the following guidelines:

irresistible impulse standard Establishes that if, by reason of the duress of a mental disease, an accused has so far lost the power to choose between right and wrong, he cannot be held criminally responsible.

Durham standard Establishes that the accused is not criminally responsible if his unlawful act was the product of mental disease or defect.

American Law Institute (ALI) standard Insanity defense that combines elements of the M'Naughten and irresistible impulse standards.

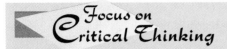

Focus on Critical Thinking

1. Do you agree with the trend over the past several decades to give mental patients many of the same rights long accorded criminal defendants? Why or why not?
2. Does the Tarasoff standard make sense to you?
3. Did Rennie v. Klein establish a patient right that you can support? Explain your answer.

■ A person is not responsible for criminal conduct if at the time of such conduct he lacks substantial capacity as a result of mental disease or defect either to appreciate the criminality of his conduct or to conform his conduct to the requirements of law. (This guideline combines the essentials of M'Naughten and Irresistible Impulse.)

■ The terms mental disease and defect do not include an abnormality manifested only by repeated criminal or otherwise antisocial conduct. (This guideline prevents the use of the diagnosis of antisocial personality disorder as a defense.)

*E*THICAL *I*SSUES

Professional Ethics

Ethical Guidelines Every organization of helping professionals—including the American Psychological Association, the American Psychiatric Association, the National Association of Social Workers, and the American Nursing Association—has an elaborate set of **ethical standards** to guide its members' professional behavior. You might wonder why intelligent, highly educated professionals need detailed instructions about what's the right thing to do. Unfortunately, as our discussion will suggest, knowing what's right and ethical isn't always as easy as it might first appear. Moreover, it's one thing to know what's right and ethical and another to do it.

The ethical guidelines of each professional association detail the association's ethical expectations of its members and discuss solutions to particularly difficult ethical problems. Such guidelines also specify the consequences for violating the guidelines, which may range from a verbal reprimand for a technical violation to expulsion from membership for a serious ethical breach.

Most professions' ethical guidelines contain two kinds of standards. Some are aspirational principles that are intended to set a high standard of conduct; if these principles are not completely fulfilled, the result isn't punishment or sanctions. For instance, the American Psychological Association's (APA) "Ethical Principles of Psychologists and Code of Conduct" (1992) list six such principles:

1. Competence
2. Integrity
3. Professional and scientific responsibility
4. Respect for people's rights and dignity
5. Concern for others' welfare
6. Social responsibility

Even the most conscientious and saintly psychologist would have trouble meeting all these principles in their entirety all the time. Nonetheless, by including these standards in its ethical guidelines, the APA establishes the aspirations it has for its members.

The second kind of ethical standards detailed in each profession's guidelines are more specific and more prescriptive. These standards establish a minimal or

ethical standards Guidelines detailing a professional association's ethical expectations of its members.

threshold level of professional behavior for a wide range of professional activities, which may only be violated at the member's peril. In the statement of ethical principles mentioned earlier, the APA (1992) both encourages and discourages professional behaviors in eight distinct areas:

1. General standards
2. Evaluation, assessment, or intervention
3. Advertising and other public statements
4. Therapy
5. Privacy and confidentiality
6. Teaching, training supervision, research, and publishing
7. Forensic (legal) activities
8. Resolving ethical issues

The states have incorporated many of these ethical guidelines into their licensing laws. (Psychologists, psychiatrists, and nurses are licensed in every state; social workers are licensed in an increasing number of states.) Thus, licensed mental health professionals can lose their licenses and be unable to practice, should they fail to observe ethical standards. Although it's embarrassing to be dropped from membership in a professional association for unethical behavior, it's a very serious matter to lose a lawsuit for malpractice or to have your license to practice taken away. These consequences threaten your livelihood.

Therapist/Patient Sexual Involvement   Section 4.05 of the APA's (1992) "Ethical Principles of Psychologists and Code of Conduct" states, "Psychologists do not engage in sexual intimacies with current patients or clients." Related sections add that psychologists do not take patients or clients into therapy with whom they have previously had sexual relationships and that psychologists do not develop sexual relationships with former patients or clients until at least 2 years after the end of therapy. Psychologists who are found to have breached these ethical guidelines are generally dropped from APA membership and in many states can be tried, convicted, and sentenced to prison.

Nonetheless, therapist/patient sexual involvement continues to be an issue for every mental health professional who provides clinical services. In fact, it's the complaint most frequently investigated by the APA and its sister associations (American Psychological Association, 1991, 1993b). Surveys have suggested that up to 12 percent of all therapists may have engaged in this behavior at least once in their professional careers.

Why is the problem of therapist/patient sexual involvement so persistent and widespread? The closeness and intimacy of counseling and psychotherapy relationships often foster sexual feelings on the parts of both therapists and patients. Most of the time, these feelings are simply discussed, just as other feelings in therapy are discussed (Rodolfa et al., 1994). But sometimes, they are acted on, and when they are, the patient is almost always harmed, sometimes severely (Stake & Oliver, 1991). The fact that therapist/patient sexual involvement most often involves an older, male therapist and a younger, female patient makes this type of misconduct an issue of gender and power, as well as ethics.

The damage that sexual involvement between a therapist and patient causes the patient is well documented (Williams, 1992). Patient self-esteem suffers, guilt is induced, depression is intensified, and suicidal thoughts and attempts may result. Therapist/patient sex almost always makes future efforts at treatment more difficult; it also decreases the likelihood that existing problems will ease, with or without therapy. More and more individuals see therapist/patient sexual involvement as a form of sexual abuse (Pope, 1990).

Common Ethical Dilemmas   Ethical issues are much easier to resolve when the difference between ethical and unethical behavior is clear cut. Certainly, a sexual relationship between a mental health professional and a client is unethical under all circumstances (and in most states, it's illegal). Other clear-cut ethical violations include formation of a business or financial relationship between a patient and a therapist, use of confidential information gained by a therapist in therapy for his own personal gain, misrepresentation of professional credentials or training, and practicing beyond one's professional competence.

Other situations involving mental health professionals aren't always so straightforward, however. That was the conclusion reached by a recent national survey of ethical dilemmas encountered by psychologists (Pope & Vetter, 1992). One psychologist faced a particularly difficult decision involving confidentiality:

> One of my clients claimed she was raped; the police did not believe her and refused to follow up (because of her mental history). Another of my clients described how he raped a woman (the same woman). (Pope & Vetter, 1992, p. 399)

Or consider the following ethical dilemma, which stems from professionals' responsibility for other professionals:

> The toughest situations I and my colleague seem to keep running into (in our small town) are ones involving obvious (to us) ethical infractions by other psychologists or professionals in the area. On 3 or more occasions he and I have personally confronted and taken to local Boards . . . issues which others would rather avoid, deal with lightly, ignore, etc., because of peer pressure in a small community. This has had the combined effect of making me doubt my reality (or experience), making me wonder why I have such moral compunctions, making me feel isolated and untrusting of professional peers, etc. (Pope & Vetter, 1992, p. 404)

Ethical Dilemmas of Correctional Psychologists   Most of the ethical dilemmas that confront correctional psychologists are created by the constant conflict in prisons between treatment concerns and security concerns. Such concerns in both state and federal prisons have heightened during the past 20 years or so, as the inmate population has increased dramatically and virtually every prison has become seriously overcrowded. More and more resources have had to be devoted to hiring additional correctional officers and building new prisons; corresponding reductions have been made in funds for and commitment to rehabilitation and treatment. With these changes have come even more substantial ethical dilemmas for prison psychologists, who still believe that treatment and rehabilitation are primary.

Who are the prison psychologist's clients? Traditionally, they have been the inmates whom the psychologist evaluates and treats. But in the present prison environment, the needs of inmates have sometimes become secondary to those of the warden and correction officers. Consider the following two cases, which illustrate different aspects of this transformation in the traditional role of the correctional psychologist:

> Inmate X has a long history of violent behavior, which has resulted in his current imprisonment. While incarcerated, he has been a model prisoner. Inmate X has now been scheduled for a parole board hearing. Upon reviewing Inmate X's central file, the warden believes that the inmate is still a dangerous individual who should not be granted parole despite his record of no institutional infractions. Accordingly, the warden requests that Dr. R evaluate Inmate X using psychological tests. The warden would like the information about the inmate's personality relating to his continued threat to public safety, and he would like this evaluation to be performed without the inmate being informed of its purpose because he believes Inmate X might otherwise refuse to participate in the evaluation. (Weinberger & Sreenivasan, 1994, p. 164)

Thinking about CONTROVERSIAL ISSUES

The Vietnam War and the Ethics of Combat Psychiatry

Those of you addicted to *M*A*S*H* reruns on late-night television might conclude that while the job of military physician—at least during the Korean conflict—required considerable skill and training, it also included lots of alcohol, fun, sex, comradeship, and patriotism. But according to someone who was a military psychiatrist during the Vietnam War, the job could not have been more different (Camp, 1993).

The fundamental mission of the military psychiatrist in combat is to "conserve the fighting strength." This purpose translates into making every effort to return as many psychiatric casualties as possible to combat, as quickly as possible. As Camp described it:

> Over the course of World War I, World War II, and the Korean conflict, combat psychiatrists empirically derived a set of clinical principles that appeared to restore quickly the affected soldier's critical physical and psychological functions, so that he could return to his military unit and comrades and resume the fight. These principles have become condensed in the mnemonic PIES: proximity, immediacy, expectancy, and simplicity. They refer to elementary physical treatments (i.e., rest, replenishment, and psychoactive medication in certain instances) and psychosocial treatments (i.e., assisted anamnesis, reassurance, and encouragement) that are applied as rapidly as possible and as close to the soldier's unit and the fighting as the tactical and clinical situations permit. (p. 1002)

The role of the combat psychiatrist and psychologist became much more conflicted during the Vietnam War. Profoundly disturbed by the morality of the war and their roles in supporting U.S. involvement in what appeared to many to be an unjust, immoral conflict, many mental health professionals questioned their duty to "conserve the fighting strength." In doing their duty, they knew they were condemning many young men to death. The ethics of doing so were a great problem for a significant number of mental health professionals. As one military psychiatrist put it, "I accepted my assignment as an obligation despite my conviction as early as 1964 that our involvement [in Vietnam] was stupid, would fail, would be a disastrous waste of wealth, power, and lives, and was unjustified politically, historically, and morally" (Camp, 1993, p. 1008).

Camp summed up the issue as follows:

> The moral dilemma for combat psychiatrists in Vietnam was no greater than that for the soldiers or military leaders. Furthermore, their service there was clearly less physically hazardous. Still, might psychiatry and the nation owe some measure of gratitude and acknowledgment to these men and women in consideration of their impossible task and the personal sacrifices they sustained in performing the duties that their country asked of them? (p. 1008)

Compared to enlisted infantrymen, many fewer military psychologists and psychiatrists were killed or wounded in the Vietnam War. But Camp has suggested that the psychological wounds they received are likely still unhealed, more than a quarter of a century later.

Think about the following questions:

1. What is the fundamental role conflict that confronts all military psychiatrists and psychologists?
2. Why was that role conflict so much more difficult to deal with during the Vietnam War?
3. How might some military psychologists and psychiatrists from the Vietnam War have chosen to resolve their role conflict?

Psychologist A receives a call in his office from the associate warden, directing him to report to Unit C, where they are short of correctional officers. Psychologist A reports to Unit C and participates in the evening count. Subsequently, he is approached by the captain and directed to perform a search for contraband of the inmates' property. The psychologist is also told he will have to "pat search" all inmates in his section. The psychologist is to seize any contraband and report all infractions to the captain. (Weinberger & Sreenivasan, 1994, p. 163)

In both instances, the psychologist is caught in conflict between the traditional role as therapist and humane advocate and the new role as enforcer of custody and security. The two roles are mutually exclusive. As long as the psychologist is seen by inmates as an agent of the correctional side of the prison, he will not be able to function as a trusted professional with a primary allegiance to the mental health and welfare of inmates.

Ethical Dilemmas of Military Psychologists   The ethical dilemmas facing military psychologists may be even greater than those of correctional psychologists. Most problems stem from the contradictory expectations of the military psychologist's two primary affiliations: the U.S. Department of Defense and the American Psychological Association.

Illustrating this conflict, Jeffrey, Rankin, and Jeffrey (1992) have told of a military psychologist that a 32-year-old army captain had been referred to for emergency evaluation because of his superior officer's concern about suicidal potential. The captain had expressed "vague suicidal ideation" in the field the preceding day; his superior worried this might be a reaction to a very stressful work environment and that suicide might be a real possibility. During the evaluation that followed, the captain expressed concern that what he said might be the basis for disciplinary action against him. The psychologist implied but did not directly say that the evaluation and the therapy that followed would remain confidential. A few months after the successful termination of therapy, the captain was transferred overseas and the military psychologist was transferred to another duty station. On receiving a formal request from the captain's supervisor for the confidential record of both evaluation and therapy, the chief of the mental health clinic found the military psychologist's confidential notes, and from them, he prepared a detailed written report for the requesting officer. Shortly thereafter, the captain's attorney lodged a formal complaint with the APA Ethics Committee for the psychologist's failure to maintain therapist/patient confidentiality.

The constant conflict between the military's need to know as much as possible about its personnel (including their mental status) and the psychologist's need to be able to reassure clients of the confidential nature of their relationship makes working within the military setting extremely difficult. Some military psychologists have solved the problem by keeping very scanty records, and others have simply warned clients at the beginning of their relationship that it's possible what they discuss will not remain confidential. Neither solution is ideal.

Thinking about Controversial Issues looks at the profound ethical dilemma faced by military psychiatrists and psychologists assigned to combat—in this case, in the Vietnam War.

Ethical Issues in Research

AIDS Research   Psychological and psychiatric research also raises important ethical and legal issues. Research on AIDS—perhaps the United States' most pressing national health problem—poses particularly troubling ethical issues. For example, consider the ethics of requiring research workers to participate in AIDS research, despite the minuscule but real possibility of their becoming infected. Also consider the ethical problems posed by researchers' inability to guarantee confidentiality to subjects with AIDS as well as the dilemma created when this disease is diagnosed but the subject refuses to share this information with his past and/or present sexual partners (Melton & Gray, 1988; Melton, Levine, Koocher, Rosenthal, & Thompson, 1988).

Animals in Research   Many people in U.S. society have become concerned over the ethical issues raised by using animals in research, especially if they must be hurt or killed. Opponents claim that the use of animals in research is rarely necessary, and when it is, far more care can and should be taken to ensure that the animals will experience the least pain possible. Supporters of animal research argue that it has saved millions of human lives, that animals are used when conducting tests on humans would be impossible, and that researchers generally care extremely well for their animal subjects. This conflict promises to rage on into the distant future.

Psychotherapy Research The ethical issues raised by controlled clinical trials of psychotherapy and other treatments for psychiatric disorders have also been widely discussed (Imber et al., 1986; Heflinger, 1987). The accepted research method of controlled clinical trials involves giving the active treatment that's being studied—for example, a new form of psychotherapy or drug—on a random basis to half the patients with the disorder. The other half of the patients are given either another treatment or a placebo (a substance that looks like the active medication but has no clinical effect). The ethical issue arises when the disorder under treatment is devastating—like AIDS or schizophrenia—and a promising treatment is withheld while being fully evaluated. In other words, this controversy concerns the ethics of giving treatment to some persons (even a treatment with unproved efficacy) and withholding it from others. Although controlled clinical trials are the foundation of treatment research, the debate continues on the ethics of their use.

Sexism and Ageism in Research Ethical concerns of ageism and sexism in psychological and psychiatric research have also been raised (Nadelson, 1993; Tangri & Kahn, 1993). Researchers studying older people or women are sometimes unfamiliar with the specialized literature on these groups of individuals. As a result, researchers may conclude that their findings were influenced by subjects' age or sex when an adequate grasp of the research literature would have led them to conclude that neither factor was responsible. Instead, variables like socioeconomic status, educational level, the nature of the research instruments, or the experimental setting were responsible. Attributing experimental effects to the wrong factors—in this case, age or sex—reinforces stereotypes about "the elderly" or "most women."

Ethics and Research Ethical lapses in research present particularly difficult dilemmas because, most of the time, researchers do not intentionally violate ethical guidelines (Blanck, Bellack, Rosnow, Rotheram-Borus, & Schooler, 1992). Of course, there are always the marginal scientists who "fudge" their data, take credit for the work of someone else, or plagiarize others' writing. Ethical violations such as these are certainly less common than the lapses we have noted, yet they must also be dealt with. Because the fact is, one of the most precious assets that scientists have to offer society is their own credibility—the assurance that colleagues reading their papers can believe what is written and, as a result, be willing to incorporate the ideas or results into their own research planning. Without credibility—which can be lost for major or minor deviations from the ethical mainstream—a scientist has nothing to offer.

Ethical Standards and the Law

In the most serious cases, professionals have violated both ethical standards and the law. Fortunately, these cases are rare. A recent report of the Ethics Committee of the American Psychological Association (1993b) summarized the ethical violations it investigated during 1991 and 1992. The distribution of the primary issues involved in investigating newly opened ethics cases in these years provides an interesting view of the range and frequency of unethical behaviors in this group of professionals:

■ *inappropriate professional practice:* 1991—53 percent; 1992—32 percent (includes inadequate handling of child custody cases; failure to respect other professionals; practicing outside area of competence; fraudulent insurance claims or exorbitant fees; breach of confidentiality; and testing abuses)

■ *dual relationship:* 1991—18 percent; 1992—32 percent (includes sexual misconduct with adult clients; sexual misconduct with minors; sexual harassment; and nonsexual dual relationships)

■ *inappropriate teaching, research, or administration:* 1991—8 percent; 1992—6 percent (includes authorship controversies; inadequacies in supervision; discrimination by age, race, or sex; improper or unsafe use of research techniques; and plagiarism)

■ *cases adjudicated in other jurisdictions:* 1991—12 percent; 1992—26 percent (includes conviction of a serious crime; loss of license for a serious crime; and expulsion from a state association for an ethical violation)

■ *inappropriate advertising and public statements:* 1991—8 percent; 1992—6 percent (includes misrepresentation and sensationalism in advertising or public statements and public allegations about colleagues)

The same report also confirms that the number of ethics cases brought to the Ethics Committee of the APA (1993b) continues to climb. Between 1983 and 1985, the total number of active cases averaged 117; between 1990 and 1992, the average was 231, almost twice as many. The "dual relationship" category of ethical violation resulted in the largest number of cases adjudicated in other jurisdictions. Psychologists who were found to have been involved in sexual misconduct with clients by the Ethics Committee were also likely to have been tried and convicted by the criminal justice system for these violations.

Focus on Critical Thinking

1. Some have urged that professional standards should be created for college and university professors that would resemble those of health care professionals. What are some of the pros and cons of this proposed plan?

2. Why do professional associations feel they need to create statements of ethical standards when criminal and civil laws governing professional practice already exist?

SUMMARY

Legal Issues

■ Mental health professionals must render expert judgments on custody, competency, and dangerousness, among other topics. Predictions of dangerousness—especially long-term dangerousness—are especially difficult.

■ The *Tarasoff* standard (based on a case rendered in 1976) established the duty of therapists to warn and protect persons threatened by their patients.

■ Today, civil commitment is indicated only for persons who represent dangers to themselves or others or who are gravely disabled and unwilling to accept voluntary hospitalization.

■ Plans for civil commitment must present the least restrictive alternative for patients' freedom and civil rights.

■ Mental patients have four specific rights: the right to treatment, the right to the least restrictive alternative, the right to refuse treatment, and the right to privacy.

■ The therapist/patient relationship is privileged; under all but very special circumstances, the contents of conversations between the two must remain confidential.

■ Over the past 150 years, four standards have guided judges and juries in deciding criminal cases involving the insanity defense: the *M'Naughten* standard, the irresistible impulse standard, the *Durham* standard, and the ALI standard.

Ethical Issues

■ Every profession has a detailed set of ethical standards that it's established to guide its members' professional behavior. These standards generally include aspirational norms, intended to set a high standard of conduct, and additional norms that are more specific and prescriptive.

■ Therapist/patient sexual involvement is one of the most common and troubling ethical violations by mental health professionals.

■ Researchers, like clinicians, must deal with a variety of ethical problems, including issues regarding AIDS, the use of animals, experimental methods, and sexism and ageism.

KEY TERMS

American Law Institute (ALI) standard, **p. 668**
civil commitment, **p. 653**
competency to stand trial, **p. 665**
confidentiality, **p. 663**
dangerousness, **p. 650**
deinstitutionalization, **p. 657**
due process, **p. 656**
Durham standard, **p. 668**

ethical standards, **p. 669**
grave disability, **p. 655**
insanity defense, **p. 665**
irresistible impulse standard, **p. 668**
least restrictive alternative, **p. 656**
malingering, **p. 650**
M'Naughten standard, **p. 667**

privileged relationships, **p. 663**
responsibility for one's actions, **p. 667**
right to least restrictive alternative, **p. 660**
right to privacy, **p. 662**
right to refuse treatment, **p. 661**
right to treatment, **p. 660**
Tarasoff standard, **p. 652**

*C*RITICAL *T*HINKING *E*XERCISE

Consider the following ethical dilemma recently reported by a psychologist:

> Six months ago a patient I had been working with for 3 years became romantically involved with my best and longest friend. I could write no less than a book on the complications of this fact! I have been getting legal and therapeutic consultations all along, and continue to do so. Currently they are living together and I referred the patient (who was furious that I did this and felt abandoned). I worked with the other psychologist for several months to provide a bridge for the patient. I told my friend soon after I found out that I would have to suspend our contact. I'm currently trying to figure out if we can ever resume our friendship and under what conditions. (Pope & Vetter, 1992, p. 401)

1. What is the nature of the ethical dilemma facing this psychologist?
2. What steps did the psychologist take to resolve this ethical dilemma?
3. Could the psychologist have resolved the ethical dilemma in another way? Explain your answer.

Glossary

A

abdominal obesity Pattern of obesity in which more body fat is carried above than below the waist; typically shown in men.

abstinence violation effect Occurs when someone on a strict diet breaks a dietary rule; she attributes the lapse to a complete inability to maintain control, abandons all attempts to regulate food intake, and overeats.

abuse Physical or sexual maltreatment or injury, or neglect; see definitions of specific types for more detail.

acetaldehyde reaction Aversive treatment for alcoholism; takes place when sufficient acetaldehyde has accumulated in the bloodstream to precipitate nausea, vomiting, and other bodily reactions.

acquired immune deficiency syndrome (AIDS) Fatal disease caused by the human immunodeficiency virus (HIV), in which cells of the immune system are attacked.

action stage Fourth stage of change; the person modifies behavior, experiences, or environment in order to overcome problems.

active or acute phase In schizophrenia, phase following the prodromal phase; individual exhibits psychotic symptoms such as delusions, hallucinations, loose associations, and unusual motor behavior.

acute cognitive disorders Cognitive disorders that last only a few minutes or a few hours; recovery from them is almost always complete.

adherence Extent to which a patient follows professional advice to take certain medications or change behavior patterns.

adoption studies Method to assess genetic predispositions for psychiatric disorders in which researchers compare the disorders of adopted children with those of their biological and adoptive parents in order to eliminate the confounding of genetic and environmental influences commonly found in traditional family studies.

adrenal gland Located just above the kidneys; consists of two parts—the inner portion (the adrenal medulla) and the outer portion (the adrenal cortex); in response to stress, the adrenal cortex secretes corticosteroids and the adrenal medulla secretes catecholamines (epinephrine and norepinephrine).

ageism Prejudicial attitudes, discriminatory practices, and institutional policies directed against certain people because of their elderly status.

agnosia Impairment in the ability to recognize or identify familiar objects.

agoraphobia Fear and avoidance of being in places or situations in which help might not be available should some incapacitating or embarrassing event occur.

alcohol expectancies Expectations of the effects of alcohol on behavior.

Alcoholics Anonymous (AA) Volunteer self-help organization designed to help individuals maintain sobriety; basic principles include anonymity, "buddy" system, and 12-step program.

alkaptonuria Disorder of amino acid formation; first genetically transmitted cause of mental retardation to be identified.

alogia Negative symptom of schizophrenia involving a speech disturbance in which the individual talks very little and gives brief, empty replies to questions.

alpha waves Regular, oscillating waves of 8 to 12 cycles a second; represent the EEG pattern of a normal, conscious, relaxed adult.

Alzheimer's disease Age-related brain disorder characterized by a profound, progressive loss in cognitive ability.

American Law Institute (ALI) standard Insanity defense that combines elements of the *M'Naughten* and irresistible impulse standards.

amnestic disorder Cognitive disorder characterized primarily by difficulty in remembering and perceiving.

amniocentesis Procedure for diagnosing hereditary conditions in fetuses; involves withdrawing a small amount of amniotic fluid to be examined for evidence of chromosomal or genetic disorder in the fetal cells suspended in it.

amniotic fluid Protective fluid the fetus is immersed in.

amotivational syndrome Condition associated with heavy use of marijuana; the individual loses motivation for virtually everything in life except continuation of heavy use of marijuana.

anal stage Second psychosexual stage, during which the child derives pleasure from the anal and urinary sphincters and learns new ways to control his parents.

anal-erotic personality Characterized by orderliness, obstinacy, and stinginess.

analogue research Experimental treatment research conducted in the laboratory under highly controlled conditions with carefully selected subjects.

angiography Medical procedure that involves inserting a catheter (fine needle) to inject a special dye into the coronary arteries; done to examine them under X-ray and determine the extent of plaque buildup.

anhedonia Marked lack of pleasure, even in reaction to things that are usually enjoyable; with depressed mood, a core symptom of a major depressive episode.

anorexia nervosa Eating disorder characterized by serious weight loss (more than 15 percent of normal body weight) and distorted body image.

Antabuse (disulfiram) Chemical that blocks the breakdown of alcohol and permits acetaldehyde to accumulate in the bloodstream whenever alcohol is consumed.

antecedents In behavioral assessment, the events and circumstances that typically precede the target behaviors.

antiandrogen drug Used to reduce testosterone level in treating males with sexual disorders.

anticipatory anxiety Anxiety over the prospect of something bad happening.

antipsychotic medications Medications used to reduce symptoms of psychosis, like hallucinations and delusions; sometimes called *major tranquilizers* because of their sedating effect.

antisocial personality disorder Characterized by frequent disregard for and violation of others' rights occurring since age 15 with evidence of conduct disorder beginning before age 15.

anxiety An uncomfortable experience of worry, fear, and apprehension accompanied by various bodily sensations, including palpitations and increased arousal.

aphasia Disturbance in the comprehension and formulation of language.

applied behavior analysis Application of the principles and procedures of operant conditioning to human problems; the analysis of environmental effects on nature.

apraxia Impairment of movement.

artifact Research finding that reflects a methodological problem, rather than a valid result.

assertion training Behavior therapy technique for helping patients express their feelings in a constructive manner that is neither submissive nor aggressive.

assertive case management Treatment approach involving multiple systems of intervention, medication, psychological services, and social services; cases are managed through a team of professionals who provide 24-hour services, often in the residence of the patient.

assessment interview Focuses on a wide range of topics, including assessment of personality, interpersonal behavior, and family functioning.

associational function Function of the cerebral cortex that links its parts, facilitating the reasoning, planning, memory, creativity, and problem-solving skills that are uniquely human.

atherosclerosis Condition in which plaque of cholesterol, fat, and calcium has built up in the coronary arteries; obstructs bloodflow and causes chest pain (angina) and heart attack (myocardial infarction).

attachment theory Theory of personality development that emphasizes the quality of the attachment relationship between the child and the primary caregiver.

attention-deficit/hyperactivity disorder (AD/HD) Childhood disorder in which the central problems are restlessness and difficulty paying attention.

attributable risk Proportion of cases in the population that are due to a particular risk factor.

attributional processes Explanations we use to explain our successes and failures to ourselves.

attributional style Cognitive style regarding beliefs about the causes of events; a particular style is characteristic of depression.

atypical features Denote a subtype of depression; characterized by mood reactivity to positive stimuli.

autistic disorder Disorder in the group of pervasive developmental disorders; characterized by marked impairment in social responsiveness, profound communication deficits, and stereotyped or bizarre habits and movements.

autistic savant Person who suffers from the full autistic disorder syndrome but also has some singular talent that usually emerges very quickly at an early age.

automatic thoughts Cognitions that pop into our minds without effort; negative automatic thoughts are associated with emotional distress, like depression and anxiety.

autonomic nervous system (ANS) Part of the peripheral nervous system that regulates the glands, heart, blood vessels, and other internal organs; responsible for the physiological events we experience as emotion.

autonomic reactivity Arousal of the autonomic nervous system in response to stress.

avoidant personality disorder Characterized by social inhibition, feelings of inadequacy, and extreme sensitivity to negative remarks.

avolition Negative symptom of schizophrenia that involves the inability to begin and sustain goal-directed activity and the expression of little or no interest in activities.

axons Extensions of the neuron that transmit nerve impulses to the dendrites of other neurons.

B

basic mistakes Adler's concept that maladaptive personal beliefs can lead to psychological problems.

Beck's cognitive therapy Form of therapy that helps patients identify and modify dysfunctional thoughts and beliefs.

behavioral activation system (BAS) Biological motivation system proposed to regulate the seeking of positive stimuli; dysregulation of the BAS may underlie mood disorder.

behavioral inhibition system (BIS) Biological motivation system proposed to underlie anxiety; acts to inhibit activity in response to potential threat.

behavioral medicine Integration of behavioral and biomedical science to better understand, prevent, and treat physical illness.

behavioral model Assigns learning the key role in the development of behavior.

bell and pad method Alarm device that awakens a bed-wetter immediately upon urination, so the child can rise and continue urination in the bathroom; the most effective and most commonly used psychological treatment for enuresis.

la belle indifference Absence of anxiety despite the presence of a somatoform disorder.

benzodiazepines Most commonly used class of antianxiety medication.

Berkson's bias Form of sampling bias in which people who have two or more medical or psychiatric problems are more likely to seek treatment than those who have only one problem; as a result, clinical samples are likely to contain more disturbed people than community samples.

binge eating Uncontrolled consumption of unusually large amounts of food.

binge-eating disorder (BED) Eating disorder characterized by recurrent binge eating but not inappropriate weight-control behaviors.

biofeedback Direct modification of physiological responses such as blood pressure by feedback that makes the person aware of the process.

biological model Assumes the principal causes of and most effective treatments for abnormal behavior are biological.

biopsychosocial perspective View stressing the vital interplay of biology, psychology, and the social environment in determining normal and abnormal behavior.

bipolar disorders Psychoses characterized generally by recurrent mood extremes, ranging from mania to severe depression; formerly called *manic-depressive disorders.*

body dysmorphic disorder Pathological preoccupation with an imaginary defect in physical appearance.

body mass index (BMI) Value used to assess healthy and unhealthy body weights; calculated as weight in kilograms divided by height in meters.

borderline personality disorder Characterized by pervasive instability in interpersonal relationships, self-image, and emotions as well as marked impulsivity.

bradykinesia Exaggeratedly slow movement because of muscle rigidity; a feature of Parkinson's disease.

brief recurrent depressive disorder Variant of major depressive disorder that lasts less than the required 2 weeks.

Broca's aphasia Disturbance of the comprehension and formulation of language; caused by dysfunction in Broca's area and neighboring brain regions.

Broca's area Posterior third of the inferior frontal convolution in the human brain; controls speech functions.

bulimia nervosa Eating disorder characterized by binge eating and extreme weight-control behaviors, such as self-induced vomiting; rooted in abnormal attitudes about the importance of body shape and weight.

C

case-control design Experimental design in which a person with an identified clinical disorder is matched with a control subject of the same sex, age, and socioeconomic status.

case study Method in which the researcher attempts to understand the unique individual by combining interview data, observations, and sometimes test scores.

catastrophic thinking In panic disorder, misinterpretation of normal physical sensations as signs of an impending disaster.

catatonic behavior Marked motor abnormalities such as bizarre postures, purposeless motor activity, and extreme degree of unawareness.

catatonic type Schizophrenia characterized by unusual patterns of motor activity, such as rigid postures and stupor or trancelike states; speech disturbances such as repetitive chatter or mutism are also common features.

catecholamines Hormones (epinephrine and norepinephrine) secreted by the adrenal medulla in response to stress.

categorical system Method of classification that separates things into distinct types; in terms of personality disorder, individuals are diagnosed according to specific disorders.

catharsis Psychological relief produced by disclosing emotionally charged thoughts and feelings.

caudate nucleus Cluster of brain cells in the basal ganglia believed to be centrally involved in anxiety disorders such as OCD.

central nervous system (CNS) The brain and spinal cord; all sensory nerve impulses are transmitted to the CNS, and all motor impulses are sent from the CNS.

cerebral cortex Outer layer of the cerebrum; this part of the brain mediates such human abilities as thinking, feeling, perceiving, and reflecting.

cerebrum Outer layer of this part of the forebrain, called the *cerebral cortex,* mediates our ability to think, feel, perceive, and reflect.

chemical aversion treatment Treatment for alcoholism; involves pairing the sight, smell, and taste of alcoholic beverages with the onset of chemically induced nausea and vomiting, producing a conditioned aversion to alcohol.

child abuse Physical abuse, sexual abuse, emotional abuse, and/or neglect directed against a child.

child emotional abuse Behavior that is harsh, critical, and overly demanding toward a child.

child sexual abuse Sexual activity imposed or forced on a child.

childhood depression Childhood disorder whose symptoms include depressed mood, low self-esteem, fatigue, somatic complaints, suicidal thoughts, and a sense of hopelessness.

chorea Involuntary, jerky movements of the face, arms, and legs; a trait of Huntington's disease.

chromosomes Humans have 46 chromosomes (23 pairs), along which millions of genes are aligned.

chronic cognitive disorders Cognitive disorders that last for a long time, often a lifetime; typically irreversible, they generally have serious behavioral consequences.

chronological age Age in years; used to determine IQ on the Binet Scales.

cingulotomy Psychosurgery that severs the pathway from the frontal lobe to the basal ganglia; used to treat OCD.

circadian rhythms Daily biological cycles of various bodily functions, such as the sleep/wake or body temperature cycles.

civil commitment Involuntary, enforced inpatient or outpatient treatment; necessary when clearly indicated for a psychiatric condition a patient refuses treatment for.

classical conditioning Form of learning in which an unconditioned stimulus and a conditioned stimulus are repeatedly paired to produce a conditioned response.

claustrophobia Fear of being confined in any space.

clinical assessment Process clinicians use to gather the information needed to diagnose a disorder, determine its causes, plan treatments for it, and predict its future course.

clinical neuropsychology Subfield of clinical psychology devoted to assessing the intellectual and emotional consequences of brain damage.

clitoris Female organ that's the main site of sexual responsiveness in women.

coercion Threats, force, and other psychological means used to attempt to control another.

cognition Uniquely human mental processes of thinking and reasoning, perceiving and recognizing, judging and conceiving.

cognitive appraisal Individual's judgment as to whether a potentially stressful event poses a personal threat.

cognitive disorders Clinically significant deficits in cognition or memory that represent significant changes from individuals' previous levels of functioning.

cognitive restructuring Technique in which patients are helped to identify, challenge, and modify dysfunctional thoughts.

cognitive symptoms Changes in content of thought or quality of thought processes, such as poor concentration or suicidal ideation.

cognitive therapy In treating anxiety disorders, a form of therapy that focuses on deliberately activating catastrophic thoughts and teaching patients to reinterpret them so that they no longer trigger panic.

cognitive triad Negative beliefs about yourself, the world, and the future; said to characterize depression, according to Beck's cognitive theory.

cognitive-behavioral therapy (CBT) Form of psychological therapy that focuses on directly modifying both cognitive processes and behavior; draws heavily on cognitive theory and research as well as more traditional classical and operant conditioning principles.

collaborative empiricism Process in cognitive therapy through which the therapist and patient together identify, analyze, and test the validity of the patient's dysfunctional cognitions.

common factors approach Approach to psychotherapy integration that emphasizes clinical strategies common to all forms of psychological therapy.

community psychology Programs designed to prevent problems and to teach new skills; examples include television messages, preventive policing, and community meetings to foster health-promoting behaviors.

comorbidity Co-occurrence of more than one clinical disorder in the same person.

comparative outcome study Treatment research in which one or more specific treatments are compared with each other.

competency to stand trial Legal concept that asks whether the accused is able to understand the charges against him and participate fully in his own defense.

compulsions Repetitive, stereotyped acts that a person with the disorder feels compelled to carry out, despite some recognition that they are unreasonable.

computerized axial tomography (CAT) Brain-imaging technique in which multiple views of the brain are X-rayed and then combined, producing a single, reconstructed image.

concordance Likelihood of individuals sharing a quality or condition; twins who both have a mental disorder are concordant for that disorder.

concurrent validity Diagnostic system's ability to identify and categorize current disorders accurately.

conditioned appetitive motivational model Classical conditioning theory explaining the craving addicted individuals experience for the substances they're dependent on.

conditioned compensatory response model Siegel's classical conditioning theory of acquired behavioral tolerance to dependency-inducing drugs.

conditioned response (CR) In classical conditioning, the response elicited by the CS.

conditioned stimulus (CS) In classical conditioning, a formerly neutral stimulus that comes to elicit the CR after repeated pairing with the UCS.

conduct disorder (CD) Repetitive and persistent pattern of conduct that violates the basic rights of others and major age-appropriate societal norms or rules.

confidentiality Legal term that refers to the very special, restricted circumstances in which a therapist can reveal the content of conversations or other information about a patient gathered during assessment or therapy.

confounds Factors other than the independent variable that could explain changes in the dependent variable.

conjoint sessions Marital therapy sessions in which both partners are present.

conscious psychological processes Thoughts, feelings, and memories we are aware of that influence our behavior.

consequences In behavioral assessment, the events and circumstances that typically follow the target behaviors.

contemplation stage Second stage of change; the person is aware a problem exists, is seriously thinking of confronting it, but has not made a commitment to do so.

content specificity Hypothesis that the focus of negative thoughts is specific to a disorder; for instance, depressive cognitions are characterized by themes of loss and failure.

control group Group of subjects that is functionally the same as the experimental group on all dimensions except the one being manipulated.

controllability Real or perceived ability to control or influence potentially threatening events.

controlled drinking goals Goals for alcoholism treatment that do not aim for abstinence, which is traditional, but for nonabusive drinking.

conversion disorder Loss or alteration of physical functioning that suggests a physical disease but for which no underlying physical cause can be found.

coronary heart disease (CHD) Partial or total obstruction of one or more of the coronary arteries due to atherosclerosis.

correlation coefficient Number describing the strength and direction of the relationship between two variables; ranges from +1 to –1.

correlational designs Research designs in which investigators gather information without altering subjects' experiences and examine relationships between variables; do not permit inferences about cause and effect.

cortical atrophy Reduction in brain volume.

corticosteroids Hormones secreted by the adrenal cortex in response to stress.

cortisol Hormone secreted by the adrenal gland that is part of the stress-response system that prepares us for emergencies.

countertransference In psychoanalytic theory, the feelings a psychotherapist develops for his patients.

course Life history of a disorder; for example, some disorders are chronic (long lasting), whereas others are episodic (come and go).

covert sensitization Behavior therapy technique used to decrease a patient's desire for negative sexual activity; patient is taught to use imagery that links a negative consequence with the activity.

culture of poverty Concept that suggests that the social and psychological traits of people who are poor maintain their poverty and contribute to their high rates of psychopathology.

cyclothymic disorder Mood disorder characterized by frequent alteration between hypomanic and depressive symptoms that don't meet criteria for a major depressive episode.

D

dangerousness Legal concept that refers to the likelihood a person is or will be a danger to herself or others.

date rape Unwanted or nonconsensual sexual activity that is forced or coerced against a person by her dating partner.

debriefing Providing a full account and justification of research activities to subjects who have participated in a study.

defense mechanism Strategy used by the ego to prevent threatening unconscious thoughts or memories from becoming conscious.

deinstitutionalization Trend started in the 1960s, in which hospitals markedly reduced the populations of psychiatric wards by returning to the community patients judged capable of functioning outside the hospital.

delinquent Individual under 18 who has committed a legal offense; may not necessarily have a diagnosable psychological or psychiatric disorder.

delirium Acute cognitive disorder characterized by a disturbance of consciousness, such that awareness of the environment is reduced; also involves changes in memory, orientation, and perception.

delirium due to HIV disease Acute cognitive disorder that can result from infection by the human immunodeficiency virus (HIV).

delirium tremens Alcohol withdrawal delirium.

delirium, dementia, and amnestic and other cognitive disorders Conditions involving deterioration in cognitive abilities such as memory, reasoning, and planning; sometimes short lived, sometimes long lasting and progressive.

delta waves EEG pattern involving a slow brainwave pattern of less than 4 cycles a second; normally recorded when a person is deeply asleep; may also signal localized brain damage.

delusions Common symptom of psychosis that involves false or unusual beliefs; common delusions include persecution, romance, grandeur, and control.

demand characteristics Cues in a situation people respond to in ways assumed to be socially appropriate.

dementia Chronic cognitive disorder characterized by memory impairment and other cognitive disturbances affecting language, motor abilities, recognition of familiar objects, and planning and organization; causes significant impairment in social or occupational functioning.

dementia due to HIV disease Chronic cognitive disorder that can result from infection by the human immunodeficiency virus (HIV).

dementia of the Alzheimer's type Age-related cognitive disorder characterized by profound, progressive losses in cognitive ability and marked changes in behavior and personality.

dementia praecox Term coined by Emil Kraepelin, meaning "premature dementia," to describe the psychotic disorder now called schizophrenia.

dendrites Extensions of neurons that receive nerve impulses from the axons of other neurons.

dependent personality disorder Characterized by a pervasive and excessive need to be taken care of, which causes submissive, clinging behavior and fears of separation.

dependent variable Variable the researcher expects to be influenced by the independent variable in an experiment.

depersonalization disorder Dissociative disorder in which the person feels unreal and disconnected from the self.

depressive pseudodementia Mood disorder in which the symptoms resemble those of dementia, but the condition is not a cognitive disorder.

depressogenic Causing depression.

detoxification Process of withdrawing an alcohol- or drug-dependent person from the substance or substances she is addicted to.

dexamethasone suppression test (DST) Test for abnormal secretion of cortisol; formerly used in diagnosis of depression.

diabetes Disorder of carbohydrate metabolism in which individuals have trouble regulating blood-sugar levels.

diagnosis Formal act of identifying and naming a disorder or disease.

Diagnostic and Statistical Manual of Mental Disorders (DSM-IV) Current authoritative listing of mental disorders in use in the United States.

diagnostic bias Biases or prejudices by diagnosticians that affect the reliability and validity of the diagnostic process.

diagnostic interview Designed to gather information on past and present behaviors that have specific value for diagnosis.

diagnostic reliability Degree to which a diagnostic system fosters diagnostic agreement among clinicians.

diagnostic validity Ability of a diagnostic system to identify and predict disorders accurately.

dialectical behavior therapy (DBT) Treatment approach that blends aspects of psychodynamic, client-centered, strategic, interpersonal, cognitive-behavioral, and crisis intervention approaches into a coherent theoretical orientation; assumes that personality disorders result from multiple causes.

diathesis-stress model Causal model for pathology in which two elements are necessary: a vulnerability (diathesis) and a negative event (stress).

dimensional system Method of descriptive classification in which things are described using a specified set of qualities or other continuous variables; in terms of personality disorder, individuals are described according to a designated set of personality traits.

discriminative stimulus (SD) In operant conditioning, the information the environment provides about the likelihood that a response will be reinforced, ignored, or punished.

disease model Suggests that metabolic brain dysfunction is the likely cause of several common mental disorders; synonymous with the *biological model.*

disorganized speech Symptom of schizophrenia in which the individual's speech is incomprehensible or remotely related to the topic of conversation (such as derailment, tangentiality).

disorganized type Schizophrenia characterized by an absence of elaborated sets of delusions and by verbal incoherence, grossly disorganized behavior, marked loosening of associations (disconnected thoughts), and inappropriate affect.

displacement Defense mechanism in which an unacceptable reaction is shifted unconsciously from the object perceived as threatening to a substitute object that is less threatening.

dissociation Process in which part of mental functioning is split from the rest of consciousness.

dissociative amnesia Disorder in which the person is suddenly unable to recall important personal information to an extent that cannot be explained by ordinary forgetfulness.

dissociative disorders Disorders in which the normal, integrated function of a person's identity or consciousness undergoes a sudden change.

dissociative fugue Disorder characterized by sudden and unexpected travel away from home and the adoption of a new identity.

dissociative identity disorder Dissociative disorder in which two or more distinctive personalities co-exist within an individual, alternately dominating functioning; previously known as multiple personality disorder.

dizygotic twins Twins who develop simultaneously from two fertilized ova; also called *fraternal twins*.

dominant gene One of a pair of genes that determines a particular physical or psychological characteristic in the phenotype.

double depression Presence of both dysthymic disorder and a major depressive episode.

double-bind hypothesis Contradictory messages from another person, often the parent, to the child; as when the parent communicates warmth but is cold and withdraws when the child approaches; the child is thus caught in a double bind.

double-blind strategy Administration of medication in an experiment in which neither the patient nor the therapist knows whether the medication is an active drug or a pill placebo.

Down syndrome Common form of mental retardation that's caused by a chromosomal mutation; generally involves moderate and severe categories of retardation.

dream interpretation Psychoanalytic treatment method in which the unconscious significance of dreams is related to the patient's current problems.

due process During commitment proceedings, mental patients must be accorded specific rights: the right to confront the person responsible for the commitment request, to have a hearing before a judge, and to be represented by an attorney at the hearing.

Durham standard Establishes that the accused is not criminally responsible if his unlawful act was the product of mental disease or defect.

dysfunctional thought records (DTRs) Records kept by patients between treatment sessions in which they identify dysfunctional thoughts (cognitions) associated with their emotional problems and challenge the validity of those thoughts.

dyslexia Term used for reading disorder; characterized by impaired word-recognition skills and reading comprehension; dyslexics often omit, add, and distort words.

dyspareunia Condition in which burning or itching sensations are felt during vaginal intercourse.

dysthymic disorder Depressive disorder that's less severe but of longer duration than major depression.

E

early stage problem drinker Person who has not developed alcohol dependence but has experienced one or more problems because of drinking.

eating disorder not otherwise specified (EDNOS) *DSM-IV* designation of disorders that are closely related to anorexia nervosa and bulimia nervosa but do not meet all the formal diagnostic criteria.

effect size (ES) Statistical index of the extent of treatment effects; calculated by subtracting the mean of the control group from that of the treatment group and dividing the difference by the standard deviation of the control group.

efficacy expectations People's feelings of confidence that they can cope with particular situations.

ego Part of the psychic apparatus that tempers and controls the id's primitive drives and impulses so they conform more closely to the realistic demands of the environment.

ego psychology Psychodynamic approach that stresses the importance of the ego and its defenses in personality development.

Electra complex In Freudian theory, a common feature of girls' efforts during the phallic stage to deal with conflicting sexual and aggressive feelings toward their parents.

electroconvulsive therapy (ECT) Treatment for depression in which electrical charges are sent through the brain to induce a generalized seizure.

electroencephalography (EEG) Technique that measures the electrical activity of the brain; EEG waves can indicate brain injury or damage.

electronic therapy Treatment delivered via the telephone or computers, such as hotlines, telephone networks, and electronic mail (e-mail).

electroshock treatment Passage of electrical current through the brain to produce a convulsion; used to alleviate severe depression; also known as electroconvulsive therapy (ECT).

empathy Ability to communicate to another person an understanding of what she's feeling and experiencing.

encephalitis Infection of the brain that, untreated, can cause brain damage and mental retardation.

endocrine organs Endocrine glands secrete hormones into the bloodstream, which stimulates a variety of physiological functions.

endocrine system Physiological system that consists of glands secreting hormones into the bloodstream; these hormones allow the brain to send chemical messages to different parts of the body in addition to direct neural transmission.

enuresis Disorder diagnosed for children of at least 5 years of age when bed-wetting or involuntary discharge of urine occurs more than once a week for at least 3 consecutive months.

epidemiological surveys Studies of the incidence, prevalence, and often causation of specific disorders in particular groups or populations.

epidemiology Study of disorders or diseases in a population.

epilepsy Chronic brain disorder manifested by recurrent seizures.

episodes Discrete periods of time in which a number of specified symptoms are present and represent a change from previous functioning; the building blocks for mood disorders.

ethical standards Guidelines detailing a professional association's ethical expectations of its members.

etiology Cause or causes of disorders and diseases, including mental disorders.

event-related potential (ERP) Electrical events that arise during information processing in the brain.

evoked potential (EP) Brain's electrical response to external stimuli.

exhibitionist Man who exposes his genitals to unsuspecting women and has strong and persistent urges and sexually arousing fantasies concerning such exposure.

explanatory style Habitual manner in which people explain the negative life events they experience.

exposure treatment Behavioral therapy technique in which patients are guided to gradually confront the situations they avoid to help overcome their phobic anxiety.

external validity Degree to which the findings of a particular experiment can be generalized to other subjects under other circumstances.

extinction In classical conditioning, the disappearance of the CR when it is no longer paired with the UCR.

extraverted personality type Jung's personality type for persons who tend to be gregarious, social, and emotionally open.

F

factitious disorder Intentional production of symptoms with an actual physiological basis.

familial aggregation Finding showing that the relatives of a person with a given disorder are more likely to have the disorder than would be expected by chance.

familial mental retardation Results from having parents who are mentally retarded.

familial transmission Transmission of a clinical disorder within a family.

family studies Genetic studies that assume that even if a mental disorder does not obey the laws of inheritance, it is hereditary if it occurs more often in the families of index cases.

family systems therapy Therapy treating the family as a dynamic system in which each member's role affects each other member and the system as a whole; relationships among family members are emphasized more than the specific difficulties of individual family members.

family therapy Therapeutic method that involves assessment and treatment of all immediate family members; emphasizes treating the family as a system.

fear of fear hypothesis Suggests that patients with panic disorder will panic if they experience anxiety or fear.

Feingold diet Special diet designed for children with AD/HD, whom Dr. Benjamin Feingold believed to be physiologically sensitive to certain substances in food, beverages, and medicines; the diet is free of food additives (like red and yellow dye) and food preservatives.

female orgasmic disorder Persistent or recurrent delay in or absence of orgasm following adequate sexual arousal.

female sexual arousal disorder Persistent or recurrent failure to be physiologically aroused until completion of sexual activity.

femoral obesity Pattern of obesity in which more fat is carried below than above the waist; typically shown by women.

fetishism Paraphilia in which an individual becomes sexually aroused by persistent fantasies about or actual use of nonliving objects, such as women's panties.

field research Research design in which subjects are randomly assigned to treatment conditions in natural settings.

"fight or flight" system Biological system that responds to unconditioned negative stimuli and directs an organism to action (fleeing or fighting) when threatened.

five-factor approach to personality Currently popular approach to personality that describes five major traits or dimensions: Neuroticism, Extraversion, Agreeableness, Conscientiousness, and Openness to Experience.

fixation Defense mechanism used to keep potentially threatening thoughts and feelings from consciousness by clinging psychologically to an earlier, less threatening stage of maturity.

flights of ideas Thoughts or speech that jumps from topic to topic with no clear direction or plan; often seen during manic episodes.

forebrain Part of the brain that controls our abilities to speak, think, plan, and remember.

fraternal twins Twins who develop simultaneously from two fertilized ova; also called *dizygotic twins.*

free association Technique in psychoanalysis in which patients are encouraged to talk in therapy about whatever thoughts or feelings they experience without any effort to censor.

free-floating anxiety Old-fashioned term used to describe the pervasive anxiety characteristic of generalized anxiety disorder.

frontal lobes Part of the cerebral cortex that enables us to solve problems flexibly; also appears to be involved in social cognition.

frotteurism Paraphilia involving touching or rubbing against a nonconsenting and unsuspecting person.

G

gamete Sperm cell or ovum.

gender-identity disorder Paraphilia in which an individual wants to be a member of the opposite sex.

gender-role identity Individual's self-perception as consistently masculine or feminine in characteristics and behavior.

generalized anxiety disorder (GAD) Unrealistic and excessive anxiety about two or more life situations.

genes Basic chemical units of heredity; millions align along the 46 human chromosomes.

genital stage Puberty marks the beginning of this psychosexual stage.

genotype Array of genes a person possesses, which is hereditary.

genuineness Ability to understand what another person is experiencing emotionally; rooted in the therapist's complete trust of his own experience of his relationships with the patient.

gestalt therapy Humanistically oriented therapy in which participants are encouraged to complete "unfinished business" by examining the past for unresolved conflicts yet deal with current life issues and make the most of each day.

gonadal gland Endocrine organ that produces sex hormones responsible for the development of secondary sexual characteristics and influential in determining the pattern of sexual behavior.

grand mal epilepsy One of the most common seizure disorders; involves loss of consciousness and a generalized convulsion of the entire body.

grave disability Principal criterion for civil commitment that depends above all on the patient's ability to care for herself.

grossly disorganized behavior Inability to persist in goal-directed behavior; inappropriate behavior in public.

group therapy Approach to therapy that brings a therapist and several patients together; after a time, the patients begin to play a therapeutic role that complements that of the therapist.

H

halfway house Facility for individuals released from a hospital or other treatment program who need more supervision and monitoring than their families can provide before they can live on their own.

hallucinations Abnormal auditory, gustatory, kinesthetic, olfactory, or visual perceptions that are common symptoms of psychosis; most common are those in which voices are heard or objects are seen that don't exist.

Halstead-Reitan Neuropsychological Battery Most widely used measure of the cognitive and behavioral consequences of brain damage; developed more than 50 years ago.

health psychology Application of psychology as a discipline to promote health and prevent and treat illness.

hemispheres Symmetrical halves of the cerebral cortex.

hierarchy of needs Concept developed by Maslow describing the hierarchy of physiological, social, and complex human emotional needs people progress through to reach self-actualization.

higher-order conditioning In classical conditioning, when a CS effectively becomes a UCS following the formation of a second-order conditioned association.

hindbrain Part of the brain that controls autonomic nervous system functions.

hippocampus Part of the limbic system that plays a major role in memory.

histrionic personality disorder Characterized by excessive expression of emotion and attention seeking.

homeostatic mechanisms Self-regulation processes in the brain that work to maintain a more-or-less steady state.

hopelessness theory Revision of the learned helplessness theory; suggests that expectancies of hopelessness are the immediate cause of depression.

hormones Chemical substances secreted into the bloodstream by endocrine organs; serve as chemical messengers in much the same way that neurons convey nerve impulses.

human immunodeficiency virus (HIV) Viral infection that causes AIDS as well as delirium and dementia due to HIV.

humanistic model Emphasizes the uniqueness of human consciousness and the importance of understanding each person's singular perception of reality; highlights the uniqueness and worth of each of us.

Huntington's disease Autosomal-dominant chronic cognitive disorder with a deteriorating course; characterized by changes in personality, intellect, memory, interpersonal behavior, and movement, typically culminating in dementia; generally begins in midlife.

hypertension Chronic, abnormally high blood pressure; measure of 140/90 is borderline hypertension and one of 160/95 is definite hypertension.

hypnosis Condition in which people behave as if they were in a trance or altered state of consciousness and appear to be highly susceptible to suggestions from a hypnotist.

hypoactive sexual desire (HSD) Absence of sexual fantasies and wish for sexual activity.

hypochondriasis Belief that an individual has a serious physical illness, despite medical judgments to the contrary.

hypomanic episode Shorter, milder variant of a manic episode.

hypothalamus With the thalamus and parts of the cerebral cortex, this part of the forebrain controls the experiences of emotion, pain and pleasure, and aggression.

hypothesis What an experiment is designed to test.

hysterical blindness Loss of vision that is not due to any physical basis.

I

id Reservoir of primitive drives and desires untouched and unaffected by the real world; strongly influences infant behavior.

identical twins Twins who develop from a single fertilized ovum; also called *monozygotic twins.*

identification Defense mechanism that protects against threatening feelings aroused by someone else's behavior; produces a strong psychological linkage with that person.

idiotism Component of Pinel's classification system; no longer used to refer to mental retardation.

imipramine (Tofranil) Antidepressant medication that is also used to treat enuresis.

immune system Physiological system that protects the body against viral and bacterial disease.

incest Sexual relations between family members; typically, sex between fathers and daughters or between siblings.

incidence Number of people within a given population who have acquired a disorder or condition within a specific time period, usually a year.

independent variable Variable manipulated by the researcher in an experiment by randomly assigning subjects to treatment conditions.

index cases Patients who suffer from the disorder being studied; synonymous with *probands.*

individual therapy interview Basic element of the therapeutic relationship; requires therapists to be good listeners and insightful and skilled commentators; requires patients to be willing to remember and reproduce past and present behaviors, feelings, and attitudes.

inept discipline Frequent and severe physical punishment (such as grabbing, hitting, or beating with an object) as well as scolding and nagging when trivial problems occur, combined with failure to follow through on threats.

inept monitoring Failure to provide adequate supervision and attention during child care.

infantile autism Term previously used for what is now called *autistic disorder.*

informed consent Authorization granted by research subjects based on their understanding of what's involved in the research; all aspects that may affect subjects' willingness to participate must be explained.

insanity Synonym for *psychosis.*

insanity defense Legal defense that asserts the defendant is not guilty of a crime by reason of insanity.

insight In psychodynamic therapy, the awareness patients develop (usually in extended treatment) of their unconscious conflicts and psychological defenses.

insulin Hormone that converts glucose into energy to store in cells.

intelligence quotient (IQ) Estimate of intelligence produced by dividing mental age by chronological age and multiplying by 100; first associated with the Binet Scales.

interactional perspective View that depression is developed and maintained, in part, by negative interpersonal cycles.

intergenerational transmission of violence Passing on of violence within a family from one generation to the next; for example, being the victim of physical abuse as a child increases the likelihood that a person will later engage in violent and/or abusive behaviors.

internal validity Degree to which change in the dependent variable is due to manipulation of the independent variable.

interpersonal psychotherapy (IPT) Time-limited treatment in which the focus is on understanding and changing interpersonal factors which are thought to maintain the patient's current problems.

interrater reliability Consistency of diagnosis or observational ratings between two or more different interviewers or raters.

intrapsychic conflict Conflict between the ego and id or the ego and superego.

introspectionism Subjective analysis of consciousness, introduced and intensively pursued by Wilhelm Wundt.

introverted personality type Jung's personality type describing persons who tend to be quiet, shy, and uncomfortable in social situations.

invalidating environments Interpersonal environments in which significant others (such as parents) negate and/or respond erratically and inappropriately to an individual's private emotional experiences.

irresistible impulse standard Establishes that if, by reason of the duress of a mental disease, an accused has so far lost the power to choose between right and wrong, he cannot be held criminally responsible.

J

Jacksonian seizures Form of epilepsy involving a variety of partial motor symptoms; initially, the involuntary movement of a finger or a toe; ultimately leading to a period of involuntary jerking of a part of an entire side of the body.

K

koro Fear that the sexual organs will retract into the body; experienced by ethnic Chinese in Singapore.

L

labile Describes a mood that's very changeable; as in a manic episode, when euphoria quickly changes to anger if the person is provoked.

latency stage Extended period of psychosexual calm; age 6 to about 12 years.

law of effect Thorndike's theory that behaviors associated with satisfying consequences are strengthened and thus more likely to be repeated whereas those linked to unsatisfying consequences are weakened and less likely to be repeated.

learned helplessness Theory that experiencing uncontrollable stress leads to depression.

learning disorders (LD) Characterized by academic, language, speech, and motor skills that are substantially lower than would be expected based on a child's intellectual capacity; subcategories include reading disorder, mathematics disorder, and disorder of written expression.

least restrictive alternative Arrangement in a plan for civil commitment that will be least restrictive of a patient's freedom and civil rights.

libido Life instinct of the id; composed primarily of sexual drives and impulses.

lifetime prevalence Percentage of individuals who have had a disorder at any time in their lives.

limbic system Composed of the thalamus and hypothalamus; along with parts of the cerebral cortex, responsible for the physical expression of emotion.

lithium Naturally occurring salt that is the drug of choice for treating bipolar disorder; normalizes mood, especially manic highs.

longitudinal design Research design in which one group of subjects is studied repeatedly at different ages.

love days or caring days Technique used in couples therapy to increase daily positive interactions between partners; each person agrees to engage in specific behaviors that please his or her partner.

lovemap Hypothesized pattern of brain functioning that determines what sexual imagery and actions an individual will find stimulating.

Luria-Nebraska Neuropsychological Battery Tests cognitive functioning in 14 areas; some, such as memory and problem solving, are also tapped by the Halstead-Reitan Battery; others, such as writing, are not.

M

M'Naughten standard Establishes that the accused cannot be held criminally responsible if, at the time the crime was committed, he was laboring under such a defect of reason from mental disorder as not to know the nature and quality of what he was doing.

magnetic resonance imaging (MRI) Noninvasive imaging technique that produces a finely detailed visual reconstruction of the brain that looks like a three-dimensional "slice"; does so by analyzing the nuclear magnetic movements of ordinary hydrogen nuclei in the body's water and fat.

maintenance stage Final stage of change; the person works to prevent relapse and consolidate gains made in the action stage.

major depressive disorders One of the main types of mood disorders; characterized by one or more major depressive episodes but no manic, mixed, or hypomanic episodes.

major depressive episode One of two main types of mood episodes; characterized by depressed mood and related changes in behavior and physical and cognitive functioning.

male erectile disorder Persistent or recurrent failure to attain or maintain an adequate erection until completion of sexual activity.

male orgasmic disorder Persistent delay in or absence of orgasm following normal arousal during sexual activity; typically means the inability to ejaculate in the vagina.

malingering Falsely claiming an illness or disorder in order to obtain some reward or to avoid an unpleasant situation.

managed care movement System of health care in which all costs, options, and procedures are tightly controlled by health maintenance organizations (HMOs).

mania Part of Pinel's classification system; today refers to periods of marked agitation, elation, and grandiose thinking.

manic episode One of two main types of mood episodes; characterized by extremely elevated mood and related changes in behavior and physical and cognitive functioning.

manic-depressive disorder Serious psychiatric disorder that (like schizophrenia) involves psychotic behavior; now called bipolar disorder.

marital therapy Intervention designed to help couples improve their communication, develop insight into their problems, and explore their feelings.

masochism Paraphilia in which an individual becomes sexually aroused by fantasizing about or engaging in being dominated, humiliated, or beaten.

masochistic personality disorder Former diagnostic label used to characterize self-defeating behavior; individuals with this personality disorder diagnosis (which no longer exists) were thought to be drawn to situations or relationships in which they would suffer.

matrilineal Describes a society in which family structure and inheritance are based on females' (wives') bloodlines.

Megan's Law A New Jersey law that requires state prisons to notify community officials when convicted rapists and sexual offenders are released from prison and are about to enter the community.

melancholia Term used by Pinel to refer to severe depression; rarely employed today to describe that condition.

melancholic features Denote a particularly severe form of major depressive episode; characterized by almost complete loss of pleasure and reactivity to positive stimuli.

meningitis Infection of the membrane covering the brain; untreated, it can cause brain damage and mental retardation.

mental age Refers to the number of age-grouped tests and problems passed in the Binet Scales; mental age divided by chronological age multiplied by 100 determines IQ.

mental disorder as biological disadvantage Behaviors that interfere with reproduction and evolution should be considered mental disorders.

mental disorder as harmful dysfunction Mental disorder is best defined as harmful dysfunction.

mental disorder as myth Mental disorders don't exist; the concept of mental disorder was invented by psychiatrists to justify their exercise of power.

mental disorder as statistical deviance Behaviors that are statistically deviant, rare, and unusual should be considered mental disorders.

mental disorder as unexpectable distress or disability Mental disorder is best defined as unexpectable distress or disability.

mental disorder as violation of social norms Mental disorder is largely a product of social norms that determine the behaviors a group finds acceptable and unacceptable.

mental disorder as whatever professionals treat Mental disorder is best defined as whatever professionals decide to treat.

mental retardation Condition characterized by subaverage intelligence beginning before the age of 18, accompanied by impairments in adaptive functioning.

meta-analysis Quantitative method of integrating the standardized results of a large number of separate studies.

methadone Synthetic opiate drug that replaces heroin in the addict's CNS opiate receptors, thereby markedly reducing heroin's reinforcing effects.

midbrain Part of the brain that contains most of the reticular activating system (RAS); the sleep-wake center; also mediates attentional processes.

Midtown Manhattan Study Investigation of mental health problems and resources in New York City between 1952 and 1960; revealed substantially more psychiatric impairment in residents than anyone expected.

mild mental retardation Characterized by IQ of between 50–55 and 70; includes 85 percent of persons with mental retardation.

milieu treatment Therapy focusing on the responsibilities of patients to seek employment, care for themselves, and participate in social activities.

Millon Clinical Multiaxial Inventory (MCMI) Objective measure of personality designed specifically for diagnostic purposes; major focus is on diagnosis of personality disorders; revised test is the MCMI-II.

minimal brain dysfunction (MBD) Term once used synonymously with AD/HD; some medical professionals believed MBD was the cause of children's hyperactivity and motor coordination problems.

Minnesota Multiphasic Personality Inventory (MMPI) Most commonly used objective, self-report measure of personality; used to explore personality and aid in diagnosis; revised test is the MMPI-2.

minor depressive disorder Variant of major depressive disorder with fewer than the required 5 symptoms.

mixed episode Mood episode characterized by alternation between full-blown depressive and manic episodes.

modeling Synonym for *observational learning.*

models Approximations of real-world phenomena designed to help clarify and explain them.

moderate mental retardation Characterized by IQ between 35–40 and 50–55; includes 10 percent of persons with mental retardation.

monoamine oxidase (MAO) Chemical that breaks down neurotransmitters into simpler compounds.

monoamine oxidase inhibitors (MAOIs) Class of drugs used to treat depression that act by increasing the amount of available norepinephrine and serotonin; prescribed less often than other antidepressant medications because of their potentially lethal interactions with certain foods.

monozygotic twins Twins who develop from a single fertilized ovum; also called *identical twins.*

mood disorders Class of mental disorders characterized primarily by disturbances in mood (for example, depression).

moral anxiety Generated by guilt and shame; product of a punitive superego.

motivational interview Interview with an alcohol- or drug-dependent person, designed to heighten motivation for change in drinking by providing direct feedback on the status and severity of his substance-related problem.

motor function Function of the cerebral cortex that controls movements of our muscles.

multiaxial diagnosis Complete *DSM-IV* multiaxial diagnosis requires the clinician to evaluate the patient along five behavioral dimensions, or axes.

multifactorial polygenic model Etiological model for psychiatric disorders involving many genes interacting with environmental influences.

multimodal therapy Approach to treatment in which seven modalities of functioning (behavior, affect, sensation, imagery, cognition, interpersonal relations, and biology) are each assessed and then targeted for intervention using an eclectic range of methods; developed by Arnold Lazarus.

multiple personality disorder Dissociative disorder now known as dissociative identity disorder.

N

naloxone Narcotic antagonist; used to treat narcotic addiction.

naltrexone Opioid antagonist; originally developed to treat opioid dependence by inducing withdrawal in opioid addicts; also appears to have a strong impact on alcoholics by reducing craving.

narcissistic personality disorder Characterized by grandiose fantasies or behavior, constant need for admiration, and lack of empathy.

narcotic antagonist Drug that precipitates immediate withdrawal from narcotics.

Narcotics Anonymous Self-help group for narcotics addicts modeled after Alcoholics Anonymous.

natural forces As causes of mental disorder, include genetic factors, disease processes, and environmental and psychological factors.

natural killer (NK) cells Part of the immune system; destroy viruses and some tumor cells; derived from bone marrow.

negative affectivity Temperamental sensitivity to negative stimuli; one of the three factors of the tripartite model.

negative effect Outcome of psychotherapy in which the patient's problems have become worse.

negative symptoms Absence of behaviors and feelings normally present; for example, little or no speech, social withdrawal, or blunted affect.

neglect Failure of a parent or caregiver to provide minimal care and support for a child.

NEO Personality Inventory (NEO-PI) Objective measure of personality designed to study normal personality development, specifically, the "big five": Extraversion, Agreeableness, Neuroticism, Conscientiousness, and Openness to Experience.

neurons Nerve cells; the brain is composed of billions of these cells.

neuropeptides Class of brain chemicals that regulate neurotransmitter activity.

neuropsychology Branch of clinical psychology devoted to the evaluation and diagnosis of brain injury.

neurotic anxiety Experienced when id impulses threaten to overwhelm the ego.

neurotic disorders Describes what the *DSM-IV* now refers to as anxiety; from the psychodynamic model.

neurotransmitter Biochemical substance in the brain that mediates transmission of electrical impulses across the synapses; excesses and deficits are believed to cause psychopathology.

NIMH Epidemiologic Catchment Area (ECA) Study Surveyed the psychiatric status of more than 20,000 persons residing in five U.S. cities and towns in the early 1980s; reported even higher rates of psychiatric disorder than the Midtown Manhattan Study.

nocturnal penile tumescence (NPT) Erection that occurs in healthy males during the rapid eye movement (REM) stage of sleep.

nonabstinent treatment goals Synonym for *controlled drinking goals for alcoholism treatment.*

NOS diagnoses Not Otherwise Specified diagnoses; used when a patient has a significant clinical problem that doesn't fit any categories in the *DSM.*

O

obesity Body weight 20 percent or more than a person's desirable weight.

object-relations theory Modern version of psychoanalytic theory that stresses the influence of early parental relationships in personality development.

objective anxiety Realistic apprehension we feel when confronted by real danger.

observational learning Mode of learning in which you watch others engaging in various kinds of behavior, without engaging in them yourself.

obsessions Repetitive, intrusive thoughts, images, or impulses that are distressing and unwanted.

obsessive-compulsive disorder (OCD) Anxiety disorder characterized by uncontrollable thoughts or images and behavioral rituals.

obsessive-compulsive personality disorder Characterized by preoccupation with orderliness, perfectionism, and mental and interpersonal control at the cost of flexibility, openness, and efficiency.

occipital lobes Division of the cerebral cortex that controls visual perception.

Oedipus complex Psychosexual challenge that boys experience during the phallic period; requires the resolution of conflicting sexual and aggressive feelings about parents.

operant conditioning Mode of learning in which behavior is acquired, maintained, and eliminated as a function of its consequences.

operant response (R) Voluntary response that operates on the environment and produces reinforcement or punishment.

operational criteria Signs and symptoms of each *DSM-IV* diagnosis are organized as a set of operational criteria, which outlines and fully describes the behaviors characteristic of the diagnosis.

operational definition Description of a construct in objective, measurable terms.

oppositional defiant disorder (ODD) Characterized by significant defiant and negative child behavior, including frequent anger, temper tantrums, swearing, and defiance of adult rules.

oral stage First stage of psychosexual development, extending from birth to about 18 months; the infant's mouth, lips, and tongue are invested with libido, so that eating gives great pleasure.

orgasm Intensely satisfying physiological reflex, releasing sexual tension.

outcome Eventual result of a disorder; for example, symptoms may go away or persist.

outcome expectations People's beliefs that their actions will result in particular outcomes.

outcome research Controlled research designed to evaluate how effective a particular treatment method is.

overanxious disorder Childhood anxiety disorder characterized by excessive worrying about new and future situations, such as being hurt, doing poorly on a test, or being criticized by others; a subclass of generalized anxiety disorder.

ovum Female gamete, when fertilized by a sperm cell, develops into an embryo.

P

pain disorder Somatoform disorder in which the person complains of severe pain that cannot be explained by known physical causes.

panic Clinical manifestation of fear; usually of sudden onset.

panic attack Sudden feeling of intense fear accompanied by physiological symptoms and thoughts of losing control or dying.

panic disorder Unexpected, recurrent attacks of intense anxiety occurring in situations that do not normally elicit anxiety.

paradoxical directive Technique in which the therapist encourages the client to do something that seems contradictory, such as prescribing the actual symptom the client wishes to eliminate.

paranoid personality disorder Characterized by ongoing feelings of distrust and suspicion of others, whose motives are seen as harmful.

paranoid type Schizophrenia characterized by a preoccupation with one or more sets of delusions organized around one or more central themes.

paraphilias Sexual disorders in which bizarre or unusual acts, imagery, or objects are required for sexual stimulation.

parasympathetic division Division of the ANS that regulates normal bodily functions, such as digestion and heartbeat; the "housekeeping" functions.

parataxic distortions Effects that problematic interpersonal relationships in childhood have on the adult's misperceptions of reality.

Parents Anonymous (PA) Voluntary program for parents who think they are abusive or have the potential for abusing their child; program is modeled after Alcoholics Anonymous, in that the individuals do not reveal their full identities.

parietal lobes Portion of the cerebral cortex that mediates touch recognition; a portion of the left parietal lobe is also involved in speech production.

Parkinson's disease Chronic cognitive disorder caused by the destruction of brain cells producing dopamine; results in a degenerative process that includes tremor, muscular rigidity, stooped posture, shuffling gait, depression, and dementia.

Parkinsonian effects Side effects of antipsychotic medications; typically include muscle rigidity, stooped posture, an unusual shuffling gait, and drooling.

partner abuse Repeated physical aggression against a partner and/or isolated acts of physical aggression against a partner that lead to fear and/or injury.

patriarchy A form of social organization in which power is held by and transferred through males.

pedigree studies Genetic research involving families in which substantial numbers of members are affected with the disorder under study.

pedophilia Paraphilia characterized by the unnatural desire to have sexual contact with a prepubescent child (age 13 or younger).

penile plethysmograph Device that measures changes in size of the penis during arousal.

peripheral nervous system Comprised of the somatic nervous system and the autonomic nervous system.

person-centered theory of personality Rogers's humanistic theory emphasizing each of our value, worth, and individuality; also stresses our potential to improve ourselves and our personal environment.

personality According to psychologists, enduring traits of character—the basic, lasting qualities that make us who we are.

personality disorder Extreme and inflexible personality traits that are distressing to the person or that cause problems in school, work, or interpersonal relationships.

personality disorder–not otherwise specified (PD–NOS) Catchall category that includes diagnoses not specific to the ten described in the *DSM-IV*; sometimes referred to as *mixed* or *atypical* personality disorder.

petit mal epilepsy Condition involving a brief disruption in consciousness, generally lasting from 2 to 10 seconds; may be overlooked by observers.

phallic stage Third stage of psychosexual development; libido is invested in the genitals, and the child works through her feelings about her parents.

phenotype Observable characteristics, such as hair color and height.

phenylketonuria (PKU) Condition that's the result of a disorder of amino acid metabolism; most intensively studied inborn error of metabolism.

phrenologist Quasi-scientists who studied the formation of the skull in the belief that it revealed a person's mental facilities and character.

physical abuse Acts of physical aggression by one individual against another, often leading to fear and/or injury.

pituitary gland Triggers the activities of many other glands by releasing hormones into the bloodstream that affect them; the "master gland."

placebo So-called sugar pill that looks just like real medication but contains no active substance.

pleasure principle To maximize pleasure and reduce tension without concern for morality or reality; the sole aim of the id.

pneumoencephalogram Diagnostic procedure that employs air as an X-ray contrast medium to demonstrate brain contours.

point prevalence Percentage of individuals with a disorder at a particular point in time.

polysubstance abuse Concurrent abuse of or dependence on more than one substance.

positive affectivity Temperamental sensitivity to positive stimuli; one of the three factors of the tripartite model.

positive symptoms Presence of behaviors and feelings normally not present, such as hallucinations, delusions, or disorganized speech/behavior.

positron emission tomography (PET scan) Brain-imaging technology that permits study of the functions of different brain areas.

postsynaptic receptors Sites on a neuron that receive released neurotransmitters and trigger the next electrical impulse.

posttraumatic stress disorder (PTSD) Syndrome that may be experienced following exposure to a traumatic stressor, such as rape; symptoms may include intrusive memories, numbing of sensations, and withdrawal.

precontemplation stage First stage of change; the person has no intention of changing behavior any time soon.

predictive validity Describes a diagnostic system's capacity to predict future mental disorders.

prefrontal lobotomy Surgical operation involving cutting fibers of the anterior portion of the frontal lobe of the brain.

premature ejaculation Disorder in which the male is unable to prevent reaching orgasm before he wants to during vaginal intercourse.

premenstrual dysphoric disorder Commonly known as *premenstrual syndrome* or *PMS*; can be diagnosed as a Mood Disorder–NOS.

preparation stage Third stage of change; the person intends to take action within a month.

preparedness hypothesis Suggests that our evolutionary history has prepared us biologically to acquire fears of objects or situations that were at one time associated with danger to the species.

pressured speech Loud, fast, nonstop talking that's hard to direct or interrupt; often seen during manic episodes.

presynaptic receptors Sites on a neuron that release neurotransmitters that provide feedback regarding the amount of neurotransmitter in the synapse.

prevalence Total number of people within a given population who suffer from a disorder or condition.

primary prevention Efforts to reduce the occurrence of new problems in a population.

primary-process thinking Characterized by sexual preoccupations and fantasies, anger, jealousy, selfishness, and envy; guides the id's impulses.

privileged relationships Therapist/patient relationships are privileged because the confidentiality of communication in them is protected by legal statute.

probands Patients who suffer from the disorder under study; synonymous with *index cases*.

problem-solving therapy Approach in which the therapist focuses on improving the family's process of solving problems by teaching family members to define each problem, generate alternative solutions, evaluate those alternatives, and implement the best alternative.

problem-solving training Treatment approach with a focus on cognitive processes, such as expectations, self-statements, taking the perspectives of others, defining problems, and evaluating alternative solutions.

process research Research designed to uncover why a particular treatment method has certain effects.

prodromal phase In schizophrenia, the phase immediately before the active phase of the disorder.

profound mental retardation Characterized by IQ below 20–25; includes 1–2 percent of persons with mental retardation.

progressive relaxation Form of relaxation training widely used to treat different stress-related disorders; involves alternate tensing and relaxing of different muscle groups.

projection Defense mechanism used to deny the existence of a fearful or threatening emotion by attributing it to another person.

projective drawings Assessment technique in which respondents are asked to draw objects; based on the assumption that they reveal important traits of character by what they draw and how they draw it.

projective tests Measures of personality based on the assumption that individuals call on enduring traits of character to structure otherwise unstructured test stimuli.

prototype Particularly good example of a category; one that has almost all the category's features and few features of other categories.

Prozac (fluoxetine) Antidepressant medication that also reduces panic and anxiety by increasing the amount of available serotonin in the brain.

psychodynamic model Based on the belief that human behavior is influenced, in large part, by unconscious factors that we are largely unaware of.

psychomotor agitation Marked increase in physical restlessness; common in major depressive episodes.

psychomotor retardation Significant slowing down of motor activity; common in major depressive episodes.

psychopathy Conceptualization of a personality disorder similar to the *DSM-IV* antisocial personality disorder; emphasizes such traits as lack of empathy, superficial charm, egocentricity and inflated self-worth, emotional unresponsiveness and irresponsibility, poor judgment, deceitfulness, and impulsive behavior.

psychopharmacology Use of drugs to treat psychopathology.

psychosis Serious form of mental disorder, involving an actual break with reality.

psychosomatic medicine Study of clinical disorders in which emotional conflicts are said to cause physical damage or symptoms such as hypertension, headaches, and ulcers.

psychostimulants Medication of choice for children with AD/HD; appear to increase certain brain functions that improve attention span and fine motor control.

psychosurgery Surgical destruction of certain neural pathways in the brain done in an effort to control a severe mental disorder.

psychotherapy integration Process of looking for commonalities among different and often conflicting systems, learning from other perspectives, and integrating divergent methods.

psychotic Out of touch with reality; showing delusions, hallucinations, and disorganized speech/behavior.

psychotropic medications Drugs used to alter feelings, thoughts, and behavior.

punishment In operant conditioning, presentation of an aversive stimulus or removal of a reinforcing stimulus following a response; decreases the probability that the response will recur.

purging Self-induced vomiting or laxative misuse designed to control weight.

Q

quasi-experimental methods Studies in which membership in a class or category defines the experimental group; for example, a case-control design.

R

random assignment Procedure for assigning subjects to treatment groups such that each subject has an equal chance of being in either the experimental or control group; improves the chances that subjects' characteristics will be equally distributed across treatment conditions in an experiment.

rape Unwanted or nonconsensual sexual activity that is forced or coerced against another.

rapid cycling Subtype of bipolar I disorder, in which 4 or more mood episodes occur per year.

rapid eye movement (REM) sleep Stage of sleep characterized by rapid eye movements and associated with dreaming.

rational-emotive therapy (RET) Therapy aimed at identifying and changing irrational cognitions that are assumed to cause emotional disorders.

rationalization Defense mechanism used to avoid confronting irrational motives for behavior by invoking an "after the fact" set of logical reasons for it.

reaction formation Defense mechanism used to avoid the turmoil aroused by conflicting feelings about someone by excluding the negative feelings and focusing on the positive ones.

reality principle To recognize society's realistic demands; guides the ego "by observing the rules."

recessive gene Gene that must be paired with one identical to it to determine a trait in the phenotype.

recidivism Rate of relapse or repeat offending (that is, return of symptoms or to criminal behavior).

reciprocal determinism Describes Bandura's belief in the reciprocal interaction of behavioral, cognitive, and environmental influences.

reframing Conceptualizing a problem in a new way.

regression Defense mechanism used to avoid painful thoughts and feelings from the past by returning psychologically to an earlier, less stressful period.

reinforcement In operant conditioning, presentation of a rewarding stimulus or removal of an aversive stimulus following a response; increases the probability that a response will recur.

reinforcing stimulus (SR) In operant conditioning, the positive or negative consequences of a response that determine its subsequent frequency.

relapse prevention model Attempts to identify the cues associated with relapse and to strengthen strategies to cope with the high-risk situations these cues refer to.

relapse prevention training Therapeutic strategy that prepares patients to cope with threats to self-control and thus to prevent relapse.

reliability Consistency or replicability of a test, measure, or finding.

remission Lessening or disappearance of symptoms of a disorder.

repression Defense mechanism used to prevent painful, potentially disruptive thoughts, feelings, memories, and impulses from reaching consciousness.

residual phase In schizophrenia, the phase following the active phase; characterized by social withdrawal, inactivity, and bizarre thoughts; negative symptoms are often predominant, along with impairment in social and vocational functioning.

residual type Schizophrenia that occurs after prominent delusions, hallucinations, or formal thought disorder are no longer displayed but when the individual still speaks very little, shows little affect, has almost no motivation, and experiences some irregular beliefs.

resistance Unwillingness on the part of a patient to cooperate fully in therapy; for instance, refusing to discuss a certain topic.

response prevention Behavior therapy technique in which phobic or compulsive behavior is prevented so the patient is exposed to anxiety-eliciting stimuli.

responsibility for one's actions Legal concept that asks whether the accused was responsible for the actions taking place at the time she committed the crime she is accused of.

reticular activating system (RAS) Brain's "sleep-wake" center; also mediates attentional processes.

reuptake Reabsorption of a neurotransmitter into the neuron it was released from.

right to least restrictive alternative People who are mentally ill cannot be confined to psychiatric hospitals for indefinite custodial periods simply because no one can or will assume responsibility for them outside the hospital; also applies to the regimens of locked wards, seclusion, and restraint by which committed patients are managed.

right to privacy People who are mentally ill have the right to decide the time, place, manner, and extent of sharing themselves with others.

right to refuse treatment People who are mentally ill have the legal right to refuse treatment (usually medication or another somatic treatment) under certain specified circumstances.

right to treatment People who are mentally ill have a right to receive treatment.

risk factor Predicts a clinical disorder and provides a clue to identifying its underlying causes; also encourages interventions to modify the risk and thus reduce the occurrence of the disorder.

Ritalin Most common psychostimulant medication prescribed to children for treating AD/HD symptoms.

Rorschach Inkblot Test Projective measure of personality that consists of 10 cards, each showing a different inkblot design.

rubella German measles; major prenatal infectious condition responsible for mental retardation.

ruminative response style Persistent focus on negative experiences that serves to maintain depression.

S

sadism Paraphilia in which an individual is aroused by fantasies or actions involving dominating or beating another person.

schema Underlying belief system about yourself or the world that filters and organizes your experiences.

schizoid personality disorder Characterized by being detached from social relationships and showing a restricted range of emotions in interpersonal exchanges.

schizophrenia Most common psychosis; characterized by hallucinations, delusions, profound problems in thinking, and bizarre behavior.

schizophrenia spectrum Range of disorders, including schizophrenia and the Cluster A (odd) personality disorders (paranoid, schizoid, schizotypal); believed to share an underlying dimension of vulnerability.

schizotypal personality disorder Characterized by social and interpersonal deficits that are shown primarily by intense discomfort in interpersonal relationships and impaired ability to form close relationships as well as cognitive or perceptual distortions and eccentric behavior.

school phobia Characterized by a child's specific reluctance or refusal to go to school due to fear of separating from parents; a subclass of separation anxiety disorder.

seasonal pattern Subtype of depression in which symptoms appear in winter and then often go away in the spring, even without specific treatment.

secondary prevention Efforts to detect problems early in their onset and to reduce their intensity.

secondary-process thinking Mode that employs reason and logic; used by the ego.

seduction theory of neurosis Early Freudian theory that neurotic disorders in women were caused primarily by having been sexually abused as children.

seizure Pathophysiological brain disturbance caused by the spontaneous and excessive discharge of neurons in the cortex.

selective serotonin reuptake inhibitors (SSRIs) Class of drugs that selectively prevent the reuptake of serotonin without affecting the uptake of other neurotransmitters.

self-actualization Term used by Abraham Maslow to describe how human beings can achieve their unrealized potential, despite the inevitable frustrations of life.

self-control Central feature of this social learning concept is the recognition that we can learn to regulate our own behavior.

self-efficacy Bandura's term for beliefs about our ability to exercise control over events that affect our lives.

self-monitoring Technique used in behavioral assessment and behavior therapy in which patients are asked to identify and record specific thoughts, feelings, and behaviors.

self-psychology Modification of psychoanalysis in which the emphasis is on the low self-esteem or vulnerability a child feels because of lack of love; therapy is directed toward restoring the patient's sense of self by providing the acceptance that was missing in childhood.

self-regulation Synonym for *self-control.*

self-reports Individual accounts of the frequency of target behaviors, along with descriptions of their antecedents and consequences.

semistructured interview Follows an outline but does not prescribe specific questions or require a particular ordering of questions.

sensate focus Therapeutic technique involving mutual, non-performance-oriented sensual interaction between partners.

sensory function Cerebral cortex function that receives information from the sense organs and processes it for later recall or immediate response.

sensory receptors Receive information from the environment for transmission to the central nervous system; for instance, the eyes, ears, and skin.

sentence-completion tests Projective devices that ask respondents to complete incomplete sentences, thereby imposing structure on unstructured test stimuli.

separation anxiety disorder Characterized by excessive anxiety concerning separation from the home or loved ones.

serotonin Neurotransmitter that plays a key role in regulating mood and eating behavior.

set-point theory Suggests that each individual has a biologically programmed weight range that the body defends against change.

severe mental retardation Characterized by IQ between 20–25 and 35–40; includes 3–4 percent of persons with mental retardation.

sex reassignment surgery Surgery performed to physically change an individual's sexual identity from male to female or vice versa; an established means of treating transsexuals.

sexual aversion disorder Paraphilia in which an individual avoids all or almost all genital sexual contact with a partner.

Sexually Violent Predators (SVP) Law Involuntary civil confinement of dangerous sex offenders after they have completed their prison sentence.

sign Characteristic feature of a disorder a patient may be unaware of.

single-case experimental design Intensive study of single subjects over time under systematically varied environmental conditions.

slow virus Viral infection so-called because it takes a very long time following infection for symptoms of disease to develop.

smooth-pursuit eye-tracking dysfunction Difficulty visually following a continuously moving target found in many schizophrenic patients; the best biological indicator of genetic liability to develop schizophrenia.

social causation hypothesis Hypothesis that factors associated with being a member of a lower socioeconomic class may contribute to the development of schizophrenia.

social cue Human discriminative stimulus that informs us whether a particular social behavior is likely to be reinforced or punished.

social learning approach Bandura's theory of complex human learning in which behavior is viewed as a product of both internal cognitive mediating processes (such as self-efficacy and self-regulation) and external stimuli (such as classical and operant conditioning).

social phobias Anxiety disorders characterized by the persistent fear and avoidance of social situations.

social selection hypothesis Hypothesis that persons genetically predisposed to schizophrenia drift downward socioeconomically; that is, persons with schizophrenia drift into poor urban neighborhoods.

social support Network of people that provides a foundation for an individual, showing concern and caring, communicating acceptance and group inclusion, giving tangible help, and offering advice.

socioeconomic status (SES) Individual's relative standing in society as a function of occupation, income, and education.

sociopathic personality disturbance Catchall diagnostic category in the *DSM-I* and *DSM-II* that included antisocial behavior and the sexual deviations as well as alcoholism and drug addiction.

sodium lactate infusion Injection of lactic acid, which tends to trigger panic attacks in people with panic disorder.

somatic nervous system Part of the peripheral nervous system that coordinates the skeletal muscles and controls voluntary movements, such as walking and talking.

somatic symptoms Changes in physical functioning, such as sleep and appetite disturbance.

somatization disorder Somatoform disorder characterized by recurrent somatic symptoms, causing the person to consult repeated doctors without finding an organic basis for the problem.

somatoform disorders Disorders characterized by the presence of symptoms typically associated with physical disease for which no known organic basis can be found.

specific phobias Anxiety disorders characterized by the fear and avoidance of particular objects or situations.

specifiers Variety of features describing subtypes of mood disorders; designed to assist in treatment selection and to improve predictions of course and outcome.

spectatoring Individual's self-conscious role during sexual activity, in which he becomes an observer of his sexual response and looks for signs of failure.

sperm cell Male gamete; when it fertilizes an ovum, develops into an embryo.

spontaneous remission Improvement in the patient's condition over time in the absence of formal therapy.

stages of change Research program on the process of behavioral change in treating addictions; has led to development of an assessment technique that places an individual at one of five stages of change.

standardization Process in which the validity of an assessment device has been analyzed for age, sex, education, socioeconomic status, or other relevant variables to yield quantifiable indices of validity.

Stanford-Binet Scales Series of intelligence tests for children originally developed by Alfred Binet at the beginning of the twentieth century; their form, content, and philosophy continue to influence the field of intellectual assessment.

stimulus generalization In classical conditioning, when a CR is linked both to the CS with which it was first associated and to similar stimuli not originally part of the conditioning.

stimulus-response approach In behavior therapy, the application of classical conditioning principles to clinical problems.

stress State of physical and psychological tension caused by pressure or strain; a complex physiological response, according to Selye.

structural family therapy Treatment approach in which the family is viewed as the unit to change; the therapist's main goal is to alter the entire family system by assessing and restructuring the roles of and relationships between family members.

structural theory of personality Divides the psyche into three parts: the ego, id, and superego; each is responsible for a distinct set of psychological operations.

structured interview Guided by a detailed set of questions prepared and tested before the interview and always presented in the same order; generally more reliable, which explains their expanding use for research purposes.

sublimation Defense mechanism that transforms the psychological energy associated with threatening sexual or aggressive feelings and impulses into socially acceptable pursuits, such as art, music, politics, or intellectual activities.

substance abuse Maladaptive pattern of substance use, characterized by recurrent and significant adverse consequences related to the repeated use of substances.

substance dependence Cluster of cognitive, behavioral, and physiological symptoms that indicate that the individual continues use of a substance despite significant substance-related problems.

substance-induced persisting amnestic disorder Chronic, profound, irreversible memory disorder caused by sustained substance abuse.

substance-induced persisting dementia Chronic cognitive disorder caused by sustained substance abuse.

substance intoxication delirium Substance-induced delirium that occurs during intoxication.

substance withdrawal delirium Substance-induced delirium that occurs during withdrawal.

successful aging Process in which elderly people deal successfully with the loss of a lifelong partner, a chronic disease, or a change in economic circumstance; concept defined by a MacArthur Foundation group.

superego Earliest source of what we call *conscience;* our ability to distinguish right from wrong.

supernatural forces Long thought responsible for mental disorder; demonic possession was an especially common explanation for psychosis.

sympathetic division Division of the ANS that energizes or activates organs to enable the body to respond in times of stress.

symptom Feature of a disease that a patient recognizes and may complain of.

symptom substitution Replacement of one symptom with another following treatment in which the underlying problem is not resolved.

Synanon Self-help group for heroin and cocaine addicts, requiring a lengthy residential stay and involving successive group confrontations to break through addicts' denial.

synapse Minute space between one neuron and another across which nerve impulses are sent.

syndrome Distinct, recognizable group of symptoms.

T

taijin kyofusho (TKS) Japanese social disorder in which people experience social anxiety about the possibility of embarrassing or offending others by their actions or appearance.

Tarasoff standard Established the duty of therapists to warn and protect persons threatened by their patients.

tardive dyskinesia Largely irreversible side effect of taking antipsychotic medications; characterized by involuntary lip smacking, tongue movements, and chin wagging.

target behaviors In behavioral assessment, the disturbed and disturbing behaviors themselves as well as the thoughts and feelings that accompany them.

technical eclecticism Form of psychological treatment in which therapists draw on techniques from other systems of psychotherapy without necessarily subscribing to the theories behind the techniques.

temporal lobe epilepsy Form of epilepsy that may lead the individual to perform unusual behaviors during the period of the attack; sometimes quite complicated and sometimes including episodic violence.

temporal lobes Part of the cerebral cortex that controls visual information processing, long-term memory, emotional experience, and sound recognition.

tension headache Painful contraction of skeletal muscles of the face, scalp, neck, and shoulders in response to psychological stress.

tertiary prevention Efforts to reduce long-term damage caused by a problem.

test-retest reliability or temporal stability Consistency of diagnosis, test scores, or observational ratings on two or more occasions.

testosterone Hormone that's critical in regulating sexual arousal in men.

tetrahydrocannabinol (THC) Psychoactive ingredient in cannabis products, such as marijuana and hashish.

thalamus With the hypothalamus and parts of the cerebral cortex, this part of the forebrain controls the experiences of emotion, pain and pleasure, and aggression.

thanatos Death instinct of the id; composed of aggressive and destructive impulses.

Thematic Apperception Test (TAT) Projective measure of personality consisting of 31 cards; 30 portray an ambiguous scene that often includes people, and the remaining card is blank.

theory Formal statement of a set of propositions designed to explain a particular phenomenon.

theory of infantile sexuality Freud's revised theory, in which he assumed that patients' reports of child sexual abuse were not real, instead reflecting their unconscious desire for sex with their fathers.

theory of multiple intelligences Conceives of seven independent intelligences that interact with the environment to determine success in it; proposed by Howard Gardner.

theory of psychosexual development Freud's portrayal of the development of personality in distinct, successive stages; each is characterized by a different means of gratifying libidinal (sexual) needs.

therapeutic community Treatment approach in which patients in an institutional setting are treated as normally as possible; they live in a family-style environment and are encouraged to develop routines and participate in chores.

therapy outcome studies Research to determine how effective a therapy is in comparison to placebo or minimal treatment controls or to other treatments.

thyroid gland Endocrine organ that produces hormones that affect the body's metabolism rate.

tolerance Consequence of addiction to a substance; over time, requires that increasing amounts be ingested in order to achieve the same subjective effects.

Tourette's syndrome Disorder characterized by intermittent bodily tics, sounds, and words.

tranquilizers Class of drugs that includes the antianxiety medications, benzodiazepines; have a calming effect on mood.

transcendental meditation (TM) Form of relaxation training in which the person adopts a passive attitude and focuses on a single object.

transference Special relationship that develops between patient and therapist in which the patient responds to the therapist as she did toward significant people (usually parents) in her childhood.

transsexual Individual with gender-identity disorder; wishes to be a member of the opposite sex.

transvestite Man who becomes sexually aroused by dressing as a woman.

triarchic theory of human intelligence Stresses the role of intelligence in helping us adjust to new situations and environments; proposed by Howard Sternberg.

tricyclic antidepressants Class of drugs with a 3-ring molecular structure that block or interfere with the reuptake of norepinephrine and serotonin.

tripartite model Theory that explains the overlap and distinction of anxiety and depression by hypothesizing the interaction of three factors: one shared factor and one unique factor for each type of problem.

trisomy 21 Common cause of Down syndrome; individuals have 3 rather than 2 chromosome 21s and thus 47 rather than the usual 46 chromosomes.

tumescence Engorgement of the penis during sexual arousal.

twin studies Genetic studies that depend on the differences in shared genetic material between monozygotic (identical) and dizygotic (fraternal) twins.

U

unconditional positive regard Therapist's nonjudgmental acceptance of the patient's feelings.

unconditioned response (UCR) In classical conditioning, the natural response elicited by a UCS.

unconditioned stimulus (UCS) In classical conditioning, a stimulus naturally capable of eliciting a UCR.

unconscious psychological processes Psychological conflicts, impulses, desires, and motives that influence behavior we are largely unaware of.

undifferentiated type Schizophrenia characterized by psychotic symptoms such as delusions, hallucinations, and incoherence; individuals in this category do not meet the specific criteria for the other subtypes.

unipolar disorder or unipolar depression Older name for *major depressive disorder.*

unstructured interview Does not follow an outline but occurs spontaneously.

V

vaginismus Involuntary tightening or spasms in the outer layer of the vagina.

validation Expressing an understanding of other family members' feelings and desires.

validity Degree to which a test or measure accurately captures what it was intended to.

vascular dementia Age-related cognitive disorder caused by a succession of small strokes.

victimized Made the target of another's aggressive behavior.

virtual reality therapy Computer-based means of manipulating the environment an individual experiences.

W

waiting-list control group Control group in which patients are promised therapy after a period of time, during which the experimental group does receive treatment.

Wechsler Adult Intelligence Scale-Revised (WAIS-R) Revision of first test to permit the separate examination of the diverse intellectual abilities that most experts believe constitute intelligence; the first intelligence test designed specifically for adults.

Wechsler Intelligence Scale for Children-III (WISC-III) Latest edition of the intelligence test designed for children between 5 and 16; based on the notion that intelligence is the sum of many separate abilities.

Wechsler Preschool and Primary Scale of Intelligence (WPPSI) Intelligence test for preschool children; based on the notion that intelligence is the sum of many separate abilities.

Wernicke-Korsakoff syndrome Substance-induced persisting amnestic disorder; associated with prolonged, heavy alcohol ingestion, and the chronic thiamine deficiency that typically accompanies it.

with physiological dependence Substance dependence that includes tolerance or withdrawal symptoms or both.

withdrawal Physical and psychological consequences that result when use of an addicting substance is stopped.

without physiological dependence Substance dependence that does not include tolerance or withdrawal symptoms.

X

Xanax (alprazolam) Potent benzodiazepine often used to treat anxiety and panic.

References

A

Abel, G. G. (1989). Behavioral treatment of child molesters. In A. J. Stunkard & A. Baum (Eds.), *Perspectives in behavioral medicine* (pp. 223–243). Hillsdale, NJ: Lawrence Erlbaum.

Abel, G. G., Barlow, D. H., Blanchard, E. B., & Guild, D. (1977). The components of rapists' sexual arousal. *Archives of General Psychiatry, 34,* 895–908.

Abel, G. G., Becker, J. V., Cunningham-Rathner, J., Mittelman, J., & Rouleau, J. L. (1988). Multiple paraphilic diagnoses among sex offenders. *Bulletin of the American Academy of Psychiatry and Law, 16,* 153–168.

Abel, G. G., Becker, J. V., Mittelman, M., Cunningham-Rathner, J., Rouleau, J. L., & Murphy, W. D. (1987). Self-reported sex crimes of nonincarcerated paraphiliacs. *Journal of Interpersonal Violence, 2,* 3–25.

Abel, G. G., Osborn, C. A., Anthony, D., & Gardos, P. (1992). Current treatments of paraphiliacs. In J. Bancroft, C. M. Davis, & H. J. Ruppel (Eds.), *Annual review of sex research* (Vol. 3, pp. 255–290). Mount Vernon, IA: Society for the Scientific Study of Sex.

Abikoff, H., & Klein, R. G. (1992). Attention-deficit/hyperactivity and conduct disorder: Comorbidity and implications for treatment. *Journal of Consulting and Clinical Psychology, 60,* 881–892.

Abma, J. C., & Mott, F. L. (1991). Substance abuse and prenatal care during pregnancy among young women. *Family Planning Perspective, 23,* 117–122.

Abraham, P. P., Lepisto, B. L., Lewis, M. G., Schultz, L., & Finkelberg, S. (1994). An outcome study: Changes in Rorschach variables of adolescents in residential treatment. *Journal of Personality Assessment, 62,* 505–514.

Abramowitz, S. I. (1986). Psychosocial outcomes of sex. *Journal of Consulting and Clinical Psychology, 54,* 183–189.

Abrams, D. B., Emmons, K. M., Niaura, R., Goldstein, M. G., & Sherman, C. B. (1991). Tobacco dependence: An integration of individual and public health perspectives. *Annual Review of Addictions Research and Treatment, 1,* 391–436.

Abrams, K. K., Allen, L. R., & Gray, J. J. (1993). Disordered eating attitudes and behaviors, psychological adjustment, and ethnic identity: A comparison of black and white female college students. *International Journal of Eating Disorders, 14,* 49–58.

Abramson, L. Y., Metalsky, G. I., & Alloy, L. B. (1989). Hopelessness depression: A theory-based subtype of depression. *Psychological Review, 96*(2), 358–372.

Abramson, L. Y., Seligman, M. E. P., & Teasdale, J. (1978). Learned helplessness in humans: Critique and reformulation. *Journal of Abnormal Psychology, 87,* 32–48.

Achenbach, T. M., & Edelbrock, C. (1986). *Manual for the teacher's report form and teacher version of the child behavior profile.* Burlington, VT: University of Vermont.

Adachi, S., Kawamura, K., & Takemoto, K. (1993). Oxidative damage of nuclear DNA in liver of rats exposed to psychological stress. *Cancer Research, 53,* 4153–4155.

Adair, J. G., Dushenko, T. W., & Lindsay, R. C. L. (1985). Ethical regulations and their impact on research practice. *American Psychologist, 40,* 59–72.

Adams, R. D., & Victor, M. (1981). *Principles of neurology.* New York: McGraw-Hill.

Adler, N. E., Boyce, T., Chesney, M. A., Cohen, S., Folkman, S., Kahn, R. L., & Syme, S. L. (1994). Socioeconomic status and health: The challenge of the gradient. *American Psychologist, 49,* 15–24.

Adler, N. E., Boyce, T., Chesney, M., Folkman, S., & Syme, L. (1993). Socioeconomic inequalities in health: No easy solution. *Journal of the American Medical Association, 269,* 3140–3145.

Adler, N. E., David, H. P., Major, B. N., Roth, S. H., Russo, N. F., & Wyatt, G. E. (1990). Psychological responses after abortion. *Science, 248,* 41–43.

Adler, N. E., David, H. P., Major, B. N., Roth, S. H., Russo, N. F., & Wyatt, G. E. (1992). Psychological factors in abortion: A review. *American Psychologist, 47,* 1194–1204.

Agras, W. S. (1982). Behavioral medicine in the 1980s: Nonrandom connections. *Journal of Consulting and Clinical Psychology, 50,* 797–803.

Agras, W. S. (1993). Short-term psychological treatments for binge eating. In C. G. Fairburn & G. T. Wilson (Eds.), *Binge eating. Nature, assessment, and treatment* (pp. 270–286). New York: Guilford Press.

Agras, W. S., Rossiter, E. M., Arnow, B., Telch, C. F., Raeburn, S. D., Schneider, J., Bruce, B., Perl, M., & Koran, L. (1992). Pharmacologic and cognitive-behavioral treatment for bulimia nervosa: A controlled comparison. *American Journal of Psychiatry, 149,* 82–87.

Aiken, L. S., West, S. G., Woodward, C. K., & Reno, R. R. (1994). Health beliefs and compliance with mammography-screening recommendations in asymptomatic women. *Health Psychology, 13,* 122–129.

Ainsworth, M. D. S., & Bowlby, J. (1991). An ethological approach to personality development. *American Psychologist, 46,* 333–341.

Akiskal, H. S. (1991). Cyclothymic, hyperthymic, and depressive temperaments as subaffective variants of mood disorders. In A. Tasman & M. B. Riba (Eds.), *Review of psychiatry* (Vol. 11, pp. 43–62). Washington, DC: American Psychiatric Press.

Akiskal, H. S., Chen, S. E., Davis, G. C., Puzantian, V. R., Kashgarian, M., & Bolinger, J. M. (1985). Borderline: An adjective in search of a noun. *Journal of Clinical Psychiatry, 46,* 41–48.

Albert, M., & Silvers, K. N. (1970). Perceptual characteristics distinguishing auditory hallucinations in schizophrenia and acute alcoholic psychoses. *American Journal of Psychiatry, 127,* 298–302.

Alcoholics Anonymous. (1993). *Alcoholics Anonymous 1992 membership survey.* New York: Alcoholics Anonymous World Services.

Alden, L. E. (1988). Behavioral self-management controlled-drinking strategies in a context of secondary prevention. *Journal of Consulting and Clinical Psychology, 56,* 280–286.

Alden, L. E., & Capreol, M. J. (1993). Avoidant personality disorder: Interpersonal problems as predictors of treatment response. *Behavior Therapy, 24,* 357–376.

Aldridge, L. (1990). We must be our own heroes. *Journal of the California Alliance for the Mentally Ill, 1*(3), 20.

Alexander, F. (1950). *Psychosomatic medicine.* New York: W. W. Norton.

Alexander, J. F., Mas, C. H., & Waldron, H. (1988). Behavioral and systems family therapies or Auld Lang Syne: Shall old perspectives be forgot? In R. deV. Peters & R. J. McMahon (Eds.), *Social learning and systems approaches to marriage and the family.* New York: Brunner/Mazel.

Alexander, J. F., & Parsons, B. V. (1973). Short-term behavioral intervention with delinquent families: Impact on family process and recidivism. *Journal of Abnormal Psychology, 81,* 219–226.

Allen, L. S., & Gorski, R. A. (1992). Biology, brain architecture, and human sexuality. *Journal of National Institute of Health Research, 4,* 53–59.

Allen, M. G. (1976). Twin studies of affective illness. *Archives of General Psychiatry, 33,* 1476–1478.

Allport, G. W., & Odbert, H. S. (1936). Trait-names: A psycho-lexical study. *Psychological Monographs, 47* (1, Whole no. 211).

Altemus, M., Pigott, T., Kalogeras, K. T., Demitrack, M., Dubbert, B., Murphy, D. L., & Gold, P. W. (1992). Abnormalities in the regulation of vasopressin and corticotrophin releasing factor secretion in obsessive-compulsive disorder. *Archives of General Psychiatry, 49,* 9–20.

Althof, S. E., & Turner, L. A. (1992). Self-injection therapy and external vacuum devices in the treatment of erectile dysfunction: Methods and outcome. In R. C. Rosen & S. R. Leiblum (Eds.), *Erectile disorders: Assessment and treatment* (pp. 283–312). New York: Guilford Press.

Althof, S. E., Turner, L. A., Levine, S. B., Risen, C., Kursh, E., Bodner, D., & Resnick, M. (1991). Long-term use of self-injection therapy of papaverine and phentolamine. *Journal of Sex and Marital Therapy, 17,* 101–112.

Altura, B. M. (1986). Symposium on cardiovascular effects of ethanol. *Alcoholism: Clinical and Experimental Research, 10,* 557–559.

Aman, M., & Singh, N. (1991). Pharmacological intervention. In J. Matson & J. Mulick (Eds.), *Handbook of mental retardation* (2nd ed., pp. 347–372). Elmsford, NY: Pergamon Press.

Amato, P. R., & Keith, B. (1991). Parental divorce and the well-being of children: A meta analysis. *Psychological Bulletin, 110,* 26–46.

Ambelas, A. (1979). Psychologically stressful events in their precipitation of manic episodes. *British Journal of Psychiatry, 115,* 883–888.

American Medical Association. (1992). Violence: A compendium for *JAMA, American Medical News,* and speciality journals of the American Medical Association. Chicago, IL: American Medical Association.

American Psychiatric Association. (1952). *Diagnostic and statistical manual of mental disorders.* Washington, DC: American Psychiatric Association.

American Psychiatric Association. (1968). *Diagnostic and statistical manual of mental disorders* (2nd ed.). Washington, DC: American Psychiatric Association.

American Psychiatric Association. (1980). *Diagnostic and statistical manual of mental disorders* (3rd ed.). Washington, DC: American Psychiatric Association.

American Psychiatric Association. (1987). *Diagnostic and statistical manual of mental disorders* (3rd ed., rev.). Washington, DC: American Psychiatric Association.

American Psychiatric Association. (1993). Practice guidelines for major depressive disorder in adults. *American Journal of Psychiatry, 150*(4 Suppl.).

American Psychiatric Association. (1994). *Diagnostic and Statistical Manual of Mental Disorders* (4th ed.). Washington, DC: American Psychiatric Association.

American Psychiatric Association. (in press). *The DSM-IV sourcebook* (Vol. 2). Washington, DC: American Psychiatric Association.

American Psychiatric Association Task Force on Electroconvulsive Therapy. (1990). *The practice of electroconvulsive therapy: Recommendations for treatment, training, and privileging.* Washington, DC: American Psychiatric Press.

American Psychological Association. (1990a). Ethical principles of psychologists. *American Psychologist, 45,* 390–395.

American Psychological Association. (1990b). *Guidelines for psychological practice with ethnic and culturally diverse populations.* Washington, DC: American Psychological Association.

American Psychological Association. (1990c). *Practitioner Focus, 4,* 7.

American Psychological Association. (1991). Report of the Ethics Committee, 1989 and 1990. *American Psychologist, 46,* 750–757.

American Psychological Association. (1992). Ethical principles of psychologists and code of conduct. *American Psychologist, 47,* 1597–1611.

American Psychological Association. (1993a). *Guidelines for ethical conduct in the care and use of animals.* Washington, DC: American Psychological Association.

American Psychological Association. (1993b). Report of the Ethics Committee, 1991 and 1992. *American Psychologist, 48,* 811–820.

American Psychological Association. (1994). *Violence and the family.* Washington, DC: American Psychological Association.

Ames, G. (1993). Research and strategies for the primary prevention of workplace alcohol problems. *Alcohol Health & Research World, 17,* 19–27.

Andersen, B. L., Kiecolt-Glaser, J. K., & Glaser, R. (1994). A biobehavioral model of cancer stress and disease course. *American Psychologist, 49,* 389–404.

Anderson, C. M., Reiss, D. J., & Hogarty, G. E. (1986). *Schizophrenia and the family.* New York: Guilford Press.

Anderson, J. C., Williams, S., McGee, R., & Silva, P. A. (1987). DSM-III disorders in preadolescent children: Prevalence in a large sample from the general population. *Archives of General Psychiatry, 44,* 69–76.

Anderson, N. B., McNeilly, M., & Myers, H. (1991). Autonomic reactivity and hypertension in Blacks: A review and proposed model. *Ethnicity and Disease, 1,* 154–170.

Andrasik, F., Holroyd, K. A., & Abell, T. (1979). Prevalence of headache within a college student population: A preliminary analysis. *Headache, 20,* 384–387.

Andreasen, N. C. (1984). *The broken brain: The biological revolution in psychiatry.* New York: Harper & Row.

Andreasen, N. C. (Ed.). (1989). *Brain imaging: Applications in psychiatry.* Washington, DC: American Psychiatric Press.

Andreasen, N. C., & Black, D. W. (1991). *Introductory textbook of psychiatry.* Washington, DC: American Psychiatric Press.

Andreasen, N. C., & Black, D. W. (1995). *Introductory textbook of psychiatry* (2nd ed.). Washington, DC: American Psychiatric Press.

Andreasen, N. C., & Carpenter, W. T. (1993). Diagnosis and classification of schizophrenia. *Schizophrenia Bulletin, 19,* 199–214.

Andreasen, N., & Flaum, M. (1994). Characteristic symptoms of schizophrenia. In *DSM-IV sourcebook* (Vol. 1, pp. 351–380). Washington, DC: American Psychiatric Association.

Andreasen, N. C., Flaum, M., Swayze, V., O'Leary, D. S., Alliger, R., Cohen, G., Ehrhardt, J., & Yuh, W. T. C. (1993). Intelligence and brain structure in normal individuals. *American Journal of Psychiatry, 150,* 130–134.

Andreasen, N. C., Hoffman, R. E., & Grove, W. M. (1985). Mapping abnormalities in language and cognition. In M. Alpert (Ed.), *Controversies in schizophrenia: Changes and constancies.* New York: Guilford Press.

Andrews, G., Stewart, G., Morris-Yates, A., Holt, P., & Henderson, S. (1990). Evidence for a general neurotic syndrome. *British Journal of Psychiatry, 157,* 6–12.

Angier, N. (1993, October 12). An old idea about genius wins new scientific support. *New York Times,* p. B5.

Angst, J. (1966). *Zur atiologie und nosologie endogener depressiver psychosen.* Monographen aus der Neurologie und Psychiatry. No. 112. Berlin, Germany: Springer-Verlag.

Angst, J. (1992). Minor depression and recurrent brief depression. In H. S. Akiskal & G. B. Cassano (Eds.), *Chronic depressions and their treatment.* New York: Guilford Press.

Annis, H. M. (1986). A relapse prevention model for treatment of alcoholics. In W. R. Miller & N. Heather (Eds.), *Treating addictive behaviors: Processes of change* (pp. 407–433). New York: Plenum.

Antoni, M., Levine, J., Tischer, P., Green, C., & Millon, T. (1987). Refining personality assessments by combining MCMI high-point profiles and MMPI codes, Part V: MMPI 78/87. *Journal of Personality Assessment, 51,* 375–387.

Aponte, H., & Hoffman, L. (1973). The open door: A structural approach to a family with an anorexic child. *Family Process, 12,* 1–44.

Appelbaum, P. S. (1985). Civil commitment. In J. O. Cavenar, Jr., R. Michels, & H. K. H. Brodie (Eds.), *Psychiatry* (Vol. 3). Philadelphia: J. B. Lippincott.

Appelbaum, P. S. (1988a). The right to refuse treatment with antipsychotic medications: Retrospect and prospect. *American Journal of Psychiatry, 145,* 413–419.

Appelbaum, P. S. (1988b). The new preventive detention: Psychiatry's problematic responsibility for the control of violence. *American Journal of Psychiatry, 145,* 779–785.

Appelbaum, P. S., & Gutheil, T. G. (1991). *Clinical handbook of psychiatry and the law* (2nd ed.). Baltimore, MD: Williams & Wilkins.

Appelbaum, P. S., & Hamm, R. M. (1982). Decision to seek commitment. *Archives of General Psychiatry, 39,* 447–451.

Appelbaum, P. S., & Rosenbaum, A. (1989). *Tarasoff* and the researcher: Does the duty to protect apply in the research setting? *American Psychologist, 44,* 885–894.

Appelstein, C. D. (1994). *The Gus chronicles: Reflections from an abused kid.* Needham, MA: Albert E. Trieschman Center.

Archer, J. (1994, June). *What can ethology offer the study of human aggression?* Paper presented at the World Meeting, International Society for Research on Aggression, Delray, FL.

Aries, P. (1962). *Centuries of childhood: A social history of family life.* New York: Knopf.

Arieti, S. (1976). The psychotherapeutic approach to schizophrenia. In D. Kemali, G. Bartholini, & D. Richter (Eds.), *Schizophrenia today* (pp. 245–257). Oxford, England: Pergamon Press.

Arkowitz, H. (1992). Integrative theories of therapy. In D. K. Freedheim (Ed.), *History of psychotherapy: A century of change* (pp. 261–303). Washington, DC: American Psychological Association.

Arlow, J. A. (1989). Psychoanalysis. In R. J. Corsini & D. Wedding (Eds.), *Current psychotherapies*, 4th ed. (pp. 19–64). Itasca, IL: F. E. Peacock.

Arnold, D. S., O'Leary, S. G., Wolff, L. S., & Acker, M. M. (1993). The Parenting Scale: A measure of dysfunctional parenting in discipline situations. *Psychological Assessment, 5,* 137–144.

Arnow, B., Taylor, C. B., Agras, W. S., & Telch, M. (1985). Enhancing agoraphobia treatment outcome by changing couple communication patterns. *Behavior Therapy, 16,* 452–467.

Atkinson, J. W. (1983). *Personality, motivation, and action.* New York: Praeger.

Avery-Leaf, S., Cano, A., Cascardi, M., & O'Leary, K. D. (1995). *Evaluation of a dating violence prevention program.* Paper presented at the Fourth International Family Violence Research Conference, Durham, NH.

Ayllon, T., & Azrin, N. H. (1965). The measurement and reinforcement of psychotics. *Journal of the Experimental Analysis of Behavior, 8,* 357–383.

Azar, S. T., & Rohrbeck, C. A. (1986). Child abuse and unrealistic expectations: Further validation of the parent opinion questionnaire. *Journal of Consulting and Clinical Psychology, 54,* 867–868.

Azrin, N. H., Sneed, T. J., & Foxx, R. M. (1973). Dry bed: A rapid method of eliminating bedwetting (enuresis) of the retarded. *Behaviour Research and Therapy, II,* 427–434.

B

Babor, T. F., Brown, J., & Del Boca, F. K. (1990). Validity of self-reports in applied research on addictive behaviors: Fact or fiction. *Behavioral Assessment, 12,* 5–32.

Bachrach, L. L. (1984). Deinstitutionalization and women: Assessing the consequences of public policy. *American Psychologist, 39,* 1171–1177.

Bailey, A., Le Couteur, A., Rutter, M., Pickles, A., Yuzda, E., Schmidt, D., & Gottesman, I. I. (1991). *Obstetric and neurodevelopmental data from the British twin study of autism.* Paper presented at the Second World Congress on Psychiatric Genetics.

Bailey, J. M., Gaulin, S., Agyei, Y., & Gladue, B. A. (1994). Effects of gender and sexual orientation on evolutionarily relevant aspects of human mating psychology. *Journal of Personality and Social Psychology, 66,* 1081–1093.

Bailey, J. M., Pillard, R. C., Neale, M. E., & Agyei, Y. (1993). Heritable factors influence sexual orientation in women. *Archives of General Psychiatry, 50,* 217–223.

Baker, T. R., Sherman, J. E., & Morse, E. (1987). The motivation to use drugs: A psychobiological analysis of urges. In C. Rivers (Ed.), *The Nebraska symposium on motivation: Alcohol use and abuse.* Lincoln, NE: University of Nebraska Press.

Baldessarini, R. J., & Cole, J. O. (1988). Chemotherapy. In A. M. Nicholi, Jr. (Ed.), *The new Harvard guide to psychiatry.* Cambridge, MA: Harvard University Press.

Ball, J. C., & Ross, A. (1991). *The effectiveness of methadone maintenance.* New York: Springer-Verlag.

Bancroft, J. (1974). *Deviant sexual behaviour.* Oxford, England: Oxford University Press.

Bancroft, J. (1992). Foreword. In R. C. Rosen & S. R. Leiblum (Eds.), *Erectile disorders: Assessment and treatment* (pp. vii–xv). New York: Guilford Press.

Bancroft, J., Skrimshire, A., Casson, J., Harvard-Watts, O., & Reynolds, F. (1977). People who deliberately poison or injure themselves: Their problems and contacts with helping agencies. *Psychological Medicine, 7,* 289–303.

Bandura, A. (1969). *Principles of behavior modification.* Englewood Cliffs, NJ: Prentice Hall.

Bandura, A. (1973). *Aggression: A social learning analysis.* Englewood Cliffs, NJ: Prentice Hall.

Bandura, A. (1977). *Social learning theory.* Englewood Cliffs, NJ: Prentice Hall.

Bandura, A. (1986). *Social foundations of thought and action: A social cognitive theory.* Englewood Cliffs, NJ: Prentice Hall.

Bandura, A. (1989). Human agency in social cognitive theory. *American Psychologist, 44,* 1175–1184.

Bandura, A., & Menlove, F. L. (1968). Factors determining vicarious extinction of avoidance behavior through symbolic modeling. *Journal of Personality and Social Psychology, 8,* 99–108.

Bandura, A., Ross, D., & Ross, S. A. (1961). Transmission of aggression through imitation of aggressive models. *Journal of Abnormal and Social Psychology, 63,* 575–582.

Bandura, A., Ross, D., & Ross, S. A. (1963). Imitation of film-mediated aggressive models. *Journal of Abnormal and Social Psychology, 66,* 3–11.

Bandura, A., & Walters, R. H. (1959). *Adolescent aggression.* New York: Ronald Press.

Bandura, A., & Walters, R. H. (1963). *Social learning and personality development.* New York: Holt, Rinehart & Winston.

Bank, L., Marlowe, J. H., Reid, J. B., Patterson, G. R., & Weinrott, M. R. (1991). A comparative evaluation of parent training for families of chronic delinquents. *Journal of Abnormal Child Psychology, 19,* 15–33.

Barbaree, H. E., & Marshall, W. L. (1991). The role of male sexual arousal in rape: Six models. *Journal of Consulting and Clinical Psychology, 59,* 621–630.

Barbaree, H. E., Marshall, W. L., & Lanthier, R. D. (1979). Deviant sexual arousal in rapists. *Behaviour Research and Therapy, 17,* 215–222.

Barefoot v. Estelle, 459 U.S. 1169 (1983).

Barefoot, J. C., Dahlstrom, W. G., & Williams, R. G. (1983). Hostility, CHD incidence and total mortality: A 25-year follow up study of 255 physicians. *Psychosomatic Medicine, 245,* 59–63.

Barkley, R. A., & Cunningham, C. E. (1978). Do stimulant drugs improve the academic performance of hyperkinetic children? *Clinical Pediatrics, 17,* 85–92.

Barkley, R. A., & Cunningham, C. E. (1979). The effects of methylphenidate on the mother-child interactions of hyperactive children. *Archives of General Psychiatry, 36,* 201–208.

Barkley, R. A., Grodzinsky, & Dupaul, G. J. (1992). Frontal lobe functions in attention deficit disorder with and without hyperactivity: A review and research report. *Journal of Abnormal Child Psychology, 20,* 163–188.

Barley, W. D., Buie, S. E., Peterson, E. W., Hollingsworth, A. S., Griva, M., Hickerson, S. C., Lawson, J. E., & Bailey, B. J. (1993). Development of an inpatient cognitive-behavioral treatment program for borderline personality disorder. *Journal of Personality Disorders, 7,* 232–240.

Barling, J. (1990). *Employment, stress and the family functioning.* New York: John Wiley.

Barlow, D. H. (1986). Causes of sexual dysfunction: The role of anxiety and cognitive interference. *Journal of Consulting and Clinical Psychology, 54,* 140–148.

Barlow, D. H. (1988). *Anxiety and its disorders.* New York: Guilford Press.

Barlow, D. H. (Ed.). (1993). *Clinical handbook of psychological disorders.* New York: Guilford Press.

Barlow, D. H. (1994). Psychological interventions in the era of managed competition. *Clinical Psychology, 1,* 109–122.

Barlow, D. H., Abel, G. G., & Blanchard, E. B. (1979). Gender identity change in transsexuals. *Archives of General Psychiatry, 36,* 1001–1007.

Barlow, D. H., O'Brien, G. T., Last, C. G., & Holder, A. E. (1983). Couples treatment of agoraphobia: Initial outcome. In K. D. Craig & R. J. McMahon (Eds.), *Advances in clinical behavior therapy.* New York: Brunner/Mazel.

Barlow, D. H., Sakheim, D. K., & Beck, J. G. (1983). Anxiety increases sexual arousal. *Journal of Abnormal Psychology, 92,* 49–54.

Barnett, P., & Gotlib, I. H. (1988). Psychosocial functioning and depression: Distinguishing between antecedents, consequents and consequences. *Psychological Bulletin, 104,* 97–126.

Baron, R., & Richardson, D. R. (1994). *Human aggression* (2nd ed.). New York: Plenum.

Barr, C. E., Mednick, S. A., & Munk-Jorgenson, P. (1990). Exposure to epidemics during gestation and adult schizophrenia. *Archives of General Psychiatry, 47,* 869–874.

Barrios, B. A., & O'Dell, S. L. (1989). Fears and anxieties. In E. J. Mash and R. A. Barkley (Eds.), *Treatment of childhood disorders* (pp. 167–221). New York: Guilford Press.

Barrowclough, C., & Tarrier, N. (1992). Interventions with families. In M. Birchwood and N. Tarrier (Eds.), *Innovations in the psychologi-*

cal management of schizophrenia: Assessment, treatment and services (pp. 79–101). Chichester, England: John Wiley.

Barsky, A. J. (1992). Amplification, somatization, and the somatoform disorders. *Psychosomatics, 33,* 28–34.

Barsky, A. J., Barnett, M. C., & Cleary, P. D. (1994). Hypochondriasis and panic disorder. *Archives of General Psychiatry, 51,* 918–925.

Barsky, A. J., & Klerman, G. L. (1983). Overview: Hypochondriasis, bodily complaints and somatic styles. *American Journal of Psychiatry, 140,* 273–281.

Barsky, A. J., Wyshak, G., & Klerman, G. L. (1986). Hypochondriasis: An evaluation of the DSM-III criteria in medical outpatients. *Archives of General Psychiatry, 43,* 493–500.

Barsky, A. J., Wyshak, G., & Klerman, G. L. (1992). Psychiatric comorbidity in DSM-III-R hypochondriasis. *Archives of General Psychiatry, 49,* 101–108.

Bartlett, L., Ferrero, F., Szigethy, L., Giddey, C., & Pellizer, G. (1990). Expressed emotion and first-admission schizophrenia. Nine month follow-up in a French cultural environment. *British Journal of Psychiatry, 16,* 327–333.

Bastarrachea, J., Hortobagyi, G. N., Smith, T. L., Kau, S. W. C., & Buzdar, A. U. (1994). Obesity as an adverse prognostic factor for patients receiving adjuvant chemotherapy for breast cancer. *Annals of Internal Medicine, 119,* 18–25.

Bateson, G., Jackson, D. D., Haley, J., & Weakland, J. (1956). Toward a theory of schizophrenia. *Behavior Science, 1,* 251–264.

Baucom, D. H., & Epstein, N. (1990). *Cognitive-behavioral marital therapy.* New York: Brunner/Mazel.

Baxter, L. R. (1991). PET studies of cerebral function in major depression and obsessive-compulsive disorder: The emerging prefrontal cortex consensus. *Annals of Clinical Psychiatry, 3,* 103–109.

Baxter, L. R., Phelps, M. E., Mazziotta, J. C., Guze, B. H., Schwartz, J. M., & Selin, C. E. (1987). Local cerebral glucose metabolic rates in obsessive-compulsive disorder. *Archives of General Psychiatry, 44,* 211–281.

Baxter, L. R., Schwartz, J. M., Bergman, K. S., Szuba, M. P., Guze, B. H., Mazziotta, J. C., Alazraki, A., Selin, C. E., Ferng, H. K. Munford, P., & Phelps, M. E. (1992). Caudate glucose metabolic rate changes with both drug and behavior therapy for obsessive-compulsive disorder. *Archives of General Psychiatry, 49,* 681–689.

Baxter, L. R., Schwartz, J. M., Guze, B. H., Bergman, K., & Szuba, M. P. (1990). PET imaging in obsessive compulsive disorder with and without depression. *Journal of Clinical Psychiatry, 51,* 61–69.

Beach, S. R. H., Arias, I., & O'Leary, K. D. (1986). The relationship of marital satisfaction and social support to depressive symptomatology. *Journal of Psychopathology and Behavior Assessment, 8,* 305–316.

Beach, S. R. H., Jouriles, E. N., & O'Leary, K. D. (1985). Extramarital sex: Impact on depression and commitment in couples seeking marital therapy. *Journal of Sex and Marital Therapy, 11,* 99–108.

Beach, S. R. H., & O'Leary, K. D. (1985). Current status of outcome research in marital therapy. In L. L'Abate (Ed.), *The handbook of family psychology and therapy* (Vol. 2). Homewood, IL: Dorsey Press.

Beach, S. R. H., & O'Leary, K. D. (1986). The treatment of depression occurring in the context of marital discord. *Behavior Therapy, 17,* 43–49.

Beach, S. R. H., & O'Leary, K. D. (1993). Dysphoria and marital discord: Are dysphoric individuals at risk for marital maladjustment? *Journal of Marital and Family Therapy, 19,* 355–368.

Beach, S. R. H., Sandeen, E., & O'Leary, K. D. (1990). *Depression in marriage.* New York: Guilford Press.

Beach, S. R. H., Smith, D. A., & Fincham, F. D. (1994). Marital interventions for depression: Empirical foundation and future prospects. *Applied and Preventive Psychology, 3,* 233–250.

Beach, S. R. H., Whisman, M., & O'Leary, K. D. (1994). Marital therapy for depression: Theoretical foundation, current status, and future directions. *Behavior Therapy, 25,* 345–371.

Beardsley, R. S., Gardocki, G. J., Larson, D. B., & Hidalgo, J. (1988). Prescribing of psychotropic medication by primary care physicians and psychiatrists. *Archives of General Psychiatry, 45,* 1117–1119.

Beasley, C. M., Dornseif, B. E., Bosomworth, J. C., & Sayler, M. E. (1992). Fluoxetine and suicide: A meta-analysis of controlled trials of treatment for depression. *International Clinical Psychopharmacology, 6*(Suppl. 6), 35–57.

Beck, A. T. (1963). Thinking and depression: I. Idiosyncratic content and cognitive distortions. *Archives of General Psychiatry, 10,* 561–571.

Beck, A. T. (1967). *Depression: Causes and treatment.* Philadelphia: University of Pennsylvania Press.

Beck, A. T. (1976). *Cognitive therapy and the emotional disorders.* New York: International Universities Press.

Beck, A. T., Brown, G., Steer, R. A., & Eidelson, J. I. (1987). Differentiating anxiety and depression: A test of the cognitive content-specificity hypothesis. *Journal of Abnormal Psychology, 96,* 179–183.

Beck, A. T., Freeman, A., & Associates. (1990). *Cognitive therapy of personality disorders.* New York: Guilford Press.

Beck, A. T., Rush, A. J., Shaw, B. F., & Emery, G. (1979). *Cognitive therapy of depression.* New York: Guilford Press.

Beck, A. T., Steer, R. A., Sanderson, W. C., & Skeie, T. M. (1991). Panic disorder and suicidal ideation and behavior: Discrepant findings in psychiatric outpatients. *American Journal of Psychiatry, 148,* 1195–1199.

Beck, S. J. (1938). Personality structure in schizophrenia: A Rorschach investigation in eighty-one patients and sixty-four controls. *Nervous and Mental Diseases Monographs.* New York: Nervous and Mental Diseases Publishing.

Becker, J. V. (1988). Adolescent sex offenders. *Behavior Therapist, 11,* 185–188.

Becker, J. V., Skinner, L. J., & Abel, G. G. (1983). Sequellae of sexual assault: The survivor's perspective. In J. G. Greer & I. R. Stuart (Eds.), *The sexual aggressor: Current perspectives on treatment* (pp. 240–266). New York: Van Nostrand.

Begleiter, H., Porjesz, B., & Bihari, B. (1987). Auditory brainstem potentials in sons of alcoholic fathers. *Alcoholism: Clinical and Experimental Research, 11,* 447–480.

Begleiter, H., Porjesz, B., Bihari, B., & Kissin, B. (1984). Event-related potentials in boys at risk for alcoholism. *Science, 225,* 1493–1496.

Beitman, B. D., Goldfried, M. R., & Norcross, J. C. (1989). The movement toward integrating the psychotherapies: An overview. *American Journal of Psychiatry, 146,* 138–147.

Belitsky, R., & McGlashan, T. H. (1993). The manifestations of schizophrenia in late life: A dearth of data. *Schizophrenia Bulletin, 19,* 683–685.

Bellack, A. S., & Hersen, M. (1988). *Behavioral assessment: A practical handbook.* Elmsford, NY: Pergamon Press.

Bellack, A. S., & Mueser, K. T. (1994). Schizophrenia. In L. W. Craighead, W. E. Craighead, A. E. Kazdin, & M. J. Mahoney (Eds.), *Cognitive and behavioral interventions: An empirical approach to mental health problems* (pp. 105–122). Boston: Allyn and Bacon.

Ben-Eliyahu, S., Yirmiya, R., Liebeskind, J. C., Taylor, A. N., & Gayle, R. P. (1991). Stress increases metastatic spread of a mammary tumor in rats: Evidence for mediation by the immune system. *Brain, Behavior & Immunology, 325,* 606–612.

Ben-Porath, Y. S., & Waller, N. G. (1992). "Normal" personality inventories in clinical assessment: General requirements and the potential for using the NEO Personality Inventory. *Psychological Assessment, 4,* 14–19.

Benjamin, L. (1993). *An interpersonal approach to the* DSM *personality disorders.* New York: Guilford Press.

Benson, H. (1975). *The relaxation response.* New York: Morrow.

Benton, A. L. (1994). Neuropsychological assessment. In L. W. Porter & M. R. Rosenzweig (Eds.), *Annual review of psychology* (Vol. 45) (pp. 1–23). Palo Alto, CA: Annual Reviews.

Berg, F. (1991). Health risks escalate for black Americans. *Obesity and Health, 5,* 1–4.

Bergeman, C. S., Plomin, R., Pederson, N. L., McClearn, G. E., & Nesselroade, J. R. (1990). Genetic and environmental influences on social support: The Swedish adoption/twin study of aging. *Journal of Gerontology, 45,* 101–106.

Bergin, A. E. (1966). Some implications of psychotherapy research for therapeutic practice. *Journal of Abnormal Psychology, 71,* 235–246.

Berk, R. A. (1993). On the average, we can do no better than arrest. In R. J. Gelles and D. R. Loseke (Eds.), *Current controversies on family violence* (pp. 323–336). Newbury Park, CA: Sage.

Berkeley Planning Associates. (1983). *The exploration of client characteristics, services, and outcomes: Evaluation of the clinical demonstration projects on child abuse and neglect* (Contract No. 105-78-1108). Washington, DC: National Center on Child Abuse and Neglect.

Berkowitz, R., Stunkard, A. J., & Stallings, D. (in press). Binge-eating disorder in obese adolescent girls. In C. L. Williams & S. Kimm (Eds.), *Prevention and treatment of childhood obesity.* New York: New York Academy of Sciences.

Berman, A. L., & Jobes, D. A. (1990). *Adolescent suicide: Assessment and intervention.* Washington, DC: American Psychological Association.

Berman, J. S., & Norton, N. C. (1985). Does professional training make a therapist more effective? *Psychological Bulletin, 98,* 401–406.

Berman, K. F., & Weinberger, D. R. (1990). Laterization of cortical functioning during cognitive tasks: Regional cerebral blood flow studies of normal individuals and patients with schizophrenia. *Journal of Neurology, Neurosurgery, and Psychiatry, 53,* 150–160.

Bernard, J. (1972). *The future of marriage.* New Haven, CT: Yale University Press.

Bernstein, J. G. (1988). *Handbook of drug therapy in psychiatry.* Littleton, MA: John Wright–PSG.

Berry, J. C. (1967). *Antecedents of schizophrenia, impulsive character, and alcoholism in males.* Paper presented at the 75th Annual Convention of the American Psychological Association, Washington, DC.

Bettelheim, B. (1974). *A home for the heart.* New York: Knopf.

Beumont, P. J. V., Garner, D. M., & Touyz, S. W. (1994). Diagnoses of eating or dieting disorders: What may we learn from past mistakes? *International Journal of Eating Disorders, 16,* 349–362.

Bieber, I., Dain, H. J., Dince, P. R., Drellich, M. G., Grand, H. G., Gundlach, R. H., Kremer, M. W., Rifkin, A. H., Wilbur, C. B., & Bieber, T. B. (1962). *Homosexuality: A psychoanalytic study.* New York: Basic Books.

Biederman, J., Faraone, S. V., Keenan, K., Benjamin, J., Krifcher, B., Moore, C., Sprich-Buckminster, S., Ugaglia, K., Jellinek, M. S., Steingard, R., Spencer, T., Norman, D., Kolodny, R., Kraus, I., Perrin, J., Keller, M. B., & Tsuang, M. T. (1992). Further evidence for family-genetic risk factors in attention-deficit/hyperactivity disorder. *Archives of General Psychiatry, 49,* 728–738.

Bigelow, G., Cohen, M., Liebson, I., & Faillace, L. (1972). Abstinence or moderation? Choice by alcoholics. *Behaviour Research and Therapy, 10,* 209–214.

Bigelow, G., Liebson, I., & Griffiths, R. R. (1974). Alcohol drinking: Suppression by a behavioral time-out procedure. *Behaviour Research and Therapy, 12,* 107–115.

Binder, R. L., & McNiel, D. E. (1991). *Involuntary patients' right to refuse medication: Impact of the Riese decision on a California inpatient unit.* Paper presented at the annual meeting of the American Academy of Psychiatry and the Law, Orlando, FL.

The biochemistry of cocaine. (1989, August 24). *New York Times,* p. B7.

Birtchnell, J. (1993). Does recollection of exposure to poor maternal care in childhood affect later ability to relate? *British Journal of Psychiatry, 162,* 335–344.

Bjorntorp, P. (1986). Fat cells and obesity. In K. D. Brownell & J. P. Foreyt (Eds.), *Handbook of eating disorders* (pp. 88–98). New York: Basic Books.

Black, D. W., Noyes, R., Goldstein, R. B., & Blum, N. (1992). A family study of obsessive-compulsive disorder. *Archives of General Psychiatry, 49,* 362–368.

Black, D. W., Warrack, G., & Winokur, G. (1985). The Iowa record-linkage study. *Archives of General Psychiatry, 42,* 78–88.

Blakeslee, S. (1992, October 27). Nerve cell rhythm may be key to consciousness. *New York Times,* p. B5.

Blakeslee, S. (1993a, June 1). Scanner pinpoints site of thought as brain sees or speaks. *New York Times,* p. B5.

Blakeslee, S. (1993b, June 2). New therapies are helping men to overcome impotence. *New York Times,* p. C10.

Blanchard, E. B. (1981). Behavioral assessment of psychophysiologic disorders. In D. H. Barlow (Ed.), *Behavioral assessment of adult disorders.* New York: Guilford Press.

Blanchard, E. B. (1982). Behavioral medicine: Past, present, and future. *Journal of Consulting and Clinical Psychology, 50,* 795–796.

Blanchard, E. B. (1992). Psychological treatment of benign headache disorders. *Journal of Consulting and Clinical Psychology, 60,* 537–551.

Blanck, P. D., Bellack, A. S., Rosnow, R. L., Rotheram-Borus, M. J., & Schooler, N. R. (1992). Scientific rewards and conflicts of ethical choices in human subjects research. *American Psychologist, 47,* 959–965.

Bland, K., & Hallam, R. (1981). Relationship between response to graded exposure and marital satisfaction in agoraphobics. *Behaviour Research and Therapy. 19,* 335–338.

Blatt, S. (1974). Levels of object representation in anaclitic and introjective depression. *Psychoanalytic Study of the Child, 24,* 107–157.

Blatt, S. (1986). Where have we been and where are we going? Reflections on fifty years of personality assessment. *Journal of Personality Assessment, 50,* 343–346.

Blatt, S. (1992). The differential effect of psychotherapy and psychoanalysis with anaclitic and introjective patients: The Menninger psychotherapy research project revisited. *Journal of the American Psychoanalytic Association, 40,* 691–724.

Blatt, S., & Zuroff, D. (1992). Interpersonal relatedness and self-definition: Two prototypes for depression. *Clinical Psychology Review, 12,* 527–562.

Blazer, D. G., George, L. K., Landerman, R., Pennybacker, M., Melville, M. L., Woodbury, M., Manton, K. G., Jordan, K., & Locke, B. Z. (1985). Psychiatric disorders: A rural urban comparison. *Archives of General Psychiatry, 42,* 651–656.

Blazer, D. G., Kessler, R. C., McGonagle, K. A., & Swartz, M. S. (1994). The prevalence and distribution of major depression in a national community sample: The National Comorbidity Survey. *American Journal of Psychiatry, 151,* 979–986.

Bleuler, E. (1950). *Dementia praecox or the group of schizophrenias* (J. Zinkin, Trans.). New York: International University Press. (Original work published 1911)

Bleuler, M. (1974). The long-term course of schizophrenic psychoses. *Psychological Medicine, 4,* 244–254.

Bleuler, M. (1978). *The schizophrenic disorders: Long term patient and family studies.* New Haven: Yale University Press.

Bleuler, M. (1984). Different forms of childhood stress and patterns of adult psychiatric outcome. In N. F. Watt, E. J. Anthony, L. C. Wynne, & J. E. Rolf (Eds.), *Children at risk for schizophrenia: A longitudinal perspective.* New York: Cambridge University Press.

Blumenthal, J. A., Williams, R. B., Kong, Y., Schanberg, S. M., & Thompson, L. W. (1978). Type A behavior pattern and coronary arteriosclerosis. *Circulation, 258,* 63–69.

Boelens, W., Emmelkamp, P., MacGillavry, D., & Markvoort, M. A. (1980). A clinical evaluation of marital treatment: Reciprocity counseling versus system-theoretic counseling. *Behavioral Analysis and Modification, 4,* 85–96.

Boeringa, J. A., & Castellani, S. (1982). Reliability and validity of emotional blunting as a criterion for diagnosis of schizophrenia. *American Journal of Psychiatry, 139,* 1131–1135.

Bograd, M. (1988). Feminist perspectives on wife abuse: An introduction. In K. Yllo & M. Bograd (Eds.), *Feminist perspectives on wife abuse.* Newbury Park, CA: Sage.

Bohman, M., Cloninger, C. R., von Knorring, A. L., & Sigvardsson, S. (1984). An adoption study of somatoform disorders. III. Cross-fostering analysis and genetic relationship to alcoholism and criminality. *Archives of General Psychiatry, 41,* 872–878.

Bohman, M., Sigvardsson, S., & Cloninger, C. R. (1981). Maternal inheritance of alcohol abuse. *Archives of General Psychiatry, 38,* 965–969.

Boller, F. (1980). Mental status of patients with Parkinson's disease. *Journal of Clinical Neuropsychology, 2,* 157–172.

Böök, J. A. (1960). Genetical aspects of schizophrenic psychoses. In D. D. Jackson (Ed.), *The etiology of schizophrenia* (pp. 23–36). New York: Basic Books.

Boon, S., & Draijer, N. (1993). Multiple personality disorder in The Netherlands: A clinical investigation of 71 patients. *American Journal of Psychiatry, 150,* 489–494.

Borkovec, T. D., & Costello, E. (1993). Efficacy of applied relaxation and cognitive behavioral therapy in the treatment of generalized anxiety disorder. *Journal of Consulting and Clinical Psychology, 61,* 611–619.

Bornstein, R. A., Pace, P., Rosenberger, P., Nasrallah, H. A., Para, M. F., Whitacre, C. C., & Fass, R. J. (1993). Depression and neuropsychological performance in asymptomatic HIV infection. *American Journal of Psychiatry, 150,* 922–927.

Borod, J. C. (1992). Interhemispheric and intrahemispheric control of emotion: A focus on nonunilateral brain damage. *Journal of Consulting and Clinical Psychology, 60,* 339–348.

Borthwick-Duffy, S. A. (1994). Epidemiology and prevalence of psychopathology in people with mental retardation. *Journal of Consulting and Clinical Psychology, 62,* 17–27.

Botvin, G., Baker, E., Filazzola, A. D., & Botvin, E. M. (1990). A cognitive behavioral approach to substance abuse prevention: One-year follow-up. *Addictive Behavior, 15,* 47–63.

Bower, B. (1992). Depression boosts blood-vessel disease. *Science News, 141,* 196.

Bower, B. (1994). Assaults may amplify female alcoholism. *Science News, 146,* 5.

Bower, G. H. (1981). Mood and memory. *American Psychologist, 36,* 129–148.

Bower, G. H. (1986). Prime time in cognitive psychology. In P. Eelen & O. Fontaine (Eds.), *Behavior therapy: Beyond the conditioning framework.* Hillsdale, NJ: Lawrence Erlbaum.

Bower, G. H. (1987). Commenting on mood and memory. *Behaviour Research and Therapy, 25,* 443–456.

Bowers, T. G., & Al-Redha, M. R. (1990). A comparison of outcome with group/marital and standard/individual therapies with alcoholics. *Journal of Studies on Alcohol, 51,* 301–309.

Bowlby, J. (1973). *Attachment and loss* (Vols. 1 & 2). New York: Basic Books.

Boyer, J. L. (1990). Assuming risk in child custody evaluations. *Register Report, 16,* 13–14.

Bradbury, T. N., & Fincham, F. D. (1993). Assessing dysfunctional cognition in marriage: A reconsideration of the Relationship Belief Inventory. *Psychological Assessment, 5,* 92–101.

Braddock, D., & Fujiura, G. (1991). Politics, public policies, and the development of community services in the United States. *American Journal of Mental Retardation, 95,* 369–387.

Bradford, J. (1989). The organic treatment of violent sexual offenders. In A. J. Stunkard & A. Baum (Eds.), *Perspectives in behavioral medicine* (pp. 203–221). Hillsdale, NJ: Lawrence Erlbaum.

Bradley, C. (1937). The behavior of children receiving Benzedrine. *American Journal of Psychiatry, 94,* 577–585.

Bradsher, K. (1995, August 14). Low ranking for poor American children. *New York Times,* p. A9.

Brady, J. P. (1976). Behavior therapy and sex therapy. *American Journal of Psychiatry, 133,* 896–899.

Brakel, S. J. (1986). Involuntary institutionalization. In S. J. Brakel, J. Parry, & B. A. Weiner (Eds.), *The mentally disabled and the law.* Chicago: American Bar Foundation.

Brawman-Mintzer, O., Lydiard, R. B., Emmanuel, N., Payeur, R., Johnson, M., Roberts, J., Jarrell, M. P., & Ballenger, J. C. (1993). Psychiatric comorbidity in patients with generalized anxiety disorder. *American Journal of Psychiatry, 150,* 1216–1218.

Bray, G. A., & Gray, D. S. (1988). Obesity. Part 1—Pathogenesis. *Western Journal of Medicine, 149,* 429–441.

Breggin, P. R. (1991). *Toxic psychiatry.* New York: St. Martin's Press.

Breggin, P. R. (1994). *Talking back to Prozac.* New York: St. Martin's Press.

Bremner, J. D., Southwick, S., Johnson, D. R., Yehuda, R., & Charney, D. (1993). Childhood physical abuse and combat-related post-traumatic stress disorder in Vietnam veterans. *American Journal of Psychiatry, 150,* 235–239.

Bremner, J. D., Steinberg, M., Southwick, S. M., Johnson, D. R., & Charney, D. S. (1993). Use of the structured clinical interview for DSM-IV dissociative disorders for systematic assessment of dissociative symptoms in posttraumatic stress disorder. *American Journal of Psychiatry, 150,* 1011–1014.

Brennan, P., Mednick, S., & Kandel, E. (1991). Congenital determinants of violent and property offending. In D. J. Pepler & K. H. Rubin (Eds.), *The development and treatment of childhood aggression* (pp. 81–92). Hillside, NJ: Lawrence Erlbaum.

Breslau, N., Davis, G. C., Andreski, P., & Peterson, E. (1991). Traumatic events and posttraumatic stress disorder in an urban population of young adults. *Archives of General Psychiatry, 48,* 216–222.

Breuer, J., & Freud, S. (1895). Studies on hysteria. In J. Strachey (Ed.), *The standard edition of the complete psychological works of Sigmund Freud* (Vol. 2). London, England: Hogarth Press.

Breuer, J., & Freud, S. (1957). *Studies on hysteria.* New York: Basic Books. (Original work published 1895)

Brewer, J. A. (1995). *Introduction to early childhood education: Preschool through primary grades* (2nd ed.). Boston: Allyn and Bacon.

Briddell, D. W., Rimm, D., Caddy, G., Krawitz, G., Sholis, D., & Wunderlin, R. (1978). The effects of alcohol and expectancy set on male sexual arousal. *Journal of Abnormal Psychology, 82,* 418–430.

Brier, A., Buchanan, R. W., Irish, D., & Carpenter, W. T. (1993). Clozapine treatment of outpatients with schizophrenia: Outcome and long-term response patterns. *Hospital and Community Psychiatry, 44,* 1145–1149.

Brigham, A. (1994). The moral treatment of insanity. *American Journal of Insanity, 151*(June suppl.), 10–15. (Original work published in 1847)

Brinkman, S. D., & Largen, J. W. (1984). Changes in brain ventricular size with repeated CAT scans in suspected Alzheimer's disease. *American Journal of Psychiatry, 141,* 81–83.

Bristol-Myers Squibb. (1995). D5-K001. Princeton, NJ: Bristol-Myers Squibb.

Brody, J. E. (1994, December 14). Personal health: Prostate patients "learn to hope by sharing." *New York Times,* p. C12.

Brooks, A. D. (1994). The civil commitment of pathologically violent sex offenders. *Administration and Policy in Mental Health, 21,* 417–428.

Brown, G. W. (1959). Experiences of discharged chronic schizophrenic mental hospital patients in various types of living groups. *Millbank Memorial Fund Quarterly, 37,* 105–131.

Brown, G. W., Birley, J. L. T., & Wing, J. K. (1972). Influence of family life on the course of schizophrenic disorders: A replication. *British Journal of Psychiatry, 121,* 241–258.

Brown, G. W., Carstairs, G. M., & Topping, G. C. (1958). The post hospital adjustment of chronic mental patients. *Lancet, II,* 685–689.

Brown, G. W., & Davidson, S. (1978). Social class, psychiatric disorder of mother, and accidents to children. *Lancet, 1,* 378.

Brown, G. W., & Harris, T. (1978). *Social origins of depression: A study of psychiatric disorder in women.* New York: Free Press.

Brown, G. W., Harris, T., & Hepworth, C. (1994). Life events and endogenous depression: A puzzle reexamined. *Archives of General Psychiatry, 51,* 524–534.

Brown, G. W., Monck, E. M., Carstairs, G. M., & Wing, J. K. (1962). The influence of family life on the course of schizophrenic illness. *British Journal of Preventative Social Medicine, 16,* 55–68.

Brown, J. M., & Miller, W. R. (1993). Impact of motivational interviewing on participation and outcome in residential alcoholism treatment. *Psychology of Addictive Behaviors, 7,* 211–218.

Brown, R. (1965). *Social psychology.* New York: Free Press.

Brown, T. A., O'Leary, T. A., & Barlow, D. H. (1993). Generalized anxiety disorder. In D. H. Barlow (Ed.), *Clinical handbook of psychological disorders* (pp. 137–188). New York: Guilford Press.

Browne, A., & Williams, W. R. (1993). Gender, intimacy, and lethal violence: Trends from 1976 through 1987. *Gender and Society, 7,* 78–98.

Brownell, K. D., Hayes, S. C., & Barlow, D. H. (1977). Patterns of appropriate and deviant sexual arousal: The behavioral treatment of multiple sexual deviations. *Journal of Consulting and Clinical Psychology, 45,* 1144–1155.

Brownell, K. D., & Rodin, J. (1992). *Medical, metabolic and psychological effects of weight cycling.* Unpublished manuscript, Yale University.

Brownell, K. D., & Wadden T. A. (1992). Etiology and treatment of obesity. *Journal of Consulting and Clinical Psychology, 60,* 505–517.

Brownmiller, S. (1975). *Against our will: Men, women, and rape.* New York: Simon & Schuster.

Bruce, M. L., Takeuchi, D. T., & Leaf, P. J. (1991). Poverty and psychiatric status: Longitudinal evidence from the New Haven Epidemiologic Catchment Area Study. *Archives of General Psychiatry, 48,* 470–474.

Bruch, H. (1978). *The golden cage: The enigma of anorexia nervosa.* New York: Basic Books.

Brunk, M., Henggler, S. W., & Whelan, J. P. (1987). Comparison of multisystemic therapy and parent training in the brief treatment of child abuse and neglect. *Journal of Consulting and Clinical Psychology, 55,* 171–178.

Bryson, S. E., Clark, B. S., & Smith, I. M. (1988). First report of a Canadian epidemiological study of autistic syndromes. *Journal of Child Psychology and Psychiatry, 29,* 433–445.

Buchanan, R. D. (1994). The development of the Minnesota Multiphasic Personality Inventory. *Journal of Clinical Psychology, 30,* 148–161.

Buchsbaum, M. S. (1990). Frontal lobes, basal ganglia, temporal lobes—Three sites for schizophrenia. *Schizophrenia Bulletin, 16,* 379–389.

Bunney, W. E., Goodwin, F. K., & Murphy, D. L. (1992). Affective illness: Two decades of psychobiological investigations. *Pharmacopsychiatry, 25,* 10–13.

Burack, J. A. (1994). Selective attention deficits in persons with autism: Preliminary evidence of an inefficient attentional lens. *Journal of Abnormal Psychology, 103,* 535–543.

Burisch, M. (1984). Approaches to personality inventory construction. *American Psychologist, 39,* 214–227.

Burling, T. A., Lovett, S. B., Frederiksen, L. W., Jerome, A., & Jonske-Gubosh, L.-A. (1989). Can across-treatment changes in cumulative puff duration predict treatment outcome during nicotine fading? *Addictive Behaviors, 14,* 75–82.

Burnam, M. A., Hough, R. L., Escobar, J. I., Karno, M., Timbers, D. M., Telles, C. A., & Locke, B. Z. (1987). Six-month prevalence of specific psychiatric disorders among Mexican Americans and non-Hispanic whites in Los Angeles. *Archives of General Psychiatry, 44,* 687–694.

Burnam, M. A., Stein, J. A., Golding, J. M., Siegel, J. M., Sorenson, S. B., Forsythe, A. B., & Telles, C. A. (1988). Sexual assault and mental disorders in a community population. *Journal of Consulting and Clinical Psychology, 56,* 843–850.

Burton, R. (1973). *The anatomy of melancholia.* New York: AMA Press. (Original work published 1624)

Butcher, J. N., Dahlstrom, W. E., Graham, J. R., Teilegen, A., & Kaemmer, B. (1989). *Manual for the restandardized Minnesota Multiphasic Personality Inventory: MMPI-2.* Minneapolis, MN: University of Minnesota Press.

Butler, A. C., Hokanson, J. E., & Flynn, H. A. (1994). A comparison of self-esteem lability and low trait self-esteem as vulnerability factors for depression. *Journal of Personality & Social Psychology, 66,* 166–177.

Butler, G., Cullington, A., Munby, M., Amies, P., & Gelder, M. (1984). Exposure and anxiety management in the treatment of social phobia. *Journal of Consulting and Clinical Psychology, 52,* 642–669.

Butler, G., Fennell, M., Robson, P., & Gelder, M. (1991). Comparison of behavior therapy and cognitive-behavior therapy in the treatment of generalized anxiety disorder. *Journal of Consulting and Clinical Psychology, 59,* 167–175.

Butow, P., Beumont, P., & Touyz, S. (1993). Cognitive processes in dieting disorders. *International Journal of Eating Disorders, 14,* 319–330.

Butters, N., & Stuss, D. T. (1989). Diencephalic amnesia. In F. Bolero & J. Grafman (Eds.), *Handbook of neuropsychology* (Vol. 3, pp. 102–115). Amsterdam, The Netherlands: Elsevier.

Buvat, J., Buvat-Herbaut, M., Lemaire, A., Marcolin, G., & Quittelier, E. (1990). Recent developments in the clinical assessment and diagnosis of erectile dysfunction. *Annual Review of Sex Research, 1,* 265–308.

Byne, W., & Parsons, B. (1993). Human sexual orientation. *Archives of General Psychiatry, 50,* 228–239.

C

Cacioppo, J. T., & Berntson, G. G. (1992). Social psychological contributions to the decade of the brain. *American Psychologist, 47,* 1019–1028.

Cadoret, R. J., O'Gorman, T. W., Troughton, E., & Heywood, E. (1985). Alcoholism and antisocial personality. *Archives of General Psychiatry, 42,* 161–167.

Cadoret, R. J., & Stewart, M. A. (1991). An adoption study of attention deficit/hyperactivity/aggression and their relationship to adult antisocial personality. *Comprehensive Psychiatry, 32,* 73–82.

Cadoret, R. J., Troughton, E., O'Gorman, T. W., & Heywood, E. (1986). An adoption study of genetic and environmental factors in drug abuse. *Archives of General Psychiatry, 43,* 1131–1136.

Calhoun, K. S., & Resick, P. A. (1993). Post-traumatic stress disorder. In D. H. Barlow (Ed.), *Clinical handbook of psychological disorders: A step by step treatment manual* (2nd ed., pp. 48–98). New York: Guilford Press.

Camp, N. M. (1993). The Vietnam War and the ethics of combat psychiatry. *American Journal of Psychiatry, 150,* 1000–1010.

Campbell, M., Cohen, I. L., Perry, R., & Small, A. M. (1989). Psychopharmacological treatment. In T. H. Ollendick & M. Hersen (Eds.), *Handbook of child psychopathology* (2nd ed., pp. 473–497). New York: Plenum.

Canino, G. J., Bird, H. R., Shrout, P. E., Rubio-Stipec, M., Bravo, M., Martinez, R., Sesman, M., & Guevara, L. M. (1987). The prevalence of specific psychiatric disorders in Puerto Rico. *Archives of General Psychiatry, 44,* 727–735.

Cannon, T. D., Zorrilla, L. E., Shtasel, D., Gur, R. E., Gur, R. C., Marco, E. J., Moberg, P., & Price, R. A. (1994). Neuropsychological functioning in siblings discordant for schizophrenia and healthy volunteers. *Archives of General Psychiatry, 51,* 651–661.

Cantos, A. L., Neidig, P. H., & O'Leary, K. D. (1994). Injuries of women and men in a treatment program for domestic violence. *Journal of Family Violence, 9,* 113–124.

Cantwell, D. P. (1983). Issues in the management of childhood depression. In D. P. Cantwell & G. A. Carlson (Eds.), *Affective disorders in childhood and adolescence: An update* (pp. 354–362). New York: SP Medical & Scientific Books.

Cardon, L. R., Smith, S. D., Fulker, D. W., Kimberling, W. J., Pennington, B. F., & DeFries, J. C. (1994). Quantitative trait locus for reading disability on chromosome 6. *Science, 266,* 276–279.

Carey, G., & DiLalla, D. L. (1994). Personality and psychopathology: Genetic perspectives. *Journal of Abnormal Psychology, 103,* 32–43.

Carey, M. P., Wincze, J. P., & Meisler, A. W. (1993). Sexual dysfunction: Male erectile disorder. In D. H. Barlow (Ed.), *Clinical handbook of psychological disorders* (pp. 442–480). New York: Guilford Press.

Carlson, C. L., Pelham, W. E., Milich, R., & Dixon, J. (1992). Single and combined effects of methylphenidate and behavior therapy on the classroom performance of children with attention-deficit/hyperactivity disorder. *Journal of Abnormal Child Psychology, 20,* 213–232.

Carlson, G. A., & Cantwell, D. P. (1980). A survey of depressive symptoms, syndrome, and disorder in a child and adolescent psychiatric population. *Journal of Child Psychology and Psychiatry, 21,* 19–25.

Carmody, T. P., & Matarazzo, J. D. (1991). Health psychology. In M. Hersen, A. E. Kazdin, & A. S. Bellack (Eds.), *The clinical psychology handbook* (2nd ed.) (pp. 695–723). New York: Pergamon Press.

Carpenter, W. T., Stephens, J. H., Rey, A. C., Hanlon, T. E., & Heinrichs, D. W. (1982). Early intervention vs. continuous pharmacotherapy of schizophrenia. *Psychopharmacology Bulletin, 18,* 21–23.

Carr, E. G., Robinson, S., Taylor, J. C., & Carlson, J. I. (1990). *Positive approaches to the treatment of severe behavior problems in persons with developmental disabilities: A review and analysis of reinforcement and stimulus-based procedures* (Monograph No. 4). Seattle, WA: The Association for Persons with Severe Handicaps.

Carroll, B. J., Feinberg, M., Greden, J. F., Tarika, J., Albala, A. A., Haskett, R. F., James, N. M., Kronfol, Z., Lohr, N., Steiner, M., de Vigne, J. P., & Young, E. (1981). A specific laboratory test for the diagnosis of melancholia. *Archives of General Psychiatry, 38,* 15–22.

Cascardi, M. C., Langhinrichsen, J., & Vivian, D. (1992). Marital aggression: Impact, injury, and health correlates for husbands and wives. *Archives of Internal Medicine, 152,* 1178–1184.

Cascardi, M., O'Leary, K. D., Lawrence, E. E., & Schlee, K. A. (1995a). Characteristics of women physically abused by their spouses who seek treatment regarding marital conflict. *Journal of Consulting and Clinical Psychology, 63,* 616–623.

Cascardi, M. C., O'Leary, K. D., Schlee, K. A., & Lawrence, E. (1995b). Major depressive disorder and posttraumatic stress disorder in physically abused women. *Journal of Consulting and Clinical Psychology, 63,* 616–623.

Cascardi, M. C., & Vivian, D. (1995). Context for specific episodes of marital violence: Gender and severity of violence differences. *Journal of Family Violence.*

Cassileth, B. R., Lusk, E. J., Miller, D. S., Brown, L. L., & Miller, C. (1985). Psychosocial correlates of survival in advanced malignant disease? *New England Journal of Medicine, 312,* 1551–1555.

Caton, C. L. M., Wyatt, R. J., Felix, A., Grunberg, J., & Dominguez, M. S. (1993). Follow-up of chronically homeless mentally ill men. *American Journal of Psychiatry, 150,* 1639–1642.

Cattell, R. B., & Stice, G. F. (1957). *Handbook for the 16 Personality Factor Questionnaire.* Champaign, IL: Institute for Personality and Ability Testing.

Cavanaugh, J. C., & Park, D. C. (1993). Vitality for life: Psychological research for productive aging [Special issue, Human capital initiative, report 2]. *APS Observer.*

Cazenave, N. A., & Straus, M. A. (1992). Race, class, network embeddedness, and family violence: A search for potent support systems. In M. A. Straus & R. J. Gelles (Eds.), *Physical violence in American families: Risk factors and adaptations to violence in 8,145 families* (pp. 321–339). New Brunswick, NJ: Transaction.

Centers for Disease Control Vietnam Experience Study. (1987). Postservice mortality among Vietnam veterans. *Journal of the American Medical Association, 257,* 790–795.

Centerwall, B. S. (1992). Television and violence: The scale of the problem and where to go from here. *Journal of the American Medical Association, 267,* 3059–3063.

Cepeda-Benito, A. (1993). Meta-analytic review of the efficacy of nicotine chewing gum in smoking treatment programs. *Journal of Consulting and Clinical Psychology, 61,* 822–830.

Cermak, T. L. (1988). *A time to heal.* New York: Avon Books.

Cerreto, M. C., & Tuma, J. M. (1977). Distribution of DSM-III diagnoses in a child psychiatric setting. *Journal of Abnormal Child Psychology, 5,* 147–155.

Chambless, D. (1993). *Task force on promotion and dissemination of psychological procedures.* Unpublished manuscript, Division 12, American Psychological Association.

Chambless, D. L., & Mason, J. (1986). Sex, sex role stereotyping, and agoraphobia. *Behaviour Research and Therapy, 24,* 231–235.

Chang, S. S., & Renshaw, D. C. (1986). Psychosis and pregnancy. *Comprehensive Therapy, 12,* 36–41.

Charney, D. S., Deutch, A. Y., Krystal, J. H., Southwick, S. M., & Davis, M. (1993). Psychobiologic mechanisms of post-traumatic stress disorder. *Archives of General Psychiatry, 50,* 294–305.

Charney, D. S., Goodman, W. K., Price, L. H., Woods, S. W., Rasmussen, S. A., & Heninger, G. R. (1988). Serotonin function in obsessive-compulsive disorder. *Archives of General Psychiatry, 45,* 177–185.

Chesney, M. A. (1993). Health psychology in the 21st century: Acquired immunodeficiency syndrome as a harbinger of things to come. *Health Psychology, 12,* 259–268.

Chesney-Lind, M. (1987). Girls and violence: An exploration of the gender gap in serious delinquent behavior. In D. H. Crowell, I. M. Evand, & C. R. O'Donnell (Eds.), *Childhood aggression and violence* (pp. 211–230). New York: Plenum.

Chien, C. (1993). Ethnopsychopharmacology. In A. G. Gaw (Ed.), *Culture, ethnicity, and mental illness* (pp. 413–430). Washington, DC: American Psychiatric Association.

Children's Defense Fund. (1991). *Leave no child behind.* Washington, DC: Children's Defense Fund.

Chipuer, H. M., Rovine, M., & Plomin, R. (1990). LISREL modelling: Genetic and environmental influences on IQ revisited. *Intelligence, 14,* 11–29.

Chiu, T. M., Mendelson, J. H., Woods, B. T., Teoh, S. K., Levisohn, L., & Mello, N. K. (1994). In vivo proton magnetic resonance spectroscopy detection of human alcohol tolerance. *Magnetic Resonance Medicine, 32,* 511–516.

Chodoff, P. (1974). The diagnosis of hysteria: An overview. *American Journal of Psychiatry, 131,* 1073–1078.

Chodoff, P., & Lyons, H. (1958). Hysteria, the hysterical personality and "hysterical" conversion. *American Journal of Psychiatry, 114,* 734–740.

Christensen, A., & Jacobson, N. S. (1994). Who (or what) can do psychotherapy: The status and challenge of nonprofessional therapies. *Psychological Science, 5,* 8–14.

Christensen, A., Jacobson, N. S., & Babcock, J. C. (1995). Integrative behavioral couples therapy. In N. S. Jacobson & A. S. Gurman, *Clinical handbook of couples therapy* (pp. 31–64). New York: Guilford Press.

Christensen, J. K., Moller, I. W., Ronsted, P., Angelo, H. R., & Johansson, B. (1991). Dose-effect relationship of disulfiram in human volunteers: I. Clinical studies. *Pharmacology and Toxicology, 68,* 163–165.

Christian-Herman, J., Avery-Leaf, S., & O'Leary, K. D. (1994, August). *Impact of negative marital events on depression.* Paper presented at the American Psychological Association, Los Angeles, CA.

Christiansen, B. A., Goldman, M. S., & Inn, A. (1982). The development of alcohol-related expectancies in adolescents. *Journal of Consulting and Clinical Psychology, 50,* 336–344.

Chun, Z. F., Mitchell, J. E., Li, K., Yu, W. M., Lan, Y. D., Jun, Z., Rong, Z. Y., Huan, Z. Z., Filice, G. A., Pomeroy, C., & Pyle, R. L. (1992). The prevalence of anorexia nervosa and bulimia nervosa among freshman medical college students in China. *International Journal of Eating Disorders, 12,* 209–214.

City of Cleburne v. Cleburne Living Center Inc., 473 U.S. 432 (1985).

Clark, C. R. (1990). Agreeing to be an expert witness: Considerations of competence and role integrity. *Register Report, 16,* 16–17.

Clark, D. A., Beck, A. T., & Stewart, B. (1990). Cognitive specificity and positive-negative affectivity: Complementary or contradictory view on anxiety and depression? *Journal of Abnormal Psychology, 99,* 148–155.

Clark, D. A., Steer, R. A., & Beck, A. T. (1994). Common and specific dimensions of self-reported anxiety and depression. Implications for the cognitive and tripartite models. *Journal of Abnormal Psychology, 103,* 645–654.

Clark, D. B., Turner, S. M., Beidel, D. C., Donovan, J. E., Kirisci, L., & Jacob, R. G. (1994). Reliability and validity of the Social Phobia and Anxiety Inventory for adolescents. *Psychological Assessment, 6,* 135–140.

Clark, D. M. (1986). A cognitive approach to panic. *Behaviour Research and Therapy, 24,* 461–470.

Clark, D. M. (1988). A cognitive model of panic attacks. In S. Rachman & J. Maser (Eds.), *Panic: Cognitive views* (pp. 71–90). Hillsdale, NJ: Lawrence Erlbaum.

Clark, D. M. (1989). Anxiety states. In K. Hawton, P. M. Salkovskis, & D. M. Clark (Eds.), *Cognitive behaviour therapy for psychiatric problems* (pp. 52–96). Oxford, England: Oxford University Press.

Clark, D. M., & Ehlers, A. (1993). An overview of the cognitive theory and treatment of panic disorder. *Applied and Preventive Psychology, 2,* 131–139.

Clark, D. M., Salkovskis, P. M., Hackmann, A., Middleton, H., Anastasiades, P., & Gelder, M. (1994). A comparison of cognitive therapy, applied relaxation and imipramine in the treatment of panic disorder. *British Journal of Psychiatry, 164,* 759–769.

Clark, L. A. (1993). *Schedule for Nonadaptive and Adaptive Personality (SNAP).* Minneapolis: University of Minnesota Press.

Clark, L. A., & Livesley, W. J. (1994). Two approaches to identifying the dimensions of personality disorder: Convergence on the five-factor model. In P. T. Costa, Jr., & T. Widiger (Eds.), *Personality disorders and the five-factor model of personality* (pp. 261–278). Washington, DC: American Psychological Association.

Clark, L. A., Livesley, W. J., Schroeder, M. L., & Irish, S. L. (1995). Convergence of two systems for assessing specific traits of personality disorder. Manuscript submitted for publication.

Clark, L. A., & Watson, D. B. (1991a). General affective dispositions in physical and psychological health. In C. R. Snyder & D. R. Forsyth (Eds.). *Handbook of social and clinical psychology: The health perspective* (pp. 221–245). New York: Pergamon Press.

Clark, L. A., & Watson, D. B. (1991b). Tripartite model of anxiety and depression: Psychometric evidence and taxonomic implications. *Journal of Abnormal Psychology, 100,* 316–336.

Clark, L. A., Watson, D. B., & Mineka, S. (1994). Temperament, personality, and the mood and anxiety disorders. *Journal of Abnormal Psychology, 103,* 103–116.

Clark, L. A., Watson, D., & Reynolds, S. (1995). Diagnosis and classification of psychopathology: Challenges to the current system and future directions. *Annual Review of Psychology, 46,* 121–153.

Clark, L. P. (1933). *Lincoln: A psychobiography.* New York: Scribner.

Clavelle, P. R. (1992). Clinicians' perceptions of the comparability of the MMPI and MMPI-2. *Psychological Assessment, 4,* 466–472.

Cleckley, H. (1982). *The mask of sanity* (6th ed.). St. Louis, MO: Mosby. (Original work published 1941)

Clements, S. D. (1966). *Minimal brain dysfunction in children—terminology and identification* (USPHS Publication No. 1415). Washington, DC: U.S. Government Printing Office.

Clomipramine Collaborative Study Group, The. (1991). Clomipramine in the treatment of patients with obsessive-compulsive disorder. *Archives of General Psychiatry, 48,* 730–738.

Cloninger, C. R. (1981). Inheritance of alcohol abuse: Cross-fostering analysis of adopted men. *Archives of General Psychiatry, 38,* 861–868.

Cloninger, C. R. (1987). Neurogenetic adaptive mechanisms in alcoholism. *Science, 236,* 410–416.

Cloninger, C. R., Bohman, M., & Sigvardsson, S. (1981). Inheritance of alcohol abuse: Cross-fostering analysis of adopted men. *Archives of General Psychiatry, 38,* 861–868.

Cloninger, C. R., & Gottesman, I. I. (1987). Genetic and environmental factors in antisocial behavior disorders. In S. P. A. Mednick, T. E. Moffitt, & S. A. Stack (Eds.), *The causes of crime: New biological approaches* (pp. 92–109). New York: Cambridge University Press.

Cloninger, C. R., Svrakic, D. M., & Przybeck, T. R. (in press). A psychobiological model of temperament and character. *Archives of General Psychiatry.*

Closing the gap. (1990). Washington, DC: U.S. Department of Health and Human Services, Office of Minority Health.

Coates, T. J. (1993). Prevention of HIV infection: Accomplishments and priorities. *The Journal of NIH Research, 5,* 73–76.

Cobb, J. P., McDonald, R., Marks, I. M., & Atern, R. S. (1980). Marital versus exposure therapy: Psychological treatments of co-existing marital and phobic-obsessive problems. *European Journal of Behavioural Analysis and Modification, 4,* 3–17.

Coccaro, E. F. (1993). Psychological studies in patients with personality disorders: Review and perspective. *Journal of Personality Disorders,* Special Supplement, 181–192.

Cohen, F., Horowitz, M., Lazarus, R., Moos, R., Robins, L., Rose, R., & Rutter, M. (1982). Panel report of psychosocial assets and modifiers of stress. In G. R. Elliot & C. Eisdorfer (Eds.), *Stress and human health: Analysis and implications of research.* New York: Springer-Verlag.

Cohen, J. S., Fihn, S. D., Boyko, E. J., & Jonsen, A. R. (1994). Attitudes toward assisted suicide and euthanasia among physicians in Washington State. *New England Journal of Medicine, 331,* 89–94.

Cohen, S., Kaplan, J. R., Cunnick, J. E., Manuck, S. B., & Rabin, B. S. (1992). Chronic social stress, affiliation, and cellular immune response in nonhuman primates. *Psychological Science, 3,* 301–304.

Cohen, S., & Syme, S. L. (1985). *Social support and health.* New York: Academic Press.

Cohen, S., Tyrrell, D. A. J., Russell, M. A. H., Jarvis, M. J., & Smith, A. P. (1993). Smoking, alcohol consumption, and susceptibility to the common cold. *Annals of Behavioral Medicine, 83,* 1277–1283.

Cohen, S., Tyrrell, D. A. J., & Smith, A. P. (1991). Psychological stress and susceptibility to the common cold. *New England Journal of Medicine, 325,* 606–612.

Coie, J. D., Underwood, M., & Lochman, J. E. (1991). Programmatic intervention with aggressive children in the school setting. In D. J. Pepler & K. H. Rubin (Eds.), *The development and treatment of childhood aggression* (pp. 389–410). Hillside, NJ: Lawrence Erlbaum.

Comas-Diaz, L. (1992). The future of psychotherapy with ethnic minorities. *Psychotherapy, 29,* 88–94.

Conners, C. K. (1969). A teacher rating scale for use in drug studies with children. *American Journal of Psychiatry, 6,* 884–888.

Conners, C. K. (1980). *Food additives and hyperactive children.* New York: Plenum.

Conners, C. K. (1990). *Conners' Rating Scales Manual.* North Tonawanda, NY: Multi-Health Systems.

Conners, C. K., & Wells, K. C. (1986). *Hyperkinetic children: A neuropsychosocial approach.* Beverly Hills, CA: Sage.

Conway, M. A. (1991). In defense of everyday memory. *American Psychologist, 46,* 19–26.

Cook, M., Mineka, S., Wolkenstein, B., & Laitsch, K. (1985). Observational conditioning of snake fear in unrelated rhesus monkeys. *Journal of Abnormal Psychology, 94,* 591–610.

Cooke, P. (1991, June 23). They cried until they couldn't see. *New York Times Magazine,* pp. 25–43.

Cooklin, R., Sturgeon, D., & Leff, J. (1983). The relationship between auditory hallucinations and spontaneous fluctuations of skin conductance in schizophrenia. *British Journal of Psychiatry, 142,* 47–52.

Cooney, R. S., Rogler, L. H., Hurrell, R., & Ortiz, V. (1982). Decision making in intergenerational Puerto Rican families. *Journal of Marriage and the Family, 44,* 621–631.

Coons, P. M. (1986). Treatment progress in 20 patients with multiple personality disorder. *Journal of Nervous and Mental Disease, 174,* 715–721.

Coons, P. M. (1988). Misuse of forensic hypnosis. *The International Journal of Clinical and Experimental Hypnosis, 36,* 1–11.

Coons, P. M. (1994). Confirmation of childhood abuse in child and adolescent cases of multiple personality disorder and dissociative disorder not otherwise specified. *Journal of Nervous and Mental Disease, 182,* 461–464.

Cooper, A. M., & Ronningstam, E. (1992). Narcissistic personality disorder. In A. Tasman & M. B. Riba (Eds.). *Review of psychiatry* (Vol. 11, pp. 80–97). Washington, DC: American Psychiatric Press.

Cooper, M. L. (1994). Motivations for alcohol use among adolescents: Development and validation of a four-factor model. *Psychological Assessment, 6,* 117–128.

Cooper, M. L., Peirce, R. S., & Huselid, R. F. (1994). Substance use and sexual risk taking among black adolescents and white adolescents. *Health Psychology, 13,* 251–262.

Cooper, S. J., Scott, A. I., & Whalley, L. J. (1990). A neuroendocrine view of ECT. *British Journal of Psychiatry, 157,* 740–743.

Cornblatt, B. A., & Erlenmeyer-Kimling, L. (1985). Global attentional deviance as a marker of risk for schizophrenia: Specificity and predictive validity. *Journal of Abnormal Psychology, 94,* 470–486.

Coryell, W., & Zimmerman, M. (1988). The heritability of schizophrenia and schizoaffective disorder. *Archives of General Psychiatry, 45,* 323–327.

Costa, P. T., Jr., & McCrae, R. R. (1985). *The NEO Personality Inventory manual.* Odessa, FL: Psychological Assessment Resources.

Costa, P. T., Jr., & McCrae, R. R. (1989). *The NEO–PI/NEO–FFI manual supplement.* Odessa, FL: Psychological Assessment Resources.

Costa, P. T., Jr., & McCrae, R. R. (1992a). Normal personality assessment in clinical practice: The NEO Personality Inventory. *Personality Assessment, 4,* 5–13.

Costa, P. T., Jr., & McCrae, R. R. (1992b). *Revised NEO Personality Inventory (NEO-PI-R) and NEO Five-Factor Inventory (NEO-FFI) professional manual.* Odessa, FL: Psychological Assessment Resources.

Cottler, L. B., Schuckit, M. A., Helzer, J. E., Crowley, T., Woody, G., Nathan, P. E., & Hughes, J. (1995). The DSM-IV field trial for substance use disorders: Major results. *Alcohol and Drug Dependence, 38,* 59–69.

Courtney, J. G., Longnecker, M. P., Theorell, T., & de Verdier, M. Gerhardsson. (1993). Stressful life events and the risk of colorectal cancer. *Epidemiology, 4,* 407–414.

Cowen, P. J., Anderson, I. M., & Fairburn, C. G. (1992). Neurochemical effects of dieting: Relevance to eating and affective disorders. In G. H. Anderson & S. H. Kennedy (Eds.), *The biology of feast and famine: Relevance to eating disorders* (pp. 269–284). New York: Academic Press.

Cowley, G. (1990, February 12). Hanging up the knife. *Newsweek,* pp. 58–59.

Cowley, G., with Springen, K., Leonard, E., Robins, K., & Gordon, J. (1990, March 26). The promise of Prozac. *Newsweek,* pp. 39–44.

Cox, B. J., Swinson, R. P., Parker, J. D. A., Kuch, K., & Reichman, J. T. (1993). Confirmatory factor analysis of the Fear Questionnaire in panic disorder with agoraphobia. *Psychological Assessment, 5,* 235–237.

Cox, D. J., Goner-Frederick, L. A., Clarke, W. L., & Carter, W. R. (1988). *Effects of acute experimental stressors on insulin-dependent diabetes mellitus.* Paper presented at the meetings of the American Diabetes Association, New Orleans.

Coyne, J. C. (1976a). Depression and the response of others. *Journal of Abnormal Psychology, 55,* 186–193.

Coyne, J. C. (1976b). Toward an interactional description of depression. *Psychiatry, 39,* 28–40.

Coyne, J. C. (1986). Strategic marital therapy for depression. In N. S. Jacobson & A. S. Gurman (Eds.), *Clinical handbook of marital therapy.* New York: Guilford Press.

Coyne, J. C., Burchill, S. A. L., & Styles, W. B. (1991). An interactional perspective on depression. In C. R. Snyder & D. R. Forsyth (Eds.), *Handbook of social and clinical psychology: The health perspective* (pp. 327–349). New York: Pergamon Press.

Coyne, J. C., & Fechner-Bates, S. (1992). Depression, the family, and family therapy. *Australian & New Zealand Journal of Family Therapy, 13,* 203–208.

Craig, M. E., Kalichman, S. C., & Follingstad, D. R. (1989). Verbal coercive sexual behavior among college students. *Archives of Sexual Behavior, 18,* 421–434.

Craighead, L. W., Craighead, W. E., Kazdin, A. E., & Mahoney, M. J. (Eds.). (1994). *Cognitive and behavioral interventions.* Boston: Allyn and Bacon.

Craighead, W. E., Curry, J. F., & McMillan, D. K. (1994). Child and adolescent depression. In L. W. Craighead, W. E. Craighead, A. E. Kazdin, & M. J. Mahoney (Eds.), *Cognitive and behavioral interventions* (pp. 301–312). Boston: Allyn & Bacon.

Cranston-Cuebas, M. A., & Barlow, D. H. (1990). Cognitive and affective contributions to sexual functioning. *Annual Review of Sex Research, 1,* 119–161.

Crapper, D. R., Kirshnan, S. S., & Dalton, A. J. (1973). Brain aluminum distribution in Alzheimer's disease and experimental neurofibrillary degeneration. *Science, 180,* 511–513.

Craske, M. G., & Barlow, D. H. (1993). Panic disorder and agoraphobia. In D. H. Barlow (Ed.), *Clinical handbook of psychological disorders* (pp. 1–47). New York: Guilford Press.

Crewdson, J. (1988). *By silence betrayed.* Boston: Little Brown.

Crick, N. R., & Dodge, K. A. (1994). A review and reformulation of social information processing mechanisms in children's social adjustment. *Psychological Bulletin, 115,* 74–101.

Crits-Christoph, P. (1992). The efficacy of brief dynamic psychotherapy: A meta-analysis. *American Journal of Psychiatry, 149,* 151–158.

Crockenberg, S. B., & Covey, S. L. (1991). Marital conflict and externalizing behavior in children. In D. Cicchetti & S. Toth (Eds.), *Rochester Symposium on Developmental Psychopathology: Vol. 3. Research and clinical contributions to a theory of developmental psychopathology* (pp. 235–260). Rochester, NY: University of Rochester Press.

Cronbach, L. J. (1957). The two disciplines of scientific psychology. *American Psychologist, 12,* 671–684.

Crow, T. J. (1985). The two-syndrome concept: Origins and current status. *Schizophrenia Bulletin, 11,* 471–485.

Crow, T. J., & Johnstone, E. C. (1985). Schizophrenia: The nature of the disease process and its biological correlates. In V. B. Montcastle & F. Plum (Eds.), *Handbook of Physiology: The Nervous System* (Vol. 5). Bethesda, MD: American Psychological Society.

Crowell, C. R., Hinson, R. E., & Siegel, S. (1981). The role of conditional drug responses in tolerance to the hypothermic effects of alcohol. *Psychopharmacology, 73,* 51–54.

Crowley, T. J. (1994). The organization of intoxication and withdrawal disorders. In T. A. Widiger, A. J. Frances, H. A. Pincus, M. B. First, R. Ross, & W. Davis (Eds.), *DSM-IV sourcebook* (Vol. 1, pp. 93–108). Washington, DC: American Psychiatric Association.

Cummings, E. M., Vogel, D., Cummings, J. S., & El-Sheikh, M. (1989). Children's responses to different forms of expression of anger between adults. *Child Development, 60,* 1392–1404.

Cummings, J. L., & Mahler, M. E. (1991). Cerebrovascular dementia. In R. A. Bornstein & G. G. Brown (Eds.), *Neurobehavioral aspects of cerebrovascular disease.* New York: Oxford University Press.

Cummings, M. E., & Davies, P. (1994). *Children and marital conflict: The impact of family dispute and resolution.* New York: Guilford Press.

Cutting, J. (1985). *The psychology of schizophrenia.* New York: Churchill Livingstone.

Cypress, B. K. (1980). *Characteristics of visits to female and male physicians: The national ambulatory medical care survey, 1977.* Hyattsville, MD: National Center for Health Statistics.

D

Daly, M., & Wilson, M. (1988). Evolutionary social psychology and family homicide. *Science, 242,* 519–524.

Damasio, A. R. (1992). Aphasia. *New England Journal of Medicine, 326,* 531–539.

Damasio, A. R., & Tranel, D. (1991). Disorders of higher brain function. In R. N. Rosenberg (Ed.), *Comprehensive Neurology* (pp. 639–655). New York: Raven Press.

Damasio, H., & Frank, R. (1992). Three-dimensional in vivo mapping of brain lesions in humans. *Archives of Neurology, 49,* 137–143.

Davidson, J. R. T., Hughes, D., Blazer, D. G., & George, L. K. (1991). Post-traumatic stress disorder in the community: An epidemiological study. *Psychological Medicine, 21,* 713–721.

Davidson, W. S., II, Gottschalk, R., Gensheimer, L., & Mayer, J. (1987). Interventions with juvenile delinquents: A meta-analysis of treatment efficacy. In C. Hampton (Ed.), *Juvenile offenders.* Washington, DC: U.S. Government Printing Office.

Davidson, W. S., II, Redner, R., Blakely, C. H., Mitchell, C. M., & Emshoff, J. G. (1987). Diversion of juvenile offenders: An experimental comparison. *Journal of Consulting and Clinical Psychology, 55,* 68–75.

Davies, P., & Wolozin, B. L. (1987). Recent advances in the neurochemistry of Alzheimer's disease. *Journal of Clinical Psychiatry, 48,* 23–30.

Davis, G. E., & Leitenberg, H. (1987). Adolescent sex offenders. *Psychological Bulletin, 101,* 417–427.

Davis, H. (1992). Crossroads on the pathways to discovery. In F. G. Worden, J. P. Swazey, & G. Adelman (Eds.), *The neurosciences: Paths of discovery.* Boston: Birkhauser.

Davison, G. C. (1976). Homosexuality: The ethical challenge. *Journal of Consulting and Clinical Psychology, 44,* 157–162.

Dawber, T. R., Meadors, T. F., & Moore, F. E. (1951). Epidemiological approaches to heart disease: The Framingham Study. *American Journal of Public Health, 41,* 279–286.

Dawes, R. M. (1994). *House of cards.* New York: Free Press.

Dawidoff, N. (1994, April 24). The business of begging. *New York Times Magazine,* pp. 34–41, 50, 52.

Dawson, G., & Castelloe, P. (1992). Autism. In C. E. Walker & M. C. Roberts (Eds.), *Handbook of clinical child psychology* (2nd ed., pp. 375–397). New York: John Wiley.

Dawson, G., & Lewy, A. (1989). Arousal, attention, and the socioemotional impairments of individuals with autism. In G. Dawson (Ed.), *Autism: Nature, diagnosis, and treatment* (pp. 49–74). New York: Guilford Press.

de Zwaan, M., Mitchell, J. E., Seim, H. C., Specker, S. M., Pyle, R. L., Raymond, N. C., & Crosby, R. B. (1994). Eating related and general psychopathology in obese females with binge eating disorder. *International Journal of Eating Disorders, 15,* 43–52.

DeAngelis, T. (1994). Psychologists' expertise is often essential in court. *APA Monitor, 25*(1), 29.

Deland, F. H., & Borenstein, N. M. (1990). Medicine court, II: Rivers in practice. *American Journal of Psychiatry, 142,* 38–43.

Delay, J., & Deniker, P. (1952). Le traitement des psychoses par une méthode neurolytique dérivée de l'hibernothera pie. In P. C. Ossa (Ed.), *Congrès de medecins alienistes et neurologistes de France.* Paris, France: Maisson.

DeMonbreun, B. G., & Craighead, W. E. (1977). Distortion of perception and recall of positive and neutral feedback in depression. *Cognitive Therapy and Research, 1,* 311–330.

DeMyer, M. K., Barton, S., DeMyer, W. E., Norton, J. A., Allen, J., & Steele, R. (1973). Prognosis in autism: A follow-up study. *Journal of Autism and Childhood Schizophrenia, 3,* 199–246.

Depression Guideline Panel. (1993a). *Depression in primary care: Vol. 1. Detection and diagnosis* (AHCPR Publication, No. 93-0550, Clinical Practice Guideline No. 5). Rockville, MD: U.S. Department of Health and Human Services, Public Health Service, Agency for Health Care Policy and Research.

Depression Guideline Panel. (1993b). *Depression in primary care: Vol 2. Treatment of major depression* (AHCPR Publication, No. 93–0551, Clinical Practice Guideline No. 5). Rockville, MD: U.S. Department of Health and Human Services, Public Health Service, Agency for Health Care Policy and Research.

Depue, R. A., & Iacono, W. G. (1988). Neurobehavioral aspects of affective disorders. *Annual Review of Psychology, 40,* 457–492.

Depue, R. A., Luciana, M., Arbisi, P., Collins, P., & Leon, A. (1994). Dopamine and the structure of personality: Relation of agonist-induced dopamine activity to positive emotionality. *Journal of Personality and Social Psychology, 67,* 485–498.

DeRubeis, R. J., Hollon, S. D., Evans, M. D., & Bemis, K. M. (1982). Can psychotherapies for depression be discriminated? A systematic investigation of cognitive therapy and interpersonal therapy. *Journal of Consulting and Clinical Psychology, 50,* 744–756.

Des Jarlais, D. C. (1988). *Effectiveness of AIDS educational programs for intravenous drug users.* Unpublished manuscript, State of New York Division of Substance Abuse Services, New York.

Devanand, D. P., Dwork, A. J., Hutchinson, E. R., Bolwig, T. G., & Sackheim, H. A. (1994). Does ECT alter brain structure? *American Journal of Psychiatry, 151,* 957–970.

DeVellis, B. M., & Blalock, S. J. (1992). Illness attributions and hopelessness depression: The role of hopelessness expectancy. *Journal of Abnormal Psychology, 101,* 257–264.

Dew, M. A., Bromet, E. J., Brent, D., & Greenhouse, J. B. (1987). A quantitative literature review of the effectiveness of suicide prevention centers. *Journal of Consulting and Clinical Psychology, 55,* 239–244.

Dial, T. H., Grimes, P. E., Leibenluft, E., & Pincus, H. A. (1994). Sex differences in psychiatrists' practice patterns and incomes. *American Journal of Psychiatry, 151,* 96–101.

Dial, T. H., Pion, G., Cooney, B., Kohout, J., Kaplan, K., Ginsberg, L., Merwin, E., Fox, J., Ginsberg, M., Staton, J., Clawson, T., Wildermuth, V., Blankertz, L., & Hughes, R. (1992). Training of mental health providers. In R. Manderscheid & M. Sonnenschein (Eds.), *Mental health, United States, 1992* (pp. 142–162). Rockville, MD: U.S. Department of Health and Human Services.

Diehl, D. J., & Gershon, S. (1992). The role of dopamine in mood disorders. *Comprehensive Psychiatry, 33,* 115–120.

Dinsmoor, J. A. (1992). Setting the record straight: The social views of B. F. Skinner. *American Psychologist, 47,* 1454–1463.

Dodrill, C. B., & Matthews, C. G. (1992). The role of neuropsychology in the assessment and treatment of persons with epilepsy. *American Psychologist, 47,* 1139–1142.

Dohrenwend, B. P. (1994). The problem of validity in field studies in psychological disorders. In J. E. Mezzich, M. R. Jorge, & I. M. Salloum (Eds.), *Psychiatric epidemiology: Assessment concepts and methods* (pp. 201–222). Baltimore: Johns Hopkins University Press.

Dohrenwend, B. P., & Egri, G. (1981). Recent stressful life events and episodes of schizophrenia. *Schizophrenia Bulletin, 7,* 12–23.

Dohrenwend, B. P., Levav, I., Shrout, P. E., Schwartz, S., Naveg, G., Link, B. G., Skodal, A. E., & Stueve, A. (1992). Socioeconomic status and psychiatric disorders: The causation-selection issue. *Science, 255,* 946–952.

Dolan, B. (1991). Cross-cultural aspects of anorexia nervosa and bulimia: A review. *International Journal of Eating Disorders, 10,* 67–78.

Doleys, D. M. (1989). Enuresis and encopresis. In T. H. Ollendick & M. Hersen (Eds.), *Handbook of childhood psychopathology* (2nd ed., pp. 291–314). New York: Plenum.

Donaldson v. O'Connor, 519 F. 2d 59 (5th Cir. 1975).

Dongier, M., Vachon, L., & Schwartz, G. (1991). Bromocriptine in the treatment of alcohol dependence. *Alcoholism: Clinical and Experimental Research, 15,* 970–977.

Dorken, H. (1993). The hospital private practice of psychology: CHAMPUS 1981–1991. *Professional Psychology: Research and Practice, 24,* 409–417.

Douglas, V. I. (1983). Attentional and cognitive problems. In M. Rutter (Ed.), *Developmental neuropsychiatry* (pp. 280–329). New York: Guilford Press.

Dressler, W. W. (1985). The social and cultural context of coping. Action, gender and symptoms in a southern black community. *Social Science Medicine, 21,* 499–506.

Dubro, A. F., & Wetzler, S. (1989). An external validity study of the MMPI personality disorder scales. *Journal of Clinical Psychology, 45,* 570–575.

Dumas, J. E. (1986). Parent perception and treatment outcome in families of aggressive children: A causal model. *Behavior Therapy, 17,* 420–432.

Dumas, J. E., & Wahler, R. G. (1985). Indiscriminate mothering as a contextual factor in aggressive-oppositional child behavior: "Damned if you do damned if you don't." *Journal of Abnormal Child Psychology, 13,* 1–17.

Dunham, H. W. (1965). *Community and schizophrenia: An epidemiological analysis.* Detroit: Wayne State University Press.

Dunlap, G., Robbins, F. R., & Kern, L. (1994). Some characteristics of nonaversive intervention for severe behavior problems. In E. Schopler & G. B. Mesibov (Eds.), *Behavioral issues in autism* (pp. 227–245). New York: Plenum Press.

Dunner, D. L. (1993). A review of the diagnostic status of "bipolar II" for the *DSM-IV* work group on mood disorders. *Depression, 1,* 2–10.

Durham v. United States, 214 F. 2d 862, 874-75 (D.C. Cir. 1954).

Durkheim, E. (1951). *Suicide.* New York: Free Press. (Original work published 1897)

Dusky v. United States, 362 U.S. 402 (1960).

Dutton, D. G. (1994). Patriarchy and wife assault: The ecological fallacy. *Violence and Victims, 9,* 167–182.

Duval, S., & Wickland, R. (1972). *A theory of objective self-awareness.* New York: Academic Press.

Dyck, M. J., Jolly, J. B., & Kramer, T. (1994). An evaluation of positive affectivity, negative affectivity, and hyperarousal as markers for assessing between syndrome relationships. *Personality and Individual Differences, 17,* 637–646.

Dyck, M. J., & Stewart, B. L. (1991). Cognitive vulnerability to depression. *Journal of Cognitive Psychotherapy, 5,* 115–129.

E

Eaton, W. W., Anthony, J. C., Tepper, S., & Dryman, A. (1992). Psychopathology and attrition in the Epidemiologic Catchment Area Study. *American Journal of Epidemiology, 135,* 1051–1059.

Eaton, W. W., Holzer, C. E., Von Korff, M., Anthony, J. C., Helzer, J. E., George, L., Burnam, A., Boyd, J. H., Kessler, L. G., & Locke, B. Z. (1984). The design of the epidemiologic catchment area surveys. *Archives of General Psychiatry, 41,* 942–948.

Editorial. (1994, May 11). *Los Angeles Times,* p. B-6.

Edwards, A. L. (1967). *Edwards Personality Inventory: Manual.* Chicago: Science Research Associates.

Edwards, D. W., Morrison, T. L., & Weissman, H. N. (1993). Uniform versus linear T scores on the MMPI–2/MMPI in an outpatient psychiatric sample: Differential contributions. *Psychological Assessment, 5,* 499–500.

Edwards, G. (1992). The history of two dimensions. In M. Lader, G. Edwards, & D. C. Drummond (Eds.), *The nature of alcohol and drug related problems* (pp. 1–14). New York: Oxford University Press.

Effective treatment for treating depression. (1994, April). *Johns Hopkins Medical Letter, 6*(2), 6–7.

Eidelson, R. J., & Epstein, N. (1982). Cognitions and relationship readjustment: Development of a measure of dysfunctional relationship beliefs. *Journal of Consulting and Clinical Psychology, 50,* 715–720.

Eisenberg, L. (1968). The interaction of biological and experiential factors in schizophrenia. In D. Rosenthal & S. S. Kety (Eds.), *The transmission of schizophrenia* (pp. 403–409). Oxford, England: Pergamon Press.

Elia, J., Rapoport, J. L., & Kirby, J. (1993). Pharmacological treatment of attention deficit hyperactivity disorder. In J. L. Matson (Ed.), *Handbook of hyperactivity in children* (pp. 220–233). Boston: Allyn & Bacon.

Elkin, I., Parloff, M. B., Hadley, S. W., & Autry, J. H. (1985). NIMH treatment of Depression Collaborative Research Program: Background and research plan. *Archives of General Psychiatry, 42,* 305–316.

Elkin, I., Shea, M. T., Watkins, J. T., & Imber, S. D. (1989). National Institute of Mental Health Treatment of Depression Collaborative Research Program: General effectiveness of treatments. *Archives of General Psychiatry, 46,* 971–982.

Elkin, I., Shea, M. T., Watkins, J. T., Imber, S. D., Sotsky, S. M., Collins, J. F., Glass, D. R., Pilkonis, P. A., Leber, W. R., Docherty, J. P., Fiester, S. J., & Parloff, M. B. (1989). National Institute of Mental Health Treatment of Depression Collaborative Research Program: General effectiveness of treatments. *Archives of General Psychiatry, 46,* 971–982.

Ellenberger, H. F. (1972). The story of Anna O: A critical review with new data. *Journal of the History of Behavioral Sciences, 8,* 267–279.

Ellicott, A., Hammen, C., Gitlin, M., & Brown, G. (1990). Life events and the course of bipolar disorder. *American Journal of Psychiatry, 147,* 1194–1198.

Elliot, D. S. (1994). Serious violent offenders: Onset, developmental course, and termination. *The American Society of Criminology, 32,* 1–21.

Ellis, A. (1970). *The essence of rational psychotherapy: A comprehensive approach to treatment.* New York: Institute for Rational Living.

Ellis, A. (1995). Rational emotive behavior therapy. In R. J. Corsini & D. Wedding (Eds.), *Current psychotherapies* (5th ed., pp. 162–196). Itasca, IL: F. E. Peacock.

Ellis, L. (1991). A synthesized (biosocial) theory of rape. *Journal of Consulting and Clinical Psychology, 59*, 631–642.

Emery, R. E. (1982). Interparental conflict and the children of divorce and discord. *Psychological Bulletin, 92*, 310–330.

Emery, R. E., Weintraub, S., & Neale, J. M. (1982). Effects of marital discord on the school behavior of children of schizophrenic, affectively disordered, and normal parents. *Journal of Abnormal Child Psychology, 10*, 215–228.

Engel, G. L. (1977). The need for a new medical model: A challenge for bio-medicine. *Science, 196*, 129–136.

Entwisle, D. (1972). To dispel fantasies about fantasy-based measures of achievement motivation. *Psychological Bulletin, 77*, 377–391.

Epstein, L. H., Klein, K. R., & Wisniewski, L. (1994). Child and parent factors that influence psychological problems in obese children. *International Journal of Eating Disorders, 15*, 151–157.

Epstein, L. H., Valoski, A., Wing, R. A., & McCurley, J. (1994). Ten-year outcomes of behavioral family-based treatment for childhood obesity. *Health Psychology, 13*, 373–383.

Epstein, N., Schlesinger, S. E., & Dryden, W. (1988). Concepts and methods of cognitive-behavioral family treatment. In N. Epstein, S. E. Schlesinger, & W. Dryden (Eds.), *Cognitive-behavioral therapy with families.* New York: Brunner/Mazel.

Erikson, E. H. (1959). *Identity and the life cycle.* New York: International Universities Press.

Erwin, E. (1986). Establishing causal connections: Meta-analysis and psychotherapy. *Midwest Studies in Philosophy, 9*, 421–436.

Evans, M. D., Hollon, S. D., DeRubeis, R. J., Piasecki, J., Grove, W. M., Garvey, M. J., & Tuason, V. B. (1992). Differential relapse following cognitive therapy and pharmacotherapy for depression. *Archives of General Psychiatry, 49*, 802–808.

Exner, J. E. (1993). *The Rorschach: A comprehensive approach* (Vol. I). New York: John Wiley.

Eysenck, H. J. (1952). The effects of psychotherapy: An evaluation. *Journal of Consulting Psychology, 16*, 319–324.

Eysenck, H. J. (1959). Learning theory and behaviour therapy. *British Journal of Mental Science, 105*, 61–75.

Eysenck, H. J. (1960). *Experiments in personality.* London, England: Routledge & Paul.

Eysenck, H. J., & Eysenck, S. B. (1969). *Eysenck Personality Inventory* (rev. manual). San Diego: Educational and Industrial Testing Service.

Eysenck, H. J., & Rachman, S. (1965). *The causes and cures of neurosis.* San Diego, CA: Robert E. Knapp.

F

Fabrega, H., Mezzich, J. E., Mezzich, A. C., & Coffman, G. A. (1986). Descriptive validity of *DSM-III* depressions. *The Journal of Nervous and Mental Disease, 174*, 573–584.

Fabrega, H., Ulrich, R., Pilkonis, P., & Mezzich, J. E. (1991). Pure personality disorders in an intake psychiatric setting. *Journal of Personality Disorders, 6*, 153–161.

Fairburn, C. G. (1994, April). *The etiology of bulimia nervosa.* Keynote address, Sixth International Conference on Eating Disorders, New York, New York.

Fairburn, C. G. (1994, May). *The etiology of bulimia nervosa.* Paper presented at Sixth International Conference on Eating Disorders, New York.

Fairburn, C. G. (1995). *Overcoming binge eating.* New York: Guilford Press.

Fairburn, C. G., Agras, W. S., & Wilson, G. T. (1992). The research on the treatment of bulimia nervosa: Practical and theoretical implications. In G. H. Anderson & S. H. Kennedy (Eds.), *The biology of feast and famine: Relevance to eating disorders* (pp. 318–340). New York: Academic Press.

Fairburn, C. G., & Cooper, P. J. (1993). The eating disorder examination (12th ed.). In C. G. Fairburn & G. T. Wilson (Eds.), *Binge eating: Nature, assessment, and treatment* (pp. 317–360). New York: Guilford Press.

Fairburn, C. G., Hay, P. J., & Welch, S. L. (1993). Binge eating and bulimia nervosa: Distribution and determinants. In C. G. Fairburn & G. T. Wilson (Eds.), *Binge eating: Nature, assessment, and treatment* (pp. 123–143). New York: Guilford Press.

Fairburn, C. G., Jones, R., Peveler, R. C., Hope, R. A., & O'Connor M. (1993). Psychotherapy and bulimia nervosa: The longer-term effects of interpersonal psychotherapy, behaviour therapy and cognitive behaviour therapy. *Archives of General Psychiatry, 50*, 419–428.

Fairburn, C. G., Norman, P. A., Welch, S. L., O'Connor, M. E., Doll, H. A., & Peveler, R. C. (1995). A prospective study of outcome in bulimia nervosa and the long-term effects of three psychological treatments. *Archives of General Psychiatry, 52*, 304–312.

Fairburn, C. G., Welch, S. L., & Hay, P. J. (1993). The classification of recurrent overeating: The "Binge Eating Disorder" proposal. *International Journal of Eating Disorders, 13*, 155–160.

Fairburn, C. G., & Wilson, G. T. (Eds.). (1993). *Binge eating: Nature, assessment and treatment.* New York: Guilford Press.

Falloon, I. R. H., Boyd, J. L., McGill, C. W., Williamson, M., Ranzani, J., Moss, H. B., Gilderman, A. M., & Simpson, G. M. (1985). Family management in the prevention of morbidity of schizophrenia. *Archives of General Psychiatry, 42*, 887–896.

Faris, R. E. L., & Dunham, H. W. (1939). *Mental disorders in urban areas.* New York: Hafner.

Farquhar, J. W., Fortmann, S. P., Flora, J. A., Taylor, C. B., Haskell, W. L., Williams, P. T., Maccoby, N., & Wood, P. D. (1990). Effects of communitywide education on cardiovascular disease risk factors. *Journal of the American Medical Society, 264*, 359–365.

Fava, M., & Kaji, J. (1994). Continuation and maintenance treatments of major depressive disorder. *Psychiatric Annals, 24*, 281–290.

Feingold, B. (1975). *Why your child is hyperactive.* New York: Random House.

Feldman, H. A., Goldstein, I., Hatzichristou, D. G., Krane, R. J., & McKinlay, J. B. (1994). Impotence and its medical and psychosocial correlates: Results of the Massachusetts male aging study. *Journal of Urology, 151*, 54–61.

Feldman, M. A. (1986). Research on parenting by mentally retarded persons. *Psychiatric Clinics of North America, 9*, 777–795.

Fenton, W. S., Wyatt, R. J., & McGlashan, T. H. (1994). Risk factors for spontaneous dyskinesia in schizophrenia. *Archives of General Psychiatry, 51*, 643–650.

Fergusson, D. M., Horwood, L. J., & Lynskey, M. T. (1993). Prevalence and comorbidity of DSM-III-R disorders in a birth cohort of 15 year olds. *Journal of the American Academy of Child and Adolescent Psychiatry, 32*, 1127–1134.

Ferster, C. B. (1961). Positive reinforcement and behavioral deficits of autistic children. *Child Development, 32*, 437–456.

Ferster, C. B., & Skinner, B. F. (1957). *Schedules of reinforcement.* New York: Appleton-Century-Crofts.

Fiester, S. (1991). Self-defeating personality disorder: A review of data and recommendations for *DSM-IV. Journal of Personality Disorders, 5*, 194–209.

Fincham, F. D. (1994). Understanding the association between marital conflict and child adjustment. *Journal of Family Psychology, 8*, 123–127.

Fincham, F. D., Grych, J. H., & Osborne, L. N. (1994). Does marital conflict cause child maladjustment? Directions and challenges for longitudinal research. *Journal of Family Psychology, 8*, 128–140.

Fink, M. (1994). Can ECT be an effective treatment for adolescents? *Harvard Mental Health Letter, 10*, 8.

Fink, M., Bush, G., & Petrides, G. (1995). What is catatonia? *Harvard Mental Health Letter, 11*(8), 8.

Finkel, N. J. (1988). *Insanity on trial.* New York: Plenum.

Finkelhor, D., & Dzulba-Leatherman, J. (1994). Victimization of children. *American Psychologist, 3*, 173–183.

Finkelhor, D., & Yllo, K. (1983). Rape in marriage: A sociological view. In D. Finkelhor, R. J. Gelles, G. T. Hotaling, & M. A. Straus (Eds.), *The dark side of families* (pp. 119–130). Beverly Hills, CA: Sage.

Finn, S. E., & Butcher, J. N. (1991). Clinical objective personality assessment. In M. Hersen, A. E. Kazdin, & A. S. Bellack (Eds.), *The clinical psychology handbook* (2nd ed.) (pp. 362–373). New York: Pergamon Press.

Finn, S. E., & Tonsager, M. E. (1992). Therapeutic effects of providing MMPI-2 test feedback to college students awaiting therapy. *Psychological Assessment, 4*, 278–287.

Fischbach, G. D. (1992). Mind and brain. *Scientific American, 267*, 48–57.

Fisher, E. B., Delamater, A. M., Bertelson, A. D., & Kirkley, B. G. (1982). Psychological factors in diabetes and its treatment. *Journal of Consulting and Clinical Psychology, 50*, 993–1003.

Fisher, S., & Greenberg, R. P. (1977). *The scientific credibility of Freud's theories and therapy.* Sussex, England: Harvester Press.

Foa, E. B., Rothbaum, B. O., Riggs, D. S., & Murdock, T. B. (1991). Treatment of posttraumatic stress disorder in rape victims: A comparison between cognitive-behavioral procedures and counseling. *Journal of Consulting and Clinical Psychology, 59,* 715–723.

Foderaro, L. W. (1993, July 19). With reforms in treatment, shock therapy loses shock. *New York Times,* p. 1.

Fodor, I. S. (1974). The phobic syndrome in women: Implications for treatment. In V. Franks & V. Burtle (Eds.), *Women in therapy: New psychotherapies for a changing society.* New York: Brunner/Mazel.

Folingstad, D. R., Wright, S., Lloyd, S., & Sebastian, J. A. (1991). Sex differences in motivations and effects in dating violence. *Family Relations, 40,* 51–57.

Fontana, V. J. (1991). *Save the family, save the child.* New York: E. P. Dutton.

Forehand, R., & McMahon, R. (1981). *Helping the noncompliant child: A clinician's guide to parent training.* New York: Guilford Press.

Forgac, G. E., & Michaels, E. J. (1982). Personality characteristics of two types of male exhibitionists. *Journal of Abnormal Psychology, 91,* 287–293.

Forgatch, M. S. (1991). The clinical science vortex: A developing theory of antisocial behavior. In D. Pepler & K. Rubin (Eds.), *The development and treatment of childhood aggression* (pp. 291–315). Hillsdale, NJ: Lawrence Erlbaum.

Forsythe, W. I., & Redmond, A. (1974). Enuresis and spontaneous cure rate: Study of 1,129 neurotics. *Archives of Disease in Childhood, 49,* 259–263.

Foster, S. L., Prinz, R. J., & O'Leary, K. D. (1983). Impact of problem solving communication training and generalization procedures on family conflict. *Child and Family Behavior Therapy, 5,* 1–23.

Fotheringham, J. B. (1991). Autism: Its primary psychological and neurological deficit. *Canadian Journal of Psychiatry, 36,* 686–692.

Fowers, B. J. (1991). His and her marriage: A multivariate study of gender and marital satisfaction. *Sex Roles, 24,* 209–221.

Fowles, D. C. (1980). The three-arousal model: Implications of Gray's two-factor learning theory for heart rate, electrodermal activity, and psychopathy. *Psychophysiology, 17,* 87–104.

Fowles, D. C. (1992). Schizophrenia: Diathesis-stress revisited. *Annual Review of Psychology, 43,* 303–336.

Fowles, D. C. (1993a). A motivational theory of psychopathology. In W. Spaulding (Ed.), *Nebraska Symposium on Motivation: Integrated views of motivation, cognition and emotion* (Vol. 41). Lincoln, NE: University of Nebraska Press.

Fowles, D. C. (1993b). Electrodermal activity and antisocial behavior. In J.-C. Roy, W. Boucsein, D. Fowles, & J. Gruzelier (Eds.), *Progress in electrodermal research.* London, England: Plenum.

Fowles, D. C. (1994). A motivational theory of psychopathology. In W. Spaulding (Ed.), *Nebraska symposium on motivation: Integrated views of motivation and emotion* (Vol. 41, pp. 181–238). Lincoln: University of Nebraska Press.

Fox, H. A. (1993). Patients' fear of and objection to electroconvulsive therapy. *Hospital & Community Psychiatry, 44,* 357–360.

Foy, D. W., Cline, K. A., & Laasi, N. (1987). Assessment of alcohol and drug abuse. In T. D. Nirenberg & S. A. Maisto (Eds.), *Developments in the assessment and treatment of addictive behaviors.* Norwood, NJ: Ablex.

Foy, D. W., Donahoe, C. P., Carroll, E. M., Gallers, J., & Reno, R. (1987). Posttraumatic stress disorder. In L. Michelson & L. M. Aschner (Eds.), *Anxiety and stress disorders.* New York: Guilford Press.

Frame, C. L., Robinson, S. L., & Cuddy, E. (1992). Behavioral treatment of childhood depression. In S. M. Turner, K. S. Calhoun, & H. E. Adams (Eds.), *Handbook of clinical behavior therapy* (2nd ed., pp. 245–258). New York: John Wiley.

Frances, A. J. (1980). The *DSM-III* personality disorders section: A commentary. *American Journal Psychiatry, 137,* 1050–1054.

Frances, A. J. (1993). Dimensional classification of personality disorder: Not whether but when, and which. *Psychological Inquiry, 4,* 110–111.

Frances, A. J., Davis, W. W., & Kline, M. (in press). The DSM-IV field trials: Moving towards an empirically derived classification. *European Psychiatry.*

Frances, A. J., Pincus, H. A., Widiger, T. A., Davis, W. W., & First, M. B. (1994). *DSM-IV*: Work in progress. In J. E. Mezzich, M. R. Jorge, & I. M. Salloum (Eds.), *Psychiatric epidemiology: Assessment concepts and methods* (pp. 116–135). Baltimore: Johns Hopkins University Press.

Frances, A. J., & Widiger, T. A. (1986). The classification of personality disorders: An overview of problems and solutions. In A. J.

Frances & R. E. Hales (Eds.), *Annual review* (Vol. 5). Washington, DC: American Psychiatric Press.

Frank, E., Anderson, B., Reynolds, C. F., Ritenour, A., & Kupfer, D. J. (1994). Life events and the Research Diagnostic Criteria endogenous subtype. *Archives of General Psychiatry, 51,* 519–524.

Frank, E., Anderson, C., & Rubinstein, D. (1978). Frequency of sexual dysfunction in "normal" couples. *New England Journal of Medicine, 299,* 111–115.

Frank, E., Kupfer, D. J., Perel, J. M., Cornes, C., Jarret, D. B., Mallinger, A. G., Thase, M. E., McEachran, A. B., & Grochocinski, V. J. (1990). Three year outcomes for maintenance therapies in recurrent depression. *Archives of General Psychiatry, 47,* 1093–1099.

Frankel, F. H. (1993). Adult reconstruction of childhood events in the multiple personality literature. *American Journal of Psychiatry, 150,* 954–958.

Freeman, W., & Watts, J. W. (1942). *Psychosurgery: Intelligence, emotional and social behavior following prefrontal lobotomy for mental disorder.* Springfield, IL: Charles C Thomas.

Freud, A. (1936). *The ego and the mechanisms of defense.* New York: International Universities Press.

Freud, S. (1950). Mourning and melancholia. In *Collected Papers* (Vol. 4, pp. 152–172). London, England: Hogarth Press & the Institute of Psychoanalysis. (Original work published 1917)

Freud, S. (1953). Three essays of the theory of sexuality. In J. Strachey (Ed. and Trans.), *The standard edition of the complete psychological works of Sigmund Freud* (Vol. 7, pp. 125–221). London, England: Hogarth Press. (Original work published 1905)

Freud, S. (1955). Analysis of a phobia in a five-year-old boy. In J. Strachey (Ed. and Trans.), *The standard edition of the complete psychological works of Sigmund Freud* (Vol. 10). London, England: Hogarth Press. (Original work published 1909)

Freud, S. (1959). Character and anal-eroticism. In J. Stachey (Trans.), *The standard edition of the complete psychological works of Sigmund Freud* (Vol. 9). London, England: Hogarth Press. (Original work published 1908)

Freud, S. (1961). The ego and the id. In J. Strachey (Ed. and Trans.), *The standard edition of the complete psychological works of Sigmund Freud* (Vol. 19, pp. 12–68). London, England: Hogarth Press. (Original work published 1923)

Freud, S. (1963a). Introductory lectures on psycho-analysis: Lecture 25. Anxiety. In J. Strachey (Ed. and Trans.), *The standard edition of the complete psychological works of Sigmund Freud* (Vol. 16). London, England: Hogarth Press. (Original work published 1917)

Freud, S. (1963b). The libido theory and narcissism. Lecture XXVI. In J. Strachey (Ed. and Trans.), *Introductory lectures on psychoanalysis: The standard edition of the complete psychological works of Sigmund Freud* (Vol. 16, pp. 412–430). London, England: Hogarth Press. (Original work published 1917)

Freud, S. (1963c). The sexual life of human beings. In J. Strachey (Ed. and Trans.), *The standard edition of the complete psychological works of Sigmund Freud* (Vol. 16, pp. 303–319). London, England: Hogarth Press. (Original work published 1917)

Freud, S. (1964a). Femininity. In J. Strachey (Ed. and Trans.), *The standard edition of the complete psychological works of Sigmund Freud* (Vol. 22, pp. 112–135). London, England: Hogarth Press. (Original work published 1933)

Freud, S. (1964b). "The technique of psychoanalysis" in *The standard edition of the complete psychological works of Sigmund Freud* (Vol. 23). London, England: Hogarth Press. (Original work published 1938)

Frezza, M., DiPadova, C., Pozzato, G., Terpin, M., Baraona, E., & Lieber, C. S. (1990). High blood alcohol levels in women: Role of decreased gastric alcohol dehydrogenase activity and first pass metabolism. *New England Journal of Medicine, 322,* 95–99.

Friedman, H. S., Tucker, J. S., Schwartz, J. E., Tomlinson-Keasey, C., Martin, L. R., Wingard, D. L., & Criqui, M. H. (1995). Psychosocial and behavioral predictors of longevity: The aging and death of the "Termites." *American Psychologist, 50,* 69–78.

Friedman, M., & Rosenman, R. H. (1974). *Type A behavior and your heart.* Greenwich, CT: Fawcett Publications.

Friedman, S., Jones, J. C., Chernen, L., & Barlow, D. H. (1992). Suicidal ideation and suicide attempts among patients with panic disorder: A survey of two outpatient clinics. *American Journal of Psychiatry, 149,* 680–685.

Fromm-Reichmann, F. (1939). Transference problems in schizphrenics. *Psychoanalytic Quarterly, 8,* 412–426.

Furman, W., Rahe, D., & Hartup, W. (1979). Rehabilitation of socially withdrawn preschool children through mixed-age socialization. *Child Development, 50,* 915–922.

Fuster, V., Badimon, L., Badimon, J. J., & Chesebro, J. H. (1992). The pathogenesis of coronary artery disease and the acute coronary syndromes. *New England Journal of Medicine, 326,* 242–250.

G

Gagnon, J. (1977). *Human sexualities.* Chicago: Scott, Foresman.

Gallagher, J. J. (1994). Teaching and learning: New models. *Annual Review of Psychology, 45,* 171–195.

Gallant, D. M. (1987). The female alcoholic: Early onset of brain damage. *Alcoholism, 11,* 190–191.

Gallant, S. J., & Hamilton, J. A. (1988). On a premenstrual psychiatric diagnosis: What's in a name? *Professional Psychology: Research and Practice, 19,* 271–278.

Ganahl, G. F., Ferguson, L. R., & L'Abate, L. (1985). Training in family therapy. In L. L'Abate (Ed.), *The handbook of family psychology and therapy* (Vol. 2). Homewood, IL: Dorsey Press.

Garb, H. N. (1992). The trained psychologist as expert witness. *Clinical Psychology Review, 12,* 451–467.

Garcia, J., & Koelling, R. A. (1966). Relation of cue to consequence in avoidance learning. *Psychonomic Science, 4,* 123–124.

Gardner, H. (1974). *The shattered mind.* New York: Vintage Books.

Gardner, H. (1983). *Frames of mind: The theory of multiple intelligences.* New York: Basic Books.

Gardner, H. (1986). The waning of intelligence tests. In R. J. Sternberg & D. K. Detterman (Eds.), *What is intelligence?* Norwood, NJ: Ablex.

Gardner, H., & Hatch, T. (1989). Multiple intelligences go to school: Educational implications of the theory of multiple intelligences. *Educational Researcher, 18,* 4–10.

Garety, P. A. (1992). Assessing symptoms and behavior. In M. J. Birchwood & N. Tarrier (Eds.), *Innovations in the psychological management of schizophrenia: Assessment, treatment, and services.* New York: Wiley.

Garner, D. M. (1993). Binge eating in anorexia nervosa. In C. G. Fairburn & G. T. Wilson (Eds.), *Binge eating: Nature, assessment and treatment* (pp. 50–76). New York: Guilford Press.

Garner, D. M., Garfinkel, P. E., Schwartz, D., & Thompson, M. (1980). Cultural expectations of thinness in women. *Psychological Reports, 47,* 483–491.

Garner, D. M., & Wooley, S. C. (1991). Confronting the failure of behavioral and dietary treatments for obesity. *Clinical Psychology Review, 11,* 729–780.

Gawin, F. H., & Ellinwood, E. H. (1988). Cocaine and other stimulants: Actions, abuse, and treatment. *New England Journal of Medicine, 318,* 1173–1182.

Gelberg, L., Linn, L. S., & Leake, B. D. (1988). Mental health, alcohol and drug use, and criminal history among homeless adults. *American Journal of Psychiatry, 145,* 191–196.

Gelernter, C. S., Uhde, T. W., Cimbolic, P., Arnkoff, D. B., Vittone, B. J., Tancer, M. E., & Bartko, J. J. (1991). Cognitive-behavioral and pharmacological treatments of social phobia. *Archives of General Psychiatry, 48,* 938–945.

Gelles, R. J. (1993a). Through a sociological lens: Social structure and family violence. In R. J. Gelles & D. R. Loseke (Eds.), *Current controversies on family violence* (pp. 31–46). Newbury Park, CA: Sage.

Gelles, R. J. (1993b). Alcohol and other drugs are associated with violence—They are not its cause. In R. J. Gelles & D. R. Loseke (Eds.), *Current controversies on family violence* (pp. 182–196). Newbury Park, CA: Sage.

Gelles, R. J., & Loseke, D. R. (1993). Examining and evaluating controversies on family violence. In R. J. Gelles & D. R. Loseke (Eds.), *Current controversies on family violence* (pp. 182–196). Newbury Park, CA: Sage.

Gelman, D. (1987, May 4). Depression. *Newsweek,* p. 7.

George, L. K., Landoman, R., Blazer, D. G., & Anthony, J. C. (1991). Cognitive impairment. In L. N. Robins & D. A. Regier (Eds.), *Psychiatric Disorders in America* (pp. 291–327). New York: Free Press.

George, W. H., Gournic, S. J., & McAfee, M. P. (1988). Perceptions of post-drinking female sexuality: Effects of gender, beverage choice, and drink payment. *Journal of Applied Social Psychology, 18,* 1295–1317.

Gershon, E. S., & Rieder, R. O. (1992, September). Major disorders of mind and brain. *Scientific American,* pp. 127–133.

Gewirtz, J. L., & Pelaez-Nogueras, M. (1992). B. F. Skinner's legacy to human infant behavior and development. *American Psychologist, 47,* 1411–1422.

Gibbs, N. (1991, June 3). When is it rape? *Time,* pp. 48–54.

Gilbert, P. L., Harris, J., McAdams, L. A., & Jeste, D. V. (1995). Neuroleptic withdrawal in schizophrenic patients. *Archives of General Psychiatry, 52,* 173–188.

Giles, D. E., Etzel, B. A., & Biggs, M. M. (1989). Long-term effects of unipolar depression on cognitions. *Comprehensive Psychiatry, 30,* 225–230.

Gillberg, C. (1990). Autism and pervasive developmental disorders. *Journal of Child Psychology and Psychiatry, 31,* 99–119.

Gilligan, C. (1978). *In a different voice.* Cambridge, England: Cambridge University Press.

Gilman, A., Goodman, T., Rall, T. W., Nies, A. S., & Taylor, P. (Eds.). (1991). *The pharmacological basis of therapeutics* (Vol. 8). New York: Pergamon Press.

Gilmore, M. (1994). The road from nowhere: Walking the streets of Aberdeen, Wash. *Rolling Stone, 683,* 44–46 ff.

Gingerich, S. L., & Bellack, A. S. (1995). Research-based family interventions for the treatment of schizophrenia. *Clinical Psychologist, 48,* 24–27.

Giordani, B., Rourke, D., Berent, S., Sackellares, J. C., Seidenberg, M., Butterbaugh, G., Boll, T. J., O'Leary, D. S., & Dreifuss, F. E. (1993). Comparison of WAIS subtest performance of patients with complex partial (temporal lobe) and generalized seizures. *Psychological Assessment, 5,* 159–163.

Gitlin, M. J. (1990). *The psychotherapist's guide to pharmacology.* New York: Free Press.

Gittelman, R. (Ed.). (1986). *Anxiety disorders of childhood.* New York: Guilford Press.

Gittelman, R., & Koplewicz, H. S. (1986). Pharmacotherapy of childhood anxiety disorders. In R. Gittelman (Ed.), *Anxiety disorders of childhood* (pp. 186–203). New York: Guilford Press.

Gittelman-Klein, R., Klein, D. F., Abikoff, H., Katz, S., Gloisten, A. C., & Kates, W. (1976). Relative efficacy of methylphenidate and behavior modification in hyperactive children: An interim report. *Journal of Abnormal Child Psychology, 4,* 361–379.

Glasgow, R. E., & Lichtenstein, E. (1987). Long-term effects of behavioral smoking cessation interventions. *Behavior Therapy, 18,* 297–324.

Glynn, S. M. (1990). Token economy approaches for psychiatric patients: Progress and pitfalls over 25 years. *Behavior Modification, 14,* 383–407.

Glynn, S., Randolph, E., Eth, S., Paz, G., Leong, G., Shaner, A., & Strachan, A. (1990). Patient psychopathology and expressed emotion in schizophrenia. *British Journal of Psychiatry, 157,* 877–880.

Goetsch, V. L. (1989). Stress and blood glucose in diabetes mellitus: A review and methodological commentary. *Annals of Behavioral Medicine, 1,* 102–107.

Goffman, I. (1961). *Asylums: Essays on the social situation of mental patients and other inmates.* Garden City, New York: Doubleday Anchor.

Gold, M. S. (1991). *The good news about drugs and alcohol.* New York: Villard Books.

Goldberg, L. R. (1992). The development of markers of the Big-Five factor structure. *Psychological Assessment, 4,* 26–42.

Goldblatt, P. B., Moore, M. E., & Stunkard, A. J. (1965). Social factors in obesity. *Journal of the American Medical Association, 192,* 1039–1044.

Golden, C. J., Hammeke, T. A., & Purisch, A. D. (1980). *The Luria-Nebraska Battery manual.* Palo Alto, CA: Western Psychological Services.

Golden, R. N., Gilmore, J. H., Corrigan, M. H., Ekstrom, R. D., Knight, B. T., & Garbutt, J. C. (1991). Serotonin, suicide, and aggression. *Journal of Clinical Psychiatry, 52* (Supplement), 61–69.

Goldfried, M. R., & Castonguay, L. G. (1992). The future of psychotherapy integration. *Psychotherapy, 29,* 4–10.

Goldfried, M. R., & Davison, G. C. (1994). *Clinical behavior therapy.* New York: John Wiley.

Golding, J. M., Smith, R., & Kashner, M. (1991). Does somatization disorder occur in men? *Archives of General Psychiatry, 48,* 231–235.

Goldman, M. S., Brown, S. A., & Christiansen, B. A. (1987). Expectancy theory: Thinking about drinking. In H. T. Blane & K. E. Leonard (Eds.), *Psychological theories of drinking and alcoholism* (pp. 181–226). New York: Guilford Press.

Goldstein, M. J. (1984). Family intervention programs. In A. S. Bellack (Ed.), *Schizophrenia: Treatment, management, and rehabilitation.* New York: Grune & Stratton.

Goldstein, M. J. (1995, May 6). *Family interventions with schizophrenia.* Paper presented at the Marital and Family Therapy Outcome and Process Research Conference, Temple University, Philadelphia, PA.

Goleman, D. (1987, March 10). Researcher reports progress against autism. *New York Times,* p. C1.

Goleman, D. (1989, August 29). When the rapist is not a stranger: Studies seek new understanding. *New York Times,* p. C1.

Goleman, D. (1990, May 10). Why girls are prone to depression. *New York Times,* p. B15.

Goleman, D. (1992a, February 19). The children of alcoholics suffer problems that afflict others, too. *New York Times,* p. B5.

Goleman, D. (1992b, April 14). Therapies offer hope for sex offenders. *New York Times,* p. C1-3.

Goleman, D. (1992c, October 14). Study ties genes to alcoholism in women. *New York Times,* p. B7.

Goleman, D. (1993a, March 17). More than 1 in 4 U. S. adults suffers a mental disorder each year. *New York Times,* p. B7.

Goleman, D. (1993b, September 22). Scientists trace "voices" in schizophrenia. *New York Times,* p. B9.

Goleman, D. (1994a, April 19). Revamping psychiatrists' Bible. *New York Times,* pp. B5, B8.

Goleman, D. (1994b, May 31). Miscoding seen as the root of false memories. *New York Times,* p. C1.

Goleman, D. (1994c, June 22). Standard therapies may help only impulsive spouse abuse. *New York Times,* p. C11.

Golomb, A., Ludolph, P., Westen, D., & Block, M. J. (1994). Maternal empathy, family chaos, and the etiology of borderline personality disorder. *Journal of the American Psychoanalytic Association, 42,* 525–548.

Goodheart, C. D., & Markham, B. (1992). The feminization of psychology: Implications for psychotherapy. *Psychotherapy, 29,* 130–138.

Gooding, D. C., & Iacono, W. G. (1995). Schizophrenia through the lens of a developmental psychopathology perspective. In D. Cicchetti & D. J. Cohen (Eds.), *Manual of developmental psychopathology.* New York: Cambridge.

Goodman, W., Price, L., Delgado, P., Palumbo, J., Krystal, J., Nagy, L., Rasmussen, S., Heninger, G., & Charney, D. (1990). Specificity of serotonin reuptake inhibitors in the treatment of obsessive-compulsive disorder: Comparison of fluvoxamine and despiramine. *Archives of General Psychiatry, 47,* 577–588.

Goodwin, D. W. (1976). *Is alcoholism hereditary?* New York: Oxford University Press.

Goodwin, D. W. (1979). Alcoholism and heredity. *Archives of General Psychiatry, 36,* 57–61.

Goodwin, D. W. (1985). Genetic determinants of alcoholism. In J. H. Mendelson & N. K. Mello (Eds.), *The diagnosis and treatment of alcoholism* (pp. 65–87). New York: McGraw-Hill.

Goodwin, D. W. (1986). *Anxiety.* New York: Ballantine Books.

Goodwin, D. W., Schulsinger, F., Hermansen, L., Guze, S. B., & Winokur, G. (1973). Alcohol problems in adoptees raised apart from alcoholic biological parents. *Archives of General Psychiatry, 28,* 238–243.

Goodwin, F. K., & Jamison, K. R. (1990). *Manic-depressive illness.* New York: Oxford University Press.

Goodwin, G. M. (1994). Recurrence of mania after lithium withdrawal: Implications for the use of lithium in the treatment of bipolar affective disorder. *British Journal of Psychiatry, 164,* 149–152.

Gorman, J. (1994). New and experimental pharmacological treatments for panic disorder. In B. E. Wolfe & J. D. Maser (Eds.), *Treatment of panic disorder.* Washington, DC: American Psychiatric Press.

Gotlib, I. H. (1992). Interpersonal and cognitive aspects of depression. *Current Directions in Psychological Science, 1,* 149–154.

Gotlib, I. H., & McCabe, S. B. (1990). Marriage and psychopathology. In F. F. Fincham & T. N. Brabury (Eds.), *The psychology of marriage* (pp. 226–257). New York: Guilford Press.

Gotlib, I. H., & Robinson, L. A. (1982). Responses to depressed individuals: Discrepancies between self-report and observer rated behavior. *Journal of Abnormal Psychology, 91,* 231–240.

Gotlib, I. H., & Whiffen, V. E. (1991). The interpersonal context of depression: Implications for theory and research. In W. H. Jones & D. Perlman (Eds.). *Advances in personal relationships* (Vol. 3, pp. 177–206). London, England: Jessica Kingsley.

Gottesman, I. I. (1991). *Schizophrenia genesis: The origins of madness.* New York: Freeman.

Gottesman, I. I. (1993). Origins of schizophrenia: Past as prologue. In R. Plomin & G. E. McClearn (Eds.), *Nature, nurture and psychology* (pp. 2231–2244). Washington, DC: American Psychological Association.

Gottesman, I. I., McGuffin, P., & Farmer, A. (1987). Clinical genetics as clues to the "real" genetics of schizophrenia. *Schizophrenia Bulletin, 13,* 23–47.

Gottesman, I. I., & Shields, J. (1972). *Schizophrenia and genetics: A twin study vantage point.* New York: Academic Press.

Gottman, J. M., Gonso, J., & Rasmussen, B. (1975). Social interaction, social competence, and friendship in children. *Child Development, 46,* 709–718.

Gottman, J. M., Jacobson, N. S., Rushe, R. H., Short, J. W., Babcock, J., La Taillade, J. J., & Waltz, J. (1995). The relationship between heart rate reactivity, emotionally aggressive behavior and general violence in batterers. *Journal of Family Psychology, 9,* 227–248.

Gough, H. G. (1969). *California Psychological Inventory* (rev. manual). Palo Alto, CA: Consulting Psychologists Press.

Gowers, S., Norton, K., Halek, C., & Crisp, A. H. (1994). Outcome of outpatient psychotherapy in a random allocation treatment study of anorexia nervosa. *International Journal of Eating Disorders, 15,* 165–178.

Graham, S. (1992). "Most of the subjects were white and middle class": Trends in published research on African Americans in selected APA journals, 1970–1989. *American Psychologist, 47,* 629–639.

Grandin, T. (1987). Motivating autistic children. *Academic Therapy, 22,* 142–148.

Gray, J. (1970). The psychophysiological basis of introversion-extraversion. *Behavior Research and Therapy, 8,* 249–266.

Gray, J. A. (1982). *The neuropsychology of anxiety: An enquiry into the functions of the septo-hippocampal system.* Oxford, England: Oxford University Press.

Gray, J. A. (1985). Issues in the neuropsychology of anxiety. In A. H. Tuma & J. D. Maser (Eds.), *Anxiety and the anxiety disorders.* Hillsdale, NJ: Lawrence Erlbaum.

Gray, J. A. (1987). *The psychology of fear and stress* (2nd ed.). Cambridge, England: Cambridge University Press.

Gray, J. N., & Melton, G. B. (1985). The law and ethics of psychosocial research on AIDS. *Nebraska Law Review, 64,* 637–688.

Graziano, A. M., DeGiovanni, I. S., & Garcia, K. A. (1979). Behavioral treatment of children's fear: A review. *Psychological Bulletin, 86,* 804–830.

Graziano, A. M., & Mooney, K. (1980). Family self-control instruction for children's nighttime fear reduction. *Journal of Consulting and Clinical Psychology, 48,* 206–213.

Green, M. F., & Kinsbourne, M. (1990). Subvocal activity and auditory hallucinations: Clues for behavioral treatments. *Schizophrenia Bulletin, 16,* 617–625.

Green, R. (1978). Sexual identity of 37 children raised by homosexual or transsexual parents. *American Journal of Psychiatry, 135,* 692–697.

Green, R. G. (1987). *The "sissy boy syndrome" and the development of homosexuality.* New Haven, CT: Yale University Press.

Greenbaum, P. E., Dedrick, R. F., Prange, M. E., & Friedman, R. M. (1994). Parent, teacher, and child ratings of problem behaviors of youngsters with serious emotional disturbances. *Psychological Assessment, 6,* 141–148.

Greenberg, L. S. (1986). Change process research. *Journal of Consulting and Clinical Psychology, 54,* 4–9.

Greenberg, L. S., & Johnson, S. M. (1988). *Emotionally focused therapy for couples.* New York: Guilford Press.

Greenberg, L. S., Rice, L. N., & Elliot, R. (1993). *Facilitating emotional change.* New York: Guilford Press.

Greenberg, R. P., Bornstein, R. F., Greenberg, M. D., & Fisher, S. (1992). A meta-analysis of antidepressant outcome under blinder conditions. *Journal of Consulting and Clinical Psychology, 60,* 664–669.

Greenfield, J. (1972). *A child called Noah*. New York: Holt, Rinehart & Winston.

Greenfield, J. (1978). *A place for Noah*. New York: Holt, Rinehart & Winston.

Greenwood, C. R., Carta, J. J., Hart, B., Kamps, D., Terry, B., Arreaga-Mayer, C., Atwater, J., Walker, D., Risley, T., & Delquadri, J. C. (1992). Out of the laboratory and into the community. *American Psychologist, 47,* 1464–1474.

Greenwood, M. R. C. (1989). Sexual dimorphism and obesity. In A. J. Stunkard & A. Baum (Eds.), *Perspectives in behavioral medicine* (pp. 31–38). Hillsdale, NJ: Lawrence Erlbaum.

Greiner, N., & Nunno, V. J. (1994). Psychopaths at Nuremberg? A Rorschach analysis of the records of the Nazi war criminals. *Journal of Clinical Psychology, 50,* 415–429.

Griest, J. H., & Jefferson, J. W. (1992). Depression and its treatment. Washington, DC: American Psychiatric Press.

Grisso, T. (1987). The economic and scientific future of forensic psychological assessment. *American Psychologist, 42,* 831–839.

Group therapy—Part 1. (1989, January). *Harvard Medical School Mental Health Letter, 5,* 1–4.

Grunhaus, L., Zelnick, T., Albala, A., Rabin, D., Haskett, R. F., Zis, A. P., & Greden, F., Jr. (1987). Serial dexamethasone suppression tests in depressed patients treated only with electroconvulsive therapy. *Journal of Affective Disorders 13,* 233–240.

Grych, J. H., & Fincham, F. D. (1990). Marital conflict and children's adjustment: A cognitive-contextual framework. *Psychological Bulletin, 108,* 267–290.

Gull, W. W. (1873). Anorexia hysterica (apepsia hysteria). *British Medical Journal, 2,* 527.

Gunderson, J. G. (1984). *Borderline personality disorder*. Washington, DC: American Psychiatric Press.

Gunderson, J. G. (1988). Personality disorders. In A. Nicholi, Jr. (Ed.), *The new Harvard guide to psychiatry* (pp. 337–357). Cambridge, MA: Harvard University Press.

Gunderson, J. G. (1991). Diagnostic controversies. In A. Tasman & M. B. Riba (Eds.), *Review of Psychiatry* (Vol. 11, pp. 9–24). Washington, DC: American Psychiatric Press.

Gunderson, J. G., Ronningstam, E., & Smith, L. E. (1993). Narcissistic personality disorder: A review of data on *DSM-III-R* descriptions. *Journal of Personality Disorders, 5,* 167–177.

Gunderson, J. G., Zanarini, M. C., & Kisiel, C. L. (1991). Borderline personality disorder: A review of data on *DSM-III-R* descriptions. *Journal of Personality Disorders, 5,* 340–352.

Gur, R. E., & Pearlson, G. D. (1993). Neuroimaging in schizophrenia research. *Schizophrenia 1993: Special report* (pp. 163–179). Washington, DC: National Institute of Mental Health, Schizophrenia Research Branch.

Gurman, A. S., & Kniskern, D. P. (1986). Research on marital and family therapy: Progress perspective and prospect. In S. L. Garfield & A. E. Bergin (Eds.), *Handbook of psychotherapy and behavior change.* New York: John Wiley.

Guttman, M. (1994, May 9). Violence in entertainment. *US News and World Report,* pp. 39–46.

Guze, S. B., Cloninger, C. R., Martin, R. L., & Clayton, P. J. (1986). A follow-up and family study of Briquet's syndrome. *British Journal of Psychiatry, 149,* 17–23.

Gynther, M. D., & Gynther, R. A. (1983). Personality inventories. In I. B. Weiner (Ed.), *Clinical methods in psychology* (2nd ed.). New York: Wiley-Interscience.

H

Haaga, D. A. F., Dyck, M. J., & Ernst, D. (1991). Empirical status of cognitive theory of depression. *Psychological Bulletin, 110,* 215–236.

Haaland, K. Y. (1992). Introduction to the special section on the emotional concomitants of brain damage. *Journal of Consulting and Clinical Psychology, 60,* 327–328.

Hafner, R. J. (1986). *Marriage & mental illness: A sex roles perspective*. New York: Guilford Press.

Haggloff, B., Blom, L., Dahlquist, G., Lonnberg, G., & Sahlin, B. (1991). The Swedish childhood diabetes study: Indications of severe psychological stress as a risk factor for Type I (insulin-dependent) diabetes mellitus in childhood. *Diabetologia, 34,* 579–583.

Hagman, C. (1932). A study of fears of children in preschool age. *Journal of Experimental Psychology, 1,* 110–130.

Hahlweg, K. (1988, September). *Behavioural marital therapy: The state of the art*. Paper presented at the Behaviour Therapy World Congress, Edinburgh, Scotland.

Hall, A., & Hay, A. (1991). The prevalence of eating disorders in recently admitted psychiatric in-patients. *British Journal of Psychiatry, 159,* 562–565.

Hall, G. C. N. (1991). Prediction of sexual aggression. *Clinical Psychology Review, 10,* 229–245.

Hall, G. C. N. (1995). Sexual offender recidivism revisited: A meta-analysis of recent treatment studies. *Journal of Consulting and Clinical Psychology, 63,* 802–809.

Hall, G. C. N., & Hirschman, R. (1991). Toward a theory of sexual aggression: A quadripartite model. *Journal of Consulting and Clinical Psychology, 59,* 662–669.

Hall, M. (1994, August 17). Furor brews over release of sex offender. *USA Today.*

Halmi, K. A. (Ed.). (1993). *Psychobiology and treatment of anorexia nervosa and bulimia nervosa*. Washington, DC: American Psychiatric Press.

Halmi, K. A., Eckert, E., Marchi, P., Sampugnaro, V., Apple, R., & Cohen, J. (1991). Comorbidity of psychiatric diagnoses in anorexia nervosa. *Archives of General Psychiatry, 48,* 712–718.

Halstead, W. C. (1947). *Brain and intelligence: A quantitative study of the frontal lobes*. Chicago: University of Chicago Press.

Hamberger, L. K., & Hastings, J. E. (1991). Personality correlates of men who batter and nonviolent men: Some continuities and discontinuities. *Journal of Family Violence, 6,* 131–147.

Hamer, D. H., Hu, S., Magnuson, V. L., Hu, N., Pattatucci, A. M. L. (1993). A linkage between DNA markers on the X chromosome and male sexual orientation. *Science, 261,* 321–327.

Hammen, C. L. (1985). Predicting depression: A cognitive behavioral perspective. In P. Kendall (Ed.), *Advances in cognitive-behavioral research* (pp. 29–71). New York: Academic Press.

Hammen, C. L. (1991). Generation of stress in the course of unipolar depression. *Journal of Abnormal Psychology, 100,* 555–561.

Hammen, C. L., Ellicott, A., & Gitlin, M. J. (1992). Stressors and sociotropy/autonomy: A longitudinal study of their relationship to the course of bipolar disorder. *Cognitive Therapy and Research, 16,* 409–418.

Hammen, C. L., Ellicott, A., Gitlin, M. J., & Jamison, K. R. (1989). Sociotropy/autonomy and vulnerability to specific life events in patients with unipolar and bipolar disorders. *Journal of Abnormal Psychology, 98,* 154–160.

Hampton, R. L., & Gelles, R. J. (1994). Violence toward black women in a nationally representative sample of black families. *Journal of Comparative Family Studies, 25,* 105–119.

Hanneke, C. R., Shields, N. M., & McCall, G. J. (1986). Assessing the prevalence of marital rape. *Journal of Interpersonal Violence, 1,* 350–362.

Hansen, D. J., Conaway, L. P., & Christopher, J. S. (1990). Victims of child abuse. In R. T. Ammerman & M. Hersen (Eds.), *Treatment of family violence* (pp. 17–49). New York: John Wiley.

Hansen, W. B. (in press). School-based substance abuse prevention: A review of the state of the art in curriculum, 1980–1990. *Health Education Research.*

Harding, C. M., Brooks, G. W., Ashikakga, T., Strauss, J., & Brier, A. (1987). The Vermont longitudinal study of persons with severe mental illness, II: Long-term outcome of subjects who retrospectively met DSM-III criteria for schizophrenia. *American Journal of Psychiatry, 144,* 727–735.

Hardman, M. L., Drew, C. J., Egan, M. W., & Wolf, B. (1993). *Human exceptionality: Society, school, and family* (4th ed.). Boston: Allyn and Bacon.

Hare, R. D. (1991). *The Hare Psychopathy Checklist–Revised*. Toronto, Ontario, Canada: Multi-Health Systems.

Harford, T. C., Parker, D. A., Grant, B. F., & Dawson, D. A. (1992). Alcohol use and dependence among employed men and women in the United States in 1988. *Alcoholism: Clinical and Experimental Research, 16,* 146–148.

Hargrave, G. E., Hiatt, D., Ogard, E. M., & Karr, C. (1994). Comparison of the MMPI and the MMPI-2 for a sample of peace officers. *Psychological Assessment, 6,* 27–32.

Harkness, A. R. (1992). Fundamental topics in the personality disorders: Candidate trait dimensions from lower regions of the hierarchy. *Psychological Assessment, 4,* 251–259.

Harpur, T. J., & Hare, R. D. (1994). Assessment of psychopathy as a function of age. *Journal of Abnormal Psychology, 103,* 604–609.

Harris, E. L., Noyes, R., Crowe, R. R., & Chaundry, D. R. (1983). Family study of agoraphobia. *Archives of General Psychiatry, 40,* 1061–1064.

Harrow, M., Goldberg, J. F., Grossman, L. S., & Meltzer, H. Y. (1990). Outcome in manic disorders: A naturalistic follow-up study. *Archives of General Psychiatry, 47,* 665–671.

Hartmann, H. (1958). *Ego psychology and the problem of adaptation.* New York: International Universities Press.

Hartvig, P., & Sterner, G. (1985). Childhood psychologic environmental exposure in women with diagnosed somatoform disorders. *Scandinavian Journal of Social Medicine, 13,* 153–157.

Haskell, W. L., Alderman, E. L., Fair, J. M., Maron, D. J., Mackey, S. F., Superko, H. R., Williams, P. T., Johnstone, I. M., Champagne, M. A., & Krauss, R. M. (1994). Effects of intensive multiple risk factor reduction on coronary atherosclerosis and clinical cardiac events in men and women with coronary artery disease: The Stanford Coronary Risk Intervention Project (SCRIP). *Circulation, 89,* 975–990.

Hathaway, S. R., & McKinley, J. C. (1943). *Manual for the Minnesota Multiphasic Personality Inventory.* New York: Psychological Corporation.

Hathaway, S. R., & McKinley, J. C. (1951). *Minnesota Multiphasic Personality Inventory: Manual.* New York: Psychological Corporation.

Hawkins, J. D., Catalano, R. F., & Kent, L. A. (1991). Combining broadcast media and parent education to prevent teenage drug abuse. In L. Donohew, H. E. Sypher, & W. J. Bukoski (Eds.), *Persuasive communication and drug abuse education.* Hillsdale, NJ: Lawrence Erlbaum.

Hawkins, R. P., Kashden, J., Hansen, D. J., & Sadd, D. L. (1992). The increasing reference to "cognitive" variables in behavior therapy: A 20-year empirical analysis. *The Behavior Therapist, 15,* 115–118.

Hawton, K., Salkovskis, P., & Clark, D. (Eds.). (1989). *Cognitive behaviour therapy.* New York: Oxford University Press.

Hay, P. J., Fairburn, C. G., & Doll, H. A. (1995). *Towards the re-classification of bulimic eating disorders: A community-based cluster analytic study.* Unpublished manuscript, Oxford University, England.

Haynes, S. N. (1991). Behavioral assessment. In M. Hersen, A. E. Kazdin, & A. S. Bellack (Eds.), *The clinical psychology handbook* (2nd ed.) (pp. 430–464). New York: Pergamon Press.

Haynes, S. N., Falkin, S., & Sexton-Radek, K. (1989). Psychophysiological measurement in behavior therapy. In G. Turpin (Ed.), *Handbook of clinical psychophysiology.* London: John Wiley.

Haynes, S. N., Spain, E. H., & Oliveira, J. (1993). Identifying causal relationships in clinical assessment. *Psychological Assessment, 5,* 281–291.

Hays, R. B., Turner, H., & Coates, T. J. (1992). Social support, AIDS-related symptoms, and depression among gay men. *Journal of Consulting and Clinical Psychology, 60,* 463–469.

Hayward, C., Killen, J. D., Hammer, L. D., Litt, I. F., Wilson, D. M., Simmonds, B., & Taylor, C. B. (1992). Pubertal stage and panic attack history in sixth- and seventh-grade girls. *American Journal of Psychiatry, 149,* 1239–1243.

Hayward, P., Wardle, J., & Higgitt, A. (1989). Benzodiazepine research: Current findings and practical consequences. *British Journal of Psychiatry, 28,* 307–327.

Healy, D., & Williams, J. M. G. (1988). Dysrhythmia, dysphoria, and depression: The interaction of learned helplessness and circadian dysrhythmia in the pathogenesis of depression. *Psychological Bulletin, 103,* 163–178.

Heath, A. C., Cates, R., Martin, N. G., Meyer, J., Hewitt, J. K., Neale, M. C., & Eaves, L. J. (1993). Genetic contribution to risk of smoking initiation: Comparisons across birth cohorts and across cultures. *Journal of Substance Abuse, 5,* 221–246.

Heath, A. C., & Martin, N. G. (1993). Genetic models for the natural history of smoking: Evidence for a genetic influence on smoking persistence. *Addictive Behaviors, 18,* 19–34.

Heath, L., Bresolin, L. B., & Rinaldi, R. C. (1989). Effects of media violence on children. *Archives of General Psychiatry, 46,* 376–379.

Heaton, R., Paulsen, J. S., McAdams, L. A., Kuck, J., Zisook, S., Braff, D., Harris, M. J., & Jeste, D. V. (1994). Neuropsychological deficits in schizophrenics: Relationship to age, chronicity, and dementia. *Archives of General Psychiatry, 51,* 469–476.

Hechtman, L., Weiss, G., Perlman, T., & Amsel, R. (1984). Hyperactives as young adults: Initial predictors of adult outcome. *American Academy of Child Psychiatry, 23,* 250–260.

Heffernan, K. (1994). Sexual orientation as a factor in risk for binge eating and bulimia nervosa: A review. *International Journal of Eating Disorders, 16,* 335–347.

Heffernan, K. (in press). Eating disorders and weight concerns among lesbians. *International Journal of Eating Disorders.*

Heflinger, C. A. (1987). Psychotherapy research ethics: Continuing the debate on controlled clinical trials. *American Psychologist, 42,* 956–957.

Heiman, J., LoPiccolo, L., & LoPiccolo, J. (1976). *Becoming orgasmic: A sexual growth program for women.* Englewood Cliffs, NJ: Prentice Hall.

Heimberg, R. G., & Barlow, D. H. (1991). New developments in cognitive-behavioral therapy for social phobia. *Journal of Clinical Psychiatry, 52*(Suppl.), 21–30.

Heller, K., & Monahan, J. (1977). *Psychology and community change.* Homewood, IL: Dorsey Press.

Helmes, E., & Reddon, J. R. (1993). A perspective on developments in assessing psychopathology: A critical review of the MMPI and MMPI-2. *Psychological Bulletin, 3,* 453–471.

Helms, J. E. (1992). Why is there no study of cultural equivalence in standardized cognitive ability testing? *American Psychologist, 47,* 1083–1101.

Helzer, J. E. (1994). Psychoactive substance abuse and its relation to dependence. In T. A. Widiger, A. J. Frances, H. A. Pincus, M. B. First, R. Ross, & W. Davis (Eds.), DSM-IV *sourcebook* (Vol. 1, pp. 21–32). Washington, DC: American Psychiatric Association.

Helzer, J. E., Canino, G. J., Yeh, E.-K., Bland, R. C., Lee, C. K., Hwu, H.-G., & Newman, S. (1990). Alcoholism—North America and Asia. *Archives of General Psychiatry, 47,* 313–319.

Helzer, J. E., & Pryzbeck, T. R. (1988). The co-occurrence of alcoholism with other psychiatric disorders in the general population and its impact on treatment. *Journal of Studies on Alcohol, 49,* 219–224.

Helzer, J. E., Robins, L. N., & McEvoy, L. (1987). Post-traumatic stress disorder in the general population. *The New England Journal of Medicine, 317,* 1630–1634.

Henderson, S., Byrne, D. G., & Duncan-Jones, P. (1981). *Neurosis and the social environment.* London, England: Academic Press.

Henggler, S. W., Melton, G. B., & Smith, L. A. (1992). Family preservation using multisystemic therapy: An effective alternative to incarcerating juvenile offenders. *Journal of Consulting and Clinical Psychology, 60,* 953–961.

Henry, J. A. (1992). Toxicity of antidepressants: Comparisons with fluoxetine. *International Clinical Psychopharmacology, 6*(Suppl. 6), 22–27.

Herbert, J. D., Hope, D. A., & Bellack, A. S. (1992). Validity of the distinction between generalized social phobia and avoidant personality disorder. *Journal of Abnormal Psychology, 101,* 332–339.

Hermann, B., & Whitman, S. (1992). Psychopathology in epilepsy. *American Psychologist, 47,* 1134–1138.

Herrnstein, R., & Murray, C. (1994). *The bell curve.* New York: Free Press.

Herron, W. G., Schultz, C. L., & Welt, A. G. (1992). A comparison of 16 systems to diagnose schizophrenia. *Journal of Clinical Psychology, 48,* 711–721.

Heston, L. L. (1966). Psychiatric disorders in foster home reared children of schizophrenic mothers. *British Journal of Psychiatry, 112,* 819–825.

Hetherington, E. M., Cox, M., & Cox, R. (1982). Effects of divorce on parents and children. In M. Lamb (Ed.), *Nontraditional families* (pp. 233–288). Hillsdale, NJ: Lawrence Erlbaum.

Hewitt, P. L., & Flett, G. L. (1993). Dimensions of perfectionism, daily stress, and depression: A test of the specific vulnerability hypothesis. *Journal of Abnormal Psychology, 102,* 58–65.

Hiday, V. A., & Scheid-Cook, T. L. (1991). Outpatient commitment for "revolving door" patients: Compliance and treatment. *Journal of Nervous and Mental Disease, 179,* 83–88.

High anxiety. (1993, January). *Consumer Reports,* pp. 19–24.

Higuchi, S., Suzuki, K., Yamada, K., Parrish, K., & Kono, H. (1993). Alcoholics with eating disorders: Prevalence and clinical course, a study from Japan. *British Journal of Psychiatry, 162,* 403–406.

Hill, S. Y. (1995). Event-related potentials. *Alcohol Health & Research World, 19,* 54–55.

Hill, S. Y., & Steinhauer, S. R. (1993). Assessment of prepubertal and postpubertal boys and girls at risk for developing alcohol with P300 from a visual discrimination task. *Journal of Studies on Alcohol, 54,* 350–358.

Hilts, P. J. (1994a, June 16). Cigarette makers debated the risks they denied. *New York Times,* pp. A1, A12.

Hilts, P. J. (1994b, June 17). Tobacco maker studied risk but did little about results. *New York Times,* pp. A1, C16.

Hilts, P. J. (1994c, June 18). Grim findings scuttle hope for "safer" cigarette. *New York Times,* pp. 1, 10.

Hilts, P. J. (1994d, August 2). Is nicotine addictive? It depends on whose criteria you use. *New York Times,* p. B6.

Hingson, R. (1993). Prevention of alcohol-impaired driving. *Alcohol Health & Research World, 17,* 28–34.

Hirschfeld, R. M. A., & Shea, M. T. (1992). Personality. In E. S. Paykel (Ed.), *Handbook of affective disorders* (2nd ed., pp. 185–194). New York: Guilford Press.

Hirschfeld, R. M. A., Shea, M. T., & Weise, R. (1991). Dependent personality disorder: Perspectives for *DSM-IV. Journal of Personality Disorders, 5,* 135–149.

Hitzemann, R., Volkow, N., Wang, G. J., Fowler, J., Wolf, J., Burr, G., & Piscani, K. (1992, June). *Brain metabolic activity in chronic alcoholics.* Paper presented at the annual meeting of the Research Society on Alcoholism, San Diego, CA.

Hoban, P. (1989, February 20). Getting clean. *New York Magazine,* pp. 38–40.

Hoch, P. H., & Polatin, P. (1949). Pseudoneurotic forms of schizophrenia. *Psychiatry Quarterly, 23,* 248–276.

Hochschild, A. (1989). *The second shift.* New York: Avon Books.

Hoek, H. W. (1993). Review of the epidemiological studies of eating disorders. *International Review of Psychiatry, 5,* 61–74.

Hogarty, G. E. (1984). Depot neuroleptics: The relevance of psychosocial factors. A United States perspective. *Journal of Clinical Psychology, 34,* 36–42.

Hogarty, G., Anderson, C., Reiss, D., Kornblith, S., Greenwald, D., Javna, C., & Madonia, M. (1986). Family psychoeducation, social skills training, and maintenance chemotherapy in the aftercare treatment of schizophrenia: I. One-year effects of a controlled study on relapse and expressed emotion. *Archives of General Psychiatry, 33,* 633–642.

Hogarty, G., Anderson, C., Reiss, D., Kornblith, S., Greenwald, D., Ulrich, R., Carter, M., & EPICS Research Group. (1991). Family psychoeducation, social skills training, and maintenance chemotherapy in the aftercare treatment of schizophrenia: II. Two-year effects of a controlled study on relapse and adjustment. *Archives of General Psychiatry, 48,* 340–347.

Hoge, S. K., Appelbaum, P. S., & Greer, A. (1989). An empirical comparison of the Stone and dangerousness criteria for civil commitment. *American Journal of Psychiatry, 146,* 170–175.

Hoge, S. K., Sachs, G., Appelbaum, P. S., Greer, A., & Gordon, C. (1988). Limitations on psychiatrists' discretionary civil commitment authority by the Stone and dangerousness criteria. *Archives of General Psychiatry, 45,* 764–769.

Hohmann, A. A., Larson, D. B., Thompson, J. W., & Beardsley, R. S. (1988, November). *Psychotropic medication prescription in U.S. ambulatory medical care.* Paper presented at the American Public Health Association Annual Meeting, Boston, MA.

Holland, A. J., Sicotte, N., & Treasure, J. (1988). Anorexia nervosa: Evidence for a genetic basis. *Journal of Psychosomatic Research, 32,* 561–571.

Hollingshead, A. B., & Redlich, F. C. (1958). *Social class and mental illness.* New York: John Wiley.

Hollon, S. D. (1990). Cognitive therapy and pharmacotherapy for depression. *Psychiatric Annals, 20,* 249–258.

Hollon, S. D., & Beck, A. T. (1994). Cognitive and cognitive-behavioral therapies. In A. E. Bergin & S. L. Garfield (Eds.), *Handbook of psychotherapy and behavior change* (4th ed.). New York: John Wiley.

Hollon, S. D., & Carter, M. M. (1994). Depression in adults. In L. W. Craighead, W. E. Craighead, A. E. Kazdin, & M. J. Mahoney (Eds.), *Cognitive and behavioral interventions* (pp. 89–104). Boston: Allyn and Bacon.

Hollon, S. D., DeRubeis, R. J., & Seligman, M. E. P. (1992). Cognitive therapy and the prevention of depression. *Applied and Preventative Psychology, 1,* 89–95.

Hollon, S. D., Shelton, R. C., & Davis, D. D. (1993). Cognitive therapy for depression: Conceptual issues and clinical efficacy. *Journal of Consulting and Clinical Psychology, 61,* 270–275.

Hollon, S. D., Shelton, R. C., & Loosen, P. T. (1991). Cognitive therapy and pharmacotherapy for depression. *Journal of Consulting and Clinical Psychology, 59,* 88–99.

Holmes, D. (1990). The evidence of repression: An examination of sixty years of research. In J. Singer (Ed.), *Repression and dissociation: Implications for personality, theory, psychopathology, and health* (pp. 85–102). Chicago: University of Chicago Press.

Holmes, T. H., & Rahe, R. H. (1967). The social readjustment rating scale. *Journal of Psychosomatic Research, 11,* 213–218.

Holroyd, K., Penzien, D., Hursey, K., Tobin, D., Rogers, L., Holm, J., Marcille, P., Hall, J., & Chila, A. (1984). Change mechanisms in EMG biofeedback training: Cognitive changes underlying improvements in tension headache. *Journal of Consulting and Clinical Psychology, 52,* 1039–1053.

Holt, P. E., & Andrews, G. (1989). Provocation of panic: Three elements of the panic reaction in four anxiety disorders. *Behaviour Research and Therapy, 27,* 253–262.

Holtzworth-Munroe, A., & Stuart, G. L. (1994). Typologies of male batterers: Three subtypes and the differences among them. *Psychological Bulletin, 116,* 476–497.

Hooley, J. (1985). Expressed emotion: A review of the literature. *Clinical Psychology Review, 5,* 119–140.

Hooper, C. (1991). Hypotheses on homosexuality. *Journal of NIH Research, 3,* 20.

Hops, S., & Greenwood, C. R. (1981). Social skills deficits. In E. J. Mash & L. G. Terdal (Eds.), *Behavioral assessment of childhood disorders* (pp. 347–396). New York: Guilford Press.

Horgan, C. (1993). *Substance abuse: The nation's number one health problem—Key indicators for policy.* Princeton, NJ: Robert Wood Johnson Foundation.

Hornstein, G. A. (1992). The return of the repressed. *American Psychologist, 47,* 254–263.

Horowitz, M. J. (1989). Posttraumatic stress disorders. In *American Psychiatric Association Task Force on Treatments of Psychiatric Disorders* (Vol. 3). Washington, DC: American Psychiatric Association.

Horwath, E., Lish, J. D., Johnson, J., Hornig, C. D., & Weissman M. M. (1993). Agoraphobia without panic: Clinical reappraisal of an epidemiologic finding. *American Journal of Psychiatry, 10,* 1496–1501.

Horwitz, R. I., & Horwitz, S. M. (1993). Adherence to treatment and health outcomes. *Archives of Internal Medicine, 153,* 1863–1868.

House, J. S., Robbins, C., & Metzner, H. M. (1982). The association of social relationships and activities with mortality: Prospective evidence from the Tecumseh community health study. *American Journal of Epidemiology, 116,* 123–140.

Houskamp, B. M., & Foy, D. W. (1991). The assessment of post-traumatic stress disorder in battered women. *Journal of Interpersonal Violence, 6,* 367–375.

Houts, A. C., Berman, J. S., & Abramson, H. (1994). Effectiveness of psychological and pharmacological treatments for nocturnal enuresis. *Journal of Consulting and Clinical Psychology, 62,* 737–745.

Houts, A. C., & Liebert, R. M. (1984). *Bedwetting: A guide for parents and children.* Springfield, IL: Charles C Thomas.

Houts, A. C., Peterson, J. K., & Liebert, R. M. (1984). The effect of prior imipramine treatment on the results of conditioning therapy in children with enuresis. *Journal of Pediatric Psychology, 9,* 505–509.

Howard, M., & McCabe, J. B. (1990). Helping teenagers postpone sexual involvement. *Family Planning Perspective, 22,* 21–26.

Howell, T. H. (1981). Multiple lesions in stroke patients: A study in morbid anatomy. *Journal of the American Geriatric Society, 19,* 246–250.

Hoyt, M. F., & Austad, C. S. (1992). Psychotherapy in a staff model health maintenance organization: Providing and assuring quality care in the future. *Psychotherapy, 29,* 119–129.

Hsiao, J. K., Agren, H., Bartko, J. J., Rudorfer, M. V., Linnoila, M., & Potter, W. Z. (1987). Monoamine neurotransmitter interactions and the prediction of antidepressant response. *Archives of General Psychiatry, 44,* 1078–1083.

Hsu, L. K. G. (1990). *Eating disorders.* New York: Guilford Press.

Hudson, J. I., & Pope, H. G. (1990). Affective spectrum disorder: Does antidepressant response identify a family of disorders with a common pathophysiology? *American Journal of Psychiatry, 147,* 552–564.

Huesman, L. R., & Miller, L. S. (1994). Long-term effects of repeated exposure to media violence in childhood. In L. R. Huesman (Ed.), *Aggressive behavior: Current perspectives* (pp. 153–186). New York: Plenum.

Hugdahl, K. (1978). Electrodermal conditioning to potentially phobic stimuli: Effects of instructed extinction. *Behaviour Research and Therapy, 16,* 315–321.

Hugdahl, K., & Johnsen, B. H. (1989). Preparedness and electrodermal fear-conditioning: Ontogenetic vs. phylogenetic explanations. *Behaviour Research and Therapy, 27,* 269–278.

Hughes, C., & Rusch, F. R. (1990). Teaching supported employees with severe mental retardation to solve problems. *Journal of Applied Behavior Analysis, 22,* 365–372.

Hughes, C. C., Tremblay, M., Rapaport, R. N., & Leighton, A. H. (1960). *People of cove and woodlot.* New York: Basic Books.

Hughes, J. O., & Sandler, B. R. (1987). *"Friends" raping friends.* Washington, DC: Association of American Colleges, Project on the Status and Education of Women.

Hughes, J. R. (1993). Pharmacotherapy for smoking cessation: Unvalidated assumptions, anomalies, and suggestions for future research. *Journal of Consulting and Clinical Psychology, 61,* 751–760.

Hughes, J. R. (1994a). Caffeine withdrawal, dependence, and abuse. In T. A. Widiger, A. J. Frances, H. A. Pincus, M. B. First, R. Ross, & W. Davis (Eds.), DSM-IV *sourcebook* (Vol. 1, pp. 129–134). Washington, DC: American Psychiatric Association.

Hughes, J. R. (1994b). Nicotine withdrawal, dependence, and abuse. In T. A. Widiger, A. J. Frances, H. A. Pincus, M. B. First, R. Ross, & W. Davis (Eds.), DSM-IV *sourcebook* (Vol. 1, pp. 109–116). Washington, DC: American Psychiatric Association.

Humphrey, L. L. (1989). Observed family interactions among subtypes of eating disorders using structural analysis of social behavior. *Journal of Consulting and Clinical Psychology, 57,* 206–214.

Humphries, L. L., & Gruber, J. J. (1986). Nutrition behaviors of university majorettes. *Physician Sports Medicine, 14,* 91–98.

Hunt, W. A., & Nixon, S. J. (Eds.). (1993). *Alcohol-induced brain damage.* Washington, DC: National Institute on Alcohol Abuse and Alcoholism.

Huntingford, F., & Turner, A. (1987). *Animal conflict.* New York: Chapman & Hall.

Hynd, G., & Cohen, M. (1983). *Dyslexia.* New York: Grune & Stratton.

I

Iacono, W. G., & Clementz, B. A. (1992). A strategy for elucidating genetic influences on complex psychopathological syndromes (with special reference to ocular motor functioning and schizophrenia). In L. J. Chapman, J. P. Chapman, & D. W. Fowles (Eds.), *Progress in experimental personality and psychopathology research: Vol. 16. Frontiers of psychopathology* (pp. 11–65). New York: Springer.

Imber, S. D., Glanz, L. M., Elkin, I., Sotsky, S. M., Boyer, J. L., & Leber, W. R. (1986). Ethical issues in psychotherapy research: Problems in a collaborative clinical trials study. *American Psychologist, 41,* 137–146.

Imber, S. D., Pilkonis, P. A., Sotsky, S. M., Elkin, I., Watkins, J. T., Collins, J. F., Shea, M. T., Leber, W. R., & Glass, D. R. (1990). Mode-specific effects among three treatments for depression. *Journal of Consulting and Clinical Psychology, 58,* 352–359.

Ingram, R. E., Lumrey, A. B., Cruet, D., & Seiber, W. (1987). Attentional processes in depressive disorders. *Cognitive Therapy and Research, 11,* 351–360.

Ingram, R. E., Slater, M. A., Atkinson, J. H., & Scott, W. (1990). Positive automatic cognition in major affective disorder. *Psychological Assessment, 2,* 209–211.

Irwin, M., Patterson, T., Smith, T. L., Caldwell, C., Brown, S. A., Gillian, C., & Grant, I. (1990). Reduction of immune function on life stress and depression. *Biological Psychiatry, 27,* 22–30.

Iwata, B. A., Zarcone, J. R., Vollmer, T. R., & Smith, R. G. (1994). Assessment and treatment of self-injurious behavior. In E. Schopler & G. B. Mesibov (Eds.), *Behavioral issues in autism* (pp. 131–159). New York: Plenum Press.

J

Jablensky, A. (1989). Epidemiology and cross-cultural aspects of schizophrenia. *Psychiatric Annals, 19,* 516–524.

Jacob, R. G., O'Leary, K. D., & Rosenblad, C. (1978). Formal and informal class settings: Effects on hyperactivity. *Journal of Abnormal Child Psychology, 6,* 47–59.

Jacobsen, F. M. (1992). Fluoxetine-induced sexual dysfunction and an open trial of yohimbine. *Journal of Clinical Psychiatry, 53,* 119–122.

Jacobsen, R. (1986). Female alcoholics: A controlled CT brain scan and clinical study. *British Journal of Addiction, 81,* 661–669.

Jacobson, E. (1938). *Progressive relaxation.* Chicago: University of Chicago Press.

Jacobson, N. S., & Addis, M. E. (1993). Research on couples and couples therapy: What do we know? Where are we going? *Journal of Consulting and Clinical Psychology, 61,* 85–93.

Jacobson, N. S., Gottman, J. M., Waltz, J., Rushe, R., & Babcock, J. (1994). Affect, verbal content, and psychophysiology in the arguments of couples with a violent husband. *Journal of Consulting and Clinical Psychology, 62,* 982–988.

Jacobvitz, D., Sroufe, L. A., Stewart, M., & Leffert, N. (1990). Treatment of attentional and hyperactive problems in children with sympathomimetic drugs: A follow-up review. *Journal of the American Academy of Child and Adolescent Psychiatry, 29,* 677–688.

Jaenicke, C., Hammen, C., Zupan, B., Hiroto, D., Gordon, D., Adrian, C., & Burge, D. (1987). Cognitive vulnerability in children at risk for depression. *Journal of Abnormal Child Psychology, 15,* 559–572.

Jamison, K. R. (1993). *Touched with fire: Manic depressive illness and temperament.* New York: Free Press.

Jarrett, R. B., & Rush, A. J. (1994). Short-term psychotherapy of depressive disorders: Current status and future directions. *Psychiatry: Interpersonal and biological processes, 57,* 115–132.

Jarvis, E. (1971). *Insanity and idiocy in Massachusetts: Report of the Commission on Lunacy.* Cambridge, MA: Harvard University Press. (Original work published 1855)

Jeffrey, T. B., Rankin, R. J., & Jeffrey, L. K. (1992). In service of two masters: The ethical-legal dilemmas faced by military psychologists. *Professional Psychology: Research and Practice, 23,* 91–95.

Jemmott, J. B., & Magliore, K. (1988). Academic stress, social support, and secretory immunoglobulin A. *Journal of Personality and Social Psychology, 55,* 803–810.

Jenike, M. A., Baer, L., Ballantine, H. T., Martuza, R. L., Tynes, S., Girunas, I., Buttolph, M. L., & Cassem, N. H. (1991). Cingulotomy for refractory obsessive compulsive disorder: A long-term follow-up of 33 cases. *Archives of General Psychiatry, 48,* 548–557.

Jenkins, J. H., Kleinman, A., & Good, B. J. (1991). Cross-cultural studies of depression. In J. Becker & A. Kleinman (Eds.), *Psychosocial aspects of depression* (pp. 67–99). Hillsdale, NJ: Lawrence Erlbaum.

Jersild, A. T., & Holmes, F. B. (1935). Children's fears. *Child Development Monographs, 20,* 1–358.

Jeste, D. V., & Caligiuri, M. P. (1993). Tardive dyskinesia. *Schizophrenia 1993: Special report* (pp. 128–149). Washington, DC: National Institute of Mental Health, Schizophrenia Research Branch.

Jeste, D., & Heaton, S. (1994). How does late-onset compare with early-onset schizophrenia? *Harvard Mental Health Letter, 10*(8).

Jimerson, D. C., Lesem, M. D., Kaye, W. H., & Brewerton, T. D. (1992). Low serotonin and dopamine metabolite concentrations in cerebrospinal fluid from bulimic patients with frequent binge episodes. *Archives of General Psychiatry, 49,* 132–139.

Jimerson, D. C., Lesem, M. D., Kaye, W. H., Hegg, A. P., & Brewerton, T. D. (1990). Eating disorders and depression: Is there a serotonin connection? *Biological Psychiatry, 28,* 443–454.

Johnson, C. (Ed.). (1991). *Psychodynamic treatment of anorexia nervosa and bulimia.* New York: Guilford Press.

Johnson, J., Weissman, M. M., & Klerman, G. L. (1990). Panic disorder, comorbidity, and suicide attempts. *Archives of General Psychiatry, 47,* 805–808.

Johnson, R. C., Nagoshi, C. T., Danko, G. P., Honbo, K. A. M., & Chau, L. L. (1990). Familial transmission of alcohol use norms and expectancies and reported alcohol use. *Alcoholism: Clinical and Experimental Research, 14,* 216–220.

Johnson, S. B., & Melamed, D. G. (1979). The assessment and treatment of children's fears. In B. Lahey & A. E. Kazdin (Eds.), *Advances in clinical child psychology* (Vol. 2, pp. 107–139). New York: Plenum.

Jolly, J. B., Dyck, M. J., Kramer, T. A., & Wherry, J. N. (1994). Integration of positive and negative affectivity and cognitive content-specificity: Improved discrimination of anxious and depressive symptoms. *Journal of Abnormal Psychology, 103,* 544–552.

Jones, B. (1993). Schizophrenia: Into the next millennium. *Canadian Journal of Psychiatry, 38*(Suppl. 3), 67–69.

Jones, B. P., & Butters, N. (1991). Neuropsychological assessment. In M. Hersen, A. E. Kazdin, & A. S. Bellack (Eds.), *The clinical psychology handbook* (2nd ed.) (pp. 406–429). New York: Pergamon Press.

Jones, E. (1953). *The life and work of Sigmund Freud, Vol. 1: The formative years and the great discoveries.* New York: Basic Books.

Jones, M. C. (1924). The elimination of children's fears. *Journal of Experimental Psychology, 7,* 383–390.

Jones, R. R., Weinrott, M. R., & Howard, J. R. (1981). *The national evaluation of the teaching family model: Final report to the Center for Studies of Antisocial and Violent Behavior.* Bethesda, MD: National Institute of Mental Health.

Jouriles, E. N., Bourg, W. J., & Farris, A. M. (1991). Marital adjustment and child conduct problems: A comparison of the correlation across subsamples. *Journal of Consulting and Clinical Psychology, 59,* 354–357.

Joyce, C. R. B., & Welldon, R. M. C. (1965). The objective efficacy of prayer. *Journal of Chronic Disease, 18,* 367–377.

Judd, P. H., & Ruff, R. M. (1993). Neuropsychological dysfunction in borderline personality disorder. *Journal of Personality Disorders, 7,* 275–284.

Julien, R. M. (1995). *A primer of drug action* (7th ed.). New York: W. H. Freeman.

Jung, C. G. (1923). *Psychological types.* New York: Harcourt.

K

Kafka, M., & Prentky, R. (1991). Current treatments of paraphiliacs. *Annual Review of Sex Research, 3,* 255–290.

Kagan, J. (1989a). Temperamental contributions to social behavior. *American Psychologist, 44,* 668–674.

Kagan, J. (1989b). *Unstable ideas: Temperament, cognition, and self.* Cambridge, MA: Harvard University Press.

Kagan, J., Snidman, N., & Arcus, D. M. (1992). Initial reactions to unfamiliarity. *Current Directions in Psychological Science, 1,* 171–174.

Kaij, J. (1960). *Studies on the etiology and sequels of abuse of alcohol.* Lund, Sweden: University of Lund.

Kalat, J. W. (1992). *Biological psychology.* Belmont, CA: Wadsworth.

Kalichman, S. C., Kelly, J. A., Hunter, T. L., Murphy, D. A., & Tyler, R. (1993). Culturally tailored HIV-AIDS risk-reduction messages targeted to African-American urban women: Impact on risk sensitization and risk reduction. *Journal of Consulting and Clinical Psychology, 61,* 291–295.

Kallmann, F. J. (1953). *Heredity in health and mental disorder.* New York: W. W. Norton.

Kandel, D. B., Davies, M., Karns, D., & Yamaguchi, K. (1986). The consequences in young adulthood of adolescent drug involvement. *Archives of General Psychiatry, 43,* 746–754.

Kandel, E. R., & Schwartz, J. H. (1985). *Principles of neural science* (2nd ed.). New York: Elsevier.

Kandel, E. R., Schwartz, J. H., & Jessell, T. M. (1991). *Principles of neural science* (3rd ed.). East Norwalk, CT: Appleton & Lange.

Kane, J., Honigfeld, G., Singer, J., Meltzer, H., & the Clozaril Collaborative Study Group. (1988). Clozapine for the treatment-resistant schizophrenic. *Archives of General Psychiatry, 45,* 789–796.

Kane, J. M., & Marder, S. R. (1993). Psychopharmacologic treatment of schizophrenia. *Schizophrenia 1993: Special report* (pp. 113–128). Washington, DC: National Institute of Mental Health, Schizophrenia Research Branch.

Kane, J., Woerner, M., Weinhold, P., Wegner, B., & Kinon, B. (1982). A prospective study of tardive dyskinesia development: Preliminary results. *Journal of Clinical Psychology, 2,* 345–349.

Kanfer, F. H. (1977). The many faces of self-control, or behavior modification changes its focus. In R. B. Stuart (Ed.), *Behavioral self-management.* New York: Brunner/Mazel.

Kanin, E. J. (1985). Date rapists: Differential sexual socialization and relative deprivation. *Archives of Sexual Behavior, 14,* 219–231.

Kanner, A. D., Coyne, J. C., Schaefer, C., & Lazarus, R. S. (1981). Comparison of two modes of stress measurement: Daily hassles and uplifts versus major life events. *Journal of Behavioral Medicine, 4,* 1–39.

Kanner, L. (1943). Autistic disturbances of affective contact. *Nervous Child, 2,* 217–230.

Kanner, L. (1971). Follow-up study of eleven autistic children originally reported in 1943. *Journal of Autism and Childhood Schizophrenia, 1,* 119–145.

Kanner, L., & Eisenberg, L. (1955). Notes on the follow-up studies of autistic children. In P. Hoch & J. Zubin (Eds.), *Psychopathology of childhood* (pp. 143–150). New York: Grune & Stratton.

Kantor, G. K., & Straus, M. A. (1990). "The drunken bum" theory of wife beating. In M. A. Straus & R. J. Gelles (Eds.), *Physical violence in American families: Risk factors and adaptations to violence in 8,145 families* (pp. 203–224). New Brunswick, NJ: Transaction.

Kaplan, H. I., & Sadock, B. J. (1991). *Synopsis of psychiatry: Behavioral sciences and clinical psychiatry* (6th ed.). Baltimore, MD: Williams & Wilkins.

Kaplan, H. I., & Sadock, B. J. (1993). *Pocket handbook of psychiatric drug treatment.* Baltimore, MD: Williams & Wilkins.

Kaplan, H. S. (1979). *Disorders of sexual desire.* New York: Brunner/Mazel.

Kaplan, J. R., Adams, M. R., Clarkson, T. B., Manuck, S. B., & Shively, C. A. (1991). Social behavior and gender in biomedical investigations using monkeys: Studies in atherogenesis. *Laboratory Animal Science, 41,* 1–9.

Kapur, S., & Mann, J. J. (1992). Role of the dopaminergic system in depression. *Biological Psychiatry, 32,* 1–17.

Kapur, S., Mieczkowski, T., & Mann, J. J. (1992). Antidepressant medications and the relative risk of suicide attempt and suicide. *Journal of the American Medical Association, 268,* 3441–3445.

Karasu, T. B., Docherty, J. P., Gelenberg, A., Kupfer, D. J., Merriam, A. E., & Shadoan, R. (1993). Practice guidelines for major depressive disorder in adults. *American Journal of Psychiatry, 150*(Suppl.), 1–26.

Karno, M., Golding, J. M., Sorenson, S. B., & Burnam, M. A. (1988). The epidemiology of obsessive-compulsive disorder in five U. S. communities. *Archives of General Psychiatry, 45,* 1094–1099.

Karno, M., Hough, R. L., Burnam, M. A., Escobar, J. I., Timbers, D. M., Santana, F., & Boyd, J. H. (1987). Lifetime prevalence of specific psychiatric disorders among Mexican Americans and non-Hispanic whites in Los Angeles. *Archives of General Psychiatry, 44,* 695–701.

Kass, D. J., Silvers, F. M., & Abroms, G. M. (1972). Behavioral group treatment of hysteria. *Archives of General Psychiatry, 26,* 42–50.

Kaszniak, A. W., Nussbaum, P. D., Berren, M. R., & Santiago, J. (1988). Amnesia as a consequence of male rape: A case report. *Journal of Abnormal Psychology, 97,* 100–104.

Katon, W., Lin, E., Von Korff, M., Russo, J., Lipscomb, P., & Bush, T. (1991). Somatization: A spectrum of severity. *American Journal of Psychiatry, 148,* 34–40.

Katon, W., & Schulberg, H. C. (1992). Epidemiology of depression in primary care. *General Hospital Psychiatry, 14,* 237–247.

Katona, C. L., Robertson, M. M., Abou-Saleh, M. T., & Nairac, B. L. (1993). Placebo-controlled trial of lithium augmentation of fluoxetine and lofepramine. *International Clinical Psychopharmacology, 8,* 323.

Katz, R., & McGuffin, P. (1993). The genetics of affective disorders. In L. J. Chapman, J. P. Chapman, & D. Fowles (Eds.), *Progress in experimental personality and psychopathology research* (pp. 200–221). New York: Springer-Verlag.

Kaufman, B. N. (1983). *A sense of warning: The stranger than fiction true story by Barry Neil Kaufman.* New York: Delacorte Press.

Kaufman, B. N. (1994). *Son-rise: The miracle continues.* Tiburon, CA: H. J. Kramer.

Kaufmann, P., & Lilly, M. (1979). A recovering alcoholic speaks and her family therapist introduces her. In E. Kaufmann & P. N. Kaufmann (Eds.), *Family therapy of drug and alcohol abuse* (pp. 243–254). New York: Gardner Press.

Kaye, W. H., & Weltzin, T. E. (1991). Neurochemistry of bulimia nervosa. *Journal of Clinical Psychiatry, 52,* 617–622.

Kaye, W. H., Weltzin, T., & Hsu, L. K. G. (1993). Relationship between anorexia nervosa and obsessive compulsive behaviors. *Psychiatric Annals, 23*, 365–373.

Kazdin, A. E. (1981). Drawing valid inferences from case studies. *Journal of Consulting and Clinical Psychology, 49*, 183.

Kazdin, A. E. (1984). *Behavior modification in applied settings.* Homewood, IL: Dorsey Press.

Kazdin, A. E. (1987). *Conduct disorders in childhood and adolescence.* Newbury Park, CA: Sage.

Kazdin, A. E. (1989). Childhood depression. In E. J. Mash & R. A. Barkley (Eds.), *Treatment of childhood disorders* (pp. 135–166). New York: Guilford Press.

Kazdin, A. E. (1994). Antisocial behavior and conduct disorder. In L. W. Craighead, W. E. Craighead, A. E. Kazdin, & M. J. Mahoney (Eds.), *Cognitive and behavioral interventions* (pp. 267–300). Boston: Allyn and Bacon.

Kazdin, A. E., & Wilson, G. T. (1978). *Evaluation of behavior therapy: Issues, evidence, and research strategies.* Cambridge, MA: Ballinger.

Keller, M. B., Lavori, P. W., Coryell, W., Endicott, J., & Mueller, T. I. (1993). Bipolar I: A five-year prospective study. *Journal of Nervous and Mental Disease, 181*, 238–245.

Kelly, J. A., & Murphy, D. A. (1992). Psychological interventions with AIDS and HIV: Prevention and treatment. *Journal of Consulting and Clinical Psychology, 60*, 576–585.

Kelly, J. A., Murphy, D. A., Sikkema, K. J., & Kalichman, S. C. (1993). Psychological interventions to prevent HIV infection are urgently needed: New priorities for behavioral research in the second decade of AIDS. *American Psychologist, 48*, 1023–1034.

Kemeny, M. E., Cohen, F., Zegans, L. S., & Conant, M. A. (1989). Psychological and immunological predictors of genital herpes recurrence. *Psychosomatic Medicine, 51*, 195–208.

Kemp, S. (1990). *Medieval psychology.* New York: Greenwood Press.

Kendall, P. C., Kortlander, E., Chansky, T., & Brady, E. (1992). Comorbidity of anxiety and depression in youth: Treatment implications. *Journal of Consulting and Clinical Psychology, 60*, 869–880.

Kendall, P. C., & Panichelli-Mindel, S. M. (1995). Cognitive-behavioral treatments. *Journal of Abnormal Child Psychology, 23*, 107–124.

Kendler, K. S., & Diehl, S. R. (1993). The genetics of schizophrenia: A current, genetic-epidemiologic perspective. In D. Shore (Ed.), *Special report: Schizophrenia 1993* (pp. 87–111). Rockville, MD: U.S. Department of Health and Human Services.

Kendler, K. S., Gruenberg, A. M., & Kinney, D. K. (1994). Independent diagnoses of adoptees and relatives as defined by DSM-III in the provincial and national samples of the Danish Adoption Study of schizophrenia. *Archives of General Psychiatry, 51*, 456–468.

Kendler, K. S., Heath, A. C., Martin, N. G., & Eaves, L. J. (1987). Symptoms of anxiety and symptoms of depression. *Archives of General Psychiatry, 44*, 451–457.

Kendler, K. S., Heath, A. C., Neale, M. C., Kessler, R. C., & Eaves, L. J. (1992). A population-based twin study of alcoholism in women. *Journal of the American Medical Association, 268*, 1877–1882.

Kendler, K. S., Kessler, R. C., Neale, M. C., Heath, A. C., & Eaves, L. J. (1993). The prediction of major depression in women: Toward an integrated etiologic model. *American Journal Psychiatry, 150*, 1139–1148.

Kendler, K. S., MacLean, C., Neale, M., Kessler, R., Heath, A., & Eaves, L. (1991). The genetic epidemiology of bulimia nervosa. *American Journal of Psychiatry, 148*, 1627–1637.

Kendler, K. S., Neale, M. C., Kessler, R. C., Heath, A. C., & Eaves, L. J. (1992a). Generalized anxiety disorder in women. *Archives of General Psychiatry, 49*, 267–272.

Kendler, K. S., Neale, M. C., Kessler, R. C., Heath, A. C., & Eaves, L. J. (1992b). The genetic epidemiology of phobias in women. *Archives of General Psychiatry, 49*, 273–281.

Kendziora, K., & O'Leary, S. G. (1993). Dysfunctional parenting as a focus for prevention and treatment of child behavior problems. In H. Ollendick & R. J. Prinz (Eds.), *Advances in child clinical psychology* (Vol. 15, pp. 175–206). New York: Plenum.

Kennedy, S., Thomson, R., Strancer, H. C., Roy, A., & Persad, E. (1983). Life events precipitating mania. *British Journal of Psychiatry, 142*, 398–403.

Kennedy, W. A. (1965). School phobia: Rapid treatment of fifty cases. *Journal of Abnormal Psychology, 70*, 285–289.

Kernberg, O. (1993). The psychotherapeutic treatment of borderline patients. In J. Paris (Ed.), *Borderline personality disorder* (pp. 261–284). Washington, DC: American Psychiatric Press.

Kessler, R. C., Foster, C., Joseph, J., Ostrow, D., Wortman, C., Phair, J., & Chmiel, J. (1991). Stressful life events and symptom onset in HIV infection. *American Journal of Psychiatry, 148*, 733–750.

Kessler, R. C., McGonagle, K. A., Zhao, S., Nelson, C. B., Hughes, M., Eshelman, S., Wittchen, H., & Kendler, K. S. (1994). Lifetime and 12 month prevalence of DSM-III-R psychiatric disorders in the United States: Results from a national comorbidity survey. *Archives of General Psychiatry, 51*, 8–20.

Kety, S. S., Wender, P. H., Jacobsen, B., Ingraham, L. J., Jansson, L., Faber, B., & Kinney, D. K. (1994). Mental illness in the biological and adoptive relatives of schizophrenic adoptees. *Archives of General Psychiatry, 51*, 442–455.

Keys, A., Brozek, J., Henschel, A., Mickelsen, O., & Taylor, H. (1950). *The biology of human starvation.* Minneapolis: University of Minnesota Press.

Khanna, S., Desai, N. G., & Channabasavanna, S. M. (1987). A treatment package for transsexualism. *Behavior Therapy, 18*, 193–199.

Khantzian, E. J. (1985). The self-medication hypothesis of addictive disorders: Focus on heroin and cocaine dependence. *American Journal of Psychiatry, 142*, 1259–1264.

Kiecolt-Glaser, J. K., & Glaser, R. (1987). Psychosocial moderators of immune function. *Annals of Behavioral Medicine, 9*, 16–20.

Kiecolt-Glaser, J. K., & Glaser, R. (1992). Psychoneuroimmunology: Can psychological interventions modulate immunity? *Journal of Consulting and Clinical Psychology, 60*, 569–575.

Kiesler, C. A., & Sibulkin, A. E. (1987). *Mental hospitals: Myths and facts about a national crisis.* Newbury Park, CA: Sage.

Kilmann, P. R., Boland, J. P., Norton, S. P., Davidson, E., & Caird, C. (1986). Perspectives on sex therapy outcome: A survey of ASSECT providers. *Journal of Sex and Marital Therapy, 12*, 116–138.

King, M. B., & Mezey, G. (1987). Eating behaviour of male racing jockeys. *Psychological Medicine, 17*, 249–253.

King, N. J. (1993). Simple and social phobias. In H. Ollendick & R. J. Prinz (Eds.), *Advances in child clinical psychology* (Vol. 15, pp. 305–341). New York: Plenum.

King, N. J., Ollendick, T., & Gullone, E. (1991). Negative affectivity in children and adolescents: Relations between anxiety and depression. *Clinical Psychology Review, 11*, 441–459.

Kinsey, A. C., Pomeroy, W. B., & Martin, C. E. (1948). *Sexual behavior in the human male.* Philadelphia: Saunders.

Kinsey, A. C., Pomeroy, W. B., Martin, C. E., & Gebhard, P. H. (1953). *Sexual behavior in the human male.* Philadelphia: Saunders.

Kirk, S. A., & Kutchins, H. (1994, May 28). Is bad writing a mental disorder? *New York Times*, p. A12.

Kitzman, K. M., & Emery, R. E. (1994). Child and family coping one year after mediated and litigated child custody disputes. *Journal of Family Psychology, 8*, 150–159.

Kivlahan, D. R., Marlatt, G. A., Fromme, K., Coppel, D. B., & Williams, E. (1990). Secondary prevention with college drinkers: Evaluation of an alcohol skills training program. *Journal of Consulting and Clinical Psychology, 58*, 805–810.

Klatsky, A. L., & Armstrong, M. A. (1993). Alcohol use, other traits, and risk of unnatural death: A prospective study. *Alcoholism: Clinical and Experimental Research, 17*, 1156–1162.

Klausner, J., Sweeney, J., Deck, M., Hass, G., & Kelly, A. B. (1992). Clinical correlates of cerebral ventricular enlargement on schizophrenia. Further evidence for frontal lobe disease. *Journal of Nervous and Mental Disease, 180*, 407–412.

Klein, D. F., & Ross, D. C. (1993). Reanalysis of the National Institute of Mental Health Treatment of Depression Collaborative Research Program General Effectiveness Report. *Neuropsychopharmacology, 8*, 241–251.

Klein, D. F., Ross, D. C., & Cohen, P. (1987). Panic and avoidance in agoraphobia. *Archives of General Psychiatry, 44*, 377–385.

Klein, D. F., Zitrin, C. M., Woerner, M. G., & Ross, D. C. (1983). Treatment of phobias. *Archives of General Psychiatry, 40*, 139–145.

Klein, D. N., Taylor, E. B., Dickstein, S., & Harding, K. (1988). The early-late onset distinction in *DSM-III-R* dysthymia. *Journal of Affective Disorders, 14*, 25–33.

Klein, N. C., Alexander, J., & Parsons, B. V. (1977). Impact of family systems intervention on recidivism and sibling delinquency: A model of primary prevention and program evaluation. *Journal of Consulting and Clinical Psychology, 45*, 469–474.

Klein, R. G. (1995). The role of methylphenidate in psychiatry. *Archives of General Psychiatry, 52*, 429–433.

Klein, R. G., & Last, C. G. (1989). *Anxiety disorders in children.* Newbury Park, CA: Sage.

Kleinknecht, R. A., Dinnel, D. L., Tanouye-Wilson, S., & Lonner, W. J. (1994). Cultural variation in social anxiety: A study of Taijin Kyofusho. *The Behavior Therapist, 17*, 175–178.

Klerman, G. L. (1987, May 4). The suicide link. *Newsweek*, p. 52.

Klerman, G. L., & Weissman, M. M. (1990). Increasing rates of depression. *Journal of the American Medical Association, 61*, 2229–2235.

Klerman, G. L., & Weissman, M. M. (Eds.). (1993). *New applications of interpersonal psychotherapy.* Washington, DC: American Psychiatric Association.

Klerman, G. L., Weissman, M. M., Rounsaville, B., & Chevron, E. (1984). *Interpersonal psychotherapy of depression (IPT).* New York: Basic Books.

Klinger, L. G., & Dawson, G. (1992). Facilitating early social and communicative development in children with autism. In S. F. Warren & J. Reichle (Eds.), *Causes and effects in communication and language intervention* (pp. 157–186). Baltimore: Paul H. Brookes.

Klitzner, M., Stewart, K., & Fisher, D. (1993). Reducing underage drinking and its consequences. *Alcohol Health & Research World, 17*, 12–18.

Klosko, J. S., Barlow, D. H., Tassinari, R., & Cerny, J. A. (1990). A comparison of alprazolam and behavior therapy in treatment of panic disorder. *Journal of Consulting and Clinical Psychology, 58*, 77–84.

Kluft, R. P. (1986). High-functioning multiple personality patients. *The Journal of Nervous and Mental Disease, 174*, 722–726.

Kluft, R. P. (1987a). An update on multiple personality disorder. *Hospital and Community Psychiatry, 38*, 363–373.

Kluft, R. P. (1987b). First-rank symptoms as a diagnostic clue to multiple personality disorder. *American Journal of Psychiatry, 144*, 293–298.

Klug, W. S., & Cummings, M. R. (1986). *Concepts of genetics.* Glenview, IL: Scott Foresman.

Knapezyk, D. R. (1989). Generalization of student question asking from special class to regular class settings. *Journal of Applied Behavior Analysis, 22*, 77–84.

Knapp, S., & VandeCreek, L. (1990). Application of the duty to protect to HIV-positive patients. *Professional Psychology: Research and Practice, 21*, 161–166.

Kochanska, G. (1995). Children's temperament, mothers' discipline, and security of attachment: Multiple pathways to emerging internalization. *Child Development, 66*, 597–615.

Kog, E., Vandereycken, W., & Vertommen, H. (1985). Towards a verification of the psychosomatic family model: A pilot study of ten families with an anorexia/bulimia nervosa patient. *International Journal of Eating Disorders, 4*, 525–538.

Kohlenberg, R. J. (1973). Behavior approach to multiple personality: A case study. *Behavior Therapy, 4*, 137–140.

Kohn, M. L. (1968). Social class and schizophrenia: A critical review. In D. Rosenthal & S. S. Kety (Eds.), *The transmission of schizophrenia* (pp. 155–173). Elmsford, NY: Pergamon Press.

Kohut, H. (1971). *The analysis of the self.* Monograph Series of the Psychoanalytic Study of the Child. New York: International Universities Press.

Kohut, H. (1990). *The search for self: Selected writings of Heinz Kohut: 1978–1981* (Vol. 3, P. H. Ornstein, Ed.). Madison, WI: International Universities Press.

Kolata, G. (1993, May 25). Brain researcher makes it look easy. *New York Times*, pp. B5, B7.

Koop, C. E. (1985). *The Surgeon General's workshop on violence and public health, source book.* Leesburg, VA: U.S. Public Health Service/Department of Health and Human Services.

Koranyi, E. K. (1986). Mental retardation: Medical aspects. *Psychiatric Clinics of North America, 9*, 635–645.

Korb, M. P., Gorrell, J., & Van De Reit, V. (1989). *Gestalt therapy: Practice and theory.* New York: Guilford Press.

Koss, M. P. (1993). Rape: Scope, impact, interventions, and public policy responses. *American Psychologist, 48*, 1062–1069.

Koss, M. P., Gidycz, C. A., & Wisniewski, N. (1987). The scope of rape: Incidence and prevalence of sexual aggression and victimization in a national sample of higher education students. *Journal of Consulting and Clinical Psychology, 55*, 162–170.

Koss, M. P., Goodman, L. A., Browne, A., Fitzgerald, L. F., Keita, G. P., & Russo, N. F. (1994). *No safe haven: Male violence against women at home, at work, and in the community.* Washington, DC: American Psychological Association.

Kosson, D. S., & Newman, J. P. (1986). Psychopathy and the allocation of attentional capacity in a divided-attention situation. *Journal of Abnormal Psychology, 95*, 257–263.

Kosten, T. R., Mason, J. W., Giller, E. L., Ostroff, R. B., & Harkness, L. (1987). Sustained urinary norepinephrine and epinephrine elevation in post-traumatic stress disorder. *Psychoneuroendocrinology, 12*, 13–20.

Kovacs, M., & Beck, A. T. (1977). An empirical clinical approach toward definition of childhood depression. In J. B. Schulterbrandt (Ed.), *Depression in childhood: Diagnosis, treatment, and conceptual models* (pp. 1–25). New York: Raven Press.

Kovacs, M., & Beck, A. T. (1978). Maladaptive cognitive structures in depression. *American Journal of Psychiatry, 135*, 525–533.

Kovacs, M., Beck, A. T., & Weissman, M. M. (1975). The use of suicidal motives in the psychotherapy of attempted suicides. *American Journal of Psychiatry, 29*, 363–368.

Kraepelin, E. (1896). *Dementia praecox and paraphrenia.* Edinburgh: Livingston.

Kraepelin, E. (1913). *Psychiatry: A textbook.* Leipzig, Germany: Barth.

Kraepelin, E. (1915). *Clinical psychiatry.* New York: Macmillan.

Kraepelin, E. (1921). *Manic depressive insanity and paranoia.* Edinburgh, Scotland: Livingstone.

Krafft-Ebing, R. von. (1965). *Psychopathica sexualis.* New York: Putnam. (Original work published 1886)

Kramer, J. H. (1990). Guidelines for interpreting WAIS-R subtest scores. *Psychological Assessment, 2*, 202–205.

Kramer, P. D. (1993). *Listening to Prozac.* New York: Viking Press.

Krane, R. J., Goldstein, I., & DeTejada, I. S. (1989). Impotence. *New England Journal of Medicine, 321*, 1648–1657.

Krauthammer, C., & Klerman, G. L. (1979). The epidemiology of mania. In B. Shopsin (Ed.), *Manic illness* (pp. 11–18). New York: Raven Press.

Kring, A. M., Kerr, S. L., Smith, D. A., & Neale, J. M. (1993). Flat affect in schizophrenia does not reflect diminished subjective experience of emotion. *Journal of Abnormal Psychology, 102*, 507–517.

Kuczmarski, R. J., Flegal, K., Campbell, S. M., & Johnson, C. L. (1994). Increasing prevalence of overweight among U.S. adults. *Journal of the American Medical Association, 272*, 205–211.

Kuhn, R. (1958). The treatment of depressive states with G 22355 (imipramine hydrochloride). *American Journal of Psychiatry, 115*, 459–464.

Kumanyika, S. (1987). Obesity in black women. *Epidemiologic Reviews, 9*, 31–50.

Kupfer, D. J. (1993). Management of recurrent depression. *Journal of Clinical Psychiatry, 54*(Suppl.), 29–33.

Kupfer, D. J., Buysse, D. J., Nofzinger, E. A., & Reynolds, C. F. (1994). Sleep disorders. In T. A. Widiger, A. J. Frances, H. A. Pincus, M. B. First, R. Ross, & W. Davis (Eds.), *DSM-IV sourcebook* (pp. 597–606). Washington, DC: American Psychiatric Press.

Kushner, M. G., Sher, K. J., & Beitman, B. D. (1990). The relation between alcohol problems and the anxiety disorders. *American Journal of Psychiatry, 147*, 685–695.

L

Laan, E., Everaerd, W., Van Aanhold, M. T., & Rebel M. (1993). Performance demand and sexual arousal in women. *Behaviour Research and Therapy, 31*, 25–36.

Laborit, H. (1950). Le phenomene de potentialisation des anesthetiques generaux. *Noux Presse Med, 58*, 416.

Lacey, J. H. (1992). The treatment demand for bulimia: A catchment area report of referral rates and demography. *Psychiatric Bulletin, 16*, 204–205.

Lader, M., & Sartorius, N. (1968). Anxiety in patients with hysterical conversion symptoms. *Journal of Neurology, Neurosurgery and Psychiatry, 31,* 490–495.

LaGreca, A. M., & Santogrossi, D. A. (1981). Social skills training with elementary school students: A behavioral group approach. *Journal of Consulting and Clinical Psychology, 48,* 220–227.

Lahey, B. B., Hart, E. L., Pliszka, S., & Applegate, B. (1993). Neurophysiological correlates of conduct disorder: A rationale and a review of research. *Journal of Clinical Child Psychology, 22,* 141–153.

Lahey, B. B., Loeber, R., Hart, E. L., Frick, P. J., Applegate, B., Zhang, Q., Green, S. M., & Russo, M. F. (1995). Four-year longitudinal study of conduct disorder in boys: Patterns and predictors of prevalence. *Journal of Abnormal Psychology, 104,* 83–93.

Laing, R. D. (1967). *The politics of experience.* New York: Pantheon Books.

Lamb, H. R., Weinberger, L. E., & Gross, B. H. (1988). Court-mandated community outpatient treatment for persons found not guilty by reason of insanity: A five-year follow-up. *American Journal of Psychiatry, 145,* 450–456.

Lambert, M. C., Weisz, J. R., Knight, F., Desrosiers, M., Overly, K., & Thesiger, C. (1992). Jamaican and American adult perspectives on child psychopathology: Further exploration of the threshold model. *Journal of Consulting and Clinical Psychology, 60,* 146–149.

Lambert, M. J., & Bergin, A. E. (1994). The effectiveness of psychotherapy. In A. E. Bergin & S. L. Garfield (Eds.), *Handbook of psychotherapy and behavior change* (4th ed.). New York: John Wiley.

Lambert, M. J., Shapiro, D. A., & Bergin, A. E. (1986). The effectiveness of psychotherapy. In S. L. Garfield & A. E. Bergin (Eds.), *Handbook of psychotherapy and behavior change* (3rd ed.). New York: John Wiley.

Lane, K. E., & Gwartney-Gibbs, P. A. (1985). Violence in the context of dating and sex. *Journal of Family Issues, 6,* 45–59.

Laner, M. R. (1983). Courtship abuse and aggression: Contextual aspects. *Sociological Spectrum, 3,* 69–83.

Lang, P. J. (1969). The mechanics of desensitization and the laboratory study of fear. In C. M. Franks (Ed.), *Behavior therapy: Appraisal and status.* New York: McGraw-Hill.

Lang, P. J. (1985). The cognitive psychophysiology of emotion: Fear and anxiety. In A. H. Tuma & J. D. Maser (Eds.), *Anxiety and the anxiety disorders.* Hillsdale, NJ: Lawrence Erlbaum.

Langenbucher, J. W., McCrady, B. S., Brick, J., & Esterly, R. (1993). *Socioeconomic evaluations of addictions treatment.* New Brunswick, NJ: Rutgers Center of Alcohol Studies.

Lanyon, R. I. (1984). Personality assessment. *Annual Review of Psychology, 35,* 667–701.

Lanyon, R. I., & Lanyon, B. P. (1980). Behavioral assessment and decision making: The design of strategies for therapeutic behavior change. In M. P. Feldman & A. Broadhurst (Eds.), *Theoretical and experimental bases of the behavior therapies.* London: John Wiley.

Lapousse, R., & Monk, M. A. (1959). Fears and worries of a representative sample of children. *American Journal of Orthopsychiatry, 29,* 803–818.

Larimer, M. E., & Marlatt, G. A. (1994). Addictive behaviors. In L. W. Craighead, W. E. Craighead, A. E. Kazdin, & M. J. Mahoney (Eds.), *Cognitive and behavioral interventions* (pp. 157–168). Boston: Allyn and Bacon.

Larkin, M. (1992, May/June). The tools of cognitive therapy. *Headlines,* pp. 17–20.

Lashley, K. S. (1951). Discussion of W. C. Halstead; Brain and intelligence. In L. A. Jeffress (Ed.), *Cerebral mechanisms in behavior* (pp. 272–273). New York: John Wiley.

Last, C. G. (1989). Anxiety disorders. In T. H. Ollendick & M. Hersen (Eds.), *Handbook of child psychopathology* (2nd ed., pp. 219–228). New York: Plenum.

Last, C. G., Hersen, M., Kazdin, A. E., Francis, G., & Grubb, H. J. (1987). Psychiatric illness in the mothers of anxious children. *American Journal of Psychiatry, 144,* 1580–1583.

Lattal, K. A. (1992). B. F. Skinner and psychology: Introduction to the special issue. *American Psychologist, 47,* 1269–1272.

Laudenslager, M. L., Ryan, S. M., Drugan, R. C., Hyson, R. L., & Maier, S. F. (1979). Coping and immunosuppression: Inescapable but not escapable shock suppresses lymphocytes proliferation. *Science, 221,* 568–570.

Laumann, E. O., Gagnon, J. H., Michael, R. T., & Michaels, S. (1994). *The social organization of sexuality: Sexual practices in the United States.* Chicago: University of Chicago Press.

Laurence, L., & Weinhouse, B. (1994). Outrageous practices: The alarming truth about how medicine mistreats women. New York: Ballantine Books.

Laurent, J., Swerdlik, M., & Ryburn, M. (1992). Review of validity research on the Stanford-Binet Intelligence Scale: Fourth Edition. *Psychological Assessment, 4,* 102–112.

Laws, D. R. (Ed.). (1989). *Relapse prevention with sex offenders.* New York: Guilford Press.

Lazarus, A. A. (1981). *The practice of multimodal therapy.* New York: McGraw-Hill.

Lazarus, A. A. (1989). Why I am an eclectic (not an integrationist). *British Journal of Guidance and Counseling, 17,* 248–258.

Lazarus, A. A., Beutler, L. E., & Norcross, J. C. (1992). The future of technical eclecticism. *Psychotherapy, 29,* 11–20.

Lazarus, R. S. (1991). *Emotion and adaptation.* New York: Oxford Press.

LeFebvre, R. C., Cobb, G. D., Goreczny, A. J., & Carleton, R. A. (1990). Efficacy of an incentive-based community smoking cessation program. *Addictive Behaviors, 15,* 403–411.

Leff, J., & Vaughn, C. (1985). *Expressed emotion in families.* New York: Guilford.

Leff, J., & Vaughn, C. (1989). The interaction of life events and relatives' expressed emotion in schizophrenia and depressive neuroses. In T. W. Miller (Ed.), *Stressful life events* (pp. 377–391). Madison, CT: International Universities Press.

Lefkowitz, M. M., Eron, L. D., Walden, L. O., & Heusmann, L. R. (1977). *Growing up to be violent.* New York: Pergamon Press.

Lehrer, P. M., & Woolfolk, R. L. (1984). Are stress reduction techniques interchangeable, or do they have specific effects? A review of the comparative empirical literature. In R. L. Woolfolk & P. M. Lehrer (Eds.), *Principles and practices of stress management* (pp. 404–477). New York: Guilford Press.

Leigh, B. C. (1990). Relationship of substance use during sex to high-risk sexual behavior. *Journal of Sex Research, 27,* 199–213.

Leitenberg, H., Greenwald, E., & Cado, S. (1992). A retrospective study of long-term methods of coping with having been sexually abused in childhood. *Childhood Abuse and Neglect, 16,* 399–407.

Lelliot, P. T., Noshirvani, H. F., Basoglu, M., Marks, I. M., & Monterio, W. O. (1988). Obsessive-compulsive beliefs and treatment outcome. *Psychological Medicine, 18,* 697–702.

Leohlin, J. C. (1977). An analysis of alcohol-related questionnaire items from the National Merit twin study. In F. A. Seixas, G. S. Omenn, E. D. Burk, & S. Eggleston (Eds.), *Annals of the New York Academy of Sciences, 197,* 117–120.

Leonard, H. L., Lenane, M. C., Swedo, S. E., Rettew, D. C., Gershon, E. S., & Rapoport, J. L. (1992). *American Journal of Psychiatry, 149,* 1244–1251.

Leonard, H. L., Swedo, S. E., Rapoport, J. L., Koby, E. V., Lenane, M. C., Cheslow, D. L., & Hamburger, S. D. (1989). Treatment of obsessive-compulsive disorder with clomipramine and desipramine in children and adolescents. *Archives of General Psychiatry, 46,* 1088–1092.

Leonard, K. E. (1993). Drinking patterns and intoxication in marital violence: Review, critique, and future directions for research. In S. E. Martin (Ed.), *Alcohol and interpersonal violence: Fostering multidisciplinary perspectives* (pp. 253–280). Washington, DC: National Institute on Alcohol Abuse and Alcoholism.

Lepine, J. P., Chignon, J. M., & Teherani, M. (1993). Suicide attempts in patients with panic disorder. *Archives of General Psychiatry, 50,* 144–149.

Lerer, R. J., Lerer, P. M., & Artner, J. (1977). The effects of methylphenidate on the handwriting of children with minimal brain dysfunction. *Journal of Pediatrics, 91,* 121–132.

Lesage, A. D., Boyer, R., Grunberg, F., Vanier, C., Morissette, R., Menard-Buteau, C., & Loyer, M. (1994). Suicide and mental disorders: A case control study of young men. *American Journal of Psychiatry, 151,* 1063–1068.

LeVay, S. (1991). A difference in hypothalamic structure between heterosexual and homosexual men. *Science, 253,* 1–36.

Levin, A. P., Schneier, F. R., & Liebowitz, M. (1989). Social phobia: Biology and pharmacology. *Clinical Psychology Review, 9,* 129–140.

Levin, S., & Stava, L. (1987). Personality characteristics of sex offenders: A review. *Archives of Sexual Behavior, 16*, 57–79.

Levine, M., Toro, P. A., & Perkins, D. V. (1993). Social and community interventions. *Annual Review of Psychology, 44*, 525–558.

Levy, A. B., Dixon, K. N., & Stern, S. I. (1989). How are depression and bulimia related? *American Journal of Psychiatry, 146*, 162–169.

Lewin, K. (1935). *Principles of topological psychology.* New York: McGraw-Hill.

Lewinsohn, P. M., & Lee, W. M. L. (1981). Assessment of affective disorders. In D. H. Barlow (Ed.), *Behavioral assessment of adult disorders.* New York: Guilford Press.

Lewinsohn, P. M., & Libet, J. M. (1972). Pleasant events, activity schedules, and depression. *Journal of Abnormal Psychology, 79*, 291–295.

Lewis, O. (1961). *The children of Sanchez.* New York: Random House.

Lewis, O. (1969). A Puerto Rican boy. In J. C. Finney (Ed.), *Culture change, mental health, and poverty.* New York: Simon and Schuster.

Lex, B. W. (1985). Alcohol problems in special populations. In J. H. Mendelson & N. K. Mello (Eds.), *The diagnosis and treatment of alcoholism* (2nd ed.) (pp. 89–187). New York: McGraw-Hill.

Ley, P. (1977). Psychological studies of doctor-patient communication. In S. Rachman (Ed.), *Contributions to medical psychology* (pp. 9–42). London, England: Pergamon Press.

Liberman, R. P., Kopelowicz, A., & Young, A. S. (1994). Biobehavioral treatment and the rehabilitation of schizophrenia. *Behavior Therapy, 25*, 89–107.

Lichtenstein, E., & Glasgow, R. E. (1992). Smoking cessation: What have we learned over the past decade? *Journal of Consulting and Clinical Psychology, 60*, 518–527.

Lidz, C. W., Mulvey, E. P., Appelbaum, P. S., & Cleveland, S. (1989). Commitment: The consistency of clinicians and the use of legal standards. *American Journal of Psychiatry, 146*, 176–181.

Lieberman, J. A. (1994). Clinical biological studies of atypical antipsychotics: Focus on the Serotonin/Dopamine systems. *Journal of Clinical Psychiatry: Monograph Series, 12*, 24–28.

Lieberman, J. A., & Koreen, A. R. (1993). Neurochemistry and neuroendocrinology of schizophrenia. *Schizophrenia 1993: Special report* (pp. 197–256). Washington, DC: National Institute of Mental Health, Schizophrenia Research Branch.

Liebowitz, M. R., Fyer, A. J., Gorman, J. M., Dillon, D., Appleby, I. L., Levy, G., Anderson, S., Levitt, M., Palij, M., Davies, S. O., & Klein, D. F. (1984). Lactate provocation of panic attacks, I. Clinical and behavioural findings. *Archives of General Psychiatry, 41*, 764–770.

Liebowitz, M. R., Schneier, F. R., Hollander, E., & Welkowitz, L. A. (1991). Treatment of social phobia with drugs other than benzodiazepines. *Journal of Clinical Psychiatry, 52* (Suppl.), 10–15.

Liff, Z. A. (1992). Psychoanalysis and dynamic techniques. In D. K. Freedheim (Ed.), *History of psychotherapy: A century of change* (pp. 571–586). Washington, DC: American Psychological Association.

Lilienfeld, S. O. (1992). The association between antisocial personality and somatization disorders: A review and integration of theoretical models. *Clinical Psychology Review, 12*, 641–662.

Lilienfeld, S. O., Van Valkenburg, C., Larntz, K., & Akiskal, H. S. (1986). The relationship of histrionic personality disorder to antisocial personality and somatization disorders. *American Journal of Psychiatry, 143*, 718–722.

Lilienfeld, S. O., & Waldman, I. D. (1990). The relation between childhood attention-deficit hyperactivity disorder and adult antisocial behavior reexamined: The problem of heterogeneity. *Clinical Psychology Review, 10*, 699–726.

Lillard, L. A., & Waite, L. J. (1995). 'Til death do us part: Marital disruption and mortality. *American Journal of Sociology, 100*, 1131–1156.

Lin, K. M., & Finder, E. (1983). Neuroleptic dosage in Asians. *American Journal of Psychiatry, 140*, 490–491.

Linehan, M. M. (1993). *Cognitive-behavioral treatment of borderline personality disorder.* New York: Guilford Press.

Linehan, M. M., Armstrong, H. E., Suarez, A., Allmon, D., & Heard, H. L. (1991). Cognitive-behavioral treatment of chronically parasuicidal borderline patients. *Archives of General Psychiatry, 48*, 1060–1064.

Linehan, M. M., & Kehrer, C. A. (1993). Borderline personality disorder. In D. H. Barlow (Ed.), *Clinical handbook of psychological disorders* (2nd ed., pp. 396–441). New York: Guilford Press.

Linehan, M. M., Tutek, D. A., Heard, H. L., & Armstrong, H. E. (1994). Interpersonal outcome of cognitive-behavioral treatment of chronically suicidal borderline patients. *American Journal of Psychiatry, 151*, 1771–1776.

Lipscomb, G. H., Murman, D., Speck, P. M., & Mercer, B. M. (1992). Male victims of sexual assault. *Journal of the American Medical Association, 267*, 3064–3066.

Litt, M. D., Babor, T. F., DelBoca, F. K., Kadden, R. M., & Cooney, N. (1992). Types of alcoholics: II. Application of an empirically derived typology to treatment matching. *Archives of General Psychiatry, 49*, 609–614.

Livesley, W. J., & Jackson, D. N. (in press). *Dimensional assessment of personality problems (DAPP).* Port Huron, MI: Sigma Assessment Systems.

Livesley, W. J., Jang, K L., Jackson, D. N., & Vernon, P. A. (1993). Genetic and environmental contributions to dimensions of personality disorder. *American Journal of Psychiatry, 150*, 1826–1831.

Livesley, W. J., Schroeder, M. L., & Jackson, D. (1990). Dependent personality disorder and attachment problems. *Journal of Personality Disorders, 4*, 131–140.

Livesley, W. J., Schroeder, M. L., Jackson, D., & Jang, K. L. (1994). Categorical distinctions in the study of personality disorder: Implications for classification. *Journal of Abnormal Psychology, 103*, 6–17.

Lloyd, C. (1980). Life events and depressive disorder reviewed: II. Events as precipitating factors. *Archives of General Psychiatry, 37*, 541–548.

Lochman, J. E., Coie, J. D., Underwood, M. K., & Terry, R. (1993). Effectiveness of a social relations intervention program for aggressive and nonaggressive, rejected children. *Journal of Consulting and Clinical Psychology, 61*, 1053–1058.

Lochman, J. E., Lampron, L. B., Burch, P. R., & Curry, J. E. (1985). Client characteristics associated with behavior change for treated and untreated boys. *Journal of Abnormal Child Psychology, 13*, 527–538.

Loehlin, J. C. (1989). Partitioning environmental and genetic contributions to behavioral development. *American Psychologist, 44*, 1285–1292.

Loevinger, J. (1993). Measurement of personality: True or false. *Psychological Inquiry, 4*, 1–16.

Loftus, E. F. (1993). The reality of repressed memories. *American Psychologist, 48*, 518–537.

Loney, J. (1987). Hyperactivity and aggression in the diagnosis of attention deficit disorder. In B. B. Lahey & A. E. Kazdin (Eds.), *Advances in clinical psychology.* New York: Plenum.

Long, J. W., & Rybacki, J. J. (1994). *The essential guide to prescription drugs.* New York: HarperCollins.

Long, N., Slater, E., Forehand, R., & Fauber, R. (1988). Continued high or reduced interparental conflict following divorce: Relation to young adolescent adjustment. *Journal of Consulting and Clinical Psychology, 56*, 467–469.

Lopez, F. G., & Wambach, C. A. (1982). Effects of paradoxical and self-control directives in counseling. *Journal of Counseling Psychology, 29*, 115–124.

LoPiccolo, J. K., & Friedman, J. M. (1989). Broad-spectrum treatment of low sexual desire: Integration of cognitive, behavioral, and systemic therapy. In S. R. Leiblum & R. C. Rosen (Eds.), *Principles and practice of sex therapy: Update for the 1990s* (pp. 107–144). New York: Guilford Press.

Loranger, A. W. (1988). *Personality Disorder Examination (PDE) manual.* Yonkers, New York: DV Communications.

Loranger, A. W., Hirschfeld, R. M. A., Sartorius, N., & Regier, D. A. (1991). The WHO/ADAMHA International Pilot Study of Personality Disorders: Background and purpose. *Journal of Personality Disorders, 5*, 296–306.

Loranger, A. W., Lenzenweger, M. F., Gartner, A. F., Susman, V. L., Herzig, J., Zammit, G. K., Gartner, J. D., Abrams, R. C., & Young, R. C. (1991). Trait-state artifacts and the diagnosis of personality disorders. *Archives of General Psychiatry, 48*, 720–728.

Loranger, A. W., Sartorius, N., Andreoli, A., & Berger, P. (1994). The International Personality Disorder Examination: The WHO/ADAMHA International Pilot Study of Personality Disorders. *Archives of General Psychiatry, 51*, 215–224.

Lord, C., Bristol, M. M., & Schopler, E. (1993). Early intervention for children with autism and related developmental disorders. In E. Schopler, M. E. Van Bourgondien, & M. M. Bristol (Eds.), *Preschool issues in autism* (pp. 61–94). New York: Plenum Press.

Lorys-Vernon, A. R., Hynd, G. W., Lyytinen, H., & Hern, K. (1993). Etiology of attention-deficit/hyperactivity disorder. In J. L. Matson (Ed.), *Handbook of hyperactivity in children* (pp. 47–65). Boston: Allyn & Bacon.

Los Angeles Times, August 25 and 26, 1985.

Losche, G. (1990). Sensorimotor and action development in autistic children from infancy to early childhood. *Journal of Child Psychology and Psychiatry, 31,* 749–762.

Lothstein, L. M. (1982). Sex reassignment surgery. *American Journal of Psychiatry, 139,* 417–426.

Lou, H. C., Henriksen, L., & Bruhn, P. (1984). Focal cerebral hypoperfusion in children with dysphasia and or attention deficit disorder. *Archives of Neurology, 41,* 825–829.

Lovaas, O. I. (1987). Behavioral treatment and normal educational and intellectual functioning in young autistic children. *Journal of Consulting and Clinical Psychology, 55,* 3–9.

Lovaas, O. I. (1993). The development of a treatment-research project for developmentally disabled and autistic children. *Journal of Applied Behavior Analysis, 26,* 617–630.

Lovitt, R. (1993). A strategy for integrating a normal MMPI-2 and dysfunctional Rorschach in a severely compromised patient. *Journal of Personality Assessment, 60,* 141–147.

Luborsky, L. (1987). Research can now affect clinical practice: A happy turnabout. *Clinical Psychologist, 40,* 56–60.

Luborsky, L., Crits-Christoph, P., & Mellon, J. (1986). Advent of objective measures of the transference concept. *Journal of Consulting and Clinical Psychology, 54,* 39–47.

Ludwig, A. M. (1994). *The price of greatness.* New York: Guilford Press.

Lundy, A. (1985). The reliability of the Thematic Apperception Test. *Journal of Personality Assessment, 49,* 141–145.

Lutzker, J. R., & Rice, J. M. (1984). Project 12 Ways: Measuring outcome of a large in-home service for treatment and prevention of child abuse and neglect. *Child Abuse and Neglect, 8,* 519–524.

Lyketsos, C. G., Hoover, D. R., Guccione, M., Senterfitt, W., Dew, M. A., Wesch, J., van Raden, M. J., Treisman, G. J., & Morgenstern, H. (1993). Depressive symptoms as predictors of medical outcomes in HIV infection. *Journal of the American Medical Association, 270,* 2563–2567.

Lykken, D. T. (1957). A study of anxiety in the sociopathic personality. *Journal of Abnormal and Social Psychology, 55,* 6–10.

Lyman, R. D., & Hembree-Kigin, T. L. (1994). *Mental health interventions with preschool children.* New York: Plenum Press.

M

M'Naughten, 8 Eng. Rep. 715, 722–723 (1843).

MacAndrew, C., & Edgerton, R. B. (1969). *Drunken comportment: A social explanation.* Chicago: Aldine.

Mackinnon, A., Henderson, A. S., & Andrews, G. (1993). Parental "affectionless control" as an antecedent to adult depression: A risk factor refined. *Psychological Medicine, 23,* 135-141.

Madden, J. (1984). *Hey wait a minute, I wrote a book.* New York: Villard Books.

Madsen, C. H., & Madsen, C. K. (1970). *Teaching discipline.* Boston: Allyn & Bacon.

Maier, W., & Lichtermann, D. (1993). The genetic epidemiology of unipolar depression and panic disorder. *International Clinical Psychopharmacology, 8*(Suppl. 1), 27–33.

Maier, W., Lichterman, D., Klingler, T., Heun, R., & Hallmayer, J. (1992). Prevalences of personality disorders (*DSM-III-R*) in the community. *Journal of Personality Disorders, 6,* 187–196.

Main, M., & Goldwyn, R. (1984). Predicting rejection of her infant from mother's representation of her own experience: Implications for the abused-abusing intergenerational cycle. *Child Abuse & Neglect, 8,* 203–217.

Malamuth, N. M., Sockloskie, R. J., Koss, M. P., & Tanaka, J. S. (1991). Characteristics of aggressors against women: Testing a model using a national sample of college students. *Journal of Consulting and Clinical Psychology, 59,* 670–681.

Malcolm X. (1964). *The autobiography of Malcolm X.* New York: Ballantine Books.

Maletzky, B. (1980). Self-referred versus court-referred sexually deviant patients: Success with assisted covert sensitization. *Behavior Therapy, 11,* 302–314.

Mann, C. (1990). Meta-analysis in the breech. *Science, 249,* 476–480.

Mannuzza, S., Klein, R. G., Bessler, A., & Malloy, P. (1993). Adult outcome of hyperactive boys: Educational achievement, occupational rank, and psychiatric status. *Archives of General Psychiatry, 50,* 565–576.

Mannuzza, S., Klein, R. G., Bessler, A., Malloy, P., & LaPadula, M. (1993). Adult outcome of hyperactive boys: Educational achievement, occupational rank, and psychiatric status. *Archives of General Psychiatry, 50,* 565–576.

Mannuzza, S., Klein, R. G., Bonagura, N., Malloy, P., Giampino, T. L., & Addalli, K. A. (1991). Hyperactive boys almost grown up: V: Replication of psychiatric status. *Archives of General Psychiatry, 48,* 77–83.

Manson, J. E., Colditz, G., Stampfer, M., Willell, W., Rosner, B., Mortson, R., Speizer, F., & Hennekens, C. (1990). A prospective study of obesity and risk of coronary heart disease in women. *New England Journal of Medicine, 322,* 882–889.

Manson, S., Shore, J., & Bloom, J. (1985). The depressive experience in American Indian communities: A challenge for psychiatric theory and diagnosis. In A. Kleinman & B. Good (Eds.), *Culture and depression: Studies in the anthropology and cross-culture psychiatry of affect and disorder.* Berkeley: University of California Press.

Mapou, R. L., & Law, W. A. (1994). Neurobehavioral aspects of HIV disease and AIDS: An update. *Professional Psychology: Research and Practice, 25,* 132–140.

Marcus, M. D. (1993). Binge eating in obesity. In C. F. Fairburn & G. T. Wilson (Eds.), *Binge eating: Nature, assessment, and treatment* (pp. 77–96). New York: Guilford Press.

Marder, S. R., & Van Putten, T. (1988). Who should receive clozapine? *Archives of General Psychiatry, 45,* 865–867.

Marecek, J. (1987). Counseling adolescents with problem pregnancies. *American Psychologist, 42,* 89–93.

Margo, A., Hemsley, D. R., & Slade, P. D. (1981). The effects of varying auditory input on schizophrenic hallucinations. *British Journal of Psychiatry, 139,* 122–127.

Margolick, D. (1994, January 28). At the bar. *New York Times,* p. B11.

Margolin, G., Sibner, L. G., & Gleberman, L. (1988). Wife battering. In V. B. Van Hasselt, R. L. Morrison, A. S. Belleck, and M. Hersen (Eds.), *Handbook of family violence.* New York: Plenum.

Margolin, G., Talovic, S., & Weinstein, C. D. (1983). Areas of change questionnaire: A practical approach to marital assessment. *Journal of Consulting and Clinical Psychology, 57,* 920–931.

Margraf, J., Ehlers, A., Roth, W. T., Clark, D. B., Sheikh, J., Agras, W. S., & Taylor, C. B. (1991). How "blind" are double-blind studies? *Journal of Consulting and Clinical Psychology, 59,* 184–187.

Markovitz, J. H., Matthews, K. A., Kannel, W. B., Cobb, J. L., & D'Agostino, R. B. (1993). Psychological predictors of hypertension in the Framingham Study. Is there tension in hypertension? *Journal of the American Medical Association, 270,* 2439–2443.

Marks, I. M. (1987). Comment on S. Lloyd Williams' "On anxiety and phobia." *Journal of Anxiety Disorders, 1,* 181–196.

Marks, I. M., & Swinson, R. (1993). Alprazolam and exposure alone and combined in panic disorder with agoraphobia. *British Journal of Psychiatry, 162,* 776–787.

Marks, M. N., Wieck, A., Checkley, S. A., & Kumar, R. (1992). Contribution of psychological and social factors to psychotic and nonpsychotic relapse after childbirth in women with previous histories of affective disorder. *Journal of Affective Disorders, 24,* 253–263.

Markus, E., Lange, A., & Pettigrew, T. F. (1990). Effectiveness of family therapy: A meta-analysis. *Journal of Family Therapy, 12,* 205–211.

Marlatt, G. A., & Gordon, J. R. (Eds.). (1985). *Relapse prevention.* New York: Guilford Press.

Marlatt, G. A., & Rohsenow, D. J. (1980). Cognitive processes in alcohol use: Expectancy and the balanced placebo design. In N. K. Mello (Ed.), *Advances in substance abuse: Behavioral and biological research* (Vol. 1) (pp. 159–199). Greenwich, CT: JAI Press.

Marshall, W. L., Seidman, B. T., & Barbaree, H. E. (1991). The effects of prior exposure to erotic and nonerotic stimuli on the rape index. *Annals of Sex Research, 4,* 209–220.

Martin, J. L. (1987). The impact of AIDS on gay male sexual behavior patterns in New York City. *American Journal of Public Health, 77,* 578–580.

Martin, S. E. (1992). The epidemiology of alcohol-related interpersonal violence. *Alcohol Health & Research World, 16,* 230–237.

Mash, E. J., & Hunsley, J. (1993). Assessment considerations in the identification of failing psychotherapy: Bringing the negatives out of the darkroom. *Psychological Assessment, 5,* 292–301.

Mash, E. J., & Johnston, C. (1983). Sibling interactions of hyperactive children and their relationship to reports of maternal stress and self-esteem. *Journal of Consulting and Clinical Psychology, 12,* 91–99.

Maslow, A. H. (1954). *Motivation and personality.* New York: Harper & Row.

Masson, J. M. (1984). *The assault on truth: Freud's suppression of the seduction theory.* New York: Farrar, Straus, & Giroux.

Masters, W. H., & Johnson, V. (1966). *Human sexual response.* Boston: Little, Brown.

Masters, W. H., & Johnson, V. (1970). *Human sexual inadequacy.* Boston: Little, Brown.

Masters, W. H., & Johnson, V. (1979). *Homosexuality in perspective.* Boston: Little, Brown.

Matarazzo, J. D. (1992). Psychological testing and assessment in the 21st century. *American Psychologist, 47,* 1007–1018.

Matson, J. L., & Sevin, J. A. (1994a). Theories of dual diagnosis in mental retardation. *Journal of Consulting and Clinical Psychology, 62,* 6–16.

Matson, J. L., & Sevin, J. A. (1994b). Issues in the use of aversives: Factors associated with behavior modification for autistic and other developmentally disabled people. In E. Schopler & G. B. Mesibov (Eds.), *Behavioral issues in autism* (pp. 211–225). New York: Plenum Press.

Matthews, K. A. (1989). Interactive effects of behavior and reproductive hormones on sex differences in risk for coronary heart disease. *Health Psychology, 8,* 373–387.

Matthews, K. A., Glass, D. C., Rosenman, R. H., & Bortner, R. W. (1977). Competitive drive, pattern A, and coronary heart disease: A further analysis of some data from the Western Collaborative Group. *Journal of Chronic Disease, 230,* 489–498.

Matthews, K., & Haynes, S. G. (1986). Type A behavior pattern and coronary risk: Update and critical evaluation. *American Journal of Epidemiology, 123,* 923–960.

Mattick, R. P., & Newman, C. R. (1991). Social phobia and avoidant personality disorder. *International Review of Psychiatry, 3,* 163–173.

Mattson, M. E., & Allen, J. P. (1991). Research on matching alcoholic patients to treatments: Findings, issues, and implications. *Journal of Addictive Disorders, 11,* 33–49.

Mauri, M., Sarno, N., Rossi, V. M., Armani, A., Zambotto, S., Cassano, G. B., & Akiskal, H. S. (1992). Personality disorders associated with generalized anxiety, panic, and recurrent depressive disorders. *Journal of Personality Disorders, 6,* 162–167.

May, P. R. A. (1968). *Treatment of schizophrenia: A comparative study of five treatment methods.* New York: Science House.

May, P. R. A., Tuma, A. H., & Dixon, W. J. (1981). Schizophrenia: A follow-up study of the results of treatment. *Archives of General Psychiatry, 38,* 776–784.

McAllister, T. W., & Price, T. R. P. (1982). Severe depressive pseudodementia with and without dementia. *American Journal of Psychiatry, 139,* 626–629.

McCabe, S. B., & Gotlib, I. H. (1995). Selective attention and clinical depression: Performance on a deployment-of-attention task. *Journal of Abnormal Psychology, 104,* 241–245.

McCafferty, G., & Dooley, J. (1990). Involuntary outpatient commitment: An update. *MDPLR, 14,* 277–287.

McCaffrey, R. J., & Isaac, W. (1985). Preliminary data on the presence of neuro-psychological deficits in adults who are mentally retarded. *Mental Retardation, 23,* 63–66.

McCarthy, B. W. (1992). Treatment of erectile dysfunction with single men. In R. C. Rosen & S. R. Leiblum (Eds.), *Erectile disorders: Assessment and treatment* (pp. 313–340). New York: Guilford Press.

McClearn, G. E. (1993). Behavioral genetics: The last century and the next. In R. Plomin & G. E. McClearn (Eds.), *Nature, nurture and psychology* (pp. 27–51). Washington, DC: American Psychological Association.

McClelland, D. C. (1980). Motive dispositions: The merits of operant and respondent measures. In L. Wheeler (Ed.), *Review of personality and social psychology* (Vol. 1). Beverly Hills, CA: Sage.

McCord, J., & Tremblay, R. E. (1992). *Preventing antisocial behavior: Interventions from birth through adolescence.* New York: Guilford Press.

McCrady, B. S., & Miller, W. R. (1993). *Research on Alcoholics Anonymous: Opportunities and alternatives.* New Brunswick, NJ: Rutgers Center of Alcohol Studies.

McDonald, K. A. (1994, September 14). Biology and behavior. *Chronicle of Higher Education,* p. A10.

McElroy, S. L., & Keck, P. E. (1995). Misattribution of eating and obsessive-compulsive disorder symptoms to repressed memories of childhood sexual or physical abuse. *Biological Psychiatry, 37,* 48–51.

McEwen, B. S., & Stellar, E. (1993). Stress and the individual: Mechanisms leading to disease. *Archives of Internal Medicine, 153,* 2093–2101.

McGlashan, T. H. (1993). Implications of outcome research for the treatment of borderline personality disorder. In J. Paris (Ed.), *Borderline personality disorder* (pp. 235–260). Washington, DC: American Psychiatric Press.

McGue, M. (1993). From proteins to cognitions: The behavioral genetics of alcoholism. In R. Plomin & G. E. McClearn (Eds.), *Nature, nurture and psychology* (pp. 245–268). Washington, DC: American Psychological Association.

McGue, M., & Lykken, D. T. (1992). Genetic influence on risk of divorce. *Psychological Science, 3,* 368–373.

McGue, M., Pickens, R. W., & Svikis, D. S. (1992). Sex and age effects on the inheritance of alcohol problems. *Journal of Abnormal Psychology, 101,* 3–17.

McGuffin, P., & Katz, R. (1993). Genes, adversity, and depression. In R. Plomin & G. E. McClearn (Eds.), *Nature, nurture and psychology* (pp. 217–230). Washington, DC: American Psychological Association.

McGuire, P. K., Shah, G. M. S., & Murray, R. M. (1993). Increased blood pressure flow in the Broca's area during auditory hallucinations in schizophrenia. *Lancet, 342,* 703–706.

McKeon, P., & Murray, R. (1987). Familial aspects of obsessive-compulsive neurosis. *British Journal of Psychiatry, 151,* 528–534.

McLean, P., & Taylor, S. (1992). Severity of unipolar depression and choice of treatment. *Behavior Research and Therapy, 30,* 443–451.

McLellan, A. T., Alterman, A. I., Metzger, D. S., Grissom, G. R., Woody, G. E., Luborsky, L., & O'Brien, C. P. (1994). Similarity of outcome predictors across opiate, cocaine, and alcohol treatments: Role of treatment services. *Journal of Consulting and Clinical Psychology, 62,* 1141–1158.

McLeod, J. D. (1991). Childhood parental loss and adult depression. *Journal of Health & Social Behavior, 32,* 205–220.

McNally, R. J. (1987). Preparedness and phobias: A review. *Psychological Bulletin, 101,* 283–303.

McNiel, D. E., & Binder, R. L. (1987). Predictive validity of judgments of dangerousness in emergency civil commitment. *American Journal of Psychiatry, 144,* 197–200.

McNiel, D. E., & Binder, R. L. (1991). Clinical assessment of the risk of violence among psychiatric inpatients. *American Journal of Psychiatry, 148,* 1317–1321.

McRae, J. A., & Brody, C. J. (1989). The differential importance of marital experiences for the well-being of women and men: A research note. *Social Science Research, 18,* 237–248.

McReynolds, P. (1986). History of assessment in clinical and educational settings. In R. O. Nelson & S. D. Hayes (Eds.), *Conceptual foundations of behavioral assessment* (pp. 42–80). New York: Guilford Press.

Mechanic, D., & Aiken, L. A. (1987). Improving the care of patients with chronic mental illness. *New England Journal of Medicine, 317,* 1634–1638.

Mednick, S. A., & Schulsinger, F. (1968). Some premorbid characteristics related to breakdown in children with schizophrenic mothers. *Journal of Psychosomatic Research, 6,* 354–362.

Meehl, P. E. (1962). Schizotaxia, schizotypy, schizophrenia. *American Psychologist, 17,* 827–838.

Meehl, P. E. (1992). Factors and taxa, traits and types, differences of degree and differences in kind. *Journal of Personality, 60,* 117–174.

Meichenbaum, D. (1994). *A clinical handbook/practical therapist manual for assessing and treating adults with post-traumatic stress disorder.* Waterloo, Canada: Institute Press.

Meichenbaum, D. H., & Turk, D. (1988). *Facilitating treatment adherence.* New York: Plenum Press.

Meisel, A. (1982). The rights of the mentally ill under state constitutions. *Law and Contemporary Problems, 45,* 7–40.

Melamed, B. G., & Siegel, L. J. (1975). Reduction of anxiety in children facing hospitalization and surgery by use of filmed modeling. *Journal of Consulting and Clinical Psychology, 43,* 511–521.

Meleshko, K. G. A., & Alden, L. E. (1993). Anxiety and self-disclosure: Toward a motivational model. *Journal of Personality and Social Psychology, 64,* 1000–1009.

Melman, A., & Tiefer, L. (1992). Surgery for erectile disorders: Operative procedures and psychological issues. In R. C. Rosen & S. R. Leiblum (Eds.), *Erectile disorders: Assessment and treatment* (pp. 255–282). New York: Guilford Press.

Melton, G. B. (1987). Adolescent abortion: Psychological and legal issues. *American Psychologist, 42,* 73–78.

Melton, G. B., & Gray, J. N. (1988). Ethical dilemmas in AIDS research: Individual privacy and public health. *American Psychologist, 45,* 60–64.

Melton, G. B., Levine, R. J., Koocher, G. P., Rosenthal, R., & Thompson, W. C. (1988). Community consultation in socially sensitive research. *American Psychologist, 15,* 573–581.

Melton, G. B., & Limber, S. (1991). Caution in child maltreatment cases. *American Psychologist, 46,* 82–84.

Meltzer, H. Y. (1993). Clozapine: A major advance in the treatment of schizophrenia. *Harvard Mental Health Letter, 10,* 4–6.

Meltzer, H. Y. (1993, August). Clozapine: A major advance in the treatment of schizophrenia. *Harvard Mental Health Letter, 10,* 4–6.

Menaghan, E. C. (1989). Role changes and psychological well-being: Variations in effects by gender and role repertoire. *Social Forces, 67,* 693–714.

Mendlewicz, J., & Rainer, J. D. (1977). Adoption study supporting genetic transmission in manic-depressive illness. *Nature, 268,* 327–329.

Mendoza, R., Smith, M. W., Poland, R. E., Lin, K. M., & Strickland, T. L. (1991). Ethnic psychopharmacology. *Psychopharmacology Bulletin, 27,* 449–461.

Menkes, M. S., Matthews, K. A., Krantz, D. S., Lundberg, U., Mead, L. A., Qaqish, B., Liang, K. Y., Thomas, C. B., & Pearson, T. A. (1989). Cardiovascular reactivity to the cold pressor test as a predictor of hypertension. *Hypertension, 14,* 524-530.

Merskey, H. (1992). Anna O. had a severe depressive illness. *British Journal of Psychiatry, 161,* 185–194.

Messick, S. (1992). Multiple intelligences or multilevel intelligence? Selective emphasis on distinctive properties of hierarchy: On Gardner's Frames of Mind and Sternberg's Beyond IQ in the context of theory and research on the structure of human abilities. *Psychological Inquiry, 3,* 365–384.

Meyer, A. (1994). A short sketch of the problems of psychiatry. *American Journal of Psychiatry, 151*(June suppl.), 42–47. (Original work published in 1897)

Meyer, A., Nash, J., McAlister, A., Maccoby, N., & Farquhar, J. (1980). Skills training in a cardiovascular health education campaign. *Journal of Consulting and Clinical Psychology, 48,* 129–142.

Meyer, G. J. (1992). The Rorschach's factor structure: A contemporary investigation and historical review. *Journal of Personality Assessment, 59,* 117–136.

Meyer, G. J. (1993). The impact of response frequency on the Rorschach confabulation indices and on their validity with diagnostic and MMPI-2 criteria. *Journal of Personality Assessment, 60,* 153–160.

Meyer, J. K., & Reter, D. J. (1979). Sex reassignment. *Archives of General Psychiatry, 36,* 1010–1015.

Mezzich, J. E., Fabrega, H., & Kleinman, A. (in press). On enhancing the cultural sensitivity of the *DSM-IV. Journal of Nervous and Mental Disease.*

Michaelis, E. K., & Michaelis, M. L. (1994). Cellular and molecular bases of alcohol's teratogenic effects. *Alcohol Health & Research World, 18,* 17–21.

Midanik, L. T., & Room, R. (1992). The epidemiology of alcohol consumption. *Alcohol Health & Research World, 16,* 183–190.

Miklowitz, D. J., & Goldstein, M. J. (1990). Behavioral family treatment for patients with bipolar affective disorder. *Behavior Modification, 14,* 457–489.

Miklowitz, D. J., Goldstein, M. J., Neuchterlein, K. S., Snyder, K. S., & Mintz, J. (1988). Family factors and bipolar depression. *Archives of General Psychiatry, 45,* 225–231.

Miller, E. (1987). Hysteria: Its nature and explanation. *British Journal of Clinical Psychology, 26,* 163–173.

Miller, G. E., & Prinz, R. J. (1990). Enhancement of social learning family interventions for childhood conduct disorder. *Psychological Bulletin, 108,* 291–307.

Miller, I., Norman, W., & Keitner, G. (1989). Cognitive-behavioral treatment of depressed inpatients: Six- and twelve-month follow-up. *American Journal of Psychiatry, 146,* 1274–1279.

Miller, N. E. (1969). Learning of visceral and glandular responses. *Science, 163,* 434–445.

Miller, R. D. (1987). *Involuntary civil commitment of the mentally ill in the post-reform era.* Springfield, IL: Charles C Thomas.

Miller, R. D. (1991). Involuntary civil commitment. In R. I. Simon (Ed.), *American Psychiatric Press Review of Clinical Psychiatry and the Law* (Vol. 2, pp. 95–172). Washington, DC: American Psychiatric Press.

Miller, T. W. (1989). *Stressful life events.* Connecticut: International University Press.

Miller, W. R., Benefield, R. G., & Tonigan, J. S. (1993). Enhancing motivation for change in problem drinking: A controlled comparison of two therapist styles. *Journal of Consulting and Clinical Psychology, 61,* 455–461.

Miller, W. R., Leckman, A. L., Delaney, H. D., & Tinkcom, M. (1992). Long-term follow-up of behavioral self-control training. *Journal of Studies on Alcohol, 53,* 249–261.

Millon, T. (1983). *Millon Clinical Multiaxial Inventory manual* (3rd ed.). Minneapolis, MN: Interpretive Scoring Systems.

Millon, T. (1987). *Millon Clinical Multiaxial Inventory-II: Manual for the MCMI-II* (2nd ed.). Minneapolis, MN: National Computer Systems.

Mills, M. J., Sullivan, G., & Eth, S. (1987). Protecting third parties: A decade after *Tarasoff. American Journal of Psychiatry, 144,* 68–74.

Mineka, S. (1988). A primate model of phobic fears. In H. Eysenck and I. Martin (Eds.), *Theoretical foundations of behavior therapy.* New York: Plenum Press.

Mineka, S., & Cook, M. (1986). Immunization against the observational conditioning of snake fear in rhesus monkeys. *Journal of Abnormal Psychology, 95,* 307–318.

Mineka, S., Davidson, M., Cook M., & Keir, R. (1984). Observational conditioning of snake fear in rhesus monkeys. *Journal of Abnormal Psychology, 93,* 355–372.

Mineka, S., Gunnar, M., & Champoux, M. (1986). Control and early socioemotional development: Infant rhesus monkeys reared in controllable versus uncontrollable environments. *Child Development, 57,* 1241–1256.

Mineka, S., & Sutton, S. K. (1992). Cognitive biases and the emotional disorders. *Psychological Science, 3,* 65–69.

Mintz, J. (1983). Integrating research evidence. *Journal of Consulting and Clinical Psychology, 51,* 71–75.

Minuchin, S., Rosman, B. L., & Baker, L. (1978). *Psychosomatic families: Anorexia nervosa in context.* Cambridge, MA: Harvard University Press.

Mitchell, J. E., & de Zwaan, M. (1993). Pharmacological treatments of binge eating. In C. G. Fairburn & G. T. Wilson (Eds.), *Binge eating: Nature, assessment, and treatment* (pp. 250–269). New York: Guilford Press.

Mitchell, J. E., Pyle, R. L., Eckert, E. D., Hatsukami, D., Pomeroy, C., & Zimmerman, R. (1990). A comparison study of antidepressants and structured intensive group psychotherapy in the treatment of bulimia nervosa. *Archives of General Psychiatry, 47,* 149–157.

Mitchell, P., Mackinnon, A. J., & Waters, B. (1993). The genetics of bipolar disorder. *Australian & New Zealand Journal of Psychiatry, 27,* 560–580.

Mittenberg, W., Azrin, R., Millsaps, C., & Heilbronner, R. (1993). Identification of malingered head injury on the Wechsler Memory Scale—Revised. *Psychological Assessment, 5,* 34–40.

Moffatt, R. J., & Owens, S. G. (1991). Cessation from cigarette smoking: Changes in body weight, body composition, resting metabolism and energy consumption. *Metabolism, 40,* 465–470.

Moffitt, T. M. (1993). The neuropsychology of conduct disorder. *Development and Psychopathology, 5,* 135–151.

Moline, K. (1992, May/June). Cognitive-enhancing drugs. *Headlines,* pp. 22–23.

Monahan, J. (1993). Limiting therapist exposure to *Tarasoff* liability. *American Psychologist, 48,* 242–250.

Money, J., & Lamacz, M. (1989). *Vandalized lovemaps.* New York: Prometheus Books.

Moos, R. H., Finney, J. W., & Cronkite, R. C. (1990). *Alcoholism treatment: Context, process, and outcome.* New York: Oxford University Press.

Morey, L. C. (1988). The categorical representation of personality disorder: A cluster analysis of *DSM-III-R* personality features. *Journal of Abnormal Psychology, 97,* 314–321.

Morey, L. C., & Levine, D. J. (1988). A multitrait-multimethod examination of Minnesota Multiphasic Personality Inventory (MMPI) and Millon Clinical Multiaxial Inventory (MCMI). *Journal of Psychopathology and Behavioral Assessment, 10,* 333–344.

Morey, L. C., & Ochoa, E. S. (1989). An investigation of adherence to diagnostic criteria: Clinical diagnosis of the *DSM-III* personality disorders. *Journal of Personality Disorders, 3,* 180–192.

Morey, L. C., & Skinner, H. A. (1986). Empirically derived classifications of alcohol-related problems. In M. Galanter (Ed.), *Recent developments in alcoholism* (Vol. 4, pp. 144–168). New York: Plenum.

Morganthau, T. (1986, March 23). Getting high on crack. Teens fall prey to new cocaine. *Anchorage Daily News,* pp. E1, E4, E5.

Morokoff, P. J., & LoPiccolo, J. (1986). A comparative evaluation of minimal therapist contact and 15-session treatment for female orgasmic dysfunction. *Journal of Consulting and Clinical Psychology, 54,* 294–300.

Mosak, H. H. (1995). Adlerian psychotherapy. In R. J. Corsini & D. Wedding (Eds.), *Current psychotherapies* (5th ed., pp. 51–94). Itasca, IL: F. E. Peacock.

Mowrer, O. H., & Mowrer, W. M. (1938). Enuresis—a method for its study and treatment. *American Journal of Orthopsychiatry, 8,* 436–459.

Muehlenhard, C. L., & Cook, S. W. (1988). Men's self-reports of unwanted sexual activity. *Journal of Sex Research, 24,* 58–72.

Muehlenhard, C. L., Julsonnet, S., Carlson, M. I., & Flarity-White, L. A. (1989). A cognitive-behavioral program for preventing sexual coercion. *Behavior Therapist, 12,* 211–214.

Mueser, K. T., & Berenbaum, H. (1990). Psychodynamic treatment of schizophrenia: Is there a future? *Psychological Medicine, 20,* 253–262.

Mueser, K. T., & Gingerich, S. (1994). *Coping with schizophrenia: A guide for families.* Oakland, CA: Harbinger Publications.

Mueser, K. T., & Glynn, S. M. (1995). *Behavioral family therapy for psychiatric disorders.* Boston: Allyn & Bacon.

Mumford, D. B. (1993). Somatization: A transcultural perspective. *International Review of Psychiatry, 5,* 231–242.

Mumford, D. B., Whitehouse, A. M., & Choudry, I. Y. (1992). Survey of eating disorders in English-medium schools in Lahore, Pakistan. *International Journal of Eating Disorders, 11,* 173–184.

Mumford, D. B., Whitehouse, A. M., & Platts, M. (1991). Sociocultural correlates of eating disorders among Asian schoolgirls in Bradford. *British Journal of Psychiatry, 158,* 222–228.

Muñoz, R. G., Hollon, S. D., McGrath, E., Rehm, L. P., & Vandenbos, G. R. (1994). On the AHCPR *Depression in Primary Care* guidelines. *American Psychologist, 49,* 42–61.

Munro, J. D. (1986). Epidemiology and the extent of mental retardation. *Psychiatric Clinics of North America, 9,* 591–624.

Murphy, C. M., Meyer, S., & O'Leary, K. O. (1994). Dependency characteristics of partner assaultive men. *Journal of Abnormal Psychology, 103,* 729–735.

Murphy, G. E., Simons, A. D., Wetzel, R. D., & Lustman, P. J. (1984). Cognitive therapy and pharmacotherapy. *Archives of General Psychiatry, 41,* 33–41.

Murray, H. A. (1938). *Explorations in personality.* New York: Oxford Press.

Myers, J. K., Weissman, M. M., Tischler, G. L., Holzer, C. E., III, Leaf, P. J., Orvaschel, H., Anthony, J. C., Boyd, J. H., Burke, J. D., Kramer, M., & Stoltzman, R. (1984). Six-month prevalence of psychiatric disorders in three communities. *Archives of General Psychiatry, 41,* 959–967.

Myers, P. I., & Hammil, D. D. (1990). *Learning disabilities: Basic concepts, assessment practices, and instructional strategies* (4th ed.). Austin, TX: Pro-Ed.

N

Nadelson, C. C. (1993). Ethics, empathy, and gender in health care. *American Journal of Psychiatry, 150,* 1307–1314.

Naranjo, C. (1993). *Gestalt therapy.* Nevada City, CA: Gateways.

Naranjo, C. A., Kadlec, K. E., Sanhueza, P., Woodley-Remus, D., & Sellers, E. M. (1990). Fluoxetine differentially alters alcohol intake and other consummatory behaviors in problem drinkers. *Clinical Pharmacological Therapy, 47,* 490–498.

Nasar, S. (1994, November 13). The lost years of a Nobel Laureate. *New York Times,* p. III-1.

Nash, M. R., Hulsey, T. L., Sexton, M. C., Harralson, T. L., & Lambert, W. (1993). Long-term sequelae of childhood sexual abuse: Perceived family environment, psychopathology, and dissociation. *Journal of Consulting and Clinical Psychology, 61,* 276–283.

Nathan, P. E. (1981). Nonproblem drinking outcomes: The data on controlled drinking treatments. *Advances in Alcoholism, 2,* 13.

Nathan, P. E. (1983). Failures in prevention: Why we can't prevent the devastating effect of alcoholism and drug abuse on American productivity. *American Psychologist, 38,* 459–468.

Nathan, P. E. (1988). The addictive personality is the behavior of the addict. *Journal of Consulting and Clinical Psychology, 56,* 183–188.

Nathan, P. E. (1994a). *DSM-IV*: Empirical, accessible, not yet ideal. *Journal of Clinical Psychology, 50,* 103–110.

Nathan, P. E. (1994b). Psychoactive substance dependence. In T. A. Widiger, A. J. Frances, H. A. Pincus, M. B. First, R. Ross, & W. Davis (Eds.), DSM-IV *sourcebook* (Vol. 1, pp. 33–44). Washington, DC: American Psychiatric Association.

Nathan, P. E., & O'Brien, J. S. (1971). An experimental analysis of the behavior of alcoholic and nonalcoholics during prolonged experimental drinking. *Behavior Therapy, 2,* 455–476.

Nathan, P. E., & Skinstad, A.-H. (1987). Outcomes of treatment for alcohol problems: Current methods, problems, and results. *Journal of Consulting and Clinical Psychology, 55,* 332–340.

National Highway Safety Administration. (1992). *FARS fatal accident reporting system, annual report, 1992.* Washington, DC: U.S. Department of Transportation.

National Institute of Alcohol Abuse and Alcoholism (NIAAA). (1993). *Eighth special report to the U.S. Congress on alcohol and health.* Washington, DC: U.S. Department of Health and Human Services.

National Institute of Health (NIH), Technology Assessment Conference Panel. (1992). Methods for voluntary weight loss and control. *Annals of Internal Medicine, 116,* 942–949.

National Institute of Mental Health (NIMH) Consensus Statement. (1985). *Electroconvulsive therapy* (Vol. 5, No. 11). Bethesda, MD: National Institute of Mental Health.

National Institute of Mental Health (NIMH). (1989). *Depressive illnesses: Treatments bring new hope* (DHHS Pub. No. 89-1491). Rockville, MD: NIMH Office of Scientific Information.

National Institute of Mental Health (NIMH). (1991, September). Treatment of panic disorder. *NIH Consensus Development Conference Consensus Statement, 9*(2), 1–24.

National Institute on Drug Abuse (NIDA). (1991). *Third triennial report to Congress on drug abuse and drug abuse research.* Washington, DC: U.S. Department of Health and Human Services.

Nay, W. R. (1986). Analogue measures. In A. R. Ciminaro, C. S. Calhoun, & H. E. Adams (Eds.), *Handbook of behavioral assessment* (pp. 223–252). New York: John Wiley.

Needleman, H. L., Gunnoe, C., Leviton, A., Reed, R., Peresie, H., Maher, C., & Barret, B. S. (1979). Deficits in psychological and classroom performance of children with elevated dentine lead levels. *New England Journal of Medicine, 300,* 689–695.

Needleman, H. L., Schell, A., Bellinger, D., Leviton, A., & Allred, E. N. (1990). The long term effects of exposure to low dosages of lead in childhood: An 11-year follow-up report. *New England Journal of Medicine, 322,* 83–88.

Needles, D. J., & Abramson, L. Y. (1990). Positive life events, attributional style, and hopefulness: Testing a model of recovery from depression. *Journal of Abnormal Psychology, 99,* 156–165.

Neff, J. A., Holaman, B., & Schluter, T. D. (1995). Spousal violence among Anglos, Blacks, and Mexican Americans: The role of demographic variables, psychosocial predictors, and alcohol consumption. *Journal of Family Violence, 10,* 1–21.

Neidig, P. H., & Friedman, D. H. (1984). *Spouse abuse: A treatment program for couples.* Champaign, IL: Research Press.

Neighbors, B., Kempton, T., & Forehand, R. (1992). Co-occurrence of substance abuse with conduct, anxiety, and depression disorders in juvenile delinquents. *Addictive Behaviors, 17,* 379–386.

Neitzel, M. T., & Harris, M. J. (1990). Relationship of dependency and achievement/autonomy to depression. *Clinical Psychology Review, 10,* 279–298.

Nelson, R. E., & Craighead, W. E. (1977). Selective recall of positive and negative feedback, self-control behaviors, and depression. *Journal of Abnormal Psychology, 86,* 379–388.

Newman, J. P., & Kosson, D. S. (1986). Passive avoidance learning in psychopathic and nonpsychopathic offenders. *Journal of Abnormal Psychology, 95,* 252–256.

Newman, R. (1994, August). Electronic therapy raises issues, risks. *American Psychological Association Monitor,* p. 25.

Nezu, A. M., & Nezu, C. M. (1993). Identifying and selecting target problems for clinical interventions: A problem-solving model. *Psychological Assessment, 5,* 254–263.

Nezu, C. M., & Nezu, A. M. (1994). Outpatient psychotherapy for adults with mental retardation and concomitant psychopathology: Research and clinical imperatives. *Journal of Consulting and Clinical Psychology, 62,* 34–42.

Nezu, C. M., Nezu, A. M., & Gill-Weiss, M. J. (1992). *Psychopathology in persons with mental retardation: Clinical guidelines for assessment and treatment.* Champaign, IL: Research Press.

Nichols, M. P., & Schwartz, R. C. (1991). *Family therapy: Concepts and methods* (2nd ed.). Boston: Allyn and Bacon.

Nigg, J. T., & Goldsmith, H. H. (1994). Genetics of personality disorders: Perspective from personality and psychopathology research. *Psychological Bulletin, 115,* 346–380.

Nigg, J. T., Lohr, N. E., Westen, D., Gold, L. J., & Silk, K. R. (1992). Malevolent object representations in borderline personality disorder and major depression. *Journal of Abnormal Psychology, 101,* 61–67.

Nisbett, R., & Ross, L. (1980). *Human inference: Strategies and shortcomings of social judgment.* Englewood Cliffs, NJ: Prentice Hall.

Noden, M. (1994, August 8). Dying to win. *Sports Illustrated,* pp. 52–60.

Nolen-Hoeksema, S. (1990). *Sex differences in depression.* Stanford, CA: Stanford University Press.

Nolen-Hoeksema, S. (1991). Responses to depression and their effects on the duration of depressive episodes. *Journal of Abnormal Psychology, 100,* 569–582.

Nolen-Hoeksema, S., & Girgus, J. S. (1994). The emergence of gender differences in depression during adolescence. *Psychological Bulletin, 115,* 424–443.

Nolen-Hoeksema, S., Morrow, J., & Fredrickson, B. L. (1993). Response styles and the duration of episodes of depressed mood. *Journal of Abnormal Psychology, 102,* 20–28.

Nolen-Hoeksema, S., Parker, L. E., & Larson, J. (1994). Ruminative coping with depressed mood following loss. *Journal of Personality and Social Psychology, 67,* 92–104.

Norcross, J. C., Alford, B. A., & DeMichele, J. T. (1992). The future of psychotherapy: Delphi data and concluding observations. *Psychotherapy, 29,* 150–158.

Nordahl, T. E., Semple, W. E., Gross, M., Mellman, T. A., Stein, M. B., Goyer, P., King, A. C., Uhde, T. W., & Cohen, R. M. (1990). Cerebral glucose metabolic differences in patients with panic disorder. *Neuropsychopharmacology, 3,* 261–272.

Nordentoft, M., & Rubin, P. (1993). Mental illness and social integration among suicide attempters in Copenhagen: Comparison with the general population and a four-year follow-up study of 100 patients. *Acta Psychiatrica Scandinavica, 88,* 278–285.

Nordheimer, J. (1994, November 2). New look at jail unit housing sex offenders. *New York Times,* p. B6.

Norton, A. J., & Miller, L. F. (1992). *Marriage, divorce and remarriage in the 1990s.* Washington, DC: U.S. Department of Commerce, Economics, and Statistics Administration, Bureau of the Census.

Novak, M. A., & Suomi, S. J. (1988). Psychological well-being of primates in captivity. *American Psychologist, 43,* 765–773.

Noyes, R., Clarkson, C., Crowe, R. R., Yates, W. R., & McChesney, C. M. (1987). A family study of generalized anxiety disorder. *American Journal of Psychiatry, 144,* 1019–1024.

Nuechterlein, K. H., Dawson, M. E., Gitlin, M., Ventura, J., Goldstein, M. J., Snyder, K. S., Yee, C. M., & Mintz, J. (1992). Developmental processes in schizophrenic disorders: Longitudinal studies of vulnerability and stress. *Schizophrenia Bulletin, 18,* 397–425.

Nunnally, J. C. (1984). Self-report measures of personality traits. In N. S. Endler & J. M. Hunt (Eds.), *Personality and the behavior disorders.* New York: John Wiley.

Nurnberger, J. I., & Gershon, E. S. (1982). In E. S. Paykel (Ed.), *Handbook of affective disorders* (pp. 126–145). Edinburgh, Scotland: Livingstone.

O

O'Connor, A. A. (1987). Female sex offenders. *British Journal of Psychiatry, 150,* 615–620.

O'Keefe, M. (1995). Predictors of child abuse in maritally violent families. *Journal of Interpersonal Violence, 10,* 3–25.

O'Leary, A. (1990). Stress, emotion, and immune function. *Psychological Bulletin, 108,* 363–382.

O'Leary, A., Raffaelli, M., & Allende-Ramos, C. (in press). Preventing the sexual transmission of AIDS: Current status and future directions. In S. Maes, M. Johnston, & H. Leventhal (Eds.), *International yearbook of health psychology.* New York: Wiley.

O'Leary, A., Temoshok, L., Jenkins, S. R., & Sweet, D. M. (1989, October). *Autonomic reactivity and immune function in men with AIDS.* Paper presented at the annual meeting of the Society for Psychophysiological Research, New Orleans.

O'Leary, K. D. (1980). Pills or skills for hyperactive children? *Journal of Applied Behavior Analysis, 13,* 191–204.

O'Leary, K. D. (1984). *Mommy, I can't sit still: Coping with hyperactive and aggressive children.* New York: New Horizon Press.

O'Leary, K. D. (1988). Physical aggression between spouses: A social learning theory perspective. In V. B. Van Hasselt, R. L. Morrison, A. S. Belleck, & M. Hersen (Eds.), *Handbook of family violence* (pp. 31–55). New York: Plenum.

O'Leary, K. D. (1993). Through a psychological lens: Personality traits, personality disorders, and levels of violence. In R. J. Gelles & D. R. Loseke, *Current controversies on family violence* (pp. 7–30). Newbury Park, CA: Sage.

O'Leary, K. D., & Arias, I. (1983). The influence of marital therapy on sexual satisfaction. *Journal of Sex and Marital Therapy, 9,* 171–181.

O'Leary, K. D., Barling, J., Arias, I., Rosenbaum, A., Malone, J., & Tyree, A. (1989). Prevalence and stability of physical aggression between spouses: A longitudinal analysis. *Journal of Consulting and Clinical Psychology, 57,* 263–268.

O'Leary, K. D., & Beach, S. R. H. (1990). Marital therapy: A viable treatment for depression. *American Journal of Psychiatry, 147,* 183–186.

O'Leary, K. D., Christian, J. L., & Mendell, N. R. (1994). A closer look at the link between marital discord and depressive symptomatology. *Journal of Social and Clinical Psychology, 13,* 33–41.

O'Leary, K. D., & Emery, R. E. (1984). Marital discord and childhood behavior problems. In M. Levine & P. Satz (Eds.), *Middle childhood: Development and dysfunction* (pp. 345–364). Baltimore: University Park Press.

O'Leary, K. D., & Jacobson, N. S. (in press). Partner relational problems with physical abuse: *DSM-IV* literature summary. DSM-IV *sourcebook* (Vol. 3). Washington, DC: American Psychiatric Press.

O'Leary, K. D., & Neidig, P. H. (1993, November). *Treatment of wife abuse: A comparison of gender specific and couples approaches.* Paper presented at the annual meeting of the Association for the Advancement of Behavior Therapy, Atlanta, GA.

O'Leary, K. D., Vivian, D., & Malone, J. (1992). Assessment of physical aggression in marriage: The need for multimodal assessment. *Behaviour Research and Therapy, 14,* 1–10.

O'Leary, K. D., Vivian, D., & Nisi, A. (1985). Assessment and treatment of "hyperactivity" in Italy and the United States. *Journal of Abnormal Child Psychology, 13,* 485–500.

O'Leary, K. D., & Wilson, G. T. (1987). *Behavior therapy: Application and outcome* (2nd ed.). Englewood Cliffs, NJ: Prentice Hall.

O'Leary, S. G., & Pelham, W. E. (1978). Behavioral therapy and withdrawal of stimulant medication with hyperactive children. *Pediatrics, 61,* 211–217.

O'Leary, S. G., Pelham, W. E., Rosenbaum, A., & Price, G. H. (1976). Behavioral treatment of hyperkinetic children. *The Clinical Psychologist, 15,* 510–515.

O'Malley, S. S., Jaffe, A., Chang, G., Witte, G., Schottenfeld, R. S., & Rounsaville, B. J. (1992). Naltrexone in the treatment of alcohol dependence: Preliminary findings. In C. A. Naranjo & E. M. Sellars (Eds.), *Novel pharmacological interventions for alcoholism* (pp. 148–157). New York: Springer-Verlag.

O'Reilly, J., & Sales, B. (1987). Privacy for the institutionalized mentally ill: Are court-ordered standards effective? *Law and Human Behavior, 11,* 41–53.

Offord, D. R., Boyle, M. H., & Racine, Y. A. (1991). The epidemiology of antisocial behavior in childhood and adolescence. In D. J. Pepler

& K. H. Rubin (Eds.), *The development and treatment of childhood aggression* (pp. 31–54). Hillside, NJ: Lawrence Erlbaum.

Öhman, A. (1986). Face the beast and fear the face: Animal and social fears as prototypes for evolutionary analyses of emotion. *Psychophysiology, 23,* 123–145.

Ohno, M., Arai, K., Tsukahara, S., Miura, J., Yokoyama, J., & Ikeda, Y. (1991). Long-term effectiveness of combined therapy by behaviour modification and VLCD—a three-year follow-up. In Y. Oomura, S. Tarui, S. Inoue, & T. Shimazu (Eds.), *Progress in obesity research 1990* (pp. 523–530). London, England: John Libbey.

Oken, B. S. (1989). Endogenous event-related potentials. In K. H. Chiappa (Ed.), *Evoked potentials in clinical medicine* (pp. 563–592). New York: Raven Press.

Olfson, M., Pincus, H. A., & Dial, T. H. (1994). Professional practice patterns of U.S. psychiatrists. *American Journal of Psychiatry, 151,* 89–95.

Ollendick, T. H., & King, N. J. (1994). Diagnosis, assessment and treatment of internalizing problems in children: The role of longitudinal data. *Journal of Consulting and Clinical Psychology, 62,* 918–927.

Ollendick, T. H., King, N. J., & Frary, R. B. (1989). Fears in children and adolescents: Reliability and generalizability across gender, age and nationality. *Behavior Research and Therapy, 27,* 19–26.

Orne, M. T. (1962). On the social psychology of the psychological experiment: With particular reference to demand characteristics and their implications. *American Psychologist, 17,* 776–783.

Orvaschel, H., & Weissman, M. A. (1986). Epidemiology of anxiety disorders in children: A review. In R. Gittelman (Ed.), *Anxiety disorders of childhood* (pp. 58–72). New York: Guilford Press.

Otto, M. W., Pollack, M. D., Sachs, G. S., Reiter, S. R., Meltzer-Brody, S., & Rosenbaum, J. F. (1993). Discontinuation of benzodiazepine treatment: Efficacy of cognitive-behavioral therapy for patients with panic disorder. *American Journal of Psychiatry, 150,* 1485–1490.

Owen, E. (1994). *Personality pathology in patients with chronic low back disability: Assessment and treatment effects.* Unpublished doctoral dissertation, University of Texas Southwestern Medical Center, Dallas.

P

Paff, B. A. (1985). Sexual dysfunction in gay men requesting treatment. *Journal of Sex and Marital Therapy, 11,* 3–18.

Palace, E. M., & Gorzalka, B. B. (1990). The enhancing effects of anxiety on arousal in sexually dysfunctional and functional women. *Journal of Abnormal Psychology, 99,* 403–411.

Palinkas, L. A., Petterson, J. S., Russell, J., & Downs, M. A. (1993). Community patterns of psychiatric disorders after the *Exxon Valdez* oil spill. *American Journal of Psychiatry, 150,* 1517–1523.

Pan, H. S., Neidig, P. H., & O'Leary, K. D. (1994). Predicting mild and severe husband-to-wife physical aggression. *Journal of Consulting and Clinical Psychology, 62,* 975–988.

Pardes, H., Kaufman, C. A., Pincus, H. A., & West, A. (1989). Genetics and psychiatry: Past discoveries, current dilemmas, and future directions. *American Journal of Psychiatry, 146,* 435–443.

Paris, J. (1993a). *Borderline personality disorder.* Washington, DC: American Psychiatric Press.

Paris, J. (1993b). Personality disorders: A biospsychosocial model. *Journal of Personality Disorders, 7,* 255–264.

Park, D. C. (1994). Research on aging deserves top priority. *Chronicle of Higher Education, 41,* A40.

Park, H., & Gaylord-Ross, R. (1989). A problem-solving approach to social skills training in employment settings with mentally retarded youth. *Journal of Applied Behavior Analysis, 22,* 373–380.

Parker, G., & Hadzi-Pavlovic, D. (1992). Parental representations of melancholic and non-melancholic depressives: Examining for specificity to depressive type and for evidence of additive effects. *Psychological Medicine, 22,* 657–665.

Parker, G., Johnston, P., & Hayward, L. (1988). Parental "expressed emotion" as a predictor of schizophrenic relapse. *Archives of General Psychiatry, 45,* 806–813.

Parker, K. C. H., Hanson, R. K., & Hunsley, J. (1988). MMPI, Rorschach, and WAIS: A meta-analytic comparison of reliability, stability, and validity. *Psychological Bulletin, 103,* 367–373.

Parsons v. State, 2 So. 854, 866-867 (Ala. 1886).

Parsons, O. A., & Hart, R. P. (1984). Behavioral disorders associated with central nervous system dysfunction. In H. E. Adams & P. B.

Sutker (Eds.), *Comprehensive handbook of psychopathology* (pp. 841–916). New York: Plenum.

Partonen, T., & Partinen, M. (1994). Light treatment for seasonal affective disorder: Theoretical considerations and clinical implications. *Acta Psychiatrica Scandinavica, 89*(377, Suppl.), 41–45.

Pasamanick, B., Toberts, D. W., Lemkau, P. V., & Krueger, D. E. (1962). A survey of mental disease in an urban population. *American Journal of Public Health, 47,* 923–929.

Paternite, C. E., & Loney, J. (1980). Childhood hyperkinesis: Relationships between symptomatology and home environment. In C. K. Whalen & B. Henker (Eds.), *Hyperactive children: The social ecology of identification and treatment* (pp. 105–141). New York: Academic Press.

Paternite, C. E., Loney, J., & Langhorne, J. E. (1976). Relationships between symptomatology and SES-related factors in hyperkinetic/MBD boys. *American Journal of Orthopsychiatry, 46,* 291–301.

Pato, M. T., Zohar-Kadouch, R., Zohar, J., & Murphy, D. L. (1988). Return of symptoms after discontinuation of clomipramine in patients with obsessive-compulsive disorder. *American Journal of Psychiatry, 145,* 1521–1525.

Patrick, C. J., Cuthbert, B. N., & Lang, P. J. (1994). Emotion in the criminal psychopath: Fear image processing. *Journal of Abnormal Psychology, 103,* 523–534.

Patrick, J. (1988). Concordance of the MCMI and the MMPI in the diagnosis of three *DSM-III* Axis I disorders. *Journal of Clinical Psychology, 44,* 186–190.

Patrick, M., Hobson, R. P., Castle, D., & Howard, R. (1994). Personality disorder and the mental representation of early social experience. *Development and Psychopathology, 6,* 375–388.

Patterson, C. M., & Newman, J. P. (1993). Reflectivity and learning from aversive events: Toward a psychological mechanism for the syndromes of disinhibition. *Psychological Review, 100,* 716–736.

Patterson, G. R. (1982). *Coercive family process.* Eugene, OR: Castalia.

Patterson, G. R., & Bank, L. (1986). Bootstrapping your way in the nomological thicket. *Behavioral Assessment, 8,* 49–73.

Patterson, G. R., Dishion, T. J., & Chamberlain, P. (1993). Outcomes and methodological issues relating to treatment of antisocial children. In T. R. Giles (Ed.), *Handbook of effective psychotherapy.* New York: Plenum.

Patterson, G. R., Littman, R. A., & Bricker, W. (1967). Assertive behavior in children: A step toward a theory of aggression. *Monographs for the Society for Research in Child Development, 32,* 1–43.

Patterson, G. R., Reid, J. B., & Dishion, T. J. (1992). *Antisocial boys.* Eugene, OR: Castalia.

Patton, G. C., Johnson-Sabine, E., Wood, K., Mann, A. H., & Wakeling, A. (1990). Abnormal eating attitudes in London schoolgirls—a prospective epidemiological study: Outcome at twelve month follow-up. *Psychological Medicine, 20,* 383–394.

Paul, G. L. (1985). Can pregnancy be a placebo effect? Terminology, designs, and conclusions in the study of psychosocial and pharmacological treatments of behavioral disorders. In L. White, B. Turksy, & G. E. Schwartz (Eds.), *Placebo: Theory, research, and mechanisms* (pp. 137–163). New York: Guilford Press.

Paul, G. L., & Lentz, R. J. (1977). *Psychosocial treatment of chronic mental patients.* Cambridge, MA: Harvard University Press.

Pauls, D. L., Towbin, K. E., Leckman, J. F., Zahner, G. E. P., & Cohen, D. J. (1986). Gilles de la Tourette's syndrome and obsessive-compulsive disorder. *Archives of General Psychiatry, 43,* 1180–1182.

Pavkov, T. W., Lewis, D. A., & Lyons, J. S. (1989). Psychiatric diagnoses and racial bias: An empirical investigation. *Professional Psychology, 20,* 364–368.

Paykel, E. S., Brayne, C., Huppert, F. A., Gill, C., Barkley, C., Gehlhaar, E., Beardsall, L., Girling, D. M., Pollitt, P., & O'Connor, D. (1994). Incidence of dementia in a population older than 75 years in the United Kingdom. *Archives of General Psychiatry, 51,* 325–332.

Paykel, E. S., & Cooper, Z. (1992). Life events and social stress. In E. S. Paykel (Ed.), *Handbook of affective disorders* (2nd ed., pp. 149–170). New York: Guilford Press.

Paykel, E. S., Myers, J. K., Dienelt, M. N., Klerman, G. L., Lindenthal, J. J., & Pepper, M. P. (1969). Life events and depression: A controlled study. *Archives of General Psychiatry, 21,* 753–760.

Pear, R. (1991, December 4). Bigger number of new mothers are unmarried. *New York Times,* p. A 20.

Pedersen, N. L., Plomin, R., Nesselroade, J. R., & McClearn, G. E. (1992). A quantitative genetic analysis of cognitive abilities during the second half of the life span. *Psychological Science, 3,* 346–353.

Pelham, W. E. (1993). Pharmacotherapy for children with attention-deficit hyperactivity disorder. *School Psychology Review, 22,* 199–227.

Pelham, W. E., Carson, C., Sams, S., Vallano, G., Dixon, J., & Hoza, B. (1991). Separate and combined effects of methylphenidate and behavior modification on boys with attention-deficit hyperactivity in the classroom. *Journal of Consulting and Clinical Psychology, 61,* 506–515.

Pelham, W. E., & Murphy, H. A. (1986). Behavioral and pharmacological treatment of attention deficit and conduct disorders. In M. Hersen (Ed.), *Pharmacological and behavioral treatment: An integrative approach* (pp. 108–148). New York: John Wiley.

Pennebaker, J. (1990). *Opening up.* New York: Morrow.

Pennebaker, J. W., Kiecolt-Glaser, J. K., & Glaser, R. (1988). Disclosure of traumas and immune function: Health implications for psychotherapy. *Journal of Consulting and Clinical Psychology, 56,* 239–245.

Peplau, L. A., Rubin, Z., & Hill, C. T. (1977). Sexual intimacy in dating relationships. *Journal of Social Issues, 33,* 86–109.

Perkins, K. A. (1993). Weight gain following smoking cessation. *Journal of Consulting and Clinical Psychology, 61,* 768–777.

Perkins, K. A., Epstein, L. H., & Pastor, S. (1990). Changes in energy balance following smoking cessation and resumption of smoking in women. *Journal of Consulting and Clinical Psychology, 58,* 121–125.

Perls, F., Hefferline, R., & Goodman, P. (1951). *Gestalt therapy.* New York: Julian Press.

Perris, C. (1966). A study of bipolar (manic depressive) and unipolar recurrent depressive psychoses. *Acta Psychiatrica et Neurologica Scandinavica* (Suppl.).

Persad, S. M., & Polivy, J. (1993). Differences between depressed and nondepressed individuals in the recognition of and response to facial cues. *Journal of Abnormal Psychology, 102,* 358–368.

Persons, J. B., Thase, M. E., & Crits-Cristoph, P. (in press). The role of psychotherapy in the treatment of depression: Review of two practice guidelines. *Archives of General Psychiatry.*

Peters, R., Miller, K. S., Schmidt, W., & Meeter, D. (1987). The effects of statutory change on the civil commitment of the mentally ill. *Law and Human Behavior, 11,* 73–99.

Peterson, C. (1988). Explanatory style as a risk factor for illness. *Cognitive Therapy and Research, 12,* 117–130.

Peterson, C., Seligman, M. E. P., & Vaillant, G. E. (1988). Pessimistic explanatory style is a risk factor for physical illness: A thirty-five-year longitudinal study. *Journal of Personality and Social Psychology, 55,* 23–27.

Peterson, L., & Brown, D. (1994). Integrating child injury and abuse-neglect research: Common histories, etiologies, and solutions. *Psychological Bulletin, 116,* 293–315.

Petronko, M. R., Harris, S. L., & Kormann, R. J. (1994). Community-based behavioral training approaches for people with mental retardation and mental illness. *Journal of Consulting and Clinical Psychology, 62,* 49–54.

Pfeiffer, S. I. (1992). Psychology and mental retardation: Emerging research and practice opportunities. *Professional Psychology: Research and Practice, 23,* 239–243.

Pfiffner, L. J., & O'Leary, S. G. (1993). School-based psychological treatments. In J. L. Matson (Ed.), *Handbook of hyperactivity in children* (pp. 234–255). Boston: Allyn & Bacon.

Pfohl, B. (1991). Histrionic personality disorder: A review of available data and recommendations for *DSM-IV. Journal of Personality Disorders, 5,* 150–166.

Pfohl, B., Black, D. W., Noyes, R., Coryell, W. H., & Barrash, J. (1991). Axis I and axis II comorbidity findings: Implications for validity. In J. M. Oldham (Ed.), *Personality disorders: New perspectives on diagnostic validity* (pp. 145–161). Washington, DC: American Psychiatric Press.

Phillips, D. P., & King, E. W. (1988). Death takes a holiday. *Lancet, ii,* 728–732.

Phillips, D. P., Ruth, T. E., & Wagner, L. M. (1993). Psychology and survival. *Lancet, 342,* 1142–1145.

Phillips, M. R., Wolf, A. S., & Coons, D. J. (1988). Psychiatry and the criminal justice system: Testing the myths. *American Journal of Psychiatry, 145,* 605–610.

Physicians' desk reference. (1994). Montvale, NJ: Medical Economics Data Production.

Piersma, H. L. (1987). Millon Clinical Multiaxial Inventory computer-generated diagnoses: How do they compare to clinician judgment? *Journal of Psychopathology and Behavioral Assessment, 9,* 305–312.

Pike, K. M., & Rodin, J. (1991). Mothers, daughters, and disordered eating. *Journal of Abnormal Psychology, 100,* 198–204.

Pinel, P. (1962). *A treatise on insanity* (D. D. David, Trans.). New York: Hafner. (Original work published 1801)

Piotrowski, C., & Keller, J. W. (1989). Psychological testing in outpatient mental health facilities: A national study. *Professional Psychology: Research and Practice, 20,* 423–425.

Piotrowski, Z. (1937). The Rorschach inkblot method in organic disturbances of the central nervous system. *Journal of Nervous and Mental Disease, 86,* 525–537.

Piper, A. (1993). Tricyclic antidepressants versus electroconvulsive therapy: A review of the evidence for efficacy in depression. *Annals of Clinical Psychiatry, 5,* 13–23.

Piper, W. E., Rosie, J. S., Azim, H. F., & Joyce, A. S. (1993). A randomized trial of psychiatric day treatment for patients with affective and personality disorders. *Hospital and Community Psychiatry, 44,* 757–763.

Pirog-Good, M. A., & Stets, J. E. (1989). *Violence in dating relationships.* New York: Praeger.

Pithers, W. D., Martin, G. R., & Cumming, G. F. (1989). Vermont treatment program for sexual aggressors. In D. R. Laws (Ed.), *Relapse prevention with sex offenders* (pp. 292–310). New York: Guilford Press.

Plomin, R. (1990). The role of inheritance in behavior. *Science, 248,* 183–188.

Plomin, R. (1993). Nature and nurture: Perspective and prospective. In R. Plomin & G. E. McClearn (Eds.), *Nature, nurture and psychology* (pp. 459–485). Washington, DC: American Psychological Association.

Plomin, R., & McClearn, G. E. (Eds.). (1993). *Nature, nurture and psychology.* Washington, DC: American Psychological Association.

Plomin, R., & Neiderhiser, J. M. (1992). Genetics and experience. *Current Directions in Psychological Science, 1,* 160–163.

Police Foundation, The. (1976). *Domestic violence and the police studies in Detroit and Kansas City.* Washington, DC: The Police Foundation.

Pomerleau, O., Pertschuk, M., Adkins, D., & D'Aquili, E. (1978). Treatment for middle income problem drinkers. In P. E. Nathan, G. A. Marlatt, & T. Loberg (Eds.), *Alcoholism: New directions in behavioral research and treatment* (pp. 143–160). New York: Plenum.

Pope, K. S. (1990). Therapist-patient sex as sexual abuse. *Professional Psychology: Research and Practice, 21,* 227–239.

Pope, K. S., & Vetter, V. A. (1992). Ethical dilemmas encountered by members of the American Psychological Association: A national survey. *American Psychologist, 47,* 397–411.

Porjesz, B., & Begleiter, H. (1983). Brain dysfunction and alcohol. In B. Kissin & H. Begleiter (Eds.), *The pathogenesis of alcoholism* (pp. 415–483). New York: Plenum.

Potthoff, J., Holahan, C., & Joiner, T. (1995). Reassurance seeking, stress generation, and depressive symptoms: An integrative model. *Journal of Personality and Social Psychology, 68,* 646–670.

Powell, D. H., & Whitla, D. K. (1994). Normal cognitive aging: Toward empirical perspectives. *Current Directions in Psychological Science, 3,* 27–31.

Preng, K. W., & Clopton, J. R. (1986). Application of the MacAndrew Alcoholism Scale to alcoholics with psychiatric diagnoses. *Journal of Personality Assessment, 50,* 113–122.

Prescott, C. A., Hewitt, J. K., Truett, K. R., Heath, A. C., Neale, M. C., & Eaves, L. J. (1994). Genetic and environmental influences on lifetime alcohol-related problems in a volunteer sample of older twins. *Journal of Studies on Alcohol, 55,* 184–202.

Pribor, E. F., Yutzy, S. H., Dean, J. T., & Wetzel, R. D. (1993). Briquet's syndrome, dissociation, and abuse. *American Journal of Psychiatry, 150,* 1507–1511.

Prichard, J. C. (1835). *A treatise on insanity and other disorders affecting the mind.* London, England: Sherwood, Gilbert, & Piper.

Prien, R. F., & Gelenberg, A. J. (1989). Alternatives to lithium for preventive treatment of bipolar disorder. *American Journal of Psychiatry, 146,* 840–848.

Prignatano, G. P. (1992). Personality disturbances associated with traumatic brain injury. *Journal of Consulting and Clinical Psychology, 60,* 360–368.

Prinz, R. J. (1985). Diet-behavior research with children: Methodological and substantive issues. *Advances in Learning and Behavioral Disabilities, 4,* 181–189.

Prinz, R. J., & Miller, G. E. (1994). Family based treatment for childhood antisocial behavior: Experimental influences on dropout and engagement. *Journal of Consulting and Clinical Psychology, 62,* 645–650.

Prioleau, L., Murdock, M., & Brody, N. (1983). An analysis of psychotherapy versus placebo studies. *The Behavioral and Brain Sciences, 6,* 275–310.

Prizant, B. M., & Wetherby, A. M. (1993). Communication in preschool autistic children. In E. Schopler, M. E. Van Bourgondien, & M. M. Bristol (Eds.), *Preschool issues in autism* (pp. 95–128). New York: Plenum Press.

Prochaska, J. O., & DiClemente, C. C. (1983). Stages and processes of self-change of smoking: Toward an integrative model of change. *Journal of Consulting and Clinical Psychology, 51,* 390–395.

Prochaska, J. O., & DiClemente, C. C. (1986). Toward a comprehensive model of change. In W. R. Miller & N. Heather (Eds.), *Treating addictive behaviors* (pp. 3–27). New York: Plenum.

Prochaska, J. O., & DiClemente, C. C. (1992). Stages of change in the modification of problem behaviors. In M. Hersen, R. M. Eisler, & P. M. Miller (Eds.), *Progress in behavior modification* (pp. 184–214). Sycamore, IL: Sycamore.

Prochaska, J. O., DiClemente, C. C., & Norcross, J. C. (1992). In search of how people change. *American Psychologist, 47,* 1102–1114.

Pugliesi, K. (1989). Social support and self-esteem as intervening variables in the relationship between social roles and women's well-being. *Community Mental Health Journal, 25,* 87–100.

Putnam, F. (1994, September). *Psychobiological sequelae of abuse and violence: Implications for symptomatology and treatment.* Paper presented at NIMH Conference, Clinical and Research Issues in the treatment of Women Who Have Experienced Physical and Sexual Violence. Washington, DC.

Putnam, F. W. (1984). The psychophysiological investigation of multiple personality: A review. *Psychiatric Clinics of North America, 7,* 31–39.

Putnam, F. W., Guroff, J. J., Silberman, E. D., Barban, L., & Post, R. M. (1986). The clinical phenomenology of multiple personality disorder: Review of 100 recent cases. *Journal of Clinical Psychology, 47,* 285–293.

Putnam, F. W., & Loewenstein, R. J. (1993). Treatment of multiple personality disorder: A survey of current practices. *American Journal of Psychiatry, 150,* 1048–1052.

Pyle, R. L., Mitchell, J. E., Eckert, E. D., Hatsukami, D., Pomeroy, C., & Zimmerman, R. (1990). Maintenance treatment and 6-month outcome for bulimic patients who respond to initial treatment. *American Journal of Psychiatry, 147,* 871–875.

Pyszczynski, T., & Greenberg, J. (1987). Self-regulatory perseveration and the depressive self-focusing style: A self-awareness theory of reactive depression. *Psychological Bulletin, 102,* 122–138.

Q

Quay, H. (1990, October). *Electrodermal responding, inhibition, and reward-seeking in undersocialized aggressive conduct disorder.* Paper presented at the annual meeting of the American Academy of Child and Adolescent Psychiatry, Chicago, IL.

Quinsey, V. L., & Chaplin, T. C. (1984). Stimulus control of rapists' and non-sex offenders' sexual arousal. *Behavioral Assessment, 6,* 169–176.

Quitkin, F. M., Stewart, J. W., McGrath, P. J., & Tricamo, E. (1993). Columbia atypical depression: A subgroup of depressives with better response to MAOI than to tricyclic antidepressants or placebo. *British Journal of Psychiatry, 163*(Suppl. 21), 30–34.

R

Rabinovitz, J. (1995, March 13). Future plight of retarded adults tied to school's uncertain fate. *New York Times,* pp. A1, A11.

Rachman, S. (1990). *Fear and courage.* New York: W. H. Freeman.

Rachman, S., & Hodgson, R. J. (1968). Experimentally induced "sexual fetishism": Replication and development. *Psychological Record, 18,* 25–27.

Rachman, S., & Hodgson, R. J. (1980). *Obsessions and compulsions.* Englewood Cliffs, NJ: Prentice Hall.

Rachman, S., & Maser, J. D. (Eds.). (1988). *Panic: Psychological perspectives.* Hillsdale, NJ: Lawrence Erlbaum.

Rachman, S., & Wilson, G. T. (1980). *The effects of the psychological therapies.* Oxford: Pergamon Press.

Ragland, D. R., & Brand, R. J. (1988). Type A behavior and mortality from coronary heart disease. *New England Journal of Medicine, 318,* 65–69.

Raloff, J. (1995). Obesity, diet linked to deadly cancers. *Science News, 147,* 39.

Ramirez, M. (1991). *Psychotherapy and counseling with minorities.* New York: Pergamon Press.

Rankin, H. (1986). Dependence and compulsion: Experimental models of change. In W. R. Miller & N. Heather (Eds.), *Treating addictive behaviors: Processes of change* (pp. 361–374). New York: Plenum.

Rao, S. M., Huber, S. J., & Bornstein, R. A. (1992). Emotional changes with multiple sclerosis and Parkinson's disease. *Journal of Consulting and Clinical Psychology, 60,* 369–378.

Rapoport, J. L. (1989, March). The biology of obsessions and compulsions. *Scientific American,* pp. 83–89.

Rapoport, J. L., Buchsbaum, M. S., Zahn, T. P., Weingartner, H., Ludow, C., & Mikkelsen, E. (1978). Dextroamphetamine: Cognitive and behavioral effects in normal prepubertal boys. *Science, 199,* 560–563.

Raskin, N. J., & Rogers, C. R. (1995). Person-centered therapy. In R. J. Corsini & D. Wedding (Eds.), *Current psychotherapies* (5th ed., pp. 128–161). Itasca, IL: F. E. Peacock.

Rasmussen, S. A., & Eisen, J. L. (1990). Epidemiology of obsessive-compulsive disorder. *Journal of Clinical Psychiatry, 51,* 10–14.

Ravussin, E., Lillioja, S., Knowler, W. C., Christin, L., Freymond, D., Abbott, W. G. H., Boyce, U., Howard, B. U., & Bogardus, C. (1988). Reduced rate of energy expenditure as a risk factor for body-weight gain. *New England Journal of Medicine, 318,* 467–472.

Ray, O., & Ksir, C. (1990). Behavioral effects of blood alcohol levels. In *Drugs, Society, and Human Behavior* (5th ed.). St. Louis, MO: Times Mirror/Mosby College.

Ray, W. A., Fought, R. L., & Decker, M. D. (1992). Psychoactive drugs and the risk of injurious motor vehicle crashes in elderly drivers. *American Journal of Epidemiology, 136,* 873–883.

Rebok, G. W., & Folstein, M. F. (1994). Dementia. In T. A. Widiger, A. J. Frances, H. A. Pincus, M. B. First, R. Ross, & W. Davis (Eds.), *DSM-IV sourcebook* (pp. 213–236). Washington, DC: American Psychiatric Press.

Redd, W., & Andrykowski, M. A. (1982). Behavioral intervention in cancer treatment: Controlling aversion reactions to chemotherapy. *Journal of Consulting and Clinical Psychology, 50,* 1018–1029.

Ree, M. J., & Earles, J. A. (1992). Intelligence is the best predictor of job performance. *Current Directions in Psychological Science, 1,* 86–89.

Reed, T. E., & Jensen, A. R. (1991). Arm nerve conduction velocity (NCV), brain NCV, reaction time, and intelligence. *Intelligence, 15,* 33–47.

Regestein, Q. R. (1994). Primary hypersomnia. In T. A. Widiger, A. J. Frances, H. A. Pincus, M. B. First, R. Ross, & W. Davis (Eds.), *DSM-IV sourcebook* (pp. 619–626). Washington, DC: American Psychiatric Press.

Regier, D. A., & Burke, J. D. (1987). Psychiatric disorders in the community: The Epidemiologic Catchment Area study. In R. E. Hales & A. J. Frances (Eds.), *American Psychiatric Association Annual Review* (Vol. 6). Washington, DC: American Psychiatric Press.

Regier, D. A., Myers, J. K., Kramer, M., Robins, L. N., Blazer, D. G., Hough, R. L., Eaton, W. W., & Locke, B. Z. (1984). The NIMH epidemiologic catchment area program. *Archives of General Psychiatry, 41,* 934–941.

Rehm, L. P. (1988). Self-management and cognitive processes in depression. In L. B. Alloy (Ed.), *Cognitive processes in depression* (pp. 143–176). New York: Guilford Press.

Reich, J., Noyes, R., Jr., Hirshfeld, R., Coryell, W., & O'Gorman, T. (1987). State and personality in depressed and panic patients. *American Journal of Psychiatry, 144,* 181–187.

Reich, J. H., & Vasile, R. G. (1993). Effect of personality disorders on the treatment outcome of Axis I conditions: An update. *Journal of Nervous and Mental Disease, 181*, 475–484.

Reiman, E. M., Fusselman, M. J., Fox, P. T., & Raichle, M. E. (1989). Neuroanatomical correlates of anticipatory anxiety. *Science, 243*, 1071–1074.

Reiss, D., Plomin, R., & Hetherington, E. M. (1991). Genetics and psychiatry: An unheralded window on the environment. *American Journal of Psychiatry, 148*, 283–291.

Reitan, R. M. (1959). The comparative effects of brain damage on the Halstead impairment index and the Wechsler-Bellevue scale. *Journal of Clinical Psychology, 25*, 281–285.

Reitan, R. M. (1994). Ward Halstead's contribution to neuropsychology and the Halstead-Reitan Neuropsychological Test Battery. *Journal of Clinical Psychology, 50*, 47–70.

Reitan, R. M., & Davison, I. A. (1974). *Clinical neuropsychology: Current status and applications.* Washington, DC: V. H. Winston.

Reitan, R. M., & Wolfson, D. (1992). Conventional intelligence measurements and neuropsychological concepts of adaptive abilities. *Journal of Clinical Psychology, 48*, 521–529.

Rekers, G. A. (1982). *Growing up straight: What every family should know about homosexuality.* Chicago: Moody Press.

Rekers, G. A., & Lovaas, O. I. (1974). Behavioral treatment of deviant sex role behaviors in a male child. *Journal of Applied Behavior Analysis, 7*, 173–190.

Rennie v. Klein, 462 F. Supp. 1131 (D. N.J. 1978).

Repp, A., & Singh, N. (1990). *Perspectives on the use of nonaversive and aversive interventions for persons with developmental disabilities.* Sycamore, IL: Sycamore.

Rescorla, R. A. (1988). Pavlovian conditioning: It's not what you think it is. *American Psychologist, 43*, 151–160.

Rescorla, R. A. (1992). Hierarchical associative relations in Pavlovian conditioning and instrumental training. *Current Directions in Psychological Science, 1*, 66–70.

Resick, P. A., & Schnicke, M. K. (1992). Cognitive processing therapy for sexual assault victims. *Journal of Consulting and Clinical Psychology, 60*, 748–756.

Resick, P. A., & Schnicke, M. K. (1993). *Cognitive processing therapy for rape victims: A treatment manual.* Newbury Park, CA: Sage.

Resnick, H. S., Kilpatrick, D. G., Dansky, B. S., Saunders, B. E., & Best, C. L. (1993). Prevalence of civilian trauma and posttraumatic stress disorder in a representative national sample of women. *Journal of Consulting and Clinical Psychology, 61*, 984–991.

Resnick, S. M. (1992). Positron emission tomography in psychiatric illness. *Current Directions in Psychological Science, 1*, 92–98.

Retzlaff, P. D., Ofman, P., Hyer, L., & Matheson, S. (1994). MCMI-II highpoint codes: Severe personality disorder and clinical syndrome extensions. *Journal of Clinical Psychology, 50*, 228–234.

Rice, L. N., & Greenberg, L. S. (1992). Humanistic approaches to psychotherapy. In D. K. Freedheim (Ed.), *History of psychotherapy: A century of change* (pp. 197–224). Washington, DC: American Psychological Association.

Rickels, K., Case, W. G., Downing, R. W., & Winoker, A. (1983). Long-term diazepam therapy and clinical outcome. *Journal of the American Medical Association, 250*, 767–771.

Rickels, K., Downing, R., Schweizer, E., & Hassman, H. (1993). Antidepressants for the treatment of generalized anxiety disorder. *Archives of General Psychiatry, 50*, 884–895.

Riggs, D. S., & Foa, E. B. (1993). Obsessive compulsive disorder. In D. H. Barlow (Ed.), *Clinical handbook of psychological disorders* (pp. 189–239). New York: Guilford Press.

Rittenhouse v. Superior Court, 1 Cal. Rptr. 20 595 (Cal. Ct. App. 1991).

Ritvo, E. R., Freeman, B. J., & Yuwiler, A., et al. (1986). Fenfluramine treatment of autism: UCLA collaborative study of 81 patients at nine medical centers. *Psychopharmacology Bulletin, 22*, 133–140.

Ritvo, E. R., & Ritvo, R. (1992). The UCLA-University of Utah epidemiologic survey of autism: The etiologic role of rare diseases: Reply. *American Journal of Psychiatry, 149*, 146–147.

Robbins, F. R., & Dunlap, G. (1992). Effects of task difficulty on parent teaching skills and behavior problems of young children with autism. *American Journal of Mental Retardation, 96*, 631–643.

Roberts, J. E., & Monroe, S. M. (1994). A multidimensional model of self-esteem in depression. *Clinical Psychology Review, 14*, 161–181.

Robertson, N. (1988). *A.A.: Inside Alcoholics Anonymous.* New York: Morrow.

Robin, A. L., & Foster, S. L. (1988). *Negotiating adolescence: A behavioral family systems approach to parent/teen conflict.* New York: Guilford Press.

Robins, L. N. (1966). *Deviant children grown up.* Baltimore: Williams and Wilkins.

Robins, L. N. (1978). Sturdy childhood predictors of adult antisocial behavior: Replications from longitudinal studies. *Psychological Medicine, 8*, 611–622.

Robins, L. N., Helzer, J. E., Croughan, H., & Ratcliff, K. S. (1981). National Institute of Mental Health Diagnostic Interview Schedule: Its history, characteristics, and validity. *Archives of General Psychiatry, 38*, 381–389.

Robins, L. N., Helzer, J. E., Croughan, J., & Ratcliff, K. S. (1994). The National Institute of Mental Health Diagnostic Interview Schedule. In J. E. Mezzich, M. R. Jorge, & I. M. Salloum (Eds.), *Psychiatric epidemiology: Assessment concepts and methods* (pp. 227–248). Baltimore: Johns Hopkins University Press.

Robins, L. N., Helzer, J. E., Weissman, M. M., Orvaschel, H., Gruenberg, E., Burke, J. D., & Regier, D. A. (1984). Lifetime prevalence of specific psychiatric disorders in three sites. *Archives of General Psychiatry, 41*, 949–958.

Robins, L. N., Locke, B. Z., & Regier, D. A. (1991). An overview of psychiatric disorders in America. In L. N. Robins & B. Z. Locke (Eds.), *Psychiatric disorders in America* (pp. 326–366). New York: Free Press.

Robins, L. N., & Price, R. (1991). Adult disorders predicted by childhood conduct problems: Results from the NIMH epidemiological catchment area project. *Psychiatry, 54*, 116–132.

Robins, L. N., Tipp, J., & Przybeck, T. (1991). Antisocial personality. In L. N. Robins & D. A. Regier (Eds.), *Psychiatric disorders in America.* New York: Free Press.

Rodin, J. (1993). *Body traps.* New York: Norton.

Rodin, J., & Ickovics, J. R. (1990). Review and research agenda as we approach the 21st century. *American Psychologist, 45*, 1018–1034.

Rodnick, E. H., Goldstein, M. J., Lewis, J. M., & Doane, J. A. (1984). Parental communication style, affect, and role as precursors of offspring schizophrenia. In N. F. Watt, E. J. Anthony, L. C. Wynne, & J. E. Rolf (Eds.), *Children at risk for schizophrenia: A longitudinal perspective* (pp. 81–92). New York: Cambridge University Press.

Rodolfa, E., Hall, T., Holms, V., Davena, A., Komatz, D., Antunez, M., & Hall, A. (1994). The management of sexual feelings in therapy. *Professional Psychology: Research and Practice, 25*, 168–172.

Roehrich, L., & Goldman, M. S. (1993). Experience-dependent neuropsychological recovery and the treatment of alcoholism. *Journal of Consulting and Clinical Psychology, 61*, 812–821.

Rogers v. Okin, 478 F. Supp. 1342 (D. Mass. 1979).

Rogers, C. R. (1942). *Counseling and psychotherapy.* Boston: Houghton Mifflin.

Rogers, C. R. (1961). *On becoming a person.* Boston: Houghton Mifflin.

Rogler, L. H. (1994). Culturally sensitive research in mental health. In J. E. Mezzich, M. R. Jorge, & I. M. Salloum (Eds.), *Psychiatric epidemiology: Assessment concepts and methods* (pp. 565–578). Baltimore: Johns Hopkins University Press.

Roiphe, K. (1993). *The morning after: Sex, fear, and feminism on campus.* Boston: Little, Brown.

Rose, D. T., Abramson, L. Y., Hodulik, C. J., Halberstadt, L., & Leff, G. (1994). Heterogeneity in cognitive style among depressed inpatients. *Journal of Abnormal Psychology, 103*, 419–429.

Rosen, J. C., & Gross, J. (1987). The prevalence of weight reducing and weight gaining in adolescent girls and boys. *Health Psychology, 6*, 131–147.

Rosen, L. A., O'Leary, S., Joyce, S. A., Conway, G., & Pfiffner, L. (1984). The importance of prudent negative consequences for maintaining the appropriate behavior of hyperactive students. *Journal of Abnormal Child Psychology, 12*, 581–604.

Rosen, R. C., & Hall, E. (1984). *Sexuality.* New York: Random House.

Rosen, R. C., & Leiblum, S. R. (1992). Erectile disorders: An overview of historical trends and clinical perspectives. In R. C. Rosen & S. R. Leiblum (Eds.), *Erectile disorders: Assessment and treatment* (pp. 3–26). New York: Guilford Press.

Rosen, R. C., & Leiblum, S. R. (in press). Hypoactive sexual desire. *Psychiatric Clinics of North America.*

Rosen, R. C., Leiblum, S. R., & Spector, I. P. (1994). Psychologically based treatment for male erectile disorder: A cognitive-interpersonal model. *Journal of Sex & Marital Therapy, 20*, 67–85.

Rosenbaum, A., & Hoge, S. K. (1989). Head injury and marital aggression. *American Journal of Psychiatry, 146*, 1048–1051.

Rosenbaum, A., Hoge, S. K., Adelman, S. A., Warnken, W. J., Fletcher, K. E., & Kane, R. (1994). Head injury in partner abusive men. *Journal of Consulting and Clinical Psychology, 62*, 1187–1193.

Rosenbaum, A., & Maiuro, R. (1990). Perpetrators of spouse abuse. In R. T. Ammerman & M. Hersen (Eds.), *Treatment of family violence* (pp. 280–309). New York: John Wiley.

Rosenbaum, M., & Muroff, M. (Eds.). (1984). *Anna O: Fourteen contemporary interpretations.* New York: Free Press.

Rosenheck, R., & Fontana, A. (1994). A model of homelessness among male veterans of the Vietnam war generation. *American Journal of Psychiatry, 151*, 421–427.

Rosenman, R. H., Brand, R. J., Jenkins, C. D., Friedman, M., Straus, R., & Wurm, M. (1975). Coronary heart disease in the Western Collaborative Group Study: Final follow-up experience of 8-1/2 years. *Journal of the American Medical Association, 233*, 872–877.

Rosenthal, D. (1970). Genetic research in the schizophrenic syndrome. In R. Cancro (Ed.), *The schizophrenic reactions* (pp. 245–258). New York: Brunner/Mazel.

Rosenthal, E. (1993, April 7). Who will turn violent? Hospitals have to guess. *New York Times*, pp. A1, B6.

Rosenzweig, S. (1988). The identity and idiodynamics of the multiple personality "Sally Beauchamp." *American Psychologist, 43*, 45–48.

Ross, C. E., Mirowsky, J., & Huber, J. (1983). Dividing work, sharing work, and in-between: Marriage patterns and depression. *American Sociological Review, 48*, 809–823.

Ross, D. M. (1974). *Psychological disorders of children.* New York: McGraw-Hill.

Ross, D. M., & Ross, S. A. (1976). *Hyperactivity: Research-theory-action.* New York: John Wiley.

Rossiter, L. F. (1983). Prescribed medicines: Findings from the National Medical Care Expenditure Survey. *American Journal of Public Health, 73*, 1312–1315.

Rost, K. M., Akins, R. N., Brown, F. W., & Smith, G. R. (1992). The comorbidity of *DSM-III-R* personality disorders in somatization disorder. *General Hospital Psychiatry, 14*, 322–326.

Roth, B. (1980). *Narcolepsy & hypersomnia.* New York: Krager.

Rothbaum, B. O., & Foa, E. B. (1993). Subtypes of posttraumatic stress disorder and duration of symptoms. In J. R. T. Davidson & E. B. Foa (Eds.), *Posttraumatic stress disorder: DSM-IV and beyond* (pp. 23–25). Washington, DC: American Psychiatric Press.

Rounsaville, B. J., Kosten, T. R., Williams, J. B. W., & Spitzer, R. L. (1987). A field trial of *DSM-III-R* psychoactive substance dependence disorders. *American Journal of Psychiatry, 144*, 351–355.

Rowe, J. W., & Kahn, R. L. (1987). Human aging: Usual and successful. *Science, 237*, 143–149.

Ruberman, W., Weinblatt, E., Goldberg, J. D., & Chaudhary, B. S. (1984). Psychosocial influences on mortality after myocardial infarction. *New England Journal of Medicine, 34*, 552–557.

Rucker, C. E., & Cash, T. F. (1992). Body images, body-size perceptions, and eating behaviors among African-American and white college women. *International Journal of Eating Disorders, 12*, 291–300.

Runeson, B. S., & Rich, C. L. (1992). Diagnostic comorbidity of mental disorders among young suicides. *International Review of Psychiatry, 4*, 197–203.

Rush, H. A., Beck, A. T., Kovacs, M., & Hollon, S. (1977). Comparative efficacy of cognitive therapy and pharmacotherapy in treatment of depressed outpatients. *Cognitive Research and Therapy, 1*, 17–37.

Rushton, H. G. (1993, July). Older pharmacologic therapy for nocturnal enuresis. *Clinical Pediatrics*, 10–13.

Rushton, J. P., Fulker, D. W., Neale, M. C., Nias, D. K. B., & Eysenck, H. J. (1986). Altruism and aggression: The heritability of individual differences. *Journal of Personality and Social Psychology, 50*(6), 1192–1198.

Russell, D. E. H. (1982). *Rape in marriage.* New York: Macmillan.

Russell, D. E. H. (1990). *Rape in marriage* (Rev. ed.). Bloomington: Indiana University Press.

Russell, G. F. M. (1979). Bulimia nervosa: An ominous variation of anorexia nervosa. *Psychological Medicine, 9*, 429–448.

Russell, G. F. M., Szmukler, G. I., Dare, C., & Eisler, I. (1987). An evaluation of family therapy in anorexia nervosa and bulimia nervosa. *Archives of General Psychiatry, 44*, 1047–1056.

Rutter, M. (1970). Sex differences in children's response to family stress. In E. J. Anthony & C. Koupernik (Eds.), *The child in his family* (Vol. 1, pp. 169–196). New York: John Wiley.

Rutter, M. (1994). Family discord and conduct disorder: Cause, consequence, or correlate? *Journal of Family Psychology, 8*, 170–186.

Rutter, M., Bailey, A., Bolton, P., & Le Couteur, A. (1993). Autism: Syndrome definition and possible genetic mechanisms. In R. Plomin & G. E. McClearn (Eds.), *Nature, nurture and psychology* (pp. 245–268). Washington, DC: American Psychological Association.

Rutter, M., & Garmezy, N. (1983). Developmental psychology. In P. Mussen (Ed.), *Handbook of child psychology* (Vol. 4). New York: John Wiley.

Ryan, N. D. (1993). Pharmacological treatment of child and adolescent major depression. *Encephale, 19*, 67–70.

S

Sacks, O. (1995, January 9). A neurologist's notebook: Prodigies. *New Yorker*, pp. 44–65.

Salkovskis, P. M. (1989). Somatic problems. In K. Hawton, P. M. Salkovskis, J. Kirk, & D. M. Clark (Eds.), *Cognitive behaviour therapy for psychiatric problems.* New York: Oxford University Press.

Salkovskis, P. M., & Clark, D. M. (1993). Panic disorder and hypochondriasis. *Advances in Behaviour Research and Therapy, 15*, 23–48.

Salzman, B. (1991). *The handbook of psychiatric drugs.* New York: Henry Holt.

Salzman, L. (1985). *Treatment of the obsessive personality.* New York: Jason Aronson.

Sanderson, W. C., DiNardo, P. A., Rapee, R. M., & Barlow, D. H. (1990). Syndrome comorbidity in patients diagnosed with a DSM-III-R Anxiety Disorder. *Journal of Abnormal Psychology, 99*, 308–312.

Sandor, P., & Shapiro, C. M. (1994). Sleep patterns in depression and anxiety: Theory and pharmacological effects. *Journal of Psychosomatic Research, 38*(Suppl.), 125–139.

Sartorius, N., Shapiro, R., & Jablensky, A. (1974). The international pilot study of schizophrenia. *Schizophrenia Bulletin, 11*, 21–35.

Satel, S. L., & Nelson, J. C. (1989). Stimulants in the treatment of depression. *Journal of Clinical Psychiatry, 50*, 241–249.

Satir, V. (1967). *Conjoint family therapy* (Rev. ed.). Palo Alto, CA: Science and Behavior Books.

Satterfield, J. H., Cantwell, D. P., & Satterfield, B. T. (1979). Multimodality treatment. *Archives of General Psychiatry, 36*, 965–974.

Satterfield, J. H., Satterfield, B. T., & Cantwell, D. P. (1980). Multimodality treatment: A two-year evaluation of 61 hyperactive boys. *Archives of General Psychiatry, 37*, 915–918.

Satterfield, J. H., Satterfield, B. T., & Cantwell, D. P. (1981). Three year multi-modality treatment study of 100 hyperactive boys. *Journal of Pediatrics, 98*, 650–655.

Saxe, G. N., Chinman, G., Berkowitz, R., Hall, K., Lieberg, G., Schwartz, J., & van der Kolk, B. A. (1994). Somatization in patients with dissociative disorders. *American Journal of Psychiatry, 151*, 1329–1334.

Saxe, G. N., van der Kolk, B. A., Berkowitz, R., Chinman, G., Hall, K., Lieberg, G., & Schwartz, J. (1993). Dissociative disorders in psychiatric inpatients. *American Journal of Psychiatry, 150*, 1037–1042.

Sayette, M. A., Breslin, F. C., Wilson, G. T., & Rosenblum, G. D. (1994). An evaluation of the balanced placebo design in alcohol administration research. *Addictive Behaviors, 55*, 214–223.

Schacht, T. E. (1985). *DSM-III* and the politics of truth. *American Psychologist, 40*, 513–521.

Schacht, T. E., & Nathan, P. E. (1977). But is it good for the psychologists? Appraisal and status of *DSM-III. American Psychologist, 32*, 1017–1025.

Schacter, D. L., Wang, P. L., Tulving, E., & Freedman, M. (1982). Functional retrograde amnesia: A quantitative case study. *Neuropsychologia, 20*, 523–532.

Schalling, D. (1978). Psychopathy-related personality variables and the psychophysiology of socialization. In R. D. Hare & D. Schalling (Eds.), *Psychopathic behavior: Approaches to research* (pp. 85–106). New York: John Wiley.

Schechter, S. (1988). A framework for understanding and empowering battered women. In M. Straus (Ed.), *Abuse and victimization across the life span* (pp. 240–253). Baltimore: Johns Hopkins University Press.

Schiavi, R. C., Schreiner-Engel, P., White, D., & Mandeli, J. (1988). Pituitary-gonadal function during sleep in men with hypoactive sexual desire and in normal controls. *Psychosomatic Medicine, 50*, 304–318.

Schildkraut, J. J. (1965). The catecholamine hypothesis of affective disorders. *American Journal of Psychiatry, 122*, 509–522.

Schildkraut, J. J., Hirshfeld, A. J., & Murphy, J. M. (1994). Mind and mood in modern art, II: Depressive disorders, spirituality, and early deaths in the Abstract Expressionist artists of the New York School. *American Journal of Psychiatry, 151*, 482–488.

Schildkraut, J. J., & Kety, S. S. (1967). Biogenic amines and emotion. *Science, 156*, 21–30.

Schleifer, S. J., & Keller, S. E. (1989). Immunity and major depressive disorder. In A. E. Miller (Ed.), *Depressive disorders and immunity* (pp. 65–84). Washington, DC: American Psychiatric Press.

Schmauk, F. J. (1970). Punishment, arousal, and avoidance learning in sociopaths. *Journal of Abnormal Psychology, 76*, 325–335.

Schmittling, G. (Ed.). (1993). *Facts about family practice.* Kansas City, MO: American Academy of Family Physicians.

Schneck, M. K., Reisberg, B., & Ferris, S. H. (1982). An overview of current concepts of Alzheimer's disease. *American Journal of Psychiatry, 139*, 165–173.

Schneider, K. (1958). *Psychopathic personalities* (M. W. Hamilton, Trans.). London, England: Cassell. (Original work published 1934)

Schneidman, E. S. (1985). *Definition of suicide.* New York: John Wiley.

Schneidman, E. S., & Farberow, N. L. (1957). *Clues to suicide.* New York: McGraw-Hill.

Schneier, F. R., Johnson, J., Hornig, C. D., Liebowitz, M. R., & Weissman, M. M. (1992). Social phobia. Comorbidity and morbidity in an epidemiologic sample. *Archives of General Psychiatry, 49*, 282–288.

Schopler, E. (1987). Lovaas study questioned. *Autism Research Review, 1*, 6–7.

Schor, J. B. (1991). *The overworked American: The unexpected decline of leisure.* New York: Basic Books.

Schreibman, L. (1994). Autism. In L. W. Craighead, W. E. Craighead, A. E. Kazdin, & M. J. Mahoney (Eds.), *Cognitive and behavioral interventions* (pp. 335–358). Boston: Allyn and Bacon.

Schreiner-Engel, P., & Schiavi, R. C. (1986). Lifetime psychopathology in individuals with low sexual desire. *Journal of Nervous Mental Disease, 174*, 646–651.

Schuckit, M. A. (1994a). A clinical model of genetic influence in alcohol dependence. *Journal of Studies on Alcohol, 55*, 5–17.

Schuckit, M. A. (1994b, June). DSM-IV: *Was it worth all the fuss?* Paper presented at the Seventh Congress of the International Society for Biomedical Research on Alcoholism, Queensland, Australia.

Schuckit, M. A. (1994c). The relationship between alcohol problems, substance abuse, and psychiatric syndromes. In T. A. Widiger, A. J. Frances, H. A. Pincus, M. B. First, R. Ross, & W. Davis (Eds.), *DSM-IV sourcebook* (Vol. 1, pp. 45–66). Washington, DC: American Psychiatric Association.

Schuckit, M. A. (1995). *Drug and alcohol abuse* (5th ed.). New York: Plenum.

Schulberg, H. C., & Rush, A. J. (1994). Clinical practice guidelines for managing major depression in primary care practice: Implications for psychologists. *American Psychologist, 49*, 34–41.

Schuler, C. E., Snibbe, J. R., & Buckwalter, J. G. (1994). Validity of the MMPI personality disorder scales (MMPI-PD). *Journal of Clinical Psychology, 50*, 220–227.

Schwalberg, M. D., Barlow, D. H., Alger, S. A., & Howard, L. J. (1992). Comparison of bulimics, obese binge eaters, social phobics, and individuals with panic disorder on comorbidity across DSM-III-R anxiety disorders. *Journal of Abnormal Psychology, 101*, 675–681.

Schwartz, G. E., & Beatty, J. (1977). *Biofeedback: Theory and research.* New York: Academic Press.

Schwartz, G. E., & Weiss, S. M. (1978). Behavioral medicine revisited: An amended definition. *Journal of Behavioral Medicine, 1*, 249–252.

Schwartz, H. J. (Ed.). (1988). *Bulimia: Psychoanalytic treatment and theory.* Madison, CT: International Universities Press.

Schweizer, E., & Rickels, K. (1991). Pharmacotherapy of generalized anxiety disorder. In R. M. Rapee & D. H. Barlow (Eds.), *Chronic anxiety* (pp. 172–186). New York: Guilford Press.

Searles, J. S. (1985). A methodological and empirical critique of psychotherapy outcome meta-analysis. *Behavior Research and Therapy, 23*, 453–464.

Segal, J. H. (1989). Erotomania revisited: From Kraepelin to DSM-III-R. *American Journal of Psychiatry, 146*, 1261–1266.

Segal, N. L. (1993). Twin, sibling, and adoption methods. *American Psychologist, 48*, 943–956.

Segal, S. P., Watson, M. A., Goldfinger, S. M., & Averbuck, D. S. (1988a). Civil commitment in the psychiatric emergency room. I. The assessment of dangerousness by emergency room clinicians. *Archives of General Psychiatry, 45*, 748–752.

Segal, S. P., Watson, M. A., Goldfinger, S. M., & Averbuck, D. S. (1988b). Civil commitment in the psychiatric emergency room. II. Mental disorder indicators and three dangerousness criteria. *Archives of General Psychiatry, 45*, 753–758.

Segal, S. P., Watson, M. A., Goldfinger, S. M., & Averbuck, D. S. (1988c). Civil commitment in the psychiatric emergency room. III. Disposition as a function of mental disorder and dangerousness indicators. *Archives of General Psychiatry, 45*, 759–763.

Segal, Z. V., Shaw, B., Vella, D., & Katz, R. (1992). Cognitive life stress predictors of relapse in remitted unipolar depressed patients: Test of the congruency hypothesis. *Journal of Abnormal Psychology, 101*, 26–36.

Segal, Z. V., & Vella, D. D. (1990). Self-schema in major depression: Replication and extension of a priming methodology. *Cognitive Therapy & Research, 14*, 161–176.

Segraves, K. B., & Segraves, R. T. (1991). Hypoactive sexual desire disorder: Prevalence and comorbidity in 906 subjects. *Journal of Sex Marital Therapy, 17*, 55–58.

Segrin, C., & Abramson, L. Y. (1994). Negative reactions to depressive behaviors: A communication theory analysis. *Journal of Abnormal Psychology, 103*, 655–668.

Seligman, M. E. P. (1971). Phobias and preparedness. *Behavior Therapy, 2*, 307–320.

Seligman, M. E. P. (1975). *Helplessness: On depression, development, and death.* San Francisco: W. H. Freeman.

Seligman, M. E. P. (1991). *Learned optimism.* New York: Knopf.

Seligman, M. E. P. (1994). *What you can change and what you can't.* New York: Knopf.

Seligman, M. E. P., & Maier, S. (1967). Failure to escape traumatic shock. *Journal of Experimental Psychology, 74*, 1–9.

Selkoe, D. J. (1992). Aging brain, aging mind. *Scientific American, 267*, 135–142.

Selye, H. (1956). *The stress of life.* New York: McGraw-Hill.

Sevush, S., & Leve, N. (1993). Denial of memory deficit in Alzheimer's disease. *American Journal of Psychiatry, 150*, 748–751.

Sewell, D. D., Jeste, D. V., Atkinson, J. H., Heaton, R. K., Hesselink, J. R., Wiley, C., Thal, L., Chandler, J. L., & Grant, I. (1994). HIV-associated psychosis: A study of 20 cases. *American Journal of Psychiatry, 151*, 237–242.

Shadish, W. R. (1984). Policy research: Lessons from the implementation of deinstitutionalization. *American Psychologist, 39*, 725–738.

Shadish, W. R., Montgomery, L. M., Wilson, P., Wilson, M. R., Bright, I., & Okwumabua, T. (1993). The effects of family and marital therapies: A meta-analysis. *Journal of Consulting and Clinical Psychology, 61*, 992–1002.

Shah, M., & Jeffery, R. W. (1991). Is obesity due to overeating and inactivity, or to a defective metabolic rate? A review. *Annals of Behavioral Medicine, 13*, 73–81.

Shah, S., & McGarry, A. (1986). Legal psychiatry and psychology: Review of programs, training and qualifications. In W. Curran, A. McGarry, & S. Shah (Eds.), *Forensic psychiatry and psychology.* Philadelphia: Davis.

Shapiro, B. K., Palmer, F. B., & Capute, A. J. (1987). The early detection of mental retardation. *Clinical Pediatrics, 26*, 215–220.

Shea, M. T. (1993). Psychosocial treatment of personality disorders. *Journal of Personality Disorders, 7*(Suppl.), 167–180.

Shea, M. T., Elkin, I., Imber, S. D., Sotsky, S. M., Watkins, J. T., Collins, J. F., Pilkonis, P. A., Beckham, E., Glass, D. R., Dolan, R. T., & Parloff, M. B. (1992). Course of depressive symptoms over follow-up: Findings from the National Institute of Mental Health Treatment of Depression Collaborative Research Program. *Archives of General Psychiatry, 49,* 782–787.

Shea, M. T., Pilkonis, P. A., Beckham, E., Collins, J. F., Elkin, I., Sotsky, S. M., & Docherty, J. P. (1990). Personality disorders and treatment outcome in the NIMH Treatment of Depression Collaborative Research Program. *American Journal of Psychiatry, 147,* 711–718.

Shearin, E. N., & Linehan, M. M. (1992). Patient-therapist ratings and relationship to progress in dialectical behavior therapy for borderline personality disorder. *Behavior Therapy, 23,* 730–741.

Sheehan, D. V. (1983). *The anxiety disease.* New York: Charles Scribner.

Sheehan, D. V., Ballenger, J., & Jacobson, G. (1980). Treatment of endogenous anxiety with phobic hysterical and hypochondriacal symptoms. *Archives of General Psychiatry, 37,* 51–59.

Sher, K. J. (1985). Excluding problem drinkers in high-risk studies of alcoholism: Effect of screening criteria on high-risk versus low-risk comparisons. *Journal of Abnormal Psychology, 92,* 106–109.

Sher, K. J. (1991). *Children of alcoholics: A critical appraisal of theory and research.* Chicago: University of Chicago Press.

Sher, K. J., & Trull, T. J. (1994). Personality and disinhibitory psychopathology: Alcoholism and antisocial personality disorder. *Journal of Abnormal Psychology, 103,* 92–102.

Sherman, J., Factor, D. C., Swinson, R., & Darjes, R. W. (1989). The effects of fenfluramine (Hydrochloride) on the behaviors of fifteen autistic children. *Journal of Autism and Developmental Disabilities, 19,* 533–543.

Shields, N. M., Resick, P. A., & Hanneke, C. R. (1990). Victims of marital rape. In R. T. Ammerman & M. Hersen (Eds.), *Treatment of family violence* (pp. 165–182). New York: John Wiley.

Shiffman, S., Kassel, J. D., Paty, J., Gnys, M., & Zettler-Segal, M. (1994). Smoking typology profiles of chippers and regular smokers. *Journal of Substance Abuse, 6,* 21–35.

Shiffman, S., Read, L., Maltese, J., Rapkin, D., & Jarvik, M. E. (1985). Preventing relapse in ex-smokers: A self-management approach. In G. A. Marlatt & J. R. Gordon (Eds.), *Relapse prevention* (pp. 472–520). New York: Guilford Press.

Shore, D. (1993). *Special report: Schizophrenia 1993.* Rockville, MD: U.S. Department of Health and Human Services.

Shrout, P. E., Spitzer, R. E., & Fleiss, J. L. (1994). The quantification of agreement in psychiatric diagnosis. In J. E. Mezzich, M. R. Jorge, & I. M. Salloum (Eds.), *Psychiatric epidemiology: Assessment concepts and methods* (pp. 185–200). Baltimore: Johns Hopkins University Press.

Shulruff, L. I. (1990, August 10). In sex case, focus is on multiple personalities. *New York Times,* pp. 00–00.

Sieber, W. J., Rodin, J., Lareson, L., Ortega, S., Cummings, N., Levy S., Whiteside, T., & Herberman, R. (1992). Modulation of human natural killer cell activity by exposure to uncontrollable stress. *Brain, Behavior, and Immunity, 6,* 141–156.

Siegel, B. S. (1986). *Love, medicine, and miracles: Lessons learned about self-healing from a surgeon's experience with exceptional patients.* New York: Harper & Row.

Siegel, S. (1978). A Pavlovian conditioning analysis of morphine tolerance. In N. A. Krasnegor (Ed.), *Behavioral tolerance.* Washington, DC: National Institute on Drug Abuse.

Siever, L. J. (1992). Schizophrenia spectrum personality disorders. In A. Tasman & M. B. Riba (Eds.), *Review of psychiatry* (Vol. 11, pp. 25–42). Washington, DC: American Psychiatric Press.

Siever, L. J., Bernstein, D. P., & Silverman, J. M. (1991). Schizotypal personality disorder: A review of its current status. *Journal of Personality Disorders, 5,* 178–193.

Siever, L. J., & Davis, K. L. (1991). A psychobiological perspective on the personality disorders. *American Journal Psychiatry, 148,* 1647–1658.

Siever, L. J., Keefe, R., Bernstein, D. P., Coccaro, E. F., Klar, H. M., Zemishlany, Z., Peterson, A. E., Davidson, M., Mahon, T., Horvath, T., & Mohs, R. (1990). Eyetracking impairment in clinically identified patients with schizotypal personality disorder. *American Journal Psychiatry, 147,* 740–745.

Sigmund, B. B. (1989, December 30). I didn't give myself cancer. *New York Times,* p. 25.

Sigvardsson, S., Von Knorring, A. L., Bohman, M., & Cloninger, C. R. (1984). An adoption study of somatoform disorders. *Archives of General Psychiatry, 41,* 853–859.

Silva, R. R., Ernst, M., & Campbell, M. (1993). Lithium and conduct disorder. *Encephale, 19,* 585–590.

Simon, G. E., & Von Korff, M. (1991). Somatization and psychiatric disorder in the NIMH epidemiologic catchment area study. *American Journal of Psychiatry, 148,* 1494–1500.

Simon, R. I. (1992). *Clinical psychiatry and the law* (2nd ed.). Washington, DC: American Psychiatric Press.

Simons, A. D., Levine, J. L., Lustman, P. J., & Murphy, G. E. (1984). Patient attrition in a comparative outcome study of depression: A follow-up report. *Journal of Affective Disorders, 6,* 163–173.

Sims, E., Goldman, R., Gluck, C., Horton, E., Kelleher, P., & Rowe, D. (1968). Experimental obesity in man. *Transcript of American Physicians, 81,* 153.

Singer, M. I., Anglin, T. M., Song, L., & Lunghofer, L. (1995). Adolescents' exposure to violence and associated symptoms of psychological trauma. *Journal of the American Medical Association, 273,* 477–482.

Sizemore, C. C. (1986). On my life with multiple personalities. *Art Therapy,* 18–21.

Sizemore, C. C. (1989). *A mind of my own.* New York: William Morrow.

Sizemore, C. C., & Pittillo, E. S. (1977). *I'm Eve.* Garden City, NY: Doubleday.

Skinner, B. F. (1938). *The behavior of organisms.* New York: Appleton-Century-Crofts.

Skinner, H. A., & Jackson, D. N. (1978). A model of psychopathology based on an integration of MMPI actuarial systems. *Journal of Consulting and Clinical Psychology, 46,* 231–238.

Skodol, A., Oldham, J., Gallaher, P. E., & Bezirganian, S. (1994). Validity of self-defeating personality disorder. *American Journal Psychiatry, 151,* 560–567.

Skodol, A. E., Oldham, J. M., Hyler, S. E., Kellman, H. D., Dodge, N., & Davies, M. (1993). Comorbidity of DSM-III-R eating disorders and personality disorders. *International Journal of Eating Disorders, 14,* 403–416.

Skodol, A., Oldham, J., Rosnick, L., Kellman, H. D., & Hyler, S. (1991). Diagnosis of *DSM-III-R* personality disorders: A comparison of two structured interviews. *International Journal of Methods in Psychiatry Research, 1,* 13–26.

Skodol, A. E., & Spitzer, R. L. (1987). *An annotated bibliography of DSM-III.* Washington, DC: American Psychiatric Press.

Slater, E. (1953). *Psychotic and neurotic illness in twins.* London, England: MRC Special Publication 278, H.M.S.O.

Slater, E. T. O. (1965). Diagnosis of "hysteria." *British Medical Journal, 1,* 1395–1399.

Slater, E. T. O., & Glithero, E. (1965). A follow-up of patients diagnosed as suffering from "hysteria." *Journal of Psychosomatic Research, 9,* 9–13.

Sleek, S. (1994). Girls who've been molested can later become molesters. *APA Monitor, 25,* 34–35.

Small, J. G. (1990). Anticonvulsants in affective disorders. *Psychopharmacology Bulletin, 26,* 25–36.

Smith, D. (1982). Trends in counseling and psychotherapy. *American Psychologist, 37,* 802–809.

Smith, D., Carroll, J. L., & Fuller, G. B. (1988). The relationship between the Millon Clinical Multiaxial Inventory and the MMPI in a private outpatient mental health clinic population. *Journal of Clinical Psychology, 44,* 165–174.

Smith, G. R., Monson, R. A., & Ray, D. B. (1986). Psychiatric consultation is somatization disorder. *The New England Journal of Medicine, 314,* 1407–1413.

Smith, I. M., & Bryson, S. E. (1994). Imitation and action in autism: A critical review. *Psychological Bulletin, 116,* 259–273.

Smith, J. (1994). Neuroendocrine and clinical effects of electroconvulsive therapy and their relationship to treatment outcome. *Psychological Medicine, 24,* 547–555.

Smith, J., Frawler, P. J., & Polissar, L. (1991). Six- and twelve-month abstinence rates in inpatient alcoholics treated with aversion therapy compared with matched inpatients from a treatment registry. *Alcoholism: Clinical and Experimental Research, 15,* 862–870.

Smith, M. L., Glass, G., & Miller, T. (1980). *The benefits of psychotherapy.* Baltimore: Johns Hopkins University Press.

Smith, S. S., Arnett, P. A., & Newman, J. P. (1992). Neuropsychological differentiation of psychopathic and nonpsychopathic criminal offenders. *Personality and Individual Differences, 13,* 1233–1243.

Smyrnios, K. X., & Kirby, R. J. (1993). Long-term comparison of brief versus unlimited psychodynamic treatments with children and their parents. *Journal of Consulting and Clinical Psychology, 61,* 1020–1027.

Snell, J. E., Rosenwald, R. J., & Robey, A. (1964). The wife beaters wife: A study of family interaction. *Archives of General Psychiatry, 11,* 107–113.

Snow, M. G., Prochaska, J. O., & Rossi, J. S. (1992). Stages of change for smoking cessation among former problem drinkers: A cross-sectional analysis. *Journal of Substance Abuse, 4,* 107–116.

Snyder, D. K., & Wills, R. M. (1989). Behavioral versus insight-oriented marital therapy: Effects on individual and interspousal functioning. *Journal of Consulting and Clinical Psychology, 57,* 39–46.

Snyder, D. K., Wills, R. M., & Grady-Fletcher, A. (1991). Long-term effectiveness of behavioral versus insight-oriented marital therapy: A four-year follow-up study. *Journal of Consulting and Clinical Psychology, 59,* 138–141.

Snyder, J., Edwards, P., McGraw, K., Kilgore, K., & Holton, A. (1994). Escalation and reinforcement in mother-child conflict: Social processes associated with the development of physical aggression. *Development and Psychopathology, 6,* 305–321.

Sobell, L. C., & Sobell, M. B. (1990). Self-reports across addictive behaviors. *Behavioral Assessment, 12,* 1–14.

Sobell, M. B., & Sobell, L. C. (1973). Alcoholics treated by individualized behavior therapy: One year treatment outcome. *Behaviour Research and Therapy, 11,* 599–618.

Sobell, M. B., & Sobell, L. C. (1976). Second year treatment outcome of alcoholics treated by individualized behavior therapy: Results. *Behaviour Research and Therapy, 14,* 195–215.

Soloff, P. H. (1993). Is there any drug treatment of choice for the borderline patient? *Acta Psychiatric Scandinavica, 89* (379, Suppl.), 50–55.

Soloff, P. H., Cornelius, J. R., & George, A. (1991). The depressed borderline: One disorder or two? *Psychopharmacology Bulletin, 27,* 23–30.

Soloff, P. H., Lis, J. A., Kelly, T., & Cornelius, J. (1994). Risk factors for suicidal behavior in borderline personality disorder. *American Journal of Psychiatry, 151,* 1316–1323.

Solomon, G. F. (1989). Psychoneuroimmunology and human immuno-deficiency virus infection. *Psychiatric Medicine, 81,* 153.

Solomon, G. F., Temoshok, L., O'Leary, A., & Zich, J. (1987). An intensive psychoimmunologic study of long surviving persons with AIDS. *Annals of the New York Academy of Sciences, 496,* 647–655.

Solomon, R. L., Kamin, L. J., & Wynne, L. C. (1953). Traumatic avoidance learning: The outcomes of several extinction procedures. *Journal of Abnormal and Social Psychology, 48,* 291–302.

Solomon, S. D., Gerrity, E. T., & Muff, A. M. (1992). Efficacy of treatments for posttraumatic stress disorder. *Journal of the American Medical Association, 268,* 633–638.

Sontag, S. (1977). *Illness as metaphor.* New York: Random House.

Southwick, S. M., Krystal, J. H., Morgan, C. A., Johnson, D., Nagy, L. M., Nicolaou, A., Heninger, G., & Charney, D. S. (1993). Abnormal noradrenergic function in post-traumatic stress disorder. *Archives of General Psychiatry, 50,* 266–274.

Souza, F. G., & Goodwin, G. M. (1991). Lithium treatment and prophylaxis in unipolar depression: A meta-analysis. *British Journal of Psychiatry, 158,* 666–675.

Souza, F. G., Mander, A. J., & Goodwin, G. M. (1990). The efficacy of lithium in prophylaxis of unipolar depression: Evidence from its discontinuation. *British Journal of Psychiatry, 157,* 718–722.

Spaccarelli, S. (1994). Stress, appraisal, and coping in child sexual abuse: A theoretical and empirical review. *Psychological Bulletin, 116,* 340–362.

Spanos, N., Weekes, J. R., & Bertrand, L. D. (1985). Multiple personality: A social psychological perspective. *Journal of Abnormal Psychology, 94,* 362–376.

Spiegel, D. (1986). Dissociating damage. *American Journal of Clinical Hypnosis, 29,* 123–131.

Spiegel, D., Bloom, J. R., Kraemer, H., & Gottheil, E. (1989). Effect of psychosocial treatment on survival of patients with metastatic breast cancer. *Lancet, 14,* 888–891.

Spitzer, R. L., Devlin, M., Walsh, B. T., Hasin, D., Wing, R., Marcus, M., Stunkard, A., Wadden, T., Yanovski, S., Agras, S., Mitchell, J., & Nonas, C. (1992). Binge eating disorder: A multisite field trial of the diagnostic criteria. *International Journal of Eating Disorders, 11,* 191–203.

Spitzer, R. L., Forman, J. B. W., & Nee, J. (1979). *DSM-III* field trials: I. Initial interrater diagnostic reliability. *American Journal of Psychiatry, 136,* 815–817.

Spitzer, R. L., Skodol, A. E., Gibbon, M., & Williams, J. B. W. (1981). DSM-III *case book.* Washington, DC: American Psychiatric Association.

Spitzer, R. L., Skodol, A. E., Gibbon, M., & Williams, J. B. W. (1983). *Psychopathology: A case book.* New York: McGraw-Hill.

Spitzer, R. L., Yanovski, S., Wadden, T., Wing, R., Marcus, M., Stunkard, A., Devlin, M., Mitchell, J., Hasin, D., & Horne, R. L. (1993). Binge eating disorder: Its further validation in a multisite study. *International Journal of Eating Disorders, 13,* 137–153.

Spivack, G., & Shure, M. B. (1982). The cognition of social adjustment: Interpersonal cognitive problem-solving thinking. In B. B. Lahey & A. E. Kazdin (Eds.), *Advances in clinical child psychology* (Vol. 5). New York: Plenum.

Spreat, S., & Behar, D. (1994). Trends in the residential (inpatient) treatment of individuals with a dual diagnosis. *Journal of Consulting and Clinical Psychology, 62,* 43–48.

Spreen, O., & Strauss, E. (1991). *A compendium of neuropsychological tests.* New York: Oxford University Press.

Sprock, J., & Blashfield, R. K. (1991). Classification and nosology. In M. Hersen, A. E. Kazdin, & A. S. Bellack (Eds.), *The clinical psychology handbook* (2nd ed.) (pp. 329–344). New York: Pergamon Press.

Srole, L., Langner, T. S., Michael, S. T., Opler, M. K., & Rennie, T. A. C. (1962). *Mental health in the metropolis: The midtown Manhattan study.* New York: McGraw-Hill.

Stake, J., & Oliver, J. (1991). Sexual contact and touching between therapists and clients: A survey of psychologists' attitudes and behavior. *Professional Psychology: Research and Practice, 22,* 297–307.

Stallone, D. D., & Stunkard, A. J. (1991). The regulation of body weight: Evidence and clinical implications. *Annals of Behavioral Medicine, 13,* 220–230.

Stanley, B., Sieber, J. E., & Melton, G. B. (1987). Empirical studies of ethical issues in research. *American Psychologist, 42,* 735–741.

Stanton, M. D., & Todd, T. C. (1982). *The family therapy of drug abuse and addiction.* New York: Guilford Press.

Stark, K. D., Rouse, L. W., & Livingston, R. (1991). Treatment of depression during childhood: Cognitive-behavioral procedures for the individual and family. In P. C. Kendall (Ed.), *Child and adolescent therapy: Cognitive and behavioral procedures* (pp. 165–208). New York: Guilford Press.

Steadman, H. J., Monahan, J., Hartstone, E., Davis, S. K., & Robbins, P. C. (1982). Mentally disordered offenders: A national survey of patients and facilities. *Law and Human Behavior, 6,* 31–38.

Steege, J. F., Stout, A. L., & Carson, C. C. (1986). Patient satisfaction in Scott and Small-Carrion penile implant recipients: A study of 52 patients. *Archives of Sexual Behavior, 15,* 393–399.

Steffenberg, S. (1991). Neuropsychiatric assessment of children with autism: A population-based study. *Developmental Medicine and Child Neurology, 33,* 495–511.

Stein, G. (1992). Drug treatment of the personality disorders. *British Journal of Psychiatry, 161,* 167–184.

Stein, M., Keller, S. E., & Schleifer, S. J. (1985). Stress and immunomodulation: The role of depression and neuroendocrine function. *Journal of Immunology, 135,* 827–833.

Stein, M., Miller, A. H., & Trestman, R. L. (1991). Depression, the immune system, and health and illness: Findings in search of meaning. *Archives of General Psychiatry, 48,* 171–177.

Stein, M. M., Tancer, M. E., & Uhde, T. W. (1990). Major depression in patients with panic disorder: Factors associated with course and recurrence. *Journal of Affective Disorders, 19,* 287–296.

Steinhauer, S. R., & Hill, S. Y. (1993). Auditory event-related potentials in children at high risk for alcoholism. *Journal of Studies on Alcohol, 54,* 408–421.

Steketee, G., & Foa, E. (1985). Obsessive-compulsive disorder. In D. H. Barlow (Ed.), *Clinical handbook of psychological disorders: A step-by-step treatment manual.* New York: Guilford Press.

Sternberg, R. J. (1984a). A contextualist view of the nature of intelligence. *International Journal of Psychology, 19,* 307–334.

Sternberg, R. J. (1984b). Toward a triarchic theory of human intelligence. *The Behavioral and Brain Sciences, 7,* 269–315.

Sternberg, R. J. (1985). *Beyond IQ: A triarchic theory of human intelligence.* New York: Cambridge University Press.

Sternberg, R. J., & Berg, C. A. (1986). Quantitative integration: Definitions of intelligence: A comparison of the 1921 and 1986 symposia. In R. J. Sternberg & D. K. Detterman (Eds.), *What is intelligence? Contemporary viewpoints on its nature and definition.* Norwood, NJ: Ablex.

Sternberg, R. J., & Wagner, R. K. (1993). The g-ocentric view of intelligence and job performance is wrong. *Current Directions in Psychological Science, 2,* 1–4.

Steven, J. E. (1995, January 30). Virtual therapy. *Boston Globe,* p. 29.

Stevenson, J., Batten, N., & Cherner, M. (1992). Fears and fearfulness in children and adolescents: A genetic analysis of twin data. *Journal of Child Psychology and Psychiatry and Allied Disciplines, 33,* 977–985.

Stewart, J., deWit, H., & Eikelboom, R. (1984). The role of unconditioned and conditioned drug effects in the self-administration of opiates and stimulants. *Psychological Review, 91,* 251–268.

Stitzer, M. L., Iguchi, M. Y., & Felch, L. J. (1992). Contingent take-home incentive: Effects on drug use of methadone maintenance patients. *Journal of Consulting and Clinical Psychology, 60,* 927–934.

Stoller, R. J. (1967). Transvestites' women. *American Journal of Psychiatry, 124,* 333–339.

Stoller, R. J. (1979). *Sexual excitement.* New York: Pantheon Books.

Stone, M. H. (1990). Multimodal therapy: Applications to partial hospitalization in the light of long-term follow-up of borderline patients. *International Journal of Partial Hospitalization, 6,* 1–14.

Straus, M. A. (1992). Social stress and marital violence in a national sample of American families. In M. A. Straus & R. J. Gelles (Eds.), *Physical violence in American families: Risk factors and adaptations to violence in 8,145 families* (pp. 181–201). New Brunswick, NJ: Transaction.

Straus, M. A. (1994). *Beating the devil out of them: Corporal punishment in American families and its effects on children.* New York: Free Press.

Straus, M. A., & Gelles, R. J. (1992). How violent are American families? Estimates from the national family violence resurvey and other studies. In M. A. Straus & R. J. Gelles (Eds.), *Physical violence in American families: Risk factors and adaptations to violence in 8,145 families* (pp. 95–127). New Brunswick, NJ: Transaction.

Straus, M. A., & Gelles, R. J. (1992). *Physical violence in American families: Risk factors and adaptations to violence in 8,145 families.* New Brunswick, NJ: Transaction.

Straus, M. A., Gelles, R. J., & Steinmetz, S. K. (1980). *Behind closed doors: Violence in the American family.* New York: Anchor Books.

Strauss, J. S., & Carpenter, W. T., Jr. (1981). *Schizophrenia.* New York: Plenum.

Strauss, N., & Foege, A. (1994). The downward spiral: The last days of Nirvana's leader. *Rolling Stone, 683,* 35–43.

Stravynski, A., & Greenberg, D. (1992). The psychological management of depression. *Acta Psychiatrica Scandinavica, 85,* 407–414.

Streissguth, A. P. (1994). A long-term perspective of FAS. *Alcohol Health & Research World, 18,* 74–81.

Stricker, G., & Healey, B. J. (1990). Projective assessment of object relations. *Psychological Assessment, 2,* 219–230.

Strickland, B. R. (1992). Women and depression. *Current Directions in Psychological Science, 1,* 132–135.

Striegel-Moore, R. H. (1993). Etiology of binge eating: A developmental perspective. In C. G. Fairburn & G. T. Wilson (Eds.), *Binge eating: Nature, assessment, and treatment* (pp. 144–172). New York: Guilford Press.

Striegel-Moore, R. H., Silberstein, L. R., & Rodin, J. (1986). Toward an understanding of risk factors for bulimia. *American Psychologist, 41,* 246–263.

Strober, M. (1995). Family-genetic perspectives on anorexia nervosa and bulimia nervosa. In C. G. Fairburn & K. Brownell (Eds.), *Comprehensive textbook of eating disorders and obesity* (pp. 212–218). New York: Guilford Press.

Strober, M., & Katz, J. L. (1987). Do eating disorders and affective disorders share a common etiology? A dissenting opinion. *International Journal of Eating Disorders, 6,* 171–180.

Stromberg, C. (1993, April). Privacy, confidentiality and privilege. *Psychologist's Legal Update, 1,* 3–16.

Stromberg, C., Haggarty, D. J., Leibenluft, R. F., McMillian, M. H., Mishkin, B., Rubin, B. L., & Trilling, H. R. (1988). *The psychologist's legal handbook.* Washington, DC: Council for the National Register of Health Service Providers in Psychology.

Stromberg, C., Schneider, J., & Joondeph, B. (1993, August). Dealing with potentially dangerous patients. *Psychologist's Legal Update, 2,* 3–12.

Strube, M. J. (1988). The decision to leave an abusive relationship: Empirical evidence and theoretical issues. *Psychological Bulletin, 104,* 236–250.

Strunin, L., & Hingson, R. (1993). Alcohol use and risk for HIV infection. *Alcohol Health & Research World, 17,* 35–38.

Strupp, B., Weingartner, H., Goodwin, F. K., & Gold, P. W. (1983). Neurohypophyseal hormones and cognition. *Pharmacology Therapy, 23,* 267–279.

Strupp, H. H. (1980). Toward the refinement of time-limited dynamic therapy. In S. H. Budman (Ed.), *Forms of brief therapy* (pp. 219–242). New York: Guilford Press.

Strupp, H. H., & Hadley, S. W. (1979). Specific vs. nonspecific factors in psychotherapy. *Archives of General Psychiatry, 36,* 1125–1136.

Strupp, H. H., Hadley, S. W., & Gomes-Schwartz, B. (1977). *Psychotherapy for better or worse.* New York: Jason Aronson.

Stuart, R. (1967). Behavioral control of overeating. *Behaviour Research and Therapy, 5,* 357–365.

Stuart, R. B. (1980). *Helping couples change.* New York: Guilford Press.

Stunkard, A. J. (1989). Perspectives on human obesity. In A. J. Stunkard & A. Baum (Eds.), *Perspectives in behavioral medicine* (pp. 9–30). Hillsdale, NJ: Lawrence Erlbaum.

Stunkard, A. J., Foch, T. T., & Hrubec, Z. (1986). A twin study of human obesity. *Journal of the American Medical Association, 256,* 51–54.

Stunkard, A. J., Harris, J. R., Pedersen, N. L., & McClearn, G. E. (1990). The body-mass index of twins who have been reared apart. *New England Journal of Medicine, 322,* 1483–1487.

Sturgis, E. T. (1984). Anxiety disorders. In N. S. Endler & J. M. Hunt (Eds.), *Personality and the behavior disorders.* New York: John Wiley.

Suddath, R. L., Christison, G., Torrey, E. F., Casanova, M. F., & Weinberger, D. R. (1990). Anatomical abnormalities in the brains of monozygotic twins discordant for schizophrenia. *New England Journal of Medicine, 322,* 789–794.

Sue, S., Zane, N., & Young, K. (1994). Research on psychotherapy with culturally diverse populations. In A. E. Bergin & S. L. Garfield (Eds.), *Handbook of psychotherapy and behavior change* (4th ed.). New York: Wiley.

Sugarman, D. R., & Hotaling, G. T. (1989). Dating violence: Prevalence, context, and risk markers. In M. Pirog-Good & J. E. Stets (Eds.), *Violence in dating relationships* (pp. 3–32). New York: Praeger.

Sullivan, H. S. (1924). Schizophrenia: Its conservative and malignant features. *American Journal of Psychiatry, 81,* 77–91.

Sullivan, H. S. (1953). *The interpersonal theory of psychiatry.* New York: W. W. Norton.

Sullivan, H. S. (1954). *The psychiatric interview.* New York: W. W. Norton.

Sulloway, F. J. (1979). *Freud: Biologist of the mind.* New York: Basic Books.

Suls, J., Wan, C. K., & Blanchard, E. B. (1994). A multilevel data-analytic approach for evaluation of relationships between daily life stressors and symptomatology: Patients with irritable bowel syndrome. *Health Psychology, 13,* 103–113.

Sulser, F., Gillespie, D. D., Mishra, R., & Manier, D. H. (1984). Desensitization by antidepressants of central norepinephrine receptor systems coupled to adenylate cyclase. *Annals of the New York Academy of Sciences, 430,* 91–101.

Sultzer, D. L., Levin, H. S., Mahler, M. E., High, W. M., & Cummings, J. L. (1993). A comparison of psychiatric symptoms in vascular dementia and Alzheimer's disease. *American Journal of Psychiatry, 150,* 1806–1812.

Surles, R. C., Blanch, A., Shern, D., & Donahue, S. (1992). Case management as a strategy for systems change. *Health Affairs, 11,* 151–163.

Surwit, R. S., Ross, S. L., & Feingloss, M. N. (1991). Stress, behavior, and glucose control in diabetes mellitus. In P. McCabe, N. Schneidermann, T. M. Field, & J. S. Skyler (Eds.), *Stress, coping and disease* (pp. 97–117). Hillsdale, NJ: Lawrence Erlbaum.

Sutker, P. B., & Allain, A. N., Jr. (1988). Issues in personality conceptualizations of addictive behaviors. *Journal of Consulting and Clinical Psychology, 56,* 172–182.

Svrakic, D. M., Whitehead, C., Przybeck, T. R., & Cloninger, C. R. (in press). Differential diagnosis of personality disorders by the seven factor model of temperament and character. *Archives of General Psychiatry.*

Sweeney, J. A., Clarkin, J. F., & Fitzgibbon, M. L. (1987). Current practice of psychological assessment. *Professional Psychology: Research and Practice, 18,* 377–380.

Sweeney, P., Anderson, K., & Bailey, S. (1986). Attributional style in depression: A meta-analytic review. *Journal of Personality and Social Psychology, 50,* 974–991.

Szapocznik, J., Kurtines, W., Hervis, O., Rio, A. T., Faraci, A. M., & Mitrani, V. B. (1991). Assessing change in family functioning as a result of treatment: The structural family systems rating scale (SFSR). *Journal of Marriage and the Family, 17,* 295–310.

Szasz, T. S. (1960). The myth of mental illness. *American Psychologist, 15,* 113–118.

T

Takahashi, T. (1989). Social phobia syndrome in Japan. *Comprehensive Psychiatry, 30,* 45–52.

Tan, E. S. (1980). Transcultural aspects of anxiety. In G. Burrows & B. Davies (Eds.), *Handbook of studies on anxiety.* Amsterdam, The Netherlands: Elsevier.

Tangri, S. S., & Kahn, J. R. (1993). Ethical issues in the new reproductive technologies: Perspectives from feminism and the psychology profession. *Professional Psychology: Research and Practice, 24,* 271–280.

Tarasoff v. Regents of University of California, Calif. 551 P. 2d 334, 340 (1976).

Taylor, C. B. , & Arnow, B. (1988). *The nature and treatment of anxiety disorders.* New York: Free Press.

Taylor, C. B., Fortmann, S. P., Flora, J., Kayman, S., Barrett, D. C., Jatulis, D., & Farquhar, J. W. (1990). Effect of long-term community health education on body mass index. *American Journal of Epidemiology, 134,* 235–249.

Taylor, J. R., Helzer, J. E., & Robins, L. N. (1986). Moderate drinking in ex-alcoholics: Recent studies. *Journal of Studies on Alcohol, 47,* 115–121.

Teicher, M. H., Glod, C., & Cole J. O. (1990). Emergence of intense suicidal preoccupation during fluoxetine treatment. *American Journal of Psychiatry, 147,* 207–210.

Telch, M. J., Agras, W. S., Taylor, C. B., Roth, W. T., & Gallen, C. C. (1985). Combined pharmacological and behavioral treatment for agoraphobia. *Behaviour Research and Therapy, 23,* 325–336.

Telch, M. J., Brouillard, M., Telch, C. F., Agras, W. S., & Taylor, C. B. (1989). Role of cognitive appraisal in panic-related avoidance. *Behaviour Research and Therapy, 27,* 373–383.

Telch, M. J., & Lucas, R. A. (1994). Combined pharmacological and psychological treatment of panic disorder: Current status and future directions. In B. E. Wolfe & J. D. Maser (Eds.), *Treatment of panic disorder.* Washington, DC: American Psychiatric Press.

Tellegen, A. (1985). Structures of mood and personality and their relevance to assessing anxiety, with an emphasis on self-report. In A. H. Tuma & J. D. Maser (Eds.), *Anxiety and the anxiety disorders* (pp. 681–706). Hillsdale, NJ: Lawrence Erlbaum.

Tellegen, A., Lykken, D. T., Bouchard, T. J., Wilcox, K. J., Rich, S., & Segal, N. L. (1988). Personality similarity in twins reared apart and together. *Journal of Personality and Social Psychology, 54*(6), 1031–1039.

Teri, L. (1992, November). Clinical problems in older adults. *Clinician's Research Digest* (Suppl. 9).

Teri, L., & Wagner, A. (1992). Alzheimer's disease and depression. *Journal of Consulting and Clinical Psychology, 60,* 379–391.

Terman, L. M., & Merrill, M. A. (1960). *Stanford-Binet Intelligence Scale: Manual for the 2nd revision, Form-M.* Boston: Houghton Mifflin.

Terman, L. M., & Merrill, M. A. (1973). *Stanford-Binet Intelligence Scale: 1972 norms edition.* Boston: Houghton Mifflin.

Terman, M., Terman, J. S., Quitkin, F. M., & McGrath, P. J. (1989). Light therapy for seasonal affective disorder: A review of efficacy. *Neuropsychopharmacology, 2,* 1–22.

Terr, L. (1994). *Unchanged memories.* New York: Basic Books.

Terry, R. J., & Katzman, R. (1992). Alzheimer disease and cognitive loss. In R. Katzman & J. Rowe (Eds.), *Principles of geriatric neurology.* Philadelphia: F. A. Davis.

Test, M. A. (1992). Training in community living. In R. P. Liberman (Ed.), *Handbook of psychiatric rehabilitation* (pp. 153–170). New York: Macmillan.

Thase, M. E., Frank, E., & Kupfer, D. J. (1985). Biological processes in depression. In E. E. Beckman & W. R. Leber (Eds.), *Handbook of depression* (pp. 816–913). Homewood, IL: Dorsey Press.

Thase, R. G., & Moss, M. K. (1976). The relative efficacy of covert modeling on the reduction of avoidance behavior. *Journal of Behavior Therapy and Experimental Psychiatry, 7,* 7–12.

Thigpen, C. H., & Cleckley, H. M. (1954). *The three faces of Eve.* Kingsport, TN: Kingsport Press.

Thoits, P. A. (1986). Multiple identities: Examining gender and marital status differences in distress. *American Sociological Review, 51,* 259–272.

Thornberry, T. (1992). *Youth violence.* Report for National Workgroup on Violence. Bethesda, MD: National Institute of Mental Health.

Thorndike, R. L., Hagen, E. P., & Sattler, J. M. (1986). *The Stanford-Binet Intelligence Scale: Fourth Edition, Technical manual.* Chicago: Riverside.

Tofler, G. H., Muller, J. E., Stone, P. H., Davies, O., Davis, V. G., & Braunwald, E. (1993). Comparison of long-term outcome after acute myocardial infarction in patients who never graduated from high school and that in more educated patients. *American Journal of Cardiology, 71,* 1031–1035.

Tollefson, G. D., Fawcett, J., Winokur, G., & Beasley, C. M. (1993). Evaluation of suicidality during pharmacologic treatment of mood and nonmood disorders. *Annals of Clinical Psychiatry, 5,* 209–224.

Tollefson, G. D., Rampey, A. H., Potvin, J. H., Jenike, M. A., Rush, A. J., Kominquez, R. A., Koran, L. M., Shear, M. K., Goodman, W., & Genduso, L. A. (1994). A multicenter investigation of fixed-dose fluoxetine in the treatment of obsessive-compulsive disorder. *Archives of General Psychiatry, 51,* 559–567.

Toner, B. B., Garfinkel, P. E., & Garner, D. M. (1988). Affective and anxiety disorders in the long-term follow-up of anorexia nervosa. *International Journal of Psychiatry in Medicine, 18,* 357–364.

Torgersen, S. (1983). Genetic factors in anxiety disorders. *Archives of General Psychiatry, 40,* 1085–1089.

Torgersen, S. (1986). Genetic factors in moderately severe and mild affective disorders. *Archives of General Psychiatry, 43,* 222–226.

Torgersen, S., & Alnaes, R. (1992). Differential perception of parental bonding in schizotypal and borderline personality disorder patients. *Comprehensive Psychiatry, 33,* 34–38.

Torrey, E. F. (1987). Prevalence studies in schizophrenia. *British Journal of Psychiatry, 150,* 598–608.

Torrey, E. F. (1988). *Nowhere to go.* New York: Harper-Collins.

Torrey, E. F., & Bowler, A. (1990). Geographical distribution of insanity in America. *Schizophrenia Bulletin, 16,* 591–615.

Totten, G., Lamb, D. H., & Reeder, G. D. (1990). *Tarasoff* and confidentiality in AIDS-related psychotherapy. *Professional Psychology: Research and Practice, 21,* 155–160.

Touchette, N. (1992). Cowering inferno: Clearing the smoke on violence research. *The Journal of NIH Research, 4,* 31–33.

Tremblay, R. E., Pihl, R. O., Vitaro, F., & Dobkin, P. L. (1994). Predicting early onset of male antisocial behavior from preschool behavior. *Archives of General Psychiatry, 51,* 732–739.

Trice, H. M. (1992). Work-related risk factors associated with alcohol abuse. *Alcohol Health & Research World, 16,* 106–111.

True, W. R., Rice, J., Eisen, S. A., Heath, A. C., Goldberg, J., Lyons, M. J., & Nowak, J. (1993). A twin study of genetic and environmental contributions to liability for posttraumatic stress symptoms. *Archives of General Psychiatry, 50,* 257–264.

Trull, T. J. (1993). Temporal stability and validity of two personality disorder inventories. *Psychological Assessment, 5,* 11–18.

Tsuang, M. T., & Faroane, S. V. (1990). *The genetics of mood disorders.* Baltimore, MD: Johns Hopkins University Press.

Tsuang, M. T., Faraone, S. V., & Day, M. (1988). Schizophrenic disorders. In E. M. Nicholi (Ed.), *The New Harvard Guide to Psychiatry* (pp. 259–295). Cambridge, MA: Belknap.

Tuma, J. M. (1989). Traditional therapies with children. In T. H. Ollendick & M. Hersen (Eds.), *Handbook of child psychopathology* (pp. 419–437). New York: Plenum.

Turkheimer, E., & Parry, C. D. H. (1992). Why the gap? Practice and policy in civil commitment hearings. *American Psychologist, 47,* 646–655.

Turner, R. J., & Wagonfeld, M. O. (1967). Occupational mobility and schizophrenia. *American Sociological Review, 32,* 104–113.

Turner, S. M., Beidel, D. C., Cooley, M. R., & Woody, S. R. (1994). A multicomponent behavioral treatment for social phobia: Social effectiveness therapy. *Behavior Research & Therapy, 32,* 381–390.

Tutty, L. M., Bidgood, B. A., & Rothery, M. A. (1993). Support groups for battered women: Research on their efficacy. *Journal of Family Violence, 8,* 325–343.

U

U.S. Bureau of the Census. (1990). United States population estimates by age, sex, race, and Hispanic origin, 1980–1988. *Current population reports* (Series P-25, No. 1045). Washington, DC: Government Printing Office.

U.S. Department of Commerce. (1987). *Changes in the American family life (Current Population Reports Special Studies,* Series P-23, No. 163, August). Washington, DC: Government Printing Office.

U.S. Department of Health and Human Services. (1981). *Toward a national plan for the chronically mentally ill: Report to the Secretary by the Department of Health and Human Services Steering Committee on the Chronically Mentally Ill.* Washington, DC: U.S. Government Printing Office.

U.S. Department of Health and Human Services. (1993). *Depression in primary care: Vol. 1. Detection and diagnosis.* Washington, DC: Government Printing Office.

U.S. Department of Health, Education, and Welfare. (1964). *Report on smoking and health.* Washington, DC: U.S. Government Printing Office.

U.S. Department of Justice. (1993). *1991 drug use forecasting annual report.* Washington, DC: U.S. Department of Justice.

Uhlenhuth, E. H., Lipman, R. S., Balter, M. B., & Stern, M. (1974). Symptom intensity and life stress in the city. *Archives of General Psychiatry, 51,* 759–764.

Ullmann, L. P., & Krasner, L. (Eds.). (1965). *Case studies in behavior modification.* New York: Holt, Rinehart & Winston.

Ullmann, L. P., & Krasner, L. (1969). *A psychological approach to abnormal behavior.* Englewood Cliffs, NJ: Prentice-Hall.

Umberson, D. (1987). Family status and health behaviors: Social control as a dimension of social integration. *Journal of Health and Social Behavior, 28,* 306.

Unsettling report on an epidemic of rape. (1992, May 4). *Time,* p. 15.

Ursano, R. J., McCaughey, B. G., & Fullerton, C. S. (1994). *Individual and community responses to trauma and disaster: The structure of human chaos.* New York: Cambridge University Press.

V

Vaillant, G. E. (1977). *Adaptation to life.* Boston: Little, Brown.

Vaillant, G. E. (1979). Natural history of male psychological health. *New England Journal of Medicine, 301,* 1249–1254.

Vaillant, G. E. (1988). The alcohol-dependent and drug-dependent person. In A. M. Nicholi (Ed.), *The new Harvard guide to psychiatry.* Cambridge, MA: Harvard University Press.

Vaillant, G. E. (1992). *Ego mechanisms of defense.* Washington, DC: American Psychiatric Press.

Vaillant, G. E. (1994). Ego mechanisms of defense and personality psychopathology. *Journal of Abnormal Psychology, 103,* 44–50.

Vaillant, G. E., Bond, M., & Vaillant, C. O. (1986). An empirically validated hierarchy of defense mechanisms. *Archives of General Psychiatry, 43,* 786–794.

Vaillant, G. E., & Schnurr, P. (1988). What is a case? A 45-year study of psychiatric impairment within a college sample selected for mental health. *Archives of General Psychiatry, 45,* 313–319.

Van Biema, D. (1994, November 14). Parents who kill. *Time,* pp. 50–51.

Van der Kolk, B. A., Perry, J. C., & Herman, J. L. (1991). Childhood origins of self-destructive behavior. *American Journal of Psychiatry, 148,* 1665–1671.

Vaughn, C. E., & Leff, J. P. (1976). The influence of family and social factors in the course of psychiatric illness. *British Journal of Psychiatry, 129,* 125–137.

Vaughn, C. E., Snyder, K. S., Jones, S., Freeman, W. B., & Falloon, I. R. H. (1984). Family factors in schizophrenic relapse. *Archives of General Psychiatry, 41,* 1169–1177.

Vega, W. A. (1990). Hispanic families in the 1980s: A decade of research. *Journal of Marriage and the Family, 52,* 1015–1024.

Venn, J. R., & Short, J. G. (1973). Vicarious classical conditioning of emotional responses in nursery school children. *Journal of Personality and Social Psychology, 28,* 249–255.

Venter, A., Lord, C., & Schopler, E. (1992). A follow-up study of high-functioning autistic children. *Journal of Child Psychology and Psychiatry, 33,* 489–507.

Verbrugge, L. (1989). The twain meet: Empirical explanations of sex differences in health and mortality. *Journal of Health and Social Behavior, 30,* 282–304.

Verhulst, F. C., & van der Ende, J. (1992). Six-year stability of parent-reported problem behavior in an epidemiological sample. *Journal of Abnormal Child Psychology, 20,* 595–610.

Vernon, D. J., & Bailey, W. C. (1974). The use of motion pictures in the psychological preparation of children for induction of anesthesia. *Anesthesiology, 40,* 68–72.

Vetter, H., Ramsey, L. E., Luscher, T. F., Schrey, A., & Vetter, W. (1985). Symposium on compliance—improving strategies in hypertension. *Journal of Hypertension, 3*(Suppl.), 1–99.

Vivian, D., Fischel, J. E., & Liebert, R. M. (1987). Effect of "wet nights" on daytime behavior during concurrent treatment of enuresis and conduct problems. *Journal of Behavior Therapy and Experimental Psychiatry, 17,* 301–303.

Vivian, D., & Langhinrichsen-Rohling, J. (1994). Are bi-directionally violent couples mutually victimized? A gender sensitive comparison. *Violence and Victims, 8,* 107–124.

Vivian, D., & O'Leary, K. D. (1987, July). *Communication patterns in physically aggressive couples.* Paper presented at the Third National Family Violence Research Conference, University of New Hampshire, Durham, NH.

Voegtlin, W. L. (1940). The treatment of alcoholism by establishing a conditional reflex. *American Journal of Medical Science, 199,* 802–809.

W

Wadden, T. A., Sternberg, J. A., Letizia, K. A., Stunkard, A. J., & Foster, G. D. (1989). Treatment of obesity by very low calorie diet, behavior therapy, and their combination: A five-year perspective. *International Journal of Obesity, 13,* 39–46.

Wadden, T. A., & VanItallie, T. B. (Eds.). (1992). *Treatment of the seriously obese patient.* New York: Guilford Press.

Wade, P., & Bernstein, B. (1991). Culture sensitivity training and counsellors' race: Effects on Black female clients' perceptions and attrition. *Journal of Counseling Psychology, 38,* 9–15.

Wakefield, J. C. (1992). The concept of mental disorder: On the boundary between biological facts and social values. *American Psychologist, 47,* 373–388.

Wald, M. L. (1995, February 12). Lead paint: New rules, old questions. *New York Times,* sect. 9, p. 1.

Walker, L. (1993). The battered woman syndrome is a psychological consequence of abuse. In R. J. Gelles & D. R. Loseke (Eds.), *Current controversies on family violence* (pp. 133–153). Newbury Park, CA: Sage.

Walker, L. E., Norton, J. R., Fox, R. E., Geffner, R. A., Hammond, R., Sanchez, J., Stahly, G., Dutton, M. A., Courtois, C., & Hatcher, J. C. (in press). *APA presidential task force on violence and the family.* Washington, DC: American Psychological Association.

Walker, P. W., Cole, J. O., Gardner, E. A., Hughes, A. R., Johnston, J. A., & Batey, S. R. (1993). Improvement in fluoxetine-associated sexual dysfunction in patients switched to bupropion. *Journal of Clinical Psychiatry, 54,* 459–465.

Waller, N. G., & Waldman, I. D. (1990). A reexamination of the WAIS-R factor structure. *Psychological Assessment, 2,* 139–144.

Wallerstein, J. S., & Kelly, J. B. (1980). *Surviving the breakup: How children and parents cope with divorce.* New York: Basic Books.

Wallis, C. (1994, July). Life in overdrive. *Time,* pp. 43–50.

Walsh, B. T. (1993). Binge eating in bulimia nervosa. In C. G. Fairburn & G. T. Wilson (Eds.), *Binge eating: Nature, assessment, and treatment* (pp. 37–49). New York: Guilford Press.

Walsh, D. C., Hingson, R. W., Merrigan, D. M., Levenson, S. M., Cupples, L. A., Heeren, T., Coffman, G., Becker, C. A., Barker, T. A., Hamilton, S. K., McGuire, T. G., & Kelly, C. A. (1991). A randomized trial of treatment options for alcohol-abusing workers. *New England Journal of Medicine, 325,* 775–782.

Walters, E. E., Neale, M. C., Eaves, L. J., Health, A. C., Kessler, R. C., & Kendler, K. S. (1992). Bulimia nervosa and major depression: A study of common genetic and environmental factors. *Psychological Medicine, 22*, 617–622.

Warner, R. (1978). The diagnosis of antisocial and hysterical personality disorders: An example of sex bias. *Journal of Nervous and Mental Disease, 166*, 839–845.

Wartenburg, A. A., Nirenberg, T. D., Liepman, M. R., Silvia, L. Y., Begin, A. M., & Monti, P. M. (1990). Detoxification of alcoholics: Improving care by symptom-triggered sedation. *Alcoholism: Clinical and Experimental Research, 14*, 71–75.

Watson, C. G., & Buranen, C. (1979). The frequency and identification of false positive conversion reactions. *Journal of Nervous and Mental Disease, 167*, 243–247.

Watson, D., & Clark, L. A. (1984). Negative affectivity: The disposition to experience unpleasant emotional states. *Psychological Bulletin, 95*, 465–490.

Watson, D., & Clark, L. A. (1994). Personality and psychopathology [Special issue]. *Journal of Abnormal Psychology, 103* (1).

Watson, D., Clark, L. A., & Carey, G. (1988). Positive and negative affectivity and their relation to anxiety and depressive disorders. *Journal of Abnormal Psychology, 97*, 346–353.

Watson, D., Clark, L. A., & Harkness, A. R. (1994). Structures of personality and their relevance to psychopathology. *Journal of Abnormal Psychology, 103*, 18–31.

Watson, J. B. (1913). Psychology as the behaviorist views it. *Psychological Review, 20*, 158–177.

Watson, J. B., & Rayner, R. (1920). Conditioned emotional reactions. *Journal of Experimental Psychology, 3*, 1–14.

Wearing, B. (1989). Leisure, unpaid labour, lifestyles and the mental and general health of suburban mothers in Sydney, Australia. *Australian Journal of Sex, Marriage & Family, 10*, 118–132.

Webster-Stratton, C. (1985). Predictors of treatment outcome in parent training for conduct problem children. *Behavior Therapy, 20*, 103–115.

Wechsler, D. (1939). *The measurement of adult intelligence.* Baltimore, MD: Williams and Wilkins.

Wechsler, D. (1955). *Manual for the Wechsler Adult Intelligence Scale.* New York: Psychological Corporation.

Wechsler, D. (1958). *The measurement and appraisal of adult intelligence* (4th ed.). Baltimore, MD: Williams and Wilkins.

Wechsler, D. (1967). *Manual: Wechsler Preschool and Primary Scale of Intelligence.* New York: Psychological Corporation.

Wechsler, D. (1974). *Manual: Wechsler Adult Intelligence Scale-Revised.* New York: Psychological Corporation.

Wechsler, D. (1991). *Manual: Wechsler Intelligence Scale for Children-III.* San Antonio, TX: Psychological Corporation.

Wegner, J. T., Catalano, F., Gilbralter, J., & Kane, J. M. (1985). Schizophrenia with tardive dyskinesia. *Archives of General Psychiatry, 42*, 860–865.

Weinberger, D. R. (1994). Biological basis of schizophrenia: Structural/functional considerations relevant to potential for antipsychotic drug response. *Journal of Clinical Psychiatry: Monograph Series, 12*, 4–7.

Weinberger, L. E., & Sreenivasan, S. (1994). Ethical and professional conflicts in correctional psychology. *Professional Psychology: Research and Practice, 25*, 161–167.

Weiner, H. (1977). *Psychobiology and human disease.* New York: Elsevier.

Weiner, I. B. (1983). The future of psychodiagnosis revisited. *Journal of Personality Assessment, 47*, 451–459.

Weiner, I. B. (1993). Clinical considerations in the conjoint use of the Rorschach and the MMPI. *Journal of Personality Assessment, 60*, 148–152.

Weinstein, E. A. (1981). *Woodrow Wilson: A medical and psychological biography.* Princeton, NJ: Princeton University Press.

Weintraub, S., & Neale, J. M. (1984). Social behavior of children at risk for schizophrenia. In N. F. Watt, J. Anthony, L. C. Wynne, & J. E. Rolf (Eds.), *Children at risk for schizophrenia* (pp. 279–285). New York: Cambridge University Press.

Weiss, G., & Hechtman, L. T. (1986). *Hyperactive children grown up.* New York: Guilford Press.

Weiss, G., Hechtman, L., Perlman, T., Hopkins, J., & Wener, A. (1979). Hyperactives as young adults. *Archives of General Psychiatry, 36*, 675–681.

Weiss, G., Minde, K., Werry, J. S., Douglas, V. I., & Nemeth, E. (1971). Studies on the hyperactive child, VIII: Five-year follow-up. *Archives of General Psychiatry, 24*, 409–414.

Weiss, J. M. (1995, April). *Stress-induced depression: What we have found and where we are going.* Paper presented at the Wisconsin Symposium on Emotion, Inaugural Meeting, Madison, WI.

Weiss, R. L., Hops, H., & Patterson, G. R. (1973). A framework for conceptualizing marital conflict, a technology for altering it, some data for evaluating it. In L. A. Hamerlynck, L. C. Handy, & E. J. Mash (Eds.), *Behavior change: Methodology, concepts, and practice* (pp. 309–342). Champaign, IL: Research Press.

Weissman, M. (1993). The epidemiology of personality disorders: A 1990 update. *Journal of Personality Disorders, 7*(Suppl.), 44–62.

Weissman, M. M. (1987). Advances in psychiatric epidemiology: Rates and risks for major depression. *American Journal of Public Health, 77*, 445–451.

Weissman, M. M., Bruce, M. L., Leaf, P. J., Florio, L. P., & Holzer, C. (1991). Affective disorders. In L. N. Robins & D. A. Regier (Eds.), *Psychiatric disorders in America: The Epidemiological Catchment Area study* (pp. 53–80). New York: Free Press.

Weissman, M. M., Gammon, G. D., John, K., Merikangas, K. R., Warner, V., Prusoff, B. A., & Sholomskas, D. (1987). Children of depressed parents. *Archives of General Psychiatry, 44*, 847–853.

Weissman, M. M., & Klerman, G. L. (1977). Sex differences and the epidemiology of depression. *Archives of General Psychiatry, 34*, 98–111.

Weissman, M. M., Klerman, G. L., Markowitz, J. S., & Pihl, R. O. (1989). Suicidal ideation and suicide attempts in panic disorder and attacks. *New England Journal of Medicine, 321*, 1209–1214.

Weissman, M. M., Leaf, P. J., Blazer, D. G., Boyd, J. H., & Florio, L. (1986). The relationship between panic disorder and agoraphobia: An epidemiologic perspective. *Psychopharmacology Bulletin, 43*, 787–791.

Weissman, M. M., & Markowitz, J. C. (1994). Interpersonal psychotherapy: Current status. *Archives of General Psychiatry, 51*, 599–606.

Weissman, M. M., Myers, J. K., & Harding, P. S. (1978). Psychiatric disorders in a U.S. urban community: 1975–1976. *American Journal of Psychiatry, 135*, 459–462.

Weissman, M. M., Wickramaratne, P., Adams, P. B., Lish, J. D., Horwath, E., Charney, D., Woods, S. W., Leeman, E., & Frosch, E. (1993). The relationship between panic disorder and major depression. *Archives of General Psychiatry, 50*, 767–780.

Weisz, J. R., Weiss, B., Alicke, M. D., & Klotz, M. L. (1987). Effectiveness of psychotherapy with children and adolescents: A meta-analysis for clinicians. *Journal of Consulting and Clinical Psychology, 55*, 542–549.

Weizman, R., Laor, N., Barber, Y., Selman, A., Schujovizky, A., Wolmer, L., Laron, Z., & Gil-Ad, I. (1994). Impact of the Gulf War on the anxiety, cortisol, and growth hormone levels of Israeli citizens. *American Journal of Psychiatry, 151*, 71–75.

Weller, R. A., & Halikas, J. A. (1985). Marijuana use and psychiatric illness: A follow-up study. *American Journal of Psychiatry, 142*, 848–850.

Wells, K. B., Burnam, M. A., Rogers, W., & Hays, R. (1992). The course of depression in adult outpatients: Results from the Medical Outcomes Study. *Archives of General Psychiatry, 49*, 788–794.

Wells, R. A., & Dezen, A. G. (1978). The results of family therapy revisited: The non-behavioral methods. *Family Process, 17*, 251–274.

Wender, P. H. (1971). *Minimal brain dysfunction in children.* New York: John Wiley-Interscience.

Wender, P. H. (1987). *The hyperactive child, adolescent, and adult: Attention deficit disorder through the lifespan.* New York: Oxford University Press.

Wender, P. H., Kety, S. S., Rosenthal, D., Schulsinger, F., Ortmann, J., & Lunde, I. (1986). Psychiatric disorders in the biological and adoptive families of adopted individuals with affective disorders. *Archives of General Psychiatry, 43*, 923–929.

Wender, P. H., Reimherr, F. W., & Wood, D. R. (1980). Attention deficit disorder treatment. *Archives of General Psychiatry, 38*, 449–456.

Werner, E. E. (1980). Environmental interaction in brain dysfunction. In H. E. Rie & E. D. Rie (Eds.), *Handbook of minimal brain dysfunctions: A critical view* (pp. 210–231). New York: John Wiley.

Werner, P. D., & Pervin, L. A. (1986). The content of personality inventory items. *Journal of Personality and Social Psychology, 51*, 622–628.

West, D. J. (1982). *Delinquency: Its roots, careers and prospects.* Cambridge, MA: Harvard University Press.

West, M., Keller, A., Links, P. S., & Patrick, J. (1993). Borderline disorder and attachment pathology. *Canadian Journal of Psychiatry, 38* (Suppl. 1), 16–22.

Weston, D. (1991). Social cognition and object relations. *Psychological Bulletin, 3,* 429–455.

Weston, D., Lohr, N., Silk, K. R., Gold, L., & Kerber, K. (1990). Object relations and social cognition in borderlines, major depressives, and normals: A Thematic Apperception Test analysis. *Psychological Assessment, 2,* 355–364.

Whalen, C. K., & Henker, B. (Eds.). (1980). *Hyperactive children: The social ecology of identification and treatment.* New York: Academic Press.

Whatley, M. A. (1993). For better or for worse: The case of marital rape. *Violence and Victims, 8,* 29–39.

Which is the real John Hinckley? (1982, May 17). *U.S. News and World Report,* p. 15.

Whisman, M. A. (1993). Mediators and moderators of change in cognitive therapy of depression. *Psychological Bulletin, 114,* 248–265.

White, J. L., Moffitt, T. E., Caspi, A., Bartusch, D. J., Needles, D. J., & Stouthamer-Loeger, M. (1994). Measuring impulsivity and examining its relationship to delinquency. *Journal of Abnormal Psychology, 103,* 192–205.

Whitehall, J. A. (1989). A piece of mind: Wife. *Journal of the American Medical Association, 261,* 3460.

Whitman, T. L. (1994). Mental retardation. In L. W. Craighead, W. E. Craighead, A. E. Kazdin, & M. J. Mahoney (Eds.), *Cognitive and behavioral interventions* (pp. 313–334). Boston: Allyn and Bacon.

Widiger, T. A. (1992). Categorical versus dimensional classification: Implications from and for research. *Journal of Personality Disorders, 6,* 287–300.

Widiger, T. A. (1993). The *DSM-III-R* categorical personality disorder diagnoses: A critique and an alternative. *Psychological Inquiry, 4,* 75–90.

Widiger, T. A., Frances, A. J., Pincus, H. A., First, M. B., Ross, R., & Davis, W. (Eds.). (1994). DSM-IV *sourcebook* (Vol. 1). Washington, DC: American Psychiatric Association.

Widiger, T. A., & Rogers, J. H. (1989). Prevalence and comorbidity of personality disorders. *Psychiatric Annals, 19,* 132–136.

Widiger, T. A., & Sanderson, C. (1987). The convergent and discriminant validity of the MCMI as a measure of the *DSM-III* personality disorders. *Journal of Personality Assessment, 51,* 228–242.

Widiger, T. A., & Shea, T. (1991). Differentiation of Axis I and Axis II disorders. *Journal of Abnormal Psychology, 100,* 399–406.

Wiedenfeld, S. A., O'Leary, A., Bandura, A., Brown, S., Levine, S., & Raska, K. (1989). Impact of perceived self-efficacy in coping with stressors on components of the immune system. Unpublished manuscript, Stanford University.

Wiens, A. N. (1991). Diagnostic interviewing. In M. Hersen, A. E. Kazdin, & A. S. Bellack (Eds.), *The clinical psychology handbook* (2nd ed.) (pp. 345–361). New York: Pergamon Press.

Wiggins, J. G. (1994). Would you want your child to be a psychologist? *American Psychologist, 49,* 485–492.

Wiggins, J. S., & Pincus, A. L. (1989). Conceptions of personality disorders and dimensions of personality. *Psychological Assessment, 1,* 305–316.

Wilfley, D. E., Agras, W. S., Telch, C. F., Rossiter, E. M., Schneider, J. A., Cole, A. G., Sifford, L., & Raeburn, S. D. (1993). Group CBT and group interpersonal psychotherapy for non-binging bulimics: A controlled comparison. *Journal of Consulting and Clinical Psychology, 61,* 296–305.

Wilhelm, K., & Parker, G. (1994). Sex differences in lifetime depression rates: Fact or artifact? *Psychological Medicine, 24,* 97–111.

Willerman, L. (1968). Activity level and hyperactivity in twins. *Child Development, 39,* 27–34.

Willerman, L., & Cohen, D. B. (1990). *Psychopathology.* New York: McGraw-Hill.

Williams, M. H. (1992). Exploitation and inference: Mapping the damage from therapist-patient sexual involvement. *American Psychologist, 47,* 412–421.

Wilson, G. T. (1981). The effects of alcohol on human sexual behavior. In N. Mello (Ed.), *Advances in substance abuse: Behavioral and biological research* (pp. 1–40). Greenwich, CT: JAI Press.

Wilson, G. T. (1985). Limitations of meta-analysis in clinical psychology. *Clinical Psychology Review, 5,* 35–47.

Wilson, G. T. (1990). Clinical issues and strategies in the practice of behavior therapy. In C. M. Franks, G. T. Wilson, P. C. Kendall, & J. P. Foreyt (Eds.), *Review of behavior therapy* (Vol. 12, pp. 271–302). New York: Guilford Press.

Wilson, G. T. (1993a). Behavioral treatment of obesity: Thirty years and counting. *Advances in Behaviour Research and Therapy, 16,* 31–75.

Wilson, G. T. (1993b). Binge eating and addictive disorders. In C. G. Fairburn & G. T. Wilson (Eds.), *Binge eating: Nature, assessment, and treatment.* New York: Guilford Press.

Wilson, G. T. (1994). Behavioral treatment of childhood obesity: Theoretical and practical implications. *Health Psychology, 13,* 371–372.

Wilson, G. T. (1995, July). *Cognitive-behavioral treatment of bulimia nervosa: Issues and evidence.* Paper presented at the World Congress on Cognitive and Behavioral Therapies, Denmark.

Wilson, G. T., & Davison, G. C. (1971). Processes of fear-reduction in systematic desensitization: Animal studies. *Psychological Bulletin, 76,* 1–14.

Wilson, J. Q., & Hernnstein, R. J. (1985). *Crime and human nature.* New York: Simon & Schuster.

Wilson, M. (1993). DSM-III and the transformation of American psychiatry: A history. *American Journal of Psychiatry, 150,* 399–410.

Wilson-Barnett, J., & Trimble, M. R. (1985). An investigation of hysteria using the Illness Behaviour Questionnaire. *British Journal of Psychiatry, 146,* 601–608.

Wing, J. K., & Brown, D. W. (1970). *Institutionalism and schizophrenia.* Cambridge, England: Cambridge University Press.

Winkler, R. C. (1977). What types of sex-role behavior should behavior modification promote? *Journal of Applied Behavior Analysis, 10,* 549–552.

Winters, K. C., & Neale, J. M. (1985). Mania and low self-esteem. *Journal of Abnormal Psychology, 94,* 282–290.

Witelson, S. (1991). Neural sexual mosaicism: Sexual differentiation of the human temporo-parietal region for functional asymmetry. *Psychoneuroendocrinology, 16,* 131.

Wittchen, H. U., Zhao, S., Kessler, R. C., & Eaton, W. W. (1994). DSM-III-R generalized anxiety disorder in the National Comorbidity survey. *Archives of General Psychiatry, 51,* 355–364.

Wolf, L., & Goldberg, B. (1986). Autistic children group: An eight to twenty-four year follow-up study. *Canadian Journal of Psychiatry, 31,* 550–556.

Wolfe, B. E., & Maser, J. D. (1994). *Treatment of panic disorder.* Washington, DC: American Psychiatric Press.

Wolfe, D. A. (1987). *Child abuse: Implications for child development and psychopathology.* Newbury Park, CA: Sage.

Wolfe, J., Keane, T., Lyons, J., & Gerardi, R. (1987). Current trends and issues in the assessment of combat-related post-traumatic stress disorder. *The Behavior Therapist, 10,* 27–32.

Wolpe, J. (1958). *Psychotherapy by reciprocal inhibition.* Stanford, CA: Stanford University Press.

Wolpe, J., & Rachman, S. (1960). Psychoanalytic "evidence": A critique based on Freud's case of Little Hans. *Journal of Nervous and Mental Disease, 131,* 135–148.

Woodward, S. B. (1994). Observations on the medical treatment of insanity. *American Journal of Psychiatry, 151*(June suppl.), 220–230. (Original work published in 1850)

World Development Report. (1993). *Investing in health: World development indicators.* New York: Oxford University Press.

World Health Organization (WHO). (1990). *ICD-10 Chapter V. Mental and behavioral disorders: Diagnostic criteria for research.* Geneva, Switzerland: World Health Organization.

Wright, C., & Moore, R. D. (1989). Disulfiram treatment of alcoholism: Position paper of the American College of Physicians. *Annals of Internal Medicine, 111,* 943–945.

Wright, L. (1994). *Remembering Satan.* New York: Knopf.

Wyatt v. Stickney, Alabama 325 F. Supp. 781 (M.D. Ala. 1971).

Wyatt, G. E., & Newcomb, M. (1990). Internal and external mediators of women's sexual abuse in childhood. *Journal of Consulting and Clinical Psychology, 58,* 758–767.

Wyeth-Ayerst Laboratories. (1994, May 23). Effexor (Vanlafaxine HCL). Brief summary based on Cl 4193-2.

Wynne, L. C. (1984). The University of Rochester child and family study: Overview of research plan. In N. F. Watt, E. J. Anthony, L.

C. Wynne, & J. E. Rolf (Eds.), *Children at risk for schizophrenia: A longitudinal perspective* (pp. 335–347). New York: Cambridge University Press.

Y

Yalom, I. D. (1985). *The theory and practice of group therapy*. New York: Basic Books.

Yalom, I. D., Green, R., & Fisk, N. (1973). Prenatal exposure to female hormones: Effect on psychosexual development in boys. *Archives of General Psychiatry, 28*, 554–561.

Yanovski, S. Z., Leet, M., Yanovski, J. A., Flood, M., Gold, P. W., Kissileff, H. R., & Walsh, B. T. (1992). Food selection and intake of obese women with binge eating disorder. *American Journal of Clinical Nutrition, 56*, 975–980.

Yanovski, S. Z., & Sebring, N. G. (1994). Recorded food intake of obese women with binge eating disorders before and after weight loss. *International Journal of Eating Disorders, 15*, 135–150.

Yapko, M. D. (1994). *Suggestions of abuse*. New York: Simon & Schuster.

Yassa, R., Nastase, C., Dupont, D., & Thibeau, M. (1992). Tardive dyskinesia in elderly psychiatric patients: A five-year study. *American Journal of Psychiatry, 149*, 1206–1211.

Yehuda, R., Southwick, S. M., Nussbaum, G., Wahby, V., Giller, E. L., & Mason, J. W. (1990). Low urinary cortisol excretion in patients with posttraumatic stress disorder. *The Journal of Nervous and Mental Disease, 178*, 366–369.

Yeomans, F. E., Gutfreund, J., Selzer, M. A., & Clarkin, J. F. (1994). Factors related to drop-outs by borderline patients: Treatment contract and therapeutic alliance. *Journal of Psychotherapy Practice and Research, 3*, 16–24.

Yesavage, J. A., Brooks, J. O., Taylor, J., & Tinklenberg, J. (1993). Development of aphasia, apraxia, and agnosia and decline in Alzheimer's disease. *American Journal of Psychiatry, 150*, 742–747.

Yirmiya, N., & Sigman, M. (1991). High functioning individuals with autism: Diagnosis, empirical findings, and theoretical issues. *Clinical Psychology Review, 11*, 669–683.

Yllo, K. A. (1993). Through a feminist lens: Gender, power, and violence. In R. J. Gelles & D. R. Loseke (Eds.), *Current controversies on family violence* (pp. 47–62). Newbury Park, CA: Sage.

Yontef, G. M., & Simkin, J. S. (1989). Gestalt therapy. In R. Corsini & D. Wedding (Eds.), *Current psychotherapies*, 4th ed. (pp. 323–362). Itasca, IL: F. E. Peacock.

Young, J. E., & Beck, A. T. (1982). Cognitive therapy: Clinical applications. In A. J. Rush (Ed.), *Short term psychotherapies for depression*. New York: Guilford Press.

Young, L. T., Warsh, J. J., Kish, S. J., & Shannak, K. (1994). Reduced brain 5-HT and elevated NE turnover and metabolites in bipolar affective disorder. *Biological Psychiatry, 35*, 121–127.

Young, R. C. (1972). Clinical judgement as a means of improving actuarial prediction from the MMPI. *Journal of Consulting and Clinical Psychology, 38*, 457–459.

Youngblood v. Romeo, 457 U.S. 307 (1982).

Youngjohn, J. R., Larrabee, G. J., & Crook, T. H. (1992). Discriminating age-associated memory impairment from Alzheimer's disease. *Psychological Assessment, 4*, 54–59.

Yudofsky, S., Hales, R. E., & Ferguson, T. (1991). *What you need to know about psychiatric drugs*. New York: Grove Weidenfeld.

Z

Zametkin, A. J., Nordahl, T. E., Gross, M., King, C., Semple, W. E., Rumsey, J., Hamburger, S., & Cohen, R. M. (1990). Cerebral glucose metabolism in adults with hyperactivity of childhood onset. *New England Journal of Medicine, 323*, 1361–1366.

Zautra, A. J., Guenther, R. T., & Chartier, G. M. (1985). Attributions for real and hypothetical events: Their relation to self-esteem and depression. *Journal of Abnormal Psychology, 94*, 530–540.

Zayas, L. H., & Palleja, J. (1988). Puerto Rican familism: Considerations for family therapy. *Family Relations, 37*, 260–264.

Zigler, E., & Levine, J. (1981). Age of first hospitalization of schizophrenics: A development approach. *Journal of Abnormal Psychology, 90*, 458–467.

Zilbergeld, B. (1992). The man behind the broken penis: Social and psychological determinants of erectile failure. In R. C. Rosen & S. R. Leiblum (Eds.), *Erectile disorders: Assessment and treatment* (pp. 27–54). New York: Guilford Press.

Zilbergeld, B., & Ellison, C. R. (1980). Desire discrepancies and arousal problems in sex therapy. In S. Leiblum & L. Pervin (Eds.), *Principles and practice of sex therapy*. New York: Plenum Press.

Zilbergeld, B., & Evans, M. (1980). The inadequacy of Masters and Johnson. *Psychology Today, 14*, 28–43.

Zimmerman, M. (1994). Diagnosing personality disorders: A review of issues and research methods. *Archives of General Psychiatry, 51*, 225–245.

Zimring, F. M., & Raskin, N. J. (1992). Carl Rogers and client/person-centered therapy. In D. K. Freedheim (Ed.), *History of psychotherapy: A century of change* (pp. 629–656). Washington, DC: American Psychological Association.

Zinbarg, R. E., Barlow, D. H., Brown, T. A., & Hertz, R. M. (1992). Cognitive-behavioral approaches to the nature and treatment of anxiety disorders. In M. R. Rosenzweig & L. W. Porter (Eds.), *Annual review of psychology* (Vol. 43) (pp. 235–268). Palo Alto, CA: Annual Reviews.

Zivney, O. A., Nash, M. R., & Hulsey, T. L. (1988). Sexual abuse in early versus late childhood: Differing patterns of pathology as revealed on the Rorschach. *Psychotherapy, 25*, 99–106.

Zohar, J., Foa, E. B., & Insel, T. R. (1989). Behavior therapy and pharmacotherapy. In *American Psychiatric Association Task Force on Treatments of Psychiatric Disorders* (Vol. 3). Washington, DC: American Psychiatric Association.

Zohar, J., & Insel, T. R. (1987). Obsessive-compulsive disorder. *Biological Psychiatry, 22*, 667–687.

Zohar, J., Insel, T. R., Zohar-Kadouch, R. C., Hill, J. L., & Murphy, D. L. (1988). Serotonin function in obsessive-compulsive disorder. *Archives of General Psychiatry, 45*, 167–172.

Zubin, J., & Spring, B. (1977). Vulnerability: A new view of schizophrenia. *Journal of Abnormal Psychology, 86*, 103–126.

Zucker, K. J., Finegan, J. K., Deering, R. W., & Bradley, S. J. (1984). Two subgroups of gender-problem children. *Archives of Sexual Behavior, 13*, 27–39.

Zuckerman, M. (1991). *Psychobiology of personality*. New York: Cambridge University Press.

Author Index

Subject Index

12" x 18"; Chapter 8, p. 234, *Untitled* by James Prendergast. Watercolor on paper, 11" x 14"; Chapter 9, p. 270, *Birds with a Cup of Coffee* by Kenny McKay. Watercolor, marker, and crayon on paper, 10" x 13"; Chapter 10, p. 320, *God Bless America* by Helen Kossoff. Watercolor and marker on paper, 11" x 14-7/8". Collection of Ellin and Baron Gordon; Chapter 11, p. 354, *Untitled* by Wally C. Nicholson. Crayon on paper, 14"x 16-7/8"; Chapter 12, p. 378, *Head First* by William Gonzalez. Acrylic on canvas, 24" x 36"; Chapter 13, p. 410, *Untitled* by Helen Kossoff. Watercolor on paper, 11" x 14-3/4"; Chapter 14, p. 450, *Clown Songs* by Carl Greenberg. Acrylic on paper, 14" x 16-5/8"; Chapter 15, p. 484, *Train at Night* by George Knerr. Watercolor on paper, 8-1/4" x 10-1/4"; Chapter 16, p. 512, *Woman* by Donna Caesar. Acrylic on paper, 14" x 17"; Chapter 17, p. 542, *Man and Fish* by Ray Hamilton. Watercolor and marker on paper, 11-7/8" x 17-7/8"; Chapter 18, p. 570, *Untitled* by Ray Hamilton. Mixed media on paper, 14" x 17"; Chapter 20, p. 622, *Untitled* by Wally C. Nicholson. Crayon on paper, 14-3/4" x 18-1/8".

Interior Photo Credits

Chapter 1: p. 2, Reuters/Bettmann; p. 5 *top*, UPI/Bettmann; p. 5 *bottom*, Frank Ockenfels/Outline; p. 6, The Bettmann Archive; p. 10, UPI/Bettmann Newsphotos; pp. 14, 15, 16, North Wind Picture Archives; p. 20, The Bettmann Archive.

Chapter 2: p. 39, Library of Congress; p. 40, National Library of Medicine; p. 42, George Goodwin/Monkmeyer; p. 43, Topham/The Image Works; p. 44, Keystone/The Image Works; p. 47, Library of Congress; p. 49, Courtesy of Carl Rogers Memorial Library; pp. 51, 52 *top*, Lyrl Ahern; p. 52 *bottom*, National Library of Medicine; p. 54, Fabian Bachrach/National Library of Medicine; p. 56, Lyrl Ahern.

Chapter 3: p. 70, CLEO/The Picture Cube; p. 77, David Young-Wolff/Tony Stone Images; p. 78, Blair Seitz/Photo Researchers; p. 81 *top*, Peter Vandermark/Stock, Boston; p. 81 *bottom*, John Coletti; p. 86, Will Faller.

Chapter 4: p. 106, Courtesy of Allure. Copyright © 1993 by the Conde Nast Publications, Inc.; p. 109, Courtesy of Martin Seligman; p. 116, Dan McCoy/Rainbow; p. 117, Stephen Frisch/Stock, Boston; p. 128, Chuck Nacke/Woodfin Camp & Associates.

Chapter 5: p. 134, AP/Wide World Photos; p. 135, Courtesy of David Barlow; p. 137, Dion Ogust/The Image Works; p. 145, Lev Nisnevich/Tony Stone Images; p. 153, AP/Wide World Photos; p. 156, Rick Reinhard/Impact Visuals.

Chapter 6: p. 168, The Granger Collection; p. 170, Steve Smith/Onyx; pp. 182, 185, AP/Wide World Photos.

Chapter 7: p. 193, Arthur Tress/Photo Researchers; pp. 198, 199, The Bettmann Archive; p. 202, E. Williamson/The Picture Cube; p. 205, AP/Wide World Photos; p. 206, Larry Mulvehill/Science Source/Photo Researchers; p. 214, Andy Sacks/Tony Stone Images; p. 225, Wally McNamara/Woodfin Camp & Associates; p. 228, Catherine Karnow/Woodfin Camp & Associates.

Chapter 8: p. 236, UPI/Bettmann Newsphotos; p. 237, AP/Wide World Photos; p. 241, Courtesy of Raymond S. Rosen; p. 255, AP/Wide World Photos; p. 256, S. McCurry/Magnum Photos; p. 266, Chris Kleponis/Woodfin Camp & Associates.

Chapter 9: p. 272, Gilles Peress/Magnum Photos; p. 273 *top*, Library of Congress; p. 273 *bottom*, Mark Walker/The Picture Cube; p. 298, David Young-Wolff/Tony Stone Images; p. 303, Rob Schoenbaum/Black Star; p. 304, Shackman/Monkmeyer; p. 310, Hank Morgan/Rainbow.

Chapter 10: p. 322, UPI/Bettmann; p. 343, Tony Neste; p. 345, Bob Daemmrich/Stock, Boston; p. 346, Reuters/Bettmann; p. 347, Steve Leonard/Black Star; p. 348, Dan McCoy/Rainbow.

Chapter 11: p. 358, AP/Wide World Photos; p. 359, Paul Fusco/Magnum Photos; p. 362, John Harrington/Black Star; p. 371 *top*, AP/Wide World Photos; p. 371 *bottom left*, Topham/The Image Works; p. 371 *bottom right*, AP/Wide World Photos.

Chapter 12: p. 384, UPI/Bettmann; p. 385, Photofest; p. 386, © Capital Features/The Image Works; p. 387, Thomas Hoepker/Magnum Photos; p. 388, Bill Stanton/Rainbow; p. 403, Courtesy of Dr. Graznya Kochanska.

Chapter 13: p. 412 *top*, Reuters/Bettmann; p. 412 *bottom*, The Granger Collection; p. 419, UPI/Bettmann; p. 429 *top*, William Strode/Woodfin Camp & Associates; p. 429 *bottom*, Hank Morgan/Rainbow; p. 441, AP/Wide World Photos; 447, UPI/Bettmann;

Chapter 14: p. 452, The Granger Collection; p. 455, Reuters/Bettmann; p. 458, Byron/ Monkmeyer; p. 459, AP/Wide World Photos; p. 460, Courtesy of Dr. G. R. Patterson; p. 465, Betsy Cole/The Picture Cube; p. 472, Robert Harbison; p. 476, Palco Laboratories, 8030 Sequel Ave., Santa Cruz, NM 95062-2032; p. 478, UPI/Bettmann.

Chapter 15: p. 486, Robin Laurance/Photo Researchers; p. 487, UPI/Bettmann; p. 490, Courtesy of University of Washington FAS Research Fund; p. 491, Linda K. Moore/ Rainbow; p. 495, Stephen Marks; p. 502, The Alan Mason Chesney Archives of the Johns Hopkins Medical Institutions; p. 506, Courtesy of Ivar Lovaas; p. 509 *left*, Herb Goro/ Courtesy of The Option Institute and Fellowship; p. 509 *right*, Michelle Tully/Courtesy of The Option Institute and Fellowship.

Chapter 16: p. 514, Kindra Clineff/The Picture Cube; p. 515, Robert E. Daemmrich/ Tony Stone Images; p. 524, NIH/Science Source/Photo Researchers; p. 526, Reuters/ Bettmann; p. 529, Lester Sloan/Woodfin Camp & Associates; p. 530, Cecil Fox/Photo Re-searchers; p. 532, Thomas Craig/The Picture Cube; p. 534, North Wind Picture Archives; p. 536, Hank Morgan/Science Source/Photo Researchers; p. 537, Springer/Bettmann Film Archive.

Chapter 17: p. 544, John Harrington/Black Star; p. 545, Reuters/Bettmann; p. 548, Nik Habicht/Trenton Times; p. 554, Reuters/Bettmann; p. 559, Catherine Smith/Impact Vi-suals; p. 561, Photofest; p. 563, AP/Wide World Photos; p. 565, Nik Habicht/Trenton Times.

Chapter 18: p. 573, AP/Wide World Photos; p. 578, Courtesy of Myrna Weissman; pp. 580, 582, 587, Lyrl Ahern; p. 588, Courtesy of Aaron Beck; p. 591, Courtesy of Arnold Lazarus; p. 597, Robert Harbison.

Chapter 19: p. 605, Zigy Kaluzney/Tony Stone Images; p. 606, Dennis Brack/Black Star; p. 611, Bill Stanton/Rainbow; p. 614, David Harry Stewart/Tony Stone Images.

Chapter 20: p. 627, Jonathan Nourok/Tony Stone Images; p. 631, The Bettmann Archive; p. 633, Bruce Ayres/Tony Stone Images; p. 638, Courtesy of Dr. William Pelham; p. 641, James Wilson/Woodfin Camp & Associates; p. 642, Alexander Tsiaras/Stock, Boston.

Chapter 21: p. 648, AP/Wide World Photos; p. 649, Barbara Filet/Tony Stone Images; p. 652, UPI/Bettmann; p. 657, Robert Harbison; p. 660, Peter Southwick/Stock, Boston; p. 663, Stephen Frisch/Stock, Boston; p. 666, Owen DB/Black Star; p. 667 *left*, The Granger Collection; p. 667 *right*, North Wind Picture Archives.

TEXT CREDITS

DSM-IV Tables: Tables pp. 137, 138, 143, 144, 147, 150, 152, 158, 169, 173, 176, 181, 192, 195, 199, 238, 239, 243, 275, 323, 357, 360, 365, 380, 416, 455, 456, 463, 487, 501, 517, and 518 from American Psychiatric Association, 1994, *Diagnostic and Statistical Manual of Mental Disorders*, 4th ed., Washington, DC, American Psychiatric Association. Reprinted by permission.

Chapter 1: Quote pp. 3–4 from Spitzer et al., *Psychopathology: A Casebook*, p. 19. Copyright 1983 by McGraw-Hill, Inc. Reproduced with the permission of McGraw-Hill, Inc.

Chapter 2: Quotes pp. 27, 40, 44, and 60 from *The Autobiography of Malcolm X*, by Malcolm X, pp. 4, 19 and 21, 9–10, and 17–21, respectively. Copyright 1964. Quote p. 42 from Z. A. Liff, "Psychoanalysis and Dramatic Techniques," in D. K. Freedman (Ed.), *History of Psy-chotherapy: A Century of Change*, pp. 571–586. Copyright © 1992 by the American Psycho-logical Association. Reprinted with permission. Quote p. 50 from *On Becoming a Person*. Copyright © 1961 by Carl R. Rogers. Reprinted with permission of Houghton Mifflin Company. All rights reserved.

Chapter 4: Quote p. 119 from Clark, "Anxiety States." In K. Hawton, P. M. Salkovskis, and D. M. Clark (Eds.), *Cognitive Behavior Therapy for Psychiatric Problems*, p. 85. Copyright © 1989. Reprinted by permission of Oxford University Press.

Chapter 5: Quote pp. 149–150 from *The Nature and Treatment of Anxiety Disorders*, by C. Barr Taylor and Bruce A. Arrow. Copyright © 1988 by The Free Press, a Division of Simon & Schuster, Inc. Reprinted with permission of the publisher. Quote pp. 151–152 from Foy et al., "Posttraumatic Stress Disorder," in L. Michelson and L. M. Aschner (Eds.), *Anxiety and Stress Disorders*, 1987, pp. 369–370. Reprinted by permission of Guil-ford Publications, Inc.

Chapter 6: Dialogue p. 176 from P. M. Salkovskis (1989), "Somatic Problems," in K. Haw-ton, P. M. Salkovskis, J. Kirk, & D. M. Clark (Eds.), *Cognitive Behaviour Therapy for Psychi-atric Problems*. Reprinted by permission of Oxford University Press.

Chapter 7: Quotes pp. 193, 196, and 198 from R. L. Spitzer, A. E. Skodol, M. Gibbon, and J. B. W. Williams (1981), *DSM-III Case Book*, pp. 98, 98, and 242–243, respectively. Reprinted by permission of the American Psychiatric Association. Quote pp. 197–198 reprinted with

Schizophrenia and Other Psychotic Disorders

Schizophrenia
Paranoid Type
Disorganized Type
Catatonic Type
Undifferentiated Type
Residual Type

Schizophreniform Disorder

Schizoaffective Disorder

Delusional Disorder

Brief Psychotic Disorder

Shared Psychotic Disorder

Psychotic Disorder Due to a General Medical Condition

Substance-Induced Psychotic Disorder

Psychotic Disorder Not Otherwise Specified

Mood Disorders

Depressive Disorders
Major Depressive Disorder
Dysthymic Disorder
Depressive Disorder Not Otherwise Specified

Bipolar Disorders
Bipolar I Disorder
Bipolar II Disorder
Cyclothymic Disorder
Bipolar Disorder Not Otherwise Specified
Mood Disorder Due to a General Medical Condition
Substance-Induced Mood Disorder
Mood Disorder Not Otherwise Specified

Anxiety Disorders

Panic Disorder Without Agoraphobia

Panic Disorder With Agoraphobia

Agoraphobia Without History of Panic Disorder

Specific Phobia

Social Phobia

Obsessive-Compulsive Disorder

Posttraumatic Stress Disorder

Acute Stress Disorder

Generalized Anxiety Disorder

Anxiety Disorder Due to a General Medical Condition

Substance-Induced Anxiety Disorder

Anxiety Disorder Not Otherwise Specified

Somatoform Disorders

Somatization Disorder

Undifferentiated Somatoform Disorder

Conversion Disorder

Pain Disorder

Hypochondriasis

Body Dysmorphic Disorder

Somatoform Disorder Not Otherwise Specified

Factitious Disorders

Factitious Disorder

Factitious Disorder Not Otherwise Specified

Dissociative Disorders

Dissociative Amnesia

Dissociative Fugue

Dissociative Identity Disorder

Depersonalization Disorder

Dissociative Disorder Not Otherwise Specified

Sexual and Gender Identity Disorders

Sexual Desire Disorders
Hypoactive Sexual Desire Disorder
Sexual Aversion Disorder

Sexual Arousal Disorders
Female Sexual Arousal Disorder
Male Erectile Disorder

Orgasmic Disorders
Female Orgasmic Disorder
Male Orgasmic Disorder
Premature Ejaculation

Sexual Pain Disorders
Dyspareunia
Vaginismus

Sexual Dysfunction Due to a General Medical Condition
Female Hypoactive Sexual Desire Disorder Due to a General Medical Condition
Male Hypoactive Sexual Desire Disorder Due to a General Medical Condition
Male Erectile Disorder Due to a General Medical Condition
Female Dyspareunia Due to a General Medical Condition
Male Dyspareunia Due to a General Medical Condition
Other Female Sexual Dysfunction Due to a General Medical Condition
Other Male Sexual Dysfunction Due to a General Medical Condition
Substance-Induced Sexual Dysfunction
Sexual Dysfunction Not Otherwise Specified